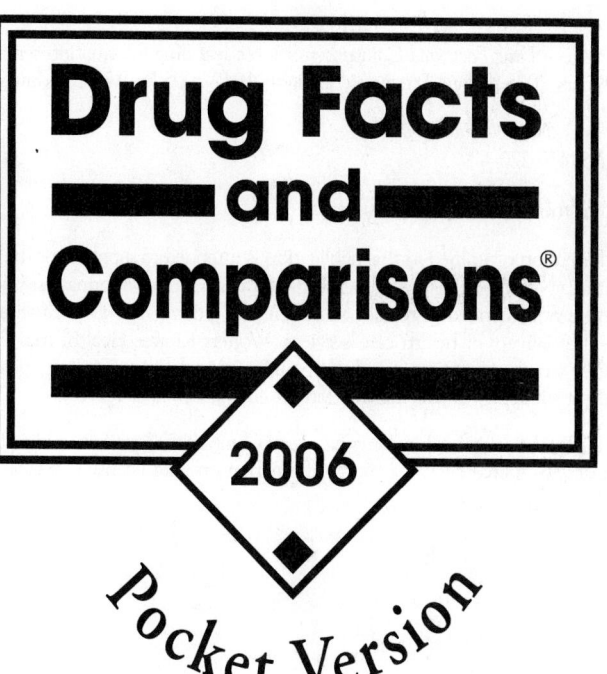

# Drug Facts
## and
# Comparisons®

### 2006

*Pocket Version*

**Drug Facts and Comparisons® Pocket Version, Tenth Edition, 2006**

Adapted from *Drug Facts and Comparisons®* loose-leaf drug information service through the February 2005 update. Previous copyrights 1947-2005 by Wolters Kluwer Health, Inc.

ISBN 1-57439-220-4

Printed in the United States of America

The information contained in *Drug Facts and Comparisons®* pocket version is available for licensing as source data. For more information on data licensing, please call 1-800-223-0554

**Facts and Comparisons®**
part of Wolters Kluwer Health
77 Westport Plaza Drive, Suite 450
St. Louis, Missouri 63146-3125
www.drugfacts.com
314/216-2100 • 800/223-0554

## FACTS AND COMPARISONS® PUBLISHING GROUP

**Kenneth H. Killion**
CEO, Clinical Tools

**Renée M. Wickersham**
Senior Managing Editor,
   Content Development

**Julie A. Scott**
Senior Managing Editor,
   Content Development

**Sara L. Schweain**
Senior Editor

**Jennifer A. Guimaraes**
**John G. Hall**
**Joseph R. Horenkamp**
Associate Editors

**Susan H. Sunderman**
Senior Quality Control Editor

**Teri Hines Burnham**
Director, Referential Product
   Management

**Cathy H. Reilly**
Vice President and Publisher

**Jill A. O'Dell**
Managing Editor

**Jennifer K. Walsh**
Senior Composition Specialist

**Linda M. Jones**
Senior SGML Specialist

**Heather L. Broad**
Purchasing Specialist

**Renée Rivard, PharmD**
Clinical Director

**Cathy A. Meives, PharmD**
Clinical Manager

**Lori A. Buss, PharmD**
**Shanti Divvela, PharmD**
**Kim S. Dufner, PharmD**
**Andrea Raftery, RPh**
Clinical Editors

## DRUG FACTS AND COMPARISONS® POCKET VERSION REVIEWERS

**Kate Farthing, PharmD**
Drug Information Coordinator
Oregon Health and Science University
   Drug Information Service
OHSU Hospitals and Clinics
Portland, Oregon

**Mary J. Ferrill, PharmD, FASHP**
Assistant Dean for Professional Affairs
Wingate University
School of Pharmacy
Wingate, North Carolina

**Joyce A. Generali, RPh, MS,
   FASHP**
Director, Drug Information Center
Clinical Professor
University of Kansas Medical Center
Kansas City, Kansas

**Beth Jones, PharmD**
Clinical Pharmacist
Missouri Baptist Medical Center
St. Louis, Missouri

**Burgunda V. Sweet, PharmD**
Director, Drug Information
Clinical Associate Professor of
   Pharmacy
University of Michigan
Ann Arbor, Michigan

**Jennifer N. Mazur, PharmD, CDE**
Clinical Specialist, Primary Care
Department of Pharmacy Services,
   Medical University of South Carolina
Clinical Assistant Professor
Department of Pharmacy Practice,
   Medical University of South Carolina

iii

iv

**Mary Beth Shirk, PharmD**
Specialty Practice
  Pharmacist
Critical Care Medicine
Clinical Assistant Professor
The Ohio State University
  Medical Center
Columbus, OH

**Udho Thadani, MD,**
  **MRCP, FRCP(C), FACC,**
  **FAHA**
Professor of Medicine
Cardiovascular Section
University of Oklahoma
  Health Sciences Center
Oklahoma City, Oklahoma

**Thom J. Zimmerman, MD,**
  **PhD**
Emeritus Professor and
  Chairman
Department of
  Ophthalmology and Visual
  Sciences
Emeritus Professor of
  Pharmacology &
  Toxicology
University of Louisville
School of Medicine
Louisville, Kentucky
Global Ophthalmic Medical
  Director
Global Medical Affairs
Pfizer Ophthalmics

# Table of Contents

Drug monographs in *Drug Facts and Comparisons®, Pocket Version* are arranged by use. Drugs with similar therapeutic or pharmacologic characteristics have been grouped together to allow the health care provider to compare these drugs easily and determine the most appropriate drug therapy. Standard sections within the monographs occur in a consistent format. Once the user is familiar with the organization of the data, the desired information can be located quickly.

## Monograph Organization

**❶** *Therapeutic class:* Drugs that share the same therapeutic class will share a common title that appears on the right-hand pages. The monograph title appears on the left-hand pages. If there is no shared class, the monograph title will repeat on the right-hand page.

**❷** *Drug name:* Generic names and any common synonyms appear in a horizontal bar that introduces a new monograph. Synonyms follow the generic name in parentheses and are separated by semicolons.

**❸** *Product table:* Doseforms and strengths of generic drugs are listed in the left column with their schedules (eg, *Rx, otc, c-ii*). If more than one generic entity is included in the monograph (eg, beta blockers), the drugs appear in all caps with specific information underneath it. The more common trade names, with their specific manufacturers/distributors, are listed in the right-hand column. If the drug is available generically, the word "Various" appears at the beginning of the trade name listing.

**❹** *Warning box:* Potentially life-threatening reactions specified in the product labeling will appear in a box. *Not included in sample.*

**❺** *Indications:* All FDA-approved indications are included. In addition, off-label uses with substantial documentation about dosing may appear under the term "Unlabeled uses."

**❻** *Administration and Dosage:* Appropriate dosage, dosage range, etc. is included. When available, specific information for administration in situations such as renal impairment, elderly patients, etc., is included.

**❼** *Actions:* This section includes a brief discussion of significant pharmacologic and pharmacokinetic information is included.

**❽** *Contraindications:* All known contraindications are included.

**❾** *Warnings:* This section includes a brief description of major warnings associated with the drug. Standard sections (eg, Pregnancy, Lactation, Children) appear at the end of this section. The Pregnancy section generally only lists the Standard Pregnancy Category (A, B, C, D, or X). A description of these categories can be found in the Appendix.

**❿** *Precautions:* Potential conditions for which the patient should be cautioned (eg, photosensitivity) are included, as well as other significant situations where caution is warranted.

**⓫** *Drug Interactions:* Drugs that may interact (affect or be affected by the interacting agent) are listed. Lab test and drug/food interactions also are included.

**⓬** *Adverse Reactions:* Where possible, reactions that occur in 3% or more of patients have been listed. When percentages are not available, significant reactions not discussed in Warnings or Precautions are included.

## CYCLOBENZAPRINE HCl

**Tablets:** 10 mg (Rx)                    Various, *Flexeril* (Merck)

### Indications

*Musculoskeletal conditions:* Adjunct to rest and physical therapy for relief of muscle spasm associated with acute painful musculoskeletal conditions.

*Unlabeled uses:* Cyclobenzaprine (10 to 40 mg/day) appears to be a useful adjunct in the management of the fibrositis syndrome.

### Administration and Dosage

Give 10 mg 3 times daily (range, 20 to 40 mg daily in divided doses). Do not exceed 60 mg/day. Do not use longer than 2 or 3 weeks.

### Actions

*Pharmacology:* Cyclobenzaprine, structurally related to the tricyclic antidepressants (TCAs), relieves skeletal muscle spasm of local origin without interfering with muscle function. It is ineffective in muscle spasm due to CNS disease. The net effect is a reduction of tonic somatic motor activity, influencing both gamma and alpha motor systems.

*Pharmacokinetics:* Cyclobenzaprine is well absorbed after oral administration, but there is a large intersubject variation in plasma levels. Peak plasma levels are reached in 4 to 6 hours. The onset of action occurs in 1 hour with a duration of 12 to 24 hours. It is highly bound to plasma proteins, extensively metabolized primarily to glucuronide-like conjugates and excreted primarily via the kidneys. Elimination half-life is 1 to 3 days.

### Contraindications

Hypersensitivity to cyclobenzaprine; concomitant use of monoamine oxidase (MAO) inhibitors or within 14 days after their discontinuation; acute recovery phase of MI and in patients with arrhythmias, heart block, or conduction disturbances or CHF; hyperthyroidism.

### Warnings

*Spasticity:* Cyclobenzaprine is not effective in the treatment of spasticity associated with cerebral or spinal cord disease, or in children with cerebral palsy.

*Duration:* Use only for short periods (up to 2 or 3 weeks); effectiveness for more prolonged use is not proven.

*Similarity to TCAs:* Cyclobenzaprine is closely related to the TCAs. In short-term studies for indications other than muscle spasm associated with acute musculoskeletal conditions, and usually at doses greater than those recommended, some of the more serious CNS reactions noted with the TCAs have occurred.

*Pregnancy: Category B.*

*Lactation:* It is not known whether cyclobenzaprine is excreted in breast milk.

*Children:* Safety and efficacy in children < 15 years of age have not been established.

### Precautions

*Anticholinergic effects:* Because of its anticholinergic action, use with caution in patients with a history of urinary retention, angle-closure glaucoma, and increased intraocular pressure.

*Hazardous tasks:* May impair mental or physical abilities required for performance of hazardous tasks; patients should observe caution while driving or performing other tasks requiring alertness, coordination, and physical dexterity.

### Drug Interactions

Drugs that may interact with cyclobenzaprine HCl include MAO inhibitors and TCAs.

### Adverse Reactions

Adverse reactions occurring in ≥ 3% of patients include drowsiness, dizziness, fatigue, tiredness, asthenia, blurred vision, headache, nervousness, confusion, dry mouth, nausea, constipation, dyspepsia, unpleasant taste, purpura, bone marrow depression, leukopenia, eosinophilia, thrombocytopenia, elevation and lowering of blood sugar levels, and weight gain or loss.

# PREFACE

The Pocket Version of *Drug Facts and Comparisons®* *(DFC)* is an abridged version of the full *DFC* publication designed for quick reference by the health care professional. The purpose of the *DFC Pocket Version* is to provide an easy-to-use, concise, portable reference that can be utilized in daily practice. It is not intended to replace the complete information found in *DFC;* however, it provides the same reliable source of drug information.

In addition to the extensive review panel for *DFC,* a separate panel of drug information specialists and hospital pharmacists was established to determine which drug monographs would be most valuable to the health care professional along with the data for each drug needed most. The book is arranged therapeutically in 13 chapters in a consistent format. Single-agent monographs have been pared down to provide the essential information that a health care provider needs to aid in drug therapy decisions. Product tables that list trade names, doseforms, strengths, and manufacturers are included at the beginning of each monograph. Group monographs contain product information and dosing instructions for each of the drugs in a specific class (eg, beta blockers). Indications, administration and dosage, actions, contraindications, warnings, drug interactions, and significant adverse reactions (those occurring in at least 3% of patients) also are included for all monographs. The useful tables that are so common to *DFC* have, for the most part, been retained in the Pocket Version.

Appendix material (eg, Management of Overdosage, FDA Pregnancy Categories) also is available for reference. A comprehensive index helps the reader reach the desired information quickly and easily.

Wolters Kluwer Health hopes health care providers find *Drug Facts and Comparisons®* *Pocket Version* a valuable tool in daily practice. As always, comments and suggestions are appreciated.

Cathy R. Reilly
Publisher

# Chapter 1
# NUTRIENTS AND NUTRITIONAL AGENTS

# RECOMMENDED DIETARY ALLOWANCES OF VITAMINS AND MINERALS

Recommended Dietary Allowances (RDA) are published by the Food and Nutrition Board, National Research Council-National Academy of Sciences, as a guide for nutritional problems and to provide standards of good nutrition for different age groups. They are revised periodically.

The RDA values are *not requirements;* they are *recommended* daily intakes of certain essential nutrients. Based on available scientific knowledge, they are believed to be adequate for known nutritional needs for most *healthy* people under usual environmental stresses. The recommended allowances vary for age and sex, with extra allowances for women during pregnancy and lactation. The most commonly used RDA values (the "reference male" and "reference female") are those of adults 23 to 50 years of age. With the exception of energy (kilocalories), the RDA provide for individual requirement variations and prevent symptoms of clinical deficiency of 97% of the population.

RDA have been established for many essential nutrients; however, present knowledge of human nutritional needs of pantothenic acid and biotin is incomplete. Therefore, to ensure adequate nutrient intake, obtain the recommended allowances from as varied a selection of foods as possible. Nutritionists suggest that dietary planning include regular intake of each of the four basic food groups:

1.) Milk, cheese, dairy products – Minimum 2 servings/day.
2.) Meat, poultry, fish, beans – Minimum 2 servings/day.
3.) Vegetables, fruit – Minimum 4 servings/day.
4.) Bread, cereal (whole-grain and enriched or fortified) – Minimum 4 servings/ day.

Such a balance, in sufficient quantities will provide about 1200 kcal, enough protein, and most of the vitamins and minerals required daily. A person may increase nutrient and energy intake by consuming larger quantities (or more servings/day) of the 4 basic food groups. Nutrient and energy intake may also be increased by selecting food from the fifth group, fats-sweets-alcohol, which provides mainly energy.

RDA quantities apply only to healthy people and are not intended to cover therapeutic nutritional requirements in disease or other abnormal states (ie, metabolic disorders, weight reduction, chronic disease, drug therapy). Although certain single nutrients in larger quantities may have pharmacologic actions, these are unrelated to nutritional functions. There is no convincing evidence that consuming excessive quantities of single nutrients will cure or prevent nonnutritional diseases.

The "official" listings of United States Recommended Daily Allowances (US-RDAs) should not be confused with the RDA values. US-RDA are derived from the 1968 RDA and serve as legal standards for nutritional labeling of food and dietary food and dietary supplement products controlled by the FDA. Generally, they represent the higher value of the male or female RDA and are grouped into only 3 age brackets plus 1 category for pregnant or lactating women. Prior to 1972, these allowances were erroneously listed as minimum daily requirements (MDR). A second fallacy perpetuated by US-RDA labeling of foods is the implication that a food is defective if it does not contain all the officially established nutrients in their full US-RDA quantities. No individual food is nutritionally complete, but several foods together should complement each other to provide maximal nutrient balance and to minimize naturally occurring toxic principles consumed from any individual foodstuff.

The RDA for adult males and adult females are included in each individual vitamin monograph. The table on the following page presents the listing of vitamin and mineral RDA values for all age groups as published in *Recommended Dietary Allowances*, 10th Edition, National Academy of Sciences, Washington, DC, 1989.

## RECOMMENDED DIETARY ALLOWANCES[1]

| Age (years) or Condition | Weight[2] (kg) | Weight[2] (lb) | Height[2] (cm) | Height[2] (in) | Protein (g) | Vitamin A (units[3]) | Vitamin D (units[4]) | Vitamin E (units[5]) | Vitamin K (mcg) | Ascorbic acid (C) (mg) | Thiamine (B1) (mg) | Riboflavin (B2) (mg) | Niacin (B3) (mg) | Pyridoxine (B6) (mg) | Folate (mcg) | Cyanocobalamin (B12) (mcg) | Calcium (mg) | Phosphorus (mg) | Magnesium (mg) | Iron (mg) | Zinc (mg) | Iodine (mcg) | Selenium (mcg) |
|---|---|---|---|---|---|---|---|---|---|---|---|---|---|---|---|---|---|---|---|---|---|---|---|
| **Infants** | | | | | | | | | | | | | | | | | | | | | | | |
| 0.0-0.5 | 6 | 13 | 60 | 24 | 13 | 1249 | 300 | 4 | 5 | 30 | 0.3 | 0.4 | 5 | 0.3 | 25 | 0.3 | 400 | 300 | 40 | 6 | 5 | 40 | 10 |
| 0.5-1 | 9 | 20 | 71 | 28 | 14 | 1249 | 400 | 6 | 10 | 35 | 0.4 | 0.5 | 6 | 0.6 | 35 | 0.5 | 600 | 500 | 60 | 10 | 5 | 50 | 15 |
| **Children** | | | | | | | | | | | | | | | | | | | | | | | |
| 1-3 | 13 | 29 | 90 | 35 | 16 | 1332 | 400 | 9 | 15 | 40 | 0.7 | 0.8 | 9 | 1 | 50 | 0.7 | 800 | 800 | 80 | 10 | 10 | 70 | 20 |
| 4-6 | 20 | 44 | 112 | 44 | 24 | 1665 | 400 | 10 | 20 | 45 | 0.9 | 1.1 | 12 | 1.1 | 75 | 1 | 800 | 800 | 120 | 10 | 10 | 90 | 20 |
| 7-10 | 28 | 62 | 132 | 52 | 28 | 2331 | 400 | 10 | 30 | 45 | 1 | 1.2 | 13 | 1.4 | 100 | 1.4 | 800 | 800 | 170 | 10 | 10 | 120 | 30 |
| **Males** | | | | | | | | | | | | | | | | | | | | | | | |
| 11-14 | 45 | 99 | 157 | 62 | 45 | 3330 | 400 | 15 | 45 | 50 | 1.3 | 1.5 | 17 | 1.7 | 150 | 2 | 1200 | 1200 | 270 | 12 | 15 | 150 | 40 |
| 15-18 | 66 | 145 | 176 | 69 | 59 | 3330 | 400 | 15 | 65 | 60 | 1.5 | 1.8 | 20 | 2 | 200 | 2 | 1200 | 1200 | 400 | 12 | 15 | 150 | 50 |
| 19-24 | 72 | 160 | 177 | 70 | 58 | 3330 | 400 | 15 | 70 | 60 | 1.5 | 1.7 | 19 | 2 | 200 | 2 | 1200 | 1200 | 350 | 10 | 15 | 150 | 70 |
| 25-50 | 79 | 174 | 176 | 70 | 63 | 3330 | 200 | 15 | 80 | 60 | 1.5 | 1.7 | 19 | 2 | 200 | 2 | 800 | 800 | 350 | 10 | 15 | 150 | 70 |
| 51+ | 77 | 170 | 173 | 68 | 63 | 3330 | 200 | 15 | 80 | 60 | 1.2 | 1.4 | 15 | 2 | 200 | 2 | 800 | 800 | 350 | 10 | 15 | 150 | 70 |
| **Females** | | | | | | | | | | | | | | | | | | | | | | | |
| 11-14 | 46 | 101 | 157 | 62 | 46 | 2664 | 400 | 12 | 45 | 50 | 1.1 | 1.3 | 15 | 1.4 | 150 | 2 | 1200 | 1200 | 280 | 15 | 12 | 150 | 45 |
| 15-18 | 55 | 120 | 163 | 64 | 44 | 2664 | 400 | 12 | 55 | 60 | 1.1 | 1.3 | 15 | 1.5 | 180 | 2 | 1200 | 1200 | 300 | 15 | 12 | 150 | 50 |
| 19-24 | 58 | 128 | 164 | 65 | 46 | 2664 | 400 | 12 | 60 | 60 | 1.1 | 1.3 | 15 | 1.6 | 180 | 2 | 1200 | 1200 | 280 | 15 | 12 | 150 | 55 |
| 25-50 | 63 | 138 | 163 | 64 | 50 | 2664 | 200 | 12 | 65 | 60 | 1.1 | 1.3 | 15 | 1.6 | 180 | 2 | 800 | 800 | 280 | 15 | 12 | 150 | 55 |
| 51+ | 65 | 143 | 160 | 63 | 50 | 2664 | 200 | 15 | 65 | 60 | 1 | 1.2 | 13 | 1.6 | 180 | 2 | 800 | 800 | 280 | 10 | 12 | 150 | 55 |
| **Pregnant** | | | | | 60 | 2664 | 400 | 15 | 65 | 70 | 1.5 | 1.6 | 17 | 2.2 | 400 | 2.2 | 1200 | 1200 | 320 | 30 | 15 | 175 | 65 |
| **Lactating** – 1st 6 mo. | | | | | 65 | 4329 | 400 | 18 | 65 | 95 | 1.6 | 1.8 | 20 | 2.1 | 280 | 2.6 | 1200 | 1200 | 355 | 15 | 19 | 200 | 75 |
| 2nd 6 mo. | | | | | 62 | 3996 | 400 | 16 | 65 | 90 | 1.6 | 1.7 | 20 | 2.1 | 260 | 2.6 | 1200 | 1200 | 340 | 15 | 16 | 200 | 75 |

Reproduced from: *Recommended Dietary Allowances*, 10th edition, 1989, National Academy of Sciences, National Academy Press, Washington, DC.

[1] The allowances, expressed as average daily intakes over time, are intended to provide for individual variations among most normal people as they live in the US under usual environmental stresses. Diets should be based on a variety of common foods in order to provide other nutrients for which human requirements have been less well defined.

[2] Weights and heights of Reference Adults are actual medians for the US population of the designated age, as reported by NHANES II. The median weights and heights of those younger than 19 years of age were taken from Hamill PV, et al. *Am J Clin Nutr*. 1979;32:607-629. The use of these figures does not imply that the height-to-weight ratios are ideal.

[3] Conversion of units to retinol equivalents (RE): 3.33 units = 1 mcg of retinol = 1 RE or 6 mcg, β-carotene.

[4] As cholecalciferol. 10 mcg cholecalciferol = 400 units of vitamin D.

[5] α-Tocopherol equivalents. 1 mg d-α-tocopherol = α-TE = 1.49 units.

Dietary Reference Intakes (DRIs) refer to nutrient intake values estimated to be adequate for 50% of age- and gender-specific groups. As seen in the table below, DRIs are comprised of RDAs in bold type and Adequate Intakes (AIs) in ordinary type followed by asterisk (*). These values may be used as goals for individual intake. RDAs are estimated to meet the needs of most individuals (97% to 98%). For healthy breast-fed infants, the AI represents mean intake. For all other life-stage groups, the AI is believed to cover the needs of all individuals, but a lack of data or uncertainty in the data prevent specifying with confidence with percentage of individuals covered by this intake.

**Food and Nutrition Board, Institute of Medicine – National Academy of Science Dietary Reference Intakes: Recommended Intakes for Individuals**

| Life-stage group | Calcium (mg/d) | Phosphorus (mg/d) | Magnesium (mg/d) | Vitamin A (mcg/d) | Vitamin C (mg/d) | Vitamin D (mcg/d)[a,b] | Vitamin E (mg/d) | Vitamin K (mcg/d) | Fluoride (mg/d) | Thiamine (mg/d) | Riboflavin (mg/d) | Niacin (mg/d)[c] | Vitamin B6 (mg/d) | Folate (mcg/d)[d] | Vitamin B12 (mcg/d) | Pantothenic acid (mg/d) | Biotin (mcg/d) | Choline[e] (mg/d) |
|---|---|---|---|---|---|---|---|---|---|---|---|---|---|---|---|---|---|---|
| **Infants** | | | | | | | | | | | | | | | | | | |
| 0-6 mo. | 210* | 100* | 30* | 400* | 40* | 5* | 4* | 2* | 0.01* | 0.2* | 0.3* | 2* | 0.1* | 65* | 0.4* | 1.7* | 5* | 125* |
| 7-12 mo | 270* | 275* | 75* | 500* | 50* | 5* | 5* | 2.5* | 0.5* | 0.3* | 0.4* | 4* | 0.3* | 80* | 0.5* | 1.8* | 6* | 150* |
| **Children** | | | | | | | | | | | | | | | | | | |
| 1-3 y | 500* | 460 | 80 | 300 | 15 | 5* | 6 | 30* | 0.7* | 0.5 | 0.5 | 6 | 0.5 | 150 | 0.9 | 2* | 8* | 200* |
| 4-8 y | 800* | 500 | 130 | 400 | 25 | 5* | 7 | 55* | 1* | 0.6 | 0.6 | 8 | 0.6 | 200 | 1.2 | 3* | 12* | 250* |
| **Males** | | | | | | | | | | | | | | | | | | |
| 9-13 y | 1300* | 1250 | 240 | 600 | 45 | 5* | 11 | 60* | 2* | 0.9 | 0.9 | 12 | 1.0 | 300 | 1.8 | 4* | 20* | 375* |
| 14-18 y | 1300* | 1250 | 410 | 900 | 75 | 5* | 15 | 75* | 3* | 1.2 | 1.3 | 16 | 1.3 | 400 | 2.4 | 5* | 25* | 550* |
| 19-30 y | 1000* | 700 | 400 | 900 | 90 | 5* | 15 | 120* | 4* | 1.2 | 1.3 | 16 | 1.3 | 400 | 2.4 | 5* | 30* | 550* |
| 31-50 y | 1000* | 700 | 420 | 900 | 90 | 5* | 15 | 120* | 4* | 1.2 | 1.3 | 16 | 1.3 | 400 | 2.4 | 5* | 30* | 550* |
| 51-70 y | 1200* | 700 | 420 | 900 | 90 | 10* | 15 | 120* | 4* | 1.2 | 1.3 | 16 | 1.7 | 400 | 2.4[f] | 5* | 30* | 550* |
| >70 y | 1200* | 700 | 420 | 900 | 90 | 15* | 15 | 120* | 4* | 1.2 | 1.3 | 16 | 1.7 | 400 | 2.4[f] | 5* | 30* | 550* |
| **Females** | | | | | | | | | | | | | | | | | | |
| 9-13 y | 1300* | 1250 | 240 | 600 | 45 | 5* | 11 | 60* | 2* | 0.9 | 0.9 | 12 | 1.0 | 300 | 1.8 | 4* | 20* | 375* |
| 14-18 y | 1300* | 1250 | 360 | 700 | 65 | 5* | 15 | 75* | 3* | 1 | 1 | 14 | 1.2 | 400[g] | 2.4 | 5* | 25* | 400* |
| 19-30 y | 1000* | 700 | 310 | 700 | 75 | 5* | 15 | 90* | 3* | 1.1 | 1.1 | 14 | 1.3 | 400[g] | 2.4 | 5* | 30* | 425* |
| 31-50 y | 1000* | 700 | 320 | 700 | 75 | 5* | 15 | 90* | 3* | 1.1 | 1.1 | 14 | 1.3 | 400[g] | 2.4 | 5* | 30* | 425* |
| 51-70 y | 1200* | 700 | 320 | 700 | 75 | 10* | 15 | 90* | 3* | 1.1 | 1.1 | 14 | 1.5 | 400 | 2.4[f] | 5* | 30* | 425* |
| >70 y | 1200* | 700 | 320 | 700 | 75 | 15* | 15 | 90* | 3* | 1.1 | 1.1 | 14 | 1.5 | 400 | 2.4[f] | 5* | 30* | 425* |
| **Pregnancy** | | | | | | | | | | | | | | | | | | |
| ≤18 y | 1300* | 1250 | 400 | 750 | 80 | 5* | 15 | 75* | 3* | 1.4 | 1.4 | 18 | 1.9 | 600[h] | 2.6 | 6* | 30* | 450* |
| 19-30 y | 1000* | 700 | 350 | 770 | 85 | 5* | 15 | 90* | 3* | 1.4 | 1.4 | 18 | 1.9 | 600[h] | 2.6 | 6* | 30* | 450* |
| 31-50 y | 1000* | 700 | 360 | 770 | 85 | 5* | 15 | 90* | 3* | 1.4 | 1.4 | 18 | 1.9 | 600[f] | 2.6 | 6* | 30* | 450* |

## Food and Nutrition Board, Institute of Medicine – National Academy of Science Dietary Reference Intakes: Recommended Intakes for Individuals

| Life-stage group | | Calcium (mg/d) | Phosphorus (mg/d) | Magnesium (mg/d) | Vitamin A (mcg/d) | Vitamin C (mg/d) | Vitamin D (mcg/d)[a,b] | Vitamin E (mg/d) | Vitamin K (mcg/d) | Fluoride (mg/d) | Thiamine (mg/d) | Riboflavin (mg/d) | Niacin (mg/d)[c] | Vitamin B6 (mg/d) | Folate (mcg/d)[d] | Vitamin B12 (mcg/d) | Pantothenic acid (mg/d) | Biotin (mcg/d) | Choline[e] (mg/d) |
|---|---|---|---|---|---|---|---|---|---|---|---|---|---|---|---|---|---|---|---|
| Lactation | ≤ 18 y | 1300* | 1250 | 360 | 1200 | 115 | 5* | 19 | 75* | 3* | 1.4 | 1.6 | 17 | 2 | 500 | 2.8 | 7* | 35* | 550* |
| | 19–30 y | 1000* | 700 | 310 | 1300 | 120 | 5* | 19 | 90* | 3* | 1.4 | 1.6 | 17 | 2 | 500 | 2.8 | 7* | 35* | 550* |
| | 31–50 y | 1000* | 700 | 320 | 1300 | 120 | 5* | 19 | 90* | 3* | 1.4 | 1.6 | 17 | 2 | 500 | 2.8 | 7* | 35* | 550* |

a As cholecalciferol. 1 mcg cholecalciferol = 40 units vitamin D.

b In the absence of adequate exposure to sunlight.

c As niacin equivalents (NE). 1 mg of niacin = 60 mg of tryptophan; 0 to 6 months = preformed niacin (not NE).

d As dietary folate equivalents (DFE). 1 DFE = 1 mcg food folate = 0.6 mcg of folic acid (from fortified food or supplement) consumed with food = 0.5 mcg of synthetic (supplemental) folic acid taken on an empty stomach.

e Although AIs have been set for choline, there are few data to assess whether a dietary supply of choline is needed at all stages of the life-cycle, and it may be that the choline requirement can be met by endogenous synthesis at some of these stages.

f Because 10% to 30% of older people may malabsorb food-bound $B_{12}$, it is advisable for those older than 50 years of age to meet their RDA mainly by consuming foods fortified with $B_{12}$ or a supplement containing $B_{12}$.

g In view of evidence linking folate intake with neural tube defects in the fetus, it is recommended that all women capable of becoming pregnant consume 400 mcg of synthetic folic acid from fortified foods and/or supplements in addition to intake of food folate from a varied diet.

h It is assumed that women will continue consuming 400 mcg of folic acid until their pregnancy is confirmed and they enter prenatal care, which ordinarily occurs after the end of the periconceptional period – the critical time for formation of the neural tube.

# VITAMIN C (Ascorbic Acid)

## ASCORBIC ACID

| | |
|---|---|
| **Tablets**: 25, 50, 100, 250, 500, and 1,000 mg (*otc*) | Various, *One A Day Extras Vitamin C* (Miles) |
| **Tablets, chewable**: 60, 100, 250, and 500 mg (*otc*) | Various |
| **Tablets and caplets, timed-release**: 500, 1,000, and 1,500 mg (*otc*) | Various |
| **Caplets**: 500 mg (*otc*) | *SunKist Vitamin C* (Ciba) |
| **Capsules, timed-release**: 500 mg (*otc*) | Various, *Ascorbicap* (ICN), *Cevi-Bid* (Geriatric) |
| **Lozenges**: 60 mg (*otc*) | *N'ice Vitamin C Drops* (SmithKline Beecham Consumer) |
| **Crystals**: 4 g/teaspoonful (*otc*) | *Vita-C* (Freeda) |
| **Powder**: 4 g/teaspoonful (*otc*) | *Dull-C* (Freeda) |
| **Liquid**: 35 mg/0.6 mL (*otc*) | *Ce-Vi-Sol* (Mead Johnson Nutritional) |
| **Solution**: 100 mg/mL (*otc*) | *Cecon* (Abbott) |
| **Syrup**: 500 mg/5 mL (*otc*) | Various |
| **Injection**: 250 and 500 mg/mL (*Rx*) | Various |

## CALCIUM ASCORBATE

| | |
|---|---|
| **Tablets**: 610 mg (equiv. to 500 mg ascorbic acid) (*otc*) | Various |
| **Powder**: 1 g (equiv. to 826 mg ascorbic acid)/ ¼ teaspoonful (*otc*) | Various |

## SODIUM ASCORBATE

| | |
|---|---|
| **Tablets**: 585 mg (equiv. to 500 mg ascorbic acid) (*otc*) | Various |
| **Crystals**: 1,020 mg (equiv. to 900 mg ascorbic acid)/ ¼ teaspoonful (*otc*) | Various |
| **Injection**: 250 mg/mL (equiv. to 222 mg/mL ascorbic acid) (*Rx*) | Various |
| 562.5 mg/mL (equiv. to 500 mg/mL ascorbic acid) (*Rx*) | *Cenolate* (Abbott) |

### Indications

Prevention and treatment of scurvy. Parenteral administration is desirable in an acute deficiency or when absorption of oral ascorbic acid is uncertain.

*Unlabeled uses:* Vitamin C (at least 2 g/day) may be used as a urinary acidifier in conjunction with methenamine therapy.

Vitamin C in doses of at least 150 mg has been used to control idiopathic methemoglobinemia (less effective than methylene blue).

### Administration and Dosage

*Parenteral:* Administer IV, IM, or subcutaneously. Avoid too rapid IV injection. Absorption and utilization are somewhat more efficient with the IM route, which is usually preferred.

*Infants:* Average daily protective requirement is 30 mg. The usual curative dose is 100 to 300 mg daily, continued as long as clinical symptoms persist or until saturation, as indicated by excretion tests, has been attained.

*Premature infants:* May require 75 to 100 mg/day.

*Adults:* The average protective dose is 70 to 150 mg/day. For scurvy, 300 mg to 1 g daily is recommended. However, up to 6 g/day has been administered parenterally to normal adults without evidence of toxicity.

*Enhanced wound healing* – Doses of 300 to 500 mg daily for 7 to 10 days both preoperatively and postoperatively are adequate, although considerably larger amounts have been recommended.

*Burns* – For severe burns, daily doses of 1 to 2 g are recommended.

In other conditions in which the need for vitamin C is increased, 3 to 5 times the daily optimum allowances appears adequate.

### Actions

*Pharmacology:* Vitamin C, a water-soluble vitamin, is an essential vitamin in man; however, its exact biological functions are not fully understood. It is essential for the formation and the maintenance of intercellular ground substance and collagen, for catecholamine biosynthesis, for synthesis of carnitine and steroids, for conversion of folic acid to folinic acid and for tyrosine metabolism.

The deficiency state scurvy is characterized by degenerative changes in the capillaries, bone, and connective tissues. Mild vitamin C deficiency symptoms may include faulty bone and tooth development, gingivitis, bleeding gums, and loosened teeth.

Absorption of dietary ascorbate from the intestines is nearly complete. Vitamin C is readily available in citrus fruit, tomatoes, potatoes, and leafy vegetables.

### Warnings

*Excessive vitamin C doses:* Diabetics, patients prone to recurrent renal calculi, those undergoing stool occult blood tests and those on sodium restricted diets or anticoagulant therapy should not take excessive doses of vitamin C over an extended time period.

*Pregnancy: Category* C. Do not administer ascorbic acid to pregnant women in excess of the amount needed for treatment. The possibility of the fetus adapting to high levels of the vitamin could result in a scorbutic condition after birth when the intake drops to normal levels. This action is controversial.

*Lactation:* Ascorbic acid is excreted in breast milk.

### Drug Interactions

*Contraceptives (oral) and estrogens:* Ascorbic acid increases serum levels of estrogen and estrogen contained in oral contraceptives, possibly resulting in adverse reactions.

*Warfarin:* The anticoagulant action of warfarin may be reduced.

*Drug/Lab test interactions:* Large doses (more than 500 mg) of vitamin C may cause false-negative urine glucose determinations.

No exogenous vitamin C should be ingested for 48 to 72 hours before amine-dependent stool occult blood tests are conducted because possible false-negative results may occur.

### Adverse Reactions

Large doses may cause diarrhea and precipitation of cystine, oxalate, or urate renal stones if the urine becomes acidic during therapy.

Transient mild soreness may occur at the site of IM or subcutaneous injection. Too rapid IV administration may cause temporary faintness or dizziness.

# CALCIUM

### CALCIUM ACETATE

**Tablets**: 667 elemental mg (169 mg elemental calcium) (*Rx*)  *PhosLo* (Braintree)
**Capsules**: 333.5 mg (half-size) (84.5 mg elemental calcium), 667 mg (169 mg elemental calcium) (*Rx*)
**Gelcaps**: 667 mg (169 mg elemental calcium) (*Rx*)

### CALCIUM CARBONATE

| | |
|---|---|
| **Tablets**: 648 to 650 mg (260 mg elemental calcium) (*otc*) | Various |
| 1,250 mg (500 mg elemental calcium) (*otc*) | Various, *Cal-Carb Forte* (Vitaline), *Oysco 500* (Rugby), *Oyst-Cal 500* (Goldline), *Os-Cal 500* (GlaxoSmithKline Consumer) |
| 1,500 mg (600 mg elemental calcium) (*otc*) | Various, *Calcium 600* (Rugby), *Caltrate 600* (Whitehall Robins), *Nephro-Calci* (Watson) |
| **Tablets, chewable**: 500 mg (200 mg elemental calcium) (*otc*) | *Tums* (GlaxoSmithKline Consumer), *Cal•Gest* (Rugby) |
| 750 mg (300 mg elemental calcium (*otc*) | Various, *Tums E-X* (GlaxoSmithKline Consumer), *Tums Calcium for Life PMS* (GlaxoSmithKline Consumer) |
| 1,000 mg (400 mg elemental calcium) (*otc*) | *Tums Ultra* (GlaxoSmithKline Consumer) |
| 1,250 mg (500 mg elemental calcium) (*otc*) | Various, *Cal-Carb Forte* (Vitaline), *Calci-Chew* (Watson), *Os-Cal 500*, *Tums Calcium for Life Bone Health* (GlaxoSmithKline Consumer) |
| **Capsules**: 1,250 mg (500 mg elemental calcium) (*otc*) | *Calci-Mix* (Watson) |
| **Capsules** and **tablets**: 364 mg calcium carbonate (145.6 mg elemental calcium) and 8.3 mg sodium fluoride (*otc*) | *Florical* (Mericon) |
| **Oral suspension**: 1,250 mg (500 mg elemental calcium)/5 mL (*otc*) | Various |
| **Powder** (*otc*) | Various |

### CALCIUM CHLORIDE

**Injection**: 10% (*Rx*)  Various

### CALCIUM CITRATE

| | |
|---|---|
| **Tablets**: 200 mg elemental calcium (*otc*) | *Citracal* (Mission) |
| 200 mg calcium citrate (*otc*) | *Citrus Calcium* (Rugby) |
| 250 mg elemental calcium (*otc*) | Various, *Cal-Citrate-250* (Bio-Tech) |
| 950 mg (*otc*) | Various |
| **Tablets, effervescent**: 500 mg calcium (*otc*) | *Citracal Liquitab* (Mission) |
| **Capsules**: 225 mg elemental calcium (*otc*) | *Cal-Citrate-225* (Bio-Tech) |
| **Powder for oral suspension**: 760 mg elemental calcium/ 5 mL (*otc*) | Various |

### CALCIUM GLUBIONATE

**Syrup**: 1.8 g/5 mL (*otc*)  Various, *Calciquid* (Breckenridge)

### CALCIUM GLUCEPTATE

**Injection**: 1.1 g/5 mL (*Rx*)  Various

### CALCIUM GLUCONATE

| | |
|---|---|
| **Tablets**: 500 mg (45 mg elemental calcium), 50 mg elemental calcium, 648 to 650 mg (58.5 to 60 mg elemental calcium), 972 to 975 mg (87.75 to 90 mg elemental calcium) (*otc*) | Various |
| **Powder for oral suspension**: 346.7 mg elemental calcium/ 15 mL (*otc*) | Various |
| **Injection**: 10% (*Rx*) | Various |

### CALCIUM LACTATE

| | |
|---|---|
| **Tablets**: 648 to 650 mg (84.5 mg elemental calcium), 100 mg elemental calcium (*otc*) | Various |
| **Capsules**: 500 mg (96 mg elemental calcium) (*otc*) | *Cal-Lac* (Bio-Tech) |

### CALCIUM SALT COMBINATIONS

**Injection**: 50 mg calcium glycerophosphate and 50 mg calcium lactate per 10 mL in sodium chloride solution (0.08 mEq Ca/mL) (*Rx*)  *Calphosan* (Glenwood)

### TRICALCIUM PHOSPHATE

**Tablets**: 600 mg elemental calcium (*otc*)  *Posture* (Iverness Medical)

### Indications

*Oral:* As a dietary supplement when calcium intake may be inadequate. Conditions that may be associated with calcium deficiency include the following: Vitamin D deficiency, sprue, pregnancy and lactation, achlorhydria, chronic diarrhea, hypoparathyroidism, steatorrhea, menopause, renal failure, pancreatitis, hyperphosphatemia, and alkalosis. Some diuretics and anticonvulsants may precipitate hypocalcemia, which may validate calcium replacement therapy. Calcium salt therapy should not preclude the use of other corrective measures intended to treat the underlying cause of calcium depletion.

Oral calcium may also be used in the treatment of osteoporosis, osteomalacia, rickets, and latent tetany.

Calcium taken daily may help reduce typical premenstrual syndrome (PMS) symptoms such as bloating, cramps, fatigue, and moodiness.

*Calcium acetate (PhosLo)* – Control of hyperphosphatemia in end-stage renal failure; does not promote aluminum absorption.

*Parenteral:*

*Hypocalcemia* – To correct plasma calcium levels (eg, neonatal tetany and tetany due to parathyroid deficiency, vitamin D deficiency, alkalosis); prevention of hypocalcemia during exchange transfusions; conditions associated with intestinal malabsorption.

*Calcium chloride and gluconate* – Adjunctive therapy in the treatment of insect bites or stings, such as Black Widow spider bites to relieve muscle cramping; sensitivity reactions, particularly when characterized by urticaria; depression due to overdosage of magnesium sulfate; acute symptoms of lead colic; rickets; osteomalacia.

*Calcium chloride* – To combat severe hyperkalemia pending correction of increased potassium in the extracellular fluid.

*Cardiac resuscitation:* After open heart surgery, when epinephrine fails to improve weak or ineffective myocardial contractions.

*Calcium gluconate* – To decrease capillary permeability in allergic conditions, nonthrombocytopenic purpura and exudative dermatoses such as dermatitis herpetiformis; for pruritus of eruptions caused by certain drugs; in hyperkalemia, calcium gluconate may aid in antagonizing the cardiac toxicity, provided the patient is not receiving digitalis therapy.

### Administration and Dosage

*Oral:*

*Dietary supplement* – The usual daily dose is 500 mg to 2 g, 2 to 4 times/day.

Calcium is recommended in doses of 1500 mg/day for men over 65 years of age and for postmenopausal women not taking estrogen replacement therapy.

*PhosLo* – For adult dialysis patients, the initial dose is 2 tablets/capsules/gelcaps with each meal. The dosage may be increased gradually to bring the serum phosphate value less than 6 mg/dL, as long as hypercalcemia does not develop. Most patients require 3 to 4 tablets with each meal.

The recommended initial dose of the half-size (333.5 mg) *PhosLo* for the adult dialysis patient is 4 capsules with each meal. The dosage may be increased gradually to bring the serum phosphate value below 6 mg/dL, as long as hypercalcemia does not develop. Most patients require 6 to 8 capsules with each meal.

*Florical* – 1 capsule or tablet daily.

*Parenteral:* Calcium gluconate is generally preferred over calcium chloride as it is less irritating.

*IV* – Warm solutions to body temperature and give slowly (0.5 to 2 mL/min); stop if patient complains of discomfort. Resume when symptoms disappear. Following injection, patient should remain recumbent for a short time. Repeated injections may be needed because of the rapid calcium excretion. Inject **calcium chloride** and **gluconate** through a small needle into a large vein to minimize venous irritation.

*IM administration* – IM administration of **calcium gluceptate** and **gluconate** should be reserved for emergencies when technical difficulty makes IV injection impossible. Administer **calcium gluconate** only by the IV route and **calcium chloride** by the IV or intraventricular route.

CALCIUM CHLORIDE –

*For IV use only:* Injection is irritating to veins and must not be injected into tissues. Avoid extravasation. Administer slowly (not to exceed 0.5 to 1 mL/min).

*Intraventricular administration* – In cardiac resuscitation, injection may be made into the ventricular cavity; do not inject into the myocardium. Replace the IV needle with a suitable intracardiac needle.

The intraventricular dose usually ranges from 200 to 800 mg (2 to 8 mL).

*Hypocalcemic disorders:*

*Adults* – 500 mg to 1 g at intervals of 1 to 3 days, depending on response of patient or serum calcium determinations.

*Children* – 0.2 mL/kg up to 1 to 10 mL/day.

*Magnesium intoxication:* Give 500 mg promptly; observe patient for signs of recovery before further doses are given.

*Hyperkalemic ECG disturbances of cardiac function:* Adjust dosage by constant monitoring of ECG changes during administration.

*Cardiac resuscitation:*

*Adults* – Dose ranges from 500 mg to 1 g IV or 200 to 800 mg injected into the ventricular cavity.

*Children* – 0.2 mL/kg

CALCIUM GLUCEPTATE –

*IM:* 2 to 5 mL (0.44 to 1.1 g). Inject 5 mL (1.1 g) doses in the gluteal region or, in infants, in the lateral thigh.

*IV:* 5 to 20 mL (1.1 to 4.4 g). Warm solution to body temperature and administer slowly (no more than 2 mL/min).

*Exchange transfusions in newborns:* 0.5 mL (0.11 g) after every 100 mL of blood exchanged.

CALCIUM GLUCONATE – For IV use only, either directly or by infusion. Do not exceed a rate of 0.5 to 2 mL/min. Calcium gluconate may also be administered by intermittent infusion at a rate not exceeding 200 mg/min, or by continuous infusion. Discontinue injection if the patient complains of discomfort.

*Adults:* 2.3 to 9.3 mEq (5 to 20 mL) as required. Dosage range is 4.65 to 70 mEq/day.

*Children:* 2.3 mEq/kg/day or 56 mEq/m$^2$/day, well diluted; give slowly in divided doses.

*Infants:* Not more than 0.93 mEq (2 mL).

*Emergency elevation of serum calcium:*

*Adults* – 7 to 14 mEq (15 to 30 mL) IV.

*Children* – 1 to 7 mEq (2.2 to 15 mL).

*Infants* – Less than 1 mEq (2.2 mL). Doses can be repeated every 1 to 3 days.

*Hypocalcemic tetany:*

*Adults* – 4.5 to 16 mEq of calcium (9.7 to 34.4 mL) may be given IM until therapeutic response occurs.

*Children* – 0.5 to 0.7 mEq/kg (1.1 to 1.5 mL/kg) IV 3 or 4 times/day or until tetany is controlled.

*Neonates* – 2.4 mEq/kg/day (5.2 mL/kg/day) in divided doses.

*Hyperkalemia with secondary cardiac toxicity:* Administer IV 2.25 to 14 mEq (4.8 to 30.1 mL) while monitoring ECG. If necessary, repeat doses after 1 to 2 minutes.

*Magnesium intoxication:*

*Adults* – Initial dose is 4.5 to 9 mEq (9.7 to 19.4 mL) IV. Adjust subsequent doses to patient response. If IV use is not possible, give 2 to 5 mEq (4.3 to 10.8 mL) IM.

*Exchange transfusion:*

*Adults* – Approximately 1.35 mEq (2.9 mL) IV concurrent with each 100 mL of citrated blood.

*Neonates* – Administer IV at a dosage of 0.45 mEq (1 mL) per 100 mL of exchanged citrated blood.

*Admixture incompatibilities:* Calcium salts should not generally be mixed with carbonates, phosphates, sulfates, or tartrates in parenteral admixtures; they are conditionally compatible with potassium phosphates, depending on concentration. Calcium ions will chelate tetracycline.

### Actions

*Pharmacology:* Calcium is essential for the functional integrity of the nervous and muscular systems, for normal cardiac contractility and the coagulation of blood. It also functions as an enzyme cofactor and affects the secretory activity of endocrine and exocrine glands.

Patients with advanced renal insufficiency (Ccr less than 30 mL/min) exhibit phosphate retention and some degree of hyperphosphatemia. The retention of phosphate plays a role in causing secondary hyperparathyroidism associated with osteodystrophy and soft-tissue calcification. Calcium acetate, when taken with meals, combines with dietary phosphate to form insoluble calcium phosphate, which is excreted in the feces.

| Elemental Calcium Content of Calcium Salts[1] | | |
| --- | --- | --- |
| Calcium salt | % Calcium | mEq $Ca^{++}$/g |
| Calcium glubionate | 6.5 | 3.3 |
| Calcium gluconate | 9 | 4.5 |
| Calcium lactate | 13 | 6.5 |
| Calcium citrate | 21 | 10.6 |
| Calcium acetate | 25 | 12.6 |
| Tricalcium phosphate | 39 | 19.3 |
| Calcium carbonate | 40 | 20 |

[1] 1 mEq of elemental calcium = 20 mg

*Pharmacokinetics:*

*Absorption* – Calcium is absorbed from the GI tract by passive diffusion and active transport. Calcium must be in a soluble, ionized form for absorption to occur. Vitamin D is required for calcium absorption and increases the absorptive mechanisms. Calcium absorption is increased in the presence of food. Oral bioavailability in adults ranges from 25% to 35% when given with a standardized breakfast. Absorption from milk was approximately 29% under the same conditions.

*Distribution* – Calcium is rapidly incorporated into skeletal tissue. Normal serum calcium concentrations range from 9 to 10.4 mg/dL (4.5 to 5.2 mEq/L), but only ionized calcium is active. Calcium crosses the placenta and reaches higher concentrations in fetal blood than maternal blood. Calcium also is distributed in milk.

*Excretion* – Calcium is mainly excreted in the feces. Urinary excretion does not exceed 150 mg/day in patients on low calcium diets. Urinary excretion decreases with age, in early renal failure, and during pregnancy. Calcium also is excreted by the sweat glands.

### Contraindications

*Oral:* Hypercalcemia, ventricular fibrillation.

*Parenteral:* Hypercalcemia; ventricular fibrillation; digitalized patients.

### Warnings

*Extravasation:* **Calcium chloride** and **gluconate** can cause severe necrosis, sloughing, and abscess formation with IM or subcutaneous administration.

*PhosLo:* End-stage renal failure patients may develop hypercalcemia when given calcium with meals. Do not give other calcium supplements concurrently with *PhosLo.* Monitor serum calcium levels twice weekly during the early dose adjustment period. Do not allow serum calcium times phosphate product to exceed 66.

*GI effects:* Oral calcium salts may be irritating to the GI tract and also may cause constipation.

*Hypercalcemia:* Hypercalcemia may occur when large doses of calcium are administered to patients with chronic renal failure. Mild hypercalcemia may exhibit as nausea, vomiting, anorexia, or constipation, with mental changes such as stupor, delirium, coma, or confusion.

*Renal calculi:* Recent studies show that high dietary intake of calcium decreases the risk of symptomatic renal calculi, while intake of supplemental calcium may increase the risk of symptomatic stones. This conflicts with the previous theory that high calcium intake contributes to the risk of renal calculi.

*Pregnancy:* Category C. (*PhosLo* and parenteral).

*Children:* Safety and efficacy in children have not been established (*PhosLo*).

### Precautions
*Oral:*

> *Monitoring* – Monitor serum calcium concentrations and maintain at 9 to 10.4 mg/dL (4.5 to 5.2 mEq/L). Do not allow levels to exceed 12 mg/dL.

> *Special risk patients* – Use calcium salts cautiously in patients with sarcoidosis, cardiac or renal disease, and in patients receiving cardiac glycosides.

> *Phenylketonurics* – Inform phenylketonuric patients that some of these products contain phenylalanine.

*Parenteral:*

> *Cardiovascular effects* – High concentrations of calcium may cause cardiac syncope.

### Drug Interactions
*Calcium citrate:* Avoid concurrent aluminum-containing antacids.

Drugs that may be affected by calcium include sodium polystyrene sulfonate, tetracyclines, verapamil. Iron salts and quinolones (oral only); digitalis glycosides (parenteral only).

*Drug/Lab test interactions:* Transient elevations of plasma 11-hydroxy-corticosteroid levels (Glenn-Nelson technique) may occur when IV calcium is administered, but levels return to control values after 1 hour. In addition, IV calcium gluconate can produce false-negative values for serum and urinary magnesium.

*Drug/Food interactions:* Diets high in dietary fiber have been shown to decrease absorption of calcium due to decreased transit time in the GI tract and complexing of fiber with the calcium.

> Calcium acetate, when taken with meals, combines with dietary phosphate to form insoluble calcium phosphate which is excreted in the feces.

### Adverse Reactions

> *Oral* – May cause constipation and headache. Mild hypercalcemia ($Ca^{++}$ greater than 10.5 mg/dL) may be asymptomatic or manifest itself as: Anorexia, nausea, and vomiting. More severe hypercalcemia ($Ca^{++}$ 12 mg/dL) is associated with confusion, delirium, stupor, and coma.

> *IM administration* – Mild local reactions may occur (calcium gluceptate). Local necrosis and abscess formation may occur with **calcium gluconate**. Severe necrosis and sloughing may occur with IM or subcutaneous administration of **calcium chloride**.

> *IV administration* – Rapid IV administration may cause bradycardia, sense of oppression, tingling, metallic, calcium, or chalky taste, or "heat waves". Rapid IV **calcium gluconate** may cause vasodilation, decreased blood pressure, cardiac arrhythmias, syncope, and cardiac arrest. **Calcium chloride** injections cause peripheral vasodilation and a local burning sensation; blood pressure may fall moderately.

# MAGNESIUM

| | |
|---|---|
| **Tablets:** 27.5 mg elemental magnesium, 30 mg elemental magnesium, 100 mg elemental magnesium (*otc*) | Various |
| 200 mg elemental magnesium (as oxide) (*otc*) | *Mag-200* (Optimox) |
| 400 mg magnesium oxide (241.3 mg elemental magnesium) (*otc*) | Various, *Mag-Ox 400* (Blaine) |
| 500 mg magnesium gluconate dihydrate (27 mg elemental magnesium) (*otc*) | *Almora* (Forest), *Mag-G* (Cypress), *Magonate* (Fleming) |
| 500 mg magnesium gluconate (29 mg elemental magnesium) (*otc*) | *Magtrate* (Mission) |
| **Tablets, enteric-coated:** 64 mg elemental magnesium (as chloride hexahydrate) (*otc*) | *Slow-Mag* (Shire) |
| **Tablets, sustained-release:** 84 mg elemental magnesium (as L-lactate dihydrate) (*otc*) | *Mag-Tab SR* (Niche) |
| **Capsules:** 140 mg magnesium oxide (84.5 mg elemental magnesium) (*otc*) | *Uro-Mag* (Blaine) |
| **Liquid:** 3.52 mg elemental magnesium/5 mL (as gluconate) (*otc*) | *Magonate Natal* (Fleming) |
| 1,000 mg magnesium dihydrate/5 mL (54 mg elemental magnesium/5 mL) (*otc*) | *Magonate* (Fleming) |
| **Injection:** 20% magnesium chloride (1.97 mEq/mL) (*Rx*) | Various |
| **Magnesium sulfate.** 10% (0.8 mEq/mL), 12.5% (1 mEq/mL) and 50% (4 mEq/mL) (*Rx*) | Various |

## Indications

Oral: As a dietary supplement.

Parenteral:

Hypomagnesemia – Magnesium sulfate is used as replacement therapy in magnesium deficiency especially in acute hypomagnesemia accompanied by signs of tetany similar to those observed in hypocalcemia. In such cases, the serum magnesium (Mg++) level is usually below the lower limit of normal (1.5 to 2.5 or 3 mEq/L) and the serum calcium (Ca++) level is normal (4.3 to 5.3 mEq/L) or elevated.

Total parenteral nutrition: Total parenteral nutrition patients may develop hypomagnesemia (less than 1.5 mEq/L) without supplementation. Magnesium is added to correct or prevent hypomagnesemia.

Preeclampsia/eclampsia/nephritis (magnesium sulfate) – Prevention and control of convulsions of severe preeclampsia and eclampsia and for control of hypertension, encephalopathy, and convulsions associated with acute nephritis in children.

## Administration and Dosage

Oral: 1 g magnesium = 83.3 mEq (41.1 mmol).

Dietary supplement – 40 to 400 mg/day in divided doses. Refer to product labeling. Magnesium-containing antacids may also be used.

Recommended dietary allowances (RDAs):

Adults – Males, 270 to 400 mg; females, 280 to 300 mg.

Parenteral:

IV administration – Do not exceed 1.5 mL/min of a 10% concentration (or its equivalent), except in cases of severe eclampsia with seizures. Dilute IV infusion solutions to a concentration of 20% or less prior to IV administration. The most commonly used diluents are 5% dextrose injection and 0.9% sodium chloride Injection.

IM administration – Deep IM injection of the undiluted (50%) solution is appropriate for adults, but dilute to 20% or less concentration prior to IM injection in children.

Admixture incompatibilities – Magnesium sulfate in solution may result in a precipitate formation when mixed with solutions containing: Alcohol (in high concentrations); alkali carbonates and bicarbonates; alkali hydroxides; arsenates; barium; calcium; clindamycin phosphate; heavy metals; hydrocortisone sodium succinate; phosphates; polymyxin B sulfate; procaine hydrochloride; salicylates; strontium; tartrates.

*Hyperalimentation* – Maintenance requirements are not precisely known. Maintenance dose range:

*Adults:* 8 to 24 mEq/day.

*Infants:* 2 to 10 mEq/day.

*Mild magnesium deficiency* –

*Adults:* 1 g (8.12 mEq; 2 mL of 50% solution) IM every 6 hours for 4 doses (total of 32.5 mEq/24 hours).

*Severe hypomagnesemia* –

*IM:* As much as 2 mEq/kg (0.5 mL of 50% solution) within 4 hours if necessary.

*IV:* 5 g (approximately 40 mEq)/L of 5% dextrose injection or 0.9% sodium chloride solution, infused over 3 hours. In treatment of deficiency states, observe caution to prevent exceeding renal excretory capacity.

*Seizures associated with preeclampsia/eclampsia/nephritis* – Refer to Anticonvulsants, Miscellaneous for complete dosing information.

## Actions

*Pharmacology:* Magnesium is the fourth most abundant mineral in the body and the second most abundant in muscles and other organs. Potassium cannot be retained in soft tissues if magnesium is deficient. An adequate amount of magnesium also is required for the absorption and utilization of calcium, favoring the deposition of calcium in bone and preventing deposition of calcium in the soft tissues and kidneys. Magnesium is required for the normal activity of 300 enzymes.

*Pharmacokinetics:* IM injection results in therapeutic plasma levels within 60 minutes and persists for 3 to 4 hours. IV doses provide immediate effects that last for 30 minutes. Effective anticonvulsant serum levels range from 2.5 to 7.5 mEq/L. Magnesium is excreted by the kidneys at a rate proportional to the plasma concentration and glomerular filtration.

## Contraindications

*Magnesium sulfate:* Heart block or myocardial damage; IV magnesium to patients with preeclampsia during the 2 hours preceding delivery.

*Magnesium chloride:* Renal impairment; marked myocardial disease; coma.

## Warnings

*Renal function impairment:* Use with caution. Parenteral use in the presence of renal insufficiency may lead to magnesium intoxication.

*Elderly:* Geriatric patients often require reduced dosage because of impaired renal function. In patients with severe impairment, dosage should not exceed 20 g in 48 hours. Monitor serum magnesium in such patients.

*Pregnancy:* It is unknown whether magnesium supplementation will harm an unborn child or a breast-feeding child. Do not take this mineral without speaking to a physician if pregnant, planning a pregnancy, or breast-feeding.

*Lactation:* Magnesium is distributed into milk during parenteral magnesium sulfate administration.

*Children:* Safety and efficacy in children have not been established.

## Precautions

*Monitoring:* Maintain urine output at a level of at least 100 mL every 4 hours. Monitor serum magnesium levels and clinical status to avoid overdosage in preeclampsia.

Serum magnesium levels usually sufficient to control convulsions range from 3 to 6 mg/dL (2.5 to 5 mEq/L). Keep an injectable calcium salt immediately available to counteract potential hazards of magnesium intoxication in eclampsia.

*Flushing/Sweating:* Administer with caution if flushing or sweating occurs.

*Renal disease:* Do not use without physician supervision because of potential accumulation.

*Excessive dosage:* Excessive dosage may cause diarrhea and GI irritation.

*Heart disease:* Magnesium supplements may make this condition worse.

#### Drug Interactions

Drugs that may be affected by magnesium salts include aminoquinolines, nitrofurantoin, penicillamine, and tetracyclines.

#### Adverse Reactions

Adverse effects are usually the result of magnesium intoxication and include flushing; sweating; hypotension; stupor; depressed reflexes; flaccid paralysis; hypothermia; circulatory collapse; cardiac and CNS depression proceeding to respiratory paralysis (the most life-threatening effect).

Hypocalcemia with signs of tetany secondary to magnesium sulfate therapy for eclampsia has occurred.

# POTASSIUM REPLACEMENT PRODUCTS

## POTASSIUM REPLACEMENT PRODUCTS

| | |
|---|---|
| **Tablets, controlled-release**: 6.7 mEq (500 mg) potassium chloride in a wax matrix (*Rx*) | *Kaon-Cl* (Adria) |
| 8 and 10 mEq (600 and 750 mg) potassium chloride in a wax matrix (*Rx*) | Various, *Klor-Con 8* (Upsher-Smith), *Kaon Cl-10* (Adria), *Klor-Con 10* (Upsher-Smith), *Klotrix* (Bristol), *K-Tab* (Abbott) |
| **Tablets, extended-release**: 750 mg potassium chloride equivalent to 10 mEq potassium in a wax matrix (*Rx*) | Various |
| **Tablets, controlled-release**: 750 mg microencapsulated potassium chloride equivalent to 10 mEq potassium (*Rx*) | *K-Dur 10* (Key), *Ten-K* (Summit) |
| 1,500 mg microencapsulated potassium chloride (equivalent to 20 mEq potassium) (*Rx*) | *K-Dur 20* (Key) |
| **Tablets**: 500 mg potassium gluconate (83.45 mg potassium) (*Rx*) | Various |
| 595 mg potassium gluconate (99 mg potassium) (*Rx*) | Various |
| **Tablets, effervescent**: 20 mEq potassium (from potassium bicarbonate) (*Rx*) | *K + Care ET* (Alra) |
| 20 mEq potassium (from potassium chloride and bicarbonate and lysine HCl) (*Rx*) | *Klorvess* (Sandoz) |
| 25 mEq potassium (from potassium chloride and bicarbonate and lysine HCl) (*Rx*) | *K•Lyte/Cl* (Bristol) |
| 50 mEq potassium (from potassium Cl and bicarbonate, lysine monohydrochloride and citric acid) (*Rx*) | *K•Lyte/Cl 50* (Bristol) |
| 25 mEq potassium (from potassium bicarbonate) (*Rx*) | *K + Care ET* (Alra) |
| 25 mEq potassium (as bicarbonate and citrate) (*Rx*) | Various, *Effer-K* (Nomax), *Klor-Con/EF* (Upsher-Smith), *K•Lyte* (Bristol) |
| 50 mEq potassium (from potassium bicarbonate and citrate and citric acid) (*Rx*) | *K•Lyte DS* (Bristol) |
| **Capsules, controlled-release**: 600 mg potassium chloride equivalent to 8 mEq potassium. Microencapsulated particles (*Rx*) | *Micro-K Extencaps* (Robins) |
| 10 mEq (750 mg) potassium chloride. Microencapsulated particles (*Rx*) | Various, *Micro-K 10 Extencaps* (Robins) |
| **Liquid**: 20 mEq/15 mL potassium and chloride (10% KCl) (*Rx*) | Various, *Cena-K* (Century), *Kay Ciel* (Forest), *Klorvess* (Sandoz) |
| 30 mEq/15 mL potassium and chloride (15% KCl) (*Rx*) | *Rum-K* (Fleming) |
| 40 mEq/15 mL potassium and chloride (20% KCl) (*Rx*) | Various, *Cena-K* (Century), *Kaon-Cl 20%* (Adria) |
| 20 mEq/15 mL potassium (as potassium gluconate) (*Rx*) | Various, *Kaon* (Adria), *K-G Elixir* (Geneva) |
| 45 mEq/15 mL potassium (from potassium acetate, potassium bicarbonate and potassium citrate) (*Rx*) | *Tri-K* (Century) |
| 20 mEq/15 mL potassium (as potassium gluconate and potassium citrate) (*Rx*) | *Twin-K* (Boots) |
| 20 mEq potassium and 3.4 mEq chloride/15 mL (from potassium gluconate and potassium chloride) (*Rx*) | *Kolyum* (Fiscns) |

| | |
|---|---|
| **Powder**: 15 mEq potassium chloride per packet (*Rx*) | *K + Care* (Alra) |
| 20 mEq potassium chloride per packet (*Rx*) | Various, *Gen-K* (Goldline), *Kay Ciel* (Forest), *K + Care* (Alta), *K-Lor* (Abbott), *Klor-Con* (Upsher-Smith), *Micro-K LS* (Robins) |
| 25 mEq potassium chloride per dose (*Rx*) | *K•Lyte/Cl* (Mead-J) |
| 20 mEq each potassium and chloride (potassium chloride, bicarbonate and citrate and lysine HCl)/packet (*Rx*) | *Klorvess Effervescent Granules* (Sandoz) |

### POTASSIUM ACETATE

| | |
|---|---|
| **Injection**: 2 and 4 mEq/mL (*Rx*) | Various |

### POTASSIUM CHLORIDE CONCENTRATE

| | |
|---|---|
| **Injection**: 2 mEq/mL and 10, 20, 30, 40, 60, and 90 mEq (*Rx*) | Various |

### Indications

*Oral:* Treatment of hypokalemia in the following conditions: With or without metabolic alkalosis; digitalis intoxication; familial periodic paralysis; diabetic acidosis; diarrhea and vomiting; surgical conditions accompanied by nitrogen loss, vomiting, suction drainage, diarrhea, and increased urinary excretion of potassium; certain cases of uremia; hyperadrenalism; starvation and debilitation; corticosteroid or diuretic therapy.

Prevention of potassium depletion when dietary intake is inadequate in the following conditions: Patients receiving digitalis and diuretics for CHF; significant cardiac arrhythmias; hepatic cirrhosis with ascites; states of aldosterone excess with normal renal function; potassium-losing nephropathy; certain diarrheal states.

When hypokalemia is associated with alkalosis, use potassium chloride. When acidosis is present, use the bicarbonate, citrate, acetate, or gluconate potassium salts.

*IV:*

*Potassium acetate* – Potassium acetate is useful as an additive for preparing specific IV fluid formulas when patient needs cannot be met by standard electrolyte or nutrient solutions.

Also indicated for marked loss of GI secretions by vomiting, diarrhea, GI intubation, or fistulas; prolonged diuresis; prolonged parenteral use of potassium-free fluids; diabetic acidosis, especially during vigorous insulin and dextrose treatment; metabolic alkalosis; attacks of hereditary or familial periodic paralysis; hyperadrenocorticism; primary aldosteronism; overmedication with adrenocortical steroids, testosterone, or corticotropin; healing phase of scalds or burns; cardiac arrhythmias, especially due to digitalis glycosides.

### Administration and Dosage

*Oral:* The usual dietary intake of potassium ranges between 40 to 150 mEq/day.

Individualize dosage. Usual range is 16 to 24 mEq/day for the prevention of hypokalemia to 40 to 100 mEq/day or more for the treatment of potassium depletion.

Reserve slow release potassium chloride preparations for patients who cannot tolerate liquids or effervescent potassium preparations, or for patients in whom there is a problem of compliance with these preparations.

Some studies suggest the "microencapsulated" preparations are less likely to cause GI damage; however, evidence conflicts and a specific recommendation of one solid oral product over another cannot be made. Avoid enteric coated products.

Potassium intoxication may result from any therapeutic dosage.

*IV:*

*Do not administer undiluted potassium* – Potassium preparations must be diluted with suitable large volume parenteral solutions, mixed well and given by slow IV infusion.

Too rapid infusion of hypertonic solutions may cause local pain and, rarely, vein irritation. Adjust rate of administration according to tolerance. Use of the largest peripheral vein and a small bore needle is recommended.

The usual additive dilution of potassium chloride is 40 mEq/L of IV fluid. The maximum desirable concentration is 80 mEq/L, although extreme emergencies may dictate greater concentrations.

In critical states, potassium chloride may be administered in saline (unless saline is contraindicated) because dextrose may lower serum potassium levels by producing an intracellular shift.

Avoid "layering" of potassium by proper agitation of the prepared IV solution. Do not add potassium to an IV bottle in the hanging position.

Individualize dosage. Guide dosage and rate of infusion by ECG and serum electrolyte determinations. The following may be used as a guide:

| Potassium Dosage/Rate of Infusion Guidelines | | | |
|---|---|---|---|
| Serum K+ | Maximum infusion rate | Maximum concentration | Maximum 24 hour dose |
| > 2.5 mEq/L | 10 mEq/h | 40 mEq/L | 200 mEq |
| < 2 mEq/L | 40 mEq/h | 80 mEq/L | 400 mEq |

Add electrolytes to the mixed solutions only after considering electrolytes already present and potential incompatibilities such as calcium and phosphate or sulfate.

*Children* – IV infusion up to 3 mEq/kg or 40 mEq/m$^2$/day. Adjust volume of administered fluids to body size.

### Actions

*Pharmacology:* Potassium participates in a number of essential physiological processes, such as maintenance of intracellular tonicity and a proper relationship with sodium across cell membranes, cellular metabolism, transmission of nerve impulses, contraction of cardiac, skeletal, and smooth muscle, acid-base balance, and maintenance of normal renal function. Normal potassium serum levels range from 3.5 to 5 mEq/L.

| mEq/g of Various Potassium Salts | |
|---|---|
| Potassium salt | mEq/g |
| Potassium gluconate | 4.3 |
| Potassium citrate | 9.8 |
| Potassium bicarbonate | 10 |
| Potassium acetate | 10.2 |
| Potassium chloride | 13.4 |
| Dibasic potassium phosphate[1] | 11.5 |
| Monobasic potassium phosphate | 7.3 |

[1] Commercial preparations of potassium phosphate injection contain a mixture of both mono- and dibasic salts.

Potassium participates in carbohydrate utilization and protein synthesis and is critical in regulating nerve conduction and muscle contraction, particularly in the heart.

*Pharmacokinetics:* Normally about 80% to 90% of potassium intake is excreted in urine with the remainder voided in stool and, to a small extent, in perspiration. Kidneys do not conserve potassium well; during fasting or in patients on a potassium-free diet, potassium loss from the body continues, resulting in potassium depletion. A deficiency of either potassium or chloride will lead to a deficit of the other.

### Contraindications

*Oral:* Severe renal impairment with oliguria or azotemia; untreated Addison disease; hyperkalemia from any cause; adynamia episodica hereditaria; acute dehydration; heat cramps; patients receiving potassium-sparing diuretics or aldosterone-inhibiting agents.

*IV:* Diseases where high potassium levels may be encountered; hyperkalemia; renal failure and conditions in which potassium retention is present; oliguria or azotemia; anuria; crush syndrome; severe hemolytic reactions; adrenocortical insufficiency (untreated Addison disease); adynamica episodica hereditaria; acute dehydration; heat cramps; hyperkalemia from any cause; early postoperative oliguria except during GI drainage.

### Warnings

*Hyperkalemia:* This occurs most commonly in patients given IV potassium, but also may occur in patients given oral potassium. Potentially fatal hyperkalemia can develop rapidly and may be asymptomatic.

*GI lesions:* Potassium chloride tablets have caused stenotic or ulcerative lesions of the small bowel and death. These lesions are caused by a concentration of potassium ion in the region of a rapidly dissolving tablet, which injures the bowel wall and produces obstruction, hemorrhage, or perforation. The reported frequency of small bowel lesions is much less with wax matrix tablets and microencapsulated tablets than with enteric coated tablets. Immediately discontinue either type of tablet and consider the possibility of bowel obstruction or perforation if severe vomiting, abdominal pain or distention, or GI bleeding occurs.

Patients at greatest risk for developing potassium chloride-induced GI lesions include: The elderly, the immobile and those with scleroderma, diabetes mellitus, mitral valve replacement, cardiomegaly, or esophageal stricture/compression.

*Metabolic acidosis and hyperchloremia:* Potassium depletion is rarely associated with metabolic acidosis and hyperchloremia. Replace with potassium bicarbonate, citrate, acetate, or gluconate.

*Potassium intoxication:* Do not infuse rapidly. High plasma concentrations of potassium may cause death through cardiac depression, arrhythmias, or arrest. Monitor potassium replacement therapy whenever possible by continuous or serial ECG. In addition to ECG effects, local pain, and phlebitis may result when a more than 40 mEq/L concentration is infused.

*Renal impairment or adrenal insufficiency* – Renal impairment or adrenal insufficiency may cause potassium intoxication. Potassium salts can produce hyperkalemia and cardiac arrest. Potentially fatal hyperkalemia can develop rapidly and be asymptomatic. Use with great caution, if at all.

*Concentrated:* Concentrated potassium solutions are for IV admixtures only; do not use undiluted. Direct injection may be instantaneously fatal.

*Metabolic alkalosis:* Potassium depletion is usually accompanied by an obligatory loss of chloride resulting in hypochloremic metabolic alkalosis. Treat the underlying cause of potassium depletion and administer IV potassium chloride.

Use solutions containing acetate ion carefully in metabolic or respiratory alkalosis, and when there is an increased level or impairment of utilization of this ion.

*Musculoskeletal/Cardiac effects:* When serum sodium or calcium concentration is reduced, moderate elevation of serum potassium may cause toxic effects on the heart and skeletal muscle. Weakness and later paralysis of voluntary muscles, with consequent respiratory distress and dysphagia, are generally late signs, sometimes significantly preceding dangerous or fatal cardiac toxicity.

*Renal function impairment:* Renal function impairment requires careful monitoring of the serum potassium concentration and appropriate dosage adjustment.

*Pregnancy:* Category C.

*Children:* Safety and efficacy for use in children have not been established.

### Precautions

*Monitoring:* Close medical supervision with frequent ECGs and serum potassium determinations. Plasma levels are not necessarily indicative of tissue levels.

*Fluid/Solute overload:* IV administration can cause fluid or solute overloading resulting in dilution of serum electrolyte concentrations, overhydration, congested states, or pulmonary edema.

*Special risk:* Use with caution in the presence of cardiac disease, particularly in digitalized patients or in the presence of renal disease, metabolic acidosis, Addison disease, acute dehydration, prolonged or severe diarrhea, familial periodic paralysis, hypoadrenalism, hyperkalemia, hyponatremia, and myotonia congenita.

**Drug Interactions**

Drugs that may interact include ACE inhibitors, potassium-sparing diuretics, digitalis, and potassium-containing salt substitutes.

**Adverse Reactions**

*Oral:* Adverse reactions may include nausea, vomiting, diarrhea, flatulence, and abdominal discomfort due to GI irritation. They are best managed by diluting the preparation further, by taking with meals, or by dose reduction. Severe reactions may include hyperkalemia; GI obstruction, bleeding, ulceration, or perforation.

*Parenteral:*

*Hyperkalemia:* Adverse reactions involve the possibility of potassium intoxication. Signs and symptoms include paresthesias of extremities; flaccid paralysis; muscle or respiratory paralysis; areflexia; weakness; listlessness; mental confusion; weakness and heaviness of legs; hypotension; cardiac arrhythmias; heart block; ECG abnormalities such as disappearance of P waves, spreading and slurring of the QRS complex with development of a biphasic curve and cardiac arrest.

# SODIUM CHLORIDE

| | |
|---|---|
| **Solution**: 0.45% (77 mEq/L sodium, 77 mEq/L chloride) (*Rx*) | Various |
| 0.9% (154 mEq/L sodium, 154 mEq/L chloride) (*Rx*) | Various |
| 3% (513 mEq/L sodium, 513 mEq/L chloride) (*Rx*) | Various |
| 5% (855 mEq/L sodium, 855 mEq/L chloride) (*Rx*) | Various |
| **Solution**: 0.9% sodium chloride (as bacteriostatic sodium chloride inj) (*Rx*) | Various |
| **Concentrated solution**: 14.6% and 23.4% sodium chloride (*Rx*) | Various |
| **Tablets**: 650 mg, 1 and 2.25 g (*otc*) | Various |
| **Tablets, slow-release**: 410 mg sodium chloride and 150 mg potassium chloride in wax matrix (*otc*) | *Slo-Salt-K* (Mission) |

## Indications

*IV:*

*Hyponatremia* – For parenteral restoration of sodium ion in patients with restricted oral intake. Sodium replacement is specifically indicated in patients with hyponatremia or low salt syndrome. Sodium chloride may also be added to compatible carbohydrate solutions such as dextrose in water to provide electrolytes.

*Diluents* – Sodium chloride injections are also indicated as pharmaceutic aids and diluents for the infusion of compatible drug additives.

*0.9% Sodium chloride (normal saline)* – 0.9% Sodium chloride (normal saline), which is isotonic, restores both water and sodium chloride losses. Other indications for parenteral 0.9% saline include: Diluting or dissolving drugs for IV, IM, or subcutaneous injection; flushing of IV catheters; extracellular fluid replacement; treatment of metabolic alkalosis in the presence of fluid loss and mild sodium depletion; as a priming solution in hemodialysis procedures and to initiate and terminate blood transfusions without hemolyzing red blood cells.

*0.45% Sodium chloride (hypotonic)* – 0.45% Sodium chloride (hypotonic) is primarily a hydrating solution and may be used to assess the status of the kidneys, because more water is provided than is required for salt excretion. It also may be used in the treatment of hyperosmolar diabetes where the use of dextrose is inadvisable and there is a need for large amounts of fluid without an excess of sodium ions.

*3% or 5% Sodium chloride (hypertonic)* – 3% or 5% Sodium chloride (hypertonic) is used in hyponatremia and hypochloremia due to electrolyte and fluid loss replaced with sodium-free fluids; drastic dilution of body water following excessive water intake; emergency treatment of severe salt depletion.

*Bacteriostatic sodium chloride* – Only for diluting or dissolving drugs for IV, IM, or subcutaneous injection.

*Concentrated sodium chloride* – As an additive in parenteral fluid therapy for use in patients who have special problems of sodium electrolyte intake or excretion. It is intended to meet the specific requirements of the patient with unusual fluid and electrolyte needs. After available clinical and laboratory information is considered and correlated, determine the appropriate number of milliequivalents of concentrated sodium chloride injection, USP and dilute for use.

*Oral:* Prevention or treatment of extracellular volume depletion, dehydration, or sodium depletion; aid in the prevention of heat prostration.

## Administration and Dosage

*IV:* In the average adult, daily requirements of sodium and chloride are met by the infusion of 1 L of 0.9% sodium chloride (154 mEq each of sodium and chloride). Base fluid administration on calculated maintenance or replacement fluid requirements.

*IV catheters* – Prior to and after administration of the medication, entirely flush the catheter with preservative free 0.9% sodium chloride for injection.

*Calculation of sodium deficit* – To calculate the amount of sodium that must be administered to raise serum sodium to the desired level, use the following equation (TBW = total body water): Na deficit (mEq) = TBW (desired – observed plasma Na).

Base the repletion rate on the degree of urgency in the patient. Use of hypertonic saline (eg, 3% or 5%) will correct the deficit more rapidly.

*Concentrated sodium chloride* – Not for direct infusion. Must be diluted before use.

The dosage as an additive in parenteral fluid therapy is predicated on specific requirements of the patient. The appropriate volume is then withdrawn for proper dilution. Having determined the mEq of sodium chloride to be added, divide by 4 to calculate the number of mL to be used. Withdraw this volume and transfer into appropriate IV solutions, such as 5% dextrose injection. The properly diluted solution may be given IV.

*Admixture incompatibilities* – Some additives may be incompatible. Consult a pharmacist.

To minimize the risk of possible incompatibilities arising from mixing this solution with other additives that may be prescribed, inspect the final infusate for cloudiness or precipitation immediately after mixing, prior to administration and periodically during administration. Do not store.

*Oral:* Refer to specific product labeling for dosage guidelines.

### Actions

*Pharmacology:* Normal osmolarity of the extracellular fluid ranges between 280 to 300 mOsm/L; it is primarily a function of sodium and its accompanying ions, chloride, and bicarbonate. Sodium chloride is the principal salt involved in maintenance of plasma tonicity. One gram of sodium chloride provides 17.1 mEq sodium and 17.1 mEq chloride.

### Contraindications

Hypernatremia; fluid retention; when the administration of sodium or chloride could be clinically detrimental.

*3% and 5% sodium chloride solutions:* Elevated, normal, or only slightly decreased plasma sodium and chloride concentrations.

*Bacteriostatic sodium chloride:* Newborns; for fluid or sodium chloride replacement.

### Warnings

*Fluid/Solute overload:* Excessive amounts of sodium chloride by any route may cause hypokalemia and acidosis. Administration of IV solutions can cause fluid or solute overload resulting in dilution of serum electrolyte concentrations, CHF, overhydration, congested states, or acute pulmonary edema, especially in patients with cardiovascular disease and in patients receiving corticosteroids or corticotropin or drugs that may give rise to sodium retention.

Infusion of more than 1 L of isotonic (0.9%) sodium chloride may supply more sodium and chloride than normally found in serum, resulting in hypernatremia; this may cause a loss of bicarbonate ions, resulting in an acidifying effect.

*Bacteriostatic sodium chloride:* Do not use in newborns. Benzyl alcohol as a preservative in bacteriostatic sodium chloride injection has been associated with toxicity in newborns. These solutions have not been reported to cause problems in older infants, children, and adults.

*Concentrated sodium chloride injection:* Inadvertent direct injection or absorption of concentrated sodium chloride injection may give rise to sudden hypernatremia and such complications as cardiovascular shock, CNS disorders, extensive hemolysis, cortical necrosis of the kidneys, and severe local tissue necrosis (if administered extravascularly). Do not use unless solution is clear. When administered peripherally, slowly infuse through a small bore needle placed well within the lumen of a large vein to minimize venous irritation. Carefully avoid infiltration.

*Surgical patients:* Surgical patients should seldom receive salt-containing solutions immediately following surgery unless factors producing salt depletion are present. Because of renal retention of salt during surgery, additional electrolytes given IV may result in fluid retention, edema, and overloading of the circulation.

*Renal function impairment:* Infusions of sodium ions may result in excessive sodium retention; administer with care.

*Pregnancy:* Category C.

*Children:* Safety and efficacy have not been established.

### Precautions

*Monitoring:* Monitor changes in fluid balance, electrolyte concentrations, and acid-base balance during prolonged parenteral therapy or whenever the condition of the patient warrants such evaluation. Significant deviations from normal concentrations may require tailoring of the electrolyte pattern.

*Hypokalemia:* Hypokalemia may result from excessive administration of potassium-free solutions.

*Special risk patients:* Administer cautiously to patients with decompensated cardiovascular, cirrhotic, and nephrotic disease; circulatory insufficiency; hypoproteinemia; hypervolemia; urinary tract obstruction; CHF; and to patients with concurrent edema and sodium retention; those receiving corticosteroids or corticotropin; and those retaining salt.

*Elderly or postoperative patients:* Exercise care in administering sodium-containing solutions in renal or cardiovascular insufficiency, with or without CHF.

*3% and 5% sodium chloride solutions:* Infuse very slowly and use with caution to avoid pulmonary edema; observe patients constantly.

## SODIUM BICARBONATE

| | |
|---|---|
| **Injection:** 4.2% (0.5 mEq/mL), 5% (0.6 mEq/mL), 7.5% (0.9 mEq/mL), 8.4% (1 mEq/mL) (Rx) | Various |
| **Neutralizing additive solution:** 4% (0.48 mEq/mL) (Rx) | *Neut* (Abbott) |
| 4.2% (0.5 mEq/mL) (Rx) | Various |

### Indications

*Metabolic acidosis:* In severe renal disease; uncontrolled diabetes; circulatory insufficiency due to shock, anoxia, or severe dehydration; extracorporeal circulation of blood; cardiac arrest; and severe primary lactic acidosis where a rapid increase in plasma total $CO_2$ content is crucial. Treat metabolic acidosis in addition to measures designed to control the cause of the acidosis. Because an appreciable time interval may elapse before all ancillary effects occur, bicarbonate therapy is indicated to minimize risks inherent to acidosis itself.

At one time it was suggested to administer bicarbonate during cardiopulmonary resuscitation following cardiac arrest; however, recent evidence suggests that little benefit is provided and its use may be detrimental. For treatment of acidosis in this clinical situation, concentrate efforts on restoring ventilation and blood flow. According to the American Heart Association guidelines, use as a last resort after other standard measures have been utilized.

*Urinary alkalinization:* In the treatment of certain drug intoxications (eg, salicylates, lithium) and in hemolytic reactions requiring alkalinization of the urine to diminish nephrotoxicity of blood pigments.

*Severe diarrhea:* Severe diarrhea that is often accompanied by a significant loss of bicarbonate.

*Neutralizing additive solution:* To reduce the incidence of chemical phlebitis and patient discomfort due to vein irritation at or near the infusion site by raising the pH of IV acid solutions.

### Administration and Dosage

One g sodium bicarbonate provides 11.9 mEq each of sodium and bicarbonate.

*Cardiac arrest:* Bicarbonate administration in this situation may be detrimental. Administer according to results of arterial blood pH and $PaCO_2$ and calculation of base deficit. Flush IV lines before and after use.

*Adults* – A rapid IV dose of 200 to 300 mEq of bicarbonate, given as a 7.5% or 8.4% solution.

*Infants (2 years of age or younger)* – 4.2% solution for IV administration at a rate not to exceed 8 mEq/kg/day to guard against the possibility of producing hypernatremia, decreasing CSF pressure, and inducing intracranial hemorrhage.

*Initial dose* – 1 to 2 mEq/kg/min given over 1 to 2 minutes followed by 1 mEq/kg every 10 minutes of arrest. If base deficit is known, give calculated dose of 0.3 × kg × base deficit. If only 7.5% or 8.4% sodium bicarbonate is available, dilute 1:1 with 5% dextrose in water before administration.

*Severe metabolic acidosis* – Administer 90 to 180 mEq/L (approximately 7.5 to 15 g) at a rate of 1 to 1.5 L during the first hour. Adjust to patient's needs for further management.

*Less urgent forms of metabolic acidosis* – Sodium bicarbonate injection may be added to other IV fluids. The amount of bicarbonate to be given to older children and adults over a 4- to 8-hour period is approximately 2 to 5 mEq/kg, depending on the severity of the acidosis as judged by the lowering of total $CO_2$ content, blood pH, and clinical condition. Initially, an infusion of 2 to 5 mEq/kg over 4 to 8 hours will produce improvement in the acid-base status of the blood.

Alternatively, estimates of the initial dose of sodium bicarbonate may be based on the following equation:

$$0.5 \text{ (L/kg)} \times \text{body weight (kg)} \times \text{desired increase in serum } HCO_3- \text{ (mEq/L)} = \text{bicarbonate dose (mEq)}$$

or

$$0.5 \text{ (L/kg)} \times \text{body weight (kg)} \times \text{base deficit (mEq/L)} = \text{bicarbonate dose (mEq)}.$$

The next step of therapy is dependent on the clinical response of the patient. If severe symptoms have abated, reduce frequency of administration and dose.

If the $CO_2$ plasma content is unknown, a safe average dose of sodium bicarbonate is 5 mEq (420 mg)/kg.

It is unwise to attempt full correction of a low total $CO_2$ content during the first 24 hours, because this may accompany an unrecognized alkalosis due to delayed readjustment of ventilation to normal. Thus, achieving total $CO_2$ content of about 20 mEq/L at the end of the first day will usually be associated with a normal blood pH.

*Neutralizing additive solution* – One vial of neutralizing additive solution added to 1 L of any of the commonly used parenteral solutions including dextrose, sodium chloride, Ringer's, etc, will increase the pH to a more physiologic range (specific pH may vary slightly).

*Note* – Some products such as amino acid solutions and multiple electrolyte solutions containing dextrose will not be brought to near physiologic pH by the addition of sodium bicarbonate neutralizing additive solution. This is due to the relatively high buffer capacity of these fluids.

*Admixture incompatibilities* – Avoid adding sodium bicarbonate to parenteral solutions containing calcium, except where compatibility is established; precipitation or haze may result. Norepinephrine, dopamine, and dobutamine are incompatible.

### Actions

*Pharmacology:* Increases plasma bicarbonate; buffers excess hydrogen ion concentration; raises blood pH; reverses the clinical manifestations of acidosis.

*Pharmacokinetics:* Sodium bicarbonate in water dissociates to provide sodium and bicarbonate ions. Sodium is the principal cation of extracellular fluid. Bicarbonate is a normal constituent of body fluids and normal plasma level ranges from 24 to 31 mEq/L. Plasma concentration is regulated by the kidney. Bicarbonate anion is considered "labile" because, at a proper concentration of hydrogen ion, it may be converted to carbonic acid, then to its volatile form, carbon dioxide, excreted by lungs. Normally, a ratio of 1:20 (carbonic acid: bicarbonate) is present in extracellular fluid. In a healthy adult with normal kidney function, almost all the glomerular filtered bicarbonate ion is reabsorbed; less than 1% is excreted in urine.

### Contraindications

Losing chloride by vomiting or from continuous GI suction; receiving diuretics known to produce a hypochloremic alkalosis; metabolic and respiratory alkalosis; hypocalcemia in which alkalosis may produce tetany, hypertension, convulsions, or congestive heart failure (CHF); when sodium use could be clinically detrimental.

*Neutralizing additive solution:* Do not use as a systemic alkalinizer.

## Warnings

*Cardiac effects:*

*Cardiac arrest* – The risk of rapid infusion must be weighed against the potential for fatality due to acidosis.

*CHF* – Because sodium accompanies bicarbonate, use cautiously in patients with CHF or other edematous or sodium-retaining states.

*Fluid/Solute overload:* IV administration can cause fluid or solute overloading resulting in dilution of serum electrolyte concentrations, overhydration, congested states, or pulmonary edema.

*Extravasation:* Extravasation of IV hypertonic solutions of sodium bicarbonate may cause chemical cellulitis (because of their alkalinity), with tissue necrosis, ulceration, or sloughing at the site of infiltration. Prompt elevation of the part, warmth, and local injection of lidocaine or hyaluronidase are recommended to prevent sloughing.

*Too rapid infusion:* Too rapid infusion of hypertonic solutions may cause local pain and venous irritation. Adjust the rate of administration according to tolerance. Use of the largest peripheral vein and a well placed small bore needle is recommended.

Too rapid or excessive administration may result in hypernatremia and alkalosis accompanied by hyperirritability or tetany. Hypernatremia may be associated with edema and exacerbation of CHF due to the retention of water, resulting in an expanded extracellular fluid volume.

*Renal function impairment:* Administration of solutions containing sodium ions may result in sodium retention. Use with caution. Also use cautiously in oliguria or anuria.

*Elderly:* Exercise particular care when administering sodium-containing solutions to elderly or postoperative patients with renal or cardiovascular insufficiency, with or without CHF.

*Pregnancy:* Category C.

*Children:*

*Neonates and children (younger than 2 years of age)* – Rapid injection (10 mL/min) of hypertonic sodium bicarbonate solutions may produce hypernatremia, a decrease in cerebrospinal fluid pressure and possible intracranial hemorrhage. Do not administer more than 8 mEq/kg/day. A 4.2% solution is preferred for such slow administration.

## Precautions

*Monitoring:* Adverse reactions may result from an excess or deficit of one or more of the ions in the solution; frequent monitoring of electrolyte levels is essential.

*Avoid overdosage and alkalosis:* Avoid overdosage and alkalosis by giving repeated small doses and periodic monitoring by appropriate laboratory tests.

*Potassium depletion:* Potassium depletion may predispose to metabolic alkalosis, and coexistent hypocalcemia may be associated with carpopedal spasm as the plasma pH rises. Minimize by treating electrolyte imbalances prior to or concomitantly with bicarbonate.

*Chloride loss:* Patients losing chloride by vomiting or GI intubation are more susceptible to developing severe alkalosis if given alkalinizing agents.

*Neutralizing additive solution:* Administer this solution promptly. When introducing additives, mix thoroughly, and do not store. Raising pH of IV fluids with neutralizing additive solution will reduce incidence of chemical irritation caused by infusate.

## Drug Interactions

Drugs that may interact include chlorpropamide, lithium, methotrexate, salicylates, tetracyclines, anorexiants, flecainide, mecamylamide, quinidine, and sympathomimetics.

## Adverse Reactions

Adverse reactions may include extravasation; local pain; venous irritation; hypernatremia; alkalosis.

# Chapter 2
# HEMATOLOGICAL AGENTS

# IRON-CONTAINING PRODUCTS, ORAL

### FERROUS SULFATE

**Tablets**: 325 mg (65 mg iron) (*otc*) — Various, *Feosol* (GlaxoSmithKline), *FeroSul* (Major)

**Elixir**: 220 mg per 5 mL ( 44 mg iron per 5 mL) (*otc*) — Various

**Drops**: 75 mg per 0.6 mL (15 mg iron per 0.6 mL) (*otc*) — Various, *Fer-In-So!* (Mead Johnson Nutritionals), *Fer-gen-sol* (Goldline)

### FERROUS SULFATE EXSICCATED (DRIED)

**Tablets**: 200 mg (65 mg iron) (*otc*) — *Feosol* (GlaxoSmithKline)

300 mg (60 mg iron) (*otc*) — *Feratab* (Upsher-Smith)

**Tablets, slow-release**: 160 mg (50 mg iron) (*otc*) — Various, *Slow FE* (Ciba)

### FERROUS GLUCONATE

**Tablets**: 225 mg (27 mg iron) (*otc*) — Various, *Fergon* (Bayer)

300 mg (35 mg iron), 324 mg (38 mg iron), 325 mg (36 mg iron) (*otc*) — Various

### FERROUS FUMARATE

**Tablets**: 90 mg (29.5 mg iron) (*otc*) — Various

324 mg (106 mg iron) (*otc*) — Various, *Hemocyte* (US Pharmaceutical Corp.)

325 mg (106 mg iron) (*otc*) — *Ferretts* (Pharmics)

350 mg (115 mg iron) (*otc*) — *Nephro-Fer* (Watson)

**Tablets, chewable**: 100 mg (33 mg iron) (*otc*) — *Feostat* (Forest)

**Tablets, timed-release**: 150 mg (50 mg iron) (*otc*) — *Ferro-Sequels* (Inverness)

### CARBONYL IRON

**Tablets**: 45 mg iron (*otc*) — *Feosol* (GlaxoSmithKline)

66 mg iron (*otc*) — *Ircon* (Kenwood)

**Tablets, chewable**: 15 mg carbonyl iron (*otc*) — *Icar* (Hawthorn)

**Suspension**: 15 mg carbonyl iron per 1.25 mL (*otc*)

### POLYSACCHARIDE-IRON COMPLEX

**Capsules**: 60 mg iron (*otc*) — *Niferex* (Ther-Rx)

150 mg iron (*otc*) — Various, *Ferrex 150* (Breckenridge), *Fe-Tinic 150* (Ethex Corp.), *Hytinic* (Hyrex), *Nu-Iron 150* (Merz)

**Elixir**: 100 mg iron per 5 mL (*otc*) — *Niferex* (Schwarz Pharma)

### IRON WITH VITAMIN C

**Tablets**: 66 mg iron, 125 mg ascorbic acid (*otc*) — *Vitron-C* (Heritage Consumer Products)

**Tablets, controlled-release**: 105 mg iron, 500 mg sodium ascorbate (*otc*) — *Fero-Grad-500* (Abbott)

**Capsules**: 150 mg iron, 50 mg ascorbic acid (*otc*) — *Ferrex 150 Plus* (Breckenridge)

150 mg iron, 50 mg calcium ascorbate and calcium threonate (*otc*) — *Niferex-150* (Ther-Rx)

65 mg iron, 150 mg ascorbic acid (*otc*) — *Vitelle Irospan* (Fielding)

---

**Warning:**

Accidental overdose of iron-containing products is a leading cause of fatal poisoning in children younger than 6 years of age. Keep products out of the reach of children. In case of accidental overdose, call a doctor or a poison control center immediately.

---

### Indications

*Iron deficiency:* For the prevention and treatment of iron deficiency and iron deficiency anemias.

*Iron supplement:* As a dietary supplement for iron.

*Unlabeled uses:* Iron supplementation may be required by most patients receiving epoetin therapy. Failure to administer iron supplements (oral or IV) during epoetin therapy can impair the hematologic response to epoetin.

**Administration and Dosage**

Due to the availability of multiple salt forms, close attention is warranted when administering iron. Substitution of 1 salt for another without proper adjustment may result in serious over or under dosing.

Carbonyl iron and polysaccharide-iron complex are reported to be associated with fewer GI effects and are less toxic than other forms of iron.

The length of iron therapy depends upon the cause and severity of the iron deficiency. In general, approximately 4 to 6 months of oral iron therapy is required to reverse uncomplicated iron deficiency anemias. Iron therapy should increase hemoglobin levels by 1 g/week.

*Iron replacement therapy in deficiency states:* Iron doses are given as elemental iron.

*Premature infants* – 2 to 4 mg/kg/day given in 1 to 2 divided doses. Maximum dosage is 15 mg/day.

*Children* – 3 to 6 mg/kg/day given in 1 to 3 divided doses.

*Adults* – 150 to 300 mg/day given in 3 divided doses. Alternatively, 60 mg given 2 to 4 times/day may help lessen GI effects.

*Prevention of iron deficiency:*

*Premature infants* – 2 mg/kg/day given in 1 to 3 divided doses. Maximum dosage is 15 mg/day.

*Children* – 1 to 2 mg/kg/day given in 1 to 3 divided doses. Maximum dosage is 15 mg/day.

*Adults* – 60 mg/day given in 1 to 2 divided doses.

*Recommended dietary allowances (RDAs):* For a complete listing of RDAs, refer to the RDAs section of the Nutrients and Nutritionals chapter.

| RDAs for Iron | |
| --- | --- |
| Patients | RDA for iron (mg/day) |
| Children | |
| 7 to 12 months of age | 11 |
| 1 to 3 years of age | 7 |
| 4 to 8 years of age | 10 |
| Males | |
| 9 to 13 years of age | 8 |
| 14 to 18 years of age | 11 |
| ≥ 19 years of age | 8 |
| Females | |
| 9 to 13 years of age | 8 |
| 14 to 18 years of age | 15 |
| 19 to 50 years of age | 18 |
| > 50 years of age | 8 |
| Pregnancy | 27 |
| Lactation | |
| ≤ 18 years of age | 10 |
| ≥ 19 years of age | 9 |

*Iron supplementation:*

*Pregnancy* – Elemental iron 15 to 30 mg/day should be adequate to meet the daily requirement of the last 2 trimesters.

**Actions**

*Pharmacology:* Iron, an essential mineral, is a component of hemoglobin, myoglobin, and a number of enzymes. Approximately two-thirds of total body iron is in the circulating red blood cell mass in hemoglobin, the major factor in oxygen transport.

*Pharmacokinetics:*

*Absorption/Distribution* – The average dietary intake of iron is 12 to 20 mg/day for males and 8 to 15 mg/day for females; however, only about 10% of this iron is absorbed (1 to 2 mg/day) in individuals with adequate iron stores. Absorption is enhanced (20% to 30%) when storage iron is depleted or when erythropoiesis occurs at an increased rate. Iron is primarily absorbed from the duodenum and jejunum. The ferrous salt form is absorbed 3 times more readily than the ferric form. The common ferrous salts (ie, sulfate, gluconate, fumarate) are absorbed almost on a milligram-for-milligram basis but differ in the content of elemental iron. Sustained-release or enteric-coated preparations reduce the amount of available iron; absorption from these doseforms is reduced because iron is transported beyond the duodenum. Dose also influences the amount of iron absorbed. The amount of iron absorbed increases progressively with larger doses; however, the percentage absorbed decreases. Food can decrease the absorption of iron by 40% to 66%; however, gastric intolerance may often necessitate administering the drug with food.

*Excretion* – The daily loss of iron from urine, sweat, and sloughing of intestinal mucosal cells amounts to approximately 0.5 to 1 mg in healthy men. In menstruating women, approximately 1 to 2 mg is the normal daily loss.

| Elemental Iron Content of Iron Salts | |
| --- | --- |
| Iron salt | % Iron |
| Ferrous fumarate | ≈ 33 |
| Ferrous gluconate | ≈ 12 |
| Ferrous sulfate | ≈ 20 |
| Ferrous sulfate, exsiccated | ≈ 32 |

## Contraindications

Hemochromatosis; hemosiderosis; hemolytic anemias; known hypersensitivity to any ingredients.

## Warnings

*Chronic iron intake:* Individuals with normal iron balance should not take iron chronically.

*Accidental overdose:* Accidental overdose of iron-containing products is a leading cause of fatal poisoning in children younger than 6 years of age. Keep this product out of reach of children.

*Pregnancy:* Category A.

## Precautions

*Intolerance:* Discontinue use if symptoms of intolerance appear.

*GI effects:* Occasional GI discomfort, such as nausea, may be minimized by taking with meals and by slowly increasing to the recommended dosage.

*Tartrazine/sulfite sensitivity:* Some of these products contain tartrazine or sulfites, which may cause allergic-type reactions.

## Drug Interactions

Iron salts may be affected by the following agents: AHA, antacids, ascorbic acid, calcium salts, chloramphenicol, digestive enzymes, $H_2$ antagonists, proton pump inhibitors, tetracyclines, and trientine.

Agents that may be affected by iron salts include: captopril, cephalosporins, levodopa, levothyroxine, methyldopa, mycophenolate mofetil, penicillamine, quinolones, tetracyclines, thyroid hormones, and trientine.

*Drug/Food interactions:* Administration of iron with food decreases the iron absorption by at least 50%. Administration of calcium and iron supplements with food can reduce ferrous sulfate absorption by 33%. If combined iron and calcium supplementation is required, iron absorption is not decreased if calcium carbonate is used and the supplements are taken between meals.

## Adverse Reactions

GI irritation; anorexia; nausea; vomiting; constipation; diarrhea. Stools may appear darker in color. Iron-containing liquids may cause temporary staining of the teeth.

# IRON DEXTRAN

**Injection**: 50 mg iron/mL (as dextran) (*Rx*)                    *InFeD* (Schein), *DexFerrum* (American Regent)

**Warning:**
The parenteral use of complexes of iron and carbohydrates has resulted in anaphylactic-type reactions. Deaths associated with such administration have been reported; therefore, use iron dextran injection only in those patients in whom the indications have been clearly established and laboratory investigations confirm an iron-deficient state not amenable to oral iron therapy. Because fatal anaphylactic reactions have been reported after administration of iron dextran injection, administer the drug only when resuscitation techniques and treatment of anaphylactic and anaphylactoid shock are readily available.

## Indications
For treatment of patients with documented iron deficiency in whom oral administration is unsatisfactory or impossible.

*Unlabeled uses:* Iron supplementation may be required by most patients receiving epoetin therapy. Failure to administer iron supplements (oral or IV) during epoetin therapy can impair the hematologic response to epoetin.

## Administration and Dosage
*Maximum dose:* 2 mL of undiluted iron dextran daily.

*Iron deficiency anemia:* The accompanying formula and table are applicable for dosage determinations only in patients with iron deficiency anemia; they are not to be used for dosage determinations in patients requiring iron replacement for blood loss.

The total amount of iron (in mL) required to restore hemoglobin to normal levels and to replenish iron stores may be approximated from the following formula:

$$\text{Dose (mL)} = 0.0442 \, (\text{desired Hb} - \text{observed Hb}) \times \text{Weight*} + (0.26 \times \text{Weight*})$$

*For adults and children more than 15 kg (33 lbs), use the lesser of lean body weight or actual body weight in kilograms. Lean body weight is 50 kg (for males) or 45.5 kg (for females) plus 2.3 kg for each inch over 5 feet. For children 5 to 15 kg (11 to 33 lbs), use actual weight in kilograms. Do not give iron dextran during the first 4 months of life.

| Total Amount of Iron Dextran Required (to the nearest mL) for Hemoglobin and Iron Stores Replacement[1] | | | | | | | | | |
|---|---|---|---|---|---|---|---|---|---|
| Lean body weight[2] | | Amount required (mL) based on observed hemoglobin | | | | | | | |
| kg | lb | 3 g/dL | 4 g/dL | 5 g/dL | 6 g/dL | 7 g/dL | 8 g/dL | 9 g/dL | 10 g/dL |
| 5 | 11 | 3 | 3 | 3 | 3 | 2 | 2 | 2 | 2 |
| 10 | 22 | 7 | 6 | 6 | 5 | 5 | 4 | 4 | 3 |
| 15 | 33 | 10 | 9 | 9 | 8 | 7 | 7 | 6 | 5 |
| 20 | 44 | 16 | 15 | 14 | 13 | 12 | 11 | 10 | 9 |
| 25 | 55 | 20 | 18 | 17 | 16 | 15 | 14 | 13 | 12 |
| 30 | 66 | 23 | 22 | 21 | 19 | 18 | 17 | 15 | 14 |
| 35 | 77 | 27 | 26 | 24 | 23 | 21 | 20 | 18 | 17 |
| 40 | 88 | 31 | 29 | 28 | 26 | 24 | 22 | 21 | 19 |
| 45 | 99 | 35 | 33 | 31 | 29 | 27 | 25 | 23 | 21 |
| 50 | 110 | 39 | 37 | 35 | 32 | 30 | 28 | 26 | 24 |
| 55 | 121 | 43 | 41 | 38 | 36 | 33 | 31 | 28 | 26 |
| 60 | 132 | 47 | 44 | 42 | 39 | 36 | 34 | 31 | 28 |
| 65 | 143 | 51 | 48 | 45 | 42 | 39 | 36 | 34 | 31 |
| 70 | 154 | 55 | 52 | 49 | 45 | 42 | 39 | 36 | 33 |
| 75 | 165 | 59 | 55 | 52 | 49 | 45 | 42 | 39 | 35 |
| 80 | 176 | 63 | 59 | 55 | 52 | 48 | 45 | 41 | 38 |
| 85 | 187 | 66 | 63 | 59 | 55 | 51 | 48 | 44 | 40 |
| 90 | 198 | 70 | 66 | 62 | 58 | 54 | 50 | 46 | 42 |
| 95 | 209 | 74 | 70 | 66 | 62 | 57 | 53 | 49 | 45 |

| Total Amount of Iron Dextran Required (to the nearest mL) for Hemoglobin and Iron Stores Replacement[1] | | | | | | | | | |
| Lean body weight[2] | | Amount required (mL) based on observed hemoglobin | | | | | | | |
| kg | lb | 3 g/dL | 4 g/dL | 5 g/dL | 6 g/dL | 7 g/dL | 8 g/dL | 9 g/dL | 10 g/dL |
|---|---|---|---|---|---|---|---|---|---|
| 100 | 220 | 78 | 74 | 69 | 65 | 60 | 56 | 52 | 47 |
| 105 | 231 | 82 | 77 | 73 | 68 | 63 | 59 | 54 | 50 |
| 110 | 242 | 86 | 81 | 76 | 71 | 67 | 62 | 57 | 52 |
| 115 | 253 | 90 | 85 | 80 | 75 | 70 | 65 | 59 | 54 |
| 120 | 264 | 94 | 88 | 83 | 78 | 73 | 67 | 62 | 57 |

[1] Table values were calculated based on a normal adult hemoglobin of 14.8 g/dL for weights greater than 15 kg (33 lbs) and a hemoglobin of 12 g/dL for weights 15 kg (33 lbs) or less.

[2] For adults and children older than 15 kg (33 lbs), use the lesser of lean body weight or actual body weight in kilograms. See above equation.

*Administration –*

*IV injection:* Individual doses of 2 mL or less may be given on a daily basis until the calculated total amount required has been reached. After administration, evidence of a therapeutic response can be seen in a few days as an increase in reticulocyte count.

Give undiluted and slowly (not to exceed 1 mL/min).

*Test dose –* Prior to administering the first therapeutic dose, give all patients an IV test dose of 0.5 mL. Administer the test dose at a gradual rate over at least 30 seconds (*InFeD*) or at least 5 minutes (*DexFerrum*). Although anaphylactic reactions known to occur following administration are usually evident within a few minutes or sooner, it is recommended that a period of at least 1 hour elapse before the remainder of the initial therapeutic dose is given.

Individual doses of 2 mL or less may be given on a daily basis until the calculated total amount required has been reached.

Give undiluted and slowly, not to exceed 50 mg/min (1 mL/min).

*IM injection:*

*Test dose –* Prior to administering the first therapeutic dose, give all patients an IM test dose of 0.5 mL. If no adverse reactions are observed, the injection can be given according to the following schedule until the calculated total amount required has been reached. Each day's dose should ordinarily not exceed 0.5 mL (25 mg iron) for infants less than 5 kg (11 lb), 1 mL (50 mg iron) for children less than 10 kg (22 lb) and 2 mL (100 mg iron) for other patients.

Inject only into the muscle mass of the upper outer quadrant of the buttock (never into the arm or other exposed areas) and inject deeply with a 2- or 3-inch 19- or 20-gauge needle. If the patient is standing, have them bear their weight on the leg opposite the injection site, or if in bed, have them in a lateral position with injection site uppermost. To avoid injection or leakage into the subcutaneous tissue, a Z-track technique (displacement of the skin laterally prior to injection) is recommended.

*Iron replacement for blood loss:* Direct iron therapy in these patients toward replacement of the equivalent amount of iron represented in the blood loss. The table and formula described under *Iron deficiency anemia* are not applicable for simple iron replacement values.

The following formula is based on the approximation that 1 mL of normocytic, normochromic red cells contains 1 mg elemental iron:

Replacement iron (in mg) = Blood loss (in mL) $\times$ hematocrit

**Actions**

*Pharmacology:* Iron dextran, a hematinic agent, is a complex of ferric hydroxide and dextran for IM or IV use. The iron dextran complex is dissociated by the reticuloendothelial system, and the ferric iron is transported by transferrin and incorporated into hemoglobin and storage sites.

*Pharmacokinetics:*

*Absorption/Distribution* – The major portion of IM injections of iron dextran is absorbed within 72 hours; most of the remaining iron is absorbed over the ensuing 3 to 4 weeks. Various studies have yielded half-life values ranging from 5 hours (circulating iron dextran) to more than 20 hours (total iron, both circulating and bound).

*Metabolism/Excretion* – Dextran, a polyglucose, is either metabolized or excreted. Negligible amounts of iron are lost via the urinary or alimentary pathways after administration of dextran.

## Contraindications

Hypersensitivity to the product; all anemias not associated with iron deficiency; acute phase of infectious kidney disease.

## Warnings

*Maximum dose:* 2 mL of undiluted iron dextran is the maximum recommended daily dose.

*Total dose infusion:* Large IV doses, such as those used with total dose infusions (TDI), have been associated with an increased incidence of adverse reactions. The adverse reactions frequently are delayed (1 to 2 days). Reactions are typified by one or more of the following symptoms: arthralgia, backache, chills, dizziness, moderate to high fever, headache, malaise, myalgia, nausea, vomiting.

*Accidental overdose:* Accidental overdose of iron-containing products is a leading cause of fatal poisoning in children younger than 6 years of age. Keep this product out of reach of children.

*Hypersensitivity reactions:* Anaphylaxis and other hypersensitivity reactions have been reported after uneventful test doses as well as therapeutic doses of iron dextran injection. Therefore, consider administration of subsequent test doses during therapy. Have epinephrine immediately available in the event of acute hypersensitivity reactions.

*Hepatic function impairment:* Use this preparation with extreme caution in the presence of serious impairment of liver function.

*Carcinogenesis:* A risk of carcinogenesis may attend the IM injection of iron-carbohydrate complexes.

*Pregnancy: Category C.*

*Lactation:* Traces of unmetabolized iron dextran are excreted in breast milk. Exercise caution when administering to a nursing woman.

*Children:* Not recommended for use in infants younger than 4 months of age.

## Precautions

*Monitoring:* Serum iron determinations (especially by colorimetric assays) may not be meaningful for 3 weeks; serum ferritin peaks after about 7 to 9 days and slowly returns to baseline after about 3 weeks.

*Iron overload:* Unwarranted therapy with parenteral iron will cause excess storage of iron with the consequent possibility of exogenous hemosiderosis.

*Cardiovascular disease:* Adverse reactions of iron dextran may exacerbate cardiovascular complications in patients with preexisting cardiovascular disease.

*Chronic renal dialysis:* Although serum ferritin is usually a good guide to body iron stores, the correlation of body iron stores and serum ferritin may not be valid in patients on chronic renal dialysis who are also receiving iron dextran complex.

*Allergies/Asthma:* Use with caution in patients with history of significant allergies/asthma.

*Arthritis:* Patients with rheumatoid arthritis may have an acute exacerbation of joint pain and swelling following administration of iron dextran.

## Drug Interactions

*Chloramphenicol:* Serum iron levels may be increased because of decreased iron clearance and erythropoiesis due to direct bone marrow toxicity from chloramphenicol.

*Drug/Lab test interactions:* Large doses of iron dextran (5 mL or more) give a brown color to serum from a blood sample drawn 4 hours after administration; they may cause falsely elevated values of serum bilirubin and falsely decreased values of serum calcium.

### Adverse Reactions
Anaphylactic reactions including fatal anaphylaxis; other hypersensitivity reactions including dyspnea, urticaria, other rashes, and febrile episodes; inflammation at or near injection site, including sterile abscesses (IM); brown skin discoloration at injection site (IM); flushing and hypotension with overly rapid IV administration; hypotensive reaction; arthralgia.

The following pattern of signs/symptoms has been reported as a delayed (1 to 2 days) reaction at recommended doses: Fever; chills; backache; headache; myalgia; malaise; nausea; vomiting; dizziness.

# IRON SUCROSE

| **Injection**: 20 mg elemental iron/mL (*Rx*) | *Venofer* (American Regent Labs) |
| --- | --- |

### Indications
*Iron deficiency anemia:* For the treatment of iron deficiency anemia in patients undergoing chronic hemodialysis who are receiving supplemental erythropoietin therapy.

### Administration and Dosage
The dosage of iron sucrose is expressed in terms of milligrams of elemental iron. Each 5 mL vial contains 100 mg of elemental iron (20 mg/mL).

*Iron deficiency anemia:* The recommended dosage for the repletion treatment of iron deficiency in hemodialysis patients is 5 mL of iron sucrose (100 mg of elemental iron) delivered IV during the dialysis session. Most patients will require a minimum cumulative dose of 1,000 mg of elemental iron, administered over 10 sequential dialysis sessions, to achieve a favorable hemoglobin or hematocrit response. Patients may continue to require therapy with iron sucrose or other IV iron preparations at the lowest dose necessary to maintain target levels of hemoglobin, hematocrit, and laboratory parameters of iron storage within acceptable limits.

*Adults* – 100 mg iron administered 1 to 3 times/week to a total dose of 1,000 mg in 10 doses, repeat if needed. Frequency of dosing should be no more than 3 times/week.

Iron sucrose must be only administered IV (directly into the dialysis line) either by slow injection or by infusion.

*Slow IV injection:* In chronic renal failure patients, iron sucrose may be administered by slow IV injection into the dialysis line at a rate of 1 mL (20 mg iron) undiluted solution per minute (ie, 5 min/vial) not exceeding 1 vial of iron sucrose (100 mg elemental iron) per injection. Discard any unused portion.

*Infusion:* Iron sucrose may be also administered by infusion (into the dialysis line for hemodialysis patients). This may reduce the risk of hypotensive episodes. The content of each vial must be diluted exclusively in a maximum of 100 mL of 0.9% NaCl, immediately prior to infusion. Infuse the solution at a rate of 100 mg of iron over a period of 15 minutes or more. Discard unused diluted solution.

*IV incompatibility:* Do not mix iron sucrose with other medications or add to parenteral nutrition solutions for IV infusion.

### Actions
*Pharmacology:* Iron is essential to the synthesis of hemoglobin to maintain oxygen transport and to the function and formation of other physiologically important heme and nonheme compounds.

*Pharmacokinetics:* In healthy adults treated with IV doses of iron sucrose, its iron component exhibits first order kinetics with an elimination half-life of 6 hours, total clearance of 1.2 L/h, non-steady-state apparent volume of distribution of 10 L, and steady-state apparent volume of distribution of 7.9 L.

Following IV administration of iron sucrose, it is dissociated into iron and sucrose by the reticuloendothelial system. The sucrose component is eliminated mainly by urinary excretion. Some iron also is eliminated in the urine.

**Contraindications**

Evidence of iron overload; known hypersensitivity to iron sucrose or any of its inactive components; anemia not caused by iron deficiency.

**Warnings**

*Hypotension:* Hypotension has been reported frequently in patients receiving IV iron. Hypotension following administration of iron sucrose may be related to rate of administration and total dose administered. Take caution to administer iron sucrose according to recommended guidelines.

*Hypersensitivity reactions:* Serious hypersensitivity reactions have been rarely reported in patients receiving iron sucrose. No life-threatening hypersensitivity reactions were observed in studies.

*Elderly:* In general, dose selection for an elderly patient should be cautious, usually starting at the low end of the dosing range, reflecting the greater frequency of decreased hepatic, renal, or cardiac function, and of concomitant disease or other drug therapy.

*Pregnancy: Category B.*

*Lactation:* It is not known whether this drug is excreted in human breast milk.

*Children:* Safety and efficacy of iron sucrose in pediatric patients have not been established.

**Precautions**

*Monitoring:* Exercise caution to withhold iron administration in the presence of evidence of tissue iron overload. Periodically monitor hematologic and hematinic parameters (hemoglobin, hematocrit, serum ferritin, and transferrin saturation). Withhold iron therapy in patients with evidence of iron overload. Transferrin saturation values increase rapidly after IV administration of iron sucrose; thus, serum iron values may be reliably obtained 48 hours after IV dosing.

**Drug Interactions**

Drug interactions involving iron sucrose have not been studied. However, like other parenteral iron preparations, iron sucrose may be expected to reduce the absorption of concomitantly administered oral iron preparations. Do not administer concomitantly with oral iron preparations.

**Adverse Reactions** Adverse events whether or not related to iron sucrose administration reported by more than 5% of treated patients are as follows: hypotension (36%); cramps/leg cramps (23%); nausea, headache, vomiting, and diarrhea.

*Hypersensitivity:* In clinical studies and postmarketing safety studies, several patients experienced mild or moderate hypersensitivity reactions presenting with wheezing, dyspnea, hypotension, rashes, or pruritus. No serious or life-threatening hypersensitivity reactions associated with iron sucrose administration were observed in these studies. From the postmarketing spontaneous reporting system, there were 83 reports of anaphylactoid reactions, including patients who experienced serious or life-threatening reactions (anaphylactic shock, loss of consciousness or collapse, bronchospasm with dyspnea, or convulsion).

# SODIUM FERRIC GLUCONATE COMPLEX

**Injection:** 62.5 mg/5 mL (12.5 mg/mL) elemental iron (*Rx*)     *Ferrlecit* (Watson Pharma)

### Indications

*Iron deficiency:* For the treatment of iron deficiency anemia in patients 6 years of age and older undergoing chronic hemodialysis who are receiving supplemental epoetin therapy.

### Administration and Dosage

The dosage of sodium ferric gluconate complex is expressed in milligrams of elemental iron. Each 5 mL ampule contains 62.5 mg elemental iron (12.5 mg/mL).

*Iron deficiency:*

*Adults –* 10 mL (elemental iron 125 mg), may be diluted in 100 mL 0.9% sodium chloride administered by intravenous (IV) infusion over 1 hour. It may also be administered undiluted as a slow IV injection (at a rate up to 12.5 mg/min). Most patients will require a minimum cumulative dose of 1 g elemental iron administered over 8 sessions at sequential dialysis treatments to achieve a favorable hemoglobin or hematocrit response. Patients may continue to require therapy with IV iron at the lowest dose necessary to maintain the target levels of hemoglobin, hematocrit, and laboratory parameters of iron storage within acceptable limits.

Sodium ferric gluconate complex has been administered at sequential dialysis sessions by infusion or by slow IV injection during the dialysis session itself.

*Children –* 0.12 mL/kg (1.5 mg/kg of elemental iron) diluted in 25 mL 0.9% sodium chloride and administered by IV infusion over 1 hour at 8 sequential dialysis sessions. The maximum dosage should not exceed 125 mg/dose.

*Admixture incompatibility:* The compatibility of sodium ferric gluconate complex with IV infusion vehicles other than 0.9% sodium chloride has not been evaluated.

### Actions

*Pharmacology:* Sodium ferric gluconate complex in sucrose injection is a stable macromolecular complex used to replete the total body content of iron.

*Pharmacokinetics:*

*Absorption/Distribution –* In multiple, sequential single-dose IV studies, peak drug levels ($C_{max}$) varied significantly by dosage and by rate of administration with the highest $C_{max}$ observed in the regimen in which 125 mg was administered in 7 minutes (19 mg/L). The initial volume of distribution of 6 L corresponds well to calculated blood volume. The AUC for bound iron varied by dose from 17.5 mg•h/L (62.5 mg) to 35.6 mg•h/L (125 mg). Approximately 80% of drug bound iron was delivered to transferrin as a mononuclear ionic iron species within 24 hours of administration in each dosage regimen. Mean peak transferrin saturation did not exceed 100% and returned to near baseline by 40 hours after administration of each dosage regimen.

*Metabolism/Excretion –* The terminal elimination half-life for drug bound iron was approximately 1 hour, varying by dose but not by rate of administration. Total clearance was 3.02 to 5.35 L/h. In vitro, less than 1% of the iron species within sodium ferric gluconate complex can be dialyzed through membranes with pore sizes corresponding to 12,000 to 14,000 daltons over a period of up to 270 minutes.

### Contraindications

All anemias not associated with iron deficiency; hypersensitivity to sodium ferric gluconate complex or any of its inactive components; evidence of iron overload.

### Warnings

*Hypotension:* Hypotension associated with lightheadedness, malaise, fatigue, weakness, or severe pain in the chest, back, flanks, or groin has been associated with administration of IV iron. These hypotensive reactions are not associated with signs of hypersensitivity and have usually resolved within 1 or 2 hours.

*Hypersensitivity reactions:* Serious hypersensitivity reactions have been rarely reported. One case of a life-threatening hypersensitivity reaction has been observed in a patient who received a single dose of sodium ferric gluconate complex in a postmarketing study. Three serious hypersensitivity reactions have been reported from the spontaneous reporting system.

*Mutagenesis:* A clastogenic effect was produced in an in vitro chromosomal aberration assay in Chinese hamster ovary cells.

*Elderly:* Cautiously select dose for an elderly patient, usually starting at the low end of the dosing range, reflecting the greater frequency of decreased hepatic, renal, or cardiac function and of concomitant disease or other drug therapy.

*Pregnancy: Category B.*

*Lactation:* It is not known whether this drug is excreted in breast milk.

*Children:* Safety and efficacy have not been established in pediatric patients younger than 6 years of age. Sodium ferric gluconate complex contains benzyl alcohol; therefore, do not use in neonates.

**Precautions**

*Benzyl alcohol:* This product contains benzyl alcohol, which has been associated with a fatal "gasping syndrome" in premature infants.

*Iron overload:* Unnecessary therapy with parenteral iron will cause excess storage of iron with consequent possibility of iatrogenic hemosiderosis. Do not administer sodium ferric gluconate complex to patients with iron overload.

**Drug Interactions**

*Oral iron preparations:* Coadministration of parenteral iron preparations may reduce absorption of oral iron preparations.

**Adverse Reactions**

Sodium ferric gluconate complex administered to patients during dialysis may cause transient hypotension. Administration may augment hypotension caused by dialysis.

Many chronic renal failure patients experience cramps, pain, nausea, rash, flushing, and pruritus.

*Adults* – Adverse reactions experienced by at least 5% of patients receiving sodium ferric gluconate complex include the following: abdominal pain, abnormal erythrocytes, asthenia, chest pain, cramps, diarrhea, dizziness, dyspnea, fatigue, fever, generalized edema, headache, hyperkalemia, hypertension, hypotension, injection-site reaction, leg cramps, nausea, pain, paresthesias, pruritus, syncope, tachycardia, upper respiratory tract infection, vomiting.

*Children* – Adverse reactions experienced by at least 3% of patients include the following: abdominal pain, diarrhea, fever, headache, hypertension, hypotension, infection, nausea, pharyngitis, rhinitis, tachycardia, thrombosis, vomiting.

# FOLIC ACID (Folacin; Pteroylglutamic Acid; Folate)

| | |
|---|---|
| **Tablets:** 0.4, 0.8, and 1 mg (*Rx<sup>a</sup>*) | Various |
| **Injection:** 5 mg/mL (*Rx*) | Various, *Folvite* (Lederle) |

<sup>a</sup> Although most folic acid products carry the Rx legend, products that provide no more than 0.4 mg (or 0.8 mg for pregnant or lactating women) may be *otc* items.

### Indications

*Megaloblastic anemia:* Treatment of megaloblastic anemias due to a deficiency of folic acid as seen in tropical or nontropical sprue, anemias of nutritional origin, pregnancy, infancy, or childhood.

### Administration and Dosage

Give orally, except in severe intestinal malabsorption. Although most patients with malabsorption cannot absorb food folates, they are able to absorb folic acid given orally.

Parenteral administration is not advocated but may be necessary in some individuals (eg, patients receiving parenteral or enteral alimentation). Give IM, IV, or subcutaneously if disease is very severe or GI absorption is very severely impaired. Doses greater than 0.1 mg should not be used unless anemia due to vitamin $B_{12}$ deficiency has been ruled out or is being adequately treated with cobalamin.

*Usual therapeutic dosage:* Up to 1 mg daily. Resistant cases may require larger doses.

*Maintenance:* When clinical symptoms have subsided and the blood picture has normalized, use the dosage below. Never give less than 0.1 mg/day. Keep patients under close supervision and adjust maintenance dose if relapse appears imminent. In the presence of alcoholism, hemolytic anemia, anticonvulsant therapy, or chronic infection, the maintenance level may need to be increased.

*Infants* – 0.1 mg/day.
*Children (younger than 4 years of age)* – Up to 0.3 mg/day.
*Adults and children (older than 4 years of age)* – 0.4 mg/day.
*Pregnant and lactating women* – 0.8 mg/day.

*Recommended Dietary Allowances (RDAs):* Adult males, 0.15 to 0.2 mg/day; females, 0.15 to 0.18 mg/day.

For a complete listing of RDAs by age and sex, refer to the RDA table in the Nutritionals chapter.

### Actions

*Pharmacology:* Exogenous folate is required for nucleoprotein synthesis and maintenance of normal erythropoiesis. Folic acid stimulates production of red and white blood cells and platelets in certain megaloblastic anemias.

*Pharmacokinetics:* Oral synthetic folic acid is a monoglutamate and is completely absorbed following administration, even in the presence of malabsorption syndromes.

Folic acid appears in the plasma approximately 15 to 30 minutes after an oral dose; peak levels are generally reached within 1 hour. After IV administration, the drug is rapidly cleared from the plasma. Folic acid is metabolized in the liver. Normal serum levels of total folate have been reported to be 5 to 15 ng/mL; normal CSF levels are approximately 16 to 21 ng/mL. In general, folate serum levels less than 5 ng/mL indicate folate deficiency, and levels less than 2 ng/mL usually result in megaloblastic anemia. A majority of the metabolic products appeared in the urine after 6 hours; excretion was generally complete within 24 hours.

### Contraindications

Treatment of pernicious anemia and other megaloblastic anemias where vitamin $B_{12}$ is deficient (not effective).

### Warnings

*Pernicious anemia:* Folic acid in doses greater than 0.1 mg/day may obscure pernicious anemia in that hematologic remission can occur while neurologic manifestations remain progressive.

Except during pregnancy and lactation, do not give folic acid in therapeutic doses greater than 0.4 mg/day until pernicious anemia has been ruled out. Do not include daily doses exceeding the Recommended Dietary Allowance in multivitamin preparations; if therapeutic amounts are necessary, give folic acid separately.

*Elderly:* It may be prudent to consider the status of folate in people older than 65 years of age.

*Pregnancy:* Category A.

*Lactation:* Folic acid is excreted in breast milk.

### Drug Interactions
Drugs that may interact with folic acid include aminosalicylic acid, oral contraceptives, dihydrofolate reductase inhibitors (eg, methotrexate, trimethoprim), sulfasalazine, hydantoins.

### Adverse Reactions
Adverse reactions may include erythema, skin rash, nausea, abdominal distention, altered sleep patterns, irritability, mental depression, confusion, and impaired judgement.

# LEUCOVORIN CALCIUM (Folinic Acid; Citrovorum Factor)

| | |
|---|---|
| **Tablets:** 5, 15, and 25 mg (*Rx*) | Various |
| **Injection:** 3 mg/mL (*Rx*) | Various |
| **Powder for injection:** 50, 100, and 350 mg/vial (*Rx*) | Various |

### Indications
*Oral and parenteral:* Leucovorin "rescue" after high-dose methotrexate therapy in osteosarcoma.

*Parenteral:* Treatment of megaloblastic anemias due to folic acid deficiency when oral therapy is not feasible.

In combination with 5-fluorouracil (5-FU) to prolong survival in the palliative treatment of patients with advanced colorectal cancer.

### Administration and Dosage
Oral administration of doses greater than 25 mg is not recommended.

*Advanced colorectal cancer:* Either of the following 2 regimens is recommended:
1.) Leucovorin 200 mg/m² by slow IV injection over a minimum of 3 minutes, followed by 5-FU 370 mg/m² by IV injection.
2.) Leucovorin 20 mg/m² by IV injection followed by 5-FU 425 mg/m² by IV injection.

Treatment is repeated daily for 5 days. This 5-day treatment course may be repeated at 4-week (28-day) intervals for 2 courses and then repeated at 4- to 5-week (28- to 35-day) intervals provided that the patient has completely recovered from the toxic effects of the prior treatment course.

Institute dosage modifications of 5-FU as follows, based on the most severe toxicities: If diarrhea or stomatitis are moderate, WBC/mm³ nadir is 1,000 to 1,900 or platelets/mm³ are 25,000 to 75,000, reduce the 5-FU dose by 20%; if diarrhea or stomatitis are severe, WBC/mm³ nadir is less than 1,000, or platelets/mm³ are less than 25,000, reduce the 5-FU dose by 30%.

If no toxicity occurs, the 5-FU dose may increase 10%.

Defer treatment until WBCs are 4,000/mm³ and platelets are 130,000/mm³. If blood counts do not reach these levels within 2 weeks, discontinue treatment.

*Leucovorin rescue after high-dose methotrexate therapy:* The recommendations for leucovorin rescue are based on a methotrexate dose of 12 to 15 g/m² administered by IV infusion over 4 hours. Leucovorin rescue at a dose of 15 mg (approximately 10 mg/m²) every 6 hours for 10 doses starts 24 hours after the beginning of the methotrexate infusion. In the presence of GI toxicity, nausea, or vomiting, administer leucovorin parenterally.

Determine serum creatinine and methotrexate levels at least once daily. Continue leucovorin administration, hydration, and urinary alkalinization (pH of at least 7) until the methotrexate level is less than $5 \times 10^{-8}$M (0.05 mcM).

If significant clinical toxicity is observed, extend leucovorin rescue for an additional 24 hours (total of 14 doses over 84 hours) in subsequent courses of therapy.

*Impaired methotrexate elimination or inadvertent overdosage:* Begin leucovorin rescue as soon as possible after an inadvertent overdosage and within 24 hours of methotrexate administration when there is delayed excretion (see Warnings). Administer leucovorin 10 mg/m$^2$ IV, IM, or orally every 6 hours until the serum methotrexate level is less than $10^{-8}$M. In the presence of GI toxicity, nausea, or vomiting, administer leucovorin parenterally.

Determine serum creatinine and methotrexate levels at 24-hour intervals. If the 24-hour serum creatinine has increased 50% over baseline or if the 24 or 48 hour methotrexate level is greater than $5 \times 10^{-6}$M or greater than $9 \times 10^{-7}$M, respectively, increase the dose of leucovorin to 100 mg/m$^2$ IV every 3 hours until the methotrexate level is less than $10^{-8}$M.

*Megaloblastic anemia due to folic acid deficiency:* No more than 1 mg leucovorin/day. There is no evidence that doses greater than 1 mg/day have greater efficacy than 1 mg doses.

### Actions

*Pharmacology:* Leucovorin is one of several active, chemically reduced derivatives of folic acid. It is useful as an antidote to drugs that act as folic acid antagonists. Administration of leucovorin can counteract the therapeutic and toxic effects of folic acid antagonists such as methotrexate, which act by inhibiting dihydrofolate reductase.

*Pharmacokinetics:*

| Leucovorin Pharmacokinetics[1] | | | |
|---|---|---|---|
| Parameter | IV | IM | Oral |
| Total reduced folates: | | | |
| Mean peak conc. (ng/mL) | 1259 (range, 897 to 1,625) | 436 (range, 240 to 725) | 393 (range, 160 to 550) |
| Mean time to peak | 10 min | 52 min | 2.3 h |
| Terminal half-life | 6.2 h | 6.2 h | 5.7 h |
| 5-Methyl-THF[2] | | | |
| Mean peak conc. (ng/mL) | 258 | 226 | 367 |
| Mean time to peak | 1.3 h | 2.8 h | 2.4 h |
| 5-Formyl-THF[3] | | | |
| Mean peak conc. (ng/mL) | 1,206 | 360 | 51 |
| Mean time to peak | 10 min | 28 min | 1.2 h |

[1] Following administration of a 25 mg dose.
[2] The major metabolite to which leucovorin is primarily converted in the intestinal mucosa and which becomes the predominant circulating form of the drug.
[3] The parent compound.

Following oral administration leucovorin is rapidly absorbed and expands the serum pool of reduced folates. Oral absorption of leucovorin is saturable at doses greater than 25 mg. The apparent bioavailability of leucovorin was 97% for 25 mg, 75% for 50 mg, and 37% for 100 mg.

### Contraindications

Pernicious anemia and other megaloblastic anemias secondary to lack of vitamin $B_{12}$.

### Warnings

*Anemias:* Leucovorin is improper therapy for pernicious anemia and other megaloblastic anemias secondary to the lack of vitamin $B_{12}$.

*5-FU dosage/toxicity:* Leucovorin enhances the toxicity of 5-FU.

Therapy with leucovorin/5-FU must not be initiated or continued in patients who have symptoms of GI toxicity of any severity, until those symptoms have completely resolved. Patients with diarrhea must be monitored with particular care until the diarrhea has resolved, as rapid clinical deterioration leading to death can occur.

*Methotrexate concentrations:* Monitoring of the serum methotrexate concentration is essential in determining the optimal dose and duration of treatment with leucovorin. Delayed methotrexate excretion may be caused by a third space fluid accumulation, renal insufficiency, or inadequate hydration. Under such circumstances, higher doses of leucovorin or prolonged administration may be indicated. Doses higher than those recommended for oral use must be given IV.

*Calcium content:* Because of the calcium content of the leucovorin solution, inject no more than 160 mg/min IV.

*Folic acid antagonist overdosage:* In the treatment of accidental overdosages of folic acid antagonists, administer leucovorin as promptly as possible. As the time interval between antifolate administration (eg, methotrexate) and leucovorin rescue increases, leucovorin's effectiveness in counteracting toxicity decreases.

*Elderly:* Take particular care in the treatment of elderly or debilitated colorectal cancer patients, as these patients may be at increased risk of severe toxicity.

*Pregnancy: Category* C.

*Lactation:* It is not known whether this drug is excreted in breast milk.

## Drug Interactions

Drugs that may be affected by leucovorin include anticonvulsants.

## Adverse Reactions

Allergic sensitization, including anaphylactoid reactions and urticaria, following administration of both oral and parenteral leucovorin.

The following adverse events occurred when leucovorin was administered at both high (200 mg/m$^2$) and low (20 mg/m$^2$) doses in combination with 5-FU: Leukopenia, thrombocytopenia, infection, nausea, vomiting, diarrhea, stomatitis, constipation, lethargy/malaise/fatigue, alopecia, dermatitis, anorexia.

# VITAMIN B₁₂ (Cyanocobalamin; Hydroxocobalamin)

**CYANOCOBALAMIN**

| | |
|---|---|
| **Tablets**: 500 and 1,000 mcg (*otc*) | Various |
| **Injection**: 100 and 1,000 mcg/mL (*Rx*) | Various, *Crysti 1000* (Roberts Hauck), *Cyanoject* (Mayrand) |
| **Gel, intranasal**: 500 mcg/0.1 mL (500 mcg/actuation) (*Rx*) | *Nascobal* (Nastech) |

**HYDROXOCOBALAMIN**

| | |
|---|---|
| **Injection**: 1,000 mcg/mL (*Rx*) | Various, *LA-12* (Hyrex), *Hydro-Crysti-12* (Roberts Hauck) |

## Indications

*Vitamin B₁₂ deficiency:* Vitamin B₁₂ deficiency due to malabsorption syndrome as seen in pernicious anemia; GI pathology, dysfunction or surgery; fish tapeworm infestation; malignancy of pancreas or bowel; gluten enteropathy; sprue; small bowel bacterial overgrowth; total or partial gastrectomy; accompanying folic acid deficiency.

*Increased vitamin B₁₂ requirements:* Increased vitamin B₁₂ requirements associated with pregnancy, thyrotoxicosis, hemolytic anemia, hemorrhage, malignancy, and hepatic and renal disease.

*Vitamin B₁₂ absorption test:* Vitamin B₁₂ absorption test (Schilling test).

## Administration and Dosage

CYANOCOBALAMIN, CRYSTALLINE:

*Addisonian pernicious anemia* – Parenteral therapy is required for life; oral therapy is not dependable. Administer 100 mcg daily for 6 or 7 days by IM or deep subcutaneous injection. If there is clinical improvement and a reticulocyte response, give the same amount on alternate days for 7 doses, then every 3 to 4 days for another 2 to 3 weeks. By this time, hematologic values should have become normal. Follow this regimen with 100 mcg monthly for life. Administer folic acid concomitantly if needed.

*Other patients with vitamin B₁₂ deficiency* – In seriously ill patients, administer both vitamin B₁₂ and folic acid. It is not necessary to withhold therapy until the precise cause of B₁₂ deficiency is established. For hematologic signs, children may be given 10 to 50 mcg/day for 5 to 10 days followed by 100 to 250 mcg/dose every 2 to 4 weeks; for neurologic signs, 100 mcg/day for 10 to 15 days, then once or twice weekly for several months, possibly tapering to 250 to 1000 mcg/month by 1 year.

*Oral* – Up to 1000 mcg/day. Oral vitamin B₁₂ therapy is not usually recommended for vitamin B₁₂ deficiency. The maximum amount of vitamin B₁₂ that can be absorbed from a single oral dose is 1 to 5 mcg. The percent absorbed decreases with increasing doses.

*IM or subcutaneous* – 30 mcg/day for 5 to 10 days followed by 100 to 200 mcg/month. Larger doses (eg, 1000 mcg) have been recommended, even though a larger amount is lost through excretion. However, it is possible that a greater amount is retained, allowing for fewer injections.

CYANOCOBALAMIN, INTRANASAL: Prime prior to initial use. Repriming between doses is not necessary if the unit is upright. Administer at least 1 hour before or 1 hour after ingestion of hot foods or liquids.

*Vitamin B₁₂ malabsorption in remission following injectable vitamin B₁₂ therapy* – 500 mcg intranasally once weekly.

HYDROXOCOBALAMIN, CRYSTALLINE: Administer IM only. The recommended dosage is 30 mcg/day for 5 to 10 days, followed by 100 to 200 mcg/month. Children may be given a total of 1 to 5 mg over 2 weeks or more in doses of 100 mcg, then 30 to 50 mcg every 4 weeks for maintenance. Institute concurrent folic acid therapy at the beginning of treatment if needed.

*Schilling test:* The flushing dose is 1000 mcg IM.

## Actions

*Pharmacology:* Vitamin B₁₂ is essential to growth, cell reproduction, hematopoiesis, and nucleoprotein and myelin synthesis. Its physiologic role is associated with methylation, participating in nucleic acid and protein synthesis. Cyanocobalamin participates in red blood cell formation through activation of folic acid coenzymes. Hydroxocobalamin (vitamin B$_{12a}$) functions the same as cyanocobalamin.

*Pharmacokinetics:* Absorption of vitamin B$_{12}$ depends on the presence of sufficient intrinsic factor and calcium. In general, absorption of oral B$_{12}$ is inadequate in malabsorptive states and in pernicious anemia (unless intrinsic factor is simultaneously administered).

*Cyanocobalamin* – Cyanocobalamin is rapidly absorbed from IM and subcutaneous injection sites; the plasma level peaks within 1 hour. Once absorbed, it is bound to plasma proteins, stored mainly in the liver and is slowly released when needed to carry out normal cellular metabolic functions. Within 48 hours after injection of 100 to 1000 mcg of vitamin B$_{12}$, 50% to 98% of the dose appears in the urine. The major portion is excreted within the first 8 hours. More rapid excretion occurs with IV administration; there is little opportunity for liver storage.

Peak concentration of B$_{12}$ after intranasal administration is 1 to 2 hours; Bioavailability is 8.9%.

*Hydroxocobalamin* – Hydroxocobalamin (vitamin B$_{12a}$) is more highly protein bound and is retained in the body longer than cyanocobalamin. However, it has no advantage over cyanocobalamin.

### Contraindications

Hypersensitivity to cobalt, vitamin B$_{12}$, or any component of these products.

### Warnings

*Inadequate response:* A blunted or impeded therapeutic response may be due to infection, uremia, bone marrow suppressant drugs, concurrent iron or folic acid deficiency, or misdiagnosis.

*Vitamin B$_{12}$ deficiency:* Vitamin B$_{12}$ deficiency allowed to progress for more than 3 months may produce permanent degenerative lesions of the spinal cord.

*Optic nerve atrophy:* Patients with early Leber disease (hereditary optic nerve atrophy) treated with cyanocobalamin suffer severe and swift optic atrophy.

*Hypokalemia:* Hypokalemia and sudden death may occur in severe megaloblastic anemia which is treated intensely.

*Pregnancy:* Category C (parenteral).

*Lactation:* Vitamin B$_{12}$ is excreted in breast milk in concentrations that approximate the mother's vitamin B$_{12}$ blood level. Amounts of B$_{12}$ recommended by the Food and Nutrition Board, National Academy of Sciences-National Research Council (2.6 mcg/day) should be consumed during lactation.

*Children:* The Food and Nutrition Board, National Academy of Sciences-National Research Council recommends a daily intake of 0.3 to 0.5 mcg/day for infants younger than 1 year of age and 0.7 to 1.4 mcg/day for children 1 to 10 years of age.

### Precautions

*Monitoring:* During treatment of severe megaloblastic anemia, monitor serum potassium levels closely for the first 48 hours and replace potassium if necessary. Obtain reticulocyte counts, hematocrit and vitamin B$_{12}$, iron and folic acid plasma levels prior to treatment and between the fifth and seventh days of therapy, and then frequently until the hematocrit is normal. If folate levels are low, also administer folic acid.

*Test dose:* Anaphylactic shock and death have occurred after parenteral vitamin B$_{12}$ administration. Give an intradermal test dose in patients sensitive to the cobalamins.

*Folate:* Doses greater than 10 mcg/day may produce hematologic response in patients with folate deficiency. Indiscriminate use may mask the true diagnosis of pernicious anemia.

Doses of folic acid greater than 0.1 mg/day may result in hematologic remission in patients with vitamin B$_{12}$ deficiency. Neurologic manifestations will not be prevented with folic acid, and if not treated with vitamin B$_{12}$, irreversible damage will result.

*Polycythemia vera:* Vitamin $B_{12}$ deficiency may suppress the signs of polycythemia vera.

*Vegetarian diets:* Vegetarian diets containing no animal products (including milk products or eggs) do not supply any vitamin $B_{12}$.

*Immunodeficient patients:* Vitamin $B_{12}$ malabsorption may occur in patients with AIDS or HIV infection. Consider monitoring levels.

*Nasal symptoms:* The effectiveness of intranasal cyanocobalamin in patients with nasal congestion, allergic rhinitis, and upper respiratory tract infections has not been determined. Defer treatment until symptoms have subsided.

### Drug Interactions

Drugs that may affect vitamin $B_{12}$ include aminosalicylic acid, chloramphenicol, colchicine, and alcohol.

*Drug/Lab test interactions:* Methotrexate, pyrimethamine, and most antibiotics invalidate folic acid and vitamin $B_{12}$ diagnostic microbiological blood assays.

### Adverse Reactions

The following reactions are associated with parenteral vitamin $B_{12}$: Anaphylactic shock, death, pulmonary edema, congestive heart failure early in treatment, severe and swift optic nerve atrophy.

# VITAMIN K$_1$ (Phytonadione, Phylloquinone, Methylphytyl Naphthoquinone)

**PHYTONADIONE**

| | |
|---|---|
| **Tablets:** 5 mg (*Rx*) | *Mephyton* (Merck) |
| **Injection (aqueous colloidal solution):** 2 mg/mL (*Rx*) | Various, *Konakion* (Roche) |
| **Injection (aqueous dispersion):** 10 mg/mL (*Rx*) | *Konakion* (Roche) |

**Warning:**
> *IV use:* Severe reactions, including fatalities, have occurred during and immediately after IV injection, even with precautions to dilute the injection and to avoid rapid infusion. These severe reactions resemble hypersensitivity or anaphylaxis, including shock and cardiac or respiratory arrest. Some patients exhibit these severe reactions on receiving vitamin K for the first time. Therefore, restrict the IV route to those situations where other routes are not feasible and the serious risk involved is justified.

**Indications**

*Coagulation disorders:* Coagulation disorders due to faulty formation of factors II, VII, IX, and X when caused by vitamin K deficiency or interference with vitamin K activity.

*Oral:* Anticoagulant-induced prothrombin deficiency (see Warnings); hypoprothrombinemia secondary to salicylates or antibacterial therapy; hypoprothrombinemia secondary to obstructive jaundice and biliary fistulas, but only if bile salts are administered concomitantly with phytonadione.

*Parenteral:* Anticoagulant-induced prothrombin deficiency; hypoprothrombinemia secondary to conditions limiting absorption or synthesis of vitamin K (eg, obstructive jaundice, biliary fistula, sprue, ulcerative colitis, celiac disease, intestinal resection, cystic fibrosis of the pancreas, regional enteritis); drug-induced hypoprothrombinemias due to interference with vitamin K metabolism (eg, antibiotics, salicylates); prophylaxis and therapy of hemorrhagic disease of the newborn.

**Administration and Dosage**

If possible, discontinue or reduce the dosage of drugs interfering with coagulation mechanisms (eg, salicylates, antibiotics) as an alternative to phytonadione. The severity of the coagulation disorder should determine whether the immediate administration of phytonadione is required in addition to discontinuation or reduction of interfering drugs.

Inject subcutaneously or IM when possible. In older children and adults, inject IM in the upper outer quadrant of the buttocks. In infants and young children, the anterolateral aspect of the thigh or the deltoid region is preferred. When IV administration is unavoidable, inject very slowly, not exceeding 1 mg/min.

*Anticoagulant-induced prothrombin deficiency in adults:* 2.5 to 10 mg or up to 25 mg (rarely, 50 mg) initially. Determine subsequent doses by prothrombin time (PT) response or clinical condition. If in 6 to 8 hours after parenteral administration (or 12 to 48 hours after oral administration), the PT has not been shortened satisfactorily, repeat dose. If shock or excessive blood loss occurs, transfusion of blood or fresh frozen plasma may be required.

*Hemorrhagic disease of the newborn:*
> *Prophylaxis* – Single IM dose of 0.5 to 1 mg within 1 hour after birth. This may be repeated after 2 to 3 weeks if the mother has received anticoagulant, anticonvulsant, antituberculous, or recent antibiotic therapy during her pregnancy. Twelve to 24 hours before delivery, 1 to 5 mg may be given to the mother.
> Oral doses of 2 mg have been shown to be adequate for prophylaxis.
> *Treatment* – 1 mg subcutaneously or IM. Higher doses may be necessary if the mother has been receiving oral anticoagulants. Empiric administration of vitamin K$_1$ should not replace proper laboratory evaluation. A prompt response (shorten-

ing of the PT in 2 to 4 hours) is usually diagnostic of hemorrhagic disease of the newborn; failure to respond indicates another diagnosis or coagulation disorder. Give blood or blood products such as fresh frozen plasma if bleeding is excessive. However, this therapy does not correct the underlying disorder; give phytonadione concurrently.

*Hypoprothrombinemia due to other causes in adults:* 2.5 to 25 mg (rarely, up to 50 mg); amount and route of administration depends on severity of condition and response obtained. Avoid oral route when clinical disorder would prevent proper absorption. Give bile salts with tablets when endogenous supply of bile to GI tract is deficient.

## Actions

*Pharmacology:* Vitamin K promotes the hepatic synthesis of active prothrombin (factor II), proconvertin (factor VII), plasma thromboplastin component (factor IX), and Stuart factor (factor X). The mechanism by which vitamin K promotes formation of these clotting factors involves the hepatic post-translational carboxylation of specific glutamate residues to gamma-carboxyglutamate residues in proteins involved in coagulation, thus leading to their activation.

Phytonadione (vitamin K₁) is a lipid-soluble synthetic analog of vitamin K. Phytonadione possesses essentially the same type and degree of activity as the naturally occurring vitamin K.

*Pharmacokinetics:* Phytonadione is only absorbed from the GI tract via intestinal lymphatics in the presence of bile salts. Although initially concentrated in the liver, vitamin K is rapidly metabolized, and very little tissue accumulation occurs.

Parenteral phytonadione is generally detectable within 1 to 2 hours. Phytonadione usually controls hemorrhage within 3 to 6 hours. A normal prothrombin level may be obtained in 12 to 14 hours. Oral phytonadione exerts its effect in 6 to 10 hours.

*The US daily allowances –* The US daily allowances for vitamin K have not been officially established, but have been estimated to be 10 to 20 mcg for infants, 15 to 100 mcg for children and adolescents, and 70 to 140 mcg for adults. Usually, dietary vitamin K will satisfy these requirements, except during the first 5 to 8 days of the neonatal period.

Recommended Dietary Allowances as published by the National Academy of Sciences are as follows: Adult males, 45 to 80 mcg/day; adult females, 45 to 65 mcg/day.

## Contraindications

Hypersensitivity to any component of the product.

## Warnings

*Oral anticoagulant-induced hypoprothrombinemia:* Vitamin K will not counteract the anticoagulant action of heparin.

Immediate coagulant effect should not be expected. It takes a minimum of 1 to 2 hours for a measurable improvement in the PT.

The prothrombin test is sensitive to the levels of factors II, VII, and X. Fresh plasma or blood transfusions may be required for severe blood loss or lack of response to vitamin K.

With phytonadione use and anticoagulant therapy indicated, the patient is faced with the same clotting hazards prior to starting anticoagulant therapy. Phytonadione is not a clotting agent, but overzealous therapy may restore original thromboembolic phenomena conditions. Keep dosage as low as possible and check PT regularly.

*Hepatic function impairment:* Hypoprothrombinemia due to hepatocellular damage is not corrected by administration of vitamin K. Repeated large doses of vitamin K are not warranted in liver disease if the initial response is unsatisfactory (Koller test). Failure to respond to vitamin K may indicate a coagulation defect or a condition unresponsive to vitamin K. In hepatic disease, large doses may further depress liver function.

Paradoxically, giving excessive doses of vitamin K or its analogs in an attempt to correct hypoprothrombinemia associated with severe hepatitis or cirrhosis may actually result in further depression of the prothrombin concentration.

*Pregnancy:* Category C.

*Lactation:* Vitamin K is excreted in breast milk.

*Children:* Safety and efficacy in children have not been established. Hemolysis, jaundice, and hyperbilirubinemia in newborns, particularly in premature infants, have been reported with vitamin K. These effects may be dose-related. Therefore, do not exceed recommended dose.

## Drug Interactions

Drugs that may interact include anticoagulants and mineral oil.

## Adverse Reactions

Adverse reactions from parenteral administration may include transient "flushing sensations" and "peculiar" sensations of taste. Deaths have occurred after IV administration. Hyperbilirubinemia has been observed in the newborn following administration of phytonadione. Anaphylactoid reactions may occur with either doseform.

# EPOETIN ALFA (Erythropoietin; EPO)

**Injection:** 2,000, 3,000, 4,000, 10,000, 20,000, and 40,000 units per mL (Rx)

*Epogen* (Amgen), *Procrit* (Ortho Biotech)

## Indications

*Treatment of anemia associated with chronic renal failure (CRF):* In adults and children 1 month of age and older, treatment of anemia associated with CRF, including patients on dialysis (end-stage renal disease) and patients not on dialysis, to elevate or maintain the red blood cell level (as manifested by the hematocrit or hemoglobin determinations) and to decrease the need for transfusions. Nondialysis patients with symptomatic anemia considered for therapy should have a hemoglobin less than 10 g/dL. Not intended for patients who require immediate correction of severe anemia. Epoetin alfa may obviate the need for maintenance transfusions but is not a substitute for emergency transfusion.

*Treatment of anemia related to zidovudine therapy in HIV-infected patients:* To elevate or maintain the red blood cell level (as manifested by the hematocrit or hemoglobin determinations) and to decrease the need for transfusions in these patients when the endogenous erythropoietin level is less than or equal to 500 milliunits/mL and the dose of zidovudine is less than or equal to 4200 mg/week.

*Treatment of anemia in cancer patients on chemotherapy:* Treatment of anemia in patients with nonmyeloid malignancies where anemia is due to the effect of concomitantly administered chemotherapy. It is intended to decrease the need for transfusions in patients who will be receiving chemotherapy for a minimum of 2 months.

*Reduction of allogeneic transfusion in surgery patients:* For the treatment of anemic patients (hemoglobin greater than 10 to 13 g/dL or less) scheduled to undergo elective, noncardiac, nonvascular surgery to reduce the need for allogeneic blood transfusions. Epoetin alfa is indicated for patients at high risk for perioperative transfusions with significant, anticipated blood loss.

## Administration and Dosage

*CRF patients:*

| General Therapeutic Guidelines in CRF Patients for Epoetin Alfa | |
| --- | --- |
| | Starting dose |
| Adults | 50 to 100 units/kg 3 times/week IV or subcutaneously |
| Children (on dialysis) | 50 units/kg 3 times/week IV or subcutaneously |
| Reduce dose when: | 1) Hemoglobin approaches 12 g/dL or 2) Hemoglobin increases by more than 1 g/dL in any 2-week period. |
| Increase dose if: | Hemoglobin does not increase by 2 g/dL after 8 weeks of therapy and hemoglobin is below suggested target range. |
| Maintenance dose | Individualize |
| Suggested target hemoglobin range | 10 to 12 g/dL |

*Administration* – Epoetin alfa may be given either as an IV or subcutaneous injection. In patients on hemodialysis, epoetin alfa usually has been administered as an IV bolus 3 times/week. While the administration is independent of the dialysis procedure, epoetin alfa may be administered into the venous line at the end of the dialysis procedure to obviate the need for additional venous access. In adult patients with CRF not on dialysis, epoetin alfa may be given either as an IV or subcutaneous injection.

*Pretherapy iron evaluation* – Prior to and during therapy, evaluate the patient's iron stores, including transferrin saturation and serum ferritin. Transferrin saturation should be at least 20% and ferritin should be at least 100 ng/mL. Virtually all patients will eventually require supplemental iron (see Precautions). Adequately control blood pressure prior to initiation of epoetin alfa therapy, and closely monitor and control it during therapy.

*Dose adjustment* – Adjust the dose for each patient to achieve and maintain a target hemoglobin not to exceed 12 g/dL.

Do not increase dose more frequently than once a month. If the hemoglobin is increasing and approaching 12 g/dL, reduce the dose by approximately 25%. If the hemoglobin continues to increase, temporarily withhold the dose until the hemoglobin begins to decrease, then resume therapy at that point at a dose approximately 25% below the previous dose. If the hemoglobin increases by more than 1 g/dL in a 2-week period, decrease the dose by approximately 25%.

If the increase in the hemoglobin is less than 1 g/dL over 4 weeks and iron stores are adequate, the dose of epoetin alfa may be increased by approximately 25% of the previous dose. Further increases may be made at 4-week intervals until the specified hemoglobin is obtained.

*Maintenance –*

*Hemodialysis patients:* Median dose is 75 units/kg 3 times/week (range, 12.5 to 525 units/kg 3 times/week).

*Peritoneal dialysis patients:* Median dosage of 76 units/kg/week (range, 24 to 323 units/kg/week) in divided doses 2 to 3 times/week.

*Children on hemodialysis:* Median dose of 167 units/kg/week (range, 49 to 477 units/kg/week) in divided doses, 2 to 3 times/week.

*Nondialysis CRF patients:* Dose of 75 to 150 units/kg/week has maintained hematocrits of 36% to 38% for up to 6 months.

If the hemoglobin remains below, or falls below, the suggested target range, reevaluate iron stores. If the transferrin saturation is less than 20%, administer supplemental iron. If the transferrin saturation is greater than 20%, the dose of epoetin alfa may be increased. Do not make such dose increases more frequently than once a month, unless clinically indicated, because the response time of the hemoglobin to a dose increase can be 2 to 6 weeks. Measure hemoglobin twice weekly for 2 to 6 weeks following dose increases.

*Delayed or diminished response* – Over 95% of patients with CRF responded with clinically significant increases in hematocrit, and virtually all patients were transfusion-independent within about 2 months of initiation of therapy.

If a patient fails to respond or maintain a response, consider other etiologies and evaluate as clinically indicated.

*Zidovudine-treated, HIV-infected patients:* Available evidence suggests that patients receiving zidovudine with endogenous serum erythropoietin levels greater than 500 milliunits/mL are unlikely to respond to therapy.

*Initial dose* – For patients with serum erythropoietin levels 500 milliunits/mL or less who are receiving a dose of zidovudine 4200 mg/week or less, the recommended starting dose is 100 units/kg as an IV or subcutaneous injection 3 times/week for 8 weeks.

If the response is not satisfactory in terms of reducing transfusion requirements or increasing hematocrit after 8 weeks of therapy, the dose can be increased by 50 to 100 units/kg 3 times/week. Evaluate response every 4 to 8 weeks thereafter and adjust the dose accordingly by 50 to 100 units/kg increments 3 times/week. If patients have not responded satisfactorily to a 300 units/kg dose 3 times/week, it is unlikely that they will respond to higher doses.

*Maintenance dose* – When the desired response is attained, titrate the dose to maintain the response based on factors such as variations in zidovudine dose and the presence of intercurrent infectious or inflammatory episodes. If hemoglobin exceeds 13 g/dL, stop the dose until hemoglobin drops to 12 g/dL. When resuming treatment, reduce the dose by 25%, then titrate to maintain desired hemoglobin.

*Cancer patients on chemotherapy:* Treatment of patients with grossly elevated serum erythropoietin levels (eg, greater than 200 milliunits/mL) is not recommended. Monitor hemoglobin on a weekly basis in patients receiving epoetin alfa therapy until hemoglobin becomes stable.

| Three Times Weekly Dosing for Cancer Patients on Chemotherapy | |
|---|---|
| Starting dose | |
| Adults | 150 units/kg 3 times/week subcutaneously |
| Reduce dose when: | 1) Hemoglobin approaches 12 g/dL or 2) Hemoglobin increases by more than 1 g/dL in any 2-week period. |
| Withhold dose when: | Hemoglobin exceeds 13 g/dL, until the hemoglobin falls to 12 g/dL, and then restart dose at 25% below the previous dose. |
| Increase dose if: | Response is not satisfactory (no reduction in transfusion requirements or rise in hemoglobin) after 8 weeks; increase dose to 300 units/kg 3 times/week. |
| Suggested target hemoglobin range | 10 to 12 g/dL |

| Weekly Dosing for Cancer Patients on Chemotherapy | |
|---|---|
| Starting dose | |
| Adults | 40,000 units subcutaneously weekly |
| Increase dose if: | After 4 weeks of therapy, the hemoglobin has not increased by 1 g/dL or more, in the absence of RBC transfusion; increase the dose to 60,000 units weekly. |
| If no response: | If patient has not responded satisfactorily to a dose of 60,000 units weekly after 4 weeks, it is unlikely he/she will respond to higher doses. |
| Withhold dose if: | Hemoglobin exceeds 13 g/dL, and when the hemoglobin falls to less than 12 g/dL, then restart dose at 25% below the previous dose. |
| Reduce dose when: | Treatment produces a very rapid hemoglobin response (eg, hemoglobin increases by more than 1 g/dL in any 2-week period). |

*Surgery* – Prior to initiating treatment with epoetin alfa, obtain a hemoglobin to establish that it is greater than 10 to 13 g/dL or less. The recommended dose is 300 units/kg/day subcutaneously for 10 days before surgery, on the day of surgery and for 4 days after surgery.

An alternate dose schedule is 600 units/kg subcutaneously in once-weekly doses (21, 14, and 7 days before surgery) plus a fourth dose on the day of surgery.

All patients should receive adequate iron supplementation. Initiate iron supplementation no later than the beginning of treatment with epoetin alfa and continue throughout the course of therapy.

### Actions

*Pharmacology:* Erythropoietin is a glycoprotein that stimulates red blood cell production. It is produced in the kidney and stimulates the division and differentiation of erythroid progenitors in bone marrow. Hypoxia and anemia generally increase the production of erythropoietin, which in turn stimulates erythropoiesis. In patients with CRF, erythropoietin production is impaired; this deficiency is the primary cause of their anemia. Epoetin alfa stimulates erythropoiesis in anemic patients on dialysis and those who do not require regular dialysis.

*Pharmacokinetics:* Epoetin alfa IV is eliminated via first-order kinetics with a circulating half-life of 4 to 13 hours in patients with CRF. Within the therapeutic dosage range, detectable levels of plasma erythropoietin are maintained for at least 24 hours. After subcutaneous administration of epoetin alfa to patients with CRF, peak serum levels are achieved within 5 to 24 hours after administration and decline slowly thereafter. The half-life in healthy volunteers is approximately 20% shorter than in CRF patients.

### Contraindications

Uncontrolled hypertension; hypersensitivity to mammalian cell-derived products or to human albumin.

## Warnings

*Pure red cell aplasia (PRCA):* PRCA has been reported in a limited number of patients exposed to epoetin alfa. This has been reported predominantly in patients with CRF. Evaluate any patient with loss of response to epoetin alfa for the etiology of loss of effect. Discontinue epoetin alfa in any patient with evidence of PRCA and evaluate the patient for the presence of binding and neutralizing antibodies to epoetin alfa, native erythropoietin, and any other recombinant erythropoietin administered to the patient. In patients with PRCA secondary to neutralizing antibodies to erythropoietin, do not administer epoetin alfa, and do not switch such patients to another product as anti-erythropoietin antibodies cross-react with other erythropoietins.

*Albumin (human):* Epoetin alfa contains albumin, a derivative of human blood. Based on effective donor screening and product manufacturing processes, it carries an extremely remote risk for transmission of viral diseases. No cases of transmission of viral diseases or Creutzfeldt-Jakob disease have ever been identified for albumin.

*Anemia:* Not intended for CRF patients who require correction of severe anemia; epoetin alfa may obviate the need for maintenance transfusions but is not a substitute for emergency transfusion. Not indicated for treatment of anemia in HIV-infected patients or cancer patients due to other factors such as iron or folate deficiencies, hemolysis, or GI bleeding, which should be managed appropriately.

*Hypertension:* Up to 80% of patients with CRF have a history of hypertension. Do not treat patients with uncontrolled hypertension; monitor blood pressure adequately before initiation of therapy. Hypertensive encephalopathy and seizures have occurred in patients with CRF treated with epoetin.

It is recommended that the epoetin alfa dose be decreased if the hemoglobin increase exceeds 1 g/dL in any 2-week period because of the possible association of excessive rate of rise of hemoglobin with an exacerbation of hypertension. In CRF patients on hemodialysis with clinically evident ischemic heart disease or CHF, manage the hemoglobin carefully, not to exceed 12 g/dL.

*Seizures:* There have been 47 seizures in 1,010 patients on dialysis treated with epoetin alfa in clinical trials, with an exposure of 986 patient-years for a rate of approximately 0.048 events per patient-year. Given the potential for an increased risk of seizure during the first 90 days of therapy, closely monitor blood pressure and the presence of premonitory neurologic symptoms. While the relationship between seizures and the rate of rise in hemoglobin is uncertain, it is recommended that the dose be decreased if the hemoglobin increase exceeds 1 g/dL in any 2-week period.

*Thrombotic events:* During hemodialysis, patients treated with epoetin alfa may require increased anticoagulation with heparin to prevent clotting of the artificial kidney.

*Growth factor potential:* The possibility that epoetin alfa can act as a growth factor for any tumor type, particularly myeloid malignancies, cannot be excluded.

*Hypersensitivity reactions:* Skin rashes and urticaria are rare, mild, and transient. If an anaphylactoid reaction occurs, immediately discontinue the drug and initiate appropriate therapy. Refer to Management of Acute Hypersensitivity Reactions.

*Fertility impairment:* In female rats treated IV with epoetin alfa, there was a trend for slightly increased fetal wastage at doses of 100 and 500 units/kg.

*Pregnancy:* Category C.

*Lactation:* It is not known whether epoetin alfa is excreted in breast milk.

*Children:* Safety and efficacy have not been established in patients less than 1 month of age.

## Precautions

*Monitoring:*

*Patients with CRF not requiring dialysis* – Monitor blood pressure and hematocrit no less frequently than for patients maintained on dialysis. Closely monitor renal function and fluid and electrolyte balance, as an improved sense of well-being may obscure the need to initiate dialysis in some patients.

Determine the hemoglobin twice a week until it has stabilized in the target range and the maintenance dose has been established. After any dose adjustment, determine the hemoglobin twice weekly for at least 2 to 6 weeks until the hemoglobin has stabilized; then monitor at regular intervals.

Perform complete blood count with differential and platelet counts regularly. Modest increases have occurred in platelets and white blood cell counts, but values remained within normal ranges.

Monitor serum chemistry values (including blood urea nitrogen, uric acid, creatinine, phosphorus, and potassium) regularly.

*Zidovudine-treated, HIV-infected and cancer patients* – Measure hemoglobin once a week until it is stabilized; measure periodically thereafter.

*Iron evaluation* – During therapy, absolute or functional iron deficiency may develop. Transferrin saturation should be at least 20%, and ferritin should be at least 100 ng/mL. Prior to and during therapy, evaluate the patient's iron status, including transferrin saturation (serum iron divided by iron binding capacity) and serum ferritin. Virtually all patients will eventually require supplemental iron to increase or maintain transferrin saturation to levels that will adequately support epoetin alfa-stimulated erythropoiesis.

*Hematology:* The elevated bleeding time characteristic of CRF decreases toward normal after correction of anemia in epoetin alfa-treated patients. Reduction of bleeding time also occurs after correction of anemia by transfusion. Allow sufficient time to determine a patient's responsiveness before adjusting the dose. An interval of 2 to 6 weeks may occur between the time of a dose adjustment and a significant change in hemoglobin.

*Porphyria* – Porphyria exacerbation has been observed rarely in epoetin alfa-treated patients with CRF. Use with caution in patients with known porphyria.

*Bone marrow fibrosis:* Bone marrow fibrosis is a complication of CRF and may be related to secondary hyperparathyroidism or unknown factors.

*Delayed or diminished response:* If the patient fails to respond or to maintain a response to doses within the recommended range, consider and evaluate the following etiologies:

1.) Functional iron deficiency may develop with normal ferritin levels but low transferrin saturation (less than 20%), presumably due to the inability to mobilize iron stores rapidly enough to support increased erythropoiesis.
2.) Underlying infectious, inflammatory, or malignant processes.
3.) Occult blood loss.
4.) Underlying hematologic diseases.
5.) Vitamin deficiencies: Folic acid or vitamin $B_{12}$.
6.) Hemolysis.
7.) Aluminum intoxication.
8.) Osteitis fibrosa cystica.
9.) In the absence of another etiology, evaluate the patient for evidence of PRCA and test sera for the presence of antibodies to recombinant erythropoietins.

*Diet:* As the hemoglobin increases and patients experience an improved sense of well-being, reinforce the importance of compliance with dietary guidelines and frequency of dialysis.

*Hyperkalemia* – Hyperkalemia is not uncommon in patients with CRF.

*Dialysis management:* Therapy with epoetin alfa results in an increase in hematocrit and a decrease in plasma volume that could affect dialysis efficiency.

*Benzyl alcohol:* Benzyl alcohol, which is contained in some of these products as a preservative, has been associated with an increased incidence of neurological and other complications in premature infants that are sometimes fatal.

*Drug abuse and dependence:* Epoetin alfa has been used by athletes to increase their performance by increasing hemoglobin ("blood doping"). Several deaths have resulted from this abuse.

**Adverse Reactions**

*CRF patients* – Epoetin alfa is generally well tolerated. The following adverse reactions are frequent (greater than 3%) sequelae of CRF and are not necessarily due to epoetin alfa therapy: hypertension, headache, arthralgia, nausea, edema, fatigue, diarrhea, vomiting, chest pain, asthenia, dizziness, skin reaction, and clotted vascular access.

*Zidovudine-treated HIV-infected patients* – Adverse experiences greater than 3% were consistent with the progression of HIV infection: pyrexia, fatigue, headache, cough, diarrhea, rash, nausea, respiratory congestion, shortness of breath, asthenia, skin reaction, and dizziness.

*Surgery patients* – Adverse reactions 3% or more include the following: pyrexia, nausea, constipation, skin reactions at injection site, vomiting, itching, insomnia, headache, dizziness, urinary tract infection, hypertension, anxiety, diarrhea, dyspepsia, edema, deep venous thrombosis.

*Cancer patients in chemotherapy* – Adverse reactions greater than 3% were consistent with the underlying disease state: pyrexia, diarrhea, nausea, vomiting, edema, asthenia, fatigue, shortness of breath, paresthesia, upper respiratory infection, dizziness, and trunk pain.

# DARBEPOETIN ALFA

**Solution:**[1] 25, 40, 60, 100, 200, 300, and 500 mcg/mL and    *Aranesp* (Amgen)
150 mg/0.75 mL (*Rx*)

[1] The polysorbate solution contains 0.05 mg polysorbate 80, 2.12 mg sodium phosphate monobasic monohydrate, 0.66 mg sodium phosphate dibasic anhydrous, and 8.18 mg sodium chloride. The albumin solution contains 2.5 mg albumin (human), 2.23 mg sodium phosphate monobasic monohydrate, 0.53 mg sodium phosphate dibasic anhydrous, and 8.18 mg sodium chloride.

**Indications**

*Anemia:* For the treatment of anemia associated with chronic renal failure (CRF), including patients on dialysis, and for the treatment of anemia in patients with nonmyeloid malignancies.

**Administration and Dosage**

Administer IV or subcutaneously as a single weekly injection. Start and slowly adjust the dose as described below based on hemoglobin levels. If a patient fails to respond or maintain a response, consider other etiologies. When darbepoetin therapy is initiated or adjusted, follow the hemoglobin level weekly until stabilized, and monitor at least monthly thereafter.

For patients who respond to darbepoetin with a rapid increase in hemoglobin (eg, more than 1 g/dL in any 2-week period), reduce the dose of darbepoetin.

*Correction of anemia:* The recommended starting dose of darbepoetin for the correction of anemia in chronic renal failure (CRF) patients is 0.45 mcg/kg body weight, administered as a single IV or subcutaneous injection. Titrate doses to not exceed a target hemoglobin concentration of 12 g/dL. Some patients have been treated successfully with subcutaneous darbepoetin administered once every 2 weeks.

*Conversion from epoetin alfa to darbepoetin:* Estimate the starting weekly dose of darbepoetin based on the weekly epoetin alfa dose at the time of substitution. Titrate doses to maintain the target hemoglobin. Due to the longer serum half-life, administer darbepoetin less frequently than epoetin alfa. Administer once a week if patient was receiving epoetin alfa 2 to 3 times/week. Administer darbepoetin once every 2 weeks if the patient was receiving epoetin alfa once per week. Maintain the route of administration (IV or subcutaneously).

| Estimated Darbepoetin Starting Doses (mcg/week) Based on Previous Epoetin Alfa Dose (units/week) ||
| Previous weekly epoetin alfa dose (units/week) | Weekly darbepoetin dose (mcg/week) |
| --- | --- |
| < 2500 | 6.25 |
| 2500 to 4999 | 12.5 |
| 5000 to 10,999 | 25 |
| 11,000 to 17,999 | 40 |
| 18,000 to 33,999 | 60 |
| 34,000 to 89,999 | 100 |
| ≥ 90,000 | 200 |

*Dose adjustment:* Do not increase doses more frequently than once a month. If the hemoglobin is increasing and approaching 12 g/dL, reduce the dose by approximately 25%. If the hemoglobin continues to increase, withhold doses temporarily until the hemoglobin begins to decrease, at which point therapy should be reinitiated at a dose approximately 25% below the previous dose. If the hemoglobin increases by more than 1 g/dL in a 2-week period, decrease the dose by approximately 25%.

If the increase in hemoglobin is less than 1 g/dL over 4 weeks and iron stores are adequate, the dose of darbepoetin may be increased by approximately 25% of the previous dose. Further increases may be made at 4-week intervals until the specified hemoglobin is obtained.

*Maintenance dose:* Adjust darbepoetin dosage to maintain a target hemoglobin not to exceed 12 g/dL. If the hemoglobin exceeds 12 g/dL, the dose may be adjusted as described above.

*Cancer patients receiving chemotherapy:* The recommended starting dose for darbepoetin alfa is 2.25 mcg/kg administered as a weekly subcutaneous injection.

The dose should be adjusted for each patient to achieve and maintain a target hemoglobin. If there is less than a 1 g/dL increase in hemoglobin after 6 weeks of therapy, increase the dose of darbepoetin alfa up to 4.5 mcg/kg. If hemoglobin increases by more than 1 g/dL in a 2-week period or if the hemoglobin exceeds 12 g/dL, reduce the dose by approximately 25%. If the hemoglobin exceeds 13 g/dL, temporarily withhold doses until the hemoglobin falls to 12 g/dL. Reinitiate therapy at a dose approximately 25% below the previous dose.

*Preparation:* Do not shake. Do not dilute. Do not administer darbepoetin in conjunction with other drug solutions. Darbepoetin is packaged in single-use vials and contains no preservatives. Discard any unused portion. Do not pool unused portions.

## Actions

*Pharmacology:* Darbepoetin alfa is an erythropoiesis-stimulating protein produced by recombinant DNA technology. Darbepoetin stimulates erythropoiesis by the same mechanism as endogenous erythropoietin.

*Pharmacokinetics:*

*Absorption* – Darbepoetin has an approximately 3-fold longer terminal half-life than epoetin alfa when administered by either the IV or subcutaneous route.

Following IV administration, darbepoetin has a distribution half-life of approximately 1.4 hours and mean terminal half-life of approximately 21 hours.

Following subcutaneous administration, the absorption is slow and rate-limiting and the terminal half-life is 49 hours. The peak concentration occurs at 34 hours post-subcutaneous administration in adult CRF patients, and bioavailability is approximately 37%.

*Distribution* – The distribution of darbepoetin in adult CRF patients is predominantly confined to the vascular space (approximately 60 mL/kg). With once-weekly dosing, steady-state serum levels are achieved within 4 weeks with a less than 2-fold increase in peak concentration when compared with the initial dose.

**Contraindications**

Uncontrolled hypertension; known hypersensitivity to the active substance or any of the excipients.

**Warnings**

*Cardiovascular events:* Darbepoetin and other erythropoietic therapies may increase the risk of cardiovascular events, including death, in patients with CRF. The higher risk of cardiovascular events may be associated with higher hemoglobin or higher rates of rise of hemoglobin. The hemoglobin level should be managed to avoid exceeding a target level of 12 g/dL. The dose of darbepoetin should be decreased if the hemoglobin increase exceeds 1 g/dL in any 2-week period because of the association of excessive rate of rise of hemoglobin with these events.

*Hypertension:* Do not treat patients with uncontrolled hypertension with darbepoetin; control blood pressure before initiation of therapy. Blood pressure may rise during treatment of anemia with darbepoetin or epoetin alfa.

*Seizures:* Seizures have occurred in patients with CRF participating in clinical trials of darbepoetin and epoetin alfa. During the first several months of therapy, closely monitor blood pressure and the presence of premonitory neurologic symptoms.

*Thrombotic events:* An increased incidence of thrombotic events has been observed in patients treated with erythropoietic agents.

*Pure red cell aplasia (PRCA):* PRCA, in association with neutralizing antibodies to native erythropoietin, has been observed in patients treated with recombinant erythropoietins. This has been reported predominantly in patients with CRF. Discontinue darbepoetin alfa in any patient with evidence of PRCA and evaluate the patient for the presence of binding and neutralizing antibodies to darbepoetin alfa, native erythropoietin, and any other recombinant erythropoietin administered to the patient.

*Albumin (human):* Darbepoetin formulated with albumin carries an extremely remote risk for transmission of viral diseases. A theoretical risk for transmission of Creutzfeldt-Jakob disease (CJD) also is considered extremely remote. No cases of transmission of viral disease or CJD have ever been identified for albumin.

*Pregnancy:* Category C.

*Lactation:* It is not known whether darbepoetin is excreted in human milk.

*Children:* The safety and efficacy of darbepoetin in pediatric patients have not been established.

**Precautions**

*Monitoring:* After initiating therapy, determine the hemoglobin weekly until stabilized and the maintenance dose established. After a dose adjustment, determine the hemoglobin weekly for at least 4 weeks until that the hemoglobin has stabilized in response to the dose change. Then monitor the hemoglobin at regular intervals.

Evaluate iron status for all patients before and during treatment. Supplemental iron therapy is recommended for all patients whose serum ferritin is below 100 mcg/L or whose serum transferrin saturation is below 20%.

*Compromised erythropoietic response:* A lack of response or failure to maintain a hemoglobin response with darbepoetin doses within recommended dosing range should prompt a search for causative factors.

The safety and efficacy of darbepoetin therapy have not been established in patients with underlying hematologic diseases (eg, hemolytic anemia, sickle cell anemia, thalassemia, porphyria).

*Patients with CRF not requiring dialysis:* Patients with CRF not yet requiring dialysis may require lower maintenance doses of darbepoetin than patients receiving dialysis. Predialysis patients may be more responsive to the effects of darbepoetin, and require judicious monitoring of blood pressure and hemoglobin. Also closely monitor renal function and fluid and electrolyte balance.

*Dialysis management:* Therapy with darbepoetin results in an increase in red blood cells and a decrease in plasma volume, which could reduce dialysis efficiency; patients who are marginally dialyzed may require adjustments in their dialysis prescription.

*Growth factor potential:* Darbepoetin alfa is a growth factor that primarily stimulates RBC production. The possibility that darbepoetin alfa can act as a growth factor for any tumor type, particularly myeloid malignancies, has not been evaluated.

**Adverse Reactions**

The most frequently reported serious adverse reactions with darbepoetin in CRF patients were vascular access thrombosis, CHF, sepsis, and cardiac arrhythmia. The most commonly reported adverse reactions were infection, hypertension, hypotension, myalgia, headache, and diarrhea. The most frequently reported adverse reactions resulting in clinical intervention were hypotension, hypertension, fever, myalgia, nausea, and chest pain.

The most frequently reported serious adverse events reported with cancer chemotherapy patients included death, fever, pneumonia, dehydration, vomiting, and dyspnea. The most commonly reported adverse events were fatigue, edema, nausea, vomiting, diarrhea, fever, and dyspnea. The most frequently reported reasons for discontinuation of darbepoetin alfa were progressive disease, death, discontinuation of the chemotherapy, asthenia, dyspnea, pneumonia, GI hemorrhage, thrombotic events, rash, dehydration.

Adverse reactions occurring in at least 3% of patients include the following: Hypertension, hypotension, cardiac arrhythmias/cardiac arrest, angina pectoris/cardiac chest pain, pruritus, thrombosis vascular access, CHF, headache, dizziness, diarrhea, vomiting, nausea, abdominal pain, constipation, myalgia, arthralgia, limb pain, back pain, upper respiratory tract infection, dyspnea, cough, bronchitis, infection (eg, sepsis, bacteremia, pneumonia, peritonitis, abscess), peripheral edema, fatigue, fever, death, injection site pain, unspecified chest pain, fluid overload, access infection influenza-like symptoms, access hemorrhage, asthenia.

# ANAGRELIDE

**Capsules:** 0.5 and 1 mg (*Rx*)                    *Agrylin* (Roberts)

### Indications

*Thrombocythemia:* For the treatment of patients with thrombocythemia, secondary to myeloproliferative disorders, to reduce the elevated platelet count and the risk of thrombosis and to ameliorate associated symptoms including thrombo-hemorrhagic events.

### Administration and Dosage

The recommended starting dose is 0.5 mg 4 times/day or 1 mg twice/day; maintain for at least 1 week, then adjust to the lowest dose required to reduce and maintain platelet count below 600,000/mcL ideally to the normal range. Increase the dosage by no more than 0.5 mg/day in any 1 week. Do not exceed 10 mg/day or 2.5 mg in a single dose. Platelet count begins to respond within 7 to 14 days at the proper dosage.

### Actions

*Pharmacology:* The mechanism by which anagrelide reduces blood platelet count is under investigation. In blood withdrawn from healthy volunteers treated with anagrelide, a disruption was found in the postmitotic phase of megakaryocyte development and a reduction in megakaryocyte size and ploidy. Anagrelide inhibits cyclic AMP phosphodiesterase and ADP- and collagen-induced platelet aggregation.

*Pharmacokinetics:*

*Absorption/Distribution* – Anagrelide plasma levels peaked at approximately 1 hour; the plasma half-life is 1.3 hours. Bioavailability is reduced by food.

*Metabolism/Excretion* – Anagrelide is extensively metabolized.

### Warnings

*Cardiovascular:* Use with caution in patients with known or suspected heart disease. Because of the positive inotropic effects and side effects of anagrelide, a pretreatment cardiovascular examination is recommended along with careful monitoring during treatment.

*Thrombocytopenia:* Platelet counts below 50,000/mcL occurred in patients with myeloproliferative disorders while on anagrelide therapy. Thrombocytopenia promptly recovered upon discontinuation of anagrelide.

*Renal toxicity:* Fifteen patients were found to have renal abnormalities. Eleven experienced renal failure while on anagrelide; in 4 cases, the renal failure was considered to be possibly related to anagrelide. No dose adjustment was required because of renal insufficiency.

*Renal function impairment:* Patients with renal insufficiency (creatinine 2 mg/dL or greater) can receive anagrelide when the potential benefits outweigh the potential risks. Monitor patients closely for signs of renal toxicity while receiving anagrelide.

*Hepatic function impairment:* Patients with hepatic dysfunction (ie, bilirubin, AST, or measures of liver function more than 1.5 times the upper limit of normal) receive anagrelide when the potential benefits outweigh the potential risks. Monitor patients closely for signs of hepatic toxicity while receiving anagrelide.

*Pregnancy:* Category C.

*Lactation:* It is not known whether this drug is excreted in breast milk.

*Children:* The safety and efficacy of anagrelide in patients younger than 16 years of age have not been established.

### Precautions

*Monitoring:* Perform platelet counts every 2 days during the first week of treatment and at least weekly thereafter until the maintenance dosage is reached. While the platelet count is being lowered (usually during the first 2 weeks of treatment), monitor blood counts (hemoglobin, white blood cells), liver function (AST, ALT) and renal function (serum creatinine, BUN). Closely monitor patients with known or suspected heart disease, renal insufficiency, or hepatic dysfunction.

*Blood pressure* – In 9 subjects receiving a single 5 mg dose of anagrelide, standing blood pressure fell an average of 22/15 mm Hg, usually accompanied by dizziness. Only minimal changes in blood pressure were observed following a 2 mg dose.

*Interruption of therapy* – In general, interruption of anagrelide treatment is followed by an increase in platelet count. After sudden discontinuation of therapy, the increase in platelet count can be observed within 4 days.

### Drug Interactions

*Sucralfate:* A single case report suggests sucralfate may interfere with anagrelide absorption.

*Drug/Food interactions:* Bioavailability is reduced by food.

### Adverse Reactions

Adverse reactions occurring in at least 3% of patients include the following: abdominal pain, anorexia, asthenia, back pain, chest pain, cough, diarrhea, dizziness, dyspepsia, dyspnea, edema, fever, flatulence, headache, malaise, nausea, pain, palpitations, paresthesia, peripheral edema, pharyngitis, photosensitivity, pruritus, rash (eg, urticaria), tachycardia, vomiting.

# DIPYRIDAMOLE

**Tablets**: 25, 50, and 75 mg (*Rx*)                    Various, *Persantine* (Boehringer Ingelheim)

### Indications

*Thromboembolic complications:* Adjunct to coumarin anticoagulants in the prevention of postoperative thromboembolic complications of cardiac valve replacement.

### Administration and Dosage

*Adjunctive use in prophylaxis of thromboembolism after cardiac valve replacement:* The recommended dose is 75 to 100 mg 4 times/day as an adjunct to the usual warfarin therapy.

### Actions

*Pharmacology:* Dipyridamole lengthens abnormally shortened platelet survival time in a dose-dependent manner.

Dipyridamole is a platelet adhesion inhibitor, although the mechanism of action has not been fully elucidated. The mechanism may relate to: 1) Inhibition of red blood cell uptake of adenosine, itself an inhibitor of platelet reactivity, 2) phosphodiesterase inhibition leading to increased cyclic-3', 5'-adenosine monophosphate within platelets and, 3) inhibition of thromboxane $A_2$ formation, which is a potent stimulator of platelet activation.

*Pharmacokinetics:*

*Metabolism* – Following an oral dose of dipyridamole, the average time to peak concentration is approximately 75 minutes. The decline in plasma concentration fits a two-compartment model. The $\alpha$ half-life (the initial decline following peak concentration) is approximately 40 minutes. The $\beta$ half-life (the terminal decline in plasma concentration) is approximately 10 hours. Dipyridamole is highly bound to plasma proteins. It is metabolized in the liver where it is conjugated as a glucuronide and excreted with the bile.

### Warnings

*Fertility impairment:* A significant reduction in number of corpora lutea with consequent reduction in implantations and live fetuses was observed at 155 times the maximum recommended human dose.

*Pregnancy:* Category B.

*Lactation:* Dipyridamole is excreted in breast milk.

*Children:* Safety and efficacy in children younger than 12 years of age have not been established.

### Precautions

*Hypotension:* Use with caution in patients with hypotension because it can produce peripheral vasodilation.

## Adverse Reactions

Adverse reactions at therapeutic doses are usually minimal and transient. With long-term use, initial side effects usually disappear. The following reactions were reported in 2 heart valve replacement trials comparing dipyridamole and warfarin therapy to either warfarin alone or warfarin and placebo: dizziness, abdominal distress, headache, and rash.

On those uncommon occasions when adverse reactions have been persistent or intolerable, they have ceased on withdrawal of the medication.

# DIPYRIDAMOLE AND ASPIRIN

**Capsules:** 200 mg extended-release dipyridamole/25 mg aspirin (*Rx*)          *Aggrenox* (Boehringer Ingelheim)

## Indications

*Stroke:* To reduce the risk of stroke in patients who have had transient ischemia of the brain or complete ischemic stroke due to thrombosis.

## Administration and Dosage

The recommended dose of dipyridamole and aspirin combination therapy is 1 capsule given orally twice daily, 1 in the morning and 1 in the evening. Swallow whole; do not crush or chew.

Do not interchange with individual components of aspirin and dipyridamole tablets.

## Actions

*Pharmacology:* Antithrombotic action is the result of the additive antiplatelet effects of dipyridamole and aspirin.

*Pharmacokinetics:*

*Absorption –*

*Dipyridamole:* Peak plasma levels of dipyridamole are achieved approximately 2 hours after administration of a daily dose of 400 mg dipyridamole and aspirin combination (given as 200 mg twice daily). The peak plasma concentration at steady-state is approximately 1.98 mcg/mL and the steady-state trough concentration is approximately 0.53 mcg/mL.

*Aspirin:* Peak plasma levels of aspirin are achieved approximately 0.63 hours after administration of a 50 mg/day aspirin dose from dipyridamole and aspirin combination (given as 25 mg twice/day). The peak plasma concentration at steady-state is approximately 319 ng/mL. Aspirin undergoes moderate hydrolysis to salicylic acid in the liver and the GI wall, with 50% to 75% of an administered dose reaching the systemic circulation as intact aspirin.

*Distribution –*

*Dipyridamole:* Dipyridamole is highly lipophilic; however, it has been shown that the drug does not cross the blood-brain barrier to any significant extent in animals. The steady-state volume of distribution of dipyridamole is approximately 92 L. Approximately 99% of dipyridamole is bound to plasma proteins, predominantly to α1-acid glycoprotein and albumin.

*Aspirin:* Aspirin is poorly bound to plasma proteins and its apparent volume of distribution is low (10 L). Its metabolite, salicylic acid, is highly bound to plasma proteins, but its binding is concentration-dependent (nonlinear). At low concentrations (less than 100 mcg/mL), approximately 90% of salicylic acid is bound to albumin. Salicylic acid is widely distributed to all tissues and fluids in the body, including the CNS, breast milk, and fetal tissues.

*Metabolism/Excretion –*

*Dipyridamole:* Dipyridamole is metabolized in the liver, primarily by conjugation with glucuronic acid, of which monoglucuronide, which has low pharmacodynamic activity, is the primary metabolite. In plasma, approximately 80% of the total amount is present as parent compound and 20% as monoglucuronide. Most of the glucuronide metabolite (approximately 95%) is excreted via bile into the feces, with some evidence of enterohepatic circulation. Renal excretion of parent compound is negligible and urinary excretion of the glucuronide metabolite is low (approximately 5%).

*Aspirin:* Aspirin is rapidly hydrolyzed in plasma to salicylic acid with a half-life of 20 minutes. Plasma levels of aspirin are essentially undetectable 2 to 2.5 hours after dosing, and peak salicylic acid concentration occurs 1 hour (range, 0.5 to 2 hours) after aspirin administration. Salicylic acid is primarily conjugated in the liver to form a number of minor metabolites. Salicylate metabolism is saturable and the total body clearance decreases at higher serum concentrations.

The elimination of acetylsalicylic acid follows first-order kinetics with the dipyridamole and aspirin combination and has a half-life of 0.33 hours. The half-life of salicylic acid is 1.71 hours.

### Contraindications

Hypersensitivity to dipyridamole, aspirin, or any of the other product components.

*Allergy:* Aspirin is contraindicated in patients with a known allergy to NSAIDs and in patients with asthma, rhinitis, and nasal polyps. Aspirin may cause severe urticaria, angioedema, or bronchospasms (asthma).

*Reye syndrome:* Do not use in children or teenagers with viral infections with or without fever. There is a risk of Reye syndrome with concomitant use of aspirin in certain viral illnesses.

### Warnings

*Alcohol:* Counsel patients who consume 3 or more alcoholic drinks every day about the bleeding risks involved with chronic, heavy alcohol use while taking aspirin.

*Coagulation abnormalities:* Even low doses of aspirin can inhibit platelet function leading to an increase in bleeding time. This can adversely affect patients with inherited or acquired bleeding disorders (eg, liver disease, vitamin K deficiency).

*Peptic ulcer disease:* Avoid using aspirin, which can cause gastric mucosal irritation and bleeding in patients with a history of active peptic ulcer disease.

*Renal function impairment:* No changes were observed in the pharmacokinetics of dipyridamole or its glucuronide metabolite with creatinine clearances ranging from approximately 15 mL/min to more than 100 mL/min if data were corrected for differences in age. Avoid aspirin in patients with severe renal failure (glomerular filtration rate less than 10 mL/min).

*Hepatic function impairment:* Elevations of hepatic enzymes and hepatic failure have been reported in association with dipyridamole administration. Dipyridamole can be dosed without restriction as long as there is no evidence of hepatic failure. Avoid aspirin in patients with severe hepatic insufficiency.

*Mutagenesis:* Aspirin induced chromosome aberrations in cultured human fibroblasts.

*Fertility impairment:* Aspirin inhibits ovulation in rats.

*Elderly:* Plasma concentrations (determined as AUC) of dipyridamole in healthy elderly subjects older than 65 years of age were approximately 40% higher than in subjects younger than 55 years of age receiving treatment with the dipyridamole and aspirin combination.

*Pregnancy:* Category B (dipyridamole); Category D (aspirin).

*Lactation:* Dipyridamole and aspirin are excreted in human breast milk in low concentrations.

*Children:* Safety and efficacy of dipyridamole and aspirin combination capsules in pediatric patients have not been studied. Because of the aspirin component, use of this product in the pediatric population is not recommended.

### Precautions

Dipyridamole and aspirin combination is not interchangeable with the individual components of aspirin and dipyridamole tablets.

*Coronary artery disease:* Due to the vasodilatory effect of dipyridamole, use with caution in patients with severe coronary artery disease (eg, unstable angina, recently sustained MI). Chest pain may be aggravated in patients with underlying coronary artery disease who are receiving dipyridamole. For stroke or transient ischemic attack patients for whom aspirin is indicated to prevent recurrent MI or angina pectoris, the aspirin in this product may not provide adequate treatment for the cardiac indications.

*Hypotension:* Dipyridamole can produce peripheral vasodilation; use with caution in patients with hypotension.

*Lab test abnormalities:* Aspirin has been associated with elevated hepatic enzymes, blood urea nitrogen and serum creatinine, hyperkalemia, proteinuria, and prolonged bleeding time. Dipyridamole has been associated with elevated hepatic enzymes.

### Drug Interactions

Drugs that may be affected by dipyridamole are adenosine and cholinesterase inhibitors.

Drugs that may be affected by aspirin include ACE inhibitors, acetazolamide, anticoagulants, anticonvulsants (hydantoins, valproic acid), beta blockers, diuretics, methotrexate, NSAIDs, oral hypoglycemics, and uricosuric agents (probenecid, sulfinpyrazone).

*Drug/Lab test interactions:* Over the course of 24 months, patients treated with dipyridamole and aspirin combination therapy showed a decline (mean change from baseline) in hemoglobin of 0.25 g/dL, hematocrit of 0.75%, and erythrocyte count of $0.13 \times 10^6/\text{mm}^3$.

### Adverse Reactions

Adverse reactions that occurred in at least 3% of patients included the following: headache; abdominal pain; dyspepsia; nausea; vomiting; diarrhea; hemorrhage; arthralgia; pain; fatigue; back pain

# TICLOPIDINE HCl

**Tablets**: 250 mg (Rx)                                              *Ticlid* (Syntex)

---

**Warning:**
Ticlopidine can cause life-threatening hematological adverse reactions, including neutropenia/agranulocytosis and thrombotic thrombocytopenic purpura (TTP).

*Neutropenia/agranulocytosis:* Neutropenia defined as an absolute neutrophil count (ANC) less than 1200 neutrophils/mm$^3$ occurred in 50 of 2048 (2.4%) stroke patients who received ticlopidine in clinical trials. Neutropenia is calculated as follows: ANC = WBC $\times$ % neutrophils. In 17 patients (0.8%) the neutrophil count was less than 450/mm$^3$.

*TTP:* TTP was not seen during clinical trials, but US physicians reported about 100 cases between 1992 and 1997. Based on an estimated patient exposure of 2 to 4 million, and assuming an event reporting rate of 10% (the true rate is not known), the incidence of ticlopidine-associated TTP may be as high as 1 case in every 2000 to 4000 patients exposed (see Warnings).

*Monitoring clinical and hematologic status:* Severe hematological adverse reactions may occur within a few days of initiating therapy. The incidence of TTP peaks after approximately 3 to 4 weeks of therapy and neutropenia peaks at approximately 4 to 6 weeks with both declining thereafter. Only a few cases have arisen after more than 3 months of treatment. Hematological adverse reactions cannot be reliably predicted by any identified demographic or clinical characteristics. During the first 3 months of treatment, hematologically and clinically monitor patients receiving ticlopidine for evidence of neutropenia or TTP. Immediately discontinue ticlopidine if there is any evidence of neutropenia or TTP.

## Indications
*Thrombotic stroke:* To reduce the risk of thrombotic stroke (fatal or nonfatal) in patients who have experienced stroke precursors, and in patients who have had a completed thrombotic stroke.

Because ticlopidine is associated with a risk of life-threatening blood dyscrasias including TTP and neutropenia/agranulocytosis (see Warnings), reserve for patients who are intolerant or allergic to aspirin therapy or who have failed aspirin therapy.

## Administration and Dosage
*Recommended dose:* 250 mg twice daily taken with food.

## Actions
*Pharmacology:* Ticlopidine is a platelet aggregation inhibitor. When taken orally, ticlopidine causes a time and dose-dependent inhibition of both platelet aggregation and release of platelet granule constituents, as well as a prolongation of bleeding time. Ticlopidine interferes with platelet membrane function by inhibiting ADP-induced platelet-fibrinogen binding and subsequent platelet-platelet interactions. The effect on platelet function is irreversible for the life of the platelet.

After discontinuation of ticlopidine, bleeding time and other platelet function tests return to normal within 2 weeks in the majority of patients.

*Pharmacokinetics:* Ticlopidine is rapidly absorbed (more than 80%), with peak plasma levels occurring at approximately 2 hours after dosing, and is extensively metabolized. Administration after meals results in a 20% increase in the area under the plasma concentration-time curve (AUC). Ticlopidine displays nonlinear pharmacokinetics and clearance decreases markedly on repeated dosing.

Ticlopidine binds reversibly (98%) to plasma proteins, mainly to serum albumin and lipoproteins. The binding to albumin and lipoproteins is nonsaturable over a wide concentration range. Ticlopidine also binds to alpha-1 acid glycoprotein; at concentrations attained with the recommended dose, 15% or less in plasma is bound to this protein.

Ticlopidine is metabolized extensively by the liver; only trace amounts of intact drug are detected in the urine. Following an oral dose, 60% is recovered in the urine and 23% in the feces. Approximately, 33% of the dose excreted in the feces is intact ticlopidine, possibly excreted in the bile. Approximately 40% to 50% of the metabolites circulating in plasma are covalently bound to plasma proteins, probably by acylation. Although analysis of urine and plasma indicates 20 metabolites or more, no metabolite that accounts for the activity of ticlopidine has been isolated.

### Contraindications

Hypersensitivity to the drug; presence of hematopoietic disorders such as neutropenia and thrombocytopenia or a history of TTP; presence of a hemostatic disorder or active pathological bleeding; severe liver impairment.

### Warnings

*Neutropenia:* Neutropenia may occur suddenly. Bone-marrow examination typically shows a reduction in myeloid precursors. After withdrawal of ticlopidine, the neutrophil count usually rises to more than $1200/mm^3$ within 1 to 3 weeks.

*Thrombocytopenia:* Rarely, thrombocytopenia may occur in isolation or together with neutropenia. If clinical evaluation and repeat laboratory testing confirm the presence of thrombocytopenia, discontinue the drug.

*TTP:* Clinically, fever might suggest neutropenia or TTP. Weakness, pallor, petechiae or purpura, dark urine (because of blood, bile pigments, or hemoglobin) or jaundice, or neurological changes might also suggest TTP. Have the patient discontinue ticlopidine and contact the physician immediately upon the occurrence of these findings.

*Monitoring* – Monitor patients for neutropenia, thrombocytopenia, and TTP prior to initiating ticlopidine and every 2 weeks through the third month of therapy. If therapy is stopped during this 3-month period, continue to monitor for 2 weeks after discontinuation. More frequent monitoring and monitoring after the first 3 months of therapy are necessary only in patients exhibiting clinical signs or hematological laboratory signs (eg, neutrophil count less than 70% of baseline count, decrease in hematocrit or platelet count).

Laboratory monitoring includes complete blood count, especially the absolute neutrophil count, platelet count, and the appearance of the peripheral smear. Thrombocytopenia induced by ticlopidine is occasionally unrelated to TTP. Further investigate for a diagnosis of TTP with the occurrence of any acute, unexplained reduction in hemoglobin or platelet count. Discontinue ticlopidine if there are laboratory signs of TTP or the neutrophil count is less than $1200/mm^3$.

*Cholesterol elevation:* Ticlopidine therapy causes increased serum cholesterol and triglycerides. Serum total cholesterol levels are increased 8% to 10% within 1 month of therapy and persist at that level. The ratios of lipoprotein subfractions are unchanged.

*Hematological effects:* Rare cases of pancytopenia and TTP, some of which have been fatal, have occurred.

*Anticoagulant drugs:* If a patient is switched from an anticoagulant or fibrinolytic drug to ticlopidine, discontinue the former drug prior to ticlopidine administration.

*Renal function impairment:* There is limited experience in patients with renal impairment. No unexpected problems have been encountered in patients having mild renal impairment, and there is no experience with dosage adjustment in patients with greater degrees of renal impairment. Nevertheless, for renally impaired patients it may be necessary to reduce ticlopidine dosage or discontinue it altogether if hemorrhagic or hematopoietic problems are encountered.

*Hepatic function impairment:* The average plasma concentration in patients with advanced cirrhosis was slightly higher than that seen in older subjects. Because of limited experience in patients with severe hepatic disease, who may have bleeding diatheses, the use of ticlopidine is not recommended.

*Elderly:* Clearance of ticlopidine is somewhat lower in elderly patients and trough levels are increased. No overall differences in safety or efficacy were observed between elderly patients and younger patients, but greater sensitivity of some older individuals cannot be ruled out.

*Pregnancy:* Category B.

*Lactation:* It is not known whether this drug is excreted in human breast milk.

*Children:* Safety and efficacy in patients younger than 18 years of age have not been established.

### Precautions

*Increased bleeding risk:* Use with caution in patients who may be at risk of increased bleeding from trauma, surgery, or pathological conditions. If it is desired to eliminate the antiplatelet effects of ticlopidine prior to elective surgery, discontinue the drug 10 to 14 days prior to surgery. Increased surgical blood loss has occurred in patients undergoing surgery during treatment with ticlopidine.

Prolonged bleeding time is normalized within 2 hours after administration of 20 mg methylprednisolone IV. Platelet transfusions also may be used to reverse the effect of ticlopidine on bleeding. If possible, avoid platelet transfusions because they may accelerate thrombosis in patients with TTP on ticlopidine.

*GI bleeding:* Ticlopidine prolongs template bleeding time. Use with caution in patients who have lesions with a propensity to bleed (such as ulcers). Use drugs that might induce such lesions with caution in patients on ticlopidine.

### Drug Interactions

The dose of drugs metabolized by hepatic microsomal enzymes with low therapeutic ratios, or being given to patients with hepatic impairment, may require adjustment to maintain optimal therapeutic blood levels when starting or stopping concomitant therapy with ticlopidine.

Drugs that may interact include antacids, cimetidine, aspirin, digoxin, phenytoin, and theophylline.

*Drug/Food interactions:* The oral bioavailability of ticlopidine is increased by 20% when taken after a meal. Administration with food is recommended to maximize GI tolerance.

### Adverse Reactions

Adverse reactions were relatively frequent, with more than 50% of patients reporting at least one. Most involved the GI tract. Most adverse effects are mild, but 21% of patients discontinued therapy because of an adverse event, principally diarrhea, rash, nausea, vomiting, GI pain, and neutropenia. Most adverse effects occur early in the course of treatment, but a new onset of adverse effects can occur after several months. Ticlopidine has been associated with a number of bleeding complications such as ecchymosis, epistaxis, hematuria, conjunctival hemorrhage, GI bleeding, posttraumatic bleeding, and perioperative bleeding. The incidence of elevated alkaline phosphatase (more than 2 times upper limit of normal) was 7.6% in ticlopidine patients. The incidence of elevated AST (more than 2 times upper limit of normal) was 3.1% in ticlopidine patients.

# CLOPIDOGREL

| Tablets: 75 mg (*Rx*) | *Plavix* (Bristol-Myers Squibb) |
|---|---|

### Indications

*Recent MI or stroke, or established peripheral arterial disease:* For patients with a history of recent MI, recent stroke, or established peripheral arterial disease, clopidogrel has been shown to reduce the rate of a combined endpoint of new ischemic stroke (fatal or not), new MI (fatal or not), and other vascular death.

*Acute coronary syndrome:* For patients with acute coronary syndrome (unstable angina/ non-Q-wave MI) including patients who are to be managed medically and those who are to be managed with percutaneous coronary intervention (with or without stent) or coronary artery bypass graft (CABG), clopidogrel has been shown to decrease the rate of a combined endpoint of cardiovascular death, MI, or stroke, as well as the rate of a combined endpoint of cardiovascular death, MI, stroke, or refractory ischemia.

### Administration and Dosage

*Recent MI, recent stroke, or established peripheral arterial disease:* The recommended dose of clopidogrel is 75 mg once daily with or without food.

*Acute coronary syndrome:* For patients with acute coronary syndrome (unstable angina/ non-Q-wave MI), initiate clopidogrel with a single 300 mg loading dose and then continue at 75 mg once daily. Initiate and continue aspirin (75 to 325 mg once daily) in combination with clopidogrel.

### Actions

*Pharmacology:* Clopidogrel is a thienopyridine derivative, chemically related to ticlopidine, that inhibits platelet aggregation. It acts by irreversibly modifying the platelet ADP receptor. Consequently, platelets exposed to clopidogrel are affected for the remainder of their lifespan.

Dose-dependent inhibition of platelet aggregation can be seen 2 hours after single oral doses of clopidogrel. Platelet aggregation and bleeding time gradually return to baseline values after treatment is discontinued, generally in about 5 days.

*Pharmacokinetics:*

*Absorption/Distribution* – Clopidogrel absorption is 50% or more and is rapid after oral administration. Bioavailability is unaffected by food. Both the parent compound and the main metabolite bind reversibly in vitro to plasma protein (98% and 94%, respectively).

*Metabolism/Excretion* – Clopidogrel is extensively metabolized by the liver. It undergoes rapid hydrolysis into its carboxylic acid derivative; glucuronidation also occurs.

The elimination half-life of the main circulating metabolite was 8 hours with approximately 50% excreted in the urine and approximately 46% in the feces 5 days after dosing.

### Contraindications

Hypersensitivity to the drug or any component of the product; active pathological bleeding such as peptic ulcer or intracranial hemorrhage.

### Warnings

*Thrombotic thrombocytopenic purpura (TTP):* TTP has been reported rarely following use of clopidogrel, sometimes after a short exposure (less than 2 weeks). It is characterized by thrombocytopenia, microangiopathic hemolytic anemia (schistocytes [fragmented RBCs] seen on peripheral smear), neurological findings, renal dysfunction, and fever.

*Hepatic function impairment:* Experience is limited in patients with severe hepatic disease, who may have bleeding diatheses. Use with caution in this population.

*Pregnancy:* Category B.

*Lactation:* Studies in rats have shown that clopidogrel and its metabolites are excreted in milk. It is not known whether this drug is excreted in human breast milk.

*Children:* Safety and efficacy have not been established.

**Precautions**

*Bleeding risk:* As with other antiplatelet agents, use with caution in patients who may be at risk of increased bleeding from trauma, surgery, or other pathological conditions. If a patient is to undergo elective surgery and an antiplatelet effect is not desired, discontinue clopidogrel 7 days prior to surgery.

*GI bleeding* – Clopidogrel prolongs the bleeding time. Use with caution in patients who have lesions with a propensity to bleed (eg, ulcers). Cautiously use drugs that might increase such lesions (eg, aspirin, other NSAIDs) in patients taking clopidogrel.

**Drug Interactions**

At high concentrations in vitro, clopidogrel inhibits P450 2C9. Accordingly, clopidogrel may interfere with the metabolism of phenytoin, tamoxifen, tolbutamide, warfarin, torsemide, fluvastatin, and many nonsteroidal anti-inflammatory agents, but there are no data with which to predict the magnitude of these interactions. Use caution when any of these drugs is coadministered with clopidogrel.

**Adverse Reactions**

Adverse reactions occurring in at least 3% of patients include flu-like symptoms, chest pain, edema, headache, dizziness, dyspepsia, abdominal pain, diarrhea, nausea, arthralgia, purpura, dyspnea, cough, rhinitis, rash, pruritus, depression, hypercholesteremia.

# ANTICOAGULANTS

Blood coagulation resulting in the formation of a stable fibrin clot involves a cascade of proteolytic reactions involving the interaction of clotting factors, platelets, and tissue materials. Clotting factors (see table) exist in the blood in inactive form and must be converted to an enzymatic or activated form before the next step in the clotting mechanism can be stimulated. Each factor is stimulated in turn until an insoluble fibrin clot is formed.

Two separate pathways, intrinsic and extrinsic, lead to the formation of a fibrin clot. Both pathways must function for hemostasis.

*Intrinsic pathway:* All the protein factors necessary for coagulation are present in circulating blood. Clot formation may take several minutes and is initiated by activation of factor XII.

*Extrinsic pathway:* Coagulation is activated by release of tissue thromboplastin, a factor not found in circulating blood. Clotting occurs in seconds because factor III bypasses the early reactions.

Refer to the next page for the complete coagulation pathway.

Anticoagulants used therapeutically include heparin, warfarin (a coumarin derivative), and anisindione (an indandione derivative).

| Blood Clotting Factors | | |
|---|---|---|
| Factor | Synonym | Vitamin K-dependent |
| I | Fibrinogen | no |
| II | Prothrombin | yes |
| III | Tissue thromboplastin, tissue factor | no |
| IV | Calcium | no |
| V | Labile factor, proaccelerin | no |
| VII | Proconvertin | yes |
| VIII | Antihemophilic factor, AHF | no |
| IX | Christmas factor, plasma thromboplastin component, PTC | yes |
| X | Stuart factor, Stuart-Prower factor | yes |
| XI | Plasma thromboplastin antecedent, PTA | no |
| XII | Hageman factor | no |
| XIII | Fibrin stabilizing factor, FSF | no |
| HMW-K | High molecular weight Kininogen, Fitzgerald factor | no |
| PL | Platelets or phospholipids | no |
| PK | Prekallikrein, Fletcher factor | no |
| Protein C[1] | | yes |
| Protein S[2] | | yes |

[1] Partially responsible for inhibition of the extrinsic pathway. Inactivates factors V and VIII and promotes fibrinolysis. Activity declines following warfarin administration.

[2] A cofactor to accelerate the anticoagulant activity of protein C. Decreased levels occur following warfarin administration.

## COAGULATION PATHWAY

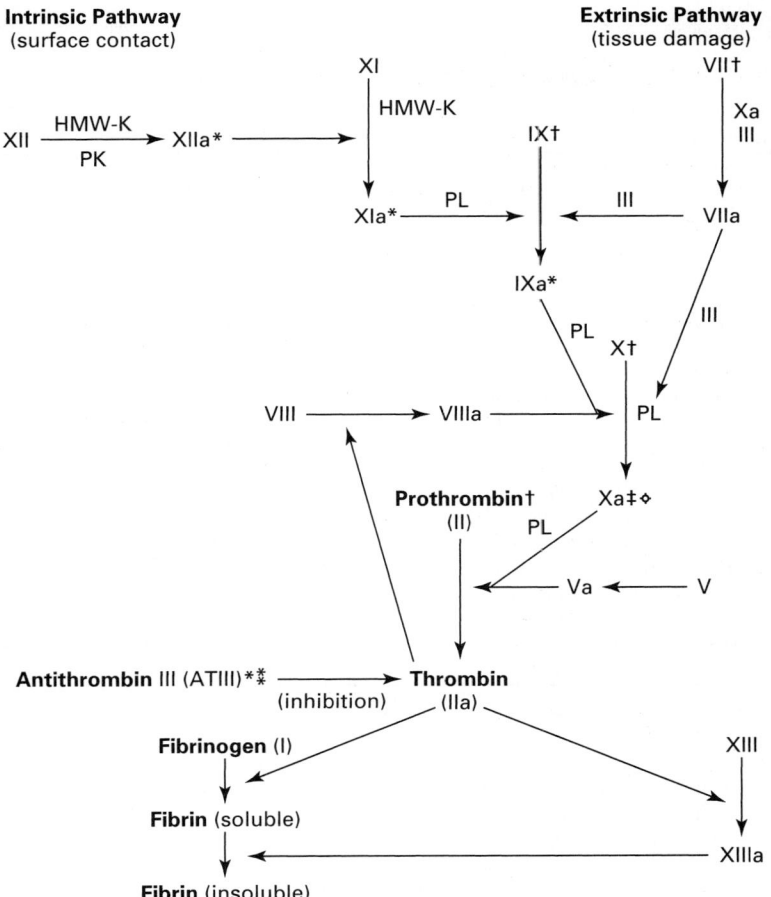

* Major site of activity for unfractionated heparin
† Site of activity for warfarin and anisindione
‡ Major site of activity for fractionated heparin
⁑ Minor site of activity for fractionated heparin
◊ Minor site of activity for unfractionated heparin

## LOW MOLECULAR WEIGHT HEPARINS

**DALTEPARIN SODIUM**

**Injection**[a]: 2,500 units/0.2 mL, 5,000 units/0.2 mL, 7,500 units/0.2 mL, 10,000 units/mL (also multidose), 25,000 units/mL (Rx)

*Fragmin* (Pfizer)

**ENOXAPARIN SODIUM**

**Injection**[b]: 30 mg/0.3 mL, 40 mg/0.4 mL, 60 mg/0.6 mL, 80 mg/0.8 mL, 100 mg/mL, 120 mg/0.8 mL, 150 mg/mL, and 300 mg/3 mL (Rx)

*Lovenox* (Aventis)

**TINZAPARIN SODIUM**

**Injection**[a]: 20,000 units/mL (Rx)

*Innohep* (Pharmion Corp)

[a] Anti-Factor Xa International Units.
[b] Approximate anti-Factor Xa activity of 100 units/1 mg enoxaparin sodium (with reference to the WHO First International Low Molecular Weight Heparin Reference Standard).

> **Warning:**
> When neuraxial anesthesia (epidural/spinal anesthesia) or spinal puncture is employed, patients who are anticoagulated or scheduled to be anticoagulated with low molecular weight heparins (LMWHs) or heparinoids for prevention of thromboembolic complications are at risk of developing an epidural or spinal hematoma, which can result in long-term or permanent paralysis.
>
> The risk of these events is increased by the use of indwelling epidural catheters for administration of analgesia or by the concomitant use of drugs affecting hemostasis, such as nonsteroidal anti-inflammatory drugs (NSAIDs), platelet inhibitors, or other anticoagulants. The risk also appears to be increased by traumatic or repeated epidural or spinal puncture.
>
> Frequently monitor patients for signs and symptoms of neurological impairment. If neurological compromise is noted, urgent treatment is necessary.
>
> The physician should consider the potential benefit versus risk before neuraxial intervention in patients anticoagulated or scheduled to be anticoagulated for thromboprophylaxis.

**Indications**

| LMWHs - Summary of Indications | | | |
|---|---|---|---|
| Indications <br><br> ✔ = labeled | Dalteparin | Enoxaparin | Tinzaparin |
| Prophylaxis of DVT that may lead to PE[a] | | | |
| In patients undergoing abdominal surgery | ✔ | ✔ | — |
| In patients undergoing hip replacement surgery | ✔ | ✔ | — |
| In patients undergoing knee replacement surgery | — | ✔ | — |
| In patients with severely restricted mobility during acute illness | ✔ | ✔ | — |
| Treatment of DVT with or without PE[b] | — | ✔ | ✔ |
| Prophylaxis of ischemic complications in unstable angina and non-Q-wave MI[c] | ✔ | ✔ | — |

[a] In patients at risk for thromboembolic complications.
[b] In conjunction with warfarin therapy.
[c] In conjunction with aspirin therapy.
DVT = Deep vein thrombosis
PE = Pulmonary embolism

### Administration and Dosage

*DALTEPARIN:*

*Administration* – Administer by subcutaneous injection; do not administer IM. Dosage adjustment and routine monitoring of coagulation parameters are not required if the dosage and administration recommendations are followed. Do not mix with other injections or infusions.

*Unstable angina/Non-Q-wave MI* – The recommended dose is 120 units/kg of body weight (but not more than 10,000 units) subcutaneously every 12 hours with concurrent oral aspirin (75 to 165 mg/day) therapy. Concurrent aspirin therapy is recommended except when contraindicated. Continue treatment until the patient is clinically stabilized. The usual duration of treatment is 5 to 8 days.

| Volume of Dalteparin to be Administered by Patient Weight | | | | | | |
|---|---|---|---|---|---|---|
| Patient weight (lb) | < 110 | 110 to 131 | 132 to 153 | 154 to 175 | 176 to 197 | ≥ 198 |
| Patient weight (kg) | < 50 | 50 to 59 | 60 to 69 | 70 to 79 | 80 to 89 | ≥ 90 |
| Volume of dalteparin (mL)[a] | 0.55 | 0.65 | 0.75 | 0.9 | 1 | 1 |

[a] Calculated volume based on the 9.5 mL multiple-dose vial (10,000 anti-Factor Xa units/mL).

*DVT, prophylaxis* –

*Abdominal surgery:* In patients undergoing abdominal surgery with a risk of thromboembolic complications, administer 2,500 units subcutaneously once daily, starting 1 to 2 hours prior to surgery and repeat once daily for 5 to 10 days postoperatively.

*High-risk patients* – In abdominal surgery in patients at high risk for thromboembolic complications (eg, malignancy), administer 5,000 units subcutaneously the evening before surgery and repeat once daily for 5 to 10 days postoperatively. Alternatively, in patients with malignancy, administer 2,500 units subcutaneously 1 to 2 hours prior to surgery with an additional 2,500 unit dose 12 hours later and then 5,000 units once daily for 5 to 10 days postoperatively.

*Hip replacement surgery:* The usual duration of administration is 5 to 10 days after surgery; up to 14 days was well tolerated in controlled clinical trials.

| Dalteparin Subcutaneous Dosing for Patients Undergoing Hip Replacement Surgery | | | | |
|---|---|---|---|---|
| Timing of first dose of dalteparin | 10 to 14 h before surgery | ≤ 2 h before surgery | 4 to 8 h after surgery[a] | Postoperative period[b] |
| Postoperative start | — | — | 2,500 units[c] | 5,000 units every day |
| Preoperative start: day of surgery | — | 2,500 units | 2,500 units[c] | 5,000 units every day |
| Preoperative start: evening before surgery[d] | 5,000 units | — | 5,000 units | 5,000 units every day |

[a] Or later, if hemostasis has not been achieved.

[b] Up to 14 days of treatment were well tolerated in controlled clinical trials, where the usual duration of treatment was 5 to 10 days postoperatively.

[c] Allow a minimum of 6 hours between this dose and the dose to be given on postoperative day 1. Adjust the timing of the dose on postoperative day 1 accordingly.

[d] Allow approximately 24 hours between doses.

*Medical patients during acute illness:* In medical patients with severely restricted mobility during acute illness, the recommended dose is 5,000 units administered by subcutaneous injection once daily. In clinical trials, the usual duration of administration was 12 to 14 days.

*Coagulation parameters:* Dosage adjustment and routine monitoring of coagulation parameters are not required if these dosage and administration recommendations are followed.

*Subcutaneous injection technique* – Administer by deep subcutaneous injection while patient is sitting or lying down. Dalteparin may be injected in a U-shaped area around the navel, the upper outer side of the thigh, or the upper outer quadrangle of the buttock. Vary the injection site daily. When the area around the navel or the thigh is used, use the thumb and forefinger to lift up a fold of skin while giving the injection. Insert the entire length of the needle at a 45- to 90-degree angle.

ENOXAPARIN:

*Administration* – Administer by subcutaneous injection only; do not administer IM. Screen patients prior to prophylactic administration to rule out a bleeding disorder. There is usually no need for daily monitoring of enoxaparin's effect in patients with normal presurgical coagulation parameters.

When using enoxaparin ampules, use a tuberculin syringe or equivalent to assure withdrawal of the appropriate volume of drug. Patients may self-inject only if their physician determines that it is appropriate and with medical follow-up as necessary. Do not mix with other injections or infusions.

*DVT, prophylaxis* –

*Hip or knee replacement surgery:* 30 mg every 12 hours by subcutaneous injection, with the initial dose given within 12 to 24 hours postoperatively provided hemostasis has been established. The average duration of administration is 7 to 10 days; up to 14 days have been well tolerated.

For hip replacement surgery, consider a dose of 40 mg once daily subcutaneously, given initially 9 to 15 hours prior to surgery. Continue prophylaxis for 3 weeks.

*Abdominal surgery:* In adults at risk for thromboembolic complications, administer 40 mg once daily subcutaneously with the initial dose given 2 hours prior to surgery. The usual duration of administration is 7 to 10 days, up to 12 days.

*Medical patients during acute illness:* In medical patients at risk for thromboembolic complications due to severely restricted mobility during acute illness, the recommended dose is 40 mg once daily subcutaneously. The usual duration of administration is 6 to 11 days; up to 14 days have been well tolerated.

*DVT with or without PE* –

*Outpatient treatment:* For patients with acute DVT without PE who can be treated at home, the recommended dose is 1 mg/kg subcutaneously every 12 hours.

*Inpatient treatment:* For patients with acute DVT with PE or patients with acute DVT without PE (who are not candidates for outpatient treatment), the recommended dose is 1 mg/kg subcutaneously every 12 hours or 1.5 mg/kg subcutaneously once daily (same time each day).

*Outpatient and inpatient treatment:* Initiate warfarin therapy when appropriate (usually within 72 hours of enoxaparin). Continue enoxaparin for a minimum of 5 days and until a therapeutic anticoagulant effect has been achieved (INR 2 to 3). The average duration is 7 days; up to 17 days have been well tolerated.

*Unstable angina/Non-Q-wave MI* – In patients with unstable angina or non-Q-wave MI, the recommended dose is 1 mg/kg subcutaneously every 12 hours in conjunction with oral aspirin therapy (100 to 325 mg once daily). Treat with enoxaparin for at least 2 days and continue until clinical stabilization. The usual duration of treatment is 2 to 8 days; up to 12.5 days have been well tolerated. To minimize the risk of bleeding following vascular instrumentation during the treatment of unstable angina, adhere precisely to the intervals recommended between doses. Leave the vascular access sheath for instrumentation in place for 6 to 8 hours following a dose of enoxaparin. Give the next scheduled dose at least 6 to 8 hours after sheath removal. Observe site for signs of bleeding or hematoma formation.

*Subcutaneous injection technique* – To avoid loss of drug, do not expel the air bubble from the syringe before the injection. The use of a tuberculin syringe or equivalent is recommended when using enoxaparin multidose vials to assure withdrawal of the appropriate volume of drug. Administer by deep subcutaneous injection while patients are lying down. Alternate administration between the left and right anterolateral and left and right posterolateral abdominal wall. Introduce the whole length of the needle into a skin fold held between the thumb and forefinger; hold the skin fold throughout the injection. To minimize bruising, do not rub the injection site. Prefilled syringes and graduated prefilled syringes are available with a system that shields the needle after injection.

*Renal function impairment* – Although no dose adjustment is recommended in patients with mild (Ccr 50 to 80 mL/min) and moderate (Ccr 30 to 50 mL/min) renal impairment, observe all such patients carefully for signs and symptoms of bleeding.

The recommended prophylaxis and treatment dosage regimens for patients with severe renal impairment (Ccr less than 30 mL/min) are described in the following table.

| Dosage Regimens for Patients with Severe Renal Impairment (Ccr < 30 mL/min) | |
| --- | --- |
| Indication | Dosage regimen |
| Prophylaxis in abdominal surgery | 30 mg subcutaneously once daily |
| Prophylaxis in hip or knee replacement surgery | 30 mg subcutaneously once daily |
| Prophylaxis in medical patients during acute illness | 30 mg subcutaneously once daily |
| Prophylaxis of ischemic complications of unstable angina and non-Q-wave MI, when concurrently administered with aspirin | 1 mg/kg subcutaneously once daily |
| Inpatient treatment of acute DVT with or without PE, when administered in conjunction with warfarin | 1 mg/kg subcutaneously once daily |
| Outpatient treatment of acute DVT without PE, when administered in conjunction with warfarin | 1 mg/kg subcutaneously once daily |

*TINZAPARIN:* Evaluate all patients for bleeding disorders before administration of tinzaparin.

*Adults* – The recommended dose for the treatment of DVT with or without PE is 175 anti-Xa units/kg of body weight, administered subcutaneously once daily for at least 6 days and until the patient is adequately anticoagulated with warfarin (INR at least 2 for 2 consecutive days). Initiate warfarin sodium therapy when appropriate (usually within 1 to 3 days of tinzaparin initiation).

As tinzaparin may theoretically affect the prothrombin time (PT)/INR, draw blood for PT/INR determination just prior to the next scheduled dose of tinzaparin for patients receiving tinzaparin and warfarin.

The following table provides tinzaparin doses for the treatment of DVT with or without PE. It is necessary to calculate the appropriate tinzaparin dose for patient weights not displayed in the table.

Use an appropriately calibrated syringe to assure withdrawal of the correct volume of drug from tinzaparin vials.

| Tinzaparin Weight-Based Dosing for Treatment of DVT With or Without Symptomatic PE | | | |
| --- | --- | --- | --- |
| | | DVT treatment | |
| | | 175 units/kg subcutaneously once daily 20,000 units/mL | |
| Body weight (lbs) | Body weight (kg) | Dose (units) | Amount (mL) |
| 68 to 80 | 31 to 36 | 6,000 | 0.3 |
| 81 to 94 | 37 to 42 | 7,000 | 0.35 |
| 95 to 107 | 43 to 48 | 8,000 | 0.4 |
| 108 to 118 | 49 to 53 | 9,000 | 0.45 |
| 119 to 131 | 54 to 59 | 10,000 | 0.5 |
| 132 to 144 | 60 to 65 | 11,000 | 0.55 |
| 145 to 155 | 66 to 70 | 12,000 | 0.6 |
| 156 to 168 | 71 to 76 | 13,000 | 0.65 |
| 169 to 182 | 77 to 82 | 14,000 | 0.7 |
| 183 to 195 | 83 to 88 | 15,000 | 0.75 |
| 196 to 206 | 89 to 93 | 16,000 | 0.8 |

| Tinzaparin Weight-Based Dosing for Treatment of DVT With or Without Symptomatic PE | | | |
|---|---|---|---|
| | | DVT treatment | |
| | | 175 units/kg subcutaneously once daily 20,000 units/mL | |
| Body weight (lbs) | Body weight (kg) | Dose (units) | Amount (mL) |
| 207 to 219 | 94 to 99 | 17,000 | 0.85 |
| 220 to 232 | 100 to 105 | 18,000 | 0.9 |
| 233 to 243 | 106 to 110 | 19,000 | 0.95 |
| 244 to 256 | 111 to 116 | 20,000 | 1 |
| 257 to 270 | 117 to 122 | 21,000 | 1.05 |
| 271 to 283 | 123 to 128 | 22,000 | 1.1 |
| 284 to 294 | 129 to 133 | 23,000 | 1.15 |
| 295 to 307 | 134 to 139 | 24,000 | 1.2 |
| 308 to 320 | 140 to 145 | 25,000 | 1.25 |
| 321 to 331 | 146 to 150 | 26,000 | 1.3 |
| 332 to 344 | 151 to 156 | 27,000 | 1.35 |
| 345 to 358 | 157 to 162 | 28,000 | 1.4 |

Use the following equation to calculate the volume (mL) of tinzaparin 175 anti-Xa units/kg subcutaneous dose for treatment of DVT:

Patient weight (kg) $\times$ 0.00875 mL/kg = volume to be given (mL) subcutaneously.

*Administration* – Administer by subcutaneous injection. Do not administer by IM or IV injection. Do not mix tinzaparin with other injections or infusions.

*Subcutaneous injection technique* – Position patients either lying down or sitting, and administer by deep subcutaneous injection. Alternate administration between left and right anterolateral and left and right posterolateral abdominal wall. Vary the injection site daily. Introduce the whole length of the needle into a skin fold held between the thumb and forefinger; hold the skin fold throughout the injection. To minimize bruising, do not rub the injection site after completion of the injection.

### Actions

*Pharmacology:* **Enoxaparin, tinzaparin,** and **dalteparin** are LMWHs. These agents enhance the inhibition of Factor Xa and thrombin by binding to and accelerating antithrombin activity. They preferentially potentiate the inhibition of Factor Xa, while only slightly affecting thrombin and clotting time (activated partial thromboplastin time [APTT] or PT).

*Pharmacokinetics:*

| LMWHs Pharmacokinetics Based on Anti-Xa Activity[a] | | | | | | |
|---|---|---|---|---|---|---|
| LMWH | Max activity (h) | Duration (h) | Bioavailability | $T_{max}$ (h) | Vd | Terminal $t\frac{1}{2}$ (h) |
| Dalteparin | — | — | $\approx$ 87% | 4 | 40 to 60 mL/kg | 3 to 5 |
| Enoxaparin | 3 to 5[b] | 12 (40 mg daily dose) | $\approx$ 100% | 3 to 4.5 | 4.3 L | 4.5 (single dose) 7 (repeated doses) |
| Tinzaparin | — | — | 86.7% | 3.7 (single dose) | 3.1 to 5 L | 3 to 4 |

[a] Information listed without regard to dosage or indication.
[b] Maximum anti-Factor Xa and antithrombin activities.

#### Contraindications

Hypersensitivity to LMWHs, heparin, or pork products; hypersensitivity to sulfites or benzyl alcohol (multidose vials); history of heparin-induced thrombocytopenia (**tinzaparin**); active major bleeding; thrombocytopenia associated with positive in vitro tests for antiplatelet antibody in the presence of a LMWH.

Do not give **dalteparin** to patients undergoing regional anesthesia for unstable angina or non-Q-wave MI because of an increased risk of bleeding associated with the dosage of dalteparin recommended for unstable angina and non-Q-wave MI.

#### Warnings

*Route of administration:* For subcutaneous administration only; do not administer IM or IV.

*Interchangeability with heparin:* LMWHs cannot be used interchangeably (unit for unit) with unfractionated heparin or other LMWHs.

*Spinal/Epidural anesthesia:* As with other anticoagulants, there have been rare cases of neuraxial, spinal, or epidural hematomas reported with the concurrent use of LMWHs and spinal/epidural anesthesia or spinal puncture resulting in long-term or permanent paralysis. The risk of these events may be higher with the use of postoperative indwelling epidural catheters or by the concomitant use of additional drugs affecting hemostasis such as NSAIDs (see Warning Box).

*Hemorrhage:* Use LMWHs, like other anticoagulants, with extreme caution in patients who have an increased risk of hemorrhage, such as those with severe uncontrolled hypertension, bleeding diathesis, diabetic retinopathy, bacterial endocarditis, congenital or acquired bleeding disorders (including hepatic failure and amyloidosis), active ulceration and angiodysplastic GI disease, hemorrhagic stroke, or shortly after brain, spinal, or ophthalmological surgery, or in patients treated concomitantly with platelet inhibitors.

*Thrombocytopenia:* The incidence of thrombocytopenia with platelet counts between 50,000/mm$^3$ and 100,000/mm$^3$ was 1.3% in patients treated with **enoxaparin**, 1% with **tinzaparin**, and less than 1% with **dalteparin**. Severe thrombocytopenia (platelet count below 50,000/mm$^3$) occurred in 0.13% of tinzaparin-treated patients and 0.1% of enoxaparin-treated patients.

*Priapism:* Priapism has been reported from postmarketing surveillance of **tinzaparin** as a rare occurrence. In some cases, surgical intervention was required.

*Renal/Hepatic function impairment:* Delayed elimination of LMWHs may occur with severe liver or kidney insufficiency. Use with caution.

In patients with renal impairment, there is an increase in exposure of **enoxaparin**. Because exposure of enoxaparin is significantly increased in patients with severe renal impairment (Ccr less than 30 mL/min), a dosage adjustment is recommended for therapeutic and prophylactic dosage ranges.

*Elderly:* Delayed elimination of **enoxaparin** and **tinzaparin** may occur.

*Pregnancy:* Category B.

*Lactation:* It is not known whether these drugs are excreted in breast milk.

*Children:* Safety and efficacy have not been established.

#### Precautions

*Monitoring:* Periodic complete blood counts, including platelet count, and stool occult blood tests are recommended during treatment. If platelet count falls below 100,000/mm$^3$, discontinue the LMWH (see Warnings). At recommended prophylaxis doses, routine coagulation tests such as PT and aPTT are relatively insensitive measures of activity and are unsuitable for monitoring. Anti-Factor Xa may be used to monitor the anticoagulant effect in patients with significant renal impairment or if abnormal coagulation parameters or bleeding should occur. Consider monitoring of elderly patients with low body weight (less than 45 kg) and those predisposed to decreased renal function.

*Benzyl alcohol:* The multiple-dose vials of **dalteparin, enoxaparin**, and **tinzaparin** contain benzyl alcohol as a preservative. Benzyl alcohol has been associated with a fatal "gasping syndrome" in premature infants. Because benzyl alcohol may cross the placenta, do not use LMWHs preserved with benzyl alcohol in pregnant women.

*Thromboembolic events:* If thromboembolic events occur despite LMWH prophylaxis, discontinue and initiate appropriate therapy.

*Mechanical prosthetic heart valves:* The use of **enoxaparin** injection has not been adequately studied for thromboprophylaxis or long-term use in patients with mechanical prosthetic heart valves. Isolated cases of prosthetic heart valve thrombosis have been reported in patients with mechanical prosthetic heart valves who have received enoxaparin for thromboprophylaxis. Some of these cases were pregnant women in whom thrombosis led to maternal and fetal deaths. Frequent monitoring of peak and trough anti-Factor Xa levels and dose adjustment may be needed.

*Low-weight patients:* An increase in exposure of **enoxaparin** with prophylactic dosages (less than 45 kg) and low-weight men (less than 57 kg) has been observed. Observe all such patients carefully for signs and symptoms of bleeding.

*Special risk:* Use with care in patients with a bleeding diathesis, uncontrolled arterial hypertension, or a history of recent GI ulceration or bleeding, diabetic retinopathy, hemorrhage, and severe liver or kidney insufficiency.

**Drug Interactions**

*Anticoagulants and platelet inhibitors:* Use LMWHs with care in patients receiving oral anticoagulants or platelet inhibitors (eg, aspirin, salicylates, NSAIDs including ketorolac tromethamine, dipyridamole, sulfinpyrazone, dextran, ticlopidine, clopidogrel) and thrombolytics because of increased risk of bleeding. Unless needed, discontinue agents that may enhance the risk of hemorrhage prior to initiation of **enoxaparin** therapy. Aspirin, unless contraindicated, is recommended in patients treated for unstable angina or non-Q-wave MI.

*Drug/Lab test interactions:* Asymptomatic reversible increases in AST and ALT aminotransferase levels have occurred in patients treated with LMWHs and heparin. Because aminotransferase determinations are important in the differential diagnosis of MI, liver disease, and PE, interpret elevations that might be caused by LMWHs with caution.

**Adverse Reactions**

Adverse reactions associated with LMWHs include anemia, clinically significant bleeding, dyspnea, hematuria, hemorrhage, injection-site hematoma, injection-site hemorrhage, nausea, pain at injection site, peripheral edema, urinary tract infection, and wound hematoma. Approximately 10% of pregnant women receiving **tinzaparin** experienced significant vaginal bleeding.

# HEPARIN

**HEPARIN SODIUM**

| | |
|---|---|
| **Injection:** 1,000, 5,000, 10,000, and 20,000 units/mL (multiple-dose vials) (*Rx*) | Various, *Liquaemin Sodium* (Organon) |
| 1,000, 5,000, 10,000, and 20,000 units/mL (single-dose amps and vials) (*Rx*) | Various, *Liquaemin Sodium Preservative Free* (Organon) |
| 1,000, 2,500, 5,000, 7,500, 10,000, and 20,000 units/mL (unit-dose vials) (*Rx*) | Various |

**HEPARIN SODIUM AND SODIUM CHLORIDE**

| | |
|---|---|
| **Injection:** 1,000 and 2,000 units (*Rx*) | *Heparin Sodium and 0.9% Sodium Chloride* (Clintec) |
| 12,500 and 25,000 units (*Rx*) | *Heparin Sodium and 0.45% Sodium Chloride* (Abbott) |

**HEPARIN SODIUM LOCK FLUSH**

| | |
|---|---|
| **Injection:** 10 and 100 units/mL (*Rx*) | Various, *Hep-Lock* (Elkins-Sinn) |

**Indications**

*Prophylaxis and treatment:* Prophylaxis and treatment of venous thrombosis and its extension; pulmonary embolism; peripheral arterial embolism; atrial fibrillation with embolization.

*Diagnosis and treatment:* Diagnosis and treatment of acute and chronic consumption coagulopathies (disseminated intravascular coagulation [DIC]).

*Postoperative:* Low dose regimen for prevention of postoperative deep venous thrombosis (DVT) and pulmonary embolism in patients undergoing major abdominothoracic surgery or patients who are at risk of developing thromboembolic disease.

According to National Institutes of Health Consensus Development Conference, low-dose heparin is treatment of choice as prophylaxis for DVT and pulmonary embolism in urology patients older than 40 years of age; pregnant patients with prior thromboembolism; stroke patients; those with heart failure, acute MI or pulmonary infection; also recommended as suggested prophylaxis in high-risk surgery patients, moderate and high-risk gynecologic patients without malignancy, neurology patients with extracranial problems, and patients with severe musculoskeletal trauma.

*Prevention:* Prevention of clotting in arterial and heart surgery, blood transfusions, extracorporeal circulation, dialysis procedures, and blood samples for laboratory purposes.

*Unlabeled uses:* As an adjunct in treatment of coronary occlusion with acute MI. Although there is some controversy regarding the efficacy of heparin therapy with concurrent antiplatelet therapy (eg, aspirin) in the prevention of rethrombosis/reocclusion after primary thrombolysis with thrombolytics during acute MI, it is recommended by the American College of Cardiology and the American Heart Association. Generally, administer heparin IV immediately after thrombolytic therapy, usually within 2 to 8 hours (depending on the thrombolytic used), and maintain the infusion for at least 24 hours. Begin aspirin therapy immediately as soon as the patient is admitted, and continue its administration.

**Administration and Dosage**

Give by intermittent IV injection, continuous IV infusion or deep subcutaneous (ie, above the iliac crest of abdominal fat layer) injection. Continuous IV infusion is generally preferable due to the higher incidence of bleeding complications with other routes. Avoid IM injection because of the danger of hematoma formation.

Adjust dosage according to coagulation test results prior to each injection. Dosage is adequate when WBCT is approximately 2.5 to 3 times control value, or when aPTT is 1.5 to 2 times normal.

When given by continuous IV infusion, perform coagulation tests every 4 hours in the early stages. When administered by intermittent IV infusion, perform coagulation tests before each dose during early stages and at appropriate intervals thereafter. After deep subcutaneous injection, perform tests 4 to 6 hours after the injections.

*General heparin dosage guidelines:* Although dosage must be individualized, the following may be used as guidelines:

| Heparin Dosage Guidelines | | |
| --- | --- | --- |
| Method of administration | Frequency | Recommended dose[1] |
| Subcutaneous[2] | Initial dose | 10,000 – 20,000 units[3] |
| | Every 8 hours | 8000 – 10,000 units |
| | Every 12 hours | 15,000 – 20,000 units |
| Intermittent IV | Initial dose | 10,000 units[4] |
| | Every 4 to 6 hours | 5000 – 10,000 units[4] |
| IV Infusion | Continuous | 20,000 – 40,000 units/day[3] |

[1] Based on a 68 kg (150 lb) patient.
[2] Use a concentrated solution.
[3] Immediately preceded by IV loading dose of 5000 units.
[4] Administer undiluted or in 50 to 100 mL 0.9% NaCl.

*Children:* In general, the following dosage schedule may be used as a guideline:

*Initial dose* – 50 units/kg IV bolus.

*Maintenance dose* – 100 units/kg/dose IV drip every 4 hours, or 20,000 units/m²/ 24 hours continuous IV infusion.

*Low-dose prophylaxis of postoperative thromboembolism:* Low-dose heparin prophylaxis, prior to and after surgery, will reduce the incidence of postoperative DVT in the legs and clinical pulmonary embolism. Give 5000 units subcutaneously 2 hours before surgery and 5000 units every 8 to 12 hours thereafter for 7 days or until the patient is fully ambulatory, whichever is longer. Administer by deep subcutaneous injection above the iliac crest or abdominal fat layer, arm, or thigh using a concentrated solution. Use a fine gauge needle (25 to 26 gauge) to minimize tissue trauma. Reserve such prophylaxis for patients older than 40 years of age undergoing major surgery. Exclude patients on oral anticoagulants or drugs that affect platelet function or in patients with bleeding disorders, brain or spinal cord injuries, spinal anesthesia, eye surgery, or potentially sanguineous operations.

If bleeding occurs during or after surgery, discontinue heparin and neutralize with protamine sulfate. If clinical evidence of thromboembolism develops despite low-dose prophylaxis, give full therapeutic doses of anticoagulants until contraindicated. Prior to heparinization, rule out bleeding disorders; perform appropriate coagulation tests just prior to surgery. Coagulation test values should be normal or only slightly elevated at these times.

*Surgery of the heart and blood vessels:* Give an initial dose of not less than 150 units/kg to patients undergoing total body perfusion for open heart surgery. Often, 300 units/kg is used for procedures less than 60 minutes and 400 units/kg is used for procedures more than 60 minutes.

*Extracorporeal dialysis:* Follow equipment manufacturers' operating directions.

*Laboratory samples:* Add 70 to 150 units per 10 to 20 mL sample of whole blood to prevent coagulation of sample.

*Clearing intermittent infusion (heparin lock) sets:* To prevent clot formation in a heparin lock set, inject dilute heparin solution (heparin lock flush solution, USP; or a 10 to 100 units/mL heparin solution) via the injection hub in a quantity sufficient to fill the entire set to the needle tip. Replace this solution each time the heparin lock is used. If the administered drug is incompatible with heparin, flush the entire heparin lock set with sterile water or normal saline before and after the medication is administered; following the second flush, the dilute heparin solution may be reinstilled into the set. Consult the set manufacturer's instructions.

*Converting to oral anticoagulant therapy:* Perform baseline coagulation tests to determine prothrombin activity when heparin activity is too low to affect PT or INR. When the results of the initial prothrombin determinations are known, initiate the oral anticoagulant in the usual amount. Thereafter, perform coagulation tests and prothrombin activity at appropriate intervals. When the prothrombin activity reaches the desired therapeutic range, discontinue heparin and continue oral anticoagulants.

## Actions

*Pharmacology:* Small amounts of heparin in combination with antithrombin III (heparin cofactor) inhibit thrombosis by inactivating factor Xa and inhibiting the conversion of prothrombin to thrombin. Once active thrombosis has developed, larger amounts of heparin can inhibit further coagulation by inactivating thrombin and preventing the conversion of fibrinogen to fibrin. In combination with antithrombin III, heparin inactivates factors IX, X, Xa, XI, XII, and thrombin, inhibiting conversion of fibrinogen to fibrin. The heparin-antithrombin III complex is 100 to 1000 times more potent as an anticoagulant than antithrombin III alone. Heparin also prevents the formation of a stable fibrin clot by inhibiting the activation of factor XIII (the fibrin stabilizing factor). Other effects include the inhibition of thrombin-induced activation of factors V and VIII.

Commercial products contain both low and high molecular weight heparin fractions. Low molecular weight heparin has a greater inhibitory effect on factor Xa, and less antithrombin activity than the high molecular weight fraction.

Heparin inhibits reactions that lead to clotting, but does not significantly alter the concentration of the normal clotting factors of blood. Although clotting time is prolonged by full therapeutic doses, in most cases it is not measurably affected by low doses of heparin. Bleeding time is usually unaffected.

Heparin also enhances lipoprotein lipase release (which clears plasma of circulating lipids), increases circulating free fatty acids, and reduces lipoprotein levels.

*Pharmacokinetics:*

*Absorption/Distribution* – Heparin is not adsorbed from the GI tract. An IV bolus results in immediate anticoagulant effects. The duration of action is dose-dependent. Peak plasma levels of heparin are achieved 2 to 4 hours following subcutaneous use. Once absorbed, heparin is distributed in plasma and is extensively protein bound.

*Metabolism/Excretion* – Following administration, heparin demonstrates a biphasic elimination curve. The lack of relationship between plasma and pharmacologic half-lives may reflect factors such as protein binding. Heparin is rapidly cleared from plasma with an average half-life of 30 to 180 minutes. Half-life is dose-dependent and may be significantly prolonged at higher doses. Heparin is partially metabolized by liver heparinase and the reticuloendothelial system. There may be a secondary site of metabolism in the kidneys. Apparent volume of distribution is 40 to 60 mL/kg. In patients with deep venous thrombosis, plasma clearance is more rapid and half-life is shorter than in patients with pulmonary embolism. Heparin is excreted in urine as unchanged drug (50% or less) particularly after large doses. Some urinary degradation products have anticoagulant activity.

## Contraindications

Hypersensitivity to heparin; severe thrombocytopenia; uncontrolled bleeding (except when it is due to DIC); any patient for whom suitable blood coagulation tests cannot be performed at the appropriate intervals (there is usually no need to monitor coagulation parameters in patients receiving low-dose heparin).

## Warnings

*Hemorrhage:* Hemorrhage can occur at virtually any site in patients receiving heparin. An unexplained fall in hematocrit, fall in blood pressure or any other unexplained symptom should lead to serious consideration of a hemorrhagic event. An overly prolonged coagulation test or bleeding can usually be controlled by withdrawing the drug. Signs and symptoms will vary according to the location and extent of bleeding and may present as paralysis, headache, chest, abdomen, joint or other pain, shortness of breath, difficulty breathing or swallowing, unexplained swelling, or unexplained shock. GI or urinary tract bleeding may indicate an underlying occult lesion. Certain hemorrhagic complications may be difficult to detect.

Use heparin with extreme caution in disease states in which there is increased danger of hemorrhage. These include:

*Cardiovascular* – Subacute bacterial endocarditis; arterial sclerosis; dissecting aneurysm; increased capillary permeability; severe hypertension.

*CNS* – During and immediately following spinal tap, spinal anesthesia, or major surgery, especially of the brain, spinal cord, or eye.

*Hematologic* – Hemophilia; some vascular purpuras; thrombocytopenia.

*GI* – Ulcerative lesions, diverticulitis or ulcerative colitis; continuous tube drainage of the stomach or small intestine.

*Obstetric* – Threatened abortion; menstruation.

*Other* – Liver disease with impaired hemostasis; severe renal disease.

*Hyperlipidemia:* Heparin may increase free fatty acid serum levels by induction of lipoprotein lipase. The catabolism of serum lipoproteins by this enzyme produces lipid fragments that are rapidly processed by the liver. Patients with dysbetalipoproteinemia (type III) are unable to catabolize the lipid fragments, resulting in hyperlipidemia.

*Resistance:* Increased resistance to the drug is frequently encountered in fever, thrombosis, thrombophlebitis, infections with thrombosing tendencies, MI, cancer, and postoperative states.

*Thrombocytopenia:* Thrombocytopenia has occurred in patients receiving heparin. The incidence of heparin-associated thrombocytopenia is higher with bovine than with porcine heparin. The severity also appears to be related to heparin dose.

*Early thrombocytopenia* – Early thrombocytopenia (Type I) develops 2 to 3 days after starting heparin, tends to be mild and is due to a direct action of heparin on platelets.

*Delayed thrombocytopenia* – Delayed thrombocytopenia (Type II) develops 7 to 12 days after either low-dose or full-dose heparin, can have serious consequences and may reflect the presence of an immunoglobulin that induces platelet aggregation.

*Mild thrombocytopenia* – Mild thrombocytopenia may remain stable or reverse even if heparin is continued. However, closely monitor thrombocytopenia of any degree. If a count falls below 100,000/mm$^3$ or if recurrent thrombosis develops, discontinue heparin. If continued heparin therapy is essential, administration of heparin from a different organ source can be reinstituted with caution.

*White clot syndrome* – Rarely, patients may develop new thrombus formation in association with thrombocytopenia resulting from irreversible aggregation of platelets induced by heparin, the so-called "white clot syndrome." The process may lead to severe thromboembolic complications. Monitor platelet counts before and during therapy. If significant thrombocytopenia occurs, immediately terminate heparin and institute other therapeutic measures.

*Hypersensitivity reactions:* Heparin is derived from animal tissue; use with caution in patients with a history of allergy. Before a therapeutic dose is given, a trial dose may be advisable. Have epinephrine 1:1000 immediately available.

*Vasospastic reactions* – Vasospastic reactions may develop 6 to 10 days after starting therapy and last 4 to 6 hours. The affected limb is painful, ischemic, and cyanotic. An artery to this limb may have been recently catheterized. After repeated injections, the reaction may gradually increase to generalized vasospasm with cyanosis, tachypnea, feeling of oppression, and headache. Itching and burning, especially on the plantar side of the feet, is possibly based on a similar allergic vasospastic reaction. Chest pain, elevated blood pressure, arthralgias, or headache also have been reported in the absence of definite peripheral vasospasm.

*Hepatic function impairment:* Heparin half-life may be prolonged in liver disease.

*Elderly:* A higher incidence of bleeding has occurred in women older than 60 years of age.

*Pregnancy:* Category C.

*Lactation:* Heparin is not excreted in breast milk.

*Children:* Safety and efficacy have not been determined in newborns; germinal matrix intraventricular hemorrhage occurs more often in low-birth-weight infants receiving heparin.

Use heparin lock-flush solution with caution in infants with disease states in which there is an increased danger of hemorrhage. The use of the 100 unit/mL concentration is not advised because of bleeding risk, especially in low-birth-weight infants.

### Precautions

*Monitoring:* The most common test used to monitor heparin's effect is aPTT. Other tests used include Activated Coagulation Time (ACT) and Lee White-Whole Blood Clotting Time (WBCT). If the coagulation test is unduly prolonged or if hemorrhage occurs, discontinue the drug promptly. Perform periodic platelet counts, hematocrit and tests for occult blood in stool during the entire course of therapy, regardless of route of administration.

*Hyperkalemia:* Hyperkalemia may develop, probably due to induced hypoaldosteronism. Use with caution in patients with diabetes or renal insufficiency. Monitor patient closely.

### Drug Interactions

Drugs that may interact include cephalosporins, nitroglycerin, penicillins, and salicylates.

*Drug/Lab test interactions:* Significant elevations of aminotransferase (AST and ALT) levels have occurred in a high percentage of patients. Cautiously interpret aminotransferase increases that might be caused by heparin.

If heparin comprises 10% or more of the total volume of a sample for blood gas analysis, errors in measurements of carbon dioxide pressure, bicarbonate concentration, and base excess may occur.

### Adverse Reactions

Adverse reactions associated with heparin include hemorrhage, chills, fever, urticaria, and thrombocytopenia.

## COUMARIN AND INDANDIONE DERIVATIVES

### WARFARIN SODIUM
**Tablets:** 1, 2, 2.5, 3, 4, 5, 6, 7.5, and 10 mg (*Rx*)          Various, *Coumadin* (DuPont)
**Powder for injection, lyophilized:** 5.4 mg (2 mg/mL when reconstituted) (*Rx*)

### Indications

Prophylaxis and/or treatment of venous thrombosis and its extension and pulmonary embolism.

Prophylaxis and/or treatment of the thromboembolic complications associated with atrial fibrillation and/or cardiac valve replacement.

To reduce the risk of death, recurrent MI, and thromboembolic events such as stroke or systemic embolization after MI.

### Administration and Dosage

*Dosage:* Individualize dosage.

*Initial dosage* – The dosing must be individualized according to patient's sensitivity to the drug as indicated by the prothrombin time (PT)/International Normalized Ratio (INR). Adjust dosage based on the patient's PT/INR. Use of a large loading dose may increase the incidence of hemorrhagic and other complications, does not offer more rapid protection against thrombi formation, and is not recommended.

*Maintenance* – Most patients are satisfactorily maintained at a dose of 2 to 10 mg/day. Gauge the individual dose and interval by the patient's prothrombin response. An INR of greater than 4 appears to provide no additional therapeutic benefit in most patients and is associated with a higher risk of bleeding.

*Duration of therapy* – Individualize the duration of therapy. Continue anticoagulant therapy until the danger of thrombosis and embolism has passed.

Recommendations from the American College of Chest Physicians (ACCP) for duration of anticoagulant therapy after venous thromboembolism (VTE) are included in the following table:

| Duration of Anticoagulant Therapy After VTE[1] | |
|---|---|
| 3 to 6 mo | First event with reversible[2] or time-limited risk factor (patient may have underlying Factor V Leiden or prothrombin 20210) |
| ≥ 6 mo | Idiopathic VTE, first event |
| 12 mo to lifetime | First event[3] with<br>Cancer, until resolved<br>Anticardiolipin antibody<br>Antithrombin deficiency<br>Recurrent event, idiopathic or with thrombophilia |

[1] All recommendations are subject to modification by individual characteristics, including patient preference, age, comorbidity, and likelihood of recurrence.
[2] Reversible or time-limited risk factors: Surgery, trauma, immobilization, estrogen use.
[3] Proper duration of therapy is unclear in first event with homozygous Factor V Leiden, homocystinemia, deficiency of protein C or S, or multiple thrombophilias; and in recurrent events with reversible risk factors.

*Missed dose* – The anticoagulant effect of warfarin persists beyond 24 hours. If the patient forgets to take the prescribed dose of warfarin at the scheduled time, the dose should be taken as soon as possible on the same day. The patient should not take the missed dose by doubling the daily dose to make up for missed doses.

*IV route of administration* – Warfarin injection provides an alternative administration route for patients who cannot receive oral drugs. The IV dosages would be the same as those that would be used orally if the patient could take the drug by the oral route. Administer as a slow bolus injection over 1 to 2 minutes into a peripheral vein. It is not recommended for IM administration.

Following are the recommended therapeutic ranges for oral anticoagulant therapy from the ACCP and the National Heart, Lung, and Blood Institute (NHLBI):

| ACCP/NHLBI Recommended Therapeutic Range for Oral Anticoagulant Therapy | | |
|---|---|---|
| Condition | PT Ratio[1] | INR |
| Acute MI[2] | 1.3 to 1.5 | 2 to 3 |
| MI, prevent recurrent | 1.4 to 1.6 | 2.5 to 3.5 |
| Atrial fibrillation[2] | 1.3 to 1.5 | 2 to 3 |
| Mechanical prosthetic valves | 1.4 to 1.6 | 2.5 to 3.5 |
| Bileaflet mechanical valve in aortic position | 1.3 to 1.5 | 2 to 3 |
| Pulmonary embolism, treatment | 1.3 to 1.5 | 2 to 3 |
| Tissue heart valves[2] | 1.3 to 1.5 | 2 to 3 |
| Valvular heart disease[2] | 1.3 to 1.5 | 2 to 3 |
| Venous thrombosis | | |
| Prophylaxis (high-risk surgery) | 1.3 to 1.5 | 2 to 3 |
| Treatment | 1.3 to 1.5 | 2 to 3 |

[1] ISI of 2.4
[2] To prevent systemic embolism

*Management of nontherapeutic INRs:* The following is a suggested approach for treatment of overanticoagulated patients:

| Management of Nontherapeutic INRs | | | |
|---|---|---|---|
| INR | Significant bleeding | Rapid reversal | Intervention |
| < 5 | No | No | Lower or omit a dose; resume therapy at lower dose when INR is in therapeutic range. If the INR is only minimally greater than the therapeutic range, no dose reduction may be required. |

| Management of Nontherapeutic INRs | | | |
|---|---|---|---|
| INR | Significant bleeding | Rapid reversal | Intervention |
| > 5 but < 9 | No | No | Omit next few doses, monitor INR more frequently, resume therapy at lower dose when INR is in therapeutic range. |
| | Yes | No | Omit dose, give 1 to 2.5 mg vitamin $K_1$ PO. |
| | Yes | Yes | Give 2 to 4 mg $K_1$ PO, decrease in INR within 24 h. If INR still high, give additional dose of 1 to 2 mg $K_1$ PO. |
| > 9 to 20 | No | No | Hold warfarin therapy, administer 3 to 5 mg $K_1$ PO; decrease in INR within 24 to 48 h; monitor INR frequently, repeat dose if necessary. Resume therapy at lower dose when INR is in therapeutic range. |
| > 20 | Yes | Yes | Hold warfarin therapy. Give 10 mg $K_1$ slow IV infusion, may repeat dose every 12 h, supplement with plasma or prothrombin complex concentrate (PCC). |
| > 20 and life-threatening | Yes | Yes | Hold warfarin therapy. Give PCC supplemented with 10 mg $K_1$ slow IV. Repeat if necessary. |

*Treatment during dentistry and surgery:* In patients who must be anticoagulated prior to, during or immediately following dental or surgical procedures, adjusting the dosage to maintain the PT at the low end of the therapeutic range (or maintain the corresponding INR value) may safely allow for continued anticoagulation. Limit the operative site to permit effective use of local measures for hemostasis. Under these conditions, dental and surgical procedures may be performed without undue risk of hemorrhage.

*Conversion from heparin therapy:* Because the anticoagulant effect of warfarin is delayed, heparin is preferred initially for rapid anticoagulation. Conversion to warfarin therapy may begin concomitantly with heparin therapy or may be delayed 3 to 6 days. To ensure continuous anticoagulation, it is advisable to continue full dose heparin therapy and that warfarin therapy be overlapped with heparin for 4 to 5 days, until warfarin therapy has produced the desired therapeutic response as determined by PT/INR. When warfarin has produced the desired PT/INR or prothrombin activity, heparin may be discontinued.

### Actions

*Pharmacology:* Anticoagulants interfere with the hepatic synthesis of vitamin K-dependent clotting factors, which results in an in vivo depletion of clotting factors VII, IX, X, and II (prothrombin). Half-lives of these clotting factors are as follows: Factor II, 60 hours; VII, 4 to 6 hours; IX, 24 hours; X, 48 to 72 hours. The half-lives of proteins C and S are approximately 8 and 30 hours, respectively. Hence, the reduction in the rate of synthesis of the clotting factors determines the clinical response. Although factor VII is quickly depleted and an initial prolongation of the

PT is seen in 8 to 12 hours, maximum anticoagulation (thus, antithrombotic effects) is not approached for 3 to 5 days as the other factors are depleted and the drug achieves steady-state.

Warfarin is available as a racemic mixture containing the R(+) and S(−) enantiomers in equal proportions; however, the S-isomer is 3 to 6 times more potent as an anticoagulant than the R-isomer.

*Pharmacokinetics:*

*Absorption* – Warfarin is completely absorbed after oral administration with peak concentration generally attained within the first 4 hours.

*Distribution* – Oral anticoagulants are highly bound to plasma proteins (97% to more than 99%), primarily albumin.

*Metabolism/Excretion* – Warfarin is metabolized by hepatic microsomal enzymes and are excreted primarily in the urine and feces as inactive metabolites.

## Contraindications

Women who are pregnant or may become pregnant (see Warnings); hemorrhagic tendencies or blood dyscrasias; recent or contemplated surgery of the CNS or eye or traumatic surgery resulting in large, open surfaces; bleeding tendencies associated with active ulceration or overt bleeding of the GI, respiratory, or GU tracts; cerebrovascular hemorrhage, aneurysm (cerebral, dissecting aorta), pericarditis and pericardial effusion, or bacterial endocarditis; threatened abortion, eclampsia and preeclampsia; inadequate laboratory facilities; unsupervised patients with senility, alcoholism, or psychosis or other lack of patient cooperation; spinal puncture and other diagnostic or therapeutic procedures with potential for uncontrollable bleeding; major regional, lumbar block anesthesia; malignant hypertension; known hypersensitivity to warfarin or any other components of the product.

## Warnings

*Hemorrhage/Necrosis:* The most serious risks associated with anticoagulant therapy are hemorrhage in any tissue or organ and, less frequently, necrosis or gangrene of skin and other tissues; this has resulted in death or permanent disability. Discontinue therapy when anticoagulants are the suspected cause of developing necrosis; consider heparin therapy.

Hemorrhagic tendency may be manifested by hematuria, skin petechiae, hemorrhage into or from a wound or ulcerating lesion, or petechial and purpuric hemorrhages throughout the body.

Bleeding during anticoagulant therapy does not always correlate with prothrombin activity. Bleeding that occurs when the PT or INR is within the therapeutic range warrants investigation because it may unmask a previously unsuspected lesion (eg, tumor, ulcer).

*"Purple toe syndrome"* – Anticoagulant therapy may enhance the release of atheromatous plaque emboli thereby increasing the risk of complications from systemic cholesterol microembolization including the "purple toe syndrome."

Excessive uterine bleeding may occur, but menstrual flow is usually normal. Women may be at risk of developing ovarian hemorrhage at the time of ovulation.

Oral anticoagulants should not be used in the treatment of acute completed strokes due to the risk of fatal cerebral hemorrhage.

*Adrenal hemorrhage* – Adrenal hemorrhage with resultant acute adrenal insufficiency has occurred.

*Atheroemboli/Microemboli:* Systemic atheroemboli and cholesterol microemboli can present with a variety of signs and symptoms including purple toes syndrome, livedo reticularis, rash, gangrene, abrupt and intense pain in the leg, foot, or toes, foot ulcers, myalgia, penile gangrene, abdominal pain, flank or back pain, hematuria, renal insufficiency, hypertension, cerebral ischemia, spinal cord infarction, pancreatitis, symptoms simulating polyarteritis, or any other sequelae of vascular compromise caused by embolic occlusion. The most commonly involved visceral organs are the kidneys, followed by the pancreas, spleen, and liver. Some cases have progressed to necrosis or death. Discontinuation of warfarin therapy is recommended when such phenomena are observed.

*Heparin-induced thrombocytopenia:* Warfarin should be used with caution in patients with heparin-induced thrombocytopenia and deep venous thrombosis.

*Nonsteroidal anti-inflammatory drugs (NSAIDs)/aspirin:* Observe caution when warfarin is administered concomitantly with NSAIDs, including aspirin, to be certain that no change in anticoagulation dosage is required. In addition to specific drug interactions that might affect PT/INR, NSAIDs, including aspirin, can inhibit platelet aggregation and can cause GI bleeding, peptic ulceration, and/or perforation.

*Special risk patients:* Exercise caution in the presence of any predisposing condition where added risk of hemorrhage, necrosis, and/or gangrene is present, as well as in the following: Severe to moderate hepatic or renal insufficiency; infectious diseases or disturbances of intestinal flora (eg, sprue, antibiotic therapy); trauma that may result in internal bleeding; surgery or trauma resulting in large exposed raw surfaces; indwelling catheters; severe to moderate hypertension; polycythemia vera; vasculitis; severe diabetes; minor and severe allergic/hypersensitivity reactions and anaphylactic reactions.

Patients with CHF may exhibit greater than expected PT/INR response to warfarin.

*Protein C deficiency:* Known or suspected hereditary, familial, or clinical deficiency in protein C has been associated with necrosis following warfarin therapy.

*Elderly:* Older patients may be more sensitive to these agents. Lower doses are recommended.

*Pregnancy:* Category X.

*Lactation:* Warfarin appears in breast milk in an inactive form. Infants nursed by warfarin-treated mothers had no change in PT.

Anisindione and dicumarol or their metabolites may be excreted in breast milk in amounts sufficient to cause a prothrombopenic state and bleeding in the newborn.

*Children:* Safety and efficacy in children younger than 18 years of age have not been established. Oral anticoagulants may be beneficial in children with rare thromboembolic disorder secondary to other disease states such as the nephrotic syndrome or congenital heart lesions. Heparin is probably the initial anticoagulant of choice because of its immediate onset of action.

## Precautions
*Monitoring:*

PT – Treatment is highly individualized. Control dosage by periodic determination of PT or other suitable coagulation tests (eg, INR). Monitor PT daily during the initiation of therapy and whenever any other drug is added to or discontinued from therapy that may alter the patient's response. Concurrent heparin therapy will elevate the PT 10% to 20%; if target PT levels are not increased by the same percentage during concurrent therapy, the patient could be inadequately anticoagulated when the heparin therapy is discontinued. Once stabilized, monitor PT every 4 to 6 weeks.

INR – INR is based on the determination of an International Normalized Ratio that provides a common basis for PT results and interpretations of therapeutic ranges. For a discussion of the relationship between PT and INR in clinical practice, refer to Administration and Dosage.

Conversion from heparin therapy – As heparin may affect the PT/INR, patients receiving both heparin and warfarin should have blood for PT/INR determination drawn at least:

- 5 hours after the last IV bolus dose of heparin, or
- 4 hours after cessation of a continuous IV infusion of heparin, or
- 24 hours after the last subcutaneous heparin injection.

*Enhanced anticoagulant effects:* Endogenous factors that may be responsible for increased PT/INR response include the following: Blood dyscrasias; cancer; collagen vascular disease; CHF; diarrhea; elevated temperature; hepatic disorders (eg, infectious hepatitis, jaundice); hyperthyroidism; poor nutritional state; steatorrhea; vitamin K deficiency.

*Patient selection:* Use care in the selection of patients to ensure cooperation, especially from alcoholic, senile, or psychotic patients.

*Decreased anticoagulant effects:* Endogenous factors that may reduce the response to the oral anticoagulants or decrease the PT or INR include: Edema; hyperlipidemia; hypothyroidism; hereditary resistance to oral anticoagulants; nephrotic syndrome.

**Drug Interactions**

Oral anticoagulants have a great potential for clinically significant drug interactions. Warn all patients about potential hazards and instruct against taking **any** drug, including nonprescription products and herbal medications, without the advice of a physician or pharmacist.

Careful monitoring and appropriate dosage adjustments usually will permit safe administration of combined therapy. Critical times during therapy occur when an interacting drug is added to or discontinued from a patient stabilized on anticoagulants.

Coumarin and indandione derivatives are affected by many drugs. Those that may significantly affect coumarin and indandione derivatives include amiodarone, 17-alkyl androgens, barbiturates, clofibrate, dextrothyroxine, erythromycin, histamine $H_2$ antagonists, metronidazole, miconazole, phenylbutazones, quinine derivatives, salicylates, sulfinpyrazone, sulfonamides, thioamines, thyroid hormones, and vitamin E.

*Drug/Food interactions:* Vitamin K-rich vegetables may decrease the anticoagulant effects of warfarin by interfering with absorption. Minimize consumption of vitamin K-rich foods (eg, spinach, seaweed, broccoli, turnip greens) or nutritional supplements. Mango has been shown to increase warfarin's effect.

**Adverse Reactions**

*Hemorrhage* – Hemorrhage is the principal adverse effect of warfarin.

Other adverse reactions include nausea; diarrhea; pyrexia; dermatitis; exfoliative dermatitis; urticaria; alopecia; sore mouth; mouth ulcers; fever; abdominal cramping; leukopenia; red-orange urine; priapism (causal relationship not established); paralytic ileus and intestinal obstruction from submucosal or intramural hemorrhage.

# LEPIRUDIN

**Powder for injection:** 50 mg (*Rx*)          *Refludan* (Hoechst-Marion Roussel)

**Indications**

*Thrombocytopenia, heparin-induced:* For anticoagulation in patients with heparin-induced thrombocytopenia (HIT) and associated thromboembolic disease in order to prevent further thromboembolic complications.

**Administration and Dosage**

*Initial dosage:* 0.4 mg/kg (110 kg or less) slowly IV (ie, over 15 to 20 seconds) as a bolus dose followed by 0.15 mg/kg (110 kg/h or less) as a continuous IV infusion for 2 to 10 days or longer if clinically needed.

Normally the initial dosage depends on the patient's body weight; this is valid for patients 110 kg or less. In patients with a body weight over 110 kg, the initial dosage should not be increased beyond the 110 kg body weight dose (maximal initial bolus dose of 44 mg, maximal initial infusion dose of 16.5 mg/h).

Determine patient baseline activated partial thromboplastin time (aPTT) prior to initiation of therapy with lepirudin, because lepirudin should not be started in patients presenting with a baseline aPTT ratio of 2.5 or more in order to avoid initial overdosing.

*Monitoring:* Adjust the dosage (infusion rate) according to the aPTT ratio.

The target range for the aPTT ratio during treatment (therapeutic window) should be 1.5 to 2.5.

The first aPTT determination for monitoring treatment should be done 4 hours after start of the lepirudin infusion. Follow-up aPTT determinations are recommended at least once daily, as long as treatment is ongoing.

More frequent aPTT monitoring is highly recommended in patients with renal impairment or serious liver injury or with an increased risk of bleeding.

*Dose modifications:* Any aPTT ratio out of the target range is to be confirmed at once before drawing conclusions with respect to dose modifications, unless there is a clinical need to react immediately.

If the confirmed aPTT ratio is above the target range, stop the infusion for 2 hours. At restart, decrease the infusion rate by 50% (no additional IV bolus should be administered). Determine the aPTT ratio again 4 hours later.

If the confirmed aPTT ratio is below the target range, increase the infusion rate in steps of 20%. Determine the aPTT ratio again 4 hours later.

Do not exceed an infusion rate of 0.21 mg/kg/h without checking for coagulation abnormalities, which might be preventive of an appropriate aPTT response.

*Renal function impairment:* As lepirudin is almost exclusively excreted in the kidneys, consider individual renal function prior to administration. In case of renal impairment, relative overdose might occur even with the standard dosing regimen.
Therefore, the bolus dose and infusion rate must be reduced in case of known or suspected renal insufficiency (Ccr less than 60 mL/min or serum creatinine more than 1.5 mg/dL).

There is only limited information on the therapeutic use of lepirudin in HIT patients with significant renal impairment. The following dosage recommendations are mainly based on single-dose studies in a small number of patients with renal impairment. Therefore, these recommendations are only tentative.

In all patients with renal insufficiency, reduce the bolus dose to 0.2 mg/kg.

The standard initial infusion rate must be reduced according to the recommendations given in the following table. Additional aPTT monitoring is highly recommended.

| Reduction of Lepirudin Infusion Rate in Patients with Renal Impairment | | | |
|---|---|---|---|
| | | Adjusted infusion rate | |
| Ccr (mL/min) | Serum creatinine (mg/dL) | % of standard initial infusion rate | mg/kg/h |
| 45 to 60 | 1.6 to 2 | 50% | 0.075 |
| 30 to 44 | 2.1 to 3 | 30% | 0.045 |
| 15 to 29 | 3.1 to 6 | 15% | 0.0225 |
| < 15[1] | > 6[1] | avoid or stop infusion[1] | |

[1] In hemodialysis patients or in case of acute renal failure (Ccr less than 15 mL/min or serum creatinine more than 6 mg/dL), avoid or stop infusion of lepirudin. Consider additional IV bolus doses of 0.1 mg/kg every other day only if the aPTT ratio falls below the lower therapeutic limit of 1.5.

*Concomitant use with thrombolytic therapy:* Clinical trials in HIT patients have provided only limited information on the combined use of lepirudin and thrombolytic agents. The following dosage regimen of lepirudin was used in 9 HIT patients in the studies who presented with TECs at baseline and were started on both lepirudin and thrombolytic therapy (alteplase, urokinase, or streptokinase).

Pay special attention to the fact that thrombolytic agents per se may increase the aPTT ratio. Therefore, aPTT ratios with a given plasma level of lepirudin are usually higher in patients who receive concomitant thrombolysis than in those who do not.

*Initial IV bolus* – 0.2 mg/kg.
*Continuous IV infusion* – 0.1 mg/kg/h.

*Patients scheduled to switch to oral anticoagulation:* If a patient is scheduled to receive coumarin for oral anticoagulation after lepirudin therapy, the dose of lepirudin should
first be gradually reduced in order to reach an aPTT ratio just above 1.5 before initiating oral anticoagulation. As soon as an international normalized ratio (INR)
of 2 is reached, stop lepirudin therapy.

*Initial IV bolus:* IV injection of the bolus is to be carried out slowly (ie, over 15 to 20 seconds).

| Standard Bolus Injection Volumes of Lepirudin According to Body Weight for a 5 mg/mL Concentration | | |
|---|---|---|
| Body weight (kg) | Injection Volume | |
| | Dosage 0.4 mg/kg | Dosage 0.2 mg/kg[1] |
| 50 | 4 mL | 2 mL |
| 60 | 4.8 mL | 2.4 mL |
| 70 | 5.6 mL | 2.8 mL |
| 80 | 6.4 mL | 3.2 mL |
| 90 | 7.2 mL | 3.6 mL |
| 100 | 8 mL | 4 mL |
| ≥ 110 | 8.8 mL | 4.4 mL |

[1] Dosage recommended for all patients with renal insufficiency.

*IV infusion:* For continuous IV infusion, solutions with concentration of 0.2 or
0.4 mg/mL may be used.

The infusion rate (mL/h) is to be set according to body weight (see following
table).

| Standard Infusion Rates of Lepirudin According to Body Weight | | |
|---|---|---|
| Body weight (kg) | Infusion rate at 0.15 mg/kg/h | |
| | 500 mL infusion bag 0.2 mg/mL | 250 mL infusion bag 0.4 mg/mL |
| 50 | 38 mL/h | 19 mL/h |
| 60 | 45 mL/h | 23 mL/h |
| 70 | 53 mL/h | 26 mL/h |
| 80 | 60 mL/h | 30 mL/h |
| 90 | 68 mL/h | 34 mL/h |
| 100 | 75 mL/h | 38 mL/h |
| ≥ 110 | 83 mL/h | 41 mL/h |

**Actions**

*Pharmacology:* Lepirudin (rDNA), a recombinant hirudin derived from yeast cells, is a
highly specific direct inhibitor of thrombin.

One molecule of lepirudin binds to one molecule of thrombin and thereby blocks
the thrombogenic activity of thrombin. As a result, all thrombin-dependent coagulation assays are affected (eg, aPTT values increase in a dose-dependent fashion).

*Pharmacokinetics:*

*Absorption/Distribution* – Following IV administration, distribution is essentially confined to extracellular fluids and is characterized by an initial half-life of about
10 minutes. Elimination follows a first-order process and is characterized by a terminal half-life of about 1.3 hours in young healthy volunteers. As the IV dose is
increased over the range of 0.1 to 0.4 mg/kg, the maximum plasma concentration
and the AUC increase proportionally.

*Metabolism/Excretion* – Lepirudin is thought to be metabolized by release of amino
acids via catabolic hydrolysis of the parent drug; however, conclusive data are not
available. Approximately 48% of the administered dose is excreted in the urine,
which consists of unchanged drug (35%) and other fragments of the parent drug.

The systemic clearance of lepirudin is proportional to the glomerular filtration rate or creatinine clearance. Dose adjustment based on creatinine clearance is recommended (see Administration and Dosage). In patients with marked renal insufficiency (creatinine clearance less than 15 mL/min) and on hemodialysis, elimination half-lives are prolonged 2 days or less.

*Special populations:* The systemic clearance of lepirudin in women is about 25% lower than in men. In elderly patients, the systemic clearance of lepirudin is 20% lower than in younger patients. This may be explained by the lower creatinine clearance in elderly patients compared with younger patients.

### Contraindications
Hypersensitivity to hirudins.

### Warnings
*Intracranial bleeding:* Following concomitant thrombolytic therapy with alteplase (tPA) or streptokinase may be life-threatening. Carefully assess the risk of lepirudin administration vs its anticipated benefit in patients with increased risk of bleeding. In particular, this includes the following conditions:

- Recent puncture of large vessels or organ biopsy
- Anomaly of vessels or organs
- Recent cerebrovascular accident, stroke, intracerebral surgery, or other neuraxial procedures
- Severe uncontrolled hypertension
- Bacterial endocarditis
- Advanced renal impairment (see Warnings)
- Hemorrhagic diathesis
- Recent major surgery
- Recent major bleeding (eg, intracranial, GI, intraocular, pulmonary)

*Renal function impairment:* With renal impairment, relative overdose might occur even with a standard dosage regimen. In patients with marked renal insufficiency (creatinine clearance less than 15 mL/min) and on hemodialysis, elimination half-lives are prolonged 2 days or less. Reduce the bolus dose and rate of infusion in patients with known or suspected renal insufficiency (see Administration and Dosage).

*Pregnancy: Category* B. Use during pregnancy only if clearly needed.

*Lactation:* It is not known whether lepirudin is excreted in breast milk. Because of the potential for serious adverse reactions in nursing infants, decide whether to discontinue nursing or to discontinue the drug, taking into account the importance of the drug to the mother.

*Children:* Safety and efficacy have not been established.

### Precautions
*Antibodies:* Formation of antihirudin antibodies was observed in approximately 40% of HIT patients treated with lepirudin. This may increase the anticoagulant effect of lepirudin possibly because of delayed renal elimination of active lepirudin-antihirudin complexes. Therefore, strict monitoring of aPTT is necessary also during prolonged therapy. No evidence of neutralization of lepirudin or of allergic reactions associated with positive antibody test results was found.

*Hepatic injury:* Serious liver injury (eg, cirrhosis) may enhance the anticoagulant effect of lepirudin caused by coagulation defects secondary to reduced generation of vitamin K-dependent coagulation factors.

*Reexposure:* There is limited information to support any recommendations for reexposure to lepirudin. Of 13 patients reexposed in 2 studies, one experienced a mild allergic skin reaction during the second treatment cycle.

*Allergic reactions:* Approximately 53% of all allergic reactions or suspected allergic reactions occurred in patients who concomitantly received thrombolytic therapy (eg, streptokinase) for acute MI or contrast media for coronary angiography (see Adverse Reactions).

*Lab test abnormalities:* In general, adjust the dosage (infusion rate) according to the aPTT ratio (patient aPTT at a given time over an aPTT reference value, usually the median of the laboratory normal range for aPTT; see Administration and Dosage). Other thrombin- dependent coagulation assays are affected by lepirudin.

## Drug Interactions

Drugs that may interact with lepirudin and increase the risk of bleeding include thrombolytics (eg, tPA, streptokinase) and coumarin derivatives (vitamin K antagonists).

## Adverse Reactions

Adverse events occurring in at least 3% of patients include the following: Abnormal liver function; allergic skin reactions; anemia or isolated drop in hemoglobin; bleeding from puncture sites and wounds; epistaxis; fever; GI and rectal bleeding; other hematoma and unclassified bleeding; hematuria; multiorgan failure; pneumonia; sepsis.

# ARGATROBAN

**Injection:** 100 mg/mL (*Rx*)                              *Argatroban* (GlaxoSmithKline)

## Indications

*Thrombosis, prophylaxis or treatment:* As an anticoagulant for prophylaxis or treatment of thrombosis in heparin-induced thrombocytopenia (HIT).

*Percutaneous coronary intervention (PCI):* As an anticoagulant in patients with or at risk for HIT undergoing PCI.

## Administration and Dosage

Argatroban, as supplied, is a concentrated drug (100 mg/mL) that must be diluted 100-fold prior to infusion. Do not mix with other drugs prior to dilution.

*Initial dosage in HIT or heparin-induced thrombocytopenia and thrombosis syndrome (HITTS):* Before administering argatroban, discontinue heparin therapy and obtain a baseline activated partial thromboplastin time (aPTT). The recommended initial dose of argatroban for adults without hepatic impairment is 2 mcg/kg/min administered as a continuous infusion (see table).

| Standard Infusion Rates for 2 mcg/kg/min Dose of Argatroban (1 mg/mL Final Concentration) | | |
| --- | --- | --- |
| Body weight (kg) | Dose (mcg/min) | Infusion rate (mL/h) |
| 50 | 100 | 6 |
| 60 | 120 | 7 |
| 70 | 140 | 8 |
| 80 | 160 | 10 |
| 90 | 180 | 11 |
| 100 | 200 | 12 |
| 110 | 220 | 13 |
| 120 | 240 | 14 |
| 130 | 260 | 16 |
| 140 | 280 | 17 |

*Monitoring therapy* – In general, argatroban therapy is monitored using aPTT. Tests of anticoagulant effects (including aPTT) typically attain steady-state levels within 1 to 3 hours following initiation of argatroban. Check the aPTT 2 hours after initiation of therapy to confirm the aPTT is within the desired therapeutic range.

*Dosage adjustment* – After the initial dose of argatroban, the dose can be adjusted as clinically indicated (not to exceed 10 mcg/kg/min), until the steady-state aPTT is 1.5 to 3 times the initial baseline value (not to exceed 100 seconds).

*PCI in HIT/HITTS patients:*

*Initial dosage* – Start an infusion of argatroban at 25 mcg/kg/min and a bolus of 350 mcg/kg administered via a large bore IV line over 3 to 5 minutes. Check activated clotting time (ACT) 5 to 10 minutes after the bolus dose is completed. Proceed with PCI if the ACT is greater than 300 seconds.

*Dosage adjustment* – If the ACT is less than 300 seconds, administer an additional IV bolus dose of 150 mcg/kg, increase the infusion dose to 30 mcg/kg/min, and check the ACT 5 to 10 minutes later. If the ACT is greater than 450 seconds, decrease the infusion rate to 15 mcg/kg/min, and check the ACT 5 to 10 minutes later. Once a therapeutic ACT (between 300 and 450 seconds) has been achieved, continue this infusion dose for the duration of the procedure.

| Recommended Doses and Infusion Rates of Argatroban for Patients Undergoing PCI | | | | | | | | |
|---|---|---|---|---|---|---|---|---|
| | For ACT 300 to 450 seconds: Initial dosage[1] 25 mcg/kg/min | | | If ACT < 300 seconds: Dosage adjustment[2] 30 mcg/kg/min | | | If ACT > 450 seconds: Dosage adjustment 15 mcg/kg/min | |
| Body weight (kg) | Bolus dose (mcg) | Infusion dose (mcg/min) | Infusion rate (mL/h) | Bolus dose (mcg) | Infusion dose (mcg/min) | Infusion rate (mL/h) | Infusion dose (mcg/min) | Infusion rate (mL/h) |
| 50 | 17,500 | 1250 | 75 | 7500 | 1500 | 90 | 750 | 45 |
| 60 | 21,000 | 1500 | 90 | 9000 | 1800 | 108 | 900 | 54 |
| 70 | 24,500 | 1750 | 105 | 10,500 | 2100 | 126 | 1050 | 63 |
| 80 | 28,000 | 2000 | 120 | 12,000 | 2400 | 144 | 1200 | 72 |
| 90 | 31,500 | 2250 | 135 | 13,500 | 2700 | 162 | 1350 | 81 |
| 100 | 35,000 | 2500 | 150 | 15,000 | 3000 | 180 | 1500 | 90 |
| 110 | 38,500 | 2750 | 165 | 16,500 | 3300 | 198 | 1650 | 99 |
| 120 | 42,000 | 3000 | 180 | 18,500 | 3600 | 216 | 1800 | 108 |
| 130 | 45,500 | 3250 | 195 | 19,500 | 3900 | 234 | 1950 | 117 |
| 140 | 49,000 | 3500 | 210 | 21,000 | 4200 | 252 | 2100 | 126 |

[1] Administer initial IV bolus dose of 350 mcg/kg.
[2] Administer additional IV bolus dose of 150 mcg/kg if ACT is less than 300 seconds.

In case of dissection, impending abrupt closure, thrombus formation during the procedure, or inability to achieve or maintain an ACT over 300 seconds, additional bolus doses of 150 mcg/kg may be administered and the infusion dose increased to 40 mcg/kg/min. Check the ACT after each additional bolus or change in the rate of infusion.

*Monitoring therapy* – Argatroban therapy is monitored using ACT. Obtain ACTs before dosing, 5 to 10 minutes after bolus dosing and after change in infusion rate, and at the end of the PCI procedure. Draw additional ACTs about every 20 to 30 minutes during a prolonged procedure.

*Continued anticoagulation after PCI* – If a patient requires anticoagulation after the procedure, argatroban may be continued at a lower infusion dose.

*Hepatically impaired patients:* For patients with moderate hepatic impairment, an initial dose of 0.5 mcg/kg/min is recommended, based on the approximate 4-fold decrease in argatroban clearance relative to those with normal hepatic function. Monitor the aPTT closely and adjust the dosage as clinically indicated.

*Conversion to oral anticoagulant therapy:*

*Initiating oral anticoagulant therapy* – Continue to monitor argatroban using aPTT. Initiate oral anticoagulation therapy (warfarin) only after substantial recovery of platelet counts. Do not use a loading dose of warfarin. Initiate therapy using the expected daily dose of warfarin. To avoid prothrombotic effects and to ensure continuous anticoagulation when initiating warfarin, it is recommended to overlap argatroban and warfarin therapy for 4 or 5 days.

*Coadministration of warfarin and argatroban at doses up to 2 mcg/kg/min* – Use of argatroban with warfarin results in prolongation of INR beyond that produced by warfarin alone. The relationship between INR obtained on combined therapy and INR obtained on warfarin alone is dependent on the dose of argatroban and the thromboplastin reagent used. The INR value on warfarin alone ($INR_w$) can be calculated from the INR value on combination argatroban and warfarin therapy. Please refer to manufacturers product labeling for calculations.

Measure INR daily while argatroban and warfarin are coadministered. In general, with doses of argatroban up to 2 mcg/kg/min, argatroban can be discontinued when the INR is greater than 4 on combined therapy. After argatroban is discontinued, repeat the INR measurement in 4 to 6 hours. If the repeat INR is below the desired therapeutic range, resume the infusion of argatroban and repeat the procedure daily until the desired therapeutic range on warfarin alone is reached.

*Coadministration of warfarin and argatroban at doses greater than 2 mcg/kg/min* – For doses greater than 2 mcg/kg/min, the relationship of INR on warfarin alone to the INR on warfarin plus argatroban is less predictable. In this case, in order to predict the INR on warfarin alone, temporarily reduce the dose of argatroban to a dose of 2 mcg/kg/min. Repeat the INR on argatroban and warfarin 4 to 6 hours after reduction of the argatroban dose and follow the process outlined above for administering argatroban at doses up to 2 mcg/kg/min.

### Actions
*Pharmacology:*

*Mechanism of action* – Argatroban is a synthetic, direct thrombin inhibitor that reversibly binds to the thrombin active site. It inhibits thrombin-catalyzed or induced reactions, including fibrin formation; activation of coagulation factors V, VIII, and XIII; protein C; and platelet aggregation.

Argatroban can inhibit the action of free and clot-associated thrombin. Argatroban does not interact with heparin-induced antibodies.

*Pharmacokinetics:*

*Distribution* – Argatroban has an apparent steady-state volume of distribution is 174 mL/kg. It is 54% bound to human serum proteins.

*Metabolism* – The main route of argatroban metabolism is in the liver by the microsomal cytochrome P450 enzymes CYP3A4/5. Data suggest that CYP3A4/5 mediated metabolism is not an important elimination pathway in vivo.

*Excretion* – Total body clearance is about 5.1 mL/min/kg (0.31 L/h/kg) for infusion doses 40 mcg/kg/min or less. The terminal elimination half-life of argatroban ranges between 39 and 51 minutes. Argatroban is excreted primarily in the feces, presumably through biliary secretion.

*Pharmacokinetic/Pharmacodynamic relationship* – Steady-state levels of drug and anticoagulant effect are typically attained within 1 to 3 hours and are maintained until the infusion is discontinued or the dosage adjusted.

*Effect on INR* – Coadministration of argatroban and warfarin produces a combined effect on the laboratory measurement of the INR. Cotherapy compared with warfarin monotherapy exerts no additional effect on vitamin K dependent factor Xa activity.

The relationship between INR on cotherapy and warfarin alone is dependent on the dose of argatroban and the thromboplastin reagent used. Thromboplastins with higher International Sensitivity Index (ISI) values result in higher INRs on combined therapy of warfarin and argatroban.

### Contraindications
Overt major bleeding; hypersensitivity to this product or any of its components (see Warnings).

### Warnings
Argatroban is intended for IV administration. Discontinue all parenteral anticoagulants before administration of argatroban.

*Hemorrhage:* Hemorrhage can occur at any site in the body in patients receiving argatroban. An unexplained fall in hematocrit or blood pressure, or any other unexplained symptom should lead to consideration of a hemorrhagic event. Use argatroban with extreme caution in disease states and other circumstances in which there is an increased danger of hemorrhage.

*Hepatic function impairment:* Exercise caution when administering argatroban to patients with hepatic disease by starting with a lower dose and carefully titrating until the desired level of anticoagulation is achieved. Also, upon cessation of argatroban infusion in the hepatically impaired patient, full reversal of anticoagulant effects may require more than 4 hours because of decreased clearance and increased elimination half-life of argatroban (see Administration and Dosage).

Avoid use of high doses of argatroban in PCI patients with clinically significant hepatic disease or AST/ALT levels at least 3 times the upper limit of normal.

*Pregnancy:* Category B.

*Lactation:* Discontinue nursing or discontinue the drug.

*Children:* The safety and effectiveness of argatroban in patients less than 18 years of age have not been established.

**Precautions**

*Lab test abnormalities:* Anticoagulation effects associated with argatroban infusion at doses 40 mcg/kg/min or less are well correlated with the aPTT. Although other global clot-based tests including PT, the INR, ACT, and TT are affected by argatroban, the therapeutic ranges for these tests have not been identified for argatroban therapy. Plasma argatroban concentrations also correlate well with anticoagulant effects (see Pharmacology).

**Drug Interactions**

The concomitant use of argatroban and warfarin results in prolongation of the PT and INR beyond that produced by warfarin alone. Alternative approaches for monitoring concurrent argatroban and warfarin therapy are described in Administration and Dosage.

*Heparin:* Heparin is contraindicated in patients with HIT. If argatroban is initiated after cessation of heparin therapy, allow sufficient time for heparin's effect on the aPTT to decrease prior to argatroban therapy.

*Oral anticoagulant agents:* The concomitant use of argatroban and warfarin has resulted in prolongation of the PT and INR.

Concomitant use of argatroban with antiplatelet agents, thrombolytics, and other anticoagulants may increase the risk of bleeding (see Warnings).

**Adverse Reactions**

Adverse reactions occurring in at least 3% of patients include the following: abdominal pain, atrial fibrillation, back pain, bradycardia, cardiac arrest, chest pain, diarrhea, dyspnea, fever, headache, hypotension, infection, MI, nausea, pain, pneumonia, sepsis, urinary tract infection, ventricular tachycardia, vomiting.

*Major hemorrhagic events:* Overall bleeding (5.3%)

*Minor hemorrhagic events:* GI (14.4%); hematuria/GU (11.6%); decreased Hgb, HCT (10.4%); groin (5.4%).

# BIVALIRUDIN

**Powder for injection, lyophilized:** 250 mg (*Rx*)          *Angiomax* (Medicines Co.)

**Indications**

*Unstable angina:* For use as an anticoagulant in patients with unstable angina undergoing percutaneous transluminal coronary angioplasty (PTCA). Bivalirudin is intended for use with aspirin and has been studied only in patients receiving concomitant aspirin.

**Administration and Dosage**

The recommended dosage of bivalirudin is an IV bolus of 1 mg/kg followed by a 4-hour IV infusion at a rate of 2.5 mg/kg/h. After completion of the initial 4-hour infusion, an additional IV infusion of bivalirudin may be initiated at a rate of 0.2 mg/kg/h for 20 hours or less, if needed. Bivalirudin is intended for use with aspirin (300 to 325 mg daily) and has been studied only in patients receiving concomitant aspirin. Initiate treatment with bivalirudin just prior to PTCA. The dose may need to be reduced, and anticoagulation status monitored, in patients with renal impairment.

*Instructions for administration:* Following product preparation, select the infusion rate to be administered from the right-hand column of the table below.

| Bivalirudin Dosing Table | | | |
|---|---|---|---|
| | Using 5 mg/mL concentration | | Using 0.5 mg/mL concentration |
| Weight (kg) | Bolus (1 mg/kg) (mL) | Initial 4-hour infusion (2.5 mg/kg/h) (mL/h) | Subsequent low-rate infusion (0.2 mg/kg/h) (mL/h) |
| 43 to 47 | 9 | 22.5 | 18 |
| 48 to 52 | 10 | 25 | 20 |
| 53 to 57 | 11 | 27.5 | 22 |
| 58 to 62 | 12 | 30 | 24 |
| 63 to 67 | 13 | 32.5 | 26 |
| 68 to 72 | 14 | 35 | 28 |
| 73 to 77 | 15 | 37.5 | 30 |
| 78 to 82 | 16 | 40 | 32 |
| 83 to 87 | 17 | 42.5 | 34 |
| 88 to 92 | 18 | 45 | 36 |
| 93 to 97 | 19 | 47.5 | 38 |
| 98 to 102 | 20 | 50 | 40 |
| 103 to 107 | 21 | 52.5 | 42 |
| 108 to 112 | 22 | 55 | 44 |
| 113 to 117 | 23 | 57.5 | 46 |
| 118 to 122 | 24 | 60 | 48 |
| 123 to 127 | 25 | 62.5 | 50 |
| 128 to 132 | 26 | 65 | 52 |
| 133 to 137 | 27 | 67.5 | 54 |
| 138 to 142 | 28 | 70 | 56 |
| 143 to 147 | 29 | 72.5 | 58 |
| 148 to 152 | 30 | 75 | 60 |

Administer bivalirudin via an IV line. Do not mix other medications with bivalirudin before or during administration. No incompatibilities have been observed with glass bottles or polyvinyl chloride bags and administration sets.

Inspect parenteral drug products visually for particulate matter and discoloration prior to administration. Do not use preparations of bivalirudin containing particulate matter.

### Actions

*Pharmacology:* Bivalirudin directly inhibits thrombin by specifically binding to the catalytic site and to the anion-binding exosite of circulating and clot-bound thrombin. The binding of bivalirudin to thrombin is reversible.

*Pharmacokinetics:* Bivalirudin exhibits linear pharmacokinetics following IV administration to patients undergoing PTCA. In these patients, a mean steady-state bivalirudin concentration of about 12.3 mcg/mL is achieved following an IV bolus of 1 mg/kg and a 4-hour 2.5 mg/kg/h IV infusion. Bivalirudin is cleared from plasma by a combination of renal mechanisms and proteolytic cleavage, with a half-life in patients with normal renal function of 25 minutes. Drug elimination is related to glomerular filtration rate (GFR). Total body clearance is similar for patients with normal renal function and with mild renal impairment (60 to 89 mL/min). Clearance is reduced about 20% in patients with moderate and severe renal impairment and reduced about 80% in dialysis-dependent patients. For patients with renal impairment, monitor the activated clotting time (ACT). Bivalirudin is hemodialyzable. Approximately 25% is cleared by hemodialysis.

Bivalirudin does not bind to plasma proteins (other than thrombin) or to red blood cells.

*Special populations –*

| Bivalirudin Pharmacokinetic Parameters and Dose Adjustments in Renal Impairment | | | |
|---|---|---|---|
| Renal function (GFR, mL/min) | Clearance (mL/min/kg) | Half-life (minutes) | Percent reduction in infusion dose |
| Normal renal function (≥ 90 mL/min) | 3.4 | 25 | 0 |
| Mild renal impairment (60 to 90 mL/min) | 3.4 | 22 | 0 |
| Moderate renal impairment (30 to 59 mL/min) | 2.7 | 34 | 20 |
| Severe renal impairment (10 to 29 mL/min) | 2.8 | 57 | 60 |
| Dialysis-dependent patients (off dialysis) | 1 | 3.5 hours | 90 |

## Contraindications
Active major bleeding; hypersensitivity to bivalirudin or any of its components.

## Warnings
*Immunogenicity/Reexposure:* Among 494 subjects who received bivalirudin in clinical trials and were tested for antibodies, 2 subjects had treatment-emergent positive bivalirudin antibody tests. Neither subject demonstrated clinical evidence of allergic or anaphylactic reactions and repeat testing was not performed. Nine additional patients who had initial positive tests were negative on repeat testing.

*Elderly:* Of the total number of patients in clinical studies of bivalirudin undergoing PTCA, 41% were 65 years of age or older, while 11% were older than 75 years of age. A difference of at least 5% between age groups was observed for heparin-treated but not bivalirudin-treated patients with regard to the percentage of patients with major bleeding events. There were no individual bleeding events that were observed with a difference of at least 5% between treatment groups, although puncture site hemorrhage and catheterization site hematoma were each observed in a higher percentage of patients 65 years of age or older than in patients younger than 65 years of age. This difference between age groups was more pronounced for heparin-treated than bivalirudin-treated patients.

*Pregnancy:* Category B.

*Lactation:* It is not known whether bivalirudin is excreted in breast milk. Exercise caution when bivalirudin is administered to a nursing woman.

*Children:* The safety and efficacy in pediatric patients have not been established.

## Precautions
*Monitoring:* An unexplained fall in blood pressure or hematocrit, or any unexplained symptom, should lead to serious consideration of a hemorrhagic event and cessation of bivalirudin administration.

*Special risk:* Clinical trials have provided limited information for use of bivalirudin in patients with heparin-induced thrombocytopenia/heparin-induced thrombocytopenia-thrombosis syndrome (HIT/HITTS) undergoing PTCA. Bivalirudin was administered to a small number of patients with a history of HIT/HITTS or active HIT/HITTS and undergoing PTCA in an uncontrolled, open-label study and in an emergency treatment program and appeared to provide adequate anticoagulation in these patients.

## Drug Interactions
The safety and efficacy of bivalirudin have not been established when used in conjunction with platelet inhibitors other than aspirin, such as glycoprotein IIb/IIIa inhibitors.

Drug interaction studies have been conducted with the adenosine diphosphate (ADP) antagonist ticlopidine and the glycoprotein IIb/IIIa inhibitor abciximab and with low molecular weight heparin. Although data are limited, the results do not suggest pharmacodynamic interactions. In patients treated with low molecular weight heparin, low molecular weight heparin was discontinued at least 8 hours prior to the procedure and administration of bivalirudin.

In clinical trials in patients undergoing PTCA, coadministration of bivalirudin with heparin, warfarin, or thrombolytics was associated with increased risks of major bleeding events compared with patients not receiving these concomitant medications. There is no experience with coadministration of bivalirudin and plasma expanders such as dextran. Use bivalirudin with caution in patients with disease states associated with an increased risk of bleeding.

**Adverse Reactions**

The most frequent adverse reactions reported were back pain, pain, nausea, headache, and hypotension. Percent of patients with major hemorrhage was 3.7%.

| Adverse Events Other Than Bleeding Occurring in ≥ 5% of Patients in Either Treatment Group in Randomized Clinical Trials | | |
|---|---|---|
| | Treatment group | |
| Adverse reaction | Bivalirudin (n = 2161) | Heparin (n = 2151) |
| *Cardiovascular* | | |
| Hypotension | 12 | 17 |
| Hypertension | 6 | 5 |
| Bradycardia | 5 | 8 |
| *CNS* | | |
| Headache | 12 | 10 |
| Insomnia | 7 | 6 |
| Anxiety | 6 | 7 |
| Nervousness | 5 | 4 |
| *GI* | | |
| Nausea | 15 | 16 |
| Vomiting | 6 | 8 |
| Abdominal pain | 5 | 5 |
| Dyspepsia | 5 | 5 |
| *Miscellaneous* | | |
| Back pain | 42 | 44 |
| Pain | 15 | 17 |
| Injection site pain | 8 | 13 |
| Pelvic pain | 6 | 8 |
| Fever | 5 | 5 |
| Urinary retention | 4 | 5 |

# FONDAPARINUX SODIUM

| | |
|---|---|
| Injection: 2.5 mg (*Rx*) | *Arixtra* (Organon/Sanofi-Synthelabo) |

**Warning:**

*Spinal/Epidural hematomas:* When neuraxial anesthesia (epidural/spinal anesthesia) or spinal puncture is employed, patients anticoagulated or scheduled to be anti-coagulated with low molecular weight heparins (LMWHs), heparinoids, or fondaparinux for prevention of thromboembolic complications are at risk of developing an epidural or spinal hematoma that can result in long-term or per-manent paralysis.

The risk of these events is increased by the use of indwelling epidural cath-eters for administration of analgesia or by the concomitant use of drugs affect-ing hemostasis, such as NSAIDs, platelet inhibitors, or other anticoagulants. The risk also appears to be increased by traumatic or repeated epidural or spinal puncture.

Frequently monitor patients for signs and symptoms of neurological impair-ment. If neurologic compromise is noted, urgent treatment is necessary.

Consider the potential benefit vs risk before neuraxial intervention in patients anticoagulated or to be anticoagulated for thromboprophylaxis (see Warnings, Precautions).

## Indications

*Prophylaxis of deep vein thrombosis:* For the prophylaxis of deep vein thrombosis, which may lead to pulmonary embolism in patients undergoing the following: hip fracture sur-gery; hip replacement surgery; or knee replacement surgery.

## Administration and Dosage

*Administration:* Administer by subcutaneous injection. Do not administer by IM injec-tion.

*Dosage:* In patients undergoing hip fracture surgery, hip replacement surgery, or knee replacement surgery, the recommended dose is 2.5 mg subcutaneously once daily. After hemostasis has been established, give the initial dose 6 to 8 hours after sur-gery. Administration before 6 hours after surgery has been associated with an increased risk of major bleeding. The usual duration of administration is 5 to 9 days, and up to 11 days of administration has been tolerated.

*Admixture incompatibilities:* Do not mix fondaparinux with other injections or infusions.

## Actions

*Pharmacology:* The antithrombotic activity is the result of antithrombin III (ATIII)-mediated selective inhibition of Factor Xa. Neutralization of Factor Xa interrupts the blood coagulation cascade and thus inhibits thrombin formation and thrombus development.

Fondaparinux does not inactivate thrombin (activated Factor II) and has no known effect on platelet function, fibrinolytic activity, or bleeding time.

*Pharmacokinetics:*

*Absorption* – Subcutaneous injection is rapidly and completely absorbed (absolute bioavailability is 100%). In patients undergoing treatment with 2.5 mg fondaparinux injection once daily, the peak steady-state plasma concentration is, on average, 0.39 to 0.5 mg/L and is reached approximately 3 hours postdose.

*Distribution* – IV or subcutaneous administration distributes mainly in blood and only to a minor extent in extravascular fluid. Apparent volume of distribution is 7 to 11 L.

*Metabolism/Excretion* – The majority of the administered dose is eliminated unchanged in urine in individuals with normal kidney function. In healthy indi-viduals up to 75 years of age, up to 77% of a single subcutaneous or IV fondaparinux dose is eliminated in urine as unchanged drug in 72 hours. The elimination half-life is 17 to 21 hours.

*Special populations –*

*Renal function impairment:* Elimination is prolonged in patients with renal impairment because the major route of elimination is urinary excretion of unchanged drug. In patients undergoing elective hip surgery or hip fracture surgery, the total clearance is approximately 25% lower in mild renal impairment (Ccr 50 to 80 mL/min), approximately 40% lower in moderate renal impairment (Ccr 30 to 50 mL/min), and approximately 55% lower in severe renal impairment (Ccr less than 30 mL/min) compared with patients with normal renal function.

*Elderly:* Elimination is prolonged in patients over 75 years of age. In studies evaluating 2.5 mg fondaparinux in hip fracture surgery or elective hip surgery, the total clearance of fondaparinux was approximately 25% lower in patients over 75 years of age as compared with patients less than 65 years of age.

*Patients weighing less than 50 kg:* Total clearance is decreased by approximately 30% in patients weighing less than 50 kg.

## Contraindications

Severe renal impairment (Ccr less than 30 mL/min); body weight less than 50 kg; active major bleeding; bacterial endocarditis; thrombocytopenia associated with a positive in vitro test for antiplatelet antibody in the presence of fondaparinux; known hypersensitivity to fondaparinux.

## Warnings

*Injection:* Not intended for IM injection.

*Interchangeability:* Do not use interchangeably (unit for unit) with heparin, LMWHs, or heparinoids, as they differ in manufacturing process, anti-Xa and anti-IIa activity, units, and dosage.

*Hemorrhage:* Use with extreme caution in conditions with increased risk of hemorrhage (eg, congenital or acquired bleeding disorders, active ulcerative and angiodysplastic GI disease), hemorrhagic stroke, or shortly after brain, spinal, or ophthalmological surgery, in patients treated concomitantly with platelet inhibitors.

*Spinal/Epidural hematomas:* See Warning Box.

*Thrombocytopenia:* Moderate thrombocytopenia (platelet counts between 100,000/mm$^3$ and 50,000/mm$^3$) occurred at a rate of 2.9% in patients given 2.5 mg fondaparinux in clinical trials. Severe thrombocytopenia (platelet counts less than 50,000/mm$^3$) occurred at a rate of 0.2% in patients given 2.5 mg fondaparinux in clinical trials.

Closely monitor thrombocytopenia of any degree. Discontinue if the platelet count falls below 100,000/mm$^3$.

*Renal function impairment:* The risk of hemorrhage increases with increasing renal impairment. Therefore, fondaparinux is contraindicated in patients with severe renal impairment (Ccr less than 30 mL/min). Use with caution in patients with moderate renal impairment (Ccr 30 to 50 mL/min).

Periodically assess renal function. Immediately discontinue in severe renal impairment or labile renal function. After discontinuation, its anticoagulant effects may persist for 2 to 4 days in patients with normal renal function and longer in patients with renal impairment.

*Elderly:* The risk of fondaparinux-associated major bleeding increased with age. Careful attention to dosing directions and concomitant medications (especially antiplatelet medication) is advised.

Fondaparinux is substantially excreted by the kidney, and the risk of toxic reactions to fondaparinux may be greater in patients with impaired renal function. Because elderly patients are more likely to have decreased renal function, it may be useful to monitor renal function.

*Pregnancy:* Category B.

*Lactation:* It is not known whether this drug is excreted in human milk. Exercise caution when administered to a nursing mother.

*Children:* Safety and efficacy of fondaparinux in pediatric patients have not been established.

### Precautions

*Monitoring:* Periodic routine CBCs (including platelet count), serum creatinine level, and stool occult blood tests are recommended during the course of treatment.

When administered at the recommended prophylaxis dose, routine coagulation tests such as prothrombin time (PT) and activated partial thromboplastin time (aPTT) are not necessary.

The anti-Factor Xa activity of fondaparinux can be measured by anti-Xa assay using the appropriate calibrator. Because the international standards of heparin or LMWH are not appropriate calibrators, the activity of fondaparinux is expressed in milligrams of the fondaparinux and cannot be compared with activities of heparin or LMWHs.

If during fondaparinux therapy unexpected changes in coagulation parameters or major bleeding occurs, discontinue fondaparinux.

*Heparin-induced thrombocytopenia:* Use fondaparinux with caution in patients with a history of heparin-induced thrombocytopenia.

*Special populations:* Use fondaparinux with care in patients with a bleeding diathesis, uncontrolled arterial hypertension, or a history of recent GI ulceration, diabetic retinopathy, and hemorrhage.

### Drug Interactions

Discontinue agents that may enhance the risk of hemorrhage prior to initiation of fondaparinux therapy. If coadministration is essential, close monitoring may be appropriate. Coumarin may be affected by fondaparinux.

### Adverse Reactions

Adverse reactions occurring in 3% or more of patients include insomnia, dizziness, confusion, rash, bullous eruption, nausea, constipation, vomiting, urinary tract infection, anemia, purpura, fever, edema, increased wound drainage, hypokalemia, hypotension.

*Hematologic:* The most common adverse reactions were bleeding complications. In knee replacement surgery, major bleeding was significantly greater in fondaparinux-treated patients than enoxaparin-treated patients. In clinical trials, major bleeding was defined as clinically overt bleeding that was (1) fatal, (2) bleeding at critical site (eg, intracranial, retroperitoneal, intraocular, pericardial, spinal, or into adrenal gland), (3) associated with reoperation at operative site, or (4) with a bleeding index (BI) of 2 or greater. BI of 2 or greater: Overt bleeding associated only with a bleeding index of 2 or greater. (Calculated as number of whole blood or packed red blood cells transfused + [(prebleeding) − (postbleeding)] hemoglobin [g/dL] values.)

*Lab test abnormalities:* Asymptomatic increases in AST and ALT levels greater than 3 times the upper limit of normal of the laboratory reference range have been reported. Such elevations are fully reversible and are rarely associated with increases in bilirubin.

Because aminotransferase determinations are important in the differential diagnosis of MI, liver disease, and pulmonary emboli, interpret with caution elevations that might be caused by drugs like fondaparinux.

*Local:* Mild local irritation (eg, injection-site bleeding, rash, pruritus) may occur following subcutaneous injection.

# Chapter 3

# ENDOCRINE AND METABOLIC AGENTS

# ESTROGENS

**ESTRADIOL TOPICAL EMULSION**
**Topical emulsion**: 2.5 mg estradiol hemihydrate/g (*Rx*) — *Estrasorb* (Novavax)

**TOPICAL ESTROGENS, MISCELLANEOUS**
**Gel**: 0.06% estradiol (0.75 mg estradiol/1.25 g unit dose) (*Rx*) — *Estrogel* (Unimed)

**ESTRADIOL TRANSDERMAL SYSTEM**

| | |
|---|---|
| **Transdermal patch**: 0.014 mg per 24 hours (*Rx*) | *Menostar* (Berlex) |
| 0.025 mg per 24 hours (*Rx*) | *Alora* (Watson), *Climara* (Berlex), *Esclim* (Women First Healthcare), *Vivelle-Dot* (Novartis) |
| 0.0375 mg per 24 hours (*Rx*) | *Esclim* (Women First Healthcare), *Climara* (Berlex), *Vivelle*, *Vivelle-Dot* (Novartis) |
| 0.05 and 0.1 mg per 24 hours (*Rx*) | *Estradiol Transdermal System* (Mylan), *Alora* (Watson), *Climara* (Berlex), *Esclim* (Women First Healthcare), *Estraderm*, *Vivelle*, *Vivelle-Dot* (Novartis) |
| 0.06 mg per 24 hours (*Rx*) | *Climara* (Berlex) |
| 0.075 mg per 24 hours (*Rx*) | *Alora* (Watson), *Climara* (Berlex), *Esclim* (Women First Healthcare), *Vivelle*, *Vivelle-Dot* (Novartis) |

**ESTRADIOL, ORAL**

| | |
|---|---|
| **Tablets**: 0.5, 1, and 2 mg micronized estradiol (*Rx*) | Various, *Estrace* (Warner Chilcott), *Gynodiol* (Fielding) |
| 1.5 mg micronized estradiol (*Rx*) | *Gynodiol* (Fielding) |

**ESTRADIOL VALERATE IN OIL**
**Injection**: 10, 20, and 40 mg/mL (*Rx*) — *Delestrogen* (Monarch)

**CONJUGATED ESTROGENS, ORAL**
**Tablets**: 0.3, 0.45, 0.625, 0.9, and 1.25 mg (*Rx*) — *Premarin* (Wyeth-Ayerst)

**CONJUGATED ESTROGENS, PARENTERAL**
**Injection**: 25 mg (*Rx*) — *Premarin Intravenous* (Wyeth-Ayerst)

**ESTERIFIED ESTROGENS**
**Tablets**: 0.3, 0.625, 1.25, and 2.5 mg (*Rx*) — *Menest* (Monarch)

**ESTROPIPATE**

| | |
|---|---|
| **Tablets**: 0.75 and 1.5 mg estropipate (*Rx*) | Various, *Ogen* (Pharmacia), *Ortho-Est* (Women First Healthcare) |
| 3 mg estropipate (*Rx*) | Various, *Ogen* (Pharmacia) |
| 6 mg estropipate (*Rx*) | Various |

**SYNTHETIC CONJUGATED ESTROGENS, A**
**Tablets**: 0.3, 0.625, 0.9, 1.25 mg (*Rx*) — *Cenestin* (Duramed)

**SYNTHETIC CONJUGATED ESTROGENS, B**
**Tablets**: 0.625 and 1.25 mg (*Rx*) — *Enjuvia* (Duramed)

**ESTRADIOL CYPIONATE IN OIL**
**Injection**: 5 mg/mL (*Rx*) — *Depo-Estradiol* (Pharmacia)

**Warning:**

*Endometrial carcinoma in postmenopausal women:* Studies have shown an increased risk of endometrial cancer in postmenopausal women exposed to exogenous estrogens for more than 1 year. The risk of endometrial cancer in estrogen users was 4.5 to 13.9 times greater than in nonusers and appears to depend on duration of treatment and dose. Therefore, when estrogens are used for the treatment of menopausal symptoms, use the lowest dose and discontinue medication as soon as possible. When prolonged treatment is indicated, reassess the patient at least semiannually by endometrial sampling to determine the need for continued therapy.

Close clinical surveillance of women taking estrogens is important. Undertake adequate diagnostic measures, including endometrial sampling when indicated, to rule out malignancy in all cases of undiagnosed persistent or recurring abnormal vaginal bleeding.

There is no evidence that natural estrogens are more or less hazardous than synthetic estrogens at equiestrogenic doses.

*Pregnancy:* Do not use estrogens during pregnancy. Estrogen therapy during pregnancy is associated with an increased risk of congenital defects in the reproductive organs of the fetus and possibly other birth defects. Studies of women who received diethylstilbestrol (DES) during pregnancy have shown that female offspring have an increased risk of vaginal adenosis, squamous cell dysplasia of the uterine cervix, and clear cell vaginal cancer later in life; male offspring have an increased risk of urogenital abnormalities and possibly testicular cancer later in life.

There is no indication for estrogen therapy during pregnancy or during the immediate postpartum period. Estrogens are ineffective for the prevention or treatment of threatened or habitual abortion. Estrogens are not indicated for the prevention of postpartum breast engorgement.

If estrogens are used during pregnancy, or if the patient becomes pregnant while taking estrogens, inform her of the potential risks to the fetus.

*Cardiovascular and other risks:* Do not use estrogens with or without progestins for the prevention of cardiovascular disease.

The Women's Health Initiative (WHI) reported increased risks of MI, stroke, invasive breast cancer, pulmonary emboli (PE), and deep vein thrombosis (DVT) in postmenopausal women during 5 years of treatment with conjugated equine estrogens (0.625 mg) combined with medroxyprogesterone acetate (2.5 mg) relative to placebo. Other doses of conjugated estrogens and medroxyprogesterone acetate and other combinations of estrogens and progestins were not studied in the WHI and, in the absence of comparable data, these risks should be assumed to be similar. Because of these risks, prescribe estrogens with or without progestins at the lowest effective doses and for the shortest duration consistent with treatment goals and risks for the individual woman.

The Women's Health Initiative Memory Study (WHIMS), a substudy of WHI, reported increased risk of developing probable dementia in postmenopausal women 65 years of age or older during 4 years of treatment with conjugated estrogens plus medroxyprogesterone acetate relative to placebo. It is unknown whether this finding applies to younger postmenopausal women or to women taking estrogen alone therapy.

**Indications**

Estrogens are most commonly used as a component of combination contraceptives or as hormone replacement therapy in postmenopausal women. Benefits in postmenopausal women include relief of moderate to severe vasomotor symptoms and decreased risk of osteoporosis. Hormone replacement therapy also may be used in vaginal and vulvar atrophy and in hypoestrogenism caused by hypogonadism, castration, or primary ovarian failure. Less commonly, select breast or prostate cancer patients with advanced disease may receive estrogens as palliative therapy. Refer to individual agents for specific indications.

### Administration and Dosage

*Moderate to severe vasomotor symptoms and/or moderate to severe symptoms of vulvar and vaginal atrophy associated with menopause:* Start at the lowest dose and discontinue as soon as possible. Make attempts to discontinue or taper medication at 3- to 6-month intervals. Therapy may be given continuously with no interruption in therapy or in cyclical regimens (eg, 25 days on drug followed by 5 days off drug) as is medically appropriate on an individualized basis.

*Hypoestrogenism caused by hypogonadism, castration, or primary ovarian failure:* Therapy usually is given cyclically (eg, 3 weeks on and 1 week off). Adjust dose depending on severity of symptoms and patient responsiveness.

*Osteoporosis prevention:* Therapy may be given continuously with no interruption in therapy or in cyclical regimens (eg, 25 days on followed by 5 days off) as is medically appropriate on an individualized basis. Discontinuation of therapy may reestablish the natural rate of bone loss.

*Prostate cancer (advanced androgen-dependent):* For palliation only. Judge efficacy of therapy by phosphatase determinations and symptomatic improvement.

*Breast cancer (metastatic):* For palliation only. Therapy usually is given for at least 3 months.

*Concomitant progestin therapy when a woman has not had a hysterectomy:* Addition of a progestin for 10 or more days of a cycle of estrogen has lowered the incidence of endometrial hyperplasia.

*ESTRADIOL TOPICAL EMULSION:*

*Moderate to severe vasomotor symptoms associated with menopause* – Use the lowest effective dose and for the shortest duration consistent with treatment goals and risks for the individual women. Periodically reevaluate patients as clinically appropriate (eg, at 3-month to 6-month intervals) to determine if treatment is still necessary. The single approved dose of estradiol topical emulsion is 3.48 g/day. The lowest effective dose for this indication has not been determined.

*Application* – Instructions for daily application of two 1.74 g foil-laminated pouches:

1.) Apply in a comfortable sitting position to clean, dry skin on both legs each morning. Open each pouch individually.

2.) Cut or tear the first pouch at the notches indicated near the top of the pouch.

3.) Apply the emulsion in the pouch to the top of the left thigh, being careful to push the entire contents from the bottom through the neck of the pouch.

4.) Using 1 or both hands, rub the emulsion into the entire left thigh and left calf for 3 minutes until thoroughly absorbed. Rub any excess material remaining on both hands on the buttocks.

5.) Cut or tear the second pouch at the notches indicated near the top of the pouch. Apply the emulsion in the pouch to the top of the right thigh, being careful to push the entire contents from the bottom through the neck of the pouch. Using 1 or both hands, rub the emulsion into the entire right thigh and right calf for 3 minutes until thoroughly absorbed. Rub any excess material remaining on both hands on the buttocks. Absorption was not studied on other parts of the body.

6.) Allow the application areas to dry completely before covering with clothing to avoid transfer to other individuals.

7.) On completion of application, wash both hands with soap and water to remove any residual estradiol.

*Concomitant progestin therapy* – When estrogen is prescribed for a postmenopausal woman with a uterus, also initiate progestin to reduce the risk of endometrial cancer. For women with a uterus, when indicated, undertake adequate diagnostic measures (eg, endometrial sampling) to rule out malignancy in cases of undiagnosed persistent or recurring abnormal vaginal bleeding.

*TOPICAL ESTROGENS, MISCELLANEOUS:*

*Moderate to severe vasomotor symptoms and/or moderate to severe symptoms of vulvar and vaginal atrophy associated with menopause –*

*Pump:* Prime the pump before using for the first time. Remove the large pump cover and fully depress the pump twice. Discard the unused gel in a manner that avoids accidental exposure or ingestion by others. To apply dose, collect the gel into the palm by pressing the pump firmly and fully with 1 fluid motion without hesitation. Apply the gel to 1 arm using the hand. Spread the gel as thinly as possible over the entire area on the inside and outside of the arm from wrist to shoulder.

Apply gel to clean, dry, unbroken skin after bath, shower, or sauna; be sure skin is completely dry before application. Try to leave as much time as possible between applying gel and going swimming. It is not necessary to massage or rub in gel. Simply allow the gel to dry for up to 5 minutes before dressing. Do not apply directly to breast.

Always place the cap back on the tip of the pump and the large pump cover over the top of the pump after each use. Wash hands with soap and water after application to avoid transfer to other individuals.

*Tube:* Gently squeeze gel from the tube to fill the applicator to the halfway mark (1.25 mark). Apply the gel to 1 arm using the applicator. Be sure to transfer all the gel from the applicator to the arm.

*ESTRADIOL TRANSDERMAL SYSTEM:*

*Initiation of therapy –*

*Treatment of menopausal symptoms:* Start with the 0.025 to 0.05 mg system applied to the skin once or twice weekly. Adjust dose as necessary to control symptoms. Use the lowest dosage necessary to control symptoms, especially in women with an intact uterus. Make attempts to taper or discontinue the drug at 3- to 6-month intervals.

*Prevention of postmenopausal osteoporosis:* Initiate with 0.025 mg/day as soon as possible after menopause. Adjust dosage if necessary. Discontinuation may reestablish natural rate of bone loss.

In women who are not taking oral estrogens, start treatment immediately. In women who are currently taking oral estrogens, start treatment 1 week after withdrawal of oral therapy or sooner if symptoms reappear in less than 1 week.

*Therapeutic regimen –* Therapy may be given continuously in patients who do not have an intact uterus. In patients with an intact uterus, therapy may be given on a cyclic schedule (eg, 3 weeks on followed by 1 week off).

*Estraderm, Alora, Esclim, Vivelle,* and *Vivelle-Dot* are applied twice a week; *Climara* lasts for 7 days.

*Application of system –* Place adhesive side of the system on a clean, dry area on the trunk of the body (including the buttocks and abdomen). Do not apply to breasts. Rotate application site with an interval of at least 1 week between applications to a particular site. The area should not be oily, damaged, or irritated. Avoid the waistline, because tight clothing may rub the system off. Apply the system immediately after opening pouch and removing protective liner. Press firmly in place with the palm for approximately 10 seconds. Make sure there is good contact, especially around the edges. In the unlikely event that a system should fall off, the same system may be reapplied. If necessary, apply a new system. In either case, continue the original treatment schedule.

*ESTRADIOL, ORAL:*

*Moderate to severe vasomotor symptoms, vulvar/vaginal atrophy associated with menopause –* Initiate treatment with 1 or 2 mg/day; adjust to control presenting symptoms. Titrate to determine the minimal effective dose for maintenance therapy. Administer cyclically (eg, 3 weeks on and 1 week off).

*Hypoestrogenism caused by hypogonadism, castration, or primary ovarian failure –* Treatment usually is initiated with a dose of 1 to 2 mg daily, adjusted as necessary to control presenting symptoms; determine the minimal effective dose for maintenance therapy by titration.

*Prostatic cancer (advanced androgen-dependent)* – For palliation only. Administer 1 to 2 mg 3 times daily. Judge efficacy of therapy by phosphatase determinations and symptomatic improvement.

*Breast cancer, metastatic* – For palliation only. The usual dose is 10 mg 3 times daily for at least 3 months.

*Osteoporosis prevention* – Administer cyclically (eg, 23 days on and 5 days off) 0.5 mg/day as soon as possible after menopause. Adjust dosage if necessary to control concurrent menopausal symptoms.

*Concomitant progestin therapy* – When estrogen is prescribed for a postmenopausal woman with a uterus, also initiate progestin to reduce the risk of endometrial cancer. A woman without a uterus does not need progestin.

ESTRADIOL VALERATE IN OIL: For IM injection only.

*Moderate to severe vasomotor symptoms, atrophic vaginitis or kraurosis vulvae associated with menopause, female hypogonadism, female castration, or primary ovarian failure* – 10 to 20 mg every 4 weeks.

*Prostatic carcinoma* – 30 mg or more every 1 or 2 weeks.

CONJUGATED ESTROGENS, ORAL: Administer cyclically (3 weeks of daily estrogen and 1 week off) for all indications except selected cases of carcinoma.

*Moderate to severe vasomotor symptoms and/or moderate to severe symptoms of vulvar and vaginal atrophy associated with menopause* – Start at the lowest dose. Therapy may be given continuously with no interruption, or in cyclical regimens (eg, 25 days on followed by 5 days off) as is medically appropriate on an individualized basis.

*Female hypogonadism* – 0.3 to 0.625 mg daily, administered cyclically (eg, 3 weeks on and 1 week off). Doses are adjusted depending on the severity of symptoms and responsiveness of the endometrium.

The dosage may be gradually titrated upward at 6- to 12-month intervals as needed to achieve appropriate bone age advancement and eventual epiphyseal closure. Chronic dosing with 0.625 mg is sufficient to induce artificial cyclic menses with sequential progestin treatment and to maintain bone mineral density after skeletal maturity is achieved.

*Female castration and primary ovarian failure* – 1.25 mg/day cyclically. Adjust according to severity of symptoms and patient response. For maintenance, adjust to lowest effective level.

*Osteoporosis prevention* – 0.625 mg/day, cyclically or continuously.

*Breast cancer, metastatic (for palliation)* – 10 mg 3 times/day for at least 3 months.

*Prostatic carcinoma (for palliation)* – 1.25 to 2.5 mg 3 times/day. Judge efficacy by phosphatase determinations and symptomatic improvement.

CONJUGATED ESTROGENS, PARENTERAL:

*Abnormal uterine bleeding caused by hormonal imbalance in the absence of organic pathology* – Usual dose is one 25 mg injection IV or IM. Repeat in 6 to 12 hours if necessary. Inject slowly to obviate the occurrence of flushes.

ESTERIFIED ESTROGENS:

*Moderate to severe vasomotor symptoms, atrophic vaginitis or kraurosis vulvae associated with menopause* – Cyclic therapy for short-term use. Average dose is 0.3 to at least 1.25 mg/day. Adjust dosage to the lowest effective level and discontinue as soon as possible.

*Female hypogonadism* – Administer 2.5 to 7.5 mg/day in divided doses for 20 days followed by a 10-day rest period. If bleeding does not occur by the end of this period, repeat the same dosage schedule. The number of courses of estrogen therapy necessary to produce bleeding varies depending on endometrial responsiveness.

If bleeding occurs before the end of the 10-day period, begin an estrogen-progestin cyclic regimen of 2.5 to 7.5 mg/day in divided doses for 20 days. During the last 5 days of estrogen therapy, give an oral progestin. If bleeding occurs before this regimen is concluded, discontinue therapy; resume on the fifth day of bleeding.

*Female castration and primary ovarian failure* – Give 1.25 mg/day, cyclically.

*Prostatic carcinoma (inoperable, progressing)* – 1.25 to 2.5 mg 3 times/day. Judge efficacy of therapy by symptomatic response and phosphatase determinations.

*Breast cancer (inoperable, progressing)* – 10 mg 3 times/day for at least 3 months.

ESTROPIPATE (Piperazine Estrone Sulfate):

*Moderate to severe vasomotor symptoms, atrophic vaginitis or kraurosis vulvae associated with meno-pause* – Give cyclically for short-term use. Choose the lowest dose and regimen that will control symptoms. Usual dosage range is 0.75 to 6 mg estropipate/day.

*Female hypogonadism, female castration, or primary ovarian failure* – Administer cyclically, 1.5 to 9 mg estropipate (calculated as 1.25 to 7.5 mg estrone sulfate)/day for the first 3 weeks, followed by a rest period of 8 to 10 days. Repeat if bleeding does not occur by the end of the rest period. The duration of therapy necessary to produce with-drawal bleeding will vary according to the responsiveness of the endometrium. If sat-isfactory withdrawal bleeding does not occur, give an oral progestin in addition to estrogen during the third week of the cycle.

*Osteoporosis prevention* – 0.75 mg/day estropipate for 25 days of a 31-day cycle per month.

SYNTHETIC CONJUGATED ESTROGENS, A:

*Menopause* – For treatment of moderate to severe vasomotor symptoms associated with menopause, choose the lowest dose and regimen that will control symptoms. Initial doses of 0.625 mg are recommended with titration up to 1.25 mg. Discon-tinue medication as soon as possible. Attempt to discontinue or taper medication at 3- to 6-month intervals.

*Vulvar and vaginal atrophy* – 0.3 mg/day.

SYNTHETIC CONJUGATED ESTROGENS, B:

*Moderate to severe vasomotor symptoms associated with menopause* – Initial dose is 0.625 mg daily. Subsequent dosage adjustment may be made based upon the individual patient response. Periodically reassess dosage.

ESTRADIOL CYPIONATE IN OIL· For IM use only.

*Moderate to severe vasomotor symptoms associated with menopause* – Usual dosage range is 1 to 5 mg IM, every 3 to 4 weeks. Attempt to discontinue or taper medication at 3- to 6-month intervals.

*Female hypogonadism* – 1.5 to 2 mg IM at monthly intervals.

## Actions

*Pharmacology:* Estrogens occur naturally in several forms. The primary source of estro-gen in normally cycling adult women is the ovarian follicle, which secretes 70 to 500 mcg of estradiol daily, depending on the phase of the menstrual cycle. This is converted primarily to estrone, which circulates in roughly equal proportion to estradiol, and to small amounts of estriol. After menopause, most endogenous estro-gen is produced by conversion of androstenedione, secreted by the adrenal cor-tex, to estrone by peripheral tissues. Thus, estrone—especially in its sulfate ester form—is the most abundant circulating estrogen in postmenopausal women. Although circulating estrogens exist in a dynamic equilibrium of metabolic inter-conversions, estradiol is the principal intracellular human estrogen and is sub-stantially more potent than estrone or estriol at the receptor.

Estrogens, important in developing and maintaining female reproductive system and secondary sex characteristics, promote growth and development of the vagina, uterus, fallopian tubes, and breasts. They affect release of pituitary gonadotro-pins; cause capillary dilatation, fluid retention, protein anabolism, and thin cervi-cal mucus; inhibit or facilitate ovulation; prevent postpartum breast discomfort. Indirectly, they contribute to: Shaping the skeleton (conserving calcium and phos-phorus and encouraging bone formation); maintenance of tone and elasticity of urogenital structures; changes in epiphyses of long bones that allow for pubertal growth spurt and its termination; growth of axillary and pubic hair; pigmentation of nipples and genitals.

*Pharmacokinetics:*

*Absorption/Distribution* – Estrogens used in therapy are well absorbed through the skin, mucous membranes, and GI tract. When applied for a local action, absorp-tion is usually sufficient to cause systemic effects. When conjugated with aryl and alkyl groups for parenteral administration, the rate of absorption of oily prepara-tions is slowed with a prolonged duration of action, such that a single IM injection of estradiol valerate or estradiol cypionate is absorbed over several weeks. Conjugated estrogens are well absorbed from the GI tract after release from the drug formulation. The tablet releases conjugated estrogens slowly over several hours. The distribution of exogenous estrogens is similar to that of endogenous estrogens.

*Transdermal system:* In contrast to oral estradiol, the skin metabolizes estradiol via the transdermal system only to a small extent. Therefore, transdermal use produces therapeutic serum levels of estradiol with lower circulating levels of estrone and estrone conjugates, and requires smaller total doses.

*Metabolism/Excretion* – Metabolism and inactivation occur primarily in the liver. During cyclic passage through the liver, estrogens are degraded to less active estrogenic compounds conjugated with sulfuric and glucuronic acids.

### Contraindications

Known or suspected breast cancer, except in appropriately selected patients being treated for metastatic disease; known or suspected estrogen-dependent neoplasia; undiagnosed abnormal genital bleeding; active DVT, PE, or a history of these conditions; active or recent (eg, within past year) arterial thromboembolic disease (eg, stroke, MI); active thrombophlebitis or thromboembolic disorders; history of thrombophlebitis, thrombosis or thromboembolic disorders associated with previous estrogen use (except when used in treatment of breast or prostatic malignancy); known or suspected pregnancy (see Warning Box); porphyria (estradiol vaginal tablets only); hypersensitivity to any product component.

### Warnings

*Induction of malignant neoplasms:* Estrogens and estrogen/progestin therapy may increase the risk of endometrial carcinoma, breast cancer, and ovarian cancer.

*Gallbladder disease:* There is a 2- to 3-fold increase in risk of gallbladder disease in women receiving postmenopausal estrogens.

*Cardiovascular disorders:* Estrogen and estrogen/progestin therapy have been associated with an increased risk of cardiovascular events (eg, MI and stroke, venous thrombosis, PE [venous thromboembolism]). Manage risk factors for cardiovascular disease (eg, hypertension, diabetes mellitus, tobacco use, hypercholesterolemia, obesity) appropriately.

*Hepatic adenoma:* Benign hepatic adenomas appear to be associated with the use of oral contraceptives (OCs).

*Dementia:* In the WHIMS, 4,532 generally healthy postmenopausal women 65 years of age and older were studied, of whom 35% were 70 to 74 years of age and 18% were 75 years of age or older. After an average follow-up of 4 years, 40 women being treated with 0.625 mg conjugated estrogens plus 2.5 mg medroxyprogesterone acetate (1.8%, n = 2,229) and 21 women in the placebo group (0.9%, n = 2,303) received diagnoses of probable dementia.

It is unknown whether these findings apply to estrogen alone therapy.

*Familial hyperlipoproteinemia:* Estrogen therapy may be associated with massive elevations of plasma triglycerides leading to pancreatitis and other complications in patients with familial defects of lipoprotein metabolism.

*Hypercalcemia:* Estrogens may lead to severe hypercalcemia in patients with breast cancer and bone metastases. If this occurs, discontinue the drug and take appropriate measures to reduce the serum calcium level.

*Glucose tolerance:* A worsening of glucose tolerance has been observed in a significant percentage of patients on estrogen-containing OCs. Carefully observe diabetic patients receiving estrogen.

*Visual abnormalities:* Retinal vascular thrombosis has been reported. Discontinue medication pending examination if there is sudden partial or complete loss of vision or a sudden onset of proptosis, diplopia, or migraine.

*Hypothyroidism:* Estrogen administration leads to increased thyroid-binding globulin (TBG) levels.

*Depression:* OCs appear to be associated with an increased incidence of mental depression.

*Uterine leiomyomata:* Preexisting uterine leiomyomata may increase in size during estrogen use.

*Hepatic function impairment:* Patients with a history of jaundice during pregnancy have an increased risk of recurrence while on estrogen-containing OCs. If jaundice develops in any patient on estrogen, discontinue medication and investigate the cause. Estrogens may be poorly metabolized in impaired liver function; use with caution.

*Pregnancy:* Category X (see Warning Box).

*Lactation:* Estrogens have been shown to decrease the quantity and quality of breast milk and may be excreted in breast milk. Administer only when clearly needed.

*Children:* Estrogen therapy has been used for the induction of puberty in adolescents with some forms of pubertal delay. Safety and efficacy in children have not otherwise been established.

### Precautions

*Elevated blood pressure:* In a small number of case reports, substantial increases in blood pressure have been attributed to idiosyncratic reactions to estrogens. Monitor blood pressure at regular intervals with estrogen use.

*Hypercoagulability:* Some studies have shown that women taking estrogen replacement therapy have hypercoagulability, primarily related to decreased antithrombin activity. This effect appears dose- and duration-dependent and is less pronounced than that associated with OC use.

*History/Physical exam:* Before initiating estrogens, take complete medical and family history. Pretreatment and periodic history and physical exams every 12 months should include blood pressure, breasts, abdomen, pelvic organs, and a Papanicolaou smear.

*Vaginal products:* Estradiol vaginal ring may not be suitable for women with narrow, short, or stenosed vaginas. Women with signs or symptoms of vaginal irritation should alert their physician.

If a vaginal infection develops during use of the estradiol vaginal ring, remove the ring and reinsert only after the infection has been appropriately treated.

Conjugated estrogens vaginal cream exposure has been reported to weaken latex condoms. Consider its potential to weaken and contribute to the failure of condoms, diaphragms, or cervical caps made of latex or rubber.

*Excessive estrogenic stimulation:* Certain patients may develop undesirable manifestations of excessive estrogenic stimulation (eg, abnormal or excessive uterine bleeding, mastodynia). Advise the pathologist of estrogen therapy when relevant specimens are submitted.

*Fluid retention:* Estrogens may cause some degree of fluid retention; conditions which might be influenced by this factor (eg, asthma, epilepsy, migraine, cardiac or renal dysfunction) require careful observation.

*Calcium and phosphorus metabolism:* Calcium and phosphorus metabolism is influenced by estrogens; use caution in patients with metabolic bone diseases associated with hypercalcemia or in renal insufficiency.

*Endometrial hyperplasia:* Prolonged unopposed estrogen therapy may increase risk of endometrial hyperplasia.

*Exacerbations of other conditions:* Endometriosis may be exacerbated with administration of estrogen therapy. Estrogen therapy also may cause an exacerbation of asthma, diabetes mellitus, epilepsy, migraine, or porphyria; use with caution in patients with these conditions.

*Benzyl alcohol:* Benzyl alcohol, contained in some of these products as a preservative, has been associated with a fatal "gasping syndrome" in premature infants.

## Drug Interactions

Drugs that may be affected by estrogens include oral anticoagulants, tricyclic antidepressants, hydantoins, corticosteroids, and thyroid hormones.

Drugs that may affect estrogens include barbiturates, rifampin, hydantoins, topiramate, and CYP 3A4 inducers and inhibitors.

*Drug/Lab test interactions:* Certain endocrine and liver function tests may be affected by estrogen-containing OCs. Expect these similar changes with larger doses:

Increased sulfobromophthalein retention.

Increased prothrombin time, partial thromboplastin time, platelet aggregation time, platelet count, and factors II, VII, VIII, IX, X, XII, VII-X complex, II-VII-X complex, and β-thromboglobulin; decreased antithrombin III, antifactor Xa; increased fibrinogen, plasminogen, norepinephrine-induced platelet aggregability.

Increased TBG leading to increased circulating total thyroid hormone, as measured by PBI, $T_4$ by column, or $T_4$ by radioimmunoassay. Free $T_3$ resin uptake is decreased, reflecting the elevated TBG; free $T_4$ concentration is unaltered.

Impaired glucose tolerance; decreased pregnanediol excretion; reduced response to metyrapone test; reduced serum folate concentration.

Increased plasma HDL and HDL-2 subfraction concentrations, reduced LDL cholesterol concentration levels, increased triglyceride levels.

## Adverse Reactions

Significant adverse reactions include abdominal cramps, aggravation of porphyria, amenorrhea during and after treatment, bloating, breakthrough bleeding, breast tenderness/enlargement/secretion, change in menstrual flow, changes in libido, chloasma or melasma (may persist when drug is discontinued), cholestatic jaundice, convulsions, dermatitis, dizziness, dysmenorrhea, edema, erythema nodosum/multiforme, headache, hemorrhagic eruption, intolerance to contact lenses, mental depression, migraine, nausea, pain at injection site, premenstrual-like syndrome, postinjection flare, redness and irritation at application site with the estradiol transdermal system (17%), spotting, steepening of corneal curvature, sterile abscess, urticaria, vomiting.

# MISCELLANEOUS ESTROGENS, VAGINAL

| | |
|---|---|
| **Tablets, vaginal:** 25 mcg estradiol (equivalent to 25.8 mcg hemihydrate) (*Rx*) | *Vagifem* (Novo Nordisk) |
| **Cream:** 1.5 mg estropipate/g (*Rx*) | *Ogen Vaginal* (Pharmacia) |
| 0.1 mg estradiol/g in a nonliquefying base (*Rx*) | *Estrace Vaginal* (Warner Chilcott) |
| 0.625 mg conjugated estrogens/g in a nonliquefying base (*Rx*) | *Premarin Vaginal* (Wyeth-Ayerst) |
| **Ring:** 2 mg estradiol[a] (*Rx*) | *Estring* (Pharmacia) |
| 0.05[b] and 0.1[c] mg/day estradiol acetate (*Rx*) | *Femring* (Galen) |

[a] Releases estradiol, approximately 7.5 mcg/24 hours, in a consistent, stable manner over 90 days. Dimensions: outer diameter, 55 mm; cross-sectional diameter, 9 mm; core diameter, 2 mm.
[b] Central core contains 12.4 mg estradiol acetate that releases 0.05 mg/day for 3 months. Dimensions: outer diameter, 56 mm; cross-sectional diameter, 7.6 mm; core diameter, 2 mm.
[c] Central core contains 24.8 mg estradiol acetate that releases 0.1 mg/day for 3 months. Dimensions: outer diameter, 56 mm; cross-sectional diameter, 7.6 mm; core diameter, 2 mm.

## Indications

*Vulvar/Vaginal atrophy:* Treatment of urogenital symptoms associated with postmenopausal atrophy of the vagina and/or the lower urinary tract.

*Atrophic vaginitis (Vagifem only):* Treatment of atrophic vaginitis.

*Vasomotor symptoms (Femring only):* Treatment of moderate to severe vasomotor symptoms associated with menopause.

## Administration and Dosage

Choose the lowest dose that will control symptoms and discontinue medication as promptly as possible. Attempt to discontinue or taper medication at 3- to 6-month intervals.

*Conjugated estrogens:* Administer cyclically; 3 weeks on and 1 week off. For short-term use only. Give 0.5 to 2 g/day intravaginally, depending on the severity of the condition.

*Estropipate:* 2 to 4 g/day intravaginally, depending on the severity of the condition.

*Estradiol:*

> *Cream* – 2 to 4 g/day for 1 or 2 weeks. Gradually reduce to 50% of initial dosage. A maintenance dose of 1 g 1 to 3 times/week may be used after restoration of the vaginal mucosa has been achieved.

> *Ring* – Press into an oval and insert as deeply as possible into the upper ⅓ of the vaginal vault. The ring is to remain in place continuously for 3 months, after which it should be removed and, if appropriate, replaced by a new ring.

> If the ring is removed or falls out at any time during the 90-day treatment period, rinse the ring in lukewarm water and re-insert.

*Estradiol hemihydrate:* Using the supplied applicator, gently insert into the vagina as far as it can comfortably go without force.

> *Initial dose* – 1 tablet inserted vaginally once daily for 2 weeks. Administer treatment at the same time each day.

> *Maintenance dose* – 1 tablet inserted vaginally twice weekly.

> The need to continue therapy should be assessed by the physician with the patient. Attempt to discontinue or taper medication at 3- to 6-month intervals.

*Concomitant progestin therapy:* When estrogen is prescribed for a postmenopausal woman with a uterus, also initiate progestin to reduce the risk of endometrial cancer. A woman without a uterus does not need progestin.

## Actions

*Pharmacology:* The signs and symptoms of vulvovaginal epithelial atrophy (atrophic vaginitis) may be alleviated by the topical application of an estrogenic hormone.

## Warnings

*Vaginal bleeding:* Uterine bleeding might be provoked by excessive administration in menopausal women. Evaluation may be required to differentiate this uterine bleeding from carcinoma. Breast tenderness and vaginal discharge may result from excessive estrogenic stimulation; endometrial withdrawal bleeding may occur if use is suddenly discontinued.

*Vaginal products:* Estradiol vaginal ring may not be suitable for women with narrow, short, or stenosed vaginas.

> If a vaginal infection develops during use of the estradiol vaginal ring, remove the ring and reinsert only after the infection has been appropriately treated.

> Conjugated estrogens vaginal cream exposure has been reported to weaken latex condoms. Consider its potential to weaken and contribute to the failure of condoms, diaphragms, or cervical caps made of latex or rubber.

# ESTROGENS AND PROGESTINS COMBINED

| | |
|---|---|
| **Tablets**: 0.45 mg conjugated estrogens/1.5 mg medroxyprogesterone, 0.625 mg conjugated estrogens/5 mg medroxyprogesterone acetate, 0.625 mg conjugated estrogens/2.5 mg medroxyprogesterone acetate (*Rx*) | *Prempro* (Wyeth-Ayerst) |
| 0.625 mg conjugated estrogens, 0.625 mg conjugated estrogens/5 mg medroxyprogesterone acetate (*Rx*) | *Premphase* (Wyeth-Ayerst) |
| 5 mcg ethinyl estradiol/1 mg norethindrone acetate (*Rx*) | *Femhrt* (Warner Chilcott) |
| 1 mg estradiol/0.5 mg norethindrone acetate (*Rx*) | *Activella* (Novo Nordisk) |
| 1 mg estradiol; 1 mg estradiol/0.09 mg norgestimate (*Rx*) | *Ortho-Prefest* (Ortho-McNeil) |
| **Transdermal patch**: 0.05 mg estradiol/0.14 mg norethindrone acetate; 0.05 mg estradiol/0.25 mg norethindrone acetate (*Rx*) | *CombiPatch* (Aventis) |

## Indications

In women with an intact uterus for the treatment of moderate to severe vasomotor symptoms associated with menopause; treatment of vulval and vaginal atrophy

(*Femhrt* excluded); osteoporosis prevention (*CombiPatch* excluded); treatment of hypoestrogenism caused by hypogonadism, castration, or primary ovarian failure (*CombiPatch* only).

*Unlabeled uses:* May be an effective alternative to treat hypercholesterolemia in post-menopausal women (0.3 to 1.25 mg conjugated estrogens with 5 mg medroxyprogesterone).

### Administration and Dosage

*Prempro:* One 0.625 mg/2.5 mg tablet once daily; can increase to 0.625 mg/5 mg once daily.

*Premphase:* One 0.625 mg conjugated estrogens tablet once daily on days 1 through 14 and one 0.625 mg conjugated estrogen/5 mg medroxyprogesterone tablet taken once daily on days 15 through 28.

*Femhrt and Activella:* One tablet/day.

*Ortho-Prefest:* One pink tablet/day for 3 days, followed by 1 white tablet/day for 3 days. This regimen is repeated continuously without interruption.

*CombiPatch:* Replace the patch system twice weekly. Advise women that monthly withdrawal bleeding often occurs.

Apply to a smooth (fold-free) clean, dry area of the skin on the lower abdomen. Do not apply to or near the breasts and avoid the waistline. The sites of application must be rotated; allow an interval of at least 1 week between applications to the same site.

*Continuous combined regimen* – Apply twice weekly during a 28-day cycle. Irregular bleeding may occur particularly in the first 6 months.

*Continuous sequential regimen* – It can be applied as a sequential regimen in combination with an estradiol-only transdermal delivery system.

*Menopause and vulval/vaginal atrophy:* Reevaluate patients at 3- to 6-month intervals to determine the need for continued treatment.

*Osteoporosis:* The mainstays of prevention and management of osteoporosis are estrogen and calcium; exercise and nutrition may be important adjuncts.

*Monitoring:* Monitor closely for signs of endometrial cancer; evaluate recurrent or persistent abnormal vaginal bleeding appropriately to rule out malignancy.

# ESTROGEN AND ANDROGEN COMBINATIONS

| | |
|---|---|
| **Tablets:** 0.625 mg esterified estrogens and 1.25 mg methyltestosterone (*Rx*) | *Estratest H.S.* (Solvay) |
| 1.25 mg esterified estrogens and 2.5 mg methyltestosterone (*Rx*) | *Estratest* (Solvay) |

**Warning:**

Estrogens have been reported to increase the risk of endometrial carcinoma.

Close clinical surveillance of all women taking estrogens is important. In all cases of undiagnosed, persistent, or recurring abnormal vaginal bleeding, adequate diagnostic measures should be undertaken to rule out malignancy.

Do not use estrogens during pregnancy.

The use of female sex hormones, estrogens and progestogens, during early pregnancy may seriously damage the offspring.

Refer to the Warning Box in the Estrogens group monograph for more information.

### Indications

*Moderate to severe vasomotor symptoms:* Moderate to severe vasomotor symptoms associated with menopause in patients not improved with estrogens alone.

**Administration and Dosage**

*Oral:* Give cyclically for short-term use only.

Use the lowest dose that will control symptoms and discontinue medication as promptly as possible.

Administer cyclically (eg, 3 weeks on and 1 week off). Make attempts to discontinue or taper medication at 3- to 6-month intervals.

*Usual dosage range –* One 1.25/2.5 mg tablet or one to two 0.625/1.25 mg tablets daily, as recommended by the physician.

Closely monitor treated patients with an intact uterus for signs of endometrial cancer and take appropriate diagnostic measures to rule out malignancy in the event of persistent or recurring abnormal vaginal bleeding.

# RALOXIFENE

**Tablets:** 60 mg *(Rx)*                                         *Evista* (Eli Lilly)

### Indications

*Osteoporosis, prevention and treatment:* Prevention and treatment of osteoporosis in postmenopausal women.

### Administration and Dosage

The recommended dosage is 60 mg/day, which may be administered any time of day
without regard to meals.

### Actions

*Pharmacology:* Raloxifene is a selective estrogen receptor modulator (SERM) that
reduces resorption of bone and decreases overall bone turnover.

*Pharmacokinetics:*

*Absorption* – Raloxifene is absorbed rapidly after oral administration with approximately 60% of an oral dose adsorbed. However, presystemic glucuronide conjugation is extensive and absolute bioavailability is only 2%.

*Distribution* – The apparent volume of distribution is 2348 L/kg and is not dose-
dependent. Raloxifene and the monoglucuronide conjugates are highly bound to
plasma proteins (95%).

*Metabolism* – Raloxifene undergoes extensive first-pass metabolism to the glucuronide conjugates. Raloxifene is not metabolized by cytochrome P450 pathways.
Plasma elimination half-life to 27.7 hours after single dose oral dosing and 32.5 after
multiple dose oral dosing.

*Excretion* – Raloxifene is primarily excreted in feces; less than 6% of the raloxifene dose is eliminated in urine as glucuronide conjugates and less than 0.2% is
excreted unchanged in urine.

### Contraindications

Women who are lactating or who are or may become pregnant (see Warnings); women
with active or a history of venous thromboembolic events, including deep vein
thrombosis, pulmonary embolism, and retinal vein thrombosis; hypersensitivity to
raloxifene or other constituents of the drug.

### Warnings

*Venous thromboembolic events:* An analysis of raloxifene-treated women showed an
increased risk of venous thromboembolic events defined as DVT and pulmonary
embolism. Other venous thromboembolic events could also occur. A less serious
event, superficial thrombophlebitis, has been reported more frequently with raloxifene. The greatest risk for DVT and pulmonary embolism occurs during the first
4 months of treatment. Discontinue raloxifene at least 72 hours prior to and during prolonged immobilization (eg, postsurgical recovery, prolonged bed rest), and
resume therapy only after the patient is fully ambulatory. Advise patients to avoid
prolonged restrictions of movement during travel.

*Premenopausal use:* There is no indication for premenopausal use of raloxifene.

*Carcinogenesis:* In long term carcinogenicity studies in animals there was an increased
incidence of ovarian tumors, testicular interstitial cell tumors, and prostatic adenocarcinomas.

*Fertility impairment:* Raloxifene delayed and disrupted embryo implantation resulting in
prolonged gestation and reduced litter size.

*Pregnancy: Category X.*

*Lactation:* Raloxifene should not be used by lactating women.

*Children:* Raloxifene should not be used in pediatric patients.

### Precautions

*Concurrent estrogen therapy:* The concurrent use of raloxifene and systemic estrogen or hormone replacement therapy (ERT or HRT) has not been studied in prospective clinical trials; therefore, concomitant use is not recommended.

> *Lipid metabolism:* Raloxifene lowers serum total and LDL cholesterol by 6% to 11% but does not affect serum concentrations of total HDL cholesterol or triglycerides. Take these effects into account in therapeutic decisions for patients who may require therapy for hyperlipidemia.
>
> Limited clinical data suggest that some women with a history of marked hypertriglyceridemia (more than 5.6 mmol/L or more than 500 mg/dL) in response to treatment with oral estrogen or estrogen plus progestin may develop increased levels of triglycerides when treated with raloxifene. Women with this medical history should have serum triglycerides monitored when taking raloxifene.

> *Endometrium:* Raloxifene has not been associated with endometrial proliferation. Investigate unexplained uterine bleeding as clinically indicated.

> *Supplemental calcium:* Add supplemental calcium to the diet if daily intake is inadequate.

### Drug Interactions

> *Highly protein-bound drugs:* In vitro, raloxifene did not affect the binding of warfarin, phenytoin, or tamoxifen. However, use caution when raloxifene is coadministered with other highly protein-bound drugs, such as diazepam, diazoxide, and lidocaine.

> Drugs that may interact with raloxifene include ampicillin and cholestyramine. Raloxifene may affect warfarin.

### Adverse Reactions

> Adverse reactions occurring in at least 3% of patients include hot flashes; depression; insomnia; vertigo; rash; sweating; nausea; diarrhea; dyspepsia; vomiting; flatulence; GI disorder; vaginitis; UTI; cystitis; leukorrhea; uterine disorder; endometrial disorder; weight gain; peripheral edema; arthralgia; myalgia; leg cramps; arthritis; tendon disorder; sinusitis; rhinitis; bronchitis; pharyngitis; increased cough; infection; flu syndrome; headache; chest pain; fever.

> *Lab test abnormalities:* Increased apolipoprotein A1; reduced serum total cholesterol, LDL cholesterol, fibrinogen, apolipoprotein B, and lipoprotein. Raloxifene modestly increases hormone-binding globulin concentrations, including sex steroid-binding globulin, thyroxine-binding globulin, and corticosteroid-binding globulin with corresponding increases in measured total hormone concentrations.
>
> There were small decreases in serum total calcium, inorganic phosphate, total protein, and albumin which were generally of lesser magnitude than decreases observed during ERT/HRT. Platelet count was also decreased slightly and was not different from ERT.

### Patient Information

> *Patient immobilization:* Discontinue raloxifene at least 72 hours prior to and during prolonged immobilization (eg, postsurgical recovery, prolonged bed rest) and advise patients to avoid prolonged restrictions of movement during travel because of the increased risk of venous thromboembolic events.

# PROGESTINS

| | |
|---|---|
| **MEDROXYPROGESTERONE** | |
| **Tablets:** 2.5 mg and 5 mg (*Rx*) | *Cycrin* (ESI Pharma), *Provera* (Upjohn) |
| 10 mg (*Rx*) | Various, *Amen* (Carnrick), *Curretab* (Solvay), *Provera* (Upjohn) |
| **MEGESTROL ACETATE** | |
| **Tablets:** 20 and 40 mg (*Rx*) | Various, *Megace* (Bristol-Myers Oncology) |
| **Suspension:** 40 mg/mL (*Rx*) | *Megace* (Bristol-Myers Oncology) |
| **NORETHINDRONE ACETATE** | |
| **Tablets:** 5 mg (*Rx*) | *Aygestin* (Barr) |
| **PROGESTERONE (MICRONIZED)** | |
| **Capsules:** 100 and 200 mg (*Rx*) | *Prometrium* (Solvay) |
| **PROGESTERONE IN OIL** | |
| **Injection:** 50 mg/mL (*Rx*) | Various |
| **PROGESTERONE POWDER** | |
| **Powder** (*Rx*) | Various |
| **PROGESTERONE GEL** | |
| **Vaginal gel:** 4% (45 mg) and 8% (90 mg) (*Rx*) | *Crinone* (Serono), *Prochieve* (Columbia) |

> **Warning:**
> *Pregnancy:* Progestins have been used beginning with the first trimester of pregnancy to prevent habitual abortion or treat threatened abortion; however, there is no adequate evidence that such use is effective. There is evidence of potential harm to the fetus when given during the first 4 months of pregnancy. Therefore, the use of such drugs during the first 4 months of pregnancy is not recommended.
>
> The cause of abortion is generally a defective ovum, which progestational agents could not be expected to influence. In addition, progestational agents have uterine relaxant properties that may cause a delay in spontaneous abortion when given to patients with fertilized defective ova.

### Indications

Amenorrhea; abnormal uterine bleeding; endometriosis (norethindrone only).

*Megestrol:* Treatment of anorexia, cachexia, or an unexplained significant weight loss in patients with a diagnosis of AIDS.

Palliative treatment of advanced carcinoma of the breast or endometrium.

*Medroxyprogesterone tablets:*

*Endometrial hyperplasia* – To reduce the incidence of endometrial hyperplasia in non-hysterectomized postmenopausal women receiving 0.625 mg conjugated estrogens.

*Secondary amenorrhea/abnormal uterine bleeding* – For secondary amenorrhea and for abnormal uterine bleeding due to hormonal imbalance in the absence of organic pathology, such as fibroids or uterine cancer.

*Progesterone capsules and gel:* Progesterone supplementation or replacement as part of an Assisted Reproductive Technology (ART) treatment for infertile women with progesterone deficiency (8% gel).

*Endometrial hyperplasia (capsules)* – For use in the prevention of endometrial hyperplasia in nonhysterectomized postmenopausal women who are receiving conjugated estrogens tablets.

*Secondary amenorrhea* – For use in secondary amenorrhea (capsules); the 4% gel is for the treatment of secondary amenorrhea, and the 8% gel is for women who have failed to respond to treatment with the 4% gel.

### Administration and Dosage

MEDROXYPROGESTERONE ACETATE: For information on parenteral medroxyprogesterone acetate, refer to monograph in Antineoplastics chapter.

*Secondary amenorrhea* – 5 to 10 mg/day for 5 to 10 days. A dose for inducing an optimum secretory transformation of an endometrium that has been adequately primed with either endogenous or exogenous estrogen is 10 mg daily for 10 days. Start therapy any time. Withdrawal bleeding usually occurs 3 to 7 days after therapy ends.

*Abnormal uterine bleeding due to hormonal imbalance in the absence of organic pathology* – 5 to 10 mg/day for 5 to 10 days, beginning on the 16th or 21st day of the menstrual cycle. To produce an optimum secretory transformation of an endometrium that has been adequately primed with either endogenous or exogenous estrogen, give 10 mg/day for 10 days, beginning on the 16th day of the cycle. Withdrawal bleeding usually occurs 3 to 7 days after discontinuing therapy. Patients with recurrent episodes of abnormal uterine bleeding may benefit from planned menstrual cycling with medroxyprogesterone acetate.

*MEGESTROL ACETATE:* Initial dose is 800 mg/day (20 mL/day); daily doses of 400 and 800 mg/day were found to be clinically effective. Shake container well before using.

*NORETHINDRONE ACETATE:* Norethindrone acetate differs from norethindrone only in potency; the acetate is approximately twice as potent.

*Secondary amenorrhea; abnormal uterine bleeding due to hormonal imbalance in the absence of organic pathology* – 2.5 to 10 mg/day for 5 to 10 days during the second half of the theoretical menstrual cycle. Withdrawal bleeding usually occurs within 3 to 7 days.

*Endometriosis* –

*Initial dose:* 5 mg/day for 2 weeks; increase in increments of 2.5 mg/day every 2 weeks until 15 mg/day is reached. Therapy may be held at this level for 6 to 9 months or until breakthrough bleeding demands temporary termination.

*PROGESTERONE:* For IM use. The drug is irritating at the injection site.

*Amenorrhea* – Administer 5 to 10 mg/day for 6 to 8 consecutive days. If ovarian activity has produced a proliferative endometrium, expect withdrawal bleeding 48 to 72 hours after the last injection. Spontaneous normal cycles may follow.

*Functional uterine bleeding* – Administer 5 to 10 mg/day for 6 doses. Bleeding should cease within 6 days. When estrogen also is given, begin progesterone after 2 weeks of estrogen therapy. Discontinue injections when menstrual flow begins.

Progesterone is available as a micronized powder for prescription compounding.

*PROGESTERONE CAPSULES:*

*Prevention of endometrial hyperplasia* – Give as a single daily dose in the evening, 200 mg orally for 12 days sequentially per 28-day cycle, to postmenopausal women with a uterus who are receiving daily conjugated estrogen tablets.

*Secondary amenorrhea* – Give as a single daily dose of 400 mg in the evening for 10 days.

*PROGESTERONE GEL:*

*Infertility* – For progesterone supplementation or replacement as part of an Assisted Reproductive Technology (ART) treatment for infertile women with progesterone deficiency. Administer 90 mg vaginally once daily in women who require progesterone supplementation. In women with partial or complete ovarian failure who require progesterone replacement, administer 90 mg vaginally twice daily. If pregnancy occurs, continue treatment until placental autonomy is achieved, no more than 10 to 12 weeks.

*Secondary amenorrhea* – Administer 45 mg (4% gel) vaginally every other day up to a total of 6 doses. For women who fail to respond, a trial of 8% gel every other day up to a total of 6 doses may be instituted. It is important to note that a dosage increase from the 4% gel can only be accomplished by using the 8% gel. Increase in the volume of gel administered does not increase the amount of progesterone absorbed.

### Actions

*Pharmacology:* Progesterone, a principle of corpus luteum, is the primary endogenous progestational substance. Progestins (progesterone and derivatives) transform proliferative endometrium into secretory endometrium. They inhibit (at the usual dose range) the secretion of pituitary gonadotropins, which in turn prevents follicular maturation and ovulation. They also inhibit spontaneous uterine contraction. Progestins may demonstrate some estrogenic, anabolic, or androgenic activity. The precise mechanism by which megestrol produces effects in anorexia and cachexia is unknown.

*Pharmacokinetics:* Absorption of oral tablets and parenteral oily solutions of progestins is rapid; however, the hormone undergoes prompt hepatic transformation.

### Contraindications

Hypersensitivity to progestins; thrombophlebitis, thromboembolic disorders, cerebral hemorrhage or patients with a history of these conditions; impaired liver function or disease; carcinoma of the breast; undiagnosed vaginal bleeding; missed abortion; as a diagnostic test for pregnancy; known or suspected pregnancy; prophylactic use to avoid weight loss (megestrol).

### Warnings

*Ophthalmologic effects:* Discontinue medication pending examination if there is a sudden partial or complete loss of vision, or if there is sudden onset of proptosis, diplopia, or migraine. If papilledema or retinal vascular lesions are present, discontinue use.

*Thrombotic disorders:* Thrombotic disorders (thrombophlebitis, cerebrovascular disorders, retinal thrombosis, pulmonary embolism) occasionally occur in patients taking progestins.

*HIV-infected women:* Although megestrol has been used extensively in women for endometrial and breast cancers, its use in HIV-infected women has been limited. All the women in the clinical trials reported breakthrough bleeding.

*Fertility impairment:* Medroxyprogesterone acetate at high doses is an antifertility drug. High doses would be expected to impair fertility until the cessation of treatment.

*Pregnancy: Category D* (progesterone injection); *Category X* (norethindrone acetate). Use is not recommended. See Warning Box.

*Lactation:* Detectable amounts of progestins enter the milk of mothers receiving these agents. The effect on the nursing infant has not been determined.

Medroxyprogesterone does not adversely affect lactation and may increase milk production and duration of lactation if given in the puerperium.

*Children:* Safety and efficacy of megestrol acetate suspension in children have not been established.

### Precautions

*Causes of weight loss:* Institute therapy with megestrol for weight loss only after treatable causes of weight loss are sought and addressed.

*Respiratory infections:* Long-term treatment may increase the risk of respiratory infections.

*Pretreatment physical examination:* Pretreatment physical examination should include breasts and pelvic organs, as well as Papanicolaou smear.

*Fluid retention:* Fluid retention may occur; therefore, conditions influenced by this factor (epilepsy, migraine, asthma, cardiac, or renal dysfunction) require careful observation.

*Depression:* Observe patients who have a history of psychic depression and discontinue the drug if the depression recurs to a serious degree.

*Glucose tolerance:* A decrease in glucose tolerance has been observed in a small percentage of patients on estrogen-progestin combination drugs. Carefully observe diabetic patients receiving progestin therapy.

*Menopause:* The age of the patient constitutes no absolute limiting factor, although treatment with progestins may mask the onset of the climacteric.

*Photosensitivity:* Photosensitization (photoallergy or phototoxicity) may occur; therefore, caution patients to take protective measures (ie, sunscreens, protective clothing) against exposure to sunlight or ultraviolet light (eg, tanning beds) until tolerance is determined.

**Drug Interactions**

Drugs that may interact with progestins include aminoglutethimide and rifampin.

*Drug/Lab test interactions:* Laboratory test results of hepatic function, coagulation tests (increase in prothrombin, Factors VII, VIII, IX, and X), thyroid, metyrapone test and endocrine functions, may be affected by progestins or estrogens. A decrease in glucose tolerance has been observed in a small percentage of patients on estrogen-progestin combination drugs. Pregnanediol determination may be altered by the use of progestins.

**Adverse Reactions**

Adverse reactions that may occur include breakthrough bleeding, spotting, change in menstrual flow, amenorrhea, changes in cervical erosion and cervical secretions; breast changes (tenderness); masculinization of the female fetus; edema; changes in weight (increase or decrease); cholestatic jaundice; rash (allergic) with and without pruritus; acne; melasma or chloasma; mental depression; alopecia; hirsutism; thromboembolic phenomena including thrombophlebitis and pulmonary embolism; sensitivity reactions ranging from pruritus and urticaria to generalized rash (medroxyprogesterone acetate).

For information concerning adverse reactions associated with combined estrogen-progestin therapy, refer to the Oral Contraceptives monograph.

*Megestrol:* Adverse reactions occurring in at least 3% of patients include diarrhea; impotence; rash; flatulence; hypertension; asthenia; insomnia; nausea; anemia; fever; libido decreased; hyperglycemia; headache.

# CONTRACEPTIVE PRODUCTS

## MONOPHASIC ORAL CONTRACEPTIVES

**Tablets:** Estrogens (ethinyl estradiol, mestranol), progestins (desogestrel, drospirenone, ethynodiol diacetate, levonorgestrel, norethindrone, norethindrone acetate, norgestimate, norgestrel) (*Rx*)

*Alesse* (Wyeth-Ayerst), *Apri, Aviane* (Barr), *Brevicon* (Watson), *Cryselle* (Barr), *Demulen* (Searle), *Desogen* (Organon), *Junel Fe, Kariva, Lessina* (Barr), *Levlen* (Berlex), *Levora* (Watson ), *Levlite* (Berlex), *Loestrin* (Warner Chilcott), *Lo/Ovral* (Wyeth Ayerst), *Low-Ogestrel* (Watson), *Microgestin Fe* (Watson), *Mircette* (Organon), *Modicon* (Ortho-McNeil), *Mononessa, Necon* (Watson), *Nordette* (Monarch), *Norinyl* (Watson), *Nortrel* (Barr), *Ogestrel* (Watson), *Ortho-Cept, Ortho-Cyclen, Ortho-Novum* (Ortho-McNeil), *Ovcon* (Warner Chilcott), *Ovral* (Wyeth-Ayerst), *Portia,* Barr), *Seasonale* (Duramed), *Sprintec* (Barr), *Yasmin* (Berlex), *Zovia* (Watson)

## BIPHASIC ORAL CONTRACEPTIVES

**Tablets:** Estrogen (ethinyl estradiol), progestin (norethindrone) (*Rx*)

*Necon 10/11* (Watson), *Ortho-Novum 10/11* (Ortho-McNeil)

## TRIPHASIC ORAL CONTRACEPTIVES

**Tablets:** Estrogen (ethinyl estradiol), progestin (desogestrel, levonorgestrel, norethindrone, norethindrone acetate, norgestimate) (*Rx*)

*Cyclessa* (Organon), *Enpresse* (Barr), *Estrostep 21, Estrostep Fe* (Warner Chilcott), *Necon 7/7/7* (Watson), *Ortho-Novum 777, Ortho Tri-Cyclen, Ortho Tri-Cyclen Lo* (Ortho-McNeil), *Tri-Levlen* (Berlex), *TriNessa* (Watson), *Tri-Norinyl* (Watson), *Triphasil* (Wyeth-Ayerst), *Tri-Sprintec* (Barr), *Trivora* (Watson), *Velivet* (Barr)

## PROGESTIN-ONLY PRODUCTS

**Tablets:** 0.35 mg norethindrone (*Rx*)

*Camila, Errin* (Barr), *Jolivette* (Watson), *Ortho-Micronor* (Ortho-McNeil), *Nor-QD, Nora-BE* (Watson)

0.075 mg norgestrel (*Rx*)

*Ovrette* (Wyeth-Ayerst)

## EMERGENCY CONTRACEPTIVES

**Tablets:** 0.75 mg levonorgestrel (*Rx*)

*Plan B* (Women's Capital Corp.)

0.25 mg levonorgestrel, 0.05 mg ethinyl estradiol (*Rx*)

*Preven* (Gynètics)

## NORELGESTROMIN/ETHINYL ESTRADIOL TRANSDERMAL SYSTEM

**Patch:** 6 mg norelgestromin, 0.75 mg ethinyl estradiol/total patch content (*Rx*)

*Ortho Evra* (Ortho-McNeil)

## ETONOGESTREL/ETHINYL ESTRADIOL VAGINAL RING

**Ring:** 11.7 mg etonogestrel, 2.7 mg ethinyl estradiol/sachet (*Rx*)

*NuvaRing* (Organon)

---

**Warning:**

*Cigarette smoking:* Cigarette smoking increases the risk of cardiovascular side effects from hormonal contraceptive use. This risk increases with age and with heavy smoking (15 or more cigarettes/day) and is quite marked in women more than 35 years of age. Women who use hormonal contraceptives should not smoke.

---

**Indications**

*Contraceptive:* For the prevention of pregnancy. Start new patients on preparations containing 35 mcg or less estrogen.

*Emergency contraception (Plan B and Preven only):* For prevention of pregnancy following unprotected intercourse or a known or suspected contraceptive failure. To obtain efficacy, take the first dose as soon as possible within 72 hours of intercourse. The second dose must be taken 12 hours later. Emergency contraceptive pills are not indicated for ongoing pregnancy protection and should not be used as a woman's routine form of contraception.

ECPs are not as effective as some other forms of contraception.

*Acne vulgaris (Ortho Tri-Cyclen and Estrostep only):* For the treatment of moderate acne vulgaris in females 15 years of age or older who have no known contraindications to oral contraceptive therapy, desire contraception, have achieved menarche, and are unresponsive to topical antiacne medications.

### Administration and Dosage

*Acne:* The timing of dosing with *Ortho Tri-Cyclen* or *Estrostep* for acne should follow the guidelines for use of *Ortho Tri-Cyclen* or *Estrostep* as an OC. The dosage regimen for treatment of facial acne uses a 21-day active and a 7-day inert schedule. Take 1 active tablet daily for 21 days followed by 1 inert for 7 days. After 28 tablets have been taken, a new course is started the next day.

*Emergency contraception:* If a positive pregnancy result is obtained, advise the patient not to take the pills in the kit.

Take the initial 1 (*Plan B*) or 2 (*Preven*) pills as soon as possible but within 72 hours of unprotected intercourse. This is followed by the second dose of 1 (*Plan B*) or 2 (*Preven*) pills 12 hours later. Emergency contraception can be used at any time during the menstrual cycle. If the user vomits 1 hour or less after taking either dose of the medication, she should contact her health care professional to discuss whether or not to repeat that dose or take an antinausea medication.

*Progestin-only contraception:* One tablet every day at the same time. Administration is continuous, with no interruption between pill packs. Every time a pill is taken late, especially if a pill is missed, pregnancy is more likely.

*Missed dose* – If the patient is more than 3 hours late or misses 1 or more tablets, she should take a missed pill as soon as remembered, then go back to taking progestin-only pills (POPs) at the regular time, but should use a backup method (such as a condom or spermicide) every time she has sexual intercourse for the next 48 hours.

If fully breast-feeding (not giving baby any food or formula), start POPs 6 weeks after delivery. If partially breast-feeding (giving baby some food or formula), start taking POPs by 3 weeks after delivery.

*Switching pills* – If switching from the combined pills to POPs, take the first POP the day after the last active combined pill is finished. Do not take any of the 7 inactive pills from the combined pill pack. Many women have irregular periods after switching to POPs; this is normal and to be expected. If switching from POPs to the combined pills, take the first active combined pill on the first day of menses, even if the POP pack is not finished. If switching to another brand of POPs, start the new brand any time. If breast-feeding, switch to another method of birth control at any time, except do not switch to the combined pills until breast-feeding is stopped or until at least 6 months after delivery.

*Combined:*

*Sunday-Start packaging* – Take the first tablet on the first Sunday after menstruation begins. If menstruation begins on Sunday, take the first tablet on that day.

*21-Day regimen* – Day 1 of the cycle is the first day of menstrual bleeding. Take 1 tablet daily for 21 days. No tablets are taken for 7 days. Whether bleeding has stopped or not, start a new course of 21 days.

*28-Day regimen* – To eliminate the need to count the days between cycles, some products contain 7 inert or iron-containing tablets to permit continuous daily dosage during the entire 28-day cycle. Take the 7 tablets on the last 7 days of the cycle.

*84-day regimen* – The dosage of *Seasonale* is 1 pink (active) tablet per day for 84 consecutive days, followed by 7 days of white (inert) tablets. Withdrawal bleeding should occur during the 7 days following discontinuation of pink active tablets. During the first cycle, the patient should not place contraceptive reliance on *Seasonale* until a pink tablet has been taken daily for 7 consecutive days; the patient should use a nonhormonal backup method of birth control (such as condoms or spermicide) during those 7 days. The patient should consider the possibility of ovulation and conception prior to initiation of medication.

*Biphasic and triphasic OCs* – Follow instructions on the dispensers or packs. As with the monophasic OCs, 1 tablet is taken each day; however, as the color of the tablet changes, the strength of the tablet also changes (ie, the estrogen/progestin ratio varies).

*Missed dose* –

*One tablet:* Take it as soon as remembered, or take 2 tablets the next day. Alternatively take 1 tablet, discard the other missed tablet, continue as scheduled and use another form of contraception until menses.

*Two consecutive tablets:* Take 2 tablets as soon as remembered with the next pill at the usual time, or take 2 tablets/day for the next 2 days, then resume the regular schedule. Use an additional form of contraception for the 7 days after pills are missed, preferably for the remainder of the cycle. If 2 active pills are missed in a row in the third week and the patient is a Sunday starter, 1 pill should be taken every day until Sunday. On Sunday, the rest of the pack should be discarded and a new pack of pills started that same day. If 2 active pills are missed in a row in the third week and the patient is a day 1 starter, the rest of the pill pack should be discarded and a new pack started that same day. Menses may not occur this month but this is expected.

*Three consecutive tablets:* If the patient is a Sunday starter, she should keep taking 1 pill every day until Sunday. On Sunday, the rest of the pack should be discarded and a new pack of pills started that same day. If she is a day 1 starter, the rest of the pill pack should be discarded and a new pack started that same day. Menses may not occur this month, but this is expected. If menses do not occur 2 months in a row, the physician or clinic should be contacted because of the possibility of pregnancy. Pregnancy may result from sexual intercourse during the 7 days after the pills are missed. Use another birth control method (eg, condoms, foam) as a back-up method for those 7 days.

*Missed menstrual period:* If the patient has not adhered to the prescribed dosage regimen, consider possible pregnancy after the first missed period; withhold OCs until ruling out pregnancy and use a nonhormonal method of contraception. If the patient has adhered to the prescribed regimen and misses 2 consecutive periods, rule out pregnancy before continuing the contraceptive regimen.

After several months of treatment, menstrual flow may reduce to a point of virtual absence. This reduced flow may occur as a result of medication and is not indicative of pregnancy.

*Postpartum administration:* Postpartum administration in non-nursing mothers may begin at the first postpartum examination (4 to 6 weeks), regardless of whether spontaneous menstruation has occurred. Also, start no earlier than 4 to 6 weeks after a midtrimester pregnancy termination.

*Dosage adjustments:* Side effects noted during the initial cycles may be transient; if they continue, dosage adjustments may be indicated. Many side effects are related to the potency of the estrogen or progestin in the products. The following table summarizes these dose-related side effects.

| Achieving Proper Hormonal Balance In An Oral Contraceptive | | | |
| --- | --- | --- | --- |
| Estrogen | | Progestin | |
| Excess | Deficiency | Excess | Deficiency |
| Nausea, bloating Cervical mucorrhea, polyposis Melasma Hypertension Migraine headache Breast fullness or tenderness Edema | Early or midcycle breakthrough bleeding Increased spotting Hypomenorrhea | Increased appetite Weight gain Tiredness, fatigue Hypomenorrhea Acne, oily scalp[1] Hair loss, hirsutism[1] Depression Monilial vaginitis Breast regression | Late breakthrough bleeding Amenorrhea Hypermenorrhea |

[1] Result of androgenic activity of progestins.

| Pharmacological Effects of Progestins Used in Oral Contraceptives[1] | | | |
|---|---|---|---|
| | Progestin | Estrogen | Androgen |
| Desogestrel | ++++ | 0 | +++ |
| Levonorgestrel | ++++ | 0 | ++++ |
| Norgestrel | +++ | 0 | +++ |
| Ethynodiol diacetate | ++ | +++ | + |
| Norgestimate | ++ | 0 | ++ |
| Norethindrone acetate | ++ | ++ | ++ |
| Norethindrone | ++ | ++ | ++ |

[1] *Symbol Key:* ++++ – *pronounced effect* +++ – *moderate effect* ++ – *low effect* + – *slight effect* 0 – *no effect*

Minimize the above effects by adjusting the estrogen/progestin balance or dosage. The following table categorizes products by their estrogenic, progestational, and androgenic activity. Because overall activity is influenced by the interaction of components, including androgenic and antiestrogenic activity, it is difficult to precisely classify products; placement in the table is only approximate. Differences between products within a group are probably not clinically significant.

| Estimated Relative Oral Contraceptive Progestin/Estrogen/Androgen Activity | | | | |
|---|---|---|---|---|
| Ingredients | Brand-name examples | Progestin activity | Estrogen activity | Androgen activity |
| 0.1 mg levonorgestrel/20 mcg EE | Alesse, Aviane, Lessina, Levlite | Low | Low | Low |
| 0.25 mg norgestimate/35 mcg EE | Ortho-Cyclen, Sprintec | | Intermediate | |
| 0.5 mg norethindrone/35 mcg EE | Brevicon, Modicon, Necon 0.5/35, Nortrel 0.5/35 | | High | |
| 0.4 mg norethindrone/35 mcg EE | Ovcon-35 | | | |
| 0.15 mg levonorgestrel/30 mcg EE | Levlen, Levora, Nordette, Portia | Intermediate | Low | Intermediate |
| 0.3 mg norgestrel/30 mcg EE | Cryselle, Lo-Ovral, Low-Ogestrel | | | |
| 1 mg norethindrone/50 mcg mestranol | Necon 1/50, Norinyl 1+50, Ortho-Novum 1/50 | | Intermediate | |
| 1 mg norethindrone/35 mcg EE | Necon 1/35, Norinyl 1+35, Nortrel 1/35, Ortho-Novum 1/35 | | High | |
| 1 mg norethindrone/50 mcg EE | Ovcon-50 | | | |
| 1 mg norethindrone acetate/20 mcg EE | Loestrin 21 1/20, Loestrin Fe 1/20, Microgestin Fe 1/20 | High | Low | |
| 1.5 mg norethindrone acetate/30 mcg EE | Loestrin 21 1.5/30, Loestrin Fe 1.5/30, Microgestin Fe 1.5/30 | | | High |
| 1 mg ethynodiol diacetate/35 mcg EE | Demulen 1/35, Zovia 1/35E | | | Low |
| Desogestrel/EE 0.15 mg-20 mcg and EE 10 mcg | Kariva, Mircette | | | |
| 0.15 mg desogestrel/30 mcg EE | Apri, Desogen, Ortho-Cept | High | Intermediate | |
| 1 mg ethynodiol diacetate/50 mcg EE | Demulen 1/50, Zovia 1/50E | | | |
| 0.5 mg norgestrel/50 mcg EE | Ovral, Ogestrel | | High | High |
| 3 mg drospirinone/30 mcg EE | Yasmin | No data | Intermediate[1] | None[1] |

Monophasic

| Estimated Relative Oral Contraceptive Progestin/Estrogen/Androgen Activity | | | | | |
|---|---|---|---|---|---|
| | Ingredients | Brand-name examples | Progestin activity | Estrogen activity | Androgen activity |
| Biphasic | Norethindrone/ EE 0.5-35/ 1-35 mg-mcg | Necon 10/11, Ortho-Novum 10/11 | Inter-mediate | High | Low |
| Triphasic | Norgestimate/EE 0.18 -25/0.215-25/0.25-25 mg-mcg | Ortho Tri-Cyclen Lo | Low | Low | |
| | Levonorgestrel/EE 0.05-30/0.075-40/ 0.125-30 mg-mcg | Enpresse, Tri-Levlen, Triphasil, Trivora | | Inter-mediate | |
| | Norgestimate/EE 0.18-35/0.215-35/ 0.25-35 mg-mcg | Ortho Tri-Cyclen | | | |
| | Norethindrone/EE 0.5-35/1-35/0.5-35 mg-mcg | Tri-Norinyl | | High | |
| | Norethindrone/EE 0.5-35/0.75-35/1-35 mg-mcg | Necon 7/7/7, Ortho-Novum 7/7/7 | Inter-mediate | | |
| | Norethindrone/EE 1-20/1-30/1-35 mg-mcg | Estrostep 21, Estrostep Fe | High | Low | Inter-mediate |
| | Desogestrel/EE 0.1-25/0.125-25/ 0.15-25 mg-mcg | Cyclessa | | | Low |

EE = ethinyl estradiol.
[1] Preclinical studies have shown that drospirenone has no androgenic, estrogenic, glucocorticoid, antiglucocorticoid, or antiandrogenic activity.

*Patch:*

  *Use* – This system uses a 28-day (4-week) cycle. A new patch is applied each week for 3 weeks (21 days total). Week 4 is patch-free. Withdrawal bleeding is expected to begin during this time.

  Apply every new patch on the same day of the week. This day is known as the "Patch Change Day."

  On the day after week 4 ends, a new 4-week cycle is started by applying a new patch. Under no circumstances should there be more than a 7 day patch-free interval between dosing cycles. If there are more than 7 patch-free days, the woman may not be protected from pregnancy and back-up contraception (eg, condoms, spermicide, diaphragm) must be used for 7 days.

  *The patient must choose 1 option:*

    *First day start* – For first day start, apply the first patch during the first 24 hours of the menstrual period. If therapy starts after day 1 of the menstrual cycle, a nonhormonal back-up contraceptive (eg, condoms, spermicide, diaphragm) should be used concurrently for the first 7 consecutive days of the first treatment cycle.

    *Sunday start* – For Sunday start, apply the first patch on the first Sunday after the menstrual period starts. Use back-up contraception for the first week of the first cycle. If the menstrual period begins on a Sunday, the first patch should be applied on that day and no back-up contraception is needed.

  *Application* – Apply the patch to clean, dry, intact, healthy skin on the buttock, abdomen, upper outer arm, or upper torso in a place where it will not be rubbed by tight clothing. The patch should not be placed on skin that is red, irritated, or cut, nor should it be placed on the breasts.

  To prevent interference with the adhesive properties of the patch, no topical products should be applied to the skin area where the patch is or will be placed.

Patch changes may occur at any time on the change day. Apply each new patch to a new spot on the skin to help avoid irritation, although they may be kept within the same anatomic area.

*If a patch is partially or completely detached –*

*For less than 1 day (up to 24 hours):* Try to reapply it to the same place or replace it with a new patch immediately. No back-up contraception is needed. The woman's "patch change day" will remain the same.

*For more than 1 day (24 hours or more) or if the woman is not sure how long the patch has been detached:* The woman may not be protected from pregnancy. Stop the current contraceptive cycle and start a new cycle immediately by applying a new patch. There is now a new "day 1" and a new "patch change day." Back-up contraception (eg, condoms, spermicide, diaphragm) must be used for the first week of the new cycle.

Do not reapply a patch if it is no longer sticky, if it has become stuck to itself or another surface, if it has other material stuck to it, or if it has previously become loose or fallen off. If a patch cannot be reapplied, a new patch should be applied immediately. Do not use supplemental adhesives or wraps to hold the patch in place.

*If the woman forgets to change her patch –*

*At the start of any patch cycle (week 1/day 1):* She may not be protected from pregnancy. Apply the first patch of the new cycle as soon as she remembers. There is now a new "patch change day" and a new "day 1." Use back-up contraception for the first week of the new cycle.

*In the middle of the patch cycle (week 2/day 8 or week 3/day 15):*

*For 1 or 2 days (up to 48 hours)* – Apply a new patch immediately. The next patch should be applied on the usual "patch change day." No back-up contraception is needed.

*For more than 2 days (48 hours or more)* – She may not be protected from pregnancy. Stop the current contraceptive cycle and start a new 4-week cycle immediately by putting on a new patch. There is now a new "patch change day" and a new "day 1." Use back-up contraception for 1 week.

*At the end of the patch cycle (week 4/day 22):* If the woman forgets to remove her patch, take it off as soon as remembered. The next cycle should be started on the usual "patch change day," which is the day after day 28. No back-up contraception is needed.

*Change day adjustment* – If the woman wishes to change her patch change day, complete the current cycle, removing the third patch on the correct day. During the patch-free week, select an earlier patch change day by applying a new patch on the desired day. In no case should there be more than 7 consecutive patch-free days.

*Switching from an oral contraceptive* – Treatment with the norelgestromin/ethinyl estradiol transdermal patch should begin on the first day of withdrawal bleeding. If there is no withdrawal bleeding within 5 days of the last active (hormone-containing) tablet, pregnancy must be ruled out. If therapy starts later than the first day of withdrawal bleeding, a nonhormonal contraceptive should be used concurrently for 7 days. If more than 7 days elapse after taking the last active oral contraceptive tablet, consider the possibility of ovulation and conception.

*Use after childbirth* – Women who elect not to breast-feed should start contraceptive therapy with the norelgestromin/ethinyl estradiol transdermal patch no sooner than 4 weeks after childbirth. If a woman begins using the patch postpartum and has not yet had a period, consider the possibility of ovulation and conception occurring prior to use of the patch, and instruct her to use an additional method of contraception (eg, condoms, spermicide, diaphragm) for the first 7 days.

*Use after abortion or miscarriage* – After an abortion or miscarriage that occurs in the first trimester, the patch may be started immediately. An additional method of contraception is not needed if the patch is started immediately. If use of the patch is not started within 5 days following a first trimester abortion, the woman should follow the instructions for a woman starting the patch for the first time. In the meantime, advise her to use a nonhormonal contraceptive method. Ovulation may occur within 10 days after an abortion or miscarriage.

Do not start the patch any earlier than 4 weeks after a second trimester abortion or miscarriage. When the patch is used postpartum or postabortion, the increased risk of thromboembolic disease must be considered.

*Breakthrough bleeding or spotting* – In the event of breakthrough bleeding or spotting (bleeding that occurs on the days that the patch is worn), continue treatment. If breakthrough bleeding persists longer than a few cycles, consider a cause other than the patch.

In the event of no withdrawal bleeding (bleeding that should occur during the patch-free week), resume treatment on the next scheduled change day. If the patch has been used correctly, the absence of withdrawal bleeding is not necessarily an indication of pregnancy. Nevertheless, consider the possibility of pregnancy, especially if absence of withdrawal bleeding occurs in 2 consecutive cycles. Discontinue the patch if pregnancy is confirmed.

*Skin irritation* – If patch use results in uncomfortable irritation, the patch may be removed and a new patch may be applied to a different location until the next change day. Only 1 patch should be worn at a time.

*Missed menstrual period* – If the woman has not adhered to the prescribed schedule, consider the possibility of pregnancy at the time of the first missed period. Discontinue hormonal contraceptive use if pregnancy is confirmed.

If the woman has adhered to the prescribed regimen and misses 1 period, she should continue using her contraceptive patches.

If the woman has adhered to the prescribed regimen and misses 2 consecutive periods, rule out pregnancy. Discontinue use of the patch if pregnancy is confirmed.

*Vaginal ring:* One etonogestrel/ethinyl vaginal ring is inserted in the vagina by the patient. The ring remains in place continuously for 3 weeks. Remove for a 1-break, during which withdrawal bleeding usually occurs. Insert a new ring 1 week after the last ring was removed on the same day of the week as it was inserted in the previous cycle. Withdrawal bleeding usually starts on day 2 to 3 after removal of the ring. To maintain contraceptive effectiveness, insert the new ring 1 week after the previous one was removed even if menstrual bleeding has not finished.

*Insertion* – Choose the insertion position that is most comfortable, for example standing with one leg up, squatting, or lying down. Compress the ring and insert into the vagina. The exact position of the ring inside the vagina is not critical for its function. Insert the contraceptive vaginal ring on the appropriate day and leave in place for 3 consecutive weeks.

*Removal* – Remove the vaginal ring by hooking the index finger under the forward rim or by grasping the rim between the index and middle finger and pulling it out. Place the used ring in the sachet (foil pouch) and discard in a waste receptacle out of the reach of children and pets. Do not flush in the toilet.

*Starting the contraceptive vaginal ring* – Consider the possibility of ovulation and conception prior to the first use of the contraceptive vaginal ring.

*No preceding hormonal contraceptive use in the past month:* Counting the first day of menstruation as day 1, insert the contraceptive vaginal ring on or prior to day 5 of the cycle, even if the patient has not finished bleeding. During the first cycle, an additional method of contraception is recommended until after the first 7 days of continuous ring use.

*Switching from a combination oral contraceptive:* Insert the contraceptive vaginal ring anytime within 7 days after the last combined (estrogen plus progestin) oral contraceptive tablet and no later than the day that a new cycle of pills would have started. No backup method is needed.

*Switching from a progestin-only method:* Insert the first contraceptive vaginal ring as follows:

- Any day of the month when switching from a progestin-only pill; do not skip any days between the last pill and the first day of contraceptive vaginal ring use;
- on the same day as contraceptive implant removal;

- on the same day as removal of a progestin-containing IUD; or
- on the day when the next contraceptive injection would be due.

In all of these cases, advise the patient to use an additional method of contraception for the first 7 days after insertion of the ring.

*Following complete first-trimester abortion:* The patient may start using the contraceptive vaginal ring within the first 5 days following a complete first trimester abortion and does not need to use an additional method of contraception. If use is not started within 5 days following a first trimester abortion, the patient should follow the instructions for "No preceding hormonal contraceptive use in the past month." Advise the patient to use a nonhormonal contraceptive method.

*Following delivery or second-trimester abortion:* Initiate the use of the contraceptive vaginal ring 4 weeks postpartum in women who elect not to breast-feed. Advise women who are breast-feeding not to use the contraceptive vaginal ring but to use other forms of contraception until the child is weaned. Initiate use of the contraceptive vaginal ring 4 weeks after a second-trimester abortion. When the contraceptive vaginal ring is used postpartum or postabortion, consider the increased risk of thromboembolic disease. If the patient begins using the contraceptive vaginal ring postpartum and has not yet had a period, consider the possibility of ovulation and conception occurring prior to initiation of the contraceptive vaginal ring. Instruct the patient to use an additional method of contraception for the first 7 days.

*Inadvertent removal, expulsion, or prolonged ring-free interval:* If the contraceptive vaginal ring has been out during the 3-week use period, rinse with cool to lukewarm water and reinsert as soon as possible, at the latest within 3 hours. If the ring has been out of the vagina for more than 3 hours, contraceptive effectiveness may be reduced. Use an additional method of contraception until the contraceptive vaginal ring has been used continuously for 7 days.

Consider the possibility of pregnancy if the ring-free interval has been extended beyond 1 week. Use an additional method of contraception until the contraceptive vaginal ring has been used continuously for 7 days.

*Prolonged use:* If the contraceptive vaginal ring has been left in place for up to 1 extra week (ie, up to 4 weeks total), remove it and insert a new ring after a 1-week ring-free interval. Rule out pregnancy if the contraceptive vaginal ring has been left in place for more than 4 weeks. Use an additional method of contraception until the contraceptive vaginal ring has been used continuously for 7 days.

*In the event of a missed menstrual period:* If the patient has not adhered to the prescribed regimen, consider the possibility of pregnancy at the time of the first missed period and discontinue the use of the contraceptive vaginal ring if pregnancy is confirmed.

Rule out pregnancy if the patient has adhered to the prescribed regimen and misses 2 consecutive periods.

### Actions

*Pharmacology:* Oral contraceptives (OCs) include estrogen-progestin combinations and progestin-only products.

*Progestin-only* – Progestin-only OCs prevent conception by suppressing ovulation in about 50% of users, thickening the cervical mucus to inhibit sperm penetration, lowering the midcycle luteinizing hormone (LH) and follicle-stimulating hormone (FSH) peaks, slowing the movement of the ovum through the fallopian tubes, and altering the endometrium.

*Combination OCs* – Combination OCs inhibit ovulation by suppressing the gonadotropins, FSH, and LH. Additionally, alterations in the genital tract, including cervical mucus (which inhibits sperm penetration) and the endometrium (which reduces the likelihood of implantation), may contribute to contraceptive effectiveness.

*Vaginal ring:* The contraceptive vaginal ring is a nonbiodegradable, flexible, transparent, colorless to almost colorless combination contraceptive vaginal ring containing etonogestrel and ethinyl estradiol. When placed in the vagina, each ring releases on average 0.12 mg/day of etonogestrel and 0.015 mg/day of ethinyl estradiol over a 3-week period of use.

There are 3 types of combination OCs: Monophasic, biphasic, and triphasic.

*Monophasic* – Fixed dosage of estrogen to progestin throughout the cycle.

*Biphasic* – Amount of estrogen remains the same for the first 21 days of the cycle. Decreased progestin:estrogen ratio in first half of cycle allows endometrial proliferation. Increased ratio in second half provides adequate secretory development.

*Triphasic* – Estrogen amount remains the same or varies throughout cycle. Progestin amount varies.

*Pharmacokinetics:*

*Estrogens* – Ethinyl estradiol is rapidly absorbed with peak concentrations attained in 1 to 2 hours. It undergoes considerable first-pass elimination. Mestranol is demethylated to ethinyl estradiol. Ethinyl estradiol is approximately 97% to 98% bound to plasma albumin. Half-life varies from 6 to 20 hours. It is excreted in bile and urine as conjugates, and undergoes some enterohepatic recirculation.

*Progestins* – Peak concentrations of norethindrone occur 0.5 to 4 hours after oral administration; it undergoes first-pass metabolism with an overall bioavailability of approximately 65%. Levonorgestrel reaches peak concentrations between 0.5 to 2 hours, does not undergo a first-pass effect, and is completely bioavailable. Norethindrone and levonorgestrel are chiefly metabolized by reduction followed by conjugation. Desogestrel is rapidly and completely absorbed and converted into 3-keto-desogestrel, the biologically active metabolite. Relative bioavailability is approximately 84%. Maximum concentrations of the metabolite are reached at approximately 1.4 hours. Norgestimate is well absorbed; peak serum concentrations are observed within 2 hours followed by a rapid decline to levels generally below assay within 5 hours. However, a major metabolite, 17-deacetyl norgestimate, appears rapidly in serum with concentrations greatly exceeding that of the parent. Both norethynodrel and ethynodiol diacetate are converted to norethindrone. Peak serum concentrations of drospirenone are reached 1 to 3 hours after administration. Progestins are bound to albumin (79% to 95%) and to sex hormone binding globulin (except drospirenone). Terminal half-life of the progestins are as follows: Norethindrone, 5 to 14 hours; levonorgestrel, 11 to 45 hours; desogestrel (metabolite), 38 $\pm$ 20 hours; norgestimate (metabolite), 12 to 30 hours; drospirenone, 30 hours. Progestin-only administration results in lower steady-state serum progestin levels and a shorter elimination half-life than coadministration with estrogens.

*Patch* – Following application, norelgestromin and ethinyl estradiol rapidly appear in the serum, plateau by about 48 hours, and are maintained at steady state throughout the wear period. The metabolites of norelgestromin and ethinyl estradiol are eliminated by renal and fecal pathways.

*Vaginal ring* – Etonogestrel and ethinyl estradiol released by the vaginal ring are rapidly absorbed. Bioavailability of etonogestrel after vaginal administration is about 100%. Bioavailability of ethinyl estradiol after vaginal administration is about 55.6%, which is comparable to that with oral administration of ethinyl estradiol. Etonogestrel is about 66% bound to albumin in blood. Ethinyl estradiol is highly bound to albumin.

In vitro data show that both etonogestrel and ethinyl estradiol are metabolized in liver microsomes by the cytochrome P450 3A4 isoenzyme. Etonogestrel and ethinyl estradiol are primarily eliminated in urine, bile, and feces.

### Contraindications

Thrombophlebitis; thromboembolic disorders; history of deep-vein thrombophlebitis; cerebral vascular disease; MI; coronary artery disease; known or suspected breast carcinoma or estrogen-dependent neoplasia; carcinoma of endometrium; hepatic adenomas/carcinomas (see Warnings); undiagnosed abnormal genital bleeding; known or suspected pregnancy (see Warnings); cholestatic jaundice of pregnancy/jaundice with prior pill use; hypersensitivity to any component of the product;

acute liver disease; uncontrolled hypertension; headaches with focal neurological symptoms; diabetes with vascular complications; major surgery with prolonged immobility.

*Yasmin:* Renal insufficiency, hepatic dysfunction, adrenal insufficiency, heavy smoking (15 or more cigarettes per day) and over 35 years of age.

**Warnings**

*Cigarette smoking:* See Warning Box.

*Hyperkalemia: Yasmin* contains the progestin drospirenone that has antimineralocorticoid activity, including the potential for hyperkalemia in high-risk patients, comparable to a 25 mg dose of spironolactone. *Yasmin* should not be used in patients with conditions that predispose to hyperkalemia. Women receiving daily, long-term treatment for chronic conditions or diseases with medications that may increase serum potassium should have their serum potassium level checked during the first treatment cycle.

*Risks of OC use:* The use of OCs is associated with increased risk of thromboembolism, stroke, MI, hypertension, hepatic neoplasia, and gallbladder disease, although risk of serious morbidity or mortality is very small in healthy women without underlying risk factors.

*Mortality:* Mortality associated with all methods of birth control is low and below that associated with childbirth, with the exception of OC use in women 35 or older who smoke and 40 and older who do not smoke. The Fertility and Maternal Health Drugs Advisory Committee recommended that the benefits of low-dose OC use by healthy nonsmoking women older than 40 years of age may outweigh the possible risks. Like all women, older women who take oral contraceptives should take an oral contraceptive that contains the least amount of estrogen and progestin that is compatible with a low failure rate and individual patient needs.

*Thromboembolism:* Be alert to the earliest symptoms of thromboembolic and thrombotic disorders. Should any of these occur or be suspected, discontinue the drug immediately.

The risk of nonfatal venous thrombosis with third-generation OCs (desogestrel, gestodene, and norgestimate) is 2 to 3 times the risk of second-generation OCs. The risk of development of deep vein thrombosis was found to be 2 to 5 times higher with low-estrogen, desogestrel-containing OCs than with second-generation monophasic and triphasic preparations.

*MI* – MI risk associated with OC use is increased. This risk is primarily in smokers or women with other underlying risk factors for coronary artery disease such as hypertension, hypercholesterolemia, morbid obesity, and diabetes. The risk is very low in women younger than 30 years of age.

*Long-term use* – Data suggest that the increased risk of MI persists after discontinuation of long-term OC use; the highest risk group includes women 40 to 49 years of age who used OCs for 5 years or more.

*Smoking* – Smoking in combination with OC use has been shown to contribute substantially to the incidence of MIs in women in their mid-30s or older, with smoking accounting for the majority of excess cases. Mortality rates associated with circulatory disease have been shown to increase substantially in smokers, especially in those 35 years of age and older who use OCs.

*Cerebrovascular diseases* – OCs increase the risks of cerebrovascular events (thrombotic and hemorrhagic strokes). In general, the risk is greatest in hypertensive women older than 35 years of age who also smoke.

*Vascular disease* – A positive association is observed between the amount of estrogen and progestin in OCs and the risk of vascular disease. A decline in serum high-density lipoproteins (HDL) has occurred with progestins and has been associated with an increased incidence of ischemic heart disease. Because estrogens increase HDL cholesterol, the net effect depends on a balance achieved between doses of estrogen and progestin and the activity of the progestin used in the contraceptives.

*Age* – The risk of cerebrovascular and circulatory disease in OC users is substantially increased in women 35 years of age and older with other risk factors (eg, smoking, uncontrolled hypertension, hypercholesterolemia [LDL 190], obesity, diabetes).

*Postsurgical thromboembolism* – Risk is increased 2- to 4-fold. If possible, discontinue OCs at least 4 weeks before and 2 weeks after surgery and during and following prolonged immobilization because OCs are associated with an increased risk of thromboembolism.

*Subarachnoid hemorrhage* – Subarachnoid hemorrhage has been increased by OC use.

*Persistence of risk* – An increased risk may persist for 6 years or more after discontinuation of OC use for cerebrovascular disease and 9 years or more for MI in users 40 to 49 years of age who had used OCs 5 years or more. This information is based on studies that used OCs containing 50 mcg estrogen or more.

NOTE – The associations between OCs and cardiovascular disease are based on epidemiological studies whose conclusions have been criticized for several reasons: National trends of cardiovascular mortality are incompatible with these risk estimates; excess deaths may not be attributable entirely to smoking; the clinical diagnosis of thromboembolism is often unreliable.

*Ocular lesions:* Ocular lesions such as optic neuritis or retinal thrombosis have been associated with the use of hormonal contraceptives.

*Risks of use immediately preceding pregnancy:* Some extensive epidemiological studies have revealed no increased risk of birth defects in OC users prior to pregnancy.

*Carcinoma:* While there are conflicting reports, the overall evidence in the literature suggests that use of OCs is not associated with an increase in the risk of developing breast cancer, regardless of age and parity of first use. Women with breast cancer should not use OCs because the role of female hormones in breast cancer has not been fully determined.

Studies have reported an increased risk of endometrial carcinoma associated with the prolonged use of estrogen in postmenopausal women. The risk appears to be decreased in OC users because of the progestin component. Users appear about half as likely to develop ovarian and endometrial cancer as women who have never used OCs. The protective effect from endometrial cancer lasts up to 15 years after the pills are stopped.

Close clinical surveillance of all women taking OCs is essential; they should be reexamined at least once a year. In all cases of undiagnosed persistent or recurrent abnormal vaginal bleeding, rule out malignancy. Monitor women with a strong family history of breast cancer or who have breast nodules, fibrocystic disease of the breast, cervical dysplasia, or abnormal mammograms.

*Hepatic lesions (adenomas, focal nodular hyperplasia, hepatocellular carcinoma, etc):* Rarely, benign and malignant hepatic adenomas have been associated with the use of hormonal contraceptives. Severe abdominal pain, shock, or death may be due to rupture and hemorrhage of a liver tumor.

*Pregnancy test:* Do not administer to induce withdrawal bleeding as a test for pregnancy.

*Carbohydrate metabolism:* Glucose tolerance may decrease. Monitor prediabetic and diabetic women closely.

*Lipid profile:* Triglycerides may increase.

*Elevated blood pressure:* Elevated blood pressure and hypertension may occur within a few months of beginning use. The prevalence increases with the duration of use and age. Incidence of hypertension may directly correlate with increasing dosages of progestin. Discontinue use if elevated blood pressure occurs. Encourage women with a history of hypertension or hypertension-related diseases during pregnancy, or renal disease to use another method of contraception.

*Headaches:* Onset or exacerbation of migraine or development of headache with a new pattern which is recurrent, persistent, or severe, requires hormonal contraceptive discontinuation and evaluation.

*Bleeding irregularities:* Breakthrough bleeding (BTB), spotting, and amenorrhea are frequent reasons for discontinuing hormonal contraceptives. Changing to an OC with a higher estrogen content may minimize menstrual irregularity, but consider the increased risk of thromboembolic disease. Consider short-term estrogen supplements.

*Seasonale* – When prescribing *Seasonale*, the convenience of fewer planned menses (4 per year instead of 13 per year) should be weighed against the inconvenience of increased intermenstrual bleeding and/or spotting.

*Progestin-only products* – Episodes of irregular, unpredictable spotting, and BTB within the first year are the most frequently encountered side effects and are the major reasons why women discontinue hormonal contraceptive use.

*Vaginal ring* – Breakthrough bleeding and spotting are sometimes encountered in women using the contraceptive vaginal ring. If abnormal bleeding persists or is severe, rule out the possibility of organic pathology or pregnancy. Rule out pregnancy in the event of amenorrhea.

*Menopause:* Treatment with hormonal contraceptives may mask the onset of the climacteric.

*Fertility impairment:* Fertility impairment may occur in women discontinuing OCs; however, impairment diminishes with time.

*Elderly:* This vaginal ring has not been studied in women 65 years of age and older and is not indicated in this population.

*Pregnancy: Category* X. Rule out pregnancy before initiating or continuing the any hormonal contraceptives, and always consider it if withdrawal bleeding does not occur or for any patient who has missed 2 consecutive periods.

Ectopic as well as intrauterine pregnancy may occur in contraceptive failures.

*Lactation:* Hormonal contraceptives may interfere with lactation, decreasing both the quantity and the quality of breast milk. A small amount of OC steroids is excreted in breast milk. A few adverse effects on the nursing infant have been reported, including jaundice and breast enlargement.

*Vaginal ring* – Advise women who are breast-feeding not to use the contraceptive vaginal ring but to use other forms of contraception until the child is weaned.

*Children:* Safety and efficacy are expected to be the same for postpubertal adolescents up to 16 years of age. Use of this product before menarche is not indicated.

### Precautions

*Monitoring:* Pretreatment and annual exams should include blood pressure, breasts, abdomen and pelvic organs, including Papanicolaou smear. Perform preventative measures and screening, which should include total and HDL cholesterol within 5-year intervals. Advise the pathologist of OC therapy when relevant specimens are submitted. Do not prescribe for more than 1 year without another physical exam.

*Lipid disorders:* Closely follow women taking OCs who are being treated for hyperlipidemias.

*Uterine fibroids:* Preexisting uterine leiomyomata (uterine fibroids) may increase in size. However, there is no evidence of this with low-dose hormonal contraceptives.

*Depression:* The incidence of depression in OC users ranges from less than 5% to 30%. Pyridoxine deficiency may be a factor in the depression. Women who become significantly depressed when using hormonal contraceptives should stop the medication and use another form of contraception.

*Fluid retention:* OCs may cause fluid retention.

*Body weight 90 kg or more (198 lbs):*
Patch – Results of clinical trials suggest that the norelgestromin/ethinyl estradiol transdermal patch may be less effective in women with body weight 90 kg or more (198 lbs) than in women with lower body weights.

*Hepatic function:* Patients with a history of jaundice during pregnancy have an increased risk of recurrence of jaundice. If jaundice develops, discontinue the medication.

*Contact lenses:* Contact lens wearers who develop changes in vision or lens tolerance should be assessed by an ophthalmologist; consider temporary or permanent cessation of wear.

*Vaginal use:* The contraceptive vaginal ring may not be suitable in conditions that make the vagina more susceptible to vaginal irritation or ulceration.

The contraceptive vaginal ring may interfere with the correct placement and position of a diaphragm. A diaphragm is not recommended as a backup method with contraceptive vaginal ring use.

*Expulsion* – The contraceptive vaginal ring can be accidentally expelled, for example, when it has not been inserted properly, or while removing a tampon, moving the bowels, straining, or with severe constipation. If this occurs, rinse the vaginal ring with cool to lukewarm (not hot) water and reinsert promptly. If the contraceptive vaginal ring is lost, insert a new vaginal ring and continue the regimen without alteration. If the ring has been out of the vagina for more than 3 hours, contraceptive effectiveness may be reduced and an additional method of contraception (eg, male condom, spermicide) must be used until the ring has been used continuously for 7 days. Vaginal stenosis, cervical prolapse, rectoceles, and cystoceles are conditions that under some circumstances may make expulsion more likely to occur.

*Serum folate levels:* Serum folate levels may be depressed by therapy.

*Acute intermittent porphyria:* Estrogens have been reported to precipitate attacks of acute intermittent porphyria.

*Vomiting/Diarrhea:* Several cases of OC failure have been reported in association with vomiting or diarrhea. If significant GI disturbance occurs, a back-up method of contraception for the remainder of the cycle is recommended.

*Sexually transmitted diseases (STDs):* Advise patients that hormonal contraceptives do not protect against HIV infection and other STDs.

## Drug Interactions

Drugs that may affect oral contraceptives include antibiotics, atorvastatin, barbiturates, carbamazepine, CYP3A4 inhibitors (eg, itraconazole, ketoconazole) felbamate, griseofulvin, hydantoins, oxcarbazepine, phenytoin, primidone, protease inhibitors, rifampin, St. John's wort, topiramate, and miconazole (vaginal ring). Drugs that may be affected by oral contraceptives include anticoagulants, benzodiazepines, beta blockers, caffeine, corticosteroids, cyclosporine, prednisolone, theophyllines, tricyclic antidepressants, lamotrigine, and selegiline.

*Drug/Lab test interactions:* Estrogen-containing hormonal contraceptives may cause the following alterations in serum, plasma or blood, unless specified otherwise.

*Increased* – Factors I (prothrombin), VII, VIII, IX, X; fibrinogen; norepinephrine-induced platelet aggregation; thyroid binding globulin (TBG), leading to increased total thyroid hormone (as measured by protein bound iodine or $T_4$); corticosteroid levels; triglycerides and phospholipids; aldosterone; amylase; gamma-glutamyl-transpeptidase; iron binding capacity; sex-hormone-binding globulins are increased and result in elevated levels of total circulating sex steroids (combination); corticoids; transferrin; prolactin; renin activity; vitamin A.

*Decreased* – Antithrombin III; free $T_3$ resin uptake; response to metyrapone test; folate; glucose tolerance; albumin; cholinesterase; haptoglobin; tissue plasminogen activator; zinc; vitamin $B_{12}$; sex-hormone-binding globulin, thyroxine due to decrease in thyroid-binding globulin (progestin-only).

## Adverse Reactions

Serious adverse reactions that may occur include thrombophlebitis and venous thrombosis with or without embolism; pulmonary embolism; coronary thrombosis; MI; cerebral thrombosis; arterial thromboembolism; cerebral hemorrhage; hypertension; gallbladder disease; hepatic adenomas or benign liver tumors; mesenteric thrombosis. Other adverse reactions that may occur include nausea and vomiting (10% to 30% of patients during the first cycle, less common with low doses, and majority resolve in 3 months); abdominal cramps; bloating; breakthrough bleeding (majority, more than 80%, resolve in 3 months); spotting; change in menstrual flow; amenorrhea during and after treatment; change in cervical erosion and cervical secretions; vaginal candidiasis; temporary infertility after discontinuation; melasma (may persist); rash (allergic); migraine; mental depression; headache; dizziness; contact lens intolerance; edema; weight change; changes in corneal curvature (steepening); neuro-ocular lesions; upper respiratory tract infection; leukorrhea; sinusitis; breast tenderness/enlargement/secretion; diminution in lactation when given immediately postpartum; cholestatic jaundice; invasive cervical cancer; prevalence of cervical chlamydia trachomatis may be increased.

*Emergency contraceptives:* The most common adverse events in the clinical trial for women receiving emergency contraceptives include nausea; abdominal pain/cramps; fatigue; headache; menstrual irregularities; dizziness; breast tenderness; vomiting; diarrhea.

*Device-related:* Device-related events (foreign body sensation, coital problems, device expulsion), vaginal symptoms (discomfort/vaginitis/leukorrhea), headache, emotional lability, and weight gain.

# LEVONORGESTREL IMPLANTS

**Kit:** 6 capsules (each contains 36 mg levonorgestrel) (*Rx*)    *Norplant System* (Wyeth)

## Indications

*Prevention of pregnancy:* The implant system is a long-term (5 years or less) reversible contraceptive system. Remove the capsules by the end of the 5th year; new capsules may be inserted at that time if continuing contraceptive protection is desired.

## Administration and Dosage

Levonorgestrel implants consist of 6 *Silastic* capsules; each capsule is 2.4 mm in diameter and 34 mm in length and contains 36 mg levonorgestrel. Total administered (implanted) dose is 216 mg. Perform implantation of all 6 capsules during the first 7 days of menses onset. Insertion is subdermal in the mid-portion of the upper arm (see literature included with the product).

## Actions

*Pharmacology:* Diffusion of levonorgestrel through the wall of each capsule provides a continuous low dose of the progestin. Because of the range of variability in blood levels and variation in individual response, blood levels alone are not predictive of the risk of pregnancy in an individual woman.

*Pharmacokinetics:* Levonorgestrel concentrations among women show considerable variation. They reach a maximum, or near maximum, within 24 hours after placement with mean values of 1600 pg/mL. Levels decline rapidly over the first month. Mean levels decline to values of around 400 pg/mL at 3 months to 258 pg/mL at 60 months.

Concentrations decrease with increasing body weight by a mean of 3.3 pg/mL/ kg. After capsule removal, mean concentrations drop to less than 100 pg/mL by 96 hours and to below assay sensitivity (50 pg/mL) by 5 to 14 days.

*Contraceptive efficacy* –

| Annual and 5-Year Cumulative Pregnancy Rates Per 100 Levonorgestrel Implant Users by Weight | | | | | | |
|---|---|---|---|---|---|---|
| | Year | | | | | |
| Weight | 1 | 2 | 3 | 4 | 5 | Cumulative |
| < 50 kg (< 110 lbs) | 0.2 | 0 | 0 | 0 | 0 | 0.2 |
| 50-59 kg (110-130 lbs) | 0.2 | 0.5 | 0.4 | 2 | 0.4 | 3.4 |
| 60-69 kg (131-153 lbs) | 0.4 | 0.5 | 1.6 | 1.7 | 0.8 | 5 |
| ≥ 70 kg (≥ 154 lbs) | 0 | 1.1 | 5.1 | 2.5 | 0 | 8.5 |
| All | 0.2 | 0.5 | 1.2 | 1.6 | 0.4 | 3.9 |

## Contraindications

Active thrombophlebitis or thromboembolic disorders; undiagnosed abnormal genital bleeding; known or suspected pregnancy; acute liver disease; benign or malignant liver tumors; known or suspected carcinoma of the breast; history of idiopathic intracranial hypertension; hypersensitivity to levonorgestrel or any component of the product.

## Warnings

*Insertion and removal complications:* A surgical incision is required to insert the capsules. Complications related to insertion (eg, pain, edema, bruising, infection) may occur. There have been reports of arm pain, numbness, and tingling following the insertion and removal procedures. There also have been reports of nerve injury, most commonly associated with deep placement and removal. Expulsion of capsules has been reported more frequently when placement of the capsules was shallow or too close to the incision or when infection was present.

*Bleeding irregularities:* Most women can expect some variation in menstrual bleeding patterns. Irregular menstrual bleeding, intermenstrual spotting, prolonged episodes of bleeding and spotting, and amenorrhea occur in some women. Overall, these irregularities diminish with continuing use. After a pattern of regular menses, 6 weeks or more of amenorrhea may signal pregnancy. If pregnancy occurs, the capsules must be removed.

*Delayed follicular atresia:* If follicular development occurs, atresia of the follicle is some-times delayed and the follicle may continue to grow beyond the size it would attain in a normal cycle.

*Ectopic pregnancies:* The risk of ectopic pregnancy may increase with the duration of use and, possibly, with increased weight of the user. Any patient who presents with lower abdominal pain must be evaluated to rule out ectopic pregnancy.

*Foreign body carcinogenesis:* Rarely, cancers have occurred at the site of foreign body intru-sions or old scars.

*Thromboembolic disorders:* Patients who develop active thrombophlebitis or thromboem-bolic disease should have the levonorgestrel capsules removed. Also consider removal in women who will be immobilized for a prolonged period due to surgery or other illnesses.

*Cerebrovascular disorders* – Combination oral contraceptives have been shown to increase the relative and attributable risks of cerebrovascular events (thrombotic and hemorrhagic strokes), although, in general, the risk is greatest among older (older than 35 years of age) hypertensive women who also smoke.

*MI* – An increased risk of MI has been attributed to combination oral contracep-tive use.

Studies indicate a significant trend toward higher rates of MI and strokes with increasing doses of progestin in combination oral contraceptives. There have been postmarketing reports of MI coincident with levonorgestrel implant system use.

*Idiopathic intracranial hypertension:* There have been reports of idiopathic intracranial hyper-tension. A cardinal sign of idiopathic intracranial hypertension is papilledema; early symptoms may include headache (associated with a change in frequency, pattern, severity, or persistence; of particular importance are those headaches that are unre-mitting in nature) and visual disturbances.

*Pregnancy:* Category X.

*Lactation:* Levonorgestrel has been identified in breast milk. No significant effects were observed on growth or health of infants whose mothers used implants beginning 6 weeks after parturition.

*Children:* Safety and efficacy are expected to be similar for postpubertal adolescents younger than 16 years of age and users 16 years of age or older. Use of this prod-uct before menarche is not indicated.

### Precautions

*Physical examination and follow-up:* Take a complete medical history and physical examina-tion prior to the implantation or re-implantation of levonorgestrel implants and at least annually during its use. Carefully monitor women with a strong family his-tory of breast cancer or who have breast nodules.

*Carbohydrate and lipid metabolism:* Effects of implants on carbohydrate metabolism appear to be minimal. Carefully observe diabetic and prediabetic patients.

Closely follow women who are being treated for hyperlipidemias.

*Liver function:* If jaundice develops consider removing the capsules.

*Fluid retention:* Prescribe with caution, and only with careful monitoring, in patients with conditions which might be aggravated by fluid retention.

*Emotional disorders:* Consider removing the capsules in women who become signifi-cantly depressed since the symptom may be drug-related. Carefully observe women with a history of depression and consider removal if depression recurs to a serious degree.

*Contact lens:* Contact lens wearers who develop changes in vision or in lens tolerance should be assessed by an ophthalmologist.

*Autoimmune disease:* There have been rare reports of various autoimmune diseases (eg, scleroderma, systemic lupus erythematosus, rheumatoid arthritis) in levonorgestrel implant users; however, the rate of reporting is significantly less than the expected incidence for these diseases.

*Insertion and removal:* To be sure that the woman is not pregnant at the time of capsule placement and to ensure contraceptive efficacy during the first cycle of use, insert capsules during the first 7 days of the cycle or immediately after an abortion. Insertion is not recommended before 6 weeks postpartum in breast-feeding women.

*Infection:* If infection occurs, institute suitable treatment. If infection persists, remove the capsules.

*Expulsion:* Expulsion of capsules occurs more frequently when placement of the capsules is extremely shallow, too close to the incision, or when infection is present. Replacement of an expelled capsule must be accomplished using a new sterile capsule. If infection is present, treat and cure before replacement. Contraceptive efficacy may be inadequate with less than 6 capsules.

*Provisions for removal:* The removal should be done on such request or at the end of 5 years of usage by personnel instructed in the removal technique.

## Drug Interactions

*Carbamazepine and phenytoin:* Reduced efficacy (pregnancy) has occurred. Warn users of the possibility of decreased efficacy with use of any related drugs.

*Drug/Lab test interactions:* Certain endocrine tests may be affected by levonorgestrel implants: Sex hormone binding globulin concentrations are decreased; thyroxine concentrations may be slightly decreased and triiodothyronine uptake increased.

## Adverse Reactions

Adverse reactions occurring in at least 3% of patients include prolonged bleeding; spotting; amenorrhea; irregular bleeding; frequent bleeding onsets; removal difficulties affecting patients; scanty bleeding; breast discharge; cervicitis; musculoskeletal pain; abdominal discomfort; leukorrhea; vaginitis; pain or itching near implant site.

# MEDROXYPROGESTERONE ACETATE

**Injection:** 150 mg/mL (*Rx*)                    *Depo-Provera* (Upjohn)

### Indications

*Prevention of pregnancy:* It is a long-term injectable contraceptive in women when administered at 3-month intervals.

### Administration and Dosage

Shake the vial vigorously just before use to ensure that the dose being administered represents a uniform suspension.

The recommended dose is 150 mg every 3 months administered by deep IM injection in the gluteal or deltoid muscle. To increase assurance that the patient is not pregnant at the time of the first administration, give this injection only during the first 5 days after the onset of a normal menstrual period; within 5 days postpartum if not breast-feeding; or, if breast-feeding, at 6 weeks postpartum. If the period between injections is more than 14 weeks, determine that the patient is not pregnant before administering the drug.

### Actions

*Pharmacology:* Medroxyprogesterone, when administered IM at the recommended dose to women every 3 months, inhibits the secretion of gonadotropins which, in turn, prevents follicular maturation and ovulation and results in endometrial thinning. These actions produce its contraceptive effect.

*Pharmacokinetics:* Following a single 150 mg IM dose, medroxyprogesterone concentrations increase for approximately 3 weeks to reach peak plasma concentrations of 1 to 7 ng/mL. The levels then decrease exponentially until they become undetectable (less than 100 pg/mL) between 120 to 200 days following injection. The apparent half-life following IM administration is approximately 50 days.

### Contraindications

Known or suspected pregnancy or as a diagnostic test for pregnancy; undiagnosed vaginal bleeding; known or suspected malignancy of breast; active thrombophlebitis, or current or past history of thromboembolic disorders, or cerebral vascular disease; liver dysfunction or disease; hypersensitivity to medroxyprogesterone or any of its other ingredients.

### Warnings

*Bleeding irregularities:* Most women experience disruption of menstrual bleeding patterns. If abnormal bleeding persists or is severe, institute appropriate investigation to rule out the possibility of organic pathology, and institute appropriate treatment when necessary.

*Bone mineral density changes:* Use of medroxyprogesterone may be considered among the risk factors for development of osteoporosis. The rate of bone loss is greatest in the early years of use and then subsequently approaches the normal rate of age-related fall.

*Thromboembolic disorders:* Be alert to the earliest manifestations of thrombotic disorders. If any of these occur or are suspected, do not readminister the drug.

*Ocular disorders:* Do not readminister pending examination if there is a sudden partial or complete loss of vision or if there is a sudden onset of proptosis, diplopia, or migraine. If examination reveals papilledema or retinal vascular lesions, do not readminister.

*Carcinogenesis:* Long-term case-controlled surveillance of users found slight or no increased overall risk of breast cancer and no overall increased risk of ovarian, liver, or cervical cancer and a prolonged, protective effect of reducing the risk of endometrial cancer in the population of users.

*Pregnancy: Category* X.

*Lactation:* Detectable amounts of the drug have been identified in the milk of mothers receiving medroxyprogesterone. In nursing mothers treated with medroxyprogesterone, milk composition, quality, and amount are not adversely affected. Infants exposed to medroxyprogesterone via breast milk have been studied for developmental and behavioral effects through puberty; no adverse effects have been noted.

**Precautions**

*Physical examination:* The pretreatment and annual history and physical examination should include special reference to breast and pelvic organs, as well as a Papanicolaou smear.

*Fluid retention:* Because progestational drugs may cause some degree of fluid retention, conditions that might be influenced by this condition require careful observation.

*Weight changes:* There is a tendency for women to gain weight while on medroxyprogesterone therapy.

*Return of fertility:* Medroxyprogesterone has a prolonged contraceptive effect. It is expected that 68% of women who do become pregnant may conceive within 12 months, 83% may conceive within 15 months and 93% may conceive within 18 months from the last injection.

*CNS disorders and convulsions:* Carefully observe patients who have a history of psychic depression; do not readminister if the depression recurs.

There have been a few reported cases of convulsions. Association with drug use or preexisting conditions is not clear.

*Carbohydrate metabolism:* A decrease in glucose tolerance has been observed in some patients. Carefully observe diabetic patients during therapy.

*Liver function:* If jaundice develops, consider not readministering the drug.

**Drug Interactions**

Drugs that may interact with medroxyprogesterone include aminoglutethimide.

*Drug/Lab test interactions:* The following laboratory tests may be affected by medroxyprogesterone: Plasma and urinary steroid levels are decreased; gonadotropin levels are decreased; sex-hormone binding globulin concentrations are decreased; protein bound iodine and butanol extractable protein bound iodine may increase; $T_3$ uptake values may decrease; coagulation test values for prothrombin (Factor II), and Factors VII, VIII, IX, and X may increase. Sulfobromophthalein and other liver function test values may be increased; the effects of medroxyprogesterone acetate on lipid metabolism are inconsistent. Both increases and decreases in total cholesterol, triglycerides, low-density lipoprotein (LDL) cholesterol, and high-density lipoprotein (HDL) cholesterol have been observed.

**Adverse Reactions**

Common (at least 3%) adverse reactions include menstrual irregularities; weight changes; headache; nervousness; abdominal pain; discomfort; asthenia; dizziness.

# ANDROGENS

| **FLUOXYMESTERONE** | |
| --- | --- |
| **Tablets**: 10 mg (*c-iii*) | Various |
| **METHYLTESTOSTERONE** | |
| **Tablets**: 10 mg (*c-iii*) | Various, *Methitest* (Global) |
| 25 mg (*c-iii*) | Various, *Methitest* (Global) |
| **Tablets (buccal)**: 10 mg (*c-iii*) | Various |
| **Capsules**: 10 mg (*c-iii*) | *Android* (ICN Pharm), *Testred* (Valeant), *Virilon* (Star) |
| **Injection**: 200 mg/mL (*c-iii*) | *Virilon IM* (Star) |
| **TESTOSTERONE, LONG-ACTING** | |
| **TESTOSTERONE ENANTHATE (IN OIL)** | |
| **Injection**: 200 mg/mL (*c-iii*) | *Delatestryl* (BTG) |
| **TESTOSTERONE CYPIONATE (IN OIL)** | |
| **Injection**: 100 mg/mL, 200 mg/mL (*c-iii*) | *Depo-Testosterone* (Pharmacia) |
| **TESTOSTERONE PELLETS** | |
| **Pellets**: 75 mg (*c-iii*) | *Testopel* (Bartor Pharmacal) |
| **TESTOSTERONE TRANSDERMAL SYSTEM** | |
| **Patch**: 24.3 mg testosterone (*c-iii*) | *Androderm* (Watson Pharma) |
| 12.2 mg testosterone (*c-iii*) | *Androderm* (Watson Pharma) |
| **TESTOSTERONE GEL** | |
| **Gel**: 1% testosterone (*c-iii*) | *AndroGel 1%* (Unimed Pharm), *Testim* (Auxilum Pharm) |
| **TESTOSTERONE, BUCCAL** | |
| **Buccal system**: 30 mg (*Rx*) | *Striant* (Columbia) |

Anabolic steroids are classified as a *c-iii* controlled substance under the anabolic steroids act of 1990.

**Indications**

*Males:*

*Replacement therapy* – Replacement therapy in hypogonadism associated with a deficiency or absence of endogenous testosterone. Prior to puberty, androgen replacement therapy is needed for development of secondary sexual characteristics. Prolonged treatment is required to maintain sexual characteristics in these and other males who develop testosterone deficiency after puberty. Appropriate adrenal cortical and thyroid hormone replacement therapy are still necessary, however, and are of primary importance.

*Primary hypogonadism (congenital or acquired):* Testicular failure due to cryptorchidism, bilateral torsion, orchitis, vanishing testis syndrome, or orchidectomy; Klinefelter syndrome, chemotherapy, or toxic damage from alcohol or heavy metals.

*Hypogonadotropic hypogonadism (congenital or acquired):* Idiopathic gonadotropin or luteinizing hormone releasing hormone (LHRH) deficiency or pituitary-hypothalamic injury from tumors, trauma, or radiation.

*Delayed puberty:* To stimulate puberty in carefully selected males with clearly delayed puberty. Brief treatment with conservative doses may be justified if these patients do not respond to psychological support.

*Females:*

*Metastatic cancer* – May be used secondarily in women with advancing inoperable metastatic (skeletal) breast cancer who are 1 to 5 years postmenopausal. Primary goals of therapy include ablation of the ovaries. This treatment has been used in premenopausal women with breast cancer who have benefited from oophorectomy and have a hormone-responsive tumor.

### Administration and Dosage

FLUOXYMESTERONE:

Males –

Hypogonadism: 5 to 20 mg/day.

Delayed puberty: Carefully titrate dosage using a low dose, appropriate skeletal monitoring, and by limiting the duration of therapy to 4 to 6 months.

Females –

Inoperable breast carcinoma: 10 to 40 mg/day in divided doses. Continue for 1 month for a subjective response and 2 to 3 months for an objective response.

METHYLTESTOSTERONE:

Males –

Replacement therapy: Replacement therapy in androgen-deficient males is 10 to 50 mg of methyltestosterone daily.

Delayed puberty – Doses used in delayed puberty generally are in the lower range of that given above, and for a limited duration, for example, 4 to 6 months.

Females –

Inoperable breast cancer: 50 to 200 mg/day orally. Follow women closely because androgen therapy occasionally appears to accelerate the disease. Shorter acting androgen preparations may be preferred rather than those with prolonged activity for treating breast carcinoma, particularly during the early stages of androgen therapy.

TESTOSTERONE, LONG-ACTING: For IM use only. Individualize dosage. In general, more than 400 mg/month is not required because of the prolonged action of the preparation.

Male hypogonadism –

Replacement therapy (eunuchism): 50 to 400 mg every 2 to 4 weeks.

Males with delayed puberty – 50 to 200 mg every 2 to 4 weeks for a limited duration.

Palliation of inoperable breast cancer in women – 200 to 400 mg every 2 to 4 weeks.

Androgen therapy occasionally appears to accelerate metastatic breast carcinoma.

TESTOSTERONE TRANSDERMAL SYSTEM:

Androderm – The usual starting dose is one 5 mg system or two 2.5 mg systems applied nightly for 24 hours, providing a total dose of 5 mg/day.

Apply the adhesive side of the system to a clean, dry area of the skin on the back, abdomen, upper arms or thighs. Avoid bony prominences, such as the shoulder and hip areas. Do NOT apply to the scrotum. Rotate the sites of application, with an interval of 7 days between applications to the same site. The area selected should not be oily, damaged, or irritated.

To ensure proper dosing, the morning serum testosterone concentration may be measured following system application the previous evening. If the serum concentration is outside the normal range, repeat sampling with assurance of proper system adhesion as well as appropriate application time. Confirmed serum concentrations outside the normal range may require increasing the dosage regimen to 7.5 mg, or decreasing the regimen to 2.5 mg, maintaining nightly application. Because of variability in analytical values among diagnostic laboratories, this laboratory work and any later analysis for assessing the effect of therapy should be performed at the same laboratory so results can be more easily compared.

Nonvirilized patient – Dosing may be initiated with 2.5 mg system nightly.

Storage/Stability – Do not store outside the pouch provided. Damaged systems should not be used. The drug reservoir may be burst by excessive pressure or heat. Discard systems in household trash in a manner that prevents accidental application or ingestion by children, pets, or others.

TESTOSTERONE PELLETS:

Replacement therapy – The dosage guideline for testosterone pellets for replacement therapy in androgen-deficient males is 150 to 450 mg subcutaneously every 3 to 6 months.

Delayed puberty – Dosages used in delayed puberty generally are in the lower range of that listed above, and for a limited time duration, for example 4 to 6 months.

*Determination of dose* – The number of pellets to be implanted depends upon the minimal daily requirement of testosterone propionate determined by a gradual reduction of the amount administered parenterally. The usual ratio is as follows: Implant two 75 mg pellets for each 25 mg testosterone propionate required weekly. It has been found that approximately 33% of the material is absorbed in the first month, 25% in the second month, and 17% in the third month. Adequate effect of the pellets ordinarily continues for 3 to 4 months, sometimes as long as 6 months.

*TESTOSTERONE GEL:* The recommended starting dose of 1% testosterone gel is 5 g (to deliver 50 mg of testosterone) applied once daily (preferably in the morning) to clean, dry, intact skin of the shoulders and upper arms or abdomen (*AndroGel* only). Upon opening the packet(s), squeeze the entire contents into the palm of the hand and immediately apply it to the application sites. Allow application sites to dry for a few minutes prior to dressing. Wash hands with soap and water after application. Cover the application sites with clothing after gel has dried.

Do not apply the gel to the genitals. Do not apply *Testim* to the abdomen.

For optimal absorption of testosterone from *AndroGel*, it appears reasonable to wait 5 to 6 hours after application prior to showering or swimming. Showering or swimming after just 1 hour should have a minimal effect on the amount absorbed if done infrequently. Do not wash the sites of application for at least 2 hours after application of *Testim*.

Measure serum testosterone levels 14 days after initiation of therapy to ensure proper dosing. If the serum testosterone concentration is below the normal range, or if the desired clinical response is not achieved, the dose may be increased from 5 to 7.5 g (*AndroGel*) or 10 g (*Testim*) and from 7.5 to 10 g (*AndroGel*), as instructed by the physician.

In order to prevent transfer to another person, instruct patients to wear clothing to cover the application sites. If direct skin-to-skin contact with another person is anticipated, the application sites must be washed thoroughly with soap and water.

In order to maintain serum testosterone levels in the normal range, instruct patients not to wash the sites of application for at least 2 hours after application.

*TESTOSTERONE, BUCCAL:* The recommended dosing schedule is the application of 1 buccal system (30 mg) to the gum region twice daily, morning and evening (about 12 hours apart). Testosterone buccal should be placed in a comfortable position just above the incisor tooth on either side of the mouth. With each application, testosterone should be rotated to alternate sides of the mouth.

Upon opening the packet, the rounded side surface of the buccal system should be placed against the gum and held firmly in place with a finger over the lip and against the product for 30 seconds to ensure adhesion. Testosterone buccal is designed to stay in position until removed. If the buccal system fails to properly adhere to the gum or falls off during the 12-hour dosing interval, the old buccal system should be removed and a new one applied. If the buccal system falls out of position within 4 hours before the next dose, a new buccal system should be applied and may remain in place until the time of next regularly scheduled dosing.

Take care to avoid dislodging the buccal system and check to see if testosterone buccal is in place following brushing of teeth, use of mouthwash, and consumption of food or beverages. Testosterone buccal should not be chewed or swallowed. To remove testosterone, gently slide it downwards from the gum toward the tooth to avoid scratching the gum.

### Actions

*Pharmacology:* Testosterone, produced by the Leydig cells of the testis, is the primary natural androgen. In women, small amounts are synthesized by the ovary and adrenal cortex.

Endogenous androgens are responsible for the normal growth and development of the male sex organs and for maintenance of secondary sex characteristics. Androgens are responsible for the growth spurt of adolescence and for the termination of linear growth by fusion of the epiphyseal growth centers. During administration of exogenous androgens, endogenous testosterone release is inhibited through feedback inhibition of pituitary luteinizing hormone (LH). Large doses of exogenous androgens may suppress spermatogenesis through feedback inhibition of pituitary follicle-stimulating hormone (FSH).

*Pharmacokinetics:*

*Absorption –*

*Oral:* Testosterone is metabolized by the gut and 44% is cleared by the liver in the first pass. The synthetic androgens are less extensively metabolized by the liver and have longer half-lives and are more suitable than testosterone for oral administration.

*IM:* Testosterone esters in oil injected IM are absorbed slowly from the lipid phase; thus, testosterone cypionate and enanthate can be given at intervals of 2 to 4 weeks.

*Topical gel:* Absorption of testosterone into the blood continues for the entire 24-hour dosing interval. Serum concentrations approximate the steady-state level by the end of the first 24 hours and are at steady state by the second or third day of dosing.

When the topical gel treatment is discontinued after achieving steady state, serum testosterone levels remain in the normal range for 24 to 48 hours but return to their pretreatment levels by the fifth day after the last application.

*Transdermal:*

*Androderm –* Following application to nonscrotal skin, testosterone is continuously absorbed during the 24-hour dosing period. Daily application of 2 systems at approximately 10:00 p.m. results in a serum testosterone concentration profile that mimics the normal circadian variation observed in healthy young men. Maximum concentrations occur in the early morning hours with minimum concentrations in the evening.

*Distribution –* Testosterone in plasma is approximately 98% bound to a specific testosterone-estradiol binding globulin. There are considerable variations in the reported half-life of testosterone, ranging from 10 to 100 minutes. The half-life of testosterone cypionate IM is approximately 8 days; for oral fluoxymesterone, it is approximately 9.2 hours; and for methyltestosterone it is 2.5 to 3 hours.

*Metabolism/Excretion –* There are considerable variations in the reported half-life of testosterone, ranging from 10 to 100 minutes. The half-life of testosterone cypionate IM is approximately 8 days; for oral fluoxymesterone, it is approximately 9.2 hours; and for methyltestosterone it is 2.5 to 3 hours. Inactivation of testosterone occurs primarily in the liver. About 90% of a testosterone dose is excreted in the urine as conjugates of testosterone and its metabolites; about 6% of a dose is excreted in the feces.

## Contraindications

Patients with serious cardiac, hepatic, or renal diseases; hypersensitivity to the drug; in men with carcinomas of the breast or prostate; pregnancy (see Warnings).

Pregnant women should avoid skin contact with *AndroGel* application sites in men. Testosterone may cause fetal harm. In the event that unwashed or unclothed skin to which *AndroGel* has been applied does come in direct contact with the skin of a pregnant woman, wash the general area of contact on the woman with soap and water as soon as possible. In vitro studies show that residual testosterone is removed from the skin surface by washing with soap and water.

## Warnings

*Athletic performance:* Although the anabolic steroids are generally the agents that are abused for enhancement of athletic performance, these agents have also been used for such purposes. However, these drugs are not safe and effective for this use and have a potential risk of serious side effects.

*Sleep apnea:* The treatment of hypogonadal men with testosterone esters may potentiate sleep apnea in some patients, especially those with risk factors such as obesity or chronic lung diseases.

*Product interchange:* Do not use testosterone cypionate interchangeably with testosterone propionate because of differences in duration of action.

*Breast cancer:* Androgen therapy may cause hypercalcemia by stimulating osteolysis.

*Hepatotoxicity:* Prolonged use of high doses of androgens has been associated with the development of potentially life-threatening peliosis hepatis, hepatic neoplasms, and hepatocellular carcinoma. Cholestatic hepatitis and jaundice occur with fluoxymesterone and methyltestosterone at relatively low doses. Drug-induced jaundice is reversible when the medication is discontinued.

*Oligospermia:* Oligospermia and reduced ejaculatory volume may occur after prolonged administration or excessive dosage.

*Edema:* Edema, with or without CHF, may be a serious complication in patients with preexisting cardiac, renal, or hepatic disease.

*Gynecomastia:* Gynecomastia frequently develops and occasionally persists in patients being treated for hypogonadism.

*Bone maturation:* Use cautiously in healthy males with delayed puberty. Monitor bone maturation by assessing bone age of the wrist and hand every 6 months.

*Carcinogenesis:* There are rare reports of hepatocellular carcinoma in patients receiving long-term therapy with androgens in high doses.

*Elderly:* Elderly males, or men in general, treated with androgens may be at an increased risk of developing prostatic hypertrophy, prostatic carcinoma, and prostatic hyperplasia.

*Pregnancy: Category X.*

*Lactation:* It is not known whether androgens are excreted in breast milk.

*Children:* Use androgens very cautiously in children; the drugs should only be given by specialists who are aware of the adverse effects on bone maturation. Androgens may accelerate bone maturation without producing compensatory gain in linear growth. This adverse effect may result in compromised adult stature. The younger the child, the greater the risk of compromising final mature height.

### Precautions

*Monitoring:* Frequently determine urine and serum calcium levels during the course of therapy in women with disseminated breast carcinoma. Periodically perform liver function tests, prostate specific antigen, cholesterol, and high-density lipoprotein. To ensure proper dosing, measure serum testosterone concentrations. Make periodic (every 6 months) x-ray examinations of bone age during treatment of prepubertal males to determine the rate of bone maturation and the effects of the androgen therapy on the epiphyseal centers. Check hemoglobin and hematocrit periodically for polycythemia in patients who are receiving high doses of androgens.

*Virilization:* Observe women for signs of virilization (deepening voice, hirsutism, acne, clitoromegaly, and menstrual irregularities). Discontinue therapy at the time of evidence of mild virilism to prevent irreversible virilization.

*Benign prostatic hypertrophy:* Patients with benign prostatic hypertrophy may develop acute urethral obstruction. Priapism or excessive sexual stimulation may develop. Oligospermia may occur after prolonged administration or excessive dosage.

*Hypercholesterolemia:* Serum cholesterol may be altered during therapy.

### Drug Interactions

Androgens may affect anticoagulants, oxyphenbutazone, insulin, propranolol, corticosteroids/ACTH, and cyclosporine.

*Drug/Lab test interactions:*

*Thyroid function tests* – Decreased levels of thyroxine-binding globulin, resulting in decreased total $T_4$ serum levels and increased resin uptake of $T_3$ and $T_4$. Free thyroid hormone levels remain unchanged, and there is no clinical evidence of thyroid dysfunction.

**Adverse Reactions**

Adverse reactions occurring in 3% or more of patients include headache, dizziness/vertigo, libido decreased, application site itching/erythema/discomfort, pruritus, burning sensation, acne, other application site reactions, burn-like blister under system, breast pain/tenderness, UTI/Prostatitis, prostate disorder, gynecomastia, abnormal lab tests (including abnormal hemoglobin, hematocrit, triglycerides, serum lipids, potassium glucose, creatinine, bilirubin, liver function tests).

*Females* – Amenorrhea and other menstrual irregularities; inhibition of gonadotropin secretion and virilization, including deepening voice and clitoral enlargement.

# FINASTERIDE

**Tablets:** 1 mg (*Rx*)
5 mg (*Rx*)

*Propecia* (Merck)
*Proscar* (Merck)

### Indications

*Benign prostatic hyperplasia (BPH):* Treatment of symptomatic BPH in men with an enlarged prostate to improve symptoms, reduce acute urinary retention risk, and reduce the risk of the need for surgery including transurethral resection of the prostate (TURP) and prostatectomy.

*Androgenetic alopecia:* Treatment of male pattern hair loss (vertex and anterior mid-scalp).

### Administration and Dosage

*Benign prostatic hyperplasia:* Recommended dose is 5 mg once/day, with or without meals. Prior to initiating therapy, perform appropriate evaluation to identify other conditions that might mimic BPH, such as infection, prostate cancer, stricture disease, hypotonic bladder, or other neurogenic disorders.

Although early improvement may be seen, at least 6 to 12 months of therapy may be necessary to assess whether a beneficial response has been achieved. Perform periodic follow-up evaluations to determine whether a clinical response has occurred.

*Androgenetic alopecia:* The recommended dosage is 1 mg once/day, with or without meals. In general, daily use for at least 3 months is necessary before benefit is observed. Continued use is recommended to sustain benefit. Withdrawal of treatment leads to reversal of effect within 12 months.

*Hepatic function impairment:* Use caution in those patients with liver function abnormalities because finasteride is metabolized extensively in the liver.

### Actions

*Pharmacology:* Finasteride, a synthetic 4-azasteroid compound, is a competitive and specific inhibitor of steroid 5α-reductase, an intracellular enzyme that converts testosterone into the potent androgen 5α-dihydrotestosterone (DHT).

*Pharmacokinetics:* Finasteride is well absorbed after oral administration, with a mean bioavailability of approximately 64%, which is unaffected by food. The half-life of finasteride is 4.8 to 6 hours following 1 and 5 mg/day dosing, respectively.

Finasteride undergoes extensive hepatic metabolism through oxidative pathways to inactive compounds that are eliminated primarily through the bile; the mean urinary recovery of the parent drug within 24 hours of a dose was only 0.04%.

Approximately 90% is bound to plasma proteins. Finasteride crosses the blood-brain barrier.

### Contraindications

Hypersensitivity to finasteride or any component of this product; use in women or children; pregnancy or use in women who may potentially be pregnant, including handling of crushed or broken tablets.

### Warnings

*Hepatic function impairment:* Use caution in those patients with liver function abnormalities since finasteride is metabolized extensively in the liver.

*Pregnancy: Category* X. Because of the potential risk to a male fetus, a woman who is pregnant or who may become pregnant should not handle crushed or broken finasteride tablets.

*Lactation:* Finasteride is not indicated for use in women. It is not known whether finasteride is excreted in breast milk.

*Children:* Finasteride is not indicated for use in children; safety and efficacy in children have not been established.

## Precautions

*Prostate cancer evaluation:* Perform digital rectal examinations, as well as other evaluations for prostate cancer, on patients with BPH prior to initiating therapy and periodically thereafter.

Finasteride causes a decrease in serum prostate specific antigen (PSA) levels in patients with BPH even in the presence of prostate cancer. Consider this reduction of PSA levels when evaluating PSA laboratory data; it does not suggest a beneficial effect of finasteride on prostate cancer.

Carefully evaluate any sustained increases in PSA levels while on finasteride, including consideration of noncompliance to therapy.

*Obstructive uropathy:* Because not all patients demonstrate a response to finasteride, carefully monitor patients with a large residual urinary volume or severely diminished urinary flow for obstructive uropathy. These patients may not be candidates for this therapy.

## Drug Interactions

Finasteride may affect theophylline.

*Drug/Lab test interactions:* When PSA laboratory determinations are evaluated, consider the fact that PSA levels are decreased in patients treated with finasteride.

## Adverse Reactions

Adverse reactions occurring in 3% or more of patients include impotence and decreased libido. Breast tenderness and enlargement; hypersensitivity reactions, including lip swelling and skin rash also have been reported with 5 mg finasteride.

# DUTASTERIDE

**Capsules:** 0.5 mg (*Rx*)                              *Avodart* (GlaxoSmithKline)

## Indications

*Benign prostatic hyperplasia (BPH):* For the treatment of symptomatic BPH in men with an enlarged prostate to improve symptoms, reduce the risk of acute urinary retention, and reduce the risk of the need for BPH-related surgery.

## Administration and Dosage

*Dose:* 0.5 mg taken orally once daily. Swallow the capsules whole. Dutasteride may be administered with or without food.

## Actions

*Pharmacology:* Dutasteride inhibits the conversion of testosterone to 5α-dihydrotestosterone (DHT), the androgen primarily responsible for the initial development and subsequent enlargement of the prostate gland. Testosterone is converted to DHT by the enzyme 5α-reductase, which exists as 2 isoforms, type 1 and type 2. The type 2 isoenzyme is primarily active in the reproductive tissues while the type 1 isoenzyme is also responsible for testosterone conversion in the skin and liver.

Dutasteride is a competitive and specific inhibitor of type 1 and type 2 5α-reductase isoenzymes.

*Effect on DHT and testosterone* – The maximum effect of daily doses of dutasteride on the reduction of DHT is dose dependent and is observed within 1 to 2 weeks.

*Pharmacokinetics:*

*Absorption* – Following administration of a single 0.5 mg dose of a soft gelatin capsule, time to peak serum concentrations ($T_{max}$) of dutasteride occurs within 2 to 3 hours. Absolute bioavailability in 5 healthy subjects is approximately 60% (range, 40% to 94%). When the drug is administered with food, the maximum serum concentrations were reduced by 10% to 15%.

*Distribution* – There is a large volume of distribution (300 to 500 L); the drug is highly bound to plasma albumin (99%) and alpha-1 acid glycoprotein (96.6%).

*Metabolism/Excretion* – Dutasteride is extensively metabolized in humans. In vitro studies showed that dutasteride is metabolized by the CYP3A4 isoenzyme to 2 minor mono-hydroxylated metabolites. Dutasteride is not metabolized in vitro by human cytochrome P450 isozymes CYP1A2, CYP2C9, CYP2C19, and CYP2D6 at 2000 ng/mL, 3 major metabolites (4'-hydroxydutasteride, 1,2-dihydrodutasteride, and 6-hydroxydutasteride), and 2 minor metabolites (6,4'-dihydroxydutasteride and 15-hydroxydutasteride) have been detected.

The terminal elimination half-life of dutasteride is approximately 5 weeks at steady state. The average steady-state serum dutasteride concentration was 40 ng/mL following 0.5 mg/day for 1 year.

*Special populations –*

*Gender:* Dutasteride is not indicated for use in women.

### Contraindications

In women and children; known hypersensitivity to dutasteride, other 5α-reductase inhibitors, or any component of the preparation.

### Warnings

*Exposure of women/risk to male fetus:* Dutasteride is absorbed through the skin. Therefore, women who are pregnant or may be pregnant should not handle dutasteride capsules because of the possibility of absorption of dutasteride and the potential risk of a fetal anomaly to a male fetus. In addition, women should use caution whenever handling dutasteride capsules. If contact is made with leaking capsules, the contact area should be washed immediately with soap and water.

*Blood donation:* Men being treated with dutasteride should not donate blood until at least 6 months have passed following their last dose. The purpose of this deferred period is to prevent administration of dutasteride to a pregnant female transfusion recipient.

*CNS toxicity:* Some animals showed signs of nonspecific, reversible, centrally mediated toxicity.

*Renal function impairment:* Less than 0.1% of a steady-state 0.5 mg dose of dutasteride is recovered in human urine, so no adjustment in dosage is anticipated for patients with renal impairment.

*Hepatic function impairment:* Because dutasteride is extensively metabolized and has a half-life of approximately 5 weeks at steady state, use caution in the administration of dutasteride to patients with liver disease.

*Pregnancy: Category X.*

*Lactation:* It is not known whether dutasteride is excreted in human breast milk.

*Children:* Safety and effectiveness in the pediatric population have not been established.

### Precautions

*Other urological diseases:* Perform digital rectal examinations, as well as other evaluations for prostate cancer, on patients with BPH prior to initiating therapy with dutasteride and periodically thereafter.

### Drug Interactions

*CYP450:* Dutasteride may increase in the presence of inhibitors of CYP3A4, such as ritonavir, ketoconazole, verapamil, diltiazem, cimetidine, and ciprofloxacin.

*Drug/Lab test interactions:*

*Effects on PSA –* PSA levels generally decrease in patients treated with dutasteride as the prostate volume decreases. Establish a new baseline PSA concentration after 3 to 6 months of treatment with dutasteride.

### Adverse Reactions

Adverse reaction occurring in 3% or more of patients included transient impotence and decreased libido within the first 6 months.

# DANAZOL

| Capsules: 50, 100, and 200 mg (Rx) | Various, *Danocrine* (Sanofi-Synthelabo) |

---

**Warning:**
Use of danazol in pregnancy is contraindicated. A sensitive test (eg, beta subunit test if available) capable of determining early pregnancy is recommended immediately prior to start of therapy. Additionally, a nonhormonal method of contraception should be used during therapy. If a patient becomes pregnant while taking danazol, discontinue administration of the drug and apprise the patient of the potential risk to the fetus.

Thromboembolism, thrombotic and thrombophlebitic events, including sagittal sinus thrombosis and life-threatening or fatal strokes have been reported.

Experience with long-term therapy with danazol is limited. Peliosis hepatis and benign hepatic adenoma have been observed with long-term use. Peliosis hepatis and hepatic adenoma may be silent until complicated by acute, potentially life-threatening intra-abdominal hemorrhage. Therefore, alert the physician to this possibility. Attempts should be made to determine the lowest dose that will provide adequate protection (see Warnings).

Danazol has been associated with several cases of benign intracranial hypertension also known as pseudotumor cerebri. Early signs and symptoms of benign intracranial hypertension include papilledema, headache, nausea, and vomiting, and visual disturbances. Screen patients with these symptoms for papilledema and, if present, advise the patients to discontinue danazol immediately and refer them to a neurologist for further diagnosis and care.

---

## Indications
*Endometriosis:* For the treatment of endometriosis amenable to hormonal management.

*Fibrocystic breast disease:* Danazol is usually effective in decreasing nodularity, pain, and tenderness, but it alters hormone levels; recurrence of symptoms is very common after cessation of therapy.

*Hereditary angioedema:* For the prevention of attacks of angioedema in males and females.

## Administration and Dosage
*Endometriosis:* Begin therapy during menstruation or make sure the patient is not pregnant. Administer 800 mg/day in 2 divided doses to best achieve amenorrhea and rapid response to painful symptoms. Downward titration to a dose sufficient to maintain amenorrhea may be considered depending upon response. Initially, for mild cases, give 200 to 400 mg in 2 divided doses.

*Fibrocystic breast disease:* Begin therapy during menstruation or make sure patient is not pregnant. Dosage ranges from 100 to 400 mg/day in 2 divided doses.

*Hereditary angioedema:* Recommended starting dose is 200 mg 2 or 3 times/day. After a favorable initial response, determine continuing dosage by decreasing the dosage by 50% or less at intervals of at least 1 to 3 months if frequency of attacks prior to treatment dictates. If an attack occurs, increase dosage by 200 mg/day or less.

## Actions
*Pharmacology:* A synthetic androgen derived from ethisterone, danazol suppresses the pituitary-ovarian axis by inhibiting the output of pituitary gonadotropins. Danazol depresses the output of both follicle-stimulating hormone (FSH) and luteinizing hormone (LH). Danazol acts by direct enzymatic inhibition of sex steroid synthesis and competitively inhibits binding of steroids to their cytoplasmic receptors in target tissues.

*Endometriosis* – In endometriosis, danazol alters the normal and ectopic endometrial tissue so that it becomes inactive and atrophic.

*Hereditary angioedema* – Danazol prevents attacks of the disease characterized by episodic edema of the abdominal viscera, extremities, face, and airway that may be disabling and, if the airway is involved, fatal. In addition, danazol partially or completely corrects the primary biochemical abnormality of hereditary angioedema. It increases the levels of the deficient C1 esterase inhibitor, thereby increasing the serum levels of the C4 component of the complement system.

*Pharmacokinetics:* Blood levels of danazol do not increase proportionately with increases in dose. When the dose is doubled, plasma levels increase only approximately 35% to 40%.

## Contraindications
Undiagnosed abnormal genital bleeding; markedly impaired hepatic, renal, or cardiac function; pregnancy and lactation; patients with porphyria.

## Warnings
*Thrombotic events:* Thromboembolism, thrombotic and thrombophlebitic events including sagittal sinus thrombosis and life-threatening or fatal strokes have been reported.

*Hepatic events:* Experience with long-term therapy with danazol is limited. Peliosis hepatis and benign hepatic adenoma have been observed with long-term use (see Black Box Warning).

*Intracranial hypertension:* Danazol has been associated with several cases of benign intracranial hypertension (also known as pseudotumor cerebri) (see Black Box Warning).

*Lipoprotein alterations:* A temporary alteration of lipoproteins in the form of decreased high density lipoproteins (HDL) and possibly increased low density lipoproteins (LDL) has been reported during danazol therapy.

*Carcinoma of the breast:* Carcinoma of the breast should be excluded before initiating therapy for fibrocystic breast disease.

*Long-term experience:* Long-term experience with danazol is limited. Long-term therapy with other steroids alkylated at the 17 position has been associated with serious toxicity (cholestatic jaundice, peliosis hepatitis). Similar toxicity may develop after long-term danazol.

*Androgenic effects:* Androgenic effects may not be reversible even when the drug is discontinued. Watch patients closely for signs of virilization.

*Pregnancy:* Category X.

*Lactation:* Breastfeeding is contraindicated in patients taking danazol.

*Children:* Safety and efficacy in pediatric patients has not been established.

## Precautions
*Fluid retention:* Conditions influenced by edema require careful observation.

*Hepatic dysfunction:* Hepatic dysfunction has been reported; perform periodic liver function tests.

*Lipoproteins:* Monitor HDL and LDL periodically.

*Semen:* Semen should be checked for volume, viscosity, sperm count, and motility every 3 to 4 months, especially in adolescents.

*Porphyria:* Danazol administration has been reported to cause exacerbation of the manifestations of acute intermittent porphyria.

## Drug Interactions
Drugs that maybe affected by danazol are carbamazepine, cyclosporine, and warfarin.

## Adverse Reactions
Significant adverse reactions include edema; vaginitis; nervousness; emotional lability; hepatic dysfunction; elevated blood pressure; pelvic pain; carpal tunnel syndrome; sleep disorders; fatigue; tremor; visual disturbances; anxiety; depression; gastroenteritis.

# GLUCOCORTICOIDS

**BETAMETHASONE**
**BETAMETHASONE, ORAL**
**Syrup:** 0.6 mg/5 mL (*Rx*)                    *Celestone* (Schering)
**BETAMETHASONE SODIUM PHOSPHATE**
**Injection:** 4 mg/mL (*Rx*)                   *Celestone Phosphate* (Schering)
**BETAMETHASONE SODIUM PHOSPHATE AND ACETATE**
**Injection:** 3 mg acetate and 3 mg sodium phosphate/mL (*Rx*)   *Celestone Soluspan* (Schering)
**BUDESONIDE**
**Capsules:** 3 mg micronized budesonide (*Rx*)   *Entocort EC* (AstraZeneca)
**CORTISONE**
**Tablets:** 25 mg (*Rx*)                       Various
**DEXAMETHASONE**
**DEXAMETHASONE, ORAL**
**Tablets:** 0.25, 1.5, 4, and 6 mg (*Rx*)       Various
0.5 and 0.75 mg (*Rx*)                          Various, *Decadron* (Merck)
1 and 2 mg (*Rx*)                               *Dexamethasone* (Roxane)
**Elixir:** 0.5 mg/5 mL (*Rx*)                   Various
**Oral solution:** 0.5 mg/5 mL (*Rx*)            Various
**Oral solution (concentrate):** 1 mg/mL (*Rx*)   *Dexamethasone Intensol* (Roxane)
**DEXAMETHASONE SODIUM PHOSPHATE**
**Injection:** 4 mg/mL (*Rx*)                   Various
10 mg/mL (*Rx*)                                 Various
**HYDROCORTISONE (CORTISOL)**
**HYDROCORTISONE**
**Tablets:** 5 mg (*Rx*)                        *Cortef* (Upjohn)
10 mg (*Rx*)                                    *Cortef* (Upjohn), *Hydrocortone* (MSD), *Hydrocortisone* (Major)
20 mg (*Rx*)                                    Various, *Cortef* (Upjohn), *Hydrocortone* (MSD)
**HYDROCORTISONE CYPIONATE**
**Oral suspension:** 10 mg/5 mL (*Rx*)          *Cortef* (Upjohn)
**HYDROCORTISONE SODIUM PHOSPHATE**
**Injection:** 50 mg/mL (*Rx*)                  *Hydrocortone Phosphate* (MSD)
**HYDROCORTISONE SODIUM SUCCINATE**
**Injection:** 100, 250, 500, and 1,000 mg per vial (*Rx*)   *A-Hydrocort* (Abbott), *Solu-Cortef* (Upjohn)
**HYDROCORTISONE ACETATE**
**Injection:** 25 mg/mL (*Rx*)                  Various, *Hydrocortone Acetate* (MSD)
50 mg/mL (*Rx*)                                 Various
**METHYLPREDNISOLONE**
**METHYLPREDNISOLONE, ORAL**
**Tablets:** 2, 24, and 32 mg (*Rx*)            *Medrol* (Upjohn)
4 and 16 mg (*Rx*)                              Various, *Medrol* (Upjohn)
8 mg (*Rx*)                                     *Medrol* (Upjohn), *Methylprednisolone* (Prasco)
**METHYLPREDNISOLONE SODIUM SUCCINATE**
**Powder for injection:** 40, 125, and 500 mg and 1 g per vial (*Rx*)   Various, *A-Methapred* (Abbott), *Solu-Medrol* (Upjohn)
2 g (*Rx*)                                      *Solu-Medrol* (Upjohn)
**METHYLPREDNISOLONE ACETATE**
**Injection:** 20 mg/mL (*Rx*)                  Various, *Depo-Medrol* (Upjohn)
40 mg/mL (*Rx*)                                 Various, *depMedalone 40* (Forest), *Depo-Medrol* (Upjohn), *Depopred-40* (Hyrex), *Duralone-40* (Hauck), *Medralone 40* (Keene)
80 mg/mL (*Rx*)                                 Various, *depMedalone 80* (Forest), *Depo-Medrol* (Upjohn), *Depopred-80* (Hyrex), *Duralone-80* (Hauck), *Medralone 80* (Keene)

## PREDNISOLONE
### PREDNISOLONE, ORAL
| | |
|---|---|
| **Tablets**: 5 mg *(Rx)* | Various |
| **Syrup**: 5 mg/5 mL *(Rx)* | *Prelone* (Aero) |
| 15 mg/5 mL *(Rx)* | Various, *Prelone* (Aero) |

### PREDNISOLONE ACETATE
| | |
|---|---|
| **Injection**: 25 mg/mL *(Rx)* | Various |
| 50 mg/mL *(Rx)* | Various, *Predalone 50* (Forest), *Predcor-50* (Hauck) |

### PREDNISOLONE TEBUTATE
| | |
|---|---|
| **Injection**: 20 mg/mL *(Rx)* | *Prednisol TBA* (Pasadena) |

### PREDNISOLONE SODIUM PHOSPHATE
| | |
|---|---|
| **Injection**: 20 mg/mL *(Rx)* | *Hydeltrasol* (MSD), *Key-Pred-SP* (Hyrex) |
| **Oral liquid**: 5 mg/5 mL *(Rx)* | *Pediapred* (Fisons) |
| **Oral solution**: 15 mg/5 mL *(Rx)* | *Orapred* (Ascent Pediatrics) |

## PREDNISONE
| | |
|---|---|
| **Tablets**: 1 mg *(Rx)* | Various, *Meticorten* (Schering), *Orasone* (Solvay), *Panasol-S* (Seatrace) |
| 2.5 mg *(Rx)* | *Deltasone* (Upjohn) |
| 5 mg *(Rx)* | Various, *Deltasone* (Upjohn), *Orasone* (Solvay), *Prednicen-M* (Central), *Sterapred* (Merz) |
| 10 mg *(Rx)* | Various, *Deltasone* (Upjohn), *Orasone* (Solvay), *Sterapred DS* (Merz) |
| 20 mg *(Rx)* | Various, *Deltasone* (Upjohn), *Orasone* (Solvay) |
| 50 mg *(Rx)* | Various, *Orasone* (Solvay) |
| **Oral solution**: 5 mg/5 mL *(Rx)* | *Prednisone*, *Prednisone Intensol Concentrate* (Roxane) |
| **Syrup**: 5 mg/5 mL *(Rx)* | *Liquid Pred* (Muro) |

## TRIAMCINOLONE
### TRIAMCINOLONE, ORAL
| | |
|---|---|
| **Tablets**: 4 mg *(Rx)* | Various, *Aristocort* (Fujisawa), *Kenacort* (Apothecon) |
| 8 mg *(Rx)* | *Aristocort* (Fujisawa), *Kenacort* (Apothecon) |
| **Syrup**: 4 mg/5 mL (as diacetate) *(Rx)* | *Kenacort* (Apothecon) |

### TRIAMCINOLONE DIACETATE
| | |
|---|---|
| **Injection**: 25 mg/mL *(Rx)* | *Aristocort Intralesional* (Fujisawa) |
| 40 mg/mL *(Rx)* | Various, *Trilone* (Hauck), *Amcort* (Keene), *Clinacort* (Clint) |

### TRIAMCINOLONE HEXACETONIDE
| | |
|---|---|
| **Injection**: 5 mg/mL *(Rx)* | *Aristospan Intralesional* (Fujisawa) |
| 20 mg/mL *(Rx)* | *Aristospan Intra-articular* (Fujisawa) |

### TRIAMCINOLONE ACETONIDE
| | |
|---|---|
| **Injection**: 3 mg/mL *(Rx)* | *Tac-3* (Herbert) |
| 10 mg/mL *(Rx)* | *Kenalog-10* (Westwood-Squibb) |
| 40 mg/mL *(Rx)* | Various, *Kenalog-40* (Westwood-Squibb), *Tac-40* (Parnell), *Triamonide 40* (Forest), *Tri-Kort* (Keene), *Trilog* (Hauck) |

### Indications

*Allergic states:* Control of severe or incapacitating allergic conditions intractable to conventional treatment in serum sickness and drug hypersensitivity reactions. Parenteral therapy is indicated for urticarial transfusion reactions and acute noninfectious laryngeal edema (epinephrine is the drug of first choice).

*Collagen diseases:* For exacerbation of maintenance therapy in selected cases of systemic lupus erythematosus, acute rheumatic carditis, or systemic dermatomyositis (polymyositis).

*Dermatologic diseases:* Pemphigus; bullous dermatitis herpetiformis; severe erythema multiforme (Stevens-Johnson syndrome); mycosis fungoides; severe psoriasis; angioedema or urticaria; exfoliative, severe seborrheic, contact, or atopic dermatitis.

*Edematous states:* To induce diuresis or remission of proteinuria in the nephrotic syndrome (without uremia) of the idiopathic type or that caused by lupus erythematosus.

*Endocrine disorders:* Primary or secondary adrenal cortical insufficiency (**hydrocortisone** or **cortisone** is the drug of choice; synthetic analogs may be used in conjunction with mineralocorticoids; in infancy, mineralocorticoid supplementation is important); congenital adrenal hyperplasia; nonsuppurative thyroiditis; hypercalcemia associated with cancer.

*Parenteral* – Acute adrenal cortical insufficiency (**hydrocortisone** or **cortisone** is drug of choice); preoperatively or in serious trauma or illness with known adrenal insufficiency or when adrenal cortical reserve is doubtful; shock unresponsive to conventional therapy if adrenal cortical insufficiency exists or is suspected.

*GI diseases:* Ulcerative colitis; regional enteritis (Crohn disease); intractable sprue.

*Hematologic disorders:* Idiopathic thrombocytopenic purpura (ITP) and secondary thrombocytopenia in adults; acquired (autoimmune) hemolytic anemia; erythroblastopenia (RBC anemia); congenital (erythroid) hypoplastic anemia.

*Intralesional administration:* Keloids; localized hypertrophic, infiltrated, inflammatory lesions of lichen planus, psoriatic plaques, granuloma annulare, lichen simplex chronicus (neurodermatitis); discoid lupus erythematosus; necrobiosis lipoidica diabeticorum; alopecia areata. May be useful in cystic tumors of an aponeurosis or tendon (ganglia).

*Neoplastic diseases:* Palliative management of leukemias and lymphomas in adults; acute leukemia in childhood.

*Ophthalmic:* Severe acute and chronic allergic and inflammatory processes involving the eye and its adnexa.

*Rheumatic disorders:* Adjunctive therapy for short-term use (acute episode or exacerbation) in psoriatic arthritis; rheumatoid arthritis (RA), including juvenile RA; ankylosing spondylitis; acute and subacute bursitis; acute, nonspecific tenosynovitis; acute gouty arthritis; posttraumatic osteoarthritis; synovitis of osteoarthritis; epicondylitis.

*Respiratory diseases:* Symptomatic sarcoidosis; Loeffler syndrome not manageable by other means; berylliosis; fulminating or disseminated pulmonary tuberculosis when used concurrently with appropriate antituberculous chemotherapy; aspiration pneumonitis.

*Nervous system:* Acute exacerbations of multiple sclerosis (MS).

*Miscellaneous:* Tuberculous meningitis with subarachnoid block or impending block when accompanied by appropriate antituberculous chemotherapy; in trichinosis with neurologic or myocardial involvement.

*Dexamethasone:* Testing of adrenal cortical hyperfunction; cerebral edema associated with primary or metastatic brain tumor, craniotomy, or head injury.

*Triamcinolone:* Treatment of pulmonary emphysema where bronchospasm or bronchial edema plays a significant role, and diffuse interstitial pulmonary fibrosis (Hamman-Rich syndrome); in conjunction with diuretic agents to induce a diuresis in refractory CHF and in cirrhosis of the liver with refractory ascites; and for postoperative dental inflammatory reactions.

## Administration and Dosage

The maximal activity of the adrenal cortex is between 2 and 8 am, and it is minimal between 4 pm and midnight. Exogenous corticosteroids suppress adrenocortical activity the least when given at the time of maximal activity (am). Therefore, administer glucocorticoids in the morning prior to 9 am.

*Maintenance therapy:* Decrease initial dosage in small amounts to the lowest dosage that maintains an adequate clinical response. If the drug is to be stopped after more than a few days of treatment, it usually should be withdrawn gradually.

*Dosage adjustment:* Changes in clinical status resulting from remissions or exacerbations of the disease, individual drug responsiveness, and the effect of stress (ie, surgery, infection, trauma) may require dosage adjustment.

*Withdrawal of therapy:* If, after long-term therapy, the drug is to be stopped, it must be withdrawn gradually. If spontaneous remission occurs in a chronic condition, discontinue treatment gradually.

*Alternate-day therapy:* Alternate-day therapy is a dosing regimen in which twice the usual daily dose is administered every other morning. The purpose is to provide the patient requiring long-term treatment with the beneficial effects of corticosteroids while minimizing pituitary-adrenal suppression, the Cushingoid state, withdrawal symptoms, and growth suppression in children. The benefits of alternate-day therapy are only achieved by using the intermediate-acting agents.

*Intra-articular injection:* Dose depends on the joint size and varies with the severity of the condition. In chronic cases, injections may be repeated at intervals of at least 1 to 5 weeks depending upon the degree of relief obtained from the initial injection. Injection must be made into the synovial space.

*Miscellaneous (tendinitis, epicondylitis, ganglion):* In tendinitis or tenosynovitis, inject into the tendon sheath rather than into the substance of the tendon. In epicondylitis, outline the area of greatest tenderness and infiltrate the drug into the area.

*Injections for local effect in dermatologic conditions:* Avoid injection of sufficient material to cause blanching, since this may be followed by a small slough. One to 4 injections are usually employed.

BETAMETHASONE:
> *Betamethasone, oral –*
>> *Initial dosage:* 0.6 to 7.2 mg/day.
> *Betamethasone sodium phosphate –*
>> *Systemic and local:* The initial dosage may vary up to 9 mg/day.
> *Betamethasone sodium phosphate and acetate –* Betamethasone sodium phosphate provides prompt activity, while betamethasone acetate affords sustained activity.
>> *Systemic:* Not for IV use.
>>> *Initial dose –* 0.5 to 9 mg/day. Dosage ranges are 33% to 50% of the oral dose given every 12 hours. In certain acute, life-threatening situations, dosages exceeding the usual may be justified and may be in multiples of oral dosages.
>> *Bursitis, tenosynovitis, peritendinitis:* 1 mL given intrabursally.
>> *RA and osteoarthritis:* 0.5 to 2 mL given intra-articularly.
>>> *Very large joints –* 1 to 2 mL.
>>> *Large joints –* 1 mL.
>>> *Medium joints –* 0.5 to 1 mL.
>>> *Small joints –* 0.25 to 0.5 mL.
>> *Dermatologic conditions:* 0.2 mL/cm$^2$ intradermally.
>>> *Maximum dose –* 1 mL/week.
>> *Foot disorders –* The following doses are recommended at 3- to 7-day intervals:
>>> *Bursitis:*
>>>> Under heloma durum or heloma molle – 0.25 to 0.5 mL.
>>>> Under calcaneal spur – 0.5 mL.
>>>> Over hallux rigidus or digiti quinti varus – 0.5 mL.
>>> *Tenosynovitis, periostitis of cuboid:* 0.5 mL.
>>> *Acute, gouty arthritis:* 0.5 to 1 mL.

BUDESONIDE:
> *Adults –* Take 9 mg once daily in the morning for up to 8 weeks. Swallow capsules whole; do not chew or break. For recurring episodes of active Crohn disease, a repeat 8-week course of budesonide can be given. Treatment with capsules can be tapered to 6 mg/day for 2 weeks prior to complete cessation.
> Patients with mild to moderately active Crohn disease involving the ileum or ascending colon have been switched from oral prednisolone to budesonide with

no reported episodes of adrenal insufficiency. Because prednisolone should not be stopped abruptly, tapering should begin concomitantly with initiating budesonide treatment.

*Hepatic insufficiency:* Consider reducing the dose of budesonide capsules in patients with hepatic insufficiency.

CORTISONE:
    *Initial dosage* – 25 to 300 mg/day. In less severe diseases, lower doses may suffice.

DEXAMETHASONE:
    *Dexamethasone, oral* –
      *Initial dosage:* 0.75 to 9 mg/day.
      *Acute, self-limited allergic disorders or acute exacerbations of chronic allergic disorders:* The following dosage schedule combining parenteral (dexamethasone sodium phosphate injection 4 mg/mL) and oral (0.75 mg tablets) therapy is suggested: First day, 1 or 2 mL IM; second day, 4 tablets in 2 divided doses; third day, 4 tablets in 2 divided doses; fourth day, 2 tablets in 2 divided doses; fifth day, 1 tablet; sixth day, 1 tablet; seventh day, no treatment; eighth day, follow-up visit.
      *Palliative management of recurrent or inoperable brain tumors:* 2 mg 2 or 3 times/day for maintenance therapy.
      *Administration of Intensol:* Mix with liquid (eg, water, juices, soda-like beverages) or semi-solid food (eg, applesauce, pudding). Use the provided calibrated dropper to administer prescribed amount of *Intensol* into a liquid or semi-solid food. Stir gently for a few seconds. Consume the entire amount of liquid or food immediately; do not store for future use.
      *Suppression tests:* For Cushing syndrome, give 1 mg at 11 pm. Draw blood for plasma cortisol determination the following day at 8 am. For greater accuracy, give 0.5 mg every 6 hours for 48 hours. Collect 24-hour urine to determine 17-hydroxycorticosteroid excretion.
        *Test to distinguish Cushing syndrome due to pituitary ACTH excess from Cushing syndrome due to other causes* – Give 2 mg every 6 hours for 48 hours. Collect 24-hour urine to determine 17-hydroxycorticosteroid excretion.
    *Dexamethasone sodium phosphate* –
      *Initial dosage:* 0.5 to 9 mg daily. When the IV route is used, dosage should usually be the same as the oral dosage. However, in certain acute, life-threatening situations, dosages exceeding the usual may be justified and may be in multiples of the oral dosages.
      *Cerebral edema:* In adults, administer an initial IV dose of 10 mg, followed by 4 mg IM every 6 hours until maximum response has been noted. Response is usually noted within 12 to 24 hours. Dosage may be reduced after 2 to 4 days and gradually discontinued over 5 to 7 days. For palliative management of patients with recurrent or inoperable brain tumors, maintenance therapy with either the injection or tablets in a dosage of 2 mg 2 or 3 times daily may be effective.
      *Unresponsive shock:* Reported regimens range from 1 to 6 mg/kg as a single IV injection, to 40 mg initially followed by repeated IV injections every 2 to 6 hours while shock persists.

HYDROCORTISONE (Cortisol):
    *Hydrocortisone, oral* –
      *Initial dosage:* 20 to 240 mg/day.
    *Hydrocortisone sodium phosphate* – Administer by IV, IM, or subcutaneous injection. Initial dose is 15 to 240 mg/day. Usually, 33% to 50% of the oral dose every 12 hours. For acute diseases, doses greater than 240 mg may be required.
    *Hydrocortisone sodium succinate* – May be administered IV or IM. The initial dose is 100 to 500 mg, and may be repeated at 2-, 4-, or 6-hour intervals depending on patient response and clinical condition.
    *Hydrocortisone acetate* – For intralesional, intra-articular, or soft tissue injection only. Not for IV use. Dosage range is 5 to 37.5 mg. If desired, a local anesthetic may be injected before hydrocortisone acetate or mixed in a syringe and given simultaneously.

METHYLPREDNISOLONE:
> Methylprednisolone, oral –
>> Initial dose: 4 to 48 mg/day; adjust until a satisfactory response is noted. Determine maintenance dose by decreasing initial dose in small decrements at appropriate intervals until reaching the lowest effective dose.
>> Dosepak 21 therapy: Six 4 mg tablets on day 1. Decrease by 1 tablet per day.
> Methylprednisolone sodium succinate –
>> Initial dose: 10 to 40 mg IV, administered over 1 to several minutes. Give subsequent doses IV or IM.
>> Infants and children: Not less than 0.5 mg/kg/24 hours.
>> For high-dose therapy, give 30 mg/kg IV, infused over 10 to 20 minutes. May repeat every 4 to 6 hours, not beyond 48 to 72 hours.
> Methylprednisolone acetate – Not for IV use. As a temporary substitute for oral therapy, administer the total daily dose as a single IM injection. For prolonged effect, give a single weekly dose.
>> Adrenogenital syndrome: A single 40 mg injection IM every 2 weeks.
>> RA: Weekly IM maintenance dose varies from 40 to 120 mg.
>> Dermatologic lesions: 40 to 120 mg IM weekly for 1 to 4 weeks. In severe dermatitis, relief may result within 8 to 12 hours of a single dose of 80 to 120 mg IM. In chronic contact dermatitis, repeated injections every 5 to 10 days may be necessary. In seborrheic dermatitis, a weekly dose of 80 mg IM may be adequate.
>> Asthma and allergic rhinitis: 80 to 120 mg IM.
>> Intra-articular and soft tissue: 4 to 80 mg.
>> Intralesional: 20 to 60 mg.

PREDNISOLONE:
> Prednisolone –
>> Initial dosage: 5 to 60 mg/day.
>> Multiple sclerosis: In treatment of acute exacerbations of MS, 200 mg daily for a week followed by 80 mg every other day for 1 month.
> Prednisolone acetate – Not for IV use.
>> Initial dosage: 4 to 60 mg/day IM.
>> Intralesional, intra-articular, or soft tissue injection: 4 mg, up to 100 mg.
>> Multiple sclerosis: 200 mg daily for a week, followed by 80 mg every other day or dexamethasone 4 to 8 mg every other day for 1 month.
> Prednisolone tebutate –
>> Intra-articular, intralesional, or soft tissue administration: 8 to 30 mg. Doses greater than 40 mg are not recommended.
> Prednisolone sodium phosphate –
>> Parenteral: For IV or IM use.
>>> Initial dosage – 4 to 60 mg/day.
>> Intra-articular, intralesional, or soft tissue administration: 2 to 30 mg.
>> Oral:
>>> Initial dosage – 5 to 60 mL (5 to 60 mg base) per day.
>>> Multiple sclerosis (acute exacerbations) – 200 mg daily for a week, followed by 80 mg every other day or dexamethasone 4 to 8 mg every other day for 1 month.

PREDNISONE: Initial dosage varies from 5 to 60 mg/day. Prednisone is inactive and must be metabolized to prednisolone. This may be impaired in patients with liver disease.

TRIAMCINOLONE:
> Triamcinolone, oral –
>> Adrenocortical insufficiency: 4 to 12 mg, in addition to mineralocorticoid therapy.
>> Rheumatic and dermatological disorders and bronchial asthma: 8 to 16 mg.
>> Allergic states: 8 to 12 mg.
>> Ophthalmological diseases: 12 to 40 mg.
>> Respiratory diseases: 16 to 48 mg.
>> Hematologic disorders: 16 to 60 mg.
>> Tuberculous meningitis: 32 to 48 mg.
>> Acute rheumatic carditis: 20 to 60 mg.

*Acute leukemia and lymphoma (adults):* 16 to 40 mg. It may be necessary to give as much as 100 mg/day in leukemia.

*Acute leukemia (children):* 1 to 2 mg/kg.

*Edematous states:* 16 to 20 mg (up to 48 mg) until diuresis occurs.

*Systemic lupus erythematosus:* 20 to 32 mg.

Triamcinolone diacetate –

*Systemic:* Not for IV use. May be administered IM for initial therapy; however, most clinicians prefer to adjust the dose orally until adequate control is attained. The average dose is 40 mg IM per week. In general, a single parenteral dose 4 to 7 times the oral daily dose controls the patient from 4 to 7 days, up to 3 to 4 weeks.

*Intra-articular and intrasynovial:* 5 to 40 mg.

*Intralesional or sublesional:* 5 to 48 mg. Do not use more than 12.5 mg/injection site. The usual average dose is 25 mg per lesion.

Triamcinolone hexacetonide – Not for IV use.

*Intra-articular:* 2 to 20 mg average.

*Intralesional or sublesional:* Up to 0.5 mg per square inch of affected area.

Triamcinolone acetonide –

*Systemic:*

*Initial IM dose* – 2.5 to 60 mg/day. Not for IV use.

*Intra-articular or intrabursal administration and for injection into tendon sheaths:*

*Initial dose* – 2.5 to 5 mg for smaller joints and 5 to 15 mg for larger joints. For adults, doses up to 10 mg for smaller areas and up to 40 mg for larger areas are usually sufficient.

*Intradermal:* Use only 3 or 10 mg/mL. Initial dose varies; limit to 1 mg per site.

## Actions

*Pharmacology:* The naturally occurring adrenal cortical steroids have both anti-inflammatory (glucocorticoid) and salt-retaining (mineralocorticoid) properties. These compounds are used as replacement therapy in adrenocortical deficiency states and may be used for their anti-inflammatory effects.

*Pharmacokinetics:* **Hydrocortisone** and most of its congeners are readily absorbed from the GI tract; altered onsets and durations are usually achieved with injections of suspensions and esters. Hydrocortisone is metabolized by the liver, which is the rate-limiting step in its clearance. The metabolism and excretion of the synthetic glucocorticoids generally parallel hydrocortisone. Induction of hepatic enzymes will increase the metabolic clearance of hydrocortisone and the synthetic glucocorticoids.

| Glucocorticoid Equivalencies, Potencies, and Half-Life | | | | |
|---|---|---|---|---|
| Glucocorticoid | Equivalent potency dose (mg)[a] | Anti-inflammatory potency[a] | Sodium-retaining potency | Half-life plasma (min) |
| *Short-acting* | | | | |
| Cortisone | 25 | 0.8 | 2 | 30 |
| Hydrocortisone | 20 | 1 | 2 | 80 to 118 |
| *Intermediate-acting* | | | | |
| Methylprednisolone | 4 | 5 | 0 | 78 to 188 |
| Prednisone | 5 | 4 | 1 | 60 |
| Prednisolone | 5 | 4 | 1 | 115 to 212 |
| Triamcinolone | 4 | 5 | 0 | 200+ |
| *Long-acting* | | | | |
| Betamethasone | 0.6 to 0.75 | 20 to 30 | 0 | 300+ |
| Dexamethasone | 0.75 | 20 to 30 | 0 | 110 to 210 |

[a] When converting doses, use only equivalent potency column, not anti-inflammatory potency column.

## Contraindications

Systemic fungal infections; hypersensitivity to the drug; IM use in ITP; administration of live virus vaccines (eg, smallpox) in patients receiving immunosuppressive corticosteroid doses (see Warnings).

## Warnings

*Infections:* Corticosteroids may mask signs of infection, and new infections may appear during their use. There may be decreased resistance and inability of the host defense mechanisms to prevent dissemination of the infection. Restrict use in active tuberculosis to cases of fulminating or disseminated disease in which the corticosteroid is used for disease management with appropriate chemotherapy. Corticosteroids may exacerbate systemic fungal infections and may activate latent amebiasis.

*Hepatitis:* Corticosteroids may be harmful in chronic active hepatitis positive for hepatitis B surface antigen.

*Ocular effects:* Prolonged use may produce posterior subcapsular cataracts, glaucoma with possible damage to the optic nerves, and may enhance the establishment of secondary ocular infections caused by fungi or viruses.

*Fluid and electrolyte balance:* Average and large doses of **hydrocortisone** or **cortisone** can cause elevation of blood pressure, salt and water retention, and increased excretion of potassium. These effects are less likely to occur with the synthetic derivatives except when used in large doses.

*Immunosuppression:* During therapy, do not use live virus vaccines (eg, smallpox). Do not immunize patients who are receiving corticosteroids, especially high doses, because of possible hazards of neurological complications and a lack of antibody response. This does not apply to patients receiving corticosteroids as replacement therapy.

*Adrenal suppression:* Prolonged therapy of pharmacologic doses may lead to hypothalamic-pituitary-adrenal suppression. The degree of adrenal suppression varies with the dosage, relative glucocorticoid activity, biological half-life, and duration of glucocorticoid therapy within each individual. Adrenal suppression may be minimized by the use of intermediate-acting glucocorticoids (**prednisone, prednisolone, methylprednisolone**) on an alternate-day schedule.

*Stress:* In patients receiving or recently withdrawn from corticosteroid therapy subjected to unusual stress, increased dosage of rapidly acting corticosteroids is indicated before, during, and after stressful situations, except in patients on high-dose therapy.

*Cardiovascular:* Reports suggest an apparent association between corticosteroid use and left ventricular free wall rupture after a recent MI.

*Hypersensitivity reactions:* Anaphylactoid reactions have occurred rarely with corticosteroid therapy.

*Renal function impairment:* Edema may occur in the presence of renal disease with a fixed or decreased glomerular filtration rate.

*Elderly:* Consider the risk/benefit factors of steroid use. Consider lower doses because of body changes caused by aging (ie, diminution of muscle mass and plasma volume).

*Pregnancy:* Corticosteroids cross the placenta (**prednisone** has the poorest transport). Chronic maternal ingestion during the first trimester has shown a 1% incidence of cleft palate in humans. Hypoadrenalism has occurred.

*Lactation:* Corticosteroids appear in breast milk and could suppress growth, interfere with endogenous corticosteroid production, or cause other unwanted effects in the nursing infant. However, large doses for short periods may not harm the infant. Alternatives to consider include waiting 3 to 4 hours after the dose before breast-feeding and using **prednisolone** rather than **prednisone**.

*Children:* Carefully observe growth and development of infants and children on prolonged corticosteroid therapy.

## Precautions

*Monitoring:* Observe patients for weight increase, edema, hypertension, and excessive potassium excretion, as well as for less obvious signs of adrenocortical steroid-induced untoward effects. Monitor for a negative nitrogen balance due to protein catabolism. Evaluate blood pressure and body weight, and do routine laboratory studies, including 2-hour postprandial blood glucose and serum potassium and a chest x-ray at regular intervals during prolonged therapy. Upper GI x-rays are desirable in patients with known or suspected peptic ulcer disease or significant dyspepsia or in patients complaining of gastric distress.

*Use the lowest possible dose:* Make a benefit/risk decision in each individual case as to the size of the dose, duration of treatment, and the use of daily or intermittent therapy because complications of treatment are dependent on these factors.

*Steroid psychosis:* Steroid psychosis is characterized by a delirious or toxic psychosis with clouded sensorium. Other symptoms may include euphoria, insomnia, mood swings, personality changes, and severe depression. The onset of symptoms usually occurs within 15 to 30 days. Predisposing factors include doses greater than **prednisone** 40 mg equivalent, female predominance, and, possibly, a family history of psychiatric illness.

*Multiple sclerosis:* Although corticosteroids are effective in speeding the resolution of acute exacerbations of MS, they do not affect the ultimate outcome or natural history of the disease.

*Repository injections:* To minimize the likelihood and severity of atrophy, do not inject subcutaneously, avoid injection into the deltoid, and avoid repeated IM injections into the same site, if possible. Repository injections are not recommended as initial therapy in acute situations.

*Local injections:* Intra-articular injection may produce systemic and local effects. A marked increase in pain accompanied by local swelling, further restriction of joint motion, fever, and malaise is suggestive of septic arthritis. Frequent intra-articular injection may damage joint tissues.

*Special risk:* Use with caution in the following situations: Nonspecific ulcerative colitis if there is a probability of impending perforation, abscess, or other pyogenic infection; diverticulitis; fresh intestinal anastomoses; hypertension; CHF; thromboembolitic tendencies; thrombophlebitis; osteoporosis; exanthema; Cushing syndrome; antibiotic-resistant infections; convulsive disorders; metastatic carcinoma; myasthenia gravis; vaccinia; varicella; diabetes mellitus; hypothyroidism, cirrhosis (enhanced effect of corticosteroids).

## Drug Interactions

Drugs that may be affected by glucocorticoids include anticholinesterases, anticoagulants, cyclosporine, digitalis glycosides, isoniazid, nondepolarizing neuromuscular blockers, potassium-depleting agents (eg, diuretics), salicylates, somatrem, and theophyllines. Drugs that may affect corticosteroids include aminoglutethimide, barbiturates, cholestyramine, oral contraceptives, ephedrine, estrogens, hydantoins, ketoconazole, macrolide antibiotics, and rifampin.

*CYP3A4 inhibitors:* If coadministration with a CYP3A4 inhibitor is indicated, closely monitor patients for increased signs or symptoms of hypercorticism. Consider reduction in **budesonide** dose.

*Drug/Lab test interactions:* Urine glucose and serum cholesterol levels may increase. Decreased serum levels of potassium, $T_3$, and a minimal decrease of $T_4$ may occur. Thyroid $I^{131}$ uptake may be decreased. False-negative results with the nitrobluetetrazolium test for bacterial infection. **Dexamethasone**, given for cerebral edema, may alter the results of a brain scan (decreased uptake of radioactive material).

## Adverse Reactions

Adverse reactions that may occur include abdominal distension, acneiform eruptions, aggravation of preexisting psychiatric conditions, allergic dermatitis, anaphylactoid/hypersensitivity reactions, cardiac arrhythmias or EKG changes caused by potassium deficiency, convulsions, development of Cushingoid state (eg, moonface, buffalo hump, supraclavicular fat pad enlargement, central obesity), erythema, fatigue, glaucoma, glycosuria, headache, hirsutism, hyperglycemia, hypertension, hypocalcemia, hypokalemia, hypotension or shock-like reactions, impaired wound healing, increased appetite and weight gain, increased IOP, increased sweating, insomnia, malaise, menstrual irregularities, metabolic alkalosis, muscle mass loss, muscle weakness, myocardial rupture following recent MI, nausea, neuritis/paresthesias, osteoporosis, pancreatitis, petechiae/ecchymoses, purpura, sodium and fluid retention, spontaneous fractures, steroid psychoses, suppression of growth in children, syncopal episodes, tendon rupture, thin fragile skin, thromboembolism or fat embolism, thrombophlebitis, ulcerative esophagitis, urticaria, vomiting, vertigo.

# MIGLITOL

| Tablets: 25, 50, and 100 mg (*Rx*) | *Glyset* (Pfizer) |
|---|---|

### Indications

*Type 2 diabetes:* Monotherapy adjunct to diet to improve glycemic control in patients with type 2 diabetes whose hyperglycemia cannot be managed by diet alone.

*Combination therapy* – In combination with a sulfonylurea when diet plus either miglitol or a sulfonylurea alone do not result in adequate glycemic control. The effect of miglitol to enhance glycemic control is additive to that of sulfonylureas when used in combination, presumably because the mechanism of action is different.

### Administration and Dosage

The use of miglitol must be viewed as a treatment in addition to diet and not as a substitute for diet or as a convenient mechanism for avoiding dietary restraint.

*Initial dosage:* The recommended starting dosage is 25 mg, given orally 3 times/day at the start (with the first bite) of each main meal. However, some patients may benefit by starting at 25 mg once daily to minimize GI adverse effects and gradually increasing the frequency of administration to 3 times/day.

*Maintenance dosage:* The usual maintenance dose of miglitol is 50 mg 3 times/day although some patients may benefit from increasing the dose to 100 mg 3 times/day. In order to allow adaptation to potential adverse effects, initiate miglitol therapy at a dosage of 25 mg 3 times/day, the lowest effective dosage, and then gradually titrate upward. After 4 to 8 weeks of the 25 mg 3 times/day regimen, increase the dosage to 50 mg 3 times/day for about 3 months if measured. Measure glycosylated hemoglobin level if not satisfactory, the dosage may be further increased to 100 mg 3 times/day, the maximum recommended dosage. If no further reduction in postprandial glucose or glycosylated hemoglobin levels is observed with titration to 100 mg 3 times/day, consider lowering the dose.

*Maximum dosage:* The maximum recommended dosage is 100 mg 3 times/day.

*Combination with sulfonylureas:* Because its mechanism of action is different, the effect of miglitol to enhance glycemic control is additive to that of sulfonyureas when used in combination. Miglitol given in combination with a sulfonylurea will cause a further lowering of blood glucose and may increase the risk of hypoglycemia caused by the additive effects of the 2 agents.

### Actions

*Pharmacology:* Miglitol is an alpha-glucoside inhibitor that delays the digestion of ingested carbohydrates resulting in a smaller rise in blood glucose concentration following meals. Miglitol reduces levels of glycosylated hemoglobin in patients with type 2 (non-insulin-dependent) diabetes mellitus.

In contrast to sulfonylureas and thiazolidinediones, miglitol does not enhance insulin secretion. Miglitol has minor inhibitory activity against lactase and, at recommended doses, would not be expected to induce lactose intolerance.

*Pharmacokinetics:*

*Absorption* – Absorption of miglitol is saturable at high doses; a dose of 25 mg is completely absorbed, whereas a dose of 100 mg is only 50% to 70% absorbed. Peak concentrations are reached in 2 to 3 hours.

*Distribution* – The protein binding of miglitol is negligible (less than 4%). Miglitol has a volume of distribution of 0.18 L/kg, consistent with distribution primarily into the extracellular fluid.

*Metabolism* – No metabolites have been detected in plasma, urine, or feces, indicating a lack of either systemic or presystemic metabolism.

*Excretion* – Miglitol is eliminated by renal excretion as unchanged drug. Following a 25 mg dose, more than 95% of the dose is recovered in the urine within 24 hours. The elimination half-life from plasma is approximately 2 hours.

## Contraindications

Diabetic ketoacidoses; inflammatory bowel disease; colonic ulceration; partial intestinal obstruction; patients predisposed to intestinal obstruction; chronic intestinal diseases associated with marked disorders of digestion or absorption or with conditions that may deteriorate as a result of increased gas formation in the intestine; hypersensitivity to the drug or any of its components.

## Warnings

*GI:* GI symptoms are the most common reactions to miglitol. The incidence of diarrhea and abdominal pain tend to diminish considerably with continued treatment.

*Renal function impairment:* Plasma concentrations of miglitol in renally impaired volunteers were proportionally increased relative to the degree of renal dysfunction. Long-term clinical trials in diabetic patients with significant renal dysfunction (serum creatinine more than 2 mg/dL) have not been conducted. Treatment of these patients with miglitol is not recommended.

*Pregnancy: Category B.*

*Lactation:* Although the levels of miglitol reached in breast milk are exceedingly low, do not administer miglitol to a nursing woman.

*Children:* Safety and efficacy have not been established.

## Precautions

*Monitoring:* Monitor therapeutic response to miglitol by periodic blood glucose tests. Measurement of glycosylated hemoglobin levels is recommended for the monitoring of long-term glycemic control.

*Hypoglycemia:* Because of its mechanism of action, miglitol, when administered alone, should not cause hypoglycemia. It may increase the hypoglycemic potential of the sulfonylurea. Use oral glucose (dextrose), whose absorption is not delayed by miglitol, instead of sucrose (cane sugar) in the treatment of mild to moderate hypoglycemia. Sucrose, whose hydrolysis to glucose and fructose is inhibited by miglitol, is unsuitable for the rapid correction of hypoglycemia. Severe hypoglycemia may require the use of either IV glucose infusion or glucagon injection.

*Blood glucose control:* When diabetic patients are exposed to stress such as fever, trauma, infection or surgery, a temporary loss of control of blood glucose may occur. At such times, temporary insulin therapy may be necessary.

## Drug Interactions

Drugs that may affect miglitol include digestive enzymes and intestinal adsorbents. Drugs that may be affected by miglitol include digoxin, glyburide, metformin, propranolol, and ranitidine.

## Adverse Reactions

Adverse reactions may include skin rash (4.3%, generally transient), flatulence (41.5%), diarrhea (28.7%), and abdominal pain (11.7%).

*Lab test abnormalities:* Low serum iron (9.2%) usually does not persist in the majority of cases and is not associated with reductions in hemoglobin or changes in other hematologic indices.

# REPAGLINIDE

**Tablets:** 0.5, 1, and 2 mg *(Rx)*                    *Prandin* (Novo Nordisk)

## Indications

*Type 2 diabetes mellitus:* As an adjunct to diet and exercise to lower the blood glucose in patients with type 2 diabetes mellitus and in combination with metformin or thiazolidinediones to lower blood glucose in patients whose hyperglycemia cannot be controlled by exercise, diet, and either agent alone.

## Administration and Dosage

Repaglinide doses are usually taken within 15 minutes of the meal, but time may vary from immediately preceding the meal to as long as 30 minutes before the meal.

*Starting dose:* For patients not previously treated or whose glycosylated hemoglobin (HbA$_{1c}$) is less than 8%, the starting dose is 0.5 mg with each meal. For patients previously treated with blood glucose-lowering agents and whose HbA$_{1c}$ is 8% or more, the initial dose is 1 or 2 mg before each meal.

*Dose adjustment:* Determine dosing adjustments by blood glucose response, usually fasting blood glucose. Double the preprandial dose up to 4 mg with each meal until satisfactory blood glucose response is achieved. At least 1 week should elapse to assess response after each dose adjustment.

*Dose range:* Dose range is 0.5 to 4 mg taken with meals. Repaglinide may be dosed preprandially 2, 3, or 4 times daily in response to changes in the patient's meal pattern. Maximum recommended daily dose is 16 mg.

*Patient management:* Monitor long-term efficacy by measurement of HbA$_{1c}$ levels approximately every 3 months. Failure to follow an appropriate dosage regimen may precipitate hypoglycemia or hyperglycemia. Patients who do not adhere to their prescribed dietary and drug regimen are more prone to exhibit unsatisfactory response to therapy including hypoglycemia. When hypoglycemia occurs in patients taking a combination of repaglinide and a thiazolidinedione or repaglinide and metformin, reduce the dose of repaglinide.

*Patients receiving other oral hypoglycemic agents:* When repaglinide is used to replace therapy with other oral hypoglycemic agents, it may be started the day after the final dose is given. Observe patients carefully for hypoglycemia. When transferred from longer half-life sulfonylureas (eg, chlorpropamide), close monitoring may be indicated for up to 1 week or more.

*Combination therapy:* If repaglinide monotherapy does not result in adequate glycemic control, metformin or a thiazolidinedione may be added. Or, if metformin or thiazolidinedione therapy does not provide adequate control, repaglinide may be added. The starting dose and dose adjustments for combination therapy are the same as repaglinide monotherapy. Carefully adjust the dose of each drug to determine the minimal dose required. Failure to do so could result in an increase in the incidence of hypoglycemic episodes. Use appropriate monitoring of fasting plasma glucose (FPG) and HbA$_{1c}$.

*Renal function impairment:* Patients with type 2 diabetes who have severe renal function impairment should initiate repaglinide with the 0.5 mg dose; subsequently, carefully titrate patients.

## Actions

*Pharmacology:* Repaglinide is a nonsulfonylurea hypoglycemic agent of the meglitinide class. It lowers blood glucose levels by stimulating the release of insulin. This action is dependent on functioning beta cells in the pancreatic islets. Insulin release is glucose-dependent and diminishes at low glucose concentrations.

*Pharmacokinetics:*

    *Absorption* – After oral administration, repaglinide is rapidly and completely absorbed from the GI tract. Peak plasma drug levels occur within 1 hour. The mean absolute bioavailability is 56%.

    *Distribution* – Protein binding and binding to human serum albumin was more than 98%.

    *Metabolism* – Repaglinide is completely metabolized by the liver. The cytochrome P450 enzyme system, specifically 3A4, is involved in the N-dealkylation of repaglinide.

    *Excretion* – Repaglinide is rapidly eliminated from the blood stream with a half-life of about 1 hour.

## Contraindications

Diabetic ketoacidosis, with or without coma (treat with insulin); type 1 diabetes; hypersensitivity to the drug or its inactive ingredients.

## Warnings

*Diet/Exercise:* Use of repaglinide must be viewed as a treatment in addition to diet and not as a substitute for diet or as a convenient mechanism for avoiding dietary restraint. Loss of blood glucose control on diet alone may be transient requiring only short-term administration of repaglinide.

*Renal function impairment:* Patients with type 2 diabetes who have severe renal function impairment should initiate repaglinide with the 0.5 mg dose. Studies were not conducted in patients with creatinine clearances lower than 20 mL/min or patients with renal failure requiring hemodialysis.

*Hepatic function impairment:* Patients with impaired liver function may be exposed to higher concentrations of repaglinide and its metabolites. Use repaglinide cautiously in patients with impaired liver function. Utilize longer intervals between dose adjustments to allow full assessment of response.

*Pregnancy: Category C.*

*Lactation:* It is not known whether repaglinide is excreted in breast milk.

*Children:* No studies have been performed in pediatric patients.

## Precautions

*Monitoring:* Periodically monitor FPG and HbA$_{1c}$ levels.

*Hypoglycemia:* Hepatic insufficiency may cause elevated repaglinide blood levels and may diminish gluconeogenic capacity, both of which increase the risk of serious hypoglycemia. Elderly, debilitated, or malnourished patients, and those with adrenal, pituitary, or hepatic insufficiency are particularly susceptible to the hypoglycemic action of glucose-lowering drugs.

The frequency of hypoglycemia is greater in patients with type 2 diabetes who have not been previously treated with oral hypoglycemic agents or whose HbA$_{1c}$ is less than 8%. Administer with meals to lessen the risk of hypoglycemia.

Patients taking repaglinide should not start taking gemfibrozil; patients taking gemfibrozil should not start taking repaglinide. Concomitant use may result in enhanced and prolonged blood glucose-lowering effects of repaglinide. Use caution in patients already on repaglinide.

Gemfibrozil and itraconazole have a synergistic metabolic inhibitory effect on repaglinide. Patients taking repaglinide and gemfibrozil should not take itraconazole.

*Secondary failure:* It may be necessary to discontinue repaglinide and administer insulin if the patient is exposed to stress (eg, fever, trauma, infection, surgery).

## Drug Interactions

Drugs that may affect repaglinide include CYP 450 inhibitors (eg, ketoconazole, macrolide antibiotics), CYP 450 inducers (eg, rifampin, barbiturates, carbamazepine, clarithromycin), beta blockers, chloramphenicol, coumarins, NSAIDs, probenecid, MAOIs, salicylates, sulfonamides, calcium channel blockers, corticosteroids, estrogens, gemfibrozil, itraconazole, isoniazid, nicotinic acid, oral contraceptives, phenothiazines, phenytoin, sympathomimetics, thiazides and other diuretics, thyroid products, levonorgestrel and ethinyl estradiol, and simvastatin. Drugs that may be affected by repaglinide include levonorgestrel and ethinyl estradiol.

*Drug/Food interactions:* When given with food, mean C$_{max}$ and AUC of repaglinide were decreased. Administer repaglinide before meals.

## Adverse Reactions

The most common adverse events leading to discontinuation during trials were hyperglycemia, hypoglycemia, and related symptoms.

Adverse reactions occurring in at least 3% of patients include: arthralgia, back pain, bronchitis, cardiovascular events, chest pain, constipation, diarrhea, dyspepsia, headache, hypoglycemia, nausea, paresthesia, rhinitis, sinusitis, URI, urinary tract infection, vomiting.

# NATEGLINIDE

**Tablets:** 60 and 120 mg (*Rx*)                    *Starlix* (Novartis)

### Indications

*Type 2 diabetes mellitus:*

    *Monotherapy* – To lower blood glucose in patients with type 2 diabetes whose hyperglycemia cannot be adequately controlled by diet and physical exercise and who have not been chronically treated with other antidiabetic agents.

    *Combination therapy* – In patients whose hyperglycemia is inadequately controlled with metformin or after a therapeutic response to a thiazolidinedione, nateglinide may be added to, but not substituted for, metformin.

Do not switch patients whose hyperglycemia is not adequately controlled with glyburide or other insulin secretagogues to nateglinide; do not add nateglinide to their treatment regimen.

### Administration and Dosage

*Monotherapy and combination with metformin or a thiazolidinedione:* The recommended starting and maintenance dose of nateglinide, alone or in combination with metformin, is 120 mg 3 times/day before meals.

    The 60 mg dose of nateglinide, alone or in combination with metformin or a thiazolidinedione, may be used in patients who are near goal $HbA_{1c}$ when treatment is initiated.

Take 1 to 30 minutes prior to meals.

### Actions

*Pharmacology:* Nateglinide lowers blood glucose levels by stimulating insulin secretion from the pancreas. This action is dependent upon functioning beta-cells in the pancreatic islets.

*Pharmacokinetics:*

    *Absorption* – Following oral administration immediately prior to a meal, nateglinide is rapidly absorbed with mean peak plasma drug concentrations ($C_{max}$) generally occurring within 1 hour ($T_{max}$) after dosing. Absolute bioavailability is estimated to be $\approx$ 73%.

    *Distribution* – Nateglinide is extensively bound (98%) to serum proteins, primarily serum albumin.

    *Metabolism* – The major routes of metabolism are hydroxylation followed by glucuronide conjugation.

    Nateglinide is predominantly metabolized by cytochrome P450 isoenzymes CYP2C9 (70%) and CYP3A4 (30%).

    *Excretion* – Nateglinide and its metabolites are rapidly and completely eliminated following oral administration, with an average elimination half-life of about 1.5 hours.

### Contraindications

Known hypersensitivity to the drug or its inactive ingredients; type 1 diabetes; diabetic ketoacidosis.

### Warnings

*Diet/Exercise:* Use of nateglinide must be viewed as a treatment in addition to diet and not as a substitute for diet or as a convenient mechanism for avoiding dietary restraint.

*Hepatic function impairment:* Use nateglinide with caution in patients with chronic liver disease. Use with caution in patients with moderate to severe liver disease because such patients have not been studied.

*Pregnancy: Category* C.

*Lactation:* It is not known whether nateglinide is excreted in human milk. Because many drugs are excreted in human milk, do not administer nateglinide to a nursing woman.

*Children:* The safety and efficacy of nateglinide in pediatric patients have not been established.

**Precautions**

*Monitoring:* Periodically assess response to therapies with glucose values and HbA$_{1c}$ levels.

*Hypoglycemia:* Geriatric patients, malnourished patients, and those with adrenal or pituitary insufficiency are more susceptible to the glucose-lowering effect of these treatments. Hypoglycemia may be difficult to recognize in patients with autonomic neuropathy or those who use beta-blockers. Administer nateglinide before meals to reduce the risk of hypoglycemia. Patients who skip meals should also skip their scheduled dose of nateglinide to reduce the risk of hypoglycemia.

*Secondary failure:* Transient loss of glycemic control may occur with fever, infection, trauma, or surgery. Insulin therapy may be needed instead of nateglinide therapy at such times. Secondary failure, or reduced effectiveness of nateglinide over a period of time, may occur.

**Drug Interactions**

Nateglinide is predominantly metabolized by the cytochrome P450 isozyme CYP2C9 (70%) and to a lesser extent CYP3A4 (30%). Nateglinide is a potential inhibitor of the CYP2C9 isoenzyme in vivo as indicated by its ability to inhibit the in vitro metabolism of tolbutamide. Inhibition of CYP3A4 metabolic reactions was not detected in in vitro experiments.

Drugs that may affect nateglinide include nonsteroidal anti-inflammatory agents (NSAIDs), salicylates, monoamine oxidase inhibitors, rifamycins, MAOIs, and nonselective beta-adrenergic blocking agents, thiazides, corticosteroids, thyroid products, and sympathomimetics.

*Drug/Food interactions:* Peak plasma levels were significantly reduced when nateglinide was administered 10 minutes prior to a liquid meal.

**Adverse Reactions**

Adverse reactions occurring in at least 3% of patients include arthropathy, back pain, diarrhea, dizziness, flu symptoms, upper respiratory tract infection.

# ACARBOSE

**Tablets:** 25, 50, and 100 mg *(Rx)*                     *Precose* (Bayer)

**Indications**

*Type 2 diabetes:* As monotherapy as an adjunct to diet to lower blood glucose in patients with type 2 diabetes whose hyperglycemia cannot be managed on diet alone.

Acarbose also may be used with a sulfonylurea when diet plus either acarbose or a sulfonylurea do not result in adequate glycemic control.

**Administration and Dosage**

Dosage of acarbose must be individualized while not exceeding the maximum recommended dose of 100 mg 3 times/day for patients more than 60 kg and 50 mg 3 times/day for patients less than 60 kg.

During treatment initiation and dose titration, use 1 hour postprandial plasma glucose to determine the therapeutic response to acarbose and identify the minimum effective dose for the patient. Thereafter, measure glycosylated hemoglobin at intervals of about 3 months.

*Initial dosage:* The recommended starting dosage is 25 mg given 3 times/day at the start (with the first bite) of each main meal. However, some patients may benefit from more gradual dose titration to minimize GI side effects. This may be achieved by initiating treatment at 25 mg once per day and subsequently increasing the frequency of administration to achieve 25 mg three times daily.

*Maintenance dosage:* Adjust dosage at 4- to 8-week intervals based on 1-hour postprandial glucose levels and on tolerance. After the initial dosage of 25 mg 3 times/day, the dosage can be increased to 50 mg 3 times/day. Some patients may benefit from further increasing the dosage to 100 mg 3 times/day. The maintenance dose ranges from 50 to 100 mg 3 times/day. However, because patients with low body weight may be at increased risk for elevated serum transaminases, consider only patients with body weight more than 60 kg for dose titration above 50 mg 3 times/day. If no further reduction in postprandial glucose or glycosylated hemoglobin levels is observed with titration to 100 mg 3 times/day, consider lowering the dose. Once an effective and tolerated dosage has been established, it should be maintained.

*Coadministration:* Acarbose given in combination with a sulfonylurea or insulin will cause a further lowering of blood glucose and may increase the hypoglycemic potential of the sulfonylurea.

### Actions

*Pharmacology:* Acarbose, an alpha-glucosidase inhibitor, is a complex oligosaccharide that delays the digestion of ingested carbohydrates, thereby resulting in a smaller rise in blood glucose concentration following meals. As a consequence of plasma glucose reduction, acarbose reduces levels of glycosylated hemoglobin.

Because its mechanism of action is different, the effect of acarbose to enhance glycemic control is additive to that of sulfonylureas when used in combination. In contrast to sulfonylureas, acarbose does not enhance insulin secretion.

*Pharmacokinetics:*

*Absorption* – Following oral dosing, peak plasma concentrations were attained 14 to 24 hours after dosing, while peak plasma concentrations of active drug were attained at about 1 hour.

*Metabolism* – Acarbose is metabolized exclusively within the GI tract, principally by intestinal bacteria, but also by digestive enzymes. A fraction of these metabolites (about 34% of the dose) was absorbed and subsequently excreted in the urine.

*Excretion* – The fraction of acarbose that is absorbed as intact drug is almost completely excreted by the kidneys. When acarbose was given IV, 89% of the dose was recovered in the urine as active drug within 48 hours. In contrast, less than 2% of an oral dose was recovered in the urine as active (ie, parent compound and active metabolite) drug. The plasma elimination half-life of acarbose activity is about 2 hours in healthy volunteers.

### Contraindications

Hypersensitivity to the drug; diabetic ketoacidosis or cirrhosis; inflammatory bowel disease; colonic ulceration; partial intestinal obstruction or predisposition to intestinal obstruction; chronic intestinal diseases associated with marked disorders of digestion or absorption; conditions that may deteriorate as a result of increased gas formation in the intestine.

### Warnings

*Diet/Physical activity:* The use of acarbose must be viewed by both the physician and patient as a treatment in addition to diet, and not as a substitute for diet or as a convenient mechanism for avoiding dietary restraint.

*Renal function impairment:* Patients with severe renal impairment (creatinine clearance [Ccr] less than 25 mL/min/1.73 $m^2$) attained about 5 times higher peak plasma concentrations of acarbose and 6 times larger AUCs than volunteers with normal renal function. Treatment of these patients with acarbose is not recommended.

*Carcinogenesis:* In rats, acarbose treatment resulted in a significant increase in the incidence of renal tumors (adenomas and adenocarcinomas) and benign Leydig cell tumors. Further studies showed that the increased incidence of renal tumors found in the original studies did not occur.

*Pregnancy:* Category B.

*Lactation:* It is not known whether this drug is excreted in breast milk. Do not administer to a nursing woman.

*Children:* Safety and efficacy have not been established.

## Precautions

*Monitoring:* Monitor therapeutic response to acarbose by periodic blood glucose tests. Measurement of glycosylated hemoglobin levels is recommended for the monitoring of long-term glycemic control. Acarbose, particularly at doses in excess of 50 mg 3 times/day may give rise to elevations of serum transaminases and, in rare instances, hyperbilirubinemia. It is recommended that serum transaminase levels be checked every 3 months during the first year of the treatment with acarbose and periodically thereafter. If elevated transaminases are observed, a reduction in dosage or withdrawal of therapy may be indicated, particularly if the elevations persist.

*Hypoglycemia:* Because of its mechanism of action, acarbose alone should not cause hypoglycemia in the fasted or postprandial state. It may increase the hypoglycemic potential of the sulfonylurea. Use oral glucose (dextrose), whose absorption is not inhibited by acarbose, instead of sucrose (cane sugar) in the treatment of mild-to-moderate hypoglycemia. Severe hypoglycemia may require the use of either IV glucose infusion or glucagon injection.

*Loss of blood glucose control:* When diabetic patients are exposed to stress such as fever, trauma, infection or surgery, a temporary loss of control of blood glucose may occur. At such times, temporary insulin therapy may be necessary.

*Hematocrit:* Small reductions in hematocrit occurred.

*Calcium/Vitamin $B_6$:* Low serum calcium and low plasma vitamin $B_6$ levels were associated with acarbose therapy but were thought to be either spurious or of no clinical significance.

*Lab test abnormalities:*

*Elevated serum transaminase levels* – Treatment-emergent elevations of serum transaminases (AST and /or ALT) above the upper limit of normal (ULN), greater than $1.8 \times$ ULN, and greater than $3 \times$ ULN occurred. These elevations were asymptomatic, reversible, more common in females, and, in general, were not associated with other evidence of liver dysfunction. In addition, these serum transaminase elevations appeared to be dose related.

A few cases of fulminant hepatitis with fatal outcome have been reported; the relationship to acarbose is unclear.

## Drug Interactions

Drugs that may interact with acarbose include digestive enzymes, intestinal adsorbents (eg, charcoal) and digoxin.

Certain drugs tend to produce hyperglycemia and may lead to loss of blood glucose control. These drugs include the thiazides and other diuretics, corticosteroids, phenothiazines, thyroid products, estrogens, oral contraceptives, phenytoin, nicotinic acid, sympathomimetics, calcium channel blocking drugs, and isoniazid.

## Adverse Reactions

GI symptoms are the most common reaction to acarbose. In trials, the incidences of abdominal pain, diarrhea, and flatulence were 21%, 33%, and 77%, respectively, with acarbose 50 to 300 mg 3 times/day. Rarely, hypersensitive skin reactions, such as rash, may occur.

# INSULIN

**INSULIN INJECTION (REGULAR)**

**Injection**: 100 units/mL (purified pork) (*otc*)
100 units/mL (human insulin [rDNA]) (*otc*)

*Regular Iletin* II (Lilly)
*Humulin* R (Lilly), *Novolin* R (Novo Nordisk), *Novolin* R *Prefilled* (Novo Nordisk), *Velosulin* BR (Novo Nordisk)

**Cartridges**: 100 units/mL (human insulin [rDNA]). For use with *NovoPen* and *Novolin Pen* (*otc*)

*Novolin* R *PenFill* (Novo Nordisk)

---

| **ISOPHANE INSULIN SUSPENSION (NPH; insulin combined with protamine and zinc)** | |
| --- | --- |
| **Injection:** 100 units/mL (purified pork) (*otc*) | *NPH Iletin II* (Lilly) |
| 100 units/mL (human insulin [rDNA]) (*otc*) | *Humulin N* (Lilly), *Novolin N* (Novo Nordisk), *Novolin N Prefilled* (Novo Nordisk) |
| **Cartridges:** 100 units/mL (human insulin [rDNA]). For use with *NovoPen* and *Novolin Pen* (*otc*) | *Novolin N PenFill* (Novo Nordisk) |

| **ISOPHANE INSULIN SUSPENSION (NPH) AND INSULIN INJECTION (REGULAR)** | |
| --- | --- |
| 70% isophane insulin and 30% insulin injection | |
| **Injection:** 100 units/mL (human insulin [rDNA]) (*otc*) | *Humulin 70/30* (Lilly), *Novolin 70/30* (Novo Nordisk), *Novolin 70/30 Prefilled* (Novo Nordisk) |
| **Cartridges:** 100 units/mL (human insulin [rDNA]). For use with *NovoPen* and *Novolin Pen* (*otc*) | *Novolin 70/30 PenFill* (Novo Nordisk) |
| 50% isophane insulin and 50% insulin injection | |
| **Injection:** 100 units/mL (human insulin [rDNA]) (*otc*) | *Humulin 50/50* (Lilly) |

| **INSULIN ZINC SUSPENSION (LENTE; 70% crystalline and 30% amorphous insulin suspension)** | |
| --- | --- |
| **Injection:** 100 units/mL (purified pork) (*otc*) | *Lente Iletin II* (Lilly) |
| 100 units/mL (human insulin [rDNA]) (*otc*) | *Humulin L* (Lilly) |

| **INSULIN ZINC SUSPENSION, EXTENDED (ULTRALENTE)** | |
| --- | --- |
| **Injection:** 100 units/mL (human insulin [rDNA]) (*otc*) | *Humulin U* (Lilly) |

| **INSULIN ANALOG INJECTION** | |
| --- | --- |
| **Injection:** 100 units/mL (human insulin lispro [rDNA]) (*Rx*) | *Humalog* (Lilly), *Humalog Mix 75/25*[a] (Lilly) |
| 100 units/mL (human insulin aspart [rDNA]) (*Rx*) | *NovoLog* (Novo Nordisk) |
| 100 units/mL (insulin aspart [rDNA]) (*Rx*) | *NovoLog Mix 70/30*[b] (Novo Nordisk) |

| **INSULIN GLARGINE** | |
| --- | --- |
| **Injection:** 100 units/mL (insulin glargine [rDNA]) (*Rx*) | *Lantus* (Aventis) |

| **INSULIN GLULISINE** | |
| --- | --- |
| **Injection:** 100 units/mL (insulin glulisine [rDNA]) (*Rx*) | *Apidra* (Aventis) |

| **INSULIN INJECTION CONCENTRATED** | |
| --- | --- |
| **Injection:** 500 units/mL (regular human insulin [rDNA]) (*Rx*) | *Humulin R Regular U-500 (Concentrated)* (Lilly) |

[a] Contains 75% insulin lispro protamine suspension and 25% insulin lispro injection (rDNA).
[b] Contains 70% insulin aspart protamine suspension and 30% insulin aspart (rDNA).

### Indications

Type 1 diabetes mellitus (insulin-dependent).

Type 2 diabetes mellitus (non-insulin-dependent) that cannot be properly controlled by diet, exercise, and weight reduction.

In hyperkalemia, infusion of glucose and insulin produces a shift of potassium into cells and lowers serum potassium levels.

*Severe ketoacidosis/diabetic coma:* Insulin injection (regular insulin) may be given IV or IM for rapid effect in severe ketoacidosis or diabetic coma.

*Highly purified (single component) and human insulins:* Local insulin allergy, immunologic insulin resistance, injection-site lipodystrophy; temporary insulin use (ie, surgery, acute stress type 2 diabetes, gestational diabetes); newly diagnosed diabetic patients.

*Insulin aspart:* Adults with diabetes mellitus for the control of hyperglycemia. Because insulin aspart has a more rapid onset and a shorter duration of action than human regular insulin, insulin aspart normally should be used in regimens together with an intermediate or long-acting insulin. *NovoLog* may be infused subcutaneously by external insulin pumps.

*Insulin lispro:* Treatment of patients with diabetes mellitus for the control of hyperglycemia. Insulin lispro has a more rapid onset and shorter duration of action than regular human insulin. Therefore, in patients with type 1 diabetes, use in regimens that include a longer-acting insulin. However, in patients with type 2 diabetes, insulin lispro may be used without a longer-acting insulin when used in combination therapy with sulfonylureas.

*Children (Humalog only)* – Safety and efficacy in children younger than 18 years of age have not been determined for *Humalog Mix.* Adjustment of basal insulin may be required. To improve accuracy of dosing in children, a diluent may be used. If the diluent is added directly to the vial, the shelf life may be reduced.

*Insulin glargine:* Once-daily subcutaneous administration for the treatment of adults and children with type 1 diabetes mellitus or adults with type 2 diabetes mellitus who require basal (long-acting) insulin for the control of hyperglycemia.

*Insulin glulisine:* Treatment of adult patients with diabetes mellitus for the control of hyperglycemia. Insulin glulisine has a more rapid onset and shorter duration of action than regular human insulin. It normally should be used in regimens that include a longer-acting insulin or basal insulin analog. Insulin glulisine also may be infused subcutaneously by external insulin infusion pumps.

*Insulin concentrated:* Treatment of diabetic patients with marked insulin resistance (requirements greater than 200 units/day), because a large dose may be administered subcutaneously in a reasonable volume.

### Administration and Dosage

The number and size of daily doses, time of administration, and diet and exercise require continuous medical supervision. Dosage adjustment may be necessary when changing types of insulin. Rotate administration sites to prevent lipodystrophy. Do not administer within 1 inch of the same site for 1 month. It may be best to rotate sites within an area rather than rotating areas.

INSULIN: Human regular insulin is best given 30 to 60 minutes before a meal. Administer maintenance doses subcutaneously.

*Children and adults* – 0.5 to 1 units/kg/day.

*Adolescents (during growth spurt)* – 0.8 to 1.2 units/kg/day.

Adjust doses to achieve premeal and bedtime blood glucose levels of 80 to 140 mg/dL (children younger than 5 years of age, 100 to 200 mg/dL).

INSULIN ASPART: Give immediately before a meal. In a meal-related treatment regimen, 50% to 70% of this requirement may be provided by insulin aspart and the remainder provided by an intermediate-acting or long-acting insulin. Patients may require more basal insulin in relation to bolus insulin and more total insulin when using insulin aspart compared with regular human insulin to prevent premeal hyperglycemia.

Because of the fast onset of action of insulin aspart, administer close to a meal (start of meal within 5 to 10 minutes after injection).

*Insulin pump* – When used in external insulin infusion pumps, approximately 50% of the total dose is given as meal-related boluses and the remainder as basal infusion. Higher basal rates in external subcutaneous infusion pumps may be necessary. Change the insulin in the infusion sets every 48 hours or sooner to assure the activity of insulin aspart and proper pump function.

INSULIN LISPRO: Insulin lispro is intended for subcutaneous administration. When used as a meal-time insulin, give insulin lispro within 15 minutes before or immediately after a meal.

*Compatibility* – Insulin lispro may be diluted with sterile diluent for *Humalog, Humulin N, Humulin 50/50, Humulin 70/30,* and *NPH Iletin* to a concentration of 1:10 (equivalent to U-10) or 1:2 (equivalent to U-50). Diluted insulin lispro may remain in patient use for 28 days when stored at 5°C (41°F) and for 14 days when stored at 30°C (86°F).

INSULIN GLARGINE: Insulin glargine is not intended for IV administration. Give insulin glargine subcutaneously once daily at the same time every day. The dose may be administered at any time during the day. IV administration of the usual subcutaneous dose could result in severe hypoglycemia.

Insulin glargine must not be diluted or mixed with any other insulin or solution. Only use if clear and colorless with no particles visible.

*Children* – Insulin glargine can be safely administered to children 6 years of age and older. Administration to children younger than 6 years of age has not been studied. The dose recommendation for changeover to insulin glargine is the same as described for adults.

*Initial dosing* – In a clinical study with insulin-naive patients treated with oral anti-diabetic drugs, insulin glargine was started at an average dose of 10 units once daily, and adjusted to a total daily dose ranging from 2 to 100 units.

*Changeover to insulin glargine* – In clinical studies, when patients were transferred from once-daily NPH human insulin or ultralente human insulin to once-daily insulin glargine, the initial dose was usually not changed. However, when patients were transferred from twice-daily NPH to insulin glargine once daily, the initial dose was usually reduced by about 20% (compared with total daily units of NPH human insulin) within the first week of treatment and then adjusted based on patient response.

INSULIN GLULISINE: Give within 15 minutes before a meal or within 20 minutes after starting a meal. Insulin glulisine is intended for subcutaneous administration and for use by external infusion pump.

Only use if the solution is clear and colorless with no particles visible.

INSULIN CONCENTRATED: Administer subcutaneously. Do not inject IM or IV. Use a tuberculin-type or insulin syringe for dosage measurement. Inadvertent overdose may result in irreversible insulin shock.

Concentrated insulin injection frequently has a duration similar to repository insulin; a single dose demonstrates activity for 24 hours.

*Dosage adjustments* – Closely observe every patient exhibiting insulin resistance who requires concentrated insulin for diabetic control until appropriate dosing is established. Some may require only 1 dose daily; others may require 2 or 3 injections per day. Insulin resistance is frequently self-limited; after several weeks or months of high dosage, responsiveness may be regained and dosage reduced.

*Hypoglycemic reactions* – Hypoglycemia when using this concentrated insulin can be prolonged and severe. Deep secondary hypoglycemic reactions may develop 18 to 24 hours after the original injection of concentrated insulin.

**Actions**

*Pharmacology:* Insulin and its analogs lower blood glucose levels by stimulating peripheral glucose uptake and inhibiting hepatic glucose production. Insulin, secreted by the beta cells of the pancreas, is the principal hormone required for proper glucose use in normal metabolic processes.

The bioavailability of the insulins is identical when given subcutaneously. The human insulins are slightly less antigenic than pork or beef insulins. Human insulin is the insulin of choice for patients with insulin allergy, insulin resistance, all pregnant patients with diabetes, and any patient who uses insulin intermittently.

| Pharmacokinetics and Compatibility of Various Insulins | | | | | | |
|---|---|---|---|---|---|---|
| Insulin preparations | | Half-life (h) | Onset (h) | Peak (h) | Duration (h) | Compatible mixed with |
| Rapid-Acting | Insulin injection (regular) | – | 0.5 to 1 | – | 8 to 12 | All |
| | Prompt insulin zinc suspension (semilente) | – | 1 to 1.5 | 5 to 10 | 12 to 16 | Lente |
| | Lispro insulin solution | 1 | 0.25 | 0.5 to 1.5 | 2 to 5 | Ultralente, NPH |
| | Insulin aspart solution | 1.5 | 0.25 | 1 to 3 | 3 to 5 | a |
| | Insulin glulisine | 0.7 | – | 0.5 to 1.5 | 1 to 2.5 | NPH |
| Intermediate-Acting | Isophane insulin suspension (NPH) | – | 1 to 1.5 | 4 to 12 | 24 | Regular |
| | Insulin zinc suspension (lente) | – | 1 to 2.5 | 7 to 15 | 24 | Regular, semilente |

| Pharmacokinetics and Compatibility of Various Insulins | | | | | |
|---|---|---|---|---|---|
| Insulin preparations | Half-life (h) | Onset (h) | Peak (h) | Duration (h) | Compatible mixed with |
| **Long-Acting** Insulin glargine solution | – | 1.1 | 5[b] | 24[c] | None |
| Protamine zinc insulin suspension (PZI) | – | 4 to 8 | 14 to 24 | 36 | Regular |
| Extended insulin zinc suspension (ultralente) | – | 4 to 8 | 10 to 30 | 20 to 36 | Regular, semilente |

[a] See below.
[b] No pronounced peak; small amounts of insulin glargine are slowly released, resulting in a relatively constant concentration/time profile over 24 hours.
[c] Studies only conducted up to 24 hours.

*Mixing of insulins* – The effects of mixing insulin aspart or lispro with insulins of animal source or insulin preparations produced by other manufacturers have not been studied (see Warnings).

Do not administer mixtures IV. Inject immediately after mixing.

When mixing 2 types of insulin, always draw clear regular insulin into the syringe first. To avoid dosage error, do not alter order of mixing insulins. Each type of insulin used must be of the same concentration (units/mL).

NPH/regular combinations of insulin are stable and are absorbed as if injected separately. Mixtures of regular insulin with lente must be mixed and injected immediately.

Manufacturer premixed formulations remain stable for 1 month at room temperature or for 3 months refrigerated. These mixtures also can be stored in prefilled plastic or glass syringes for 1 week to possibly 14 days under refrigeration. Slightly agitate to remix the insulins. Check for normal appearance.

Semilente, ultralente, and lente insulins may be mixed in any ratio. These mixtures are stable 1 month at room temperature or 3 months under refrigeration.

*Insulin aspart:* If insulin aspart is mixed with NPH human insulin, draw insulin aspart into the syringe first. Do not mix insulin aspart with crystalline zinc insulin preparations because of lack of compatibility data. When used in external subcutaneous infusion pumps for insulin, do not mix with any other insulins or diluent.

*Insulin lispro:* If insulin lispro is mixed with a longer-acting insulin such as *Humulin N* or *Humulin U*, draw lispro into the syringe first to prevent clouding of the lispro by the longer-acting insulin.

*Insulin glulisine:* If insulin glulisine is mixed with NPH human insulin, draw insulin glulisine into the syringe first. Make the injection immediately after mixing. Do not mix insulin glulisine with insulin preparations other than NPH. When it is used in a pump, do not mix insulin glulisine with other insulins or with a diluent.

## Contraindications

During episodes of hypoglycemia and in patients sensitive to any ingredient of the product.

## Warnings

*Change insulins:* Change insulins cautiously and under medical supervision. Changes in purity, strength, brand, type, or species source may require dosage adjustment.

*Hypersensitivity reactions:* May require discontinuation of insulin.

*Local* – Occasionally, redness, swelling, and itching at the injection site may develop. This reaction occurs if the injection is not properly made, if the skin is sensitive to the cleansing solution, or if the patient is allergic to insulin or insulin additives (eg, preservatives).

*Systemic* – Systemic reactions are less common and may present as a rash, shortness of breath, fast pulse, sweating, a drop in blood pressure, bronchospasm, shock, anaphylaxis, or angioedema and may be life-threatening.

*Insulin aspart, insulin glulisine* – Localized reactions and generalized myalgias have been reported with the use of cresol as an injectable excipient.

*Renal/Hepatic function impairment:* Careful glucose monitoring and dose adjustments of insulin may be necessary in these patients. Insulin requirements may be reduced in patients with renal function impairment.

*Pregnancy:* Category B; Category C (insulin glargine, insulin aspart, insulin glulisine).

*Lactation:* Lactating women may require adjustments in insulin dose and diet. It is unknown whether insulin glargine, insulin aspart, or insulin glulisine are excreted in significant amounts in breast milk.

*Children:* Safety and efficacy in patients younger than 12 years of age have not been established.

*Insulin glargine* – Safety and efficacy of insulin glargine have been established in children 6 to 15 years of age with type 1 diabetes.

*Humalog* – Humalog can be used in combination with sulfonylureas in children older than 3 years of age.

## Precautions

*Insulin resistance:* Insulin resistance occurs rarely. Insulin-resistant patients require more than 200 units of insulin/day for more than 2 days in the absence of ketoacidosis or acute infection.

*Hypoglycemia:* Hypoglycemia may result from excessive insulin dose or may be caused by: Increased work or exercise without eating; food not being absorbed in the usual manner because of postponement or omission of a meal or in illness with vomiting, fever, or diarrhea; when insulin requirements decline.

*Diabetic ketoacidosis:* Diabetic ketoacidosis may result from stress, illness, or insulin omission, or may develop slowly after a long period of insulin control. Hyperglucagonemia, hyperglycemia, and ketoacidosis may result.

| Symptoms of Hypoglycemia vs Ketoacidosis | | | | | | | |
|---|---|---|---|---|---|---|---|
| | | Urine glucose/ acetone | Symptoms | | | | |
| Reaction | Onset | | CNS | Respiration | Mouth/GI | Skin | Miscellaneous |
| Hypo-glycemic reaction (insulin reaction) | sudden | 0/0 | fatigue, weakness, nervousness, confusion, headache, diplopia, convulsions, psychoses, dizziness, unconscious-ness | rapid, shallow | numb, tingling, hunger, nausea | pallor, moist, shallow, or dry | normal or non-characteristic pulse, eyeballs normal |
| Keto-acidosis (diabetic coma) | gradual (hours or days) | +/+ | drowsiness, dim vision | air hunger | thirst, acetone breath, nausea, vomiting, abdominal pain, loss of appetite | dry, flushed | rapid pulse, soft eyeballs |

*Lipodystrophy:*

*Lipoatrophy* – Lipoatrophy is the breakdown of adipose tissue at the insulin injection site causing a depression in the skin.

*Lipohypertrophy* – Lipohypertrophy is the result of repeated insulin injection into the same site. This condition may be avoided by rotating the injection site.

*Diet:* Patients must follow a prescribed diet and exercise regularly. Determine the time, number, and amount of individual doses and distribution of food among the meals of the day. Do not change this regimen unless prescribed otherwise.

*Hyperthyroidism/Hypothyroidism:* Hyperthyroidism may cause an increase in the renal clearance of insulin. Therefore, patients may need more insulin to control their diabetes. Hypothyroidism may delay insulin turnover, requiring less insulin to control diabetes.

**Drug Interactions**

| Drugs That Decrease the Hypoglycemic Effect of Insulin | |
| --- | --- |
| Acetazolamide | Estrogens |
| AIDS antivirals | Ethacrynic acid |
| Albuterol | Glucagon |
| Antipsychotic medications | Isoniazid |
| (atypical [eg, olanzapine, clozapine) | Lithium carbonate |
| Asparaginase | Morphine sulfate |
| Calcitonin | Niacin |
| Contraceptives, oral | Nicotine |
| Corticosteroids | Phenothiazines |
| Cyclophosphamide | Phenytoin |
| Danazol | Progestogens (eg, oral contraceptives) |
| Dextrothyroxine | Protease inhibitors |
| Diazoxide | Somatropin |
| Diltiazem | Terbutaline |
| Diuretics | Thiazide diuretics |
| Dobutamine | Thyroid hormones |
| Epinephrine | |

| Drugs That Increase the Hypoglycemic Effect of Insulin | |
| --- | --- |
| ACE inhibitors | Lithium carbonate |
| Alcohol | MAO inhibitors |
| Anabolic steroids | Mebendazole |
| Antidiabetic products, oral | Pentamidine[b] |
| Beta-blockers[a] | Pentoxifylline |
| Calcium | Phenylbutazone |
| Chloroquine | Propoxyphene |
| Clofibrate | Pyridoxine |
| Clonidine | Salicylates |
| Disopyramide | Somatostatin analog (eg, octreotide) |
| Fluoxetine | Sulfinpyrazone |
| Fibrates | Sulfonamides |
| Guanethidine | Tetracyclines |

[a] Nonselective beta-blockers may delay recovery from hypoglycemic episodes and mask their signs/symptoms. Cardioselective agents may be alternatives.
[b] May sometimes be followed by hyperglycemia.

**Adverse Reactions**

*Human insulin:* Hypoglycemia and hypokalemia are among the potential clinical adverse reactions associated with the use of all insulins. Other adverse reactions commonly associated with human insulin therapy include the following:

*Dermatologic* – Injection-site reaction, lipodystrophy, pruritus, rash.

*Lab test abnormalities* – Hypoglycemia, hypokalemia.

*Miscellaneous* – Allergic reactions. Sodium retention and edema may occur, particularly if previously poor metabolic control is improved by intensified insulin therapy. Antibody production.

# INSULIN INJECTION CONCENTRATED

**Injection:** 500 units/mL (purified pork) (Rx)                    *Regular (Concentrated) Iletin II U-500 (Lilly)*

### Indications

Treatment of diabetic patients with marked insulin resistance (requirements more than 200 units/day). A large dose may be administered subcutaneously in a reasonable volume.

### Administration and Dosage

Administer subcutaneously. Do not inject IM or IV. It is inadvisable to inject concentrated insulin IV because of possible inadvertent overdosage.

Use a tuberculin-type or insulin syringe for dosage measurement. Dosage variations are frequent in the insulin-resistant patient, since the individual is unresponsive to the pharmacologic effect of the insulin. Nevertheless, encourage accuracy of measurement because of the potential danger of the preparations.

### Actions

*Pharmacology:*
  *Insulin resistance* – Diabetes can usually be controlled with daily insulin doses 40 to 60 units or less; however, an occasional patient develops such resistance or becomes so unresponsive to the effect of insulin that daily doses of several hundred or even several thousand units are required. Patients who require doses in excess of 300 to 500 units daily usually have impaired insulin receptor function.

*Pharmacokinetics:* It frequently has a duration similar to repository insulin; a single dose demonstrates activity for 24 hours.

### Contraindications

Hypoglycemia.

### Warnings

*General:* This human insulin product differs from animal-source insulins because it is structurally identical to the insulin produced by the body's pancreas and because of its unique manufacturing process.
  Make any change of insulin cautiously and only under medical supervision. Changes in purity, strength, brand (manufacturer), type (eg, regular, NPH, lente), species (beef, pork, beef-pork, human), or method of manufacturer (rDNA vs animal-source insulin) may result in the need for a change in dosage.
  Some patients taking this product may require a change in dosage from that used with animal-source insulins. If an adjustment is needed, it may occur with the first dose or during the first several weeks or months.

*Dosage adjustments:* Closely observe every patient exhibiting insulin resistance who requires concentrated insulin for diabetic control until appropriate dosing is established. Response will vary among patients. Most patients will show a "tolerance" to insulin, so that minor dosage variations will not cause untoward symptoms of insulin shock. Some may require only 1 dose daily; others may require 2 or 3 injections per day.

*Insulin shock:* Observe extreme caution in the measurement of dosage; inadvertent overdose may result in irreversible insulin shock.

*Hypoglycemic reactions:* Hypoglycemia when using this concentrated insulin can be prolonged and severe. As with other human insulin preparations, hypoglycemia reactions may be associated with the administration of concentrated insulin. However, deep secondary hypoglycemic reactions may develop 18 to 24 hours after the original injection of concentrated insulin.

*Lipodystrophy:* Rarely, administration of insulin subcutaneously can result in lipoatrophy (depression in the skin) or lipohypertrophy (enlargement or thickening of tissue).

*Hypersensitivity reactions:* Less common than local allergic reactions, but potentially more serious, is systemic insulin allergy, which may cause generalized urticaria, dyspnea, or wheezing and may, on continued use, progress to anaphylaxis.

*Pregnancy: Category B.*

*Lactation:* It is not known whether insulin is excreted in significant amounts in breast milk. Exercise caution when administering to a nursing woman.

### Precautions

*Monitoring:* Monitor blood and urine glucose, glycohemoglobin and urine ketones frequently. Monitor blood glucose closely and often until dosage is established.

*Insulin resistance:* Insulin resistance is frequently self-limited; after several weeks or months of high dosage, responsiveness may be regained and dosage reduced.

### Drug Interactions

*Oral hypoglycemic agents:* Concurrent use of oral hypoglycemic agents is not recommended; there are no data to support such use.

### Adverse Reactions

Hypoglycemic reactions (see Warnings); hypersensitivity (see Warnings).

## SULFONYLUREAS

| | |
|---|---|
| **ACETOHEXAMIDE** | |
| **Tablets**: 250 and 500 mg (*Rx*) | Various, *Dymelor* (Eli Lilly) |
| **CHLORPROPAMIDE** | |
| **Tablets**: 100 and 250 mg (*Rx*) | Various, *Diabinese* (Pfizer) |
| **GLIMEPIRIDE** | |
| **Tablets**: 1, 2, and 4 mg (*Rx*) | *Amaryl* (Hoechst Marion Roussel) |
| **GLIPIZIDE** | |
| **Tablets**: 5 and 10 mg (*Rx*) | Various, *Glucotrol* (Pfizer) |
| **Tablets, extended-release**: 2.5, 5, and 10 mg (*Rx*) | *Glucotrol XL* (Pfizer) |
| **GLYBURIDE** | |
| **Tablets**: 1.25, 2.5, and 5 mg (*Rx*) | Various, *DiaBeta* (Hoechst Marion Roussel), *Micronase* (Upjohn) |
| **Tablets, micronized**: 1.5, 3, 4.5, and 6 mg (*Rx*) | *Glynase PresTab* (Pharmacia & Upjohn) |
| **TOLAZAMIDE** | |
| **Tablets**: 100, 250, and 500 mg (*Rx*) | Various, *Tolinase* (Pharmacia & Upjohn) |
| **TOLBUTAMIDE** | |
| **Tablets**: 500 mg (*Rx*) | Various, *Orinase* (Pharmacia & Upjohn) |

### Indications

As an adjunct to diet and exercise to lower the blood glucose in patients with type 2 (non-insulin-dependent) diabetes mellitus whose hyperglycemia cannot be controlled by diet and exercise alone.

*Glimepiride:*

*Combination with insulin* – Glimepiride is also indicated for use in combination with insulin to lower blood glucose in patients whose hyperglycemia cannot be controlled by diet and exercise in conjunction with an oral hypoglycemic agent. Combined use of glimepiride and insulin may increase the potential for hypoglycemia.

*Glyburide:*

*Combination with metformin* – Glyburide also may be used concomitantly with metformin when diet and glyburide or diet and metformin alone do not result in adequate glycemic control (see Metformin monograph).

### Administration and Dosage

*Short-term administration:* Short-term administration of sulfonylureas may be sufficient during periods of transient loss of control in patients usually well controlled on diet.

*Transfer from other hypoglycemic agents:*

*Sulfonylureas* – When transferring patients from one oral hypoglycemic agent to another, no transitional period and no initial or priming dose is necessary. However, when transferring patients from chlorpropamide, exercise particular care during the first 2 weeks because the prolonged retention of chlorpropamide in the body and subsequent overlapping drug effects may provoke hypoglycemia.

*Insulin* – During insulin withdrawal period, test blood for glucose and urine for ketones 3 times/day and report results to physician daily.

| Insulin Requirement When Instituting Sulfonylurea Therapy | |
|---|---|
| Insulin dose | Insulin requirement |
| < 20 units | Start directly on oral agent and discontinue insulin abruptly. |
| 20-40 units | Initiate oral therapy with concurrent 25% to 50% reduction in insulin dose. Further reduce insulin as response is observed. With glyburide, insulin may be discontinued immediately. |
| > 40 units | Initiate oral therapy with concurrent 20% to 50% reduction in insulin dose. Further reduce insulin as response is observed. |

*Elderly patients:* Elderly patients may be particularly sensitive to these agents; therefore, start with a lower initial dose before breakfast, and check blood and urine glucose during the first 24 hours of therapy.

*Acute complications:* During the course of intercurrent complications (eg, ketoacidosis, severe trauma, major surgery, infections, severe diarrhea, nausea, vomiting), supportive therapy with insulin may be necessary.

*Combination insulin therapy:* Concurrent administration of insulin and an oral sulfonylurea (generally glipizide or glyburide) has been used with some success in type 2 diabetic patients who are difficult to control with diet and sulfonylurea therapy alone.

ACETOHEXAMIDE:
  *Initial dose* – 250 mg to 1.5 g/day. Patients on 1 g/day or less can be controlled with once daily dosage. Those receiving 1.5 g/day usually benefit from twice daily dosage before morning and evening meals. Doses greater than 1.5 g/day are not recommended.
  *Patients on other oral antidiabetic agents:* When transfer is made, the initial dose of acetohexamide should be about half the tolbutamide dose and about double the chlorpropamide dose. A transition period usually is required because of the long half-life of chlorpropamide. Make subsequent dosage adjustments according to clinical response.
  *Patients on insulin:*

| Transferal of Type 2 Diabetes Patients on Insulin to Acetohexamide Monotherapy | | |
|---|---|---|
| Insulin dose | Initial aceto-hexamide dose | Insulin withdrawal |
| < 20 | 250 mg/day | Not necessary; may be discontinued abruptly. |
| > 20 | 250 mg/day | Reduce insulin dose by 25% to 30%; further reduce as response is observed. Consider hospitalization during the transition period. |

CHLORPROPAMIDE:
  *Initial dose* – 250 mg/day in the mild to moderately severe, middle-aged, stable diabetic patient; use 100 to 125 mg/day in older, debilitated, or malnourished patients, and patients with impaired renal/hepatic function.
  *Maintenance therapy* – No more than 100 to 250 mg/day. Severe diabetics may require 500 mg/day. Avoid doses greater than 750 mg/day.
  *Patients on insulin* –

| Transferal of Type 2 Diabetes Patients on Insulin to Chlorpropamide Monotherapy | | |
|---|---|---|
| Insulin dose | Initial chlorpro-pamide dose | Insulin withdrawal |
| ≤ 40 | 250 mg/day | Not necessary; may be discontinued abruptly. |
| > 40 | 250 mg/day | Reduce insulin dose by 50%; further reduce as response is observed. Consider hospitalization during the transition period. |

GLIMEPIRIDE:

*Initial dose* – 1 to 2 mg once daily, given with breakfast or the first main meal. Patients sensitive to hypoglycemic drugs should begin at 1 mg once daily; titrate carefully.

Maximum starting dose is 2 mg or less.

*Maintenance dose* – 1 to 4 mg once daily. The maximum recommended dose is 8 mg once daily. After a dose of 2 mg is reached, increase dose at increments of no more than 2 mg at 1 to 2 week intervals based on the patient's blood glucose response. Monitor long-term efficacy by measurement of $HbA_{1c}$ levels, for example, every 3 to 6 months.

*Combination insulin therapy* – The recommended dose is 8 mg once daily with the first main meal with low-dose insulin.

*Patients on other oral antidiabetic agents* – When transferring patients to glimepiride, no transition period is necessary. No exact dosage relationship exists between glimepiride and the other oral hypoglycemic agents.

GLIPIZIDE:

*Immediate release* –

*Initial dose:* 5 mg, given approximately 30 minutes before breakfast to achieve the greatest reduction in postprandial hyperglycemia. Geriatric patients or those with liver disease may be started on 2.5 mg of the immediate-release formulation.

Adjust dosage in 2.5 to 5 mg increments, as determined by blood glucose response. Several days should elapse between titration steps. If response to a single dose is not satisfactory, dividing that dose may prove effective. The maximum recommended once daily dose is 15 mg. The maximum recommended total daily dose is 40 mg.

*Maintenance dose:* Some patients may be controlled on a once-a-day regimen, while others show better response with divided dosing. Divide total daily doses greater than 15 mg and give before meals of adequate caloric content. Total daily doses greater than 30 mg have been safely given on a twice daily basis to long-term patients.

*Extended release* –

*Initial dose:* 5 mg/day, given with breakfast. The recommended dose for geriatric patients is also 5 mg/day. $HbA_{1c}$ level measured at 3-month intervals is the preferred means of monitoring response to therapy. Measure $HbA_{1c}$ as extended release therapy is initiated at the 5 mg dose and repeated approximately 3 months later. If the first test result suggests that glycemic control over the preceding 3 months was inadequate, the dose may be increased to 10 mg. Make subsequent dosage adjustments at 3-month intervals. If no improvement is seen after 3 months of therapy with a higher dose, resume the previous dose. Base decisions that use fasting blood glucose to adjust therapy on at least 2 similar consecutive values obtained at least 7 days after the previous dose adjustment.

*Maintenance dose:* Most patients will be controlled with 5 or 10 mg taken once daily. However, some patients may require up to the maximum recommended daily dose of 20 mg. While the glycemic control of selected patients may improve with doses that exceed 10 mg, clinical studies conducted to date have not demonstrated an additional group average reduction of $HbA_{1c}$ beyond what was achieved with the 10 mg dose.

*Immediate vs extended release:* Patients receiving immediate-release glipizide may be switched safely to the extended-release tablets once a day at the nearest equivalent total daily dose. Patients receiving immediate-release tablets also may be titrated to the appropriate dose of the extended-release tablets starting with 5 mg once daily.

*Combination therapy:* When used in combination with other oral blood glucose-lowering agents, add the second agent at the lowest recommended dose and observe patients carefully.

*Patients on other oral antidiabetic agents* – No transition period is necessary when transferring patients to the extended-release tablets. Observe patients carefully (1 to

2 weeks) when being transferred from longer half-life sulfonylureas (ie, chlorpropamide) to the extended release tablets due to potential overlapping of drug effect.

*Patients on insulin* –

| Transferal of Type 2 Diabetes Patients on Insulin to Glipizide Monotherapy | | |
|---|---|---|
| Insulin dose | Initial glipizide dose | Insulin withdrawal |
| < 20 | 5 mg/day | Not necessary; may be discontinued abruptly. |
| > 20 | 5 mg/day | Reduce insulin dose by 50%; further reduce as response is observed. Consider hospitalization during the transition period. |

GLYBURIDE (Glibenclamide):

Nonmicronized (DiaBeta/Micronase) –

*Initial dose:* 2.5 to 5 mg/day, administered with breakfast or the first main meal. For patients who may be more sensitive to hypoglycemic drugs, start at 1.25 mg/day.

*Maintenance dose:* 1.25 to 20 mg/day. Give as a single dose or in divided doses. Increase in increments of 2.5 mg or less at weekly intervals based on the patient's blood glucose response. Daily doses greater than 20 mg are not recommended.

Micronized (Glynase) –

*Initial dose:* 1.5 to 3 mg/day, administered with breakfast or the first main meal. For patients who may be more sensitive to hypoglycemic drugs, start at 0.75 mg/day.

*Maintenance dose:* 0.75 to 12 mg/day. Give as a single dose or in divided doses; some patients, particularly those receiving more than 6 mg/day, may have a more satisfactory response with twice-daily dosing. Increase in increments of no more than 1.5 mg at weekly intervals based on the patient's blood glucose response. Daily doses greater than 12 mg are not recommended.

*Concomitant metformin:* Add micronized glyburide gradually to the dosing regimen of patients who have not responded to the maximum dose of metformin monotherapy after 4 weeks. (Refer to the Metformin monograph.) The desired control of blood glucose may be obtained by adjusting the dose of each drug. With concomitant therapy, the risk of hypoglycemia associated with sulfonylurea therapy continues and may be increased.

*Patients on other oral antidiabetic agents:* Transfer patients from other oral antidiabetic regimens to glyburide conservatively. When transferring patients from oral hypoglycemic agents other than chlorpropamide, no transition period and no initial priming dose is necessary. When transferring patients from chlorpropamide, exercise care during the first 2 weeks because the prolonged retention of chlorpropamide in the body and subsequent overlapping drug effects may provoke hypoglycemia.

*Patients on insulin:*

| Transferal of Type 2 Diabetes Patients on Insulin to Glyburide Monotherapy | | |
|---|---|---|
| Insulin dose | Initial glyburide dose | Insulin withdrawal |
| < 20 | 1.5-3 mg/day micronized, 2.5-5 mg/day nonmicronized | Not necessary; may be discontinued abruptly. |
| 20-40 | 3 mg/day micronized, 5 mg/day nonmicronized | Not necessary; may be discontinued abruptly. |
| > 40 | 3 mg/day micronized, 5 mg/day nonmicronized | Reduce insulin dose by 50%; further reduce as response is observed. Consider hospitalization during the transition period. |

*TOLAZAMIDE:*

*Initial dose* – 100 to 250 mg/day with breakfast or the first main meal. If fasting blood sugar (FBS) is less than 200 mg/dL, use 100 mg/day, or 250 mg/day if FBS is greater than 200 mg/dL. If patients are malnourished, underweight, elderly or not eating properly, use 100 mg once a day. Adjust dose to response. If greater than 500 mg/day is required, give in divided doses twice daily. Doses greater than 1 g/day are not likely to improve control.

*Maintenance dose* – The usual maintenance dose is 100 to 1000 mg/day with the average maintenance dose being 250 to 500 mg/day. Following initiation of therapy, dosage adjustment is made in increments of 100 to 250 mg at weekly intervals based on the patient's blood glucose response.

*Patients on other oral antidiabetic agents* – Transfer patients from other oral antidiabetes regimens to tolazamide conservatively. When transferring patients from oral hypoglycemic agents other than chlorpropamide to tolazamide, no transition period or initial priming dose is necessary. Consider 250 mg chlorpropamide to provide approximately the same degree of blood control as 250 mg tolazamide. Observe the patient carefully for hypoglycemia during the transition period from chlorpropamide to tolazamide (1 or 2 weeks) due to the prolonged retention of chlorpropamide in the body and the possibility of a subsequent overlapping drug effect. If patient is receiving less than 1 g/day tolbutamide, begin at 100 mg/day of tolazamide. If patient is receiving 1 g/day or more, initiate 250 mg/day tolazamide as a single dose. Consider 100 mg tolazamide to provide approximately the same degree of blood glucose control as 250 mg acetohexamide.

*Patients on insulin* –

| Transferal of Type 2 Diabetes Patients on Insulin to Tolazamide Monotherapy | | |
|---|---|---|
| Insulin dose | Initial tolazamide dose | Insulin withdrawal |
| < 20 | 100 mg/day | Not necessary; may be discontinued abruptly. |
| 20-40 | 250 mg/day | Not necessary; may be discontinued abruptly |
| > 40 | 250 mg/day | Reduce insulin by 50%; further reduce as response is observed. Consider hospitalization during the transition period. |

*TOLBUTAMIDE:*

*Initial dose* – 1 to 2 g/day (range, 0.25 to 3 g). A maintenance dose greater than 2 g/day is seldom required. Daily doses greater than 3 g are not recommended. Total dose may be taken in the morning, but divided doses may allow increased GI tolerance.

*Patients on other oral antidiabetic agents* – Transfer patients from other oral antidiabetes regimens to tolbutamide conservatively. When transferring patients from oral hypoglycemic agents other than chlorpropamide to tolbutamide, no transition period and no initial or priming doses are necessary. However, when transferring patients from chlorpropamide, exercise particular care during the first 2 weeks because of the prolonged retention of chlorpropamide in the body and the possibility that subsequent overlapping drug effects might provoke hypoglycemia.

*Patients on insulin* –

| Transferal of Type 2 Diabetes Patients on Insulin to Tolbutamide Monotherapy | | |
|---|---|---|
| Insulin dose | Initial tolbutamide dose | Insulin withdrawal |
| < 20 | 1-2 g/day | Not necessary; may be discontinued abruptly. |
| 20-40 | 1-2 g/day | Reduce insulin dose by 30% to 50%; further reduce as response is observed. |
| > 40 | 1-2 g/day | Reduce insulin dose by 20%; further reduce as response is observed. Consider hospitalization during the transition period. |

Occasionally, conversion to tolbutamide in the hospital may be advisable in candidates who require more than 40 units of insulin daily. During this conversion period when insulin and tolbutamide are being used, hypoglycemia rarely may occur. During insulin withdrawal, have patients test urine for glucose and acetone at least 3 times/day and report results to their physician. The appearance of persistent acetonuria with glycosuria indicates that the patient is a type 1 diabetes patient who requires insulin therapy.

## Actions

*Pharmacology:* The sulfonylurea hypoglycemic agents appear to lower blood glucose by stimulating insulin release from beta cells in the pancreatic islets possibly due to increased intracellular cAMP. These agents are only effective in patients with some capacity for endogenous insulin production. They may improve the binding between insulin and insulin receptors or increase the number of insulin receptors.

General clinical characteristics that favor successful sulfonylurea monotherapy following insulin withdrawal include the following:

- Onset of diabetes at 35 years of age or older
- Obese or normal body weight
- Duration of diabetes less than 10 years
- Absence of ketoacidosis
- Fasting serum glucose 200 mg/dL or less
- Postprandial blood glucose values less than 250 mg/dL
- Insulin requirement less than 40 units/day
- Absence of renal or hepatic dysfunction

*Pharmacokinetics:* All sulfonylureas are strongly bound to plasma proteins, primarily albumin.

| Major Pharmacokinetic Parameters of the Sulfonylureas | | | | | | | |
| --- | --- | --- | --- | --- | --- | --- | --- |
| Sulfonylureas | Approximate equivalent doses (mg) | Doses/day | Serum t½ (h) | Onset (h) | Duration (h) | Renal excretion (%) | Active metabolites |
| *First generation* | | | | | | | |
| Acetohexamide | 500-750 | 1-2 | ≈ 6-8 (parent drug + metabolite) | 1 | 12-24 | 100 | Yes |
| Chlorpropamide | 250-375 | 1 | 36 | 1 | 24-60 | 100 | Yes |
| Tolazamide | 250-375 | 1-2 | 7 | 4-6 | 12-24 | 100 | Yes |
| Tolbutamide | 1000-1500 | 2-3 | 4.5-6.5 | 1 | 6-12 | 100 | No |
| *Second generation* | | | | | | | |
| Glipizide | 10 | 1-2 | 2-4 | 1-3 | 10-24 | 80-85 | No |
| Glyburide Nonmicronized | 5 | 1-2 | 10 | 2-4 | 16-24 | 50 | Yes[1] |
| Micronized | 3 | 1-2 | ≈ 4 | 1 | 12-24 | 50 | Yes[1] |
| Glimepiride | NA[2] | 1 | ≈ 9 | 2-3 | 24 | 60 | Yes |

[1] Weakly active.
[2] Not applicable.

## Contraindications

Hypersensitivity to sulfonylureas; diabetes complicated by ketoacidosis, with or without coma; sole therapy of type 1 (insulin-dependent) diabetes mellitus; diabetes when complicated by pregnancy.

## Warnings

*The administration of oral hypoglycemic drugs:* The administration of oral hypoglycemic drugs has been associated with increased cardiovascular mortality as compared with treatment with diet alone or diet plus insulin.

Patients treated for 5 to 8 years with diet plus tolbutamide (1.5 g/day) had a rate of cardiovascular mortality approximately 2.5 times that of patients treated with diet alone. A significant increase in total mortality was not observed.

*Bioavailability:* Micronized glyburide 3 mg tablets provide serum concentrations that are not bioequivalent to those from the conventional formulation (nonmicronized) 5 mg tablets.

*Renal/Hepatic function impairment:* Hepatic impairment may result in inadequate release of glucose in response to hypoglycemia. Renal impairment may cause decreased elimination of sulfonylureas leading to accumulation producing hypoglycemia.

*Elderly:* In elderly, debilitated, or malnourished patients, and patients with impaired renal or hepatic function, the initial and maintenance dosing should be conservative to avoid hypoglycemic reactions.

*Pregnancy: Category* C; *Category* B (glyburide).

*Lactation:* Chlorpropamide and tolbutamide are excreted in breast milk. It is not known if other sulfonylureas are excreted in breast milk.

*Children:* Safety and efficacy in children have not been established.

### Precautions

*Monitoring:*

| Treatment Goals for Type 2 Diabetes Mellitus | | |
| --- | --- | --- |
| Patient population | Average preprandial glucose (mg/dL) | HbA$_{1c}$[1] (%) |
| ADA general recommendations[2] | 80-120 | < 7 |
| Healthy, relatively young | 80-120 | < 8 |
| Elderly and patients with serious medical conditions | 100-140 | < 9 |

[1] Glycosylated hemoglobin.
[2] American Diabetes Association 1999 Clinical Practice Recommendations.

During the transitional period, test the urine for glucose and acetone at least 3 times/day and have the results reviewed by a physician frequently. Measurement of glycosylated hemoglobin also is useful. It is important that patients be taught to correctly and frequently self-monitor blood glucose.

*Hypoglycemia:* All sulfonylureas may produce severe hypoglycemia. Proper patient selection, dosage and instructions are important to avoid hypoglycemic episodes.

*Asymptomatic patients:* Controlling blood glucose in type 2 diabetes with sulfonylureas has not been definitely established to be effective in preventing the long-term cardiovascular or neural complications of diabetes.

*Loss of blood glucose control:* When a patient stabilized on any diabetic regimen is exposed to stress such as fever, trauma, infection, or surgery, a loss of control may occur. At such times, it may be necessary to discontinue the drug and give insulin.

*Disulfiram-like syndrome:* A sulfonylurea-induced facial flushing or breathlessness reaction may occur when some sulfonylureas are administered with alcohol.

*Syndrome of inappropriate secretion of antidiuretic hormone (SIADH):* Water retention and dilutional hyponatremia have occurred after administration of sulfonylureas to type 2 diabetes patients, especially those with CHF or hepatic cirrhosis.

### Drug Interactions

Drugs that may affect sulfonylureas include androgens, anticoagulants, azole antifungals, barbiturates, beta blockers, calcium channel blockers, charcoal, chloramphenicol, cholestyramine, ciprofloxacin, clofibrate, corticosteroids, diazoxide, estrogens, ethanol, fluconazole, gemfibrozil, histamine H$_2$ antagonists, hydantoins, isoniazid, magnesium salts, methyldopa, MAO inhibitors, nicotinic acid, oral contraceptives, phenothiazines, probenecid, rifampin, salicylates, sulfinpyrazone, sulfonamides, sympathomimetics, thiazide diuretics, thyroid agents, tricyclic antidepressants, urinary acidifiers, and urinary alkalinizers. Drugs that may be affected by sulfonylureas include digitalis glycosides.

*Drug/Lab test interactions:* A metabolite of tolbutamide in the urine may give a false-positive reaction for albumin if measured by the acidification-after-boiling test, which causes the metabolite to precipitate. There is no interference with the sulfosalicylic acid test.

*Drug/Food interactions:* Absorption of glipizide is delayed by approximately 40 minutes when taken with food; the drug is more effective when given approximately 30 minutes before a meal. The other sulfonylureas may be taken with food.

### Adverse Reactions

GI disturbances (eg, nausea, epigastric fullness, heartburn) are the most common reactions. Other adverse reactions may include hypoglycemia, disulfiram-like reactions;

allergic skin reactions; eczema; pruritus; erythema; urticaria; photosensitivity reactions; leukopenia; thrombocytopenia; aplastic anemia; agranulocytosis; hemolytic anemia; pancytopenia; weakness; paresthesia; tinnitus; fatigue; dizziness; vertigo; malaise; elevated liver function tests.

# METFORMIN HYDROCHLORIDE

**Tablets**: 500, 850, and 1,000 mg (*Rx*)  
**Tablets, extended-release**: 500 mg (*Rx*)

750 mg (*Rx*)  
1,000 mg (*Rx*)  
**Oral solution**: 500 mg/5 mL (*Rx*)

Various, *Glucophage* (Bristol-Myers Squibb)  
*Metformin Hydrochloride ER* (PAR), *Fortamet* (Andrx), *Glucophage* XR (Bristol-Myers Squibb)  
*Glucophage* XR (Bristol-Myers Squibb)  
*Fortamet* (Andrx)  
*Riomet* (Ranbaxy)

---

**Warning:**

*Lactic acidosis:* Lactic acidosis is a rare, but serious, metabolic complication that can occur because of metformin accumulation during treatment; when it occurs, it is fatal in approximately 50% of cases. Lactic acidosis also may occur in association with a number of pathophysiologic conditions, including diabetes mellitus, and whenever there is significant tissue hypoperfusion and hypoxemia. Lactic acidosis is characterized by elevated blood lactate levels (greater than 5 mmol/L), decreased blood pH, electrolyte disturbances with an increased anion gap, and an increased lactate/pyruvate ratio. When metformin is implicated as the cause of lactic acidosis, metformin plasma levels greater than 5 mcg/mL are generally found.

The reported incidence of lactic acidosis in patients receiving metformin is very low (approximately 0.03 cases/1,000 patient-years, with approximately 0.015 fatal cases/1,000 patient-years). In more than 20,000 patient-years exposure to metformin in clinical trials, there were no reports of lactic acidosis. Reported cases have occurred primarily in diabetic patients with significant renal insufficiency, including intrinsic renal disease and renal hypoperfusion, often in the setting of multiple concomitant medical/surgical problems and multiple concomitant medications. Patients with congestive heart failure (CHF) requiring pharmacologic management, in particular those with unstable or acute CHF who are at risk of hypoperfusion and hypoxemia, are at increased risk of lactic acidosis. The risk of lactic acidosis increases with the degree of renal dysfunction and the patient's age. Therefore, the risk of lactic acidosis may be significantly decreased by regular monitoring of renal function in patients taking metformin and by use of the minimum effective dose. In particular, treatment of the elderly should be accompanied by careful monitoring of renal function. Do not initiate metformin treatment in patients 80 years of age and older unless measurement of creatinine clearance (Ccr) demonstrates that renal function is not reduced, because these patients are more susceptible to developing lactic acidosis. In addition, promptly withhold metformin in the presence of any condition associated with hypoxemia, dehydration, or sepsis. Because impaired hepatic function may significantly limit the ability to clear lactate, generally avoid using metformin in patients with clinical or laboratory evidence of hepatic disease. Caution patients against excessive alcohol intake (acute or chronic) because alcohol potentiates the effects of metformin on lactate metabolism. In addition, temporarily discontinue metformin prior to any intravascular radiocontrast study and for any surgical procedure.

**Warning: (cont.)**
The onset of lactic acidosis often is subtle and accompanied only by nonspecific symptoms such as malaise, myalgias, respiratory distress, increasing somnolence, and nonspecific abdominal distress. There may be associated hypothermia, hypotension, and resistant bradyarrhythmias with more marked acidosis. The patient and the patient's physician must be aware of the possible importance of such symptoms. Instruct the patient to notify the physician immediately if these symptoms occur. Withdraw metformin until the situation is clarified. Serum electrolytes, ketones, blood glucose, and, if indicated, blood pH, lactate levels, and blood metformin levels may be useful. Once a patient is stabilized on any dose of metformin, GI symptoms, which are common during initiation of therapy, are unlikely to be drug related. Later occurrence of GI symptoms could be caused by lactic acidosis or other serious disease.

Levels of fasting venous plasma lactate above the upper limit of normal but less than 5 mmol/L in patients taking metformin do not necessarily indicate impending lactic acidosis and may be explained by other mechanisms, such as poorly controlled diabetes or obesity, vigorous physical activity, or technical problems in sample handling.

Suspect lactic acidosis in any diabetic patient with metabolic acidosis lacking evidence of ketoacidosis (ketonuria and ketonemia).

Lactic acidosis is a medical emergency that must be treated in a hospital setting. In a patient with lactic acidosis who is taking metformin, immediately discontinue the drug and promptly institute general supportive measures. Because metformin is dialyzable (with a clearance of up to 170 mL/min under good hemodynamic conditions), prompt hemodialysis is recommended to correct the acidosis and remove the accumulated metformin. Such management often results in prompt reversal of symptoms and recovery.

**Indications**
*Type 2 diabetes:* As monotherapy, as an adjunct to diet and exercise to improve glycemic control in patients with type 2 diabetes. Metformin immediate-release (IR) tablets and oral solution are indicated in patients 10 years of age and older. Metformin extended-release (ER) tablets are indicated in patients 17 years of age and older.

Metformin IR tablets, oral solution, or ER tablets may be used concomitantly with a sulfonylurea or insulin to improve glycemic control in adults 17 years of age and older.

**Administration and Dosage**
Individualize dosage on the basis of efficacy and tolerance, while not exceeding the maximum recommended daily dose of metformin IR 2,550 mg in adults and 2,000 mg in children (10 to 16 years of age); the maximum recommended daily dose of metformin ER in adults is 2,000 mg (2,500 mg with *Fortamet*). Give metformin IR in divided doses with meals and give metformin ER once daily with the evening meal. Start at a low dose, with gradual dose escalation, to reduce GI side effects and identify the minimum dose required for adequate glycemic control of the patient.

During treatment initiation and dose titration, use fasting plasma glucose (FPG) to determine therapeutic response to metformin and to identify minimum effective dose. Thereafter, measure glycosylated hemoglobin (HbA$_{1c}$) at intervals of approximately 3 months.

Short-term administration may be sufficient during periods of transient loss of control in patients usually well controlled on diet alone.

Metformin ER must be swallowed whole and never crushed or chewed. Occasionally, the inactive ingredients will be eliminated in the feces as a soft, hydrated mass.

*Adults:*

*Metformin IR* – The usual starting dose is 500 mg twice/day or 850 mg once/day, given with meals. Make dosage increases in increments of 500 mg weekly or 850 mg every 2 weeks, up to a total of 2,000 mg/day, given in divided doses. Patients also can be titrated from 500 mg twice/day to 850 mg twice/day after 2 weeks. For those patients requiring additional glycemic control, metformin IR may be given to a maximum daily dose of 2,550 mg/day. Doses above 2,000 mg may be better tolerated given 3 times/day with meals.

*Metformin ER* – The usual starting dose is 500 mg once/day (or 1,000 mg once/day with *Fortamet*) with the evening meal. Make dosage increases in increments of 500 mg weekly, up to a maximum of 2,000 mg once/day (or 2,500 mg once/day with *Fortamet*) with the evening meal. If glycemic control is not achieved on 2,000 mg once/day, consider a trial of 1,000 mg twice/day. If higher doses of metformin are required, use metformin IR tablets at total daily doses up to 2,550 mg administered in divided daily doses.

*Conversion from metformin IR to ER* – A randomized trial's results suggest that patients receiving metformin IR may be safely switched to metformin ER once daily at the same total daily dose, up to 2,000 mg once/day. Following a switch, closely monitor glycemic control and make dosage adjustments accordingly.

*Children:* The usual starting dose of metformin IR is 500 mg twice a day, given with meals. Make dosage increases in increments of 500 mg/week up to a maximum of 2,000 mg/day given in divided doses.

*Transfer from other antidiabetic therapy:* When transferring patients from standard oral hypoglycemic agents other than chlorpropamide to metformin, generally no transition period is necessary. When transferring patients from chlorpropamide, exercise care during the first 2 weeks because of the prolonged retention of chlorpropamide leading to overlapping drug effects and possible hypoglycemia.

*Concomitant metformin and sulfonylurea therapy in adults:* If patients have not responded to 4 weeks of the maximum dose of metformin monotherapy, consider gradual addition of an oral sulfonylurea while continuing metformin at the maximum dose, even if prior primary or secondary failure to a sulfonylurea has occurred.

If patients have not satisfactorily responded to 1 to 3 months of concomitant therapy with the maximum doses of metformin and an oral sulfonylurea, consider institution of insulin therapy and discontinuation of these oral agents.

*Concomitant metformin IR or ER and insulin therapy in adults:* Continue the current insulin dose upon initiation of metformin IR or ER therapy. Initiate metformin IR or ER therapy at 500 mg once/day in patients on insulin therapy. For patients not responding adequately, increase the dose of metformin IR or ER by 500 mg after approximately 1 week and by 500 mg every week thereafter until adequate glycemic control is achieved. The maximum recommended daily dose is 2,500 mg for metformin IR and 2,000 mg for metformin ER (2,500 mg with *Fortamet*). It is recommended that the insulin dose be decreased 10% to 25% when FPG concentrations decrease to less than 120 mg/dL in patients receiving concomitant insulin and metformin IR or ER. Individualize further adjustment based on glucose-lowering response.

*Special patient populations:* Initial and maintenance dosing should be conservative in patients with advanced age because of the potential for decreased renal function. Base any dosage adjustment on a careful assessment of renal function. Generally, do not titrate elderly, debilitated, or malnourished patients to the maximum dose. Do not initiate metformin IR and ER treatment in patients 80 years of age and older unless measurement of Ccr demonstrates that renal function is not reduced.

## Actions

*Pharmacology:* Metformin improves glucose tolerance in subjects with type 2 diabetes, lowering basal and postprandial plasma glucose. Metformin decreases hepatic glucose production, decreases intestinal absorption of glucose, and improves insulin sensitivity (increases peripheral glucose uptake and utilization). Metformin does not produce hypoglycemia and does not cause hyperinsulinemia. With metformin therapy, insulin secretion remains unchanged while fasting insulin levels and day-long plasma insulin response may actually decrease.

*Pharmacokinetics:*

*Absorption/Distribution* – The absolute bioavailability of metformin IR 500 mg given under fasting conditions is approximately 50% to 60%. Food decreases the extent and slightly delays the absorption of metformin.

Metformin is negligibly bound to plasma proteins; steady-state plasma concentrations are reached within 24 to 48 hours and are generally less than 1 mcg/mL.

The extent of metformin absorption from metformin ER at 2,000 mg once-daily dose is similar to the same total daily dose administered as metformin IR 1,000 mg twice daily.

*Metabolism/Excretion* – Metformin is excreted unchanged in the urine and does not undergo hepatic metabolism or biliary excretion. Tubular secretion is the major route of elimination. The elimination half-life is approximately 17.6 hours.

## Contraindications

Renal disease or renal dysfunction (eg, as suggested by serum creatinine levels greater than or equal to 1.5 mg/dL [males], greater than or equal to 1.4 mg/dL [females], or abnormal Ccr) that may also result from conditions such as cardiovascular collapse (shock), acute myocardial infarction (MI), and septicemia; CHF requiring pharmacologic treatment; hypersensitivity to metformin; acute or chronic metabolic acidosis, including diabetic ketoacidosis, with or without coma. Treat diabetic ketoacidosis with insulin.

## Warnings

*Lactic acidosis:* Lactic acidosis is a rare, but serious, metabolic complication that can occur because of metformin accumulation during treatment; when it occurs, it is fatal in approximately 50% of cases (see Warning Box).

*Diet/Exercise:* In initiating treatment for type 2 diabetes, emphasize diet as the primary form of treatment. Caloric restriction and weight loss are essential in the obese diabetic patient. Also, stress the importance of regular physical activity and aid the patient in identifying cardiovascular risk factors and taking corrective measures where possible.

*Renal function impairment:* Metformin is known to be excreted by the kidney, and the risk of metformin accumulation and lactic acidosis increases with the degree of impairment of renal function. Do not give metformin to patients with serum creatinine levels above the upper limit of normal for their age.

*Hepatic function impairment:* Because impaired hepatic function has been associated with cases of lactic acidosis, avoid metformin in patients with clinical or laboratory evidence of hepatic disease.

*Elderly:* Because aging is associated with reduced renal function, use metformin with caution as age increases. Generally, do not titrate elderly patients to the maximum dose of metformin (see Administration and Dosage).

*Pregnancy: Category B.*

*Lactation:* Decide whether to discontinue nursing or to discontinue the drug, taking into account the importance of the drug to the mother.

*Children:* Safety and efficacy of metformin IR for the treatment of type 2 diabetes have been established in children 10 to 16 years of age who demonstrated a similar response in glycemic control to that seen in adults. Adverse effects were similar to those described in adults. A maximum daily dose of 2,000 mg is recommended. Safety and efficacy of metformin ER in children have not been established.

## Precautions

*Monitoring:* Before initiation of therapy and at least annually thereafter, assess renal function. In patients at risk of renal dysfunction, assess renal function more frequently and discontinue the drug if renal impairment is present.

Promptly evaluate patients previously well controlled on metformin who develop laboratory abnormalities or clinical illness for evidence of ketoacidosis or lactic acidosis. Evaluation should include serum electrolytes and ketones, blood glucose, and, if indicated, blood pH, lactate, pyruvate, and metformin levels. If acidosis of either form occurs, stop metformin immediately and initiate other appropriate corrective measures.

Monitor response to all diabetic therapies by periodic measurements of FPG and HbA$_{1c}$ levels. During initial dose titration, fasting glucose can be used to determine the therapeutic response. Thereafter, monitor both glucose and HbA$_{1c}$.

Perform initial and periodic monitoring of hematologic parameters and renal function at least on an annual basis.

*Hypoxic states:* Cardiovascular collapse (shock), acute CHF, acute MI, and other conditions characterized by hypoxemia have been associated with lactic acidosis and may cause prerenal azotemia. If such events occur, discontinue metformin.

*Surgical procedures:* Temporarily suspend metformin for surgical procedures (unless minor and not associated with restricted intake of food and fluids). Do not restart until the patient's oral intake has resumed and renal function is normal.

*Vitamin B$_{12}$ levels:* A decrease of previously normal serum vitamin B$_{12}$ levels has been observed in patients receiving metformin.

*Hypoglycemia:* Hypoglycemia does not occur in patients receiving metformin alone under usual circumstances, but could occur with deficient caloric intake, strenuous exercise not compensated by caloric supplementation, or during concomitant use with other glucose-lowering agents (such as sulfonylureas) or ethanol.

*Loss of blood glucose control:* When a patient stabilized on any diabetic regimen is exposed to stress such as fever, trauma, infection, or surgery, a temporary loss of glycemic control may occur. At such times, it may be necessary to withhold metformin and temporarily administer insulin. Metformin may be reinstituted after the acute episode is resolved.

Should secondary failure occur with metformin or sulfonylurea monotherapy, combined therapy with metformin and sulfonylurea may result in a response. Should secondary failure occur with combined therapy, it may be necessary to consider therapeutic alternatives, including initiation of insulin therapy.

Certain drugs tend to produce hyperglycemia and may lead to loss of glycemic control. When such drugs are administered to a patient receiving metformin, closely observe the patient for loss of blood glucose control.

*Iodinated contrast materials:* Radiologic studies involving the use of intravascular iodinated contrast materials (ie, IV urogram, IV cholangiography, angiography, and CT scans with intravascular contrast materials) can lead to acute alteration of renal function and have been associated with lactic acidosis in patients receiving metformin. Therefore, in patients in whom any such study is planned, temporarily discontinue metformin at the time of or prior to the procedure, and withhold for 48 hours subsequent to the procedure; reinstitute only after renal function has been reevaluated and found to be normal.

### Drug Interactions

Drugs that may affect metformin include alcohol, cationic drugs, cimetidine, furosemide, iodinated contrast material, and nifedipine.

Drugs that may be affected by metformin include glyburide and furosemide.

Certain drugs tend to produce hyperglycemia and may lead to loss of glycemic control. These drugs include thiazide and other diuretics, corticosteroids, phenothiazines, thyroid products, estrogens, oral contraceptives, phenytoin, nicotinic acid, sympathomimetics, calcium channel blocking drugs, and isoniazid. When such drugs are administered to a patient receiving metformin, closely observe the patient to maintain adequate glycemic control.

**Adverse Reactions**

Adverse reactions occurring in at least 3% of patients include the following:

*Metformin IR* – Abdominal discomfort, asthenia, diarrhea, flatulence, headache, ingestion, nausea, vomiting.

*Metformin ER (1% to 5%)* – Abdominal distention, abdominal pain, constipation, diarrhea, dizziness, dyspepsia/heartburn, flatulence, headache, nausea/vomiting, taste disturbance, upper respiratory tract infection.

# THIAZOLIDINEDIONES

| | |
|---|---|
| **ROSIGLITAZONE MALEATE** | |
| **Tablets: 2, 4, and 8 mg (Rx)** | *Avandia* (GlaxoSmithKline) |
| **PIOGLITAZONE HCl** | |
| **Tablets: 15, 30, and 45 mg (Rx)** | *Actos* (Takeda Pharm. North America, Inc.) |

**Indications**

*Type 2 diabetes:* Monotherapy as an adjunct to diet and exercise to improve glycemic control.

In combination with metformin, insulin, or a sulfonylurea when diet, exercise, and a single agent do not result in adequate glycemic control.

**Administration and Dosage**

*ROSIGLITAZONE MALEATE:* Take with or without food.

*Monotherapy* – Individualize the management of antidiabetic therapy. Rosiglitazone may be administered either at a starting dose of 4 mg once daily or divided and given in the morning and evening. For patients responding inadequately after 8 to 12 weeks of treatment, as determined by reduction in fasting plasma glucose, the dosing may be increased to 8 mg daily as indicated below. In clinical trials, the 4 mg twice daily regimen resulted in the greatest reduction in fasting blood glucose and HbA$_{1c}$.

*Combination therapy* – When rosiglitazone is added to existing therapy, the current dose of sulfonylurea, insulin, or metformin can be continued upon initiation of rosiglitazone therapy.

*Metformin:* The usual starting dose of rosiglitazone in combination with metformin is 4 mg given as either a single dose once daily or in divided doses twice daily. It is unlikely that the dose of metformin will require adjustment because of hypoglycemia during combination therapy with rosiglitazone.

*Insulin:* For patients stabilized on insulin, continue the insulin dose upon initiation of rosiglitazone therapy. Dose rosiglitazone at 4 mg daily. Doses greater than 4 mg daily in combination with insulin are not currently indicated. It is recommended that the insulin dose be decreased 10% to 25% if the patient reports hypoglycemia or if fasting plasma glucose concentrations decrease to less than 100 mg/dL.

*Sulfonylureas:* When used in combination with sulfonylurea, the recommended dose of rosiglitazone is 4 mg either as a single dose once daily or in divided doses twice daily. If patients report hypoglycemia, decrease the dose of sulfonylurea.

*Maximum recommended dose:* The dose of rosiglitazone should not exceed 8 mg/day as a single dose or divided twice daily.

*Renal impairment* – Metformin is contraindicated in patients with renal impairment. Therefore, concomitant administration of rosiglitazone and metformin is contraindicated in these patients. However, no dosage adjustment is necessary when rosiglitazone is used as monotherapy in patients with renal impairment.

*Hepatic function impairment* – Use with caution in patients with hepatic impairment. Do not initiate rosiglitazone therapy if the patient exhibits clinical evidence of active liver disease or increased serum transaminase levels (ALT more than 2.5 times the ULN) at start of therapy. Liver enzyme monitoring is recommended in all patients prior to initiation of therapy with rosiglitazone and periodically thereafter.

*Children* – The use of rosiglitazone in patients younger than 18 years of age is not recommended.

PIOGLITAZONE: Take without regard to meals.

*Monotherapy* – Initiate monotherapy in patients not adequately controlled with diet and exercise at 15 or 30 mg once daily. For patients who respond inadequately to the initial dose of pioglitazone, the dose can be increased in increments up to 45 mg once daily. Consider combination therapy for patients not responding adequately to monotherapy.

*Combination therapy* –

*Sulfonylureas:* Initiate pioglitazone in combination with a sulfonylurea at 15 or 30 mg once daily. Decrease the dose of the sulfonylurea if patients report hypoglycemia.

*Metformin:* Initiate pioglitazone in combination with metformin at 15 or 30 mg once daily. It is unlikely that the dose of metformin will require adjustment because of hypoglycemia during combination therapy with pioglitazone.

*Insulin:* Initiate pioglitazone in combination with insulin at 15 or 30 mg once daily. Continue the current insulin dose upon initiation of pioglitazone therapy. Decrease the insulin dose by 10% to 25% if the patient reports hypoglycemia or if plasma glucose concentrations decrease to less than 100 mg/dL.

*Maximum recommended dose* – Do not exceed more than 45 mg once daily of pioglitazone.

*Hepatic function impairment* – Do not initiate pioglitazone therapy if the patient exhibits clinical evidence of active liver disease or increased serum transaminase levels (ALT more than 2.5 times the ULN) at the start of therapy. Liver enzyme monitoring is recommended in all patients prior to initiation of therapy with pioglitazone and periodically thereafter.

## Actions

*Pharmacology:* **Rosiglitazone** and **pioglitazone**, members of the thiazolidinediones class of antidiabetic agents, improve glycemic control by improving insulin sensitivity. Studies indicate that they improve sensitivity to insulin in muscle and adipose tissue and inhibit hepatic gluconeogenesis.

*Pharmacokinetics:*

| Pharmacokinetics of Thiazolidinediones | | |
|---|---|---|
| Parameters | Pioglitazone | Rosiglitazone |
| Absorption | | |
| Bioavailability | — | 99% |
| $C_{max}$[1] | — | 1 mg[2]: 76 ng/mL<br>2 mg[2]: 156 ng/mL<br>8 mg[2]: 598 ng/mL<br>8 mg[3]: 432 ng/mL |
| $T_{max}$ | 2 h[2]<br>3-4 h[3] | 1 h |
| Food effect | Delays time to peak concentration; does not alter extent of absorption | 28% decrease in $C_{max}$ and delay in $T_{max}$ (1.75 h); no overall change in AUC |
| Distribution | | |
| Volume of distribution | ≈ 0.63 L/kg[1] | 17.6 L |
| Protein binding | > 99% | ≈ 99.8% |
| Metabolism | | |
| Mechanism | Hydroxylation, oxidation, CYP2C8, CYP3A4, CYP 1A1 | N-demethylation, hydroxylation, conjugation CYP2C8, CYP2C9 (minor) |
| Active metabolites | MII[4], MIII[5], MIV[4] | — |
| Excretion | | |
| Site | Urine (15 to 30%), feces | Urine (64%), feces (23%) |
| Elimination half-life | Pioglitazone: 3 to 7 h<br>Total pioglitazone: 16 to 24 h | 3 to 4 h |

| Pharmacokinetics of Thiazolidinediones | | |
|---|---|---|
| Parameters | Pioglitazone | Rosiglitazone |
| Oral clearance | 5 to 7 L/h | 1 mg[2]: 3.03 L/h<br>2 mg[2]: 2.89 L/h<br>8 mg[2]: 2.85 L/h<br>8 mg[3]: 2.97 L/h |

[1] Following single oral doses.
[2] In the fasting state.
[3] In the fed state.
[4] Hydroxy derivatives of pioglitazone.
[5] Keto derivative of pioglitazone.

## Contraindications

Hypersensitivity or allergy to **pioglitazone** or **rosiglitazone** or any of their components.

## Warnings

*Hepatotoxicity:* Available clinical data show no evidence of **pioglitazone**- and **rosiglitazone**-induced hepatotoxicity or ALT elevations. It is recommended that patients undergo periodic monitoring of liver enzymes. Check liver enzymes prior to the initiation of therapy in all treated patients. Do not initiate therapy in patients with increased baseline liver enzyme levels (ALT more than 2.5 times the ULN). In patients with normal baseline liver enzymes, it is recommended that liver enzymes be monitored every 2 months for the first 12 months and periodically thereafter. Evaluate patients with mildly elevated liver enzymes (ALT levels less than or equal to 2.5 times the ULN) at baseline or during therapy to determine the cause of the liver enzyme elevation. Proceed with caution in the initiation of, or continuation of, therapy in patients with mild liver enzyme elevations and include appropriate close clinical follow-up, including more frequent liver enzyme monitoring, to determine if the liver enzyme elevations resolve or worsen. If at any time ALT levels increase to more than 3 times the ULN, recheck liver enzyme levels as soon as possible. If ALT levels remain more than 3 times the ULN, discontinue therapy.

If any patient develops symptoms suggesting hepatic dysfunction, check liver enzymes. If jaundice is observed, discontinue therapy.

*Cardiac effects:* Thiazolidinediones can cause fluid retention, which may exacerbate or lead to heart failure. Discontinue therapy if any deterioration in cardiac status occurs. Rosiglitazone and pioglitazone are not recommended in patients with NYHA Class 3 and 4 cardiac status.

*Ovulation:* In premenopausal anovulatory patients with insulin resistance, thiazolidinedione treatment may result in resumption of ovulation. These patients may be at risk for pregnancy.

*Pregnancy:* Category C (**pioglitazone, rosiglitazone**).

*Lactation:* Do not administer to nursing women.

*Children:* Safety and efficacy have not been established in patients under 18 years of age.

## Precautions

*Monitoring:* See Warnings. Perform periodic fasting blood glucose and $HbA_{1c}$ measurements to monitor therapeutic response. Liver enzyme monitoring is recommended prior to initiation of therapy in all patients and periodically thereafter.

*Type 1 diabetes:* **Pioglitazone** and **rosiglitazone** are active only in the presence of insulin. Therefore, do not use in type 1 diabetes patients or for the treatment of diabetic ketoacidosis.

*Hypoglycemia:* Patients receiving **pioglitazone** or **rosiglitazone** in combination with insulin or oral hypoglycemics (eg, sulfonylureas) may be at risk for hypoglycemia; reduction in the dose of insulin or sulfonylureas may be necessary.

*Hematologic:* **Rosiglitazone** and **pioglitazone** may cause decreases in hemoglobin and hematocrit. These changes primarily occurred within the first 4 to 12 weeks for pioglitazone and the first 3 months of rosiglitazone therapy.

*Edema:* Use **pioglitazone** and **rosiglitazone** with caution in patients with edema.

Because thiazolidinediones can cause fluid retention, which can exacerbate or lead to CHF, use with caution in patients at risk for heart failure and monitor patients at risk for heart failure for signs and symptoms of heart failure.

*Weight gain:* Dose-related weight gain was seen with rosiglitazone and pioglitazone alone and combination with other hypoglycemic agents.

### Drug Interactions

Drugs that may affect **pioglitazone** include atorvastatin and ketoconazole. Drugs that may be affected by **pioglitazone** include atorvastatin, midazolam, nifedipine, and oral contraceptives.

The cytochrome P450 isoform CYP3A4 is partially responsible for the metabolism of **pioglitazone**.

### Adverse Reactions

*Pioglitazone* – Pioglitazone when used in combination with sulfonylureas, metformin, or insulin caused an increased incidence of edema.

Adverse reactions that occurred in at least 3% of patients included the following: Aggravated diabetes mellitus, edema, headache, hypoglycemia, myalgia, pharyngitis, sinusitis, tooth disorder, upper respiratory tract infection.

*Rosiglitazone* – Reports of anemia were greater in patients treated with a combination of rosiglitazone and metformin compared with rosiglitazone monotherapy. Edema was reported with higher frequency in the rosiglitazone plus insulin combination trials.

Adverse reactions that occurred in at least 3% of patients included the following: Back pain, fatigue, headache, hyperglycemia, injury, sinusitis, URI.

*Lab test abnormalities:*

*Hematologic* – Decreases in hemoglobin, hematocrit, and white blood cell counts may be related to increased plasma volume observed with thiazolidinedione treatment.

*Lipids* – **Rosiglitazone** as monotherapy was associated with increases in total cholesterol, LDL, and HDL and decreases in free fatty acids. Patients treated with **pioglitazone** had mean decreases in triglycerides, mean increases in HDL cholesterol.

*Serum transaminase levels* – 0.2% of patients treated with **rosiglitazone** had reversible elevations in ALT greater than 3 times the ULN compared with 0.2% on placebo and 0.5% on active comparators. Hyperbilirubinemia was found in 0.3% of patients treated with rosiglitazone compared with 0.9% treated with placebo and 1% in patients treated with active comparators.

During placebo-controlled clinical trials in the US, a total of 0.26% **pioglitazone**-treated patients and 0.25% placebo-treated patients had ALT values 3 times or more the ULN. During all clinical studies in the US, 0.43% pioglitazone-treated patients had ALT values 3 times or more the ULN.

# METFORMIN COMBINATION PRODUCTS

**GLYBURIDE/METFORMIN HCL**
**Tablets:** 1.25 mg/250 mg, 2.5 mg/500 mg, and 5 mg/500 mg   *Glucovance* (Bristol-Myers Squibb)
*(Rx)*

**GLIPIZIDE/METFORMIN HCL**
**Tablets:** 2.5 mg/250 mg, 2.5 mg/500 mg, 5 mg/500 mg *(Rx)*   *Metaglip* (Bristol-Myers Squibb)

**ROSIGLITAZONE MALEATE/METFORMIN HCL**
**Tablets:** 1 mg/500 mg, 2 mg/500 mg, 2 mg/1,000 mg, 4 mg/   *Avandamet* (GlaxoSmithKline)
500 mg, 4 mg/1,000 mg *(Rx)*

---

**Warning:**
    Lactic acidosis is a rare, but serious, metabolic complication that can occur because
    of metformin accumulation during treatment with glyburide/metformin. When
    it occurs, it is fatal in approximately 50% of cases.

---

**Indications**
> *Glyburide/Metformin and Glipizide/Metformin combinations:*
> > *Type 2 diabetes* – Initial and second-line therapy.
>
> *Rosiglitazone/Metformin combination:*
> > *Type 2 diabetes* – For patients already treated with combination rosiglitazone and
> > metformin.

**Administration and Dosage**
    Individualize dosage, not exceeding the maximum recommended daily dose of 20 mg
    **glyburide** or **glipizide**, 8 mg of **rosiglitazone** or 2000 mg **metformin**. Give with meals
    and initiate at a low dose with gradual dose escalation to avoid hypoglycemia, to
    reduce GI side effects, and to permit determination of the minimum effective dose
    for adequate control of blood glucose.

    Use appropriate blood glucose monitoring to determine the therapeutic response and
    to identify the minimum effective dose for the patient. Thereafter, measure HbA$_{1c}$
    at intervals of about 3 months to assess the effectiveness of therapy.

> *Specific patient populations:* Metformin combination products are not recommended for
> use during pregnancy or in pediatric patients. Initial and maintenance dosing
> should be conservative in patients with advanced age because of the potential for
> decreased renal function in this population. Dosage adjustment requires a care-
> ful assessment of renal function. Do not titrate elderly, debilitated, or malnour-
> ished patients to the maximum dose to avoid the risk of hypoglycemia.

*GLYBURIDE/METFORMIN and GLIPIZIDE/METFORMIN:*
> *Initial therapy –*
> > *Starting dose:*
> > > *Glyburide/Metformin* – 1.25 mg/250 mg once or twice daily with meals.
> > > *Glipizide/Metformin* – 2.5 mg/250 mg once a day with a meal.
> *Previously treated patients (second-line therapy) –*
> > *Starting dose:*
> > > *Glyburide/Metformin* – 2.5 mg/500 mg or 5 mg/500 mg twice daily with meals.
> > > Patients previously treated with combination therapy of glyburide (or
> another sulfonylurea) plus metformin, if switched to glyburide/metformin HCl, the
> starting dose should not exceed the daily dose of glyburide (or equivalent dose of
> another sulfonylurea) and metformin already being taken.
> > > *Glipizide/Metformin* – 2.5 mg/500 mg or 5 mg/500 mg twice daily with the
> morning and evening meals. In order to avoid hypoglycemia, the starting dose
> should not exceed the daily doses of glipizide or metformin already being taken.

*ROSIGLITAZONE/METFORMIN:*
> *Patients inadequately controlled on metformin monotherapy –* Starting dose is 4 mg rosigl-
> itazone (total daily dose) plus the dose of metformin already being taken (see table).

*Patients inadequately controlled on rosiglitazone monotherapy* – Starting dose is 1000 mg metformin (total daily dose) plus the dose of rosiglitazone already being taken (see table).

| Rosiglitazone/Metformin Starting Dose | | |
|---|---|---|
| | Usual *Avandamet* starting dose | |
| Prior therapy (total daily dose) | Tablet strength | Number of tablets |
| Metformin HCl[1] | | |
| 1000 mg/day | 2 mg/500 mg | 1 tablet bid |
| 2000 mg/day | 2 mg/1000 mg | 1 tablet bid |
| Rosiglitazone | | |
| 4 mg/day | 2 mg/500 mg | 1 tablet bid |
| 8 mg/day | 4 mg/500 mg | 1 tablet bid |

[1] For patients on doses of metformin HCl between 1000 and 2000 mg/day, initiation of rosiglitazone/metformin requires individualization of therapy.

*When switching from combination therapy of rosiglitazone plus metformin as separate tablets* – Starting dose is the dose of rosiglitazone and metformin already being taken.

*If additional glycemic control is needed* – The daily dose may be increased by increments of 4 mg rosiglitazone and/or 500 mg metformin, up to the maximum recommended total daily dose of 8 mg/2000 mg.

No studies have been performed specifically examining the safety and efficacy of rosiglitazone/metformin in patients previously treated with other oral hypoglycemic agents and switched to rosiglitazone/metformin. Any change in therapy of type 2 diabetes should be undertaken with care and appropriate monitoring as changes in glycemic control can occur.

Do not initiate therapy if the patient exhibits clinical evidence of active liver disease or increased serum transaminase levels (ALT more than 2.5 times upper limit of normal at start of therapy). Liver enzyme monitoring is recommended in all patients prior to initiation of therapy with rosiglitazone/metformin and periodically thereafter.

# THYROID HORMONES

### LEVOTHYROXINE SODIUM

| | |
|---|---|
| **Tablets**: 0.025, 0.05, 0.075, 0.088, 0.1, 0.112, 0.125, 0.137, 0.15, 0.175, 0.2, and 0.3 mg (*Rx*) | Various, *Levothroid* (Forest), *Levoxyl* (Jones Pharma), *Synthroid* (Abbott), *Thyro-Tabs* (Lloyd), *Unithroid* (Watson) |
| **Powder for injection, lyophilized**: 200 and 500 mcg (*Rx*) | Various |

### LIOTHYRONINE SODIUM

| | |
|---|---|
| **Tablets**: 5, 25, and 50 mcg (*Rx*) | Various, *Cytomel* (Monarch) |
| **Injection**: 10 mcg/mL (*Rx*) | *Triostat* (Monarch) |

### LIOTRIX (64.8 mg = 1 grain)

| | |
|---|---|
| **Tablets**: ¼, ½, 1, 2, and 3 grains ($T_4$:$T_3$ content in a 4:1 ratio, mcg-for-mcg basis) (*Rx*) | *Thyrolar* (Forest) |

### THYROID DESICCATED (64.8 mg = 1 grain)[1]

| | |
|---|---|
| **Tablets**: 15 and 30 mg (*Rx*) | *Armour Thyroid* (Forest) |
| 32.4 mg (*Rx*) | *Nature-Throid, Westhroid* (Western Research Labs) |
| 32.5 mg (*Rx*) | Various |
| 60 mg (*Rx*) | *Armour Thyroid* (Forest) |
| 64.8 mg (*Rx*) | *Nature-Throid, Westhroid* (Western Research Labs) |
| 65 mg (*Rx*) | Various |
| 90 and 120 mg (*Rx*) | *Armour Thyroid* (Forest) |
| 129.6 mg (*Rx*) | *Nature-Throid, Westhroid* (Western Research Labs) |
| 130 mg (*Rx*) | Various |
| 180 mg (*Rx*) | *Armour Thyroid* (Forest) |
| 194.4 mg (*Rx*) | *Nature-Throid, Westhroid* (Western Research Labs) |
| 195 mg (*Rx*) | Various |
| 240 and 300 mg (*Rx*) | *Armour Thyroid* (Forest) |
| **Capsules**: 7.5, 15, 30, 60, 90, 120, 150, 180, and 240 mg (*Rx*) | *Bio-Throid* (Bio-Tech) |

[1] Porcine derived.

**Warning:**
   Drugs with thyroid hormone activity, alone or with other therapeutic agents, have been used for the treatment of obesity. In euthyroid patients, doses within the range of daily hormonal requirements are ineffective for weight reduction. Larger doses may produce serious or even life-threatening manifestations of toxicity, particularly when given in association with sympathomimetic amines such as those used for their anorectic effects.

### Indications

   *Hypothyroidism:* As replacement or supplemental therapy in hypothyroidism of any etiology, except transient hypothyroidism during the recovery phase of subacute thyroiditis.

   *Pituitary TSH suppressants:* In the treatment or prevention of various types of euthyroid goiters, including thyroid nodules, subacute, or chronic lymphocytic thyroiditis (Hashimoto), multinodular goiter, and in the management of thyroid cancer (except liothyronine).

   *Diagnostic use (except levothyroxine):* Diagnostic use in suppression tests to differentiate suspected hyperthyroidism from euthyroidism.

   *Myxedema coma/precoma (injection only):* For the treatment of myxedema coma/precoma.

### Administration and Dosage

   Synthetic derivatives include levothyroxine ($T_4$), liothyronine ($T_3$), and liotrix (a 4 to 1 mixture of $T_4$ and $T_3$).

Generally, institute thyroid therapy at relatively low doses and slowly increase in small increments until the desired response is obtained. Administer thyroid as a single daily dose, preferably before breakfast.

*Treatment of choice:* Treatment of choice for hypothyroidism is $T_4$ because of its consistent potency and prolonged half-life.

*Thyroid cancer:* Exogenous thyroid hormone may produce regression of metastases from follicular and papillary carcinoma of the thyroid and is used as ancillary therapy of these conditions with radioactive iodine. Larger doses than those used for replacement therapy are required.

*Laboratory tests:* Laboratory tests useful in the diagnosis and evaluation of thyroid function are listed in the following table, indicating the alterations noted in various thyroid disorders.

| Laboratory Tests for Diagnosis and Evaluation of Thyroid Function | | | | | | |
|---|---|---|---|---|---|---|
| ↑ = Increased<br>↓ = Decreased<br>N = Normal<br>X = Contraindicated | Pregnancy | Primary hypothyroidism | Secondary hypothyroidism | Hyperthyroidism | $T_3$ thyrotoxicosis | Normal values |
| Free $T_4$ (unbound) | N | ↓ | ↓ | ↑ | N | 12 to 32 pmol/L |
| Total $T_4$ | ↑ | ↓ | ↓ | ↑ | N | 55 to 160 nmol/L |
| $T_3$ | ↑ | ↓ | ↓ | ↑ | ↑ | 0.6 to 3.1 nmol/L |
| RAIU[*] | X | ↓ | - | ↑ | – | 5% to 30% |
| Free thyroxine index (FT$_4$I) | N | ↓ | ↓ | ↑ | . | 6.5 to 12.5[1]<br>1.3 to 3.9[2] |
| TSH[*] | N | ↑ | N/↓ | ↓ | ↓ | 0.4 to 4.2 milliunits/L |

[*] RAIU = radioactive iodine uptake; TSH = thyroid-stimulating hormone
[1] $T_4$ uptake method
[2] $TT_4 \times RT_3U$ method

*Dosage equivalents of thyroid products:* In changing from one thyroid product to another, the following dosage equivalents may be used. However, each patient may still require dosage adjustments because these equivalents are only estimates.

LEVOTHYROXINE SODIUM ($T_4$; L-thyroxine): Take levothyroxine in the morning on an empty stomach, at least 30 minutes before any food is eaten. Take levothyroxine at least 4 hours apart from drugs that are known to interfere with its absorption.

*Hypothyroidism in adults and children in whom growth and puberty are complete* – The average full replacement dose of levothyroxine is approximately 1.7 mcg/kg/day (eg, 100 to 125 mcg/day for a 70 kg adult). Older patients may require less than 1 mcg/kg/day.

For most patients older than 50 years of age or for patients younger than 50 years of age with underlying cardiac disease, an initial starting dose of 25 to 50 mcg/day of levothyroxine is recommended, with gradual increments in dose at 6- to 8-week intervals, as needed. The recommended starting dose of levothyroxine sodium in elderly patients with cardiac disease is 12.5 to 25 mcg/day, with gradual dose increments at 4- to 6-week intervals.

*Dosage adjustment:* The levothyroxine dose generally is adjusted in 12.5 to 25 mcg increments until the patient with primary hypothyroidism is clinically euthyroid and the serum TSH has normalized.

*Severe hypothyroidism* – In patients with severe hypothyroidism, the recommended initial levothyroxine dose is 12.5 to 25 mcg/day with increases of 25 mcg/day every 2 to 4 weeks.

*IV or IM:* IV or IM injection can be substituted for the oral dosage form when oral ingestion is precluded for long periods of time. The initial parenteral dosage should be approximately one-half of the previously established oral dosage. A daily maintenance dose of 50 to 100 mcg parenterally should suffice to maintain the euthyroid state once established. Close observation of the patient, with individual adjustment of the dosage as needed, is recommended.

*Subclinical hypothyroidism* – If this condition is treated, a lower levothyroxine dose (eg, 1 mcg/kg/day) than that used for full replacement may be adequate to normalize the serum TSH level.

*Myxedema coma* – Oral thyroid hormone drug products are not recommended to treat this condition; administer thyroid hormone products formulated for IV.

In myxedema coma or stupor, without concomitant severe heart disease, 200 to 500 mcg of levothyroxine for injection may be administered IV as a solution containing 100 mcg/mL. Do not add to other IV fluids. Although the patient may show evidence of increased responsivity within 6 to 8 hours, full therapeutic effect may not be evident until the following day. An additional 100 to 300 mcg or more may be given on the second day if evidence of significant and progressive improvements has not occurred. Maintain continued daily administration of lesser amounts parenterally until the patient is fully capable of accepting a daily oral dose.

*TSH suppression in well-differentiated thyroid cancer and thyroid nodules* – The target level for TSH suppression in these conditions has not been established in controlled studies. In addition, the efficacy of TSH suppression for benign nodular disease is controversial. Therefore, individualize the dose of levothyroxine used for TSH suppression based on the specific disease and the patient being treated.

In the treatment of well-differentiated (papillary and follicular) thyroid cancer, levothyroxine is used as an adjunct to surgery and radioiodine therapy. Generally, TSH is suppressed to less than 0.1 milliunits/L, and this usually requires a levothyroxine dose of greater than 2 mcg/kg/day. However, in patients with high-risk tumors, the target level for TSH suppression may be less than 0.01 milliunits/L.

In the treatment of benign nodules and nontoxic multinodular goiter, TSH generally is suppressed to a higher target (eg, 0.1 to 0.5 or 1 milliunits/L).

*Special populations* – Exercise caution when administering levothyroxine to patients with underlying cardiovascular disease, to the elderly, and to those with concomitant adrenal insufficiency.

*Children* – Follow the recommendations in the following table. In infants with congenital or acquired hypothyroidism, institute therapy with full doses as soon as diagnosis is made.

Levothyroxine tablets may be given to infants and children who cannot swallow intact tablets. Crush the proper dose tablet and suspend in a small amount (5 to 10 mL) of water. The suspension can be given by spoon or dropper. Do not store the suspension for any period of time. Do not use foods that decrease absorption of levothyroxine, such as soybean infant formula, for administering levothyroxine sodium tablets.

*Infants and children:* Levothyroxine therapy usually is initiated at full replacement doses, with the recommended dose per body weight decreasing with age (see table). However, in children with chronic or severe hypothyroidism, an initial 25 mcg/day dose of levothyroxine is recommended with increments of 25 mcg every 2 to 4 weeks until the desired effect is achieved.

Hyperactivity in an older child can be minimized if the starting dose is one-fourth of the recommended full replacement dose and the dose is then increased on a weekly basis by an amount equal to one-fourth of the full-recommended replacement dose until the full recommended replacement dose is reached.

*Newborns:* The recommended starting dose is 10 to 15 mcg/kg/day. Consider a lower starting dose (eg, 25 mcg/day) in infants at risk for cardiac failure; the dose should be increased in 4 to 6 weeks as needed. In infants with very low (less than 5 mcg/dL) or undetectable serum $T_4$ concentrations, the recommended initial starting dose is 50 mcg/day of levothyroxine.

| Recommended Pediatric Dosage for Congenital Hypothyroidism | |
|---|---|
| Age | Daily dose per kg (mcg)[1] |
| 0 to 3 mo | 10 to 15 |
| 3 to 6 mo | 8 to 10 |
| 6 to 12 mo | 6 to 8 |
| 1 to 5 y | 5 to 6 |
| 6 to 12 y | 4 to 5 |
| > 12 y (growth/puberty incomplete) | 2 to 3 |
| > 12 y (growth/puberty complete) | 1.7 |

[1] The dose should be adjusted based on clinical response and laboratory parameters.

LIOTHYRONINE SODIUM ($T_3$):

*Mild hypothyroidism* – Starting dose is 25 mcg/day. Daily dosage may be increased by up to 25 mcg every 1 or 2 weeks. Usual maintenance dose is 25 to 75 mcg/day.

*Congenital hypothyroidism* – Starting dose is 5 mcg/day, with a 5 mcg increment every 3 to 4 days until the desired response is achieved. Infants a few months old may require only 20 mcg/day for maintenance. At 1 year of age, 50 mcg/day may be required. Above 3 years, full adult dosage may be necessary.

*Simple (nontoxic) goiter* – Starting dose is 5 mcg/day. Dosage may be increased every 1 to 2 weeks by 5 or 10 mcg every 1 to 2 weeks. When 25 mcg/day is reached, dosage may be increased every 1 to 2 weeks by 12.5 or 25 mcg. Usual maintenance dosage is 75 mcg/day.

*Thyroid suppression therapy* – 75 to 100 mcg/day for 7 days; radioactive iodine uptake is determined before and after administration of the hormone.

*Myxedema* – Starting dose is 5 mcg/day. This may be increased by 5 to 10 mcg/day every 1 to 2 weeks. When 25 mcg/day is reached, dosage may be increased by 5 or 25 mcg every 1 or 2 weeks. Usual maintenance dose is 50 to 100 mcg/day.

*Myxedema coma/precoma (injection only)* – For IV use only; do not give IM or subcutaneously. Give doses at least 4 hours, and not more than 12 hours, apart. Giving at least 65 mcg/day initially is associated with lower mortality.

An initial IV dose ranging from 25 to 50 mcg is recommended in the emergency treatment of myxedema complications in adults. In patients with known or suspected cardiovascular disease, an initial dose of 10 to 20 mcg is suggested.

A single dose of liothyronine administered IV produces a detectable metabolic response in as little as 2 to 4 hours and a maximum therapeutic response within 2 days.

*Switching to oral therapy:* Resume oral therapy as soon as the clinical situation has been stabilized and the patient is able to take oral medication. If oral levothyroxine is used, keep in mind that there is a delay of several days in the onset of action; discontinue IV therapy gradually.

*Elderly or children* – Start therapy with 5 mcg/day; increase only by 5 mcg increments at the recommended intervals.

*Exchange therapy* – When switching a patient to liothyronine from thyroid levothyroxine or thyroglobulin, discontinue the other medication, initiate liothyronine at a low dosage, and increase gradually according to the patient's response. Liothyronine has a rapid onset of action and that residual effects of the other thyroid preparation may persist for the first several weeks of therapy.

LIOTRIX:

*Hypothyroidism* –

*Initial dosage:* Usual starting dose is 1 tablet of *Thyrolar* ½ with increments of 1 tablet of *Thyrolar* ¼ every 2 to 3 weeks. A lower starting dose, 1 tablet/day *Thyrolar* ¼ is recommended in patients with long-standing myxedema, particularly if cardiovascular impairment is suspected.

*Maintenance dosage:* Most patients require 1 tablet *Thyrolar* 1 to 1 tablet *Thyrolar* 2 per day; failure to respond to 1 tablet *Thyrolar* 3 suggests lack of compliance or malabsorption.

*Dosage readjustment* – Readjust dosage within the first 4 weeks of therapy after proper clinical and laboratory evaluations including serum levels of $T_4$ bound and free, and TSH.

*Thyroid cancer:* Larger amounts of thyroid hormone than those used for replacement therapy are required.

*Diagnostic agent* – For adults, the usual suppressive dose of $T_4$ is 1.56 mcg/kg of body weight per day given for 7 to 10 days. These doses usually yield normal serum $T_4$ and $T_3$ levels and lack of response to TSH.

*Children* – In infants with congenital hypothyroidism, institute therapy with full doses as soon as diagnosis is made.

| Recommended Pediatric Dosage for Congenital Hypothyroidism | | | |
| --- | --- | --- | --- |
| | Dose per day in mcg | | |
| Age | $T_3/T_4$ | to | $T_3/T_4$ |
| 0 to 6 mo | 3.1/12.5 | to | 6.25/25 |
| 6 to 12 mo | 6.25/25 | to | 9.35/37.5 |
| 1 to 5 y | 9.35/37.5 | to | 12.5/50 |
| 6 to 12 y | 12.5/50 | to | 18.75/75 |
| Over 12 y | | | > 18.75/75 |

THYROID DESICCATED:

*Hypothyroidism* –

*Initial dosage:* Usual starting dose is 30 mg, with increments of 15 mg every 2 to 3 weeks. Use 15 mg/day in patients with long-standing myxedema, particularly if cardiovascular impairment is suspected.

*Maintenance dosage:* 60 to 120 mg/day; failure to respond to 180 mg doses suggests lack of compliance or malabsorption.

*Thyroid cancer* – Larger amounts of thyroid hormone than those used for replacement therapy are required.

*Diagnostic agent* – For adults, the usual suppressive dose of $T_4$ is 1.56 mcg/kg of body weight per day given for 7 to 10 days.

*Children* – In infants with congenital hypothyroidism, institute therapy with full doses as soon as diagnosis is made.

| Recommended Pediatric Dosage for Congenital Hypothyroidism | | |
| --- | --- | --- |
| Age | Dose per day (mg) | Daily dose per kg (mg) |
| 0 to 6 mo | 7.5 to 30 | 2.4 to 6 |
| 6 to 12 mo | 30 to 45 | 3.6 to 4.8 |
| 1 to 5 y | 45 to 60 | 3 to 3.6 |
| 6 to 12 y | 60 to 90 | 2.4 to 3 |
| > 12 y | > 90 | 1.2 to 1.8 |

*Special populations* – Initiate therapy in low doses (15 to 30 mg) in patients with angina pectoris or the elderly, in whom there is a greater likelihood of occult cardiac disease.

**Actions**

*Pharmacology:* Thyroid hormones enhance oxygen consumption by most tissues of the body and increase the basal metabolic rate and metabolism of carbohydrates, lipids, and proteins in the body.

*Pharmacokinetics:*

*Absorption* – Absorption of orally administered $T_4$ varies from 40% to 80%. $T_4$ absorption is increased by fasting and decreased in malabsorption syndromes and by certain foods, such as soybean infant formula. Dietary fiber decreases bioavailability of $T_4$. Absorption also may decrease with age. The hormones in natural preparations are absorbed in a manner similar to the synthetic hormones.

*Excretion* – Thyroid hormones are primarily eliminated by the kidneys.

| Various Pharmacokinetic Parameters of Thyroid Hormones | | | | |
|---|---|---|---|---|
| Hormone | Ratio in thyroglobulin | Biologic potency | Half-life (days) | Protein binding (%)[1] |
| Levothyroxine ($T_4$) | 10 to 20 | 1 | 6 to 7[2] | 99+ |
| Liothyronine ($T_3$) | 1 | 4 | ≤ 2.5 | 99+ |

[1] Includes TBG, TBPA, and TBA.
[2] 3 to 4 days in hyperthyroidism, 9 to 10 days in hypothyroidism.

**Contraindications**

Diagnosed but uncorrected adrenal cortical insufficiency; untreated thyrotoxicosis; hypersensitivity to active or extraneous constituents.

Levothyroxine is contraindicated in patients with untreated subclinical (suppressed serum TSH level with normal $T_3$ and $T_4$ levels) and in patients with acute MI.

Concomitant use of *Triostat* and artificial rewarming of patients is contraindicated.

**Warnings**

*Obesity:* In euthyroid patients, hormonal replacement doses are ineffective for weight reduction. Larger doses may produce serious or even life-threatening toxicity, particularly when given with sympathomimetic amines such as anorexiants.

*Infertility:* Thyroid hormone therapy is unjustified for the treatment of male or female infertility unless the condition is accompanied by hypothyroidism.

*Cardiovascular disease:* Use caution in suspected cardiovascular disease, particularly the coronary arteries, is suspect. This includes patients with angina or the elderly, in whom there is a greater likelihood of occult cardiac disease. Initiate therapy with low doses.

*Endocrine disorders:* Thyroid hormone therapy in patients with concomitant diabetes mellitus or insipidus or adrenal insufficiency (Addison disease) exacerbates the intensity of their symptoms.

    *Autoimmune polyglandular syndrome* – Chronic autoimmune thyroiditis may occur in association with other autoimmune disorders. Treat patients with concomitant adrenal insufficiency with replacement glucocorticoids prior to initiation of treatment. Failure to do so may precipitate an acute adrenal crisis when thyroid hormone therapy is initiated. Patients with diabetes mellitus may require upward adjustments of their antidiabetic therapeutic regimens.

*Nontoxic diffuse goiter or nodular thyroid disease:* Use caution when administering levothyroxine to patients with nontoxic diffuse goiter or nodular thyroid disease in order to prevent precipitation of thyrotoxicosis. If the serum TSH is already suppressed, do not administer levothyroxine.

*Severe and prolonged hypothyroidism:* In severe and prolonged hypothyroidism, supplemental adrenocortical steroids may be necessary.

*Morphologic hypogonadism and nephrosis:* Rule out morphologic hypogonadism and nephrosis prior to initiating therapy.

*Myxedema:* Start dosage at a very low level and increase gradually. Myxedema coma therapy requires simultaneous administration of glucocorticoids.

*Hyperthyroid effects:* In rare instances, the administration of thyroid hormone may precipitate a hyperthyroid state or may aggravate existing hyperthyroidism.

*Pregnancy:* Category A.

*Lactation:* Minimal amounts of thyroid hormones are excreted in breast milk. Thyroid is not associated with serious adverse reactions.

*Children:*

    *Congenital hypothyroidism* – The incidence of congenital hypothyroidism is relatively high (1:4000). Routine determinations of serum $T_4$ and/or TSH are strongly advised in neonates.

**Precautions**

*Monitoring:* Treatment of patients with thyroid hormones requires the periodic assessment of thyroid status by means of appropriate laboratory tests. The TSH suppression test can be used to test the effectiveness of any thyroid preparation.

The frequency of TSH monitoring during levothyroxine dose titration is generally recommended at 6- to 8-week intervals until normalization. For patients who have recently initiated levothyroxine therapy and whose serum TSH has normalized or in patients who have had their dosage or brand of levothyroxine changed, measure the serum TSH concentration after 8 to 12 weeks.

*Decreased bone density:* In women, long-term levothyroxine therapy has been associated with increased bone resorption, thereby decreasing bone mineral density, especially in postmenopausal women on greater than replacement doses or in women who are receiving suppressive doses of levothyroxine.

**Drug Interactions**

Drugs that may affect thyroid hormones include amiodarone, glucocorticoids, PTU, aluminum and magnesium containing antacids, bile acid sequestrants, calcium carbonate, iron salts, sodium polystyrene sulfonate, simethicone, sucralfate, beta blockers, carbamazepine, hydantoins, phenobarbital, rifamycins, estrogens, oral contraceptives, furosemide, heparin, hydantoins, NSAIDs, salicylates, SSRIs, tri- and tetra-cyclic antidepressants, and sympathomimetics. Drugs that may be affected by thyroid hormones include beta-blockers, tri- and tetra-cyclic antidepressants, anticoagulants, antidiabetic agents: biguanides, meglitinides, sulfonylureas, thiazolidinediones, and insulin, digitalis glycosides, growth hormones, ketamine, radiographic agents, sympathomimetics and theophylline.

*Drug/Lab test interactions:* Consider changes in TBG concentration when interpreting $T_4$ and $T_3$ values. In such cases, measure the unbound (free) hormone and/or free $T_4$ index ($FT_4I$). Pregnancy, infectious hepatitis, estrogens, estrogen-containing oral contraceptives, and acute intermittent porphyria increase TBG concentrations. Decreases in TBG concentrations are observed in nephrosis, severe hypoproteinemia, severe liver disease, and acromegaly, and after androgen or corticosteroid therapy. Familial hyper- or hypothyroxine binding globulinemias have been described.

Medicinal or dietary iodine interferes with all in vivo tests of radioiodine uptake, producing low uptakes that may not reflect a true decrease in hormone synthesis.

*Cytokines: Interferon-α and interleukin-2* – Therapy with interferon-α has been associated with the development of antithyroid microsomal antibodies in 20% of patients and some have transient hypothyroidism, hyperthyroidism, or both. Patients who have antithyroid antibodies before treatment are at higher risk of thyroid dysfunction during treatment. Interleukin-2 has been associated with transient painless thyroiditis in 20% of patients.

Drugs that may reduce TSTH secretion include dopamine and dopamine agonists, glucocorticoids, and octreotide. Drugs that may decrease thyroid hormone secretion include aminoglutethimide, amiodarone, iodine, lithium, methimazole, PTU, sulfonamides, and tolbutamide. Drugs that may increase thyroid hormone secretion may include amiodarone, and iodide. Drugs that may alter serum TBG concentrations include estrogen-containing contraceptives, oral estrogens, heroin and methadone, 5-fluorouracil, mitotane, and tamoxifen. Drugs that are associated with thyroid hormone and/or TSH level alterations by various mechanisms include chloral hydrate, diazepam, ethionamide, lovastatin, metoclopramide, 6-mercaptopurine, nitroprusside, para-aminosalicylate sodium, perphenazine, excessive topical use of resorcinol and thiazide diuretics.

*Drug/Food interactions:* Fasting increases the absorption of $T_4$ from the GI tract.

**Adverse Reactions**

Adverse reactions other than those indicating hyperthyroidism caused by therapeutic overdosage, initially or during the maintenance period, are rare. Symptoms of overdosage include the following: Palpitations; tachycardia; arrhythmias; angina; cardiac arrest; increased pulse and blood pressure; CHF; MI; tremors; headache;

nervousness; insomnia; hyperactivity; anxiety, irritability; emotional lability; diarrhea; vomiting; abdominal cramps; hypersensitivity reactions to inactive ingredients; weight loss; fatigue; increased appetite; menstrual irregularities; excessive sweating; heat intolerance; fever; muscle weakness; dyspnea; hair loss; flushing; decreased bone mineral density; impaired fertility; increase in liver function tests.

*Children* – Pseudotumor cerebri; slipped capital femoral epiphysis; craniosynostosis; premature closure of the epiphyses.

*Liothyronine injection only* – Hypotension; phlebitis; twitching.

# ANTITHYROID AGENTS

**METHIMAZOLE**
**Tablets**: 5 and 10 mg (*Rx*)                    Various, *Tapazole* (Lilly)
**PROPYLTHIOURACIL**
**Tablets**: 50 mg (*Rx*)                    Various

### Indications
*Hyperthyroidism:* Long-term therapy may lead to disease remission. Also used to ameliorate hyperthyroidism in preparation for subtotal thyroidectomy or radioactive iodine therapy.

Propylthiouracil is also used when thyroidectomy is contraindicated or not advisable.

### Administration and Dosage
METHIMAZOLE: Usually given in 3 equal doses at approximately 8 hour intervals.
*Adults –*
*Initial:* 15 mg daily for mild hyperthyroidism, 30 to 40 mg/day for moderately severe hyperthyroidism and 60 mg/day for severe hyperthyroidism.
*Maintenance:* 5 to 15 mg/day.
*Children –*
*Initial:* 0.4 mg/kg/day.
*Maintenance:* Approximately ½ the initial dose.
Another suggested dosage for children is as follows:
*Initial:* 0.5 to 0.7 mg/kg/day or 15 to 20 mg/m²/day in 3 divided doses.
*Maintenance:* ⅓ to ⅔ of initial dose beginning when the patient is euthyroid.
*Maximum:* 30 mg/24 hours.

PROPYLTHIOURACIL: Usually given in 3 equal doses at approximately 8 hour intervals.
*Adults –*
*Initial:* 300 mg/day. In patients with severe hyperthyroidism, very large goiters, or both, the initial dosage is usually 400 mg/day; an occasional patient will require 600 to 900 mg/day initially.
*Maintenance:* Usually, 100 to 150 mg/day.
*Children –*
*6 to 10 years of age:* Initial dose is 50 to 150 mg/day.
*10 years of age and older:* Initial dose is 150 to 300 mg/day.
*Maintenance:* Determined by patient response.
Another suggested dosage for children is as follows:
*Initial:* 5 to 7 mg/kg/day or 150 to 200 mg/m²/day in divided doses every 8 hours.
*Maintenance:* ⅓ to ⅔ the initial dose beginning when the patient is euthyroid.

### Actions
*Pharmacology:* Propylthiouracil and methimazole inhibit the synthesis of thyroid hormones and, thus, are effective in the treatment of hyperthyroidism. They do not inactivate existing thyroxine ($T_4$) and triiodothyronine ($T_3$) nor do they interfere with the effectiveness of exogenous thyroid hormones. Propylthiouracil partially inhibits the peripheral conversion of $T_4$ to $T_3$.

*Pharmacokinetics:*

| Various Pharmacokinetic Parameters of Antithyroid Agents | | | | | | |
|---|---|---|---|---|---|---|
| Antithyroid agent | Bioavailability (%) | Protein binding (%) | Transplacental passage | Breast milk levels (M:P)[1] | Half-life (h) | Excreted in urine (%) |
| Methimazole | 80-95 | 0 | High | High (1) | 6-13 | < 10 |
| Propylthiouracil | 80-95 | 75-80 | Low | Low (0.1) | 1-2 | < 35 |

[1] Approximate milk:plasma ratio.

### Contraindications
Hypersensitivity to antithyroid drugs; lactation.

## Warnings

*Agranulocytosis:* Agranulocytosis is potentially the most serious side effect of therapy. Leukopenia, thrombocytopenia and aplastic anemia (pancytopenia) may also occur.

*Pregnancy: Category D.* These agents, used judiciously, are effective drugs in hyperthyroidism complicated by pregnancy. Because they readily cross the placenta and can induce goiter and even cretinism in the developing fetus, it is important that a sufficient, but not excessive, dose be given. If an antithyroid agent is needed, propylthiouracil is preferred because it is less likely than methimazole to cross the placenta and induce fetal/neonatal complications.

*Lactation:* Postpartum patients receiving antithyroid preparations should not nurse their babies. However, if necessary, the preferred drug is propylthiouracil.

*Children:* In several case reports, propylthiouracil hepatotoxicity has occurred in pediatric patients.

## Precautions

*Monitoring:* Monitor thyroid function tests periodically during therapy.

*Hemorrhagic effects:* Because propylthiouracil may cause hypoprothrombinemia and bleeding, monitor prothrombin time during therapy, especially before surgical procedures.

## Drug Interactions

Drugs that may interact with antithyroid agents include anticoagulants.

## Adverse Reactions

Agranulocytosis is the most serious effect.

# BISPHOSPHONATES

| | |
|---|---|
| **ALENDRONATE SODIUM** | |
| **Tablets**: 5, 10, 35, 40, and 70 mg (*Rx*) | *Fosamax* (Merck) |
| **Oral solution**: 70 mg (*Rx*) | |
| **ETIDRONATE DISODIUM (ORAL)** | |
| **Tablets**: 200 and 400 mg (*Rx*) | *Didronel* (Procter & Gamble) |
| **PAMIDRONATE DISODIUM** | |
| **Powder for injection, lyophilized**: 30 and 90 mg (*Rx*) | *Aredia* (Novartis) |
| **Injection**: 3, 6, and 9 mg/mL (*Rx*) | Various |
| **RISEDRONATE SODIUM** | |
| **Tablets**: 5, 30, and 35 mg (*Rx*) | *Actonel* (Procter & Gamble) |
| **TILUDRONATE SODIUM** | |
| **Tablets**: 240 mg (equiv. to 200 mg tiludronic acid) (*Rx*) | *Skelid* (Sanofi-Synthelabo) |
| **ZOLEDRONIC ACID** | |
| **Powder for injection**: 4 mg zoledronic acid anhydrous (*Rx*) | *Zometa* (Novartis) |

## Indications

*Osteoporosis (alendronate, risedronate):*

*In postmenopausal women* – For the treatment and prevention of osteoporosis in postmenopausal women.

*Glucocorticoid-induced* – Treatment and prevention of glucocorticoid-induced osteoporosis in men and women who are either initiating or continuing systemic glucocorticoid treatment for chronic diseases and receiving glucocorticoids in a daily dosage equivalent to 7.5 mg or more prednisone and who have low bone mineral density.

*In men* – To increase bone mass in men with osteoporosis (alendronate).

*Paget disease of bone:* For treatment of Paget disease of bone where alkaline phosphatase is at least 2 times the upper limit of normal, or those who are symptomatic or at risk for future complications from their disease (**alendronate, risedronate, tiludronate**); treatment of symptomatic Paget disease (**etidronate**); treatment of moderate to severe Paget disease (**pamidronate**).

*Heterotopic ossification (etidronate):* Prevention and treatment of heterotopic ossification following total hip replacement or caused by spinal injury.

*Hypercalcemia of malignancy (HCM):* For the treatment of HCM (**zoledronic acid**); in conjunction with adequate hydration for the treatment of moderate or severe hypercalcemia associated with malignancy, with or without bone metastases (**pamidronate** patients with epidermoid or nonepidermoid tumors respond to pamidronate); for HCM that persists after adequate hydration has been restored (**zoledronic acid**).

*Breast cancer/Multiple myeloma (pamidronate):* In conjunction with standard antineoplastic therapy for the treatment of osteolytic bone metastases of breast cancer and osteolytic lesions of multiple myeloma.

*Multiple myeloma and bone metastases of solid tumors (zoledronic acid):* For the treatment of multiple myeloma and bone metastases from solid tumors, in conjunction with standard antineoplastic therapy.

## Administration and Dosage

ALENDRONATE: Alendronate must be taken at least 30 minutes before the first food, beverage, or medication of the day with plain water only. Any other beverages, food, and some medications are likely to reduce the absorption of alendronate. To facilitate delivery to the stomach, and reduce the potential for esophageal irritation, swallow alendronate only upon arising for the day. Take with a full glass of water (6 to 8 ounces; 180 to 240 mL) and avoid lying down for at least 30 minutes and until after the first food of the day. Do not take alendronate at bedtime or before arising for the day. To facilitate gastric emptying, follow the oral solution with at least 2 oz (¼ cup) of water. Advise patient to take tablet with a full glass of water (6 to 8 oz; 180 to 240 mL). Do not take alendronate at bedtime or before arising for the day. Failure to follow these instructions may increase the risk of esophageal adverse reactions.

Patients with Paget disease or receiving glucocorticoids should receive supplemental calcium and vitamin D if dietary intake is inadequate.

*Osteoporosis in postmenopausal women –*

*Treatment:* 70 mg once weekly or 10 mg once daily or 1 bottle of 70 mg oral solution once weekly.

*Prevention:* 35 mg once weekly or 5 mg once daily.

*Osteoporosis in men –* 10 mg once daily. Alternatively, one 70 mg tablet or 1 bottle of 70 mg oral solution once weekly may be considered.

*Glucocorticoid-induced osteoporosis –* 5 mg once daily. For postmenopausal women not receiving estrogen, the recommended dose is 10 mg once daily. Patients also should receive adequate amounts of calcium and vitamin D.

*Paget disease of bone –* 40 mg once a day for 6 months.

*Retreatment:* Retreatment with alendronate may be considered, following a 6-month posttreatment evaluation period, in patients who have relapsed based on increases in serum alkaline phosphatase. Retreatment also may be considered in those who failed to normalize their serum alkaline phosphatase.

*ETIDRONATE DISODIUM (ORAL):*

*Initiation of oral tablets –* The recommended oral dose of etidronate for patients who have had hypercalcemia is 20 mg/kg/day for 30 days.

Administer as a single dose. However, if GI discomfort occurs, divide the dose. To maximize absorption, avoid the following within 2 hours of dosing:

1.) Food, especially items high in calcium, such as milk or milk products.

2.) Vitamins with mineral supplements or antacids high in metals (eg, calcium, iron, magnesium, aluminum).

*Paget disease –*

*Initial treatment:* 5 to 10 mg/kg/day (not to exceed 6 months) or 11 to 20 mg/kg/day (not to exceed 3 months). Reserve doses higher than 10 mg/kg/day for use when lower doses are ineffective, when there is an overriding requirement for suppression of increased bone turnover or when prompt reduction of elevated cardiac output is required. Doses higher than 20 mg/kg/day are not recommended.

*Retreatment:* Initiate only after an etidronate-free period of at least 90 days and when there is biochemical, symptomatic, or other evidence of active disease process. For most patients, the original dose will be adequate for retreatment. If not, consider increasing the dose within the recommended guidelines.

*Heterotopic ossification –*

*Caused by spinal cord injury:* 20 mg/kg/day for 2 weeks, followed by 10 mg/kg/day for 10 weeks; total treatment period is 12 weeks. Institute as soon as feasible following the injury, preferably prior to evidence of heterotopic ossification.

*Complicating total hip replacement:* 20 mg/kg/day for 1 month preoperatively, then 20 mg/kg/day for 3 months postoperatively; total treatment period is 4 months.

*PAMIDRONATE DISODIUM:*

HCM –

*Moderate hypercalcemia:* The recommended dose in moderate hypercalcemia (corrected serum calcium of about 12 to 23.5 mg/dL) is 60 to 90 mg given as a *single-dose* IV infusion over at least 2 to 24 hours. Longer infusions (eg, more than 2 hours) may reduce the risk for renal toxicity, particularly in patients with pre-existing renal insufficiency.

*Severe hypercalcemia:* Recommended dose (corrected serum calcium higher than 13.5 mg/dL) is 90 mg, which must be given by initial *single-dose,* IV infusion over 2 to 24 hours. Longer infusions (eg, more than 2 hours) may reduce the risk for renal toxicity, particularly in patients with pre-existing renal insufficiency.

*Retreatment:* Retreatment in patients who show complete or partial response initially may be carried out if serum calcium does not return to normal or remain normal after initial treatment. Allow a minimum of 7 days to elapse before retreatment to allow for full response to the initial dose. Retreatment is identical to that of the initial therapy.

*Paget disease* – The recommended dose in patients with moderate to severe Paget disease of bone is 30 mg daily, given as a 4 hour infusion on 3 consecutive days for a total dose of 90 mg.

*Retreatment:* When clinically indicated, retreat at the dose of initial therapy.

*Osteolytic bone metastases of breast cancer* – 90 mg administered over a 2-hour infusion every 3 to 4 weeks.

*Osteolytic bone lesions of multiple myeloma* – The recommended dose is 90 mg given as a 4-hour infusion on a monthly basis. Patients with marked Bence-Jones proteinuria and dehydration should receive adequate hydration prior to pamidronate infusion.

*Admixture incompatibility* – Do not mix with calcium-containing infusion solutions, such as Ringer's solution. Give in a single IV solution and line separate from all other drugs.

*Hydration* – Initiate saline hydration promptly and attempt to restore the urine output to approximately 2 L/day throughout treatment. Mild or asymptomatic hypercalcemia may be treated with conservative measures (ie, saline hydration with or without loop diuretics). Adequately hydrate patients throughout the treatment, but avoid overhydration, especially in those patients who have cardiac failure. Do not employ diuretic therapy prior to correction of hypovolemia.

*Renal function impairment* – In patients receiving pamidronate for bone metastases who show evidence of deterioration in renal function, withhold treatment until renal function returns to baseline. In a clinical study, renal deterioration was defined as follows: for patients with normal baseline creatinine, an increase of 0.5 mg/dL; for patients with abnormal baseline creatinine, an increase of 1 mg/dL. In this clinical study, pamidronate treatment was resumed only when the creatinine returned to within 10% of the baseline value. In other indications, clinical judgment should determine whether the potential benefit outweighs the potential risk in such patients.

RISEDRONATE: Take once daily at least 30 minutes before the first food or drink of the day other than water.

Take while in an upright position with a full glass (6 to 8 ounces; 180 to 240 mL) of plain water and avoid lying down for 30 minutes to minimize the possibility of GI side effects.

Patients should receive supplemental calcium and vitamin D if dietary intake is inadequate. Take calcium supplements and calcium-, aluminum-, and magnesium-containing agents at a different time of the day to prevent interference with risedronate absorption.

*Paget disease* – 30 mg once daily for 2 months. Retreatment may be considered (following posttreatment observation of 2 months or more) if relapse occurs or if treatment fails to normalize serum alkaline phosphatase. For retreatment, the dose and duration of therapy are the same as for initial treatment. No data are available on more than 1 course of retreatment.

*Treatment/Prevention of postmenopausal osteoporosis* – 5 mg orally taken daily or one 35 mg tablet orally taken once weekly.

*Treatment/Prevention of glucocorticoid-induced osteoporosis* – 5 mg orally taken daily.

*Renal function impairment* – Risedronate is not recommended for use in patients with severe renal impairment (Ccr less than 30 mL/min). No dosage adjustment is necessary in patients with a Ccr 30 mL/min or more.

TILUDRONATE: Administer a single 400 mg/day oral dose, taken with 6 to 8 ounces of plain water only for a period of 3 months. Beverages other than plain water (including mineral water), food, and some medications are likely to reduce the absorption of tiludronate. Do not take within 2 hours of food. Take calcium or mineral supplements at least 2 hours before or after tiludronate. Take aluminum- magnesium-containing antacids at least 2 hours after taking tiludronate. Do not take within 2 hours of indomethacin.

*Retreatment* – Following therapy, allow an interval of 3 months to assess response.

*ZOLEDRONIC ACID:*
 HCM –
  *Dose:* The maximum recommended dose in hypercalcemia of malignancy (albumin-corrected serum calcium at least 12 mg/dL [3 mmol/L]) is 4 mg. The 4 mg dose must be given as a single dose IV infusion over not less than 15 minutes. Adequately rehydrate patients prior to administration of zoledronic acid.
  *Retreatment:* Retreatment with 4 mg zoledronic acid may be considered if serum calcium does not return to normal or remain normal after initial treatment. It is recommended that a minimum of 7 days elapse before retreatment, to allow for a full response to the initial dose.
  *Multiple myeloma and metastatic bone lesions from solid tumors* – The recommended dose of zoledronic acid in patients with multiple myeloma and metastatic bone lesions from solid tumors is 4 mg infused over 15 minutes every 3 or 4 weeks. Also give patients an oral calcium supplement of 500 mg and a multiple vitamin containing 400 units vitamin D daily.
  Measure serum creatinine before each zoledronic acid dose and withhold treatment for renal deterioration.
  In the clinical studies, zoledronic acid treatment was resumed only when the creatinine returned to within 10% of the baseline value.
  *Admixture incompatibilities* – Do not mix zoledronic acid with calcium-containing infusion solutions, such as Lactated Ringer's solution, and administer it as a single IV solution in a line separate from all other drugs.
  *Renal function deterioration* – Because of the risk of clinically significant deterioration in renal function, which may progress to renal failure, single doses of zoledronic acid should not exceed 4 mg and the duration of infusion should be no less than 15 minutes.

### Actions
*Pharmacology:* Bisphosphonates act primarily on bone. Their major pharmacologic action is the inhibition of normal and abnormal bone resorption. There is no evidence that the bisphosphonates are metabolized.

*Pharmacokinetics:*
 *Alendronate* – Mean steady-state volume of distribution (exclusive of bone) is 28 L or more. Protein binding in plasma is about 78%.
 *Etidronate* – The plasma half-life of etidronate is 1 to 6 hours. Within 24 hours, about half the absorbed dose is excreted in urine. The remainder is chemically adsorbed to bone and is slowly eliminated.
 *Pamidronate* – Pamidronate is exclusively eliminated by renal excretion. The mean half-life is approximately 28 hours.
 *Risedronate* – The mean steady-state volume of distribution is 6.3 L/kg; plasma protein binding is about 24%. Mean oral bioavailability is 0.63% and is decreased when administered with food.
 *Tiludronate* – Bioavailability is reduced by food. Tiludronic acid is approximately 90% bound to human serum protein. The mean plasma elimination half-life was approximately 150 hours.

### Contraindications
Hypersensitivity to bisphosphonates or any component of the products; hypocalcemia (**alendronate, risedronate**, see Precautions); abnormalities of the esophagus that delay esophageal emptying such as stricture or achalasia (**alendronate**); inability to stand or sit upright for at least 30 minutes (**alendronate, risedronate**); clinically overt osteomalacia (**etidronate**).

### Warnings
*GI irritation/disorders:* Bisphosphonates cause local irritation of the upper GI mucosa. Alert physicians to any signs or symptoms signaling a possible esophageal reaction and instruct patients to discontinue bisphosphonates and seek medical attention if they develop dysphagia, odynophagia, retrosternal pain, or new or worsening heartburn.

The risk of severe esophageal adverse experiences appears to be greater in patients who lie down after taking bisphosphonates or who fail to swallow it with a full glass (6 to 8 oz) of water, or who continue to take bisphosphonates after developing symptoms suggestive of esophageal irritation.

Use caution when bisphosphonates are given to patients with active upper GI problems (such as dysphagia, esophageal diseases, gastritis, duodenitis, or ulcers). **Etidronate** therapy has been withheld from patients with enterocolitis because diarrhea is seen in some patients, particularly at higher doses.

*Osteoporosis (alendronate):* Consider causes other than estrogen deficiency and aging; consider glucocorticoid use.

*Paget disease (etidronate):* Response may be slow and may continue for months after treatment discontinuation. Do not increase dosage prematurely or initiate retreatment until after at least a 90-day drug-free interval.

*Asthma (zoledronic acid):* While not observed in clinical trials with zoledronic acid, administration of other bisphosphonates has been associated with bronchoconstriction in aspirin-sensitive asthmatic patients. Use zoledronic acid with caution in patients with aspirin-sensitive asthma.

*Renal function impairment:*
  *Alendronate* – No dosage adjustment is necessary in mild to moderate renal insufficiency (Ccr 35 to 60 mL/min). Alendronate use is not recommended in more severe renal insufficiency (Ccr less than 35 mL/min).

  *Pamidronate* – Bisphosphonates, including pamidronate, have been associated with renal toxicity manifested as deterioration of renal function and potential renal failure.

  In patients receiving pamidronate for bone metastases who show evidence of deterioration in renal function, withhold treatment until renal function returns to baseline. In a clinical study, renal deterioration was defined as follows: for patients with normal baseline creatinine, an increase of 0.5 mg/dL; for patients with abnormal baseline creatinine, an increase of 1 mg/dL. In this clinical study, pamidronate treatment was resumed only when the creatinine returned to within 10% of the baseline value. In other indications, clinical judgment should determine whether the potential benefit outweighs the potential risk in such patients.

  *Risedronate* – Risedronate is not recommended for patients with severe renal impairment (Ccr less than 30 mL/min). No dosage adjustment is needed when Ccr is greater than 30 mL/min.

  *Tiludronate* – Tiludronate is not recommended for patients with severe renal failure (Ccr less than 30 mL/min).

  *Zoledronic acid* – Single doses of zoledronic acid should not exceed 4 mg and the duration of infusion should be no less than 15 minutes. Zoledronic acid treatment is not recommended in patients with bone metastases with severe renal impairment. Patients who receive zoledronic acid should have serum creatinine assessed prior to each treatment.

*Pregnancy:* Category D (zoledronic acid); Category C (alendronate, oral and IV etidronate, pamidronate, risedronate, and tiludronate).

*Lactation:* It is not known whether these drugs are excreted in breast milk. Because **zoledronic acid** binds to bone long-term, do not administer to a nursing woman.

*Children:* Safety and efficacy for use in children have not been established. Children have been treated with **etidronate** at doses recommended for adults, to prevent heterotopic ossifications or soft tissue calcifications.

**Precautions**
  *Monitoring:* Carefully monitor standard hypercalcemia-related metabolic parameters, such as serum levels of calcium, phosphate, magnesium, and potassium following **pamidronate** and **zoledronic acid** initiation. Also, closely monitor electrolytes, creatinine as well as CBC, differential and hematocrit/hemoglobin. Carefully monitor patients who have preexisting anemia, leukopenia or thrombocytopenia in the first 2 weeks following treatment.

*Hypercalcemia:* Carefully monitor standard hypercalcemia-related metabolic parameters, such as serum levels of calcium, phosphate, and magnesium, as well as serum creatinine. Do not use loop diuretics until the patient is adequately rehydrated; use with caution in combination with zoledronic acid in order to avoid hypocalcemia. Use **zoledronic acid** with caution with other nephrotoxic drugs.

*Concomitant use with estrogen/hormone replacement therapy (alendronate):* Two clinical studies have shown that the degree of suppression of bone turnover (as assessed by mineralizing surface) was significantly greater with the combination than with either component alone.

*Nutrition:* Patients should maintain adequate nutrition, particularly an adequate intake of calcium and vitamin D.

*Osteoid:* **Etidronate** suppresses bone turnover and may retard mineralization of osteoid laid down during the bone accretion process. In patients with fractures, especially of long bones, it may be advisable to delay or interrupt treatment until callus is evident.

*Fracture:* In Paget patients, treatment regimens of **etidronate** exceeding the recommended daily maximum dose of 20 mg/kg or continuous administration for periods greater than 6 months may be associated with an increased risk of fracture.

*Hypocalcemia:* Hypocalcemia has occurred with **pamidronate** therapy. Rare cases of symptomatic hypocalcemia (including tetany) occurred during pamidronate treatment. If hypocalcemia occurs, consider short-term calcium therapy.

Hypocalcemia must be corrected before therapy initiation with **alendronate** and **risedronate**. Also effectively treat other disturbances of mineral metabolism (eg, vitamin D deficiency).

### Drug Interactions

Drugs that may interact with **alendronate** include ranitidine and aspirin. Drugs that may interact with **tiludronate** include aspirin and indomethacin. Calcium supplements and antacids may interact with **alendronate**, **etidronate**, **risedronate**, or **tiludronate**. Warfarin may interact with etidronate. Drugs that may interact with **zoledronic acid** include aminoglycosides and loop diuretics.

*Drug/Food interactions:* Bioavailability of **alendronate** was decreased when given 0.5 or 1 hour before breakfast vs 2 hours before, and bioavailability was negligible when alendronate was given with or 2 hours after breakfast. Concomitant coffee or orange juice reduced bioavailability by 60%. Take alendronate in the morning at least 30 minutes before the first meal, beverage, or medication.

Absorption of **etidronate** may be reduced by foods. Take on an empty stomach 2 hours before a meal.

Bioavailability of **tiludronate** was reduced when administered with, or 2 hours after, breakfast compared with administration after an overnight fast and 4 hours before a standard breakfast.

Mean oral bioavailability of **risedronate** is decreased when given with food. Take at least 30 minutes before the first food or drink of the day other than water.

### Adverse Reactions

Adverse reactions occurring in at least 3% of patients include the following:

*Alendronate:* Abdominal pain, diarrhea, constipation, dyspepsia, nausea, bone/skeletal pain.

*Etidronate:* Convulsions, constipation, nausea, stomatitis, abnormal hepatic function, hypomagnesemia, hypophosphatemia, dyspnea, taste perversion, fever, fluid overload.

*Pamidronate:*

    *In patients receiving 90 mg for osteolytic bone metastases and osteolytic lesions:* Anxiety, headache, insomnia, abdominal pain, anorexia, constipation, diarrhea, dyspepsia, nausea, vomiting, anemia, granulocytopenia, thrombocytopenia, hypocalcemia, hypokalemia, hypomagnesemia, hypophosphatemia, serum creatinine, arthralgia, bone/skeletal pain, myalgia, coughing, dyspnea, pleural effusion, sinusitis, URI, asthenia, fatigue, fever, metastases, pain, urinary tract infection.

*In patients receiving 90 mg over 24 hours (HCM):* Atrial fibrillation, hypertension, syncope, tachycardia, somnolence, anorexia, constipation, GI hemorrhage, nausea, anemia, hypocalcemia, hypokalemia, hypomagnesemia, hypophosphatemia, rales/rhinitis, fatigue, fever, infusion site reaction, moniliasis, hypothyroidism.

*In patients receiving 60 mg over 4 hours (HCM):* Psychosis, anorexia, constipation, dyspepsia, nausea, vomiting, leukopenia, hypokalemia, hypomagnesemia, fever, uremia.

*In patients receiving 60 mg over 24 hours (HCM):* Hypokalemia, hypomagnesemia, hypophosphatemia, URI, fever, infusion site reaction.

*Risedronate (including all treatment regimens):* Chest pain, hypertension, anxiety, depression, dizziness, headache, insomnia, neuralgia, vertigo, pruritus, rash, abdominal pain, belching, colitis, constipation, diarrhea, dyspepsia, flatulence, gastroenteritis, ecchymosis, nausea, arthralgia, arthritis, back pain, bone disorder/fracture, bone/skeletal pain, bursitis, joint disorder, leg/muscle cramps, myalgia, myasthenia, tendon disorder, bronchitis, coughing, dyspnea, pharyngitis, pneumonia, rales/rhinitis, sinusitis, amblyopia, cataract, conjunctivitis, dry eye, tinnitus, accidental injury, asthenia, edema/peripheral edema, influenza-like symptoms, pain, cystitis, infection, neck pain, neoplasm, overdose, urinary tract infection.

*Tiludronate:* Dizziness, headache, paresthesia, diarrhea, dyspepsia, nausea, vomiting, back pain, rales/rhinitis, sinusitis, URI, accidental injury, influenza-like symptoms, pain.

*Zoledronic acid:* Hypotension, agitation, anxiety, confusion, depression, dizziness, headache, hypesthesia, insomnia, paresthesia, alopecia, dermatitis, abdominal pain, anorexia, decreased appetite, constipation, diarrhea, nausea, vomiting, decreased weight, anemia, neutropenia, hypokalemia, hypomagnesemia, hypophosphatemia, arthralgia, back pain, bone/skeletal pain, myalgia, coughing, dyspnea, URI, asthenia, edema/peripheral edema, fatigue, fever, moniliasis, cancer progression, dehydration, neoplasm, rigors, urinary tract infection.

# ANTIDOTES

| Various Detoxification Agents and Their Uses | |
|---|---|
| Drug (trade name) | Toxic/Overdosed substance |
| Dimercaprol (*BAL In Oil*) | Arsenic, gold, mercury, lead |
| Deferoxamine mesylate (*Desferal*) | Iron |
| Dexrazoxane (*Zinecard*) | Doxorubicin-induced cardiomyopathy |
| Digoxin immune fab (*Digibind, Digifab*) | Digoxin, digitoxin |
| Edetate calcium disodium (*Calcium Disodium Versenate*) | Lead |
| Flumazenil (*Romazicon*) | Benzodiazepines |
| Fomepizole (*Antizol*) | Ethylene glycol, methanol |
| Mesna (*Mesnex*) | Ifosfamide-induced hemorrhagic cystitis |
| Methylene blue (Various) | Nitrites |
| *Narcotic antagonists*<br>  Naloxone (*Narcan*)<br>  Nalmefene (*Revex*)<br>  Naltrexone (*ReVia*) | Opioids |
| Physostigmine salicylate (*Antilirium*) | Anticholinergics (including tricyclic antidepressants) |
| Pralidoxime Cl (*Protopam Cl*) | Organophosphates<br>Anticholinesterases |
| Sodium thiosulfate (Various) | Cyanide |
| Sodium nitrite (Various) | Cyanide<br>Hydrogen sulfide |
| Succimer (*Chemet*) | Lead |
| Trientene (*Syprine*) | Copper |
| *Other agents used additionally as antidotes:* | |
| Acetylcysteine (*Mucomyst, Mucosil*) | Acetaminophen |
| Amyl nitrite, Na Nitrite, Na Thiosulfate (*Cyanide antidote kit*) | Cyanide |
| *Anticholinesterases*<br>  Pyridostigmine Br (*Mestinon, Regonol*)<br>  Neostigmine Br (*Prostigmin*)<br>  Edrophonium Cl (*Tensilon*) | Nondepolarizing muscle relaxants |
| Atropine (Various) | Cholinergic agents: Organophosphates, carbamates, pilocarpine, physostigmine, or choline esters. |
| Glucagon | Insulin-induced hypoglycemia, beta-blockers |
| Hydroxocobalamin (Various) | Cyanide poisoning |
| Leucovorin calcium (*Wellcovorin*) | Folic acid antagonists (eg, methotrexate) |
| Protamine sulfate (Various) | Heparin |
| Pyridoxine | Isoniazid |
| Vitamin $K_1$ (Various) | Oral anticoagulants |

| Various Detoxification Agents and Their Uses | |
|---|---|
| Drug (trade name) | Toxic/Overdosed substance |
| Nonspecific therapy of overdoses include the following: | |
| Activated charcoal (Various) | Nonspecific, supportive therapies of overdoses. See also General Management of Acute Overdosage. |
| Cathartics | |
| Osmotic diuretics | |
| Polyethylene glycol electrolyte solution (GoLYTELY) | |
| Syrup of ipecac (Various) | |
| Urinary acidifiers | |
| Urinary alkalinizers | |

# TRIENTINE HCl

**Capsules**: 250 mg (Rx)                                  *Syprine* (Merck)

### Indications
*Wilson disease:* Treatment of patients with Wilson disease who are intolerant of penicillamine.

### Administration and Dosage
Take on an empty stomach at least 1 hour before or 2 hours after meals and at least 1 hour apart from any other drug, food, or milk. Swallow the capsules whole and do not open or chew.

*Adults:* Initially, 750 to 1250 mg/day in divided doses 2, 3, or 4 times/day. May increase to a maximum of 2000 mg/day.

*Children 12 years of age and under:* Initially, 500 to 750 mg/day in divided doses 2, 3, or 4 times/day. May increase to a maximum of 1500 mg/day.

Increase the daily dose only when the clinical response is not adequate or the concentration of free serum copper is persistently above 20 mcg/dL. Determine optimal long-term maintenance dosage at 6- to 12-month intervals.

### Actions
*Pharmacology:* Wilson disease (hepatolenticular degeneration) is an inherited metabolic defect resulting in excess copper accumulation, possibly because the liver lacks the mechanism to excrete free copper into the bile. Hepatocytes store excess copper, but when their capacity is exceeded, copper is released into the blood and is taken up into extrahepatic sites. Treat this condition with a low copper diet and chelating agents that bind copper to facilitate its excretion from the body. Trientine is a chelating compound for removal of excess copper from the body.

### Warnings
*Not indicated for the following:* Not indicated for cystinuria; rheumatoid arthritis; biliary cirrhosis.

*Patient supervision:* Patients should remain under regular medical supervision throughout the period of drug administration.

*Iron deficiency anemia:* Closely monitor patients (especially women) for evidence of iron deficiency anemia.

*Elderly:* In general, dose selection should be cautious, usually starting at the low end of the dosing range, reflecting the greater frequency of decreased hepatic, renal, or cardiac function, and of concomitant disease or other drug therapy.

*Pregnancy:* Category C.

*Lactation:* It is not known whether this drug is excreted in breast milk. Exercise caution when administering to a nursing woman.

*Children:* Safety and efficacy for use in children have not been established. Trientine has been used clinically in children as young as 6 years of age with no reported adverse effects.

## Precautions

*Monitoring:* The most reliable index for monitoring treatment is the determination of free copper in the serum, which equals the difference between quantitatively determined total copper and ceruloplasmin-copper. Adequately treated patients will usually have less than 10 mcg free copper/dL of serum.

Therapy may be monitored with a 24-hour urinary copper analysis periodically (ie, every 6 to 12 months). Urine must be collected in copper-free glassware. Because a low copper diet should keep copper absorption down to less than 1 mg/day, the patient probably will be in the desired state of negative copper balance if 0.5 to 1 mg of copper is present in a 24-hour collection of urine.

*Hypersensitivity:* There are no reports of hypersensitivity in patients given trientine for Wilson disease. However, there have been reports of asthma, bronchitis, and dermatitis occurring after prolonged environmental exposure in workers who use trientine as a hardener of epoxy resins. Observe patients closely for signs of possible hypersensitivity.

## Drug Interactions

*Mineral supplements:* In general, do not give mineral supplements; they may block the absorption of trientine. However, iron deficiency may develop, especially in children and menstruating or pregnant women, or as a result of the low copper diet recommended for Wilson disease. If necessary, iron may be given in short courses, but because iron and trientine each inhibit absorption of the other, allow 2 hours to elapse between administration of trientine and iron.

# SUCCIMER (DMSA)

**Capsules:** 100 mg (*Rx*)                                    *Chemet* (Sanofi-Synthelabo)

## Indications

*Lead poisoning:* Treatment of lead poisoning in children with blood lead levels above 45 mcg/dL. Not indicated for prophylaxis of lead poisoning in a lead-containing environment; always accompany succimer use with identification and removal of the source of lead exposure.

## Administration and Dosage

Start dosage at 10 mg/kg or 350 mg/m$^2$ every 8 hours for 5 days; initiation of therapy at higher doses is not recommended (see table). Reduce frequency of administration to 10 mg/kg or 350 mg/m$^2$ every 12 hours (two-thirds of initial daily dosage) for an additional 2 weeks of therapy. A course of treatment lasts 19 days. Repeated courses may be necessary if indicated by weekly monitoring of blood lead concentration. A minimum of 2 weeks between courses is recommended unless blood lead levels indicate the need for more prompt treatment.

| Succimer Pediatric Dosing Chart | | | |
|---|---|---|---|
| Weight | | Dose (mg)[1] | Number of capsules[1] |
| lbs | kg | | |
| 18-35 | 8-15 | 100 | 1 |
| 36-55 | 16-23 | 200 | 2 |
| 56-75 | 24-34 | 300 | 3 |
| 76-100 | 35-44 | 400 | 4 |
| > 100 | > 45 | 500 | 5 |

[1] To be administered every 8 hours for 5 days,
followed by dosing every 12 hours for 14 days.

In young children who cannot swallow capsules, succimer can be administered by separating the capsule and sprinkling the medicated beads on a small amount of soft food or putting them in a spoon and following with a fruit drink.

Identification of the lead source in the child's environment and its abatement are critical to successful therapy. Chelation therapy is not a substitute for preventing further exposure to lead and should not be used to permit continued exposure to lead.

Patients who have received calcium EDTA with or without dimercaprol may use succimer for subsequent treatment after an interval of 4 weeks. Data on the concomitant use of succimer with calcium EDTA with or without dimercaprol are not
available, and such use is not recommended.

Adequately hydrate all patients undergoing treatment.

### Actions

*Pharmacology:* Succimer is an orally active, heavy metal chelating agent; it forms water
soluble chelates and, consequently, increases the urinary excretion of lead.

*Pharmacokinetics:* In a study in healthy adult volunteers, after a single dose of 16, 32,
or 48 mg/kg, absorption was rapid but variable, with peak blood levels between
1 and 2 hours. Approximately 49% of the dose was excreted: 39% in the feces, 9%
in the urine, and 1% as carbon dioxide from the lungs. Because fecal excretion
probably represented nonabsorbed drug, most of the absorbed drug was excreted by
the kidneys. The apparent elimination half-life was about 2 days.

### Contraindications

History of allergy to the drug.

### Warnings

*Lead exposure:* Not a substitute for effective abatement of lead exposure.

*Neutropenia:* Mild to moderate neutropenia has been observed in some patients receiving succimer. While a causal relationship to succimer has not been definitely established, neutropenia has been reported with other drugs in the same chemical class.
Obtain a complete blood count with white blood cell differential and direct
platelet counts prior to and weekly during treatment. Withhold or discontinue
therapy if the absolute neutrophil count (ANC) is below 1200/mcL and follow the
patient closely to document recovery of the ANC to above 1500/mcL or to the
patient's baseline neutrophil count. There is limited experience with reexposure in
patients who have developed neutropenia. Therefore, rechallenge such patients
only if the benefit of succimer therapy clearly outweighs the potential risk of another
episode of neutropenia and then only with careful patient monitoring.

*Infection* – Instruct patients treated with succimer to report promptly any signs of
infection. If infection is suspected, immediately conduct the above laboratory tests.

*Pregnancy: Category C.*

*Lactation:* It is not known whether this drug is excreted in breast milk. Discourage mothers requiring therapy from nursing their infants.

*Children:* Safety and efficacy in children under 12 months of age have not been established.

### Precautions

*Rebound blood lead levels:* After therapy, monitor patients for rebound of blood lead levels
by measuring the levels at least once weekly until stable.

*Renal function:* Adequately hydrate all patients undergoing treatment. Exercise caution
in using succimer therapy in patients with compromised renal function. Limited
data suggest that succimer is dialyzable but that the lead chelates are not.

*Hepatic function:* Transient mild elevations of serum transaminases have been observed
in 6% to 10% of patients during the course of therapy. Monitor serum transaminases before the start of therapy and at least weekly during therapy. Closely monitor patients with a history of liver disease. No data are available regarding the
metabolism of succimer in patients with liver disease.

*Repeated courses:* Clinical experience is limited. The safety of uninterrupted dosing
longer than 3 weeks has not been established and is not recommended.

*Allergic reactions:* The possibility of allergic or other mucocutaneous reactions must be
borne in mind upon readministration (and during initial courses). Monitor patients
requiring repeated courses during each treatment course.

### Drug Interactions

*Chelation therapy (eg, EDTA):* Coadministration of succimer with other chelation therapy
is not recommended.

*Drug/Lab test interactions:* Succimer may interfere with serum and urinary laboratory tests.

## Adverse Reactions

The most common events were GI symptoms or increases in serum transaminases (10%) and rashes (4%). Mild to moderate neutropenia has occurred in some patients receiving succimer. The following table presents adverse events reported with the administration of succimer for the treatment of lead and other heavy metal intoxication.

| Succimer Adverse Reactions (%)[1] | | |
|---|---|---|
| Body system/adverse reaction | Children (n = 191) | Adults (n = 134) |
| *GI:* Nausea; vomiting; diarrhea; appetite loss; hemorrhoidal symptoms; loose stools; metallic taste in mouth | 12 | 20.9 |
| *Body as a whole:* Back, stomach, head, rib, flank pain; abdominal cramps; chills; fever; flu-like symptoms; heavy head/tired; head cold; headache; moniliasis | 5.2 | 15.7 |
| *Metabolic:* Elevated AST, ALT, alkaline phosphatase, serum cholesterol | 4.2 | 10.4 |
| *CNS:* Drowsiness; dizziness; sensorimotor neuropathy; sleepiness; paresthesia | 1 | 12.7 |
| *Dermatologic:* Papular rash; herpetic rash; rash; mucocutaneous eruptions; pruritus | 2.6 | 11.2 |
| *Special senses:* Cloudy film in eye; ears plugged; otitis media; watery eyes | 1 | 3.7 |
| *Respiratory:* Sore throat; rhinorrhea; nasal congestion; cough | 3.7 | 0.7 |
| *GU:* Decreased urination; voiding difficulty; proteinuria increased | 0 | 3.7 |
| *Other:* Arrhythmia | 0 | 1.8 |
| Mild to moderate neutropenia; increased platelet count; intermittent eosinophilia | 0.5 | 1.5 |
| Kneecap pain; leg pains | 0 | 3 |

[1] Incidence regardless of attribution or dosage.

# NALMEFENE HCl

**Injection:** 1 mg/mL [1] (as base), 100 mcg/mL[2] (as base) *(Rx)*   *Revex (Ohmeda)*

[1] The 1 mg/mL concentration is for management of overdose.
[2] The 100 mcg/mL concentration is for postoperative use.

## Indications

*Reversal of opioid effects:* Complete or partial reversal of opioid drug effects, including respiratory depression, induced by either natural or synthetic opioids.

*Opioid overdose:* Management of known or suspected opioid overdose.

## Administration and Dosage

*Administration:* Titrate nalmefene to reverse the undesired effects of opioids. Once adequate reversal has been established, additional administration is not required and actually may be harmful due to unwanted reversal of analgesia or precipitated withdrawal.

*Duration of action:* The duration of action of nalmefene is as long as most opioid analgesics. However, the apparent duration of action will vary depending on the half-life and plasma concentration of the narcotic being reversed, the presence or absence of other drugs affecting the brain or muscles of respiration and the dose of nalmefene administered. Partially reversing doses of nalmefene (1 mcg/kg) lose their effect as the drug is redistributed through the body, and the effects of these low doses may not last more than 30 to 60 minutes in the presence of persistent opioid effects. Fully reversing doses (1 mg/70 kg) last many hours, but may complicate the management of patients who are in pain, at high cardiovascular risk or who are physically dependent on opioids.

The recommended doses represent a compromise between a desirable controlled reversal and the need for prompt response and adequate duration of action. Using higher dosages or shorter intervals between incremental doses may increase the incidence and severity of symptoms related to acute withdrawal such as nausea, vomiting, elevated blood pressure, and anxiety.

*Patients tolerant to or physically dependent on opioids:* Nalmefene may cause acute withdrawal symptoms in individuals who have some degree of tolerance to and dependence on opioids. Closely observe these patients for symptoms of withdrawal. Administer subsequent doses with intervals of at least 2 to 5 minutes between doses to allow the full effect of each incremental dose of nalmefene to be reached.

*Reversal of postoperative opioid depression:* Use 100 mcg/mL dosage strength (blue label); refer to the following table for initial doses. The goal of treatment with nalmefene in the post-operative setting is to achieve reversal of excessive opioid effects without inducing a complete reversal and acute pain. This is best accomplished with an initial dose of 0.25 mcg/kg followed by 0.25 mcg/kg incremental doses at 2- to 5-minute intervals, stopping as soon as the desired degree of opioid reversal is obtained. A cumulative total dose more than 1 mcg/kg does not provide additional therapeutic effect.

| Nalmefene Dosage for Reversal of Postoperative Opioid Depression | |
|---|---|
| Body weight (kg) | Amount of nalmefene 100 mcg/mL solution (mL) |
| 50 | 0.125 |
| 60 | 0.15 |
| 70 | 0.175 |
| 80 | 0.2 |
| 90 | 0.225 |
| 100 | 0.25 |

*Cardiovascular risk patients:* In cases where the patient is known to be at increased cardiovascular risk, it may be desirable to dilute nalmefene 1:1 with saline or sterile water and use smaller initial and incremental doses of 0.1 mcg/kg.

*Management of known/suspected opioid overdose:* Use 1 mg/mL dosage strength (green label). The recommended initial dose of nalmefene for nonopioid dependent patients is 0.5 mg/70 kg. If needed, this may be followed by a second dose of 1 mg/70 kg, 2 to 5 minutes later. If a total dose of 1.5 mg/70 kg has been administered without clinical response, additional nalmefene is unlikely to have an effect.

If there is a reasonable suspicion of opioid dependency, initially administer a challenge dose of 0.1 mg/70 kg. If there is no evidence of withdrawal in 2 minutes, follow the recommended dosing.

*Repeated dosing:* Nalmefene is the longest acting of the currently available parenteral opioid antagonists. If recurrence of respiratory depression does occur, titrate the dose again to clinical effect using incremental doses to avoid overreversal.

*Hepatic and renal disease:* Hepatic disease and renal failure substantially reduce the clearance of nalmefene. For single episodes of opioid antagonism, adjustment of nalmefene dosage is not required. However, in patients with renal failure, slowly administer the incremental doses (over 60 seconds).

*Loss of IV access:* Should IV access be lost or not readily obtainable, a single dose of nalmefene should be effective within 5 to 15 minutes after 1 mg IM or subcutaneous doses.

### Actions

*Pharmacology:* Nalmefene, an opioid antagonist, is a 6-methylene analog of naltrexone. Nalmefene prevents or reverses the effects of opioids, including respiratory depression, sedation, and hypotension. Nalmefene has no opioid agonist activity; it does not produce respiratory depression, psychotomimetic effects or pupillary constriction, and no pharmacological activity was observed when it was administered in the absence of opioid agonists. Nalmefene can produce acute withdrawal symptoms in individuals who are opioid-dependent.

*Pharmacokinetics:*

*Absorption* – Nalmefene is completely bioavailable following IM or subcutaneous administration. Nalmefene will be administered primarily as an IV bolus; however, it can be given IM or subcutaneous if venous access cannot be established. While the time to maximum plasma concentration was 2.3 hours following IM and 1.5 hours following subcutaneous administrations, therapeutic plasma concentrations are likely to be reached within 5 to 15 minutes after a 1 mg dose in an emergency.

*Distribution* – Following a 1 mg parenteral dose, nalmefene was rapidly distributed. A 1 mg dose blocked more than 80% of brain opioid receptors within 5 minutes after administration. The apparent volumes of distribution centrally and at steady state are 3.9 and 8.6 L/kg, respectively. Over a concentration range of 0.1 to 2 mcg/mL, 45% is bound to plasma proteins.

*Metabolism* – Nalmefene is metabolized by the liver, primarily by glucuronide conjugation, and excreted in the urine; less than 5% is excreted in the urine unchanged, and 17% is excreted in the feces.

*Excretion* – After IV administration of 1 mg to healthy males, plasma concentrations declined biexponentially with a redistribution and a terminal elimination half-life of 41 ± 34 minutes and 10.8 ± 5.2 hours, respectively. The systemic clearance of nalmefene is 0.8 L/h/kg and the renal clearance is 0.08 L/h/kg.

## Contraindications

Hypersensitivity to the product.

## Warnings

*Emergency use:* Nalmefene is not the primary treatment for ventilatory failure. In most emergency settings, treatment with nalmefene should follow, not precede, the establishment of a patent airway, ventilatory assistance, administration of oxygen, and establishment of circulatory access.

*Respiratory depression:* Accidental overdose with long-acting opioids (eg, methadone, levomethadyl) may result in prolonged respiratory depression. While nalmefene has a longer duration of action than naloxone in fully reversing doses, be aware that a recurrence of respiratory depression is possible. Observe patients until there is no reasonable risk of recurrent respiratory depression.

*Renal function impairment:* There was a statistically significant 27% decrease in plasma clearance of nalmefene in the end-stage renal disease (ESRD) population during interdialysis (0.57 L/h/kg) and a 25% decreased plasma clearance in the ESRD population during intradialysis (0.59 L/h/kg) compared with controls (0.79 L/h/kg). The elimination half-life was prolonged in ESRD patients from 10.2 (controls) to 26.1 hours.

*Hepatic function impairment:* Subjects with hepatic disease had a 28.3% decrease in plasma clearance of nalmefene compared with controls (0.56 vs 0.78 L/h/kg, respectively). Elimination half-life increased from 10.2 to 11.9 hours in the hepatically impaired. No dosage adjustment is recommended because nalmefene will be administered as an acute course of therapy.

*Elderly:* Dose proportionality was observed in nalmefene AUC following 0.5 to 2 mg IV administration to elderly male subjects. There was an apparent age-related decrease in the central volume of distribution that resulted in a greater initial nalmefene concentration in the elderly group. While initial plasma concentrations were transiently higher in the elderly, it would not be anticipated that this population would require dosing adjustment.

*Pregnancy: Category B.*

*Lactation:* Exercise caution when nalmefene is administered to a nursing woman.

*Children:* Safety and efficacy have not been established. Only use nalmefene in the resuscitation of the newborn when the expected benefits outweigh the risks.

## Precautions

*Cardiovascular risks:* Although nalmefene has been used safely in patients with preexisting cardiac disease, use all drugs of this class with caution in patients at high cardiovascular risk or who have received potentially cardiotoxic drugs.

*Risk of precipitated withdrawal:* Nalmefene is known to produce acute withdrawal symptoms and, therefore, should be used with extreme caution in patients with known physical dependence on opioids or following surgery involving high uses of opioids.

*Incomplete reversal of buprenorphine:* In animals, nalmefene doses up to 10 mg/kg (437 times the maximum recommended human dose) produced incomplete reversal of buprenorphine-induced analgesia. Hence, nalmefene may not completely reverse buprenorphine-induced respiratory depression.

**Drug Interactions**

*Flumazenil:* Flumazenil and nalmefene can induce seizures in animals. Remain aware of the potential risk of seizures from agents in these classes.

**Adverse Reactions**

Adverse reactions occurring in at least 3% of patients include nausea; vomiting; tachycardia; hypertension; postoperative pain; fever; dizziness.

# NALOXONE HCl

| Injection: 0.4 and 1 mg/mL (Rx) | Various, *Narcan* (DuPont Pharm) |
| --- | --- |

**Indications**

For the complete or partial reversal of narcotic depression, including respiratory depression, induced by opioids including natural and synthetic narcotics, propoxyphene, methadone, nalbuphine, butorphanol, and pentazocine. Also indicated for the diagnosis of suspected acute opioid overdosage.

**Administration and Dosage**

Give IV, IM, or subcutaneously. The most rapid onset of action is achieved with IV use, which is recommended in emergency situations.

*Adults:*

*Narcotic overdose (known or suspected)* – Initial dose is 0.4 to 2 mg IV; may repeat IV at 2- to 3-minute intervals. If no response is observed after 10 mg has been administered, question the diagnosis of narcotic-induced or partial narcotic-induced toxicity.

*Postoperative narcotic depression (partial reversal)* – Smaller doses are usually sufficient. Titrate dose according to the patient's response.

*Initial dose:* Inject in increments of 0.1 to 0.2 mg IV at 2- to 3-minute intervals to the desired degree of reversal.

*Repeat doses:* Repeat doses may be required within 1- or 2-hour intervals depending on the amount, type (ie, short- or long-acting) and time interval since last administration of narcotic. Supplemental IM doses have produced a longer lasting effect.

*Children:*

*Narcotic overdose (known or suspected)* – Initial dose is 0.01 mg/kg IV; give a subsequent dose of 0.1 mg/kg if needed. If an IV route is not available, may be given IM or subcutaneously in divided doses.

*Postoperative narcotic depression* – Follow the recommendations and cautions under adult administration guidelines. For initial reversal of respiratory depression, inject in increments of 0.005 to 0.01 mg IV at 2- to 3-minute intervals to desired degree of reversal.

*Neonates:*

*Narcotic-induced depression* – Initial dose is 0.01 mg/kg IV, IM, or subcutaneously; may be repeated in accordance with adult administration guidelines.

**Actions**

*Pharmacology:* The mechanism of action is not fully understood; evidence suggests that it antagonizes the opioid effects by competing for the same receptor sites.

*Pharmacokinetics:*

*Distribution* – After parenteral use, naloxone is rapidly distributed in the body. It is metabolized in the liver, primarily by glucuronide conjugation.

*Excretion* – Naloxone is excreted in the urine. The serum half-life in adults ranged from 30 to 81 minutes; in neonates, 3.1 ± 0.5 hours.

*Onset, peak, and duration* – Onset of action of IV naloxone is generally apparent within 2 minutes; it is only slightly less rapid when given subcutaneously or IM. Duration of action of 1 to 4 hours depends upon dose and route. IM use produces a more prolonged effect than IV use.

## Contraindications
Hypersensitivity to these agents.

## Warnings
*Drug dependence:* Administer cautiously to people who are known or suspected to be physically dependent on opioids, including newborns of mothers with narcotic dependence. Reversal of narcotic effect will precipitate acute abstinence syndrome.

*Repeat administration:* The patient who has satisfactorily responded should be kept under continued surveillance. Administer repeated doses as necessary, because the duration of action of some narcotics may exceed that of the narcotic antagonist.

*Respiratory depression:* Not effective against respiratory depression due to nonopioid drugs.

*Pregnancy:* Category B.

*Lactation:* It is not known whether the drug is excreted in breast milk.

## Precautions
*Other supportive therapy:* Maintain a free airway and provide artificial ventilation, cardiac massage, and vasopressor agents; employ when necessary to counteract acute narcotic overdosage.

*Cardiovascular effects:* Several instances of hypotension, hypertension, pulmonary edema, and ventricular tachycardia and fibrillation have been reported in postoperative patients.

## Adverse Reactions
Abrupt reversal of narcotic depression may result in nausea, vomiting, sweating, tachycardia, increased blood pressure, and tremulousness.

In postoperative patients, excessive dosage may result in excitement and significant reversal of analgesia, hypotension, hypertension, pulmonary edema, and ventricular tachycardia and fibrillation.

# NALTREXONE HCl

| Tablets: 50 mg (*Rx*) | Various, *ReVia* (Barr) |
| --- | --- |

---

**Warning:**

*Hepatotoxicity:* Naltrexone has the capacity to cause hepatocellular injury when given in excessive doses.

Naltrexone is contraindicated in acute hepatitis or liver failure. Carefully consider its use in patients with active liver disease in light of its hepatotoxic effects.

The margin of separation between the apparently safe dose of naltrexone and the dose causing hepatic injury appears to be only 5-fold or less. Naltrexone does not appear to be a hepatotoxin at the recommended doses.

Warn patients of the risk of hepatic injury and advise them to stop the use of naltrexone and seek medical attention if they experience symptoms of acute hepatitis.

---

## Indications
*Narcotic addiction:* Blockade of the effects of exogenously administered opioids.

*Alcoholism:* Treatment of alcohol dependence.

## Administration and Dosage
If there is any question of occult opioid dependence, perform a naloxone challenge test. Do not attempt treatment until naloxone challenge is negative.

*Alcoholism:* A dose of 50 mg once daily is recommended for most patients.

*Narcotic dependence:* Initiate treatment using the following guidelines:

1.) Do not attempt treatment until the patient has remained opioid-free for 7 to 10 days.

2.) Administer a naloxone challenge test (see below). If signs of opioid with-drawal are still observed following challenge, do not treat with naltrexone. The naloxone challenge can be repeated in 24 hours.

3.) Initiate treatment carefully, with an initial dose of 25 mg of naltrexone. If no withdrawal signs occur, start the patient on 50 mg/day thereafter.

*Maintenance treatment:* Once the patient has been started on naltrexone, 50 mg every 24 hours will produce adequate clinical blockade of the actions of parenterally administered opioids. A flexible dosing regimen may be employed. Thus, patients may receive 50 mg every weekday with a 100 mg dose on Saturday, 100 mg every other day, or 150 mg every third day.

## Actions

*Pharmacology:* Naltrexone is a pure opioid antagonist. It markedly attenuates or com-pletely blocks, reversibly, the subjective effects of IV administered opioids.

*Pharmacokinetics:*

*Absorption* – Although well absorbed orally, naltrexone is subject to significant first-pass metabolism with oral bioavailability estimates ranging from 5% to 40%. Fol-lowing oral administration, naltrexone undergoes rapid and nearly complete absorption with approximately 96% of the dose absorbed from the GI tract. Peak plasma levels of naltrexone and 6-β-naltrexol occur within 1 hour of dosing.

*Distribution* – The volume of distribution for naltrexone after IV administration is estimated to be 1350 L. In vitro, naltrexone is 21% bound to plasma proteins.

*Metabolism/Excretion* – The major metabolite of naltrexone is 6-β-naltrexol. The activity of naltrexone is believed to be due to both parent and the 6-β-naltrexol metabolite. The mean elimination half-life values for naltrexone and 6-β-naltrexol are 4 and 13 hours, respectively.

Renal elimination is primarily by glomerular filtration. Parent drug and metabolites are excreted primarily by the kidney; however, urinary excretion of unchanged naltrexone accounts for less than 2% of an oral dose and fecal excretion is a minor elimination path-way. The urinary excretion of unchanged and conjugated 6-β-naltrexone accounts for 43% of an oral dose. Naltrexone and its metabolites may undergo enterohepatic recycling.

## Contraindications

Patients receiving opioid analgesics; opioid-dependent patients; patients in acute opi-oid withdrawal; failed naloxone challenge; positive urine screen for opioids; his-tory of sensitivity to naltrexone; acute hepatitis or liver failure.

## Warnings

*Hepatotoxicity:* Naltrexone has the capacity to cause direct hepatocellular injury when given in excessive doses. It is contraindicated in acute hepatitis or liver failure, and its use in patients with active liver disease must be carefully considered in light of its hepatotoxic effects.

Warn patients of the risk of hepatic injury and advise them to stop naltrexone and seek medical attention if they experience symptoms of acute hepatitis.

Although no cases of hepatic failure have ever been reported, consider this as a possible risk of treatment.

*Abstinence precipitation/syndrome:* Unintended precipitation of abstinence or exacerbation of a preexisting subclinical abstinence syndrome may occur; therefore, patients should remain opioid-free for a minimum of 7 to 10 days before starting naltrexone.

*Severe opioid withdrawal syndromes:* Severe opioid withdrawal syndromes precipitated by acciden-tal naltrexone ingestion have occurred in opioid-dependent individuals. Withdrawal symp-toms usually appear within 5 minutes or less of ingestion and may last up to 48 hours.

*Surmountable blockade:* While naltrexone is a potent antagonist with a prolonged pharmaco-logic effect (24 to 72 hours), the blockade produced by naltrexone is surmountable. This poses a potential risk to individuals who attempt to overcome the blockade by self-administering large amounts of opioids. Any attempt by a patient to overcome the antagonism by taking opioids is very dangerous and may lead to fatal overdose.

*Use with narcotics:* Patients taking naltrexone may not benefit from opioid-containing medicines. Use a nonopioid-containing alternative, if available.

*Pregnancy:* Category C.

*Lactation:* It is not known if naltrexone is excreted in breast milk.

*Children:* Safety for use in children younger than 18 years of age has not been established.

### Precautions

*Monitoring:* A high index of suspicion for drug-related hepatic injury is critical if the occurrence of liver damage induced by naltrexone is to be detected at the earliest possible time.

*Suicide:* The risk of suicide is increased in patients with substance abuse with or without concomitant depression. This risk is not abated by treatment with naltrexone.

### Drug Interactions

Drugs that may be affected by naltrexone include opioid-containing products and thioridazine.

### Adverse Reactions

Adverse reactions associated with treatment of alcoholism include nausea, headache, dizziness, nervousness, fatigue, insomnia, and vomiting.

Reactions associated with treatment of narcotic addiction include difficulty sleeping, anxiety, nervousness, headache, low energy, irritability, increased energy, dizziness, abdominal cramps/pain, nausea, vomiting, loss of appetite, diarrhea, constipation, joint/muscle pain, delayed ejaculation, decreased potency, skin rash, chills, and increased thirst.

# FLUMAZENIL

**Injection:** 0.1 mg/mL (*Rx*)                    *Romazicon* (Hoffman-La Roche)

### Indications

*Reversal of benzodiazepine sedation:* For the complete or partial reversal of the sedative effects of benzodiazepines in cases where general anesthesia has been induced or maintained with benzodiazepines, where sedation has been produced with benzodiazepines for diagnostic and therapeutic procedures, and for the management of benzodiazepine overdose.

### Administration and Dosage

For IV use only. To minimize the likelihood of pain at the injection site, administer flumazenil through a freely running IV infusion into a large vein.

*Individualization of dosage:* In high-risk patients, it is important to administer the smallest amount of flumazenil that is effective. The 1-minute wait between individual doses in the dose-titration recommended for general clinical populations may be too short for high-risk patients because it takes 6 to 10 minutes for any single dose of flumazenil to reach full effects. Slow the rate of administration of flumazenil administered to high-risk patients.

*Reversal of conscious sedation or in general anesthesia:* The recommended initial dose is 0.2 mg (2 mL) administered IV over 15 seconds. If the desired level of consciousness is not obtained after waiting an additional 45 seconds, a further dose of 0.2 mg (2 mL) can be injected and repeated at 60 second intervals where necessary (up to a maximum of 4 additional times) to a maximum total dose of 1 mg (10 mL). Individualize the dose based on the patient's response, with most patients responding to doses of 0.6 to 1 mg.

In the event of resedation, repeated doses may be administered at 20-minute intervals as needed. For repeat treatment, administer no more than 1 mg (given as 0.2 mg/min) at any one time, and give no more than 3 mg in any 1 hour.

*Suspected benzodiazepine overdose:* The recommended initial dose is 0.2 mg (2 mL) administered IV over 30 seconds. If the desired level of consciousness is not obtained after waiting 30 seconds, a further dose of 0.3 mg (3 mL) can be administered over another 30 seconds. Further doses of 0.5 mg (5 mL) can be administered over 30 seconds at 1-minute intervals up to a cumulative dose of 3 mg.

Most patients with benzodiazepine overdose will respond to a cumulative dose of 1 to 3 mg, and doses beyond 3 mg do not reliably produce additional effects.

If a patient has not responded 5 minutes after receiving a cumulative dose of 5 mg, the major cause of sedation is likely not to be due to benzodiazepines, and additional flumazenil is likely to have no effect.

In the event of resedation, repeated doses may be given at 20-minute intervals if needed. For repeat treatment, give no more than 1 mg (given as 0.5 mg/min) at any one time and give no more than 3 mg in any 1 hour.

## Actions

*Pharmacology:* Flumazenil antagonizes the actions of benzodiazepines on the CNS and competitively inhibits the activity at the benzodiazepine recognition site on the GABA/benzodiazepine receptor complex.

The duration and degree of reversal of benzodiazepine effects are related to the dose and plasma concentrations of flumazenil. The onset of reversal is usually evident within 1 to 2 minutes after the injection is completed. Within 3 minutes, 80% response will be reached, with the peak effect occurring at 6 to 10 minutes.

*Pharmacokinetics:* After IV administration, flumazenil has an initial distribution half-life of 7 to 15 minutes and a terminal half-life of 41 to 79 minutes. Peak concentrations of flumazenil are proportional to dose, with an apparent initial volume of distribution of 0.5 L/kg. After redistribution the apparent volume of distribution ranges from 0.77 to 1.6 L/kg. Protein binding is approximately 50%.

Flumazenil is a highly extracted drug. Clearance of flumazenil occurs primarily by hepatic metabolism and is dependent on hepatic blood flow. In healthy volunteers, total clearance ranges from 0.7 to 1.3 L/h/kg, with less than 1% of the administered dose eliminated unchanged in urine. Elimination of drug is essentially complete within 72 hours, with 90% to 95% appearing in urine and 5% to 10% in feces.

## Contraindications

Hypersensitivity to flumazenil or to benzodiazepines; benzodiazepine use for control of a potentially life-threatening condition; in patients who are showing signs of serious cyclic antidepressant overdose.

## Warnings

*Seizures:* The use of flumazenil has been associated with the occurrence of seizures. These are most frequent in patients who have been on benzodiazepines for long-term sedation or in overdose cases where patients are showing signs of serious cyclic antidepressant overdose. Individualize the dosage of flumazenil and be prepared to manage seizures.

*Seizure risk:* The reversal of benzodiazepine effects may be associated with the onset of seizures in certain high-risk populations.

Most convulsions associated with flumazenil administration require treatment and have been successfully managed with benzodiazepines, phenytoin, or barbiturates.

*Hypoventilation:* Monitor patients who have received flumazenil for the reversal of benzodiazepine effects (after conscious sedation or general anesthesia) for resedation, respiratory depression or other residual benzodiazepine effects for an appropriate period (120 minutes or less) based on the dose and duration of effect of the benzodiazepine employed, because flumazenil has not been established as an effective treatment for hypoventilation due to benzodiazepine administration.

Flumazenil may not fully reverse postoperative airway problems or ventilatory insufficiency induced by benzodiazepines. In addition, even if flumazenil is initially effective, such problems may recur because the effects of flumazenil wear off before the effects of many benzodiazepines.

*Hepatic function impairment:* Mean total clearance is decreased to 40% to 60% of normal in patients with moderate liver dysfunction and to 25% of normal in patients with severe liver dysfunction compared with age-matched healthy subjects. This results in a prolongation of the half-life from 0.8 hours in healthy subjects to 1.3 hours in patients with moderate hepatic impairment and 2.4 hours in severely impaired patients.

*Pregnancy: Category C.*

*Labor and delivery* – The use of flumazenil to reverse the effects of benzodiazepines used during labor and delivery is not recommended because the effects of the drug in the newborn are unknown.

*Lactation:* It is not known whether flumazenil is excreted in breast milk.

*Children:* Flumazenil is not recommended for use in children.

**Precautions**

*Monitoring:* Monitor patients for resedation, respiratory depression, or other persistent or recurrent agonist effects for an adequate period of time after administration of flumazenil.

*Return of sedation:* Resedation is least likely in cases where flumazenil is administered to reverse a low dose of a short-acting benzodiazepine. It is most likely in cases where a large single or cumulative dose of a benzodiazepine has been given in the course of a long procedure along with neuromuscular blocking agents and multiple anesthetic agents.

*Intensive Care Unit (ICU):* Use with caution in the ICU because of the increased risk of unrecognized benzodiazepine dependence in such settings.

*Overdose situations:* Flumazenil is intended as an adjunct to, not as a substitute for, proper management of airway, assisted breathing, circulatory access and support, internal decontamination by lavage and charcoal, and adequate clinical evaluation.

*Head injury:* Use with caution in patients with head injury as flumazenil may be capable of precipitating convulsions or altering cerebral blood flow in patients receiving benzodiazepines.

*Neuromuscular blocking agents:* Do not use flumazenil until the effects of neuromuscular blockade have been fully reversed.

*Psychiatric patients:* Flumazenil may provoke panic attacks in patients with a history of panic disorder.

*Drug and alcohol dependent patients:* Use with caution in patients with alcoholism and other drug dependencies due to the increased frequency of benzodiazepine tolerance and dependence observed in these patient populations.

*Tolerance to benzodiazepines:* Flumazenil may cause benzodiazepine withdrawal symptoms in individuals who have been taking benzodiazepines long enough to have some degree of tolerance. Slower titration rates of 0.1 mg/min and lower total doses may help reduce the frequency of emergent confusion and agitation.

*Physical dependence on benzodiazepines:* Flumazenil is known to precipitate withdrawal seizures in patients who are physically dependent on benzodiazepines, even if such dependence was established in a relatively few days of high-dose sedation in ICU environments. The risk of either seizures or resedation in such cases is high and patients have experienced seizures before regaining consciousness. Use flumazenil in such settings with extreme caution, because use of flumazenil in this situation has not been studied and no information as to dose and rate of titration is available.

*Pain on injection:* To minimize the likelihood of pain or inflammation at the injection site, administer flumazenil through a freely flowing IV infusion into a large vein. Local irritation may occur following extravasation into perivascular tissues.

*Respiratory disease:* Appropriate ventilatory support is the primary treatment of patients with serious lung disease who experience serious respiratory depression due to benzodiazepines rather than the administration of flumazenil.

*Ambulatory patients:* Effects may wear off before a long-acting benzodiazepine is completely cleared from the body.

*Mixed drug overdosage:* Particular caution is necessary when using flumazenil in cases of mixed drug overdosage; toxic effects of other drugs taken in overdose (especially cyclic antidepressants) may emerge with reversal of the benzodiazepine effect by flumazenil.

**Drug Interactions**

*Drug/Food interactions:* Ingestion of food during an IV infusion of flumazenil results in a 50% increase in flumazenil clearance, most likely due to the increased hepatic blood flow that accompanies a meal.

**Adverse Reactions**

Adverse reactions may include death, convulsions, headache, injection site pain, increased sweating, fatigue, cutaneous vasodilation, nausea, vomiting, dizziness, agitation, dry mouth, tremors, palpitations, insomnia, dyspnea, hyperventilation, emotional lability, abnormal/blurred vision, and paresthesia.

# Chapter 4

# CARDIOVASCULAR AGENTS

# CARDIAC GLYCOSIDES

## DIGOXIN

**Capsules:** 0.05, 0.1, and 0.2 mg (*Rx*)                     *Lanoxicaps* (GlaxoSmithKline)

**Tablets:** 0.125 and 0.25 mg (*Rx*)                     Various, *Lanoxin* (GlaxoSmithKline), *Digitek* (Vangard)

**Elixir, pediatric:** 0.05 mg/mL (*Rx*)                     Various, *Lanoxin* (GlaxoSmithKline)

**Injection:** 0.25 mg/mL (*Rx*)                     Various, *Lanoxin* (GlaxoSmithKline)

**Injection, pediatric:** 0.1 mg/mL (*Rx*)                     Various, *Lanoxin* (GlaxoSmithKline)

### Indications

*Congestive heart failure (CHF) all degrees:* Increased cardiac output results in diuresis and general amelioration of disturbances characteristic of right heart failure (venous congestion, edema) and left heart failure (dyspnea, orthopnea, cardiac asthma).

*Atrial flutter:* Digitalis slows the heart; normal sinus rhythm may appear. Often, flutter is converted to atrial fibrillation with a slow ventricular rate.

### Administration and Dosage

Recommended dosages of digoxin may require considerable modification because of individual sensitivity of the patient to the drug, the presence of associated conditions, or the use of concurrent medications. In selecting a dose of digoxin, the following factors must be considered:

1.) The body weight of the patient. Calculate doses based upon lean (ie, ideal) body weight.

2.) The patient's renal function, preferably evaluated on the basis of estimated creatinine clearance (Ccr).

3.) The patient's age. Infants and children require different doses of digoxin than adults.

4.) Concomitant disease states, concurrent medications, or other factors likely to alter the pharmacokinetic or pharmacodynamic profile of digoxin.

*Serum digoxin concentrations:* About 66% of adults considered adequately digitalized (without evidence of toxicity) have serum digoxin concentrations ranging from 0.8 to 2 ng/mL. Consequently, interpret the serum concentration of digoxin in the overall clinical context, and do not use an isolated measurement as the basis for increasing or decreasing the dose of the drug.

To allow adequate time for equilibration of digoxin between serum and tissue, perform sampling of serum concentrations just before the next scheduled dose of the drug. If this is not possible, perform sampling at least 6 to 8 hours after the last dose, regardless of the route of administration or the formulation used.

*Heart failure:*

*Adults* – Digitalization may be accomplished by either of 2 general approaches that vary in dosage and frequency of administration but reach the same endpoint in terms of total amount of digoxin accumulated in the body.

1.) If rapid digitalization is considered medically appropriate, it may be achieved by administering a loading dose based upon projected peak digoxin body stores. Calculate maintenance dose as a percentage of the loading dose.

2.) Obtain more gradual digitalization beginning an appropriate maintenance dose, thus allowing digoxin body stores to accumulate slowly. Steady-state serum digoxin concentration will be achieved in approximately 5 half-lives of the drug for the individual patient. Depending upon the patient's renal function, this will take between 1 and 3 weeks.

*Atrial fibrillation:* Peak digoxin body stores larger than the 8 to 12 mcg/kg required for most patients with heart failure and normal sinus rhythm have been used for control of ventricular rate in patients with atrial fibrillation. Titrate doses of digoxin used for the treatment of chronic atrial fibrillation to the minimum dose that achieves the desired ventricular rate control without causing undesirable side effects. Data are not available to establish the appropriate resting or exercise target rates that should be achieved.

*Renal function impairment:* In children with renal disease, digoxin must be carefully titrated based upon clinical response.

*Rapid digitalization with a loading dose:* Peak digoxin body stores of 8 to 12 mcg/kg should provide therapeutic effect with minimum risk of toxicity in most patients with heart failure and normal sinus rhythm. Because of altered digoxin distribution and elimination, projected peak body stores for patients with renal insufficiency should be conservative (ie, 6 to 10 mcg/kg; see Precautions).

Administer the loading dose in several portions, with roughly half the total given as the first dose. Additional fractions of this planned total dose may be given at 6- to 8-hour intervals, with careful assessment of clinical response before each additional dose.

If the patient's clinical response necessitates a change from the calculated loading dose of digoxin, then base calculation of the maintenance dose upon the amount actually given.

Digoxin injection is frequently used to achieve rapid digitalization, with conversion to digoxin tablets or capsules for maintenance therapy. If patients are switched from IV to oral digoxin formulations, make allowances for differences in bioavailability when calculating maintenance dosages (see Pharmacology).

*Tablets –* A single initial dose of 500 to 750 mcg (0.5 to 0.75 mg) of digoxin tablets usually produces a detectable effect in 0.5 to 2 hours that becomes maximal in 2 to 6 hours. Additional doses of 125 to 375 mcg (0.125 to 0.375 mg) may be given cautiously at 6- to 8-hour intervals until clinical evidence of an adequate effect is noted. The usual amount of digoxin tablets that a 70 kg patient requires to achieve 8 to 12 mcg/kg peak body stores is 750 to 1250 mcg (0.75 to 1.25 mg).

*Capsules –* A single initial dose of 400 to 600 mcg (0.4 to 0.6 mg) digoxin capsules usually produces a detectable effect in 0.5 to 2 hours that becomes maximal in 2 to 6 hours. Additional doses of 100 to 300 mcg (0.1 to 0.3 mg) may be given cautiously at 6- to 8-hour intervals until clinical evidence of an adequate effect is noted. The usual amount of the capsules that a 70 kg patient requires to achieve 8 to 12 mcg/kg peak body stores is 600 to 1000 mcg (0.6 to 1 mg).

*Injection –* A single initial IV dose of 400 to 600 mcg (0.4 to 0.6 mg) of injection usually produces a detectable effect in 5 to 30 minutes that becomes maximal in 1 to 4 hours. Additional doses of 100 to 300 mcg (0.1 to 0.3 mg) may be given cautiously at 6- to 8-hour intervals until clinical evidence of an adequate effect is noted. The usual amount of injection that a 70 kg patient requires to achieve 8 to 12 mcg/kg peak body stores is 600 to 1000 mcg (0.6 to 1 mg).

*Dosage adjustment when changing preparations:* The difference in bioavailability between digoxin injection or capsules and pediatric elixir or tablets must be considered when changing patients from 1 dosage form to another.

The absolute bioavailability of the capsule formulation is greater than that of the standard tablets and near that of the IV dosage form. As a result, the doses recommended for the capsules are the same as those for injection. Adjustments in dosage will seldom be necessary when converting a patient from the IV formulation to capsules.

Doses of 100 mcg (0.1 mg) and 200 mcg (0.2 mg) of digoxin capsules are approximately equivalent to 125 mcg (0.125 mg) and 250 mcg (0.25 mg) doses of tablets and pediatric elixir, respectively.

*Maintenance dosing:* The doses of digoxin used in controlled trials in patients with heart failure have ranged from 125 to 500 mcg (0.125 to 0.5 mg) once daily. In these studies, the digoxin dose has been generally titrated according to the patient's age, lean body weight, and renal function. Therapy is generally initiated at a dose of 250 mcg (0.25 mg) once daily in patients younger than 70 years of age with good renal function, at a dose of 125 mcg (0.125 mg) once daily in patients older than 70 years of age or with impaired renal function, and at a dose of 62.5 mcg (0.0625 mg) in patients with marked renal impairment. Doses may be increased every 2 weeks according to clinical response.

In a subset of approximately 1800 patients enrolled in a trial (wherein dosing was based on an algorithm similar to that in the table below) the mean ($\pm$ SD) serum digoxin concentrations at 1 month and 12 months were approximately 1.01 ng/mL and approximately 0.97 ng/mL, respectively.

Base the maintenance dose upon the percentage of the peak body stores lost each day through elimination. The following formula has had wide clinical use:

*Tablets:*

Maintenance dosing –

| Usual Digoxin Tablet Daily Maintenance Dose Requirements (mcg) for Estimated Peak Body Stores of 10 mcg/kg | | | | | | | Number of days before steady-state achieved[2] |
|---|---|---|---|---|---|---|---|
| Corrected Ccr (mL/min/70 kg)[1] | Lean Body Weight (kg/lbs) | | | | | | |
| | 50/110 | 60/132 | 70/154 | 80/176 | 90/198 | 100/220 | |
| 0 | 62.5 | 125 | 125 | 125 | 187.5 | 187.5 | 22 |
| 10 | 125 | 125 | 125 | 187.5 | 187.5 | 187.5 | 19 |
| 20 | 125 | 125 | 187.5 | 187.5 | 187.5 | 250 | 16 |
| 30 | 125 | 187.5 | 187.5 | 187.5 | 250 | 250 | 14 |
| 40 | 125 | 187.5 | 187.5 | 250 | 250 | 250 | 13 |
| 50 | 187.5 | 187.5 | 250 | 250 | 250 | 250 | 12 |
| 60 | 187.5 | 187.5 | 250 | 250 | 250 | 375 | 11 |
| 70 | 187.5 | 250 | 250 | 250 | 250 | 375 | 10 |
| 80 | 187.5 | 250 | 250 | 250 | 375 | 375 | 9 |
| 90 | 187.5 | 250 | 250 | 250 | 375 | 500 | 8 |
| 100 | 250 | 250 | 250 | 375 | 375 | 500 | 7 |

[1] Ccr is corrected to 70 kg body weight or 1.73 m$^2$ body surface area. For adults, if only serum creatinine concentrations (Scr) are available, a Ccr (corrected to 70 kg body weight) may be estimated in men as (140 − Age)/Scr. For women, multiply this result by 0.85. Note: This equation cannot be used for estimating Ccr in infants or children.
[2] If no loading dose is administered.

*Infants and children* – In general, divided daily dosing is recommended for infants and young children younger than 10 years of age. In the newborn period, renal clearance of digoxin is diminished and observe suitable dosage adjustments. This is especially pronounced in the premature infant. Beyond the immediate newborn period, children generally require proportionally larger doses than adults on the basis of body weight or body surface area. Children older than 10 years of age require adult dosages in proportion to their body weight. Some researchers have suggested that infants and young children tolerate slightly higher serum concentrations than do adults.

Daily maintenance doses for each age group are given in the table below and should provide therapeutic effects with minimum risk of toxicity in most patients with heart failure and normal sinus rhythm. These recommendations assume the presence of normal renal function:

| Daily Digoxin Maintenance Doses in Children with Normal Renal Function | |
|---|---|
| Age | Daily maintenance dose (mcg/kg) |
| 2 to 5 years | 10 to 15 |
| 5 to 10 years | 7 to 10 |
| > 10 years | 3 to 5 |

*Capsules:* Because of the more complete absorption of digoxin from soft capsules, recommended oral doses are only 80% of those for tablets and elixir. Because the significance of the higher peak serum concentrations associated with once daily capsules is not established, divided daily dosing is presently recommended for the following:

1.) Infants and children younger than 10 years of age.
2.) Patients requiring a daily dose of at least 300 mcg (0.3 mg).

3.) Patients with a history of digitalis toxicity.
4.) Patients considered likely to become toxic.
5.) Patients in whom compliance is not a problem.

| Usual Digoxin Solution-Filled Capsule Daily Maintenance Dose Requirements (mcg) for Estimated Peak Body Stores of 10 mcg/kg | | | | | | | |
|---|---|---|---|---|---|---|---|
| Corrected Ccr (mL/min/70 kg)[1] | Lean Body Weight (kg/lbs) | | | | | | Number of days before steady-state achieved[2] |
| | 50/110 | 60/132 | 70/154 | 80/176 | 90/198 | 100/220 | |
| 0 | 50 | 100 | 100 | 100 | 150 | 150 | 22 |
| 10 | 100 | 100 | 100 | 150 | 150 | 150 | 19 |
| 20 | 100 | 100 | 150 | 150 | 150 | 200 | 16 |
| 30 | 100 | 150 | 150 | 150 | 200 | 200 | 14 |
| 40 | 100 | 150 | 150 | 200 | 200 | 250 | 13 |
| 50 | 150 | 150 | 200 | 200 | 250 | 250 | 12 |
| 60 | 150 | 150 | 200 | 200 | 250 | 300 | 11 |
| 70 | 150 | 200 | 200 | 250 | 250 | 300 | 10 |
| 80 | 150 | 200 | 200 | 250 | 300 | 300 | 9 |
| 90 | 150 | 200 | 250 | 250 | 300 | 350 | 8 |
| 100 | 200 | 200 | 250 | 300 | 300 | 350 | 7 |

[1] Ccr is corrected to 70 kg body weight or 1.73 m$^2$ body surface area. For adults, if only serum creatinine concentrations (Scr) are available, a Ccr (corrected to 70 kg body weight) may be estimated in men as $(140 - \text{Age})/\text{Scr}$. For women, multiply this result by 0.85. Note: This equation cannot be used for estimating Ccr in infants or children.
[2] If no loading dose is administered.

*Infants and children* – Individualize dosage. Divided daily dosing is recommended for infants and young children younger than 10 years of age. In these patients, where dosage adjustment is frequent and outside the fixed dosages available, digoxin capsules may not be the formulation of choice. In the newborn period, renal clearance of digoxin is diminished; observe suitable dosage adjustment. This is especially pronounced in the premature infant. Beyond the immediate newborn period, children generally require proportionally larger doses than adults on the basis of body weight or body surface area. Children older than 10 years of age require adult dosages in proportion to body weight. Some researchers have suggested that infants and young children tolerate slightly higher serum concentrations than do adults.

*Maintenance dosage* – Daily maintenance doses for each age group are given below and should provide therapeutic effects with minimum risk of toxicity in most patients with heart failure and normal sinus rhythm. These recommendations assume the presence of normal renal function.

| Usual Digitalizing and Maintenance Dosages for Digoxin Capsules in Children with Normal Renal Function Based on Lean Body Weight | | |
|---|---|---|
| Age | Digitalizing[1] dose (mcg/kg) | Daily maintenance dose[2] (mcg/kg) |
| 2 to 5 years | 25 to 35 | 25% to 35% of the oral or IV digitalizing dose[3] |
| 5 to 10 years | 15 to 30 | |
| > 10 years | 8 to 12 | |

[1] IV digitalizing doses are the same as digitalizing doses of digoxin capsules.
[2] Divided daily dosing is recommended for children younger than 10 years of age.
[3] Projected or actual digitalizing dose providing desired clinical response.

*Pediatric elixir:*
   *Usual digitalizing and maintenance dosing –*

| Usual Digitalizing and Maintenance Dosages for Pediatric Elixir in Children with Normal Renal Function Based on Lean Body Weight | | |
| --- | --- | --- |
| Age | Oral digitalizing[1] dose (mcg/kg) | Daily maintenance dose[2] (mcg/kg) |
| Premature | 20 to 30 | 20% to 30% of oral digitalizing dose[3] |
| Full-term | 25 to 35 | 25% to 35% of oral digitalizing dose[3] |
| 1 to 24 months | 35 to 60 | |
| 2 to 5 years | 30 to 40 | |
| 5 to 10 years | 20 to 35 | |
| > 10 years | 10 to 15 | |

[1] IV digitalizing doses are 80% of oral digitalizing doses.
[2] Divided daily dosing is recommended for children younger than 10 years of age.
[3] Projected or actual digitalizing dose providing clinical response.

*Gradual digitalization with a maintenance dose –* More gradual digitalization also can be accomplished by beginning an appropriate maintenance dose. The range of percentages provided in the above table can be used in calculating this dose for patients with normal renal function.

*Injection:* Slow infusion of injection is preferable to bolus administration. Rapid infusion of digitalis glycosides has been shown to cause systemic and coronary arteriolar constriction, which may be clinically undesirable. Caution is thus advised and injection probably should be administered over a period of 5 minutes or more. Mixing injection with other drugs in the same container or simultaneous administration in the same intravenous line is not recommended.

Parenteral administration of digoxin should be used only when the need for rapid digitalization is urgent or when the drug cannot be taken orally. IM injection can lead to severe pain at the injection site, thus IV administration is preferred. If the drug must be administered by the IM route, inject it deep into the muscle followed by massage. Do not inject more than 500 mcg (2 mL) into a single site.

If tuberculin syringes are used to measure very small doses, one must be aware of the problem of inadvertent overadministration of digoxin. Do not flush the syringe with the parenteral solution after its contents are expelled into an indwelling vascular catheter.

*Admixture compatibility –* Digoxin injection can be administered undiluted or diluted with a 4-fold or greater volume of sterile water for injection, 0.9% sodium chloride injection, or 5% dextrose injection. The use of less than 4-fold volume of diluent could lead to precipitation of the digoxin. Immediate use of the diluted product is recommended.

   *Maintenance dose –*

| Usual Daily Maintenance Dose Requirements (mcg) of Digoxin Injection for Estimated Peak Body Stores of 10 mcg/kg[1] | | | | | | | |
| --- | --- | --- | --- | --- | --- | --- | --- |
| | Lean body weight (kg/lb) | | | | | | |
| Corrected Ccr (mL/min/70 kg)[2] | 50/110 | 60/132 | 70/154 | 80/176 | 90/198 | 100/220 | Number of days before steady-state achieved[3] |
| 0 | 75 | 75 | 100 | 100 | 125 | 150 | 22 |
| 10 | 75 | 100 | 100 | 125 | 150 | 150 | 19 |
| 20 | 100 | 100 | 125 | 150 | 150 | 175 | 16 |
| 30 | 10 | 125 | 150 | 150 | 175 | 200 | 14 |
| 40 | 100 | 125 | 150 | 175 | 200 | 225 | 13 |
| 50 | 125 | 150 | 175 | 200 | 225 | 250 | 12 |
| 60 | 125 | 150 | 175 | 200 | 225 | 250 | 11 |

| Usual Daily Maintenance Dose Requirements (mcg) of Digoxin Injection for Estimated Peak Body Stores of 10 mcg/kg[1] | | | | | | | |
|---|---|---|---|---|---|---|---|
| | Lean body weight (kg/lb) | | | | | | |
| Corrected Ccr (mL/min/70 kg)[2] | 50/110 | 60/132 | 70/154 | 80/176 | 90/198 | 100/220 | Number of days before steady-state achieved[3] |
| 70 | 150 | 175 | 200 | 225 | 250 | 275 | 10 |
| 80 | 150 | 175 | 200 | 250 | 275 | 300 | 9 |
| 90 | 150 | 200 | 225 | 250 | 300 | 325 | 8 |
| 100 | 175 | 200 | 250 | 275 | 300 | 350 | 7 |

[1] Daily maintenance doses have been rounded to the nearest 25 mcg increment.
[2] Ccr is corrected to 70 kg body weight or 1.73 m$^2$ body surface area. For adults, if only serum creatinine concentrations (Scr) are available, a Ccr (corrected to 70 kg body weight) may be estimated in men as (140 − Age)/Scr. For women, this result should be multiplied by 0.85. Note: This equation cannot be used for estimating Ccr in infants or children.
[3] If no loading dose is administered.

*Pediatric injection:*
   *Digitalizing and maintenance dosages* –

| Usual Digitalizing and Maintenance Dosages for Digoxin Pediatric Injection in Children with Normal Renal Function Based on Lean Body Weight | | |
|---|---|---|
| Age | IV digitalizing[1] dose (mcg/kg) | Daily IV maintenance dose[2] (mcg/kg) |
| Premature | 15 to 25 | 20% to 30% of the IV digitalizing dose[3] |
| Full-term | 20 to 30 | 25% to 35% of the IV digitalizing dose[3] |
| 1 to 24 months | 30 to 50 | |
| 2 to 5 years | 25 to 35 | |
| 5 to 10 years | 15 to 30 | |
| ≥ 10 years | 8 to 12 | |

[1] IV digitalizing doses are 80% of oral digitalizing doses.
[2] Divided daily dosing is recommended for children younger than 10 years of age.
[3] Projected or actual digitalizing dose providing clinical response.

   *Gradual digitalization with a maintenance dose* – More gradual digitalization also can be accomplished by beginning an appropriate maintenance dose. The range of percentages provided in the table above can be used in calculating this dose for patients with normal renal function.

## Actions

*Pharmacology:* Digoxin inhibits sodium-potassium ATPase, leading to an increase in the intracellular concentration of sodium and thus, (by stimulation of sodium-calcium exchange) an increase in the intracellular concentration of calcium. The pharmacologic consequences of these direct and indirect effects are the following: An increase in the force and velocity of myocardial systolic contraction (positive inotropic action); a decrease in the degree of activation of the sympathetic nervous system and renin-angiotensin system (neurohormonal deactivating effect); and slowing of the heart rate and decreased conduction velocity through the AV node (vagomimetic effect).

   *Hemodynamic effects* – Digoxin produces hemodynamic improvement in patients with heart failure. Short- and long-term therapy with the drug increases cardiac output and lowers pulmonary artery pressure, pulmonary capillary wedge pressure, and systemic vascular resistance.

*Pharmacokinetics:*
   *Absorption* – Following oral administration, peak serum concentrations of digoxin occur at 1 to 3 hours. Absorption of digoxin from the tablets has been demonstrated to be 60% to 80% complete compared with an identical IV dose of digoxin (absolute bioavailability) or capsules (relative bioavailability).

*Distribution* – Digoxin has a large apparent volume of distribution. Digoxin crosses the blood-brain barrier and the placenta. Approximately 25% of digoxin in the plasma is bound to protein. Serum digoxin concentrations correlate best with lean (ie, ideal) body weight, not total body weight.

*Metabolism* – Only a small percentage (16%) of a dose of digoxin is metabolized.

*Excretion* – Elimination of digoxin follows first-order kinetics. Following IV administration to healthy volunteers, 50% to 70% of a digoxin dose is excreted unchanged in the urine. Digoxin is not effectively removed from the body by dialysis, exchange transfusion, or during cardiopulmonary bypass because most of the drug is bound to tissue and does not circulate in the blood.

## Contraindications
Ventricular fibrillation; hypersensitivity to digoxin or other digitalis preparations.

## Warnings
*Sinus node disease and AV block:* The drug may cause severe sinus bradycardia or sino-atrial block in patients with preexisting sinus node disease and may cause advanced or complete heart block in patients with preexisting incomplete AV block. Consider inserting a pacemaker before treatment with digoxin.

*Accessory AV pathway (Wolff-Parkinson-White syndrome):* After IV digoxin therapy, some patients with paroxysmal atrial fibrillation or flutter and a coexisting accessory AV pathway have developed increased antegrade conduction across the accessory pathway bypassing the AV node, leading to a very rapid ventricular response or ventricular fibrillation. Unless conduction down the accessory pathway has been blocked (either pharmacologically or by surgery), do not use digoxin in such patients.

*Use in patients with preserved left ventricular systolic function:* Patients with certain disorders involving heart failure associated with preserved left ventricular ejection fraction may be particularly susceptible to toxicity of the drug.

*Renal function impairment:* Digoxin is primarily excreted by the kidneys; therefore, patients with impaired renal function require smaller than usual maintenance doses of digoxin (see Administration and Dosage).

*Pregnancy:* Category C.

*Lactation:* Exercise caution when digoxin is administered to a nursing woman.

*Children:* Newborn infants display considerable variability in tolerance. Premature and immature infants are particularly sensitive; reduce dosage and individualize digitalization according to infant's degree of maturity.

## Precautions
*Electrolyte disorders:* In patients with hypokalemia or hypomagnesemia, toxicity may occur despite serum digoxin concentrations less than 2 ng/mL, because potassium or magnesium depletion sensitizes the myocardium to digoxin. Therefore, it is desirable to maintain normal serum potassium and magnesium concentrations in patients being treated with digoxin.

Hypercalcemia from any cause predisposes the patient to digitalis toxicity. Calcium, particularly when administered rapidly by the IV route, may produce serious arrhythmias in digitalized patients. On the other hand, hypocalcemia can nullify the effects of digoxin in humans; thus, digoxin may be ineffective until serum calcium is restored to normal.

*Thyroid disorders and hypermetabolic states:* Hypothyroidism may reduce the requirements for digoxin. Heart failure or atrial arrhythmias resulting from hypermetabolic or hyperdynamic states (eg, hyperthyroidism, hypoxia, arteriovenous shunt) are best treated by addressing the underlying condition. Atrial arrhythmias associated with hypermetabolic states are particularly resistant to digoxin treatment. Care must be taken to avoid toxicity if digoxin is used.

*Acute MI:* Use digoxin with caution in patients with acute MI. The use of inotropic drugs in some patients in this setting may result in undesirable increases in myocardial oxygen demand and ischemia.

*Electrical cardioversion:* It may be desirable to reduce the dose of digoxin for 1 to 2 days prior to electrical cardioversion of atrial fibrillation to avoid the induction of ventricular arrhythmias, but physicians must consider the consequences of increasing the ventricular response if digoxin is withdrawn. If digitalis toxicity is suspected, delay elective cardioversion. If it is not prudent to delay cardioversion, select the lowest possible energy level to avoid provoking ventricular arrhythmias.

*Lab test abnormalities:* Periodically assess serum electrolytes and renal function (serum creatinine concentrations); the frequency of assessments will depend on the clinical setting.

### Drug Interactions

*Increased digoxin serum levels:* The following agents may increase digoxin serum levels, possibly increasing its therapeutic and toxic effects: Alprazolam, amiodarone, anticholinergics, benzodiazepines, bepridil, captopril, cyclosporine, diltiazem, diphenoxylate, erythromycin, esmolol, felodipine, flecainide, hydroxychloroquine, ibuprofen, indomethacin, itraconazole, nifedipine, omeprazole, propafenone, propantheline, quinidine, quinine, tetracycline, tolbutamide, and verapamil.

*Decreased GI absorption of digitalis glycosides:* May be caused by the following agents, possibly decreasing the serum levels and therapeutic effects: Aminoglutethimide, aminoglycosides (oral), aminosalicylic acid, antacids (aluminum or magnesium salts), antihistamines, antineoplastics, barbiturates, cholestyramine, colestipol, hydantoins, hypoglycemic agents (oral), kaolin/pectin, metoclopramide, neomycin, penicillamine, rifampin, sucralfate, and sulfasalazine.

Other drugs that may interact with cardiac glycosides include the following: Albuterol, amphotericin B, beta-blockers, calcium, disopyramide, loop diuretics, nondepolarizing muscle relaxants, potassium-sparing diuretics, succinylcholine, sympathomimetics, thiazide diuretics, thioamines, and thyroid hormones.

*Drug/Lab test interactions:* The use of therapeutic doses of digoxin may cause prolongation of the PR interval and depression of the ST segment on the electrocardiogram. Digoxin may produce false positive ST-T changes on the electrocardiogram during exercise testing.

*Drug/Food interactions:* When digoxin tablets are taken after meals, the rate of absorption is slowed but total amount absorbed is usually unchanged. However, when taken with meals high in bran fiber, the amount absorbed may be reduced.

### Adverse Reactions

Digoxin adverse reactions are dose-dependent and occur at doses higher than those needed to achieve a therapeutic effect. Cardiac adverse reactions accounted for approximately 50%, GI disturbances for approximately 25%, and CNS and other toxicity for approximately 25% of these adverse reactions. However, available evidence suggests that the incidence and severity of digoxin toxicity has decreased substantially in recent years.

Adverse reactions occurring in at least 3% of patients include the following: Headache, dizziness, mental disturbances, nausea, diarrhea, and death.

# NITRATES

| | |
|---|---|
| **AMYL NITRITE** | |
| **Inhalant**: 0.3 mL (*Rx*) | *Amyl Nitrite Vaporole* (GlaxoWellcome) |
| **ISOSORBIDE DINITRATE (ORAL)** | |
| **Tablets**: 5, 10, 20, 30, and 40 mg (*Rx*) | Various, *Isordil Titradose* (Wyeth-Ayerst) |
| **Tablets, sustained-release**: 40 mg (*Rx*) | Various |
| **Capsules, sustained-release**: 40 mg (*Rx*) | Various, *Isordil Tembids* (Wyeth-Ayerst), *Dilatrate-SR* (Schwarz Pharma) |
| **ISOSORBIDE DINITRATE (SUBLINGUAL)** | |
| **Tablets, sublingual**: 2.5, 5, and 10 mg (*Rx*) | Various, *Isordil* (Wyeth-Ayerst) |
| **ISOSORBIDE MONONITRATE (ORAL)** | |
| **Tablets**: 10 and 20 mg (*Rx*) | *Monoket* (Schwarz Pharma), *ISMO* (Wyeth-Ayerst) |
| **Tablets, extended-release**: 60 and 120 mg (*Rx*) | *Imdur* (Key) |
| **NITROGLYCERIN (IV)** | |
| **Injection**: 0.5 and 5 mg/mL (*Rx*) | Various, *Tridil* (Faulding) |
| **Injection solution**: 25, 50, 100, and 200 mg in 5% dextrose (*Rx*) | Various |
| **NITROGLYCERIN (SUBLINGUAL)** | |
| **Tablets, sublingual**: 0.3, 0.4, and 0.6 mg (*Rx*) | *Nitrostat* (Parke-Davis), *NitroQuick* (Ethex) |
| **NITROGLYCERIN (SUSTAINED-RELEASE)** | |
| **Capsules, sustained-release**: 2.5, 6.5, and 9 mg (*Rx*) | Various, *Nitro-Time* (Time-Cap Labs) |
| **NITROGLYCERIN (TOPICAL)** | |
| **Ointment**: 2% in a lanolin-petroleum base (*Rx*) | Various |
| **NITROGLYCERIN TRANSDERMAL SYSTEMS** | |
| **Patch**: 0.1, 0.2, 0.3, 0.4, 0.6, and 0.8 mg/h (*Rx*) | *Nitro-Dur* (Key) |
| **NITROGLYCERIN (TRANSLINGUAL)** | |
| **Spray**: 0.4 mg/dose (*Rx*) | *Nitrolingual* (Rhone-Poulenc Rorer) |
| **NITROGLYCERIN (TRANSMUCOSAL)** | |
| **Tablets, buccal, controlled-release**: 1, 2, and 3 mg (*Rx*) | *Nitrogard* (Forest) |

### Indications

*Acute angina (nitroglycerin sublingual, transmucosal or translingual spray; isosorbide dinitrate sublingual; amyl nitrite):* For relief of acute anginal episodes; prophylaxis prior to events likely to provoke an attack.

*Angina prophylaxis (nitroglycerin topical, transdermal, translingual spray, transmucosal and oral sustained release; isosorbide dinitrate; isosorbide mononitrate; erythrityl tetranitrate; pentaerythritol tetranitrate):* Prophylaxis and long-term management of recurrent angina.

*Nitroglycerin IV:* Control of blood pressure in perioperative hypertension associated with surgical procedures, especially cardiovascular procedures, such as endotracheal intubation, anesthesia, skin incision, sternotomy, cardiac bypass, and in the immediate postsurgical period.

CHF associated with acute MI; treatment of angina pectoris unresponsive to organic nitrates or β-blockers; production of controlled hypotension during surgical procedures.

### Administration and Dosage

*AMYL NITRITE:* Usual adult dose is 0.3 mL by inhalation, as required.

Crush the capsule and wave under the nose; 1 to 6 inhalations from one capsule are usually sufficient to produce the desired effect. May repeat in 3 to 5 minutes.

*ISOSORBIDE DINITRATE, ORAL:*

*Tablets* – Initial dose is 5 to 20 mg; maintenance dose is 10 to 40 mg every 6 hours.

*Sustained release* – The initial dose is 40 mg; maintenance controlled release dose is 40 to 80 mg every 8 to 12 hours. Do not crush or chew these preparations.

*Tolerance* – Tolerance to these agents may develop. Consider administering the short-acting preparations 2 or 3 times/day (last dose no later than 7 pm) and the sustained release preparations once daily or twice daily at 8 am and 2 pm.

*ISOSORBIDE DINITRATE, SUBLINGUAL:*

*Angina pectoris* – Usual starting dose is 2.5 to 5 mg for sublingual tablets.

*Acute prophylaxis* – 5 to 10 mg sublingual tablets every 2 to 3 hours. Limit use of sublingual isosorbide dinitrate for aborting an acute anginal attack in patients intolerant of or unresponsive to sublingual nitroglycerin.

Do not crush or chew sublingual tablets.

ISOSORBIDE MONONITRATE:

*Tablets* – 20 mg twice/day, with the 2 doses given 7 hours apart. A starting dose of 5 mg might be appropriate for people of particularly small stature, but should be increased to no more than 10 mg by the second or third day of therapy. Suggested regimen is to give first dose on awakening and second dose 7 hours later.

*Tablets, extended-release* – Initially, 30 or 60 mg once daily. After several days, the dosage may be increased to 120 mg once daily. Rarely 240 mg may be required. Suggested regimen is to give in the morning on arising. Do not crush or chew extended release tablets, and swallow them with a half glassful of liquid.

NITROGLYCERIN, IV:

*Dosage requirements* – Initially, 5 mcg/min delivered through an infusion pump. Titrate to the clinical situation, initially in 5 mcg/min increments with increases every 3 to 5 minutes until some response is noted. If no response occurs at 20 mcg/min, use increments of 10 to 20 mcg/min. Once a partial blood pressure response is observed, reduce the dose and lengthen the interval between increments.

NITROGLYCERIN, SUBLINGUAL: Dissolve 1 tablet under tongue or in buccal pouch (between cheek and gum) at first sign of an acute anginal attack. Repeat approximately every 5 minutes until relief is obtained. Take no more than 3 tablets in 15 minutes. May be used prophylactically 5 to 10 minutes prior to activities which might precipitate an acute attack.

NITROGLYCERIN, SUSTAINED-RELEASE: The usual starting dose is 2.5 or 2.6 mg, 3 or 4 times/day. The dose generally may be increased by 2.5 or 2.6 mg increments 2 to 4 times/day over a period of days or weeks. Doses as high as 26 mg given 4 times/day have been reported effective.

Give the smallest effective dose 2 to 4 times/day.

Capsules must be swallowed; not for chewing or sublingual use.

NITROGLYCERIN, TOPICAL:

*Usual therapeutic dose* – 1 to 2 inches (25 to 50 mm) every 8 hours, up to 4 to 5 inches (100 to 125 mm) every 4 hours. Start with ½ inch (12.5 mm) every 8 hours; increase by ½ inch with each application to achieve desired effects.

One inch (25 mm) of ointment contains approximately 15 mg nitroglycerin.

NITROGLYCERIN TRANSDERMAL SYSTEMS: Patient instructions for application are provided with products.

Apply once daily to a skin site free of hair and not subject to excessive movement. Do not apply to distal parts of extremities. Avoid areas with cuts/irritations.

*Starting dose* – 0.2 to 0.4 mg/h. Doses between 0.4 and 0.8 mg/h have shown continued effectiveness for 10 to 12 hours/day for at least 1 month of intermittent administration. Although the minimum nitrate-free interval has not been defined, data show that a nitrate-free interval of 10 to 12 hours is sufficient. Thus, an appropriate dosing schedule would include a daily "patch-on" period of 12 to 14 hours and a "patch-off" period of 10 to 12 hours. Tolerance is a major factor limiting efficacy when the system is used continuously for more than 12 hours each day.

NITROGLYCERIN, TRANSLINGUAL: At the onset of attack, spray 1 or 2 metered doses onto or under the tongue. No more than 3 metered doses are recommended within 15 minutes. May use prophylactically 5 to 10 minutes prior to activities which might precipitate an acute attack. Do not inhale spray.

NITROGLYCERIN, TRANSMUCOSAL: 1 mg every 3 to 5 hours during waking hours. Place tablet between lip and gum above incisors, or between cheek and gum.

### Actions

*Pharmacology:* Relaxation of vascular smooth muscle via stimulation of intracellular cyclic guanosine monophosphate production is the principal pharmacologic action of nitrates. Although venous effects predominate, nitroglycerin produces a dose-dependent dilation of both arterial and venous beds.

*Pharmacokinetics:*

| Doseform, Onset, and Duration of Available Nitrates | | | |
|---|---|---|---|
| Nitrates | Dosage form | Onset (minutes) | Duration |
| Amyl nitrate | Inhalant | 0.5 | 3 to 5 min |
| Nitroglycerin | IV | 1 to 2 | 3 to 5 min |
| | Sublingual | 1 to 3 | 30 to 60 min |
| | Translingual spray | 2 | 30 to 60 min |
| | Transmucosal tablet | 1 to 2 | 3 to 5 hours[1] |
| | Oral, sustained release | 20 to 45 | 3 to 8 hours |
| | Topical ointment | 30 to 60 | 2 to 12 hours[2] |
| | Transdermal | 30 to 60 | up to 24 hours[3] |
| Isosorbide dinitrate | Sublingual | 2 to 5 | 1 to 3 hours |
| | Oral | 20 to 40 | 4 to 6 hours |
| | Oral, sustained release | up to 4 hours | 6 to 8 hours |
| Isosorbide mononitrate | Oral | 30 to 60 | nd[4] |
| Erythrityl tetranitrate | Sublingual and chewable | 5 | 3 hours |
| | Oral | 15 to 30 | 6 hours |
| Pentaerythritol tetranitrate | Oral | 20 to 60 | ≈ 5 hours |
| | Oral, sustained release | 30 | up to 12 hours |

[1] A significant antianginal effect can persist for 5 hours if the tablet has not completely dissolved.
[2] Depends on total amount used per unit of surface area.
[3] Tolerance may develop after 12 hours.
[4] nd = No data.

## Contraindications

Hypersensitivity or idiosyncrasy to nitrates; severe anemia; closed-angle glaucoma; postural hypotension; early MI (sublingual nitroglycerin); head trauma or cerebral hemorrhage; allergy to adhesives (transdermal).

*Amyl nitrate:* Pregnancy.

*Nitroglycerin IV:* Hypotension or uncorrected hypovolemia; inadequate cerebral circulation; increased intracranial pressure; constrictive pericarditis; pericardial tamponade.

## Warnings

*MI:* In acute MI, use nitrates only under close clinical observation and with hemodynamic monitoring. In general, do not use a long-acting form because its effects are difficult to terminate rapidly if excessive hypotension or tachycardia develop.

*Arcing:* A cardioverter/defibrillator should not be discharged through a paddle electrode that overlies a transdermal nitroglycerin system.

*Postural hypotension:* Postural hypotension may occur, even with small doses.

*Angina:* Nitrates may aggravate angina caused by hypertrophic cardiomyopathy.

*Nitroglycerin IV:*

*Hepatic or renal disease, severe* – Use with caution.

*Hypotension* – Avoid excessive prolonged hypotension, because of possible deleterious effects on the brain, heart, liver, and kidney from poor perfusion and the attendant risk of ischemia, thrombosis, and altered organ function. Paradoxical bradycardia and increased angina pectoris may accompany nitroglycerin-induced hypotension.

*Alcohol intoxication* – Alcohol intoxication has developed in patients on high-dose IV nitroglycerin.

*Sublingual nitroglycerin:* Absorption is dependent on salivary secretion. Dry mouth decreases absorption.

*Transdermal nitroglycerin:* Transdermal nitroglycerin is not for immediate relief of anginal attacks.

*Pregnancy:* Category C; Category X (amyl nitrite).

*Lactation:* It is not know whether nitrates are excreted in breast milk.

*Children:* Safety and efficacy for use in children have not been established.

**Precautions**

*Tolerance:* Tolerance to vascular and antianginal effects of nitrates may develop. The use of a low-nitrate or nitrate-free period should be part of the therapeutic strategy.

*Glaucoma:* Intraocular pressure may be increased; therefore, caution is required in administering to patients with glaucoma.

*Excessive dosage:* Excessive dosage may produce severe headache.

*Volume depletion/hypotension:* Severe hypotension (particularly with upright posture) may occur with even small doses of isosorbide mononitrate.

*Withdrawal:* In terminating treatment of angina, gradually reduce the dosage to prevent withdrawal reactions.

**Drug Interactions**

Drugs that may interact with nitrates include alcohol, aspirin, calcium channel blockers, dihydroergotamine, and heparin.

*Drug/Lab test interactions:* Nitrates may interfere with the *Zlatkis-Zak* color reaction causing a false report of decreased serum cholesterol.

**Adverse Reactions**

*Cardiovascular:* Tachycardia; palpitations; hypotension (sometimes with paradoxical bradycardia and increased angina pectoris); postural hypotension.

*CNS:* Headache that may be severe and persistent (50% or less); apprehension; restlessness; weakness; vertigo; dizziness; agitation; anxiety; confusion; insomnia; nervousness.

*Dermatologic:* Drug rash or exfoliative dermatitis; cutaneous vasodilation with flushing; crusty skin lesions; pruritus; rash.

    *Sublingual nitroglycerin* – Sublingual nitroglycerin tablets may cause a local burning or tingling sensation in the oral cavity at the point of dissolution.

*GI:* Nausea; vomiting; diarrhea; dyspepsia; involuntary passing of urine and feces; abdominal pain.

*GU:* Dysuria; impotence; urinary frequency.

*Miscellaneous:* Arthralgia; bronchitis; muscle twitching; pallor; perspiration; cold sweat; asthenia; blurred vision; diplopia; edema; malaise; neck stiffness; increased appetite.

# ANTIARRHYTHMIC AGENTS

Optimal therapy of cardiac arrhythmias requires documentation, accurate diagnosis, and modification of precipitating causes, and if indicated, proper selection and use of anti-arrhythmic drugs. These drugs are classified according to their effects on the action potential of cardiac cells and their presumed mechanism of action.

*Class* I: Local anesthetics or membrane-stabilizing agents that depress phase 0.

IA *(quinidine, procainamide, disopyramide)* – Depress phase 0 and prolong the action potential duration.

IB *(tocainide, lidocaine, phenytoin, mexiletine)* – Depress phase 0 slightly and may shorten the action potential duration. Although arrhythmia is not a labeled indication for phenytoin, it is commonly used in treatment of digitalis-induced arrhythmias.

IC *(flecainide, encainide, propafenone)* – Marked depression of phase 0. Slight effect on repolarization. Profound slowing of conduction. Encainide was voluntarily with-drawn from the market, but is still available on a limited basis.

*Moricizine* – Moricizine is a Class I agent that shares some of the characteristics of the Class IA, B, and C agents.

*Class* II *(propranolol, esmolol, acebutolol)*: Depress phase 4 depolarization.

*Class* III *(bretylium, amiodarone)*: Produce a prolongation of phase 3 (repolarization).

*Class* IV *(verapamil)*: Depress phase 4 depolarization and lengthen phases 1 and 2 of repolarization.

*Sotalol:* Sotalol has both Class II (beta blocking) and III properties; Class III effects are seen at doses greater than 160 mg.

*Digitalis glycosides (digoxin):* Digitalis glycosides (digoxin) cause a decrease in maximal diastolic potential and action potential duration and increase the slope of phase 4 depolarization.

*Adenosine:* Adenosine slows conduction time through the AV node and can interrupt the reentry pathways through the AV node.

*Serum drug levels:* Some antiarrhythmic drugs (eg, quinidine) can produce toxic effects that can be easily confused with the symptoms for which the drug has been prescribed. Drug serum levels are important in evaluating toxic or subtherapeutic dosage regimens of most of the antiarrhythmic drugs.

*Proarrhythmic effects:* Antiarrhythmic agents may cause new or worsened arrhythmias. It is essential that each patient be evaluated electrocardiographically and clinically prior to and during therapy to determine whether the response to the drug supports continued treatment.

## Antiarrhythmic Electrophysiology/Electrocardiogram Effects

| Group | Drug | Automaticity | | Conduction velocity | | | Refractory period | | | | | ECG changes[1] | | | | |
|---|---|---|---|---|---|---|---|---|---|---|---|---|---|---|---|---|
| | | SA node | Ectopic pacemaker | Atrium | AV node | His-Purkinje | Atrium | AV node | His-Purkinje | Ventricle | Accessory pathways[2] | Heart rate | PR interval | QRS complex | QTc interval | JT interval |
| I | Moricizine[3] | 0 | ↓ | 0 | ↓ | ↓ | ± | 0 | 0 | 0-↑ | ↑ | 0-↑ | ↑ | ↑ | 0 | ↓ |
| | Quinidine | ± | ↓ | ↓ | ± | ↓ | ↑↑ | 0-↑[4] | ↑↑ | ↑ | ↑ | ± | ± | ↑ | ↑ | ↑ |
| | Procainamide | ± | ↓ | ↓ | ± | ↓ | ↑ | 0-↑[4] | ↑↑ | ↑ | ↑↑ | ±) | ± | ↑ | ↑ | ↑ |
| | Disopyramide | ± | ↓ | ↓ | ± | ↓ | ↑↑ | 0-↑[4] | ↑↑ | ↑ | ↑ | ± | ± | ↑ | ↑ | ↑ |
| | Lidocaine | 0 | ↓ | — | 0 | 0 | 0 | ± | ± | ± | ↑-↓ | 0 | 0 | 0 | 0-↓ | 0 |
| | Phenytoin | ↓-0 | ↓ | - | 0 | 0 | 0 | ± | ± | ± | - | ± | 0-↓ | 0 | ↓ | 0 |
| | Tocainide | 0-↓ | ↓ | 0 | 0 | 0 | ↓ | ↓ | ± | ↓ | ↑ | 0 | 0 | 0 | 0-↓ | 0 |
| | Mexiletine | ↓ | ↓ | 0 | 0 | 0 | 0 | ± | ↑ | ↑ | ↑ | - | 0 | 0 | 0 | 0 |
| | Flecainide | ↓ | ↓ | ↓↓ | ↓ | ↓↓ | 0 | 0 | ↑ | ↑ | ↑↑ | 0 | ↑[5] | ↑↑[5] | 0-↑[5] | 0 |
| | Encainide[6] | 0-↓ | ↓ | ↓↓ | ↓ | ↓↓ | 0-↑ | 0-↑ | ↑ | ↑ | ↑↑ | 0 | ↑[5] | ↑↑[5] | 0-↑[5] | 0 |
| | Propafenone | 0 | ↓ | 0 | ↓ | ↓ | 0 | ↑ | ↑ | ↑ | ↑ | 0 | ↑[5] | ↑ | 0-↑[5] | 0 |
| II | Propranolol | ↓ | ↓ | ± | ↓ | 0-↓ | ± | ↑ | 0 | 0 | 0-↑ | ↓ | 0-↑ | 0 | 0-↓ | 0 |
| | Esmolol | ↓ | ↓ | ± | ↓ | 0- | ± | ↑ | 0 | 0 | 0-↑ | ↓ | 0-↑ | 0 | 0-↓ | 0 |
| | Acebutolol | ↓ | ↓ | ± | ↓ | 0 | ± | ↑ | 0 | 0 | 0-↑ | ↓ | 0-↑ | 0 | 0-↓ | 0 |
| III | Bretylium | ↑ | ↑ | 0 | 0 | 0-↑ | 0 | ↓-0-↑[7] | ↑ | 0-↑ | ± | 0 | 0 | 0 | 0 | ↑ |
| | Amiodarone | ↓ | ↓ | ↓ | ↓ | ↓ | ↑ | ↑ | ↑ | ↑ | ↑ | ↓ | ↑ | ↑ | ↑↑ | ↑↑ |
| | Sotalol[8] | ↓ | ↓ | 0 | ↓ | 0 | ↑↑ | ↑ | ↑↑ | ↑↑ | ↑ | ↓ | ↑ | 0 | ↑↑ | ↑↑ |
| IV | Verapamil | ↓ | ↓ | 0 | ↓ | 0 | 0 | ↑ | 0 | 0 | 0 | ↓ | ↑ | 0 | 0 | 0 |
| — | Digoxin | 0-↓ | ↑ | ± | ↓ | 0-↓ | ± | ↑ | 0 | ↓ | ↓-↑ | ↓ | ↑ | 0 | ↓ | ↓ |
| — | Adenosine | ↓ | ↓ | 0 | ↓ | 0 | 0 | ↑ | 0 | 0 | 0 | ↑ | ↑ | 0 | 0 | — |

[1] These values assume therapeutic levels.
[2] Accessory pathways occur in Wolff-Parkinson-White syndrome (preexcitation phenomena) and possibly other abnormal conditions.
[3] Does not belong to any of the 3 subclasses (A, B or C), but does have some properties of each.
[4] Retrograde AV node RP↑; antegrade RP not affected.
[5] Dose-related increases.
[6] Withdrawn from the market; however, available on a limited basis.
[7] Due to a complex balance of direct and indirect autonomic effects.
[8] Has both Class II (beta-blocking) and III properties; Class III effects are seen at doses greater than 160 mg.

| Antiarrhythmics Group | Drug | Onset (h) (oral)[1] | Duration (h) | Half-life (h) | Protein binding (%) | Excreted unchanged (%) | Therapeutic serum level (mcg/mL) | Toxic serum levels (mcg/mL) |
|---|---|---|---|---|---|---|---|---|
| **I A** | Moricizine | 2 | 10-24 | 1.5-3.5[2] | 95 | < 1 | Not applicable | — |
| | Quinidine | 0.5 | 6-8 | 6-7 | 80-90 | 10-50 | 2-6 | > 8 |
| | Procainamide | 0.5 | 3+ | 2.5-4.7 | 14-23 | 40-70 | 4-8 | > 16 |
| | Disopyramide | 0.5 | 6-7 | 4-10 | 20-60[3] | 40-60 | 2-8 | > 9 |
| **B** | Lidocaine | — | 0.25[4] | 1-2 | 40-80 | < 3 | 1.5-6 | > 7 |
| | Phenytoin | 0.5-1 | 24+ | 22-36[5] | 87-93 | < 5 | 10-20 | > 20 |
| | Tocainide | — | — | 11-15 | 10-20 | 28-55 | 4-10 | > 10 |
| | Mexiletine | — | — | 10-12 | 50-60 | 10 | 0.5-2 | > 2 |
| **C** | Flecainide | — | — | 12-27 | 40 | 30 | 0.2-1 | > 1 |
| | Encainide[6] | — | — | 1-2[7] | 75-85 | < 5[8] | Not applicable | — |
| | MODE[9] | | | 6-12 | 92 | | wide range | — |
| | ODE[9] | | | 3-4 | 75-85 | | 0.1-0.3 | — |
| | Propafenone | — | — | 2-10[10] | 97 | < 1 | 0.06-1 | — |
| **II** | Propranolol | 0.5 | 3-5 | 2-3 | 90-95 | < 1 | 0.05-0.1 | — |
| | Esmolol | < 5 min | very short | 0.15 | 55 | < 2 | — | — |
| | Acebutolol | — | 24-30 | 3-4 | 26 | 15-20 | — | — |
| **III** | Bretylium | — | 6-8 | 5-10 | 0-8 | > 80 | 0.5-1.5 | — |
| | Amiodarone | 1-3 wks[11] | weeks to months | 26-107 days | 96 | negligible | 0.5-2.5 | > 2.5 |
| | Sotalol | — | — | 12 | 0 | 100 | — | — |
| **IV** | Verapamil | 0.5 | 6 | 3-7 | 90 | 3-4 | 0.08-0.3 | — |
| — | Digoxin | 0.5-2 | 24+ | 30-40 | 20-25 | 60 | 0.5-2 ng/mL | > 2.5 ng/mL |
| — | Adenosine | (34 sec IV) | 1-2 min | < 10 sec | — | 0 (enters body pool) | Not applicable | — |

**Antiarrhythmic Pharmacokinetics**

[1] Within 1 to 5 minutes with IV use.
[2] Half-life may be prolonged in patients after multiple dosing.
[3] Protein binding is concentration-dependent.
[4] Very short after discontinuation of IV infusion.
[5] Half-life increases with increasing dosage.
[6] Withdrawn from the market; however, available on a limited basis.
[7] Half-life 6 to 11 hours in less than 10% of patients (poor metabolizers).
[8] More than 50% in poor metabolizers.
[9] MODE (3-methoxy-O-demethyl encainide) and ODE (O-demethyl encainide), metabolites more active than encainide on a per mg basis.
[10] Half-life 10 to 32 hours in less than 10% of patients (slow metabolizers).
[11] Onset of action may occur in 2 to 3 days.

# QUINIDINE

| **QUINIDINE SULFATE** | |
|---|---|
| **Tablets**: 200 and 300 mg (*Rx*) | Various, *Quinora* (Key Pharm) |
| **Tablets, sustained-release**: 300 mg (*Rx*) | Various |
| **QUINIDINE GLUCONATE** | |
| **Tablets, sustained-release**: 324 mg (*Rx*) | Various |
| **Injection**: 80 mg/mL (*Rx*) | Various |

### Indications

*Oral*: Premature atrial, AV junctional and ventricular contractions; paroxysmal atrial (supraventricular) tachycardia; paroxysmal AV junctional rhythm; atrial flutter; paroxysmal and chronic atrial fibrillation; established atrial fibrillation when therapy is appropriate; paroxysmal ventricular tachycardia not associated with complete heart block; maintenance therapy after electrical conversion of atrial fibrillation or flutter.

*Parenteral*: When oral therapy is not feasible or when rapid therapeutic effect is required.
> *Quinidine gluconate* – Life-threatening *Plasmodium falciparum* malaria.

### Administration and Dosage

*Test dose:* Administer a single 200 mg tablet of quinidine sulfate or 200 mg IM quinidine gluconate to determine whether the patient has an idiosyncratic reaction.
> Adjust the dosage to maintain plasma concentration between 2 to 6 mcg/mL.

*Oral:*
> *Premature atrial and ventricular contractions* – 200 to 300 mg 3 or 4 times/day.
> *Paroxysmal supraventricular tachycardias* – 400 to 600 mg every 2 or 3 hours until the paroxysm is terminated.
> *Atrial flutter* – Administer quinidine after digitalization. Individualize dosage.
> *Conversion of atrial fibrillation* – 200 mg every 2 or 3 hours for 5 to 8 doses, with subsequent daily increases until sinus rhythm is restored or toxic effects occur. Do not exceed a total daily dose of 3 to 4 g in any regimen.
> *Maintenance therapy* – 200 to 300 mg 3 or 4 times/day. Other patients may require larger doses or more frequent administration than the usually recommended schedule.
> *Sustained-release forms* – 300 to 600 mg every 8 or 12 hours.

*Parenteral:*
> *IM* – In the treatment of acute tachycardia, the initial dose is 600 mg quinidine gluconate. Subsequently, 400 mg quinidine gluconate can be repeated as often as every 2 hours.
> *IV* – In approximately 50% of patients who respond successfully to quinidine, the arrhythmia can be terminated by 330 mg quinidine gluconate or less (or its equivalent in other salts); as much as 500 to 750 mg may be required. Inject slowly.
> *QUINIDINE GLUCONATE – P. falciparum malaria –* The following 2 regimens are effective empirically. As soon as practical, institute standard oral antiplasmodial therapy.
> 1.) Loading: 15 mg/kg in 250 mL normal saline infused over 4 hours followed by; Maintenance: beginning 24 hours after the beginning of the loading dose, 7.5 mg/kg infused over 4 hours, every 8 hours for 7 days or until oral therapy can be instituted.
> 2.) Loading: 10 mg/kg in 250 mL normal saline infused over 1 to 2 hours, followed immediately by; Maintenance: 0.02 mg/kg/min for up to 72 hours or until parasitemia decreases to less than 1% or oral therapy can be instituted.

*Children:*
> *Oral (quinidine sulfate)* – 30 mg/kg/day or 900 mg/m$^2$/day in 5 divided doses.
> *IV (quinidine gluconate)* – 2 to 10 mg/kg/dose every 3 to 6 hours as needed; however, this route is not recommended.

### Actions

*Pharmacology:* Quinidine, a class IA antiarrhythmic, depresses myocardial excitability, conduction velocity and contractility.

*Pharmacokinetics:*
 *Absorption/Distribution –*

| Anhydrous Quinidine Alkaloid Content in Various Salts | | | |
|---|---|---|---|
| | Quinidine content | | |
| Quinidine salts | Active drug | Absorbed | Time to peak plasma levels (hours) |
| Quinidine sulfate | 83% | 73% | 1 to 3[1] |
| Quinidine gluconate | 62% | 70% | 3-5 |

[1] 3 to 5 hours for sustained release form.

Quinidine is rapidly absorbed from the GI tract. Maximum effects of quinidine gluconate occur 30 to 90 minutes after IM administration; onset is more rapid after IV administration. Activity persists for at least 6 to 8 hours. The average therapeutic serum levels are reported to be 2 to 7 mcg/mL. Toxic reactions may occur at levels from 5 to 8 mcg/mL or more. Quinidine is 80% to 90% bound to plasma proteins; the unbound fraction may be significantly increased in patients with hepatic insufficiency.

*Metabolism/Excretion –* From 60% to 80% of a dose is metabolized via the liver into several metabolites. Quinidine is excreted unchanged (10% to 50%) in the urine within 24 hours. The elimination half-life ranges from 4 to 10 hours in healthy patients, with a mean of 6 to 7 hours. Urinary acidification facilitates quinidine elimination, and alkalinization retards it. In patients with cirrhosis, the elimination half-life may be prolonged and the volume of distribution increased.

## Contraindications

Hypersensitivity or idiosyncrasy to quinidine or other cinchona derivatives manifested by thrombocytopenia, skin eruption or febrile reactions; myasthenia gravis; history of thrombocytopenic purpura associated with quinidine administration; digitalis intoxication manifested by arrhythmias or AV conduction disorders; complete heart block; left bundle branch block or other severe intraventricular conduction defects exhibiting marked QRS widening or bizarre complexes; complete AV block with an AV nodal or idioventricular pacemaker; aberrant ectopic impulses and abnormal rhythms due to escape mechanisms; history of drug-induced torsade de pointes; history of long QT syndrome.

## Warnings

*Hepatotoxicity:* Hepatotoxicity (including granulomatous hepatitis) due to quinidine hypersensitivity has occurred.

*Atrial flutter or fibrillation:* Reversion to sinus rhythm may be preceded by a progressive reduction in degree of AV block to a 1:1 ratio, which results in an extremely rapid ventricular rate. Prior to use in atrial flutter, pretreat with digitalis preparation.

*Cardiotoxicity:* Cardiotoxicity (eg, increased PR and QT intervals, 50% widening of QRS complex, ventricular tachyarrhythmias, frequent ventricular ectopic beats, or tachycardia) dictates immediate discontinuation of quinidine; closely monitor the ECG.

Large oral doses may reduce the arterial pressure by means of peripheral vasodilation. Serious hypotension is more likely with parenteral use.

Use quinidine with extreme caution in incomplete AV block, because complete block and asystole may result. The drug may cause unpredictable dysrhythmias in digitalized patients. Use cautiously in patients with partial bundle branch block, severe CHF, and hypotensive states due to the depressant effects of quinidine on myocardial contractility and arterial pressure.

*Parenteral therapy:* The dangers of parenteral use of quinidine are increased in the presence of AV block or absence of atrial activity. Administration is more hazardous in patients with extensive myocardial damage. Use of quinidine in digitalis-induced cardiac arrhythmia is extremely dangerous because the cardiac glycoside may already have caused serious impairment of intracardiac conduction system. Too rapid IV administration of as little as 200 mg may precipitate a fall of 40 to 50 mm Hg in arterial pressure.

*Syncope:* Syncope occasionally occurs in patients on long-term quinidine therapy, usually resulting from ventricular tachycardia or fibrillation.

*Renal, hepatic, or cardiac insufficiency:* Use with caution in renal, cardiac, or hepatic insufficiency because of potential toxicity.

*Hypersensitivity reactions:* Asthma, muscle weakness, and infection with fever prior to quinidine administration may mask hypersensitivity reactions to the drug.

*Pregnancy:* Category C.

*Lactation:* Quinidine is excreted into breast milk with a milk:serum ratio of approximately 0.71. The American Academy of Pediatrics considers quinidine to be compatible with breast-feeding.

*Children:* Safety and efficacy have not been established.

**Precautions**

*Monitoring:* Perform periodic blood counts and liver and kidney function tests. Discontinue use if blood dyscrasias or signs of hepatic or renal disorders occur. Frequently measure arterial blood pressure during IV use.

*Potassium balance:* The effect of quinidine is enhanced by potassium and reduced if hypokalemia is present. The risk of drug-induced torsade de pointes is increased by concomitant hypokalemia.

**Drug Interactions**

Drugs that may affect quinidine include amiodarone, antacids, barbiturates, cholinergic drugs, cimetidine, disopyramide, hydantoins, nifedipine, rifampin, sucralfate, urinary alkalinizers and verapamil. Drugs that may be affected by quinidine include anticholinergics, anticoagulants, beta-blockers, cardiac glycosides, disopyramide, nondepolarizing neuromuscular blockers, procainamide, propafenone, succinylcholine, and tricyclic antidepressants.

*Drug/Lab test interactions:* Triamterene and quinidine have similar fluorescence spectra; thus, triamterene will interfere with the fluorescent measurement of quinidine serum levels.

**Adverse Reactions**

Adverse reactions may include nausea, vomiting, abdominal pain, diarrhea, anorexia; cinchonism (ringing in the ears, hearing loss, headache, nausea, dizziness, vertigo, light-headedness, disturbed vision); headache; fever; vertigo; apprehension; excitement; confusion; delirium; dementia; depression; acute hemolytic anemia; hypoprothrombinemia; thrombocytopenic purpura; agranulocytosis; thrombocytopenia; leukocytosis; mydriasis; blurred vision; disturbed color perception; reduced vision field; night blindness, photophobia; rash; urticaria; cutaneous flushing with intense pruritus; photosensitivity; eczema; psoriasis; abnormalities of pigmentation; arthralgia; myalgia; disturbed hearing; lupus erythematosus; hepatitis; cardiac asystole; ventricular ectopy; idioventricular rhythms; paradoxical tachycardia; arterial embolism; hypotension; ventricular extrasystoles; complete AV block; ventricular flutter.

# PROCAINAMIDE

| | |
|---|---|
| **Capsules**: 250, 375, and 500 mg (*Rx*) | Various |
| **Injection**: 500 mg/mL (*Rx*) | Various |
| **Tablets, sustained-release**: 250, 500, 750, and 1,000 mg (*Rx*) | Various, *Procanbid* (Monarch) |

**Warning:**

The prolonged administration often leads to the development of a positive anti-nuclear antibody (ANA) test, with or without symptoms of a lupus erythematosus-like syndrome. If a positive ANA titer develops, assess the benefit/risk ratio related to continued procainamide therapy.

*Mortality:* In the National Heart, Lung, and Blood Institute's Cardiac Arrhythmia Suppression Trial (CAST), a long-term, multicentered, randomized, double-blind study in patients with asymptomatic nonlife-threatening ventricular arrhythmias who had an MI more than 6 days but less than 2 years previously, an excessive mortality or nonfatal cardiac arrest rate was seen in patients treated with encainide or flecainide (7.7%) compared with that seen in patients assigned to matched placebo-treated groups (3%). The averaged duration of treatment with encainide or flecainide in this study was 10 months.

The applicability of these results to other populations (eg, those without recent MIs) is uncertain. Considering the known proarrhythmic properties of procainamide and the lack of evidence of improved survival for any antiarrhythmic drug in patients without life-threatening arrhythmias, the use of procainamide and other antiarrhythmic agents should be reserved for patients with life-threatening ventricular arrhythmias.

*Blood dyscrasias:* Agranulocytosis, bone marrow depression, neutropenia, hypoplastic anemia, and thrombocytopenia in patients receiving procainamide have been reported at a rate of approximately 0.5%. Most of these patients received procainamide within the recommended dosage range. Fatalities have occurred (with approximately 20% to 25% mortality in reported cases of agranulocytosis). Because most of these events have been noted during the first 12 weeks of therapy, it is recommended that complete blood counts (CBC), including white cell, differential, and platelet counts be performed at weekly intervals for the first 3 months of therapy, and periodically thereafter. Perform CBC promptly if the patient develops any signs of infection (eg, fever, chills, sore throat, stomatitis), bruising, or bleeding. If any of these hematologic disorders are identified, discontinue therapy. Blood counts usually return to normal within 1 month of discontinuation. Use caution in patients with preexisting marrow failure or cytopenia of any type.

## Indications

Treatment of documented ventricular arrhythmias, such as sustained ventricular tachycardia, that are judged to be life-threatening. Because of the proarrhythmic effects, use with lesser arrhythmias is generally not recommended.

Because procainamide has the potential to produce serious hematologic disorders (0.5%), particularly leukopenia or agranulocytosis (sometimes fatal), reserve its use for patients in whom the benefits of treatment clearly outweigh the risks.

Avoid treatment of patients with asymptomatic ventricular premature depolarizations.

*Unlabeled uses:*

*Atrial fibrillation/flutter* – Procainamide has been used to convert atrial fibrillation/flutter to sinus rhythm.

For the treatment of hemodynamically stable ventricular tachycardia in children, procainamide (loading dose of 15 mg/kg IV infused over 30 to 60 minutes) may be considered as an alternative agent to amiodarone.

### Administration and Dosage

*Oral:* Oral dosage forms are preferable for less urgent arrhythmias as well as for long-term maintenance after initial parenteral therapy. Individualize dosage based on clinical assessment of the degree of underlying myocardial disease, the patient's age and renal function.

As a general guide, for younger adult patients with normal renal function, an initial total daily oral dose of 50 mg/kg or less may be used, given in divided doses every 3 hours, to maintain therapeutic blood levels. For older patients, especially those older than 50 years of age, or for patients with renal, hepatic, or cardiac insufficiency, lesser amounts or longer intervals may produce adequate blood levels and decrease the probability of occurrence of dose-related adverse reactions. Administer the total daily dose in divided doses at 3-, 4-, or 6-hour intervals and adjust according to the patient's response.

| Guidelines to Provide up to 50 mg/kg/day Procainamide | | | | |
| --- | --- | --- | --- | --- |
| Weight | | Dose every 3 hours (standard formulation) | Dose every 6 hours (standard formulation and sustained release) | Dose every 12 hours (*Procanbid* sustained release tablets only) |
| lb | kg | | | |
| 88-110 | 40-50 | 250 mg | 500 mg | 1 g |
| 132-154 | 60-70 | 375 mg | 750 mg | 1.5 g |
| 176-198 | 80-90 | 500 mg | 1 g | 2 g |
| > 220 | > 100 | 625 mg | 1.25 g | 2.5 g |

[1] Initial dosage schedule guide only, to be adjusted for each patient individually, based on age, cardio-renal function, blood level (if available), and clinical response.

Sustained-release products are not recommended for initial therapy. Total dosage (50 mg/kg/day) may be given in divided doses every 6 hours.

*Parenteral:* Useful for arrhythmias that require immediate suppression and for maintenance of arrhythmia control. IV therapy allows most rapid control of serious arrhythmias, including those following MI; use in circumstances where close observation and monitoring of the patient are possible, such as in hospital or emergency facilities. IM administration is less apt to produce temporary high plasma levels but therapeutic plasma levels are not obtained as rapidly as with IV administration.

*IM administration* – IM administration may be used as an alternative to the oral route for patients with less threatening arrhythmias but who are nauseated or vomiting, who are ordered to receive nothing by mouth preoperatively, or who may have malabsorptive problems. An initial daily dose of 50 mg/kg may be estimated. Divide this amount into fractional doses of $\frac{1}{8}$ to $\frac{1}{4}$ to be injected IM every 3 to 6 hours until oral therapy is possible. If more than 3 injections are given, assess patient factors such as age and renal function, clinical response and, if available, blood levels of procainamide and NAPA in adjusting further doses for that individual. For treatment of arrhythmias associated with anesthesia or surgery, the suggested dose is 100 to 500 mg by IM injection.

*IV –*

| Dilutions and Rates for IV Infusions of Procainamide | | | | |
| --- | --- | --- | --- | --- |
| Infusion | Final concentration | Infusion volume[1] | Procainamide to be added | Infusion rate |
| Initial loading infusion | 20 mg/mL | 50 mL | 1000 mg | 1 mL/min (for up to 25 to 30 min) |
| Maintenance infusion[2] | 2 mg/mL or | 500 mL | 1000 mg | 1 to 3 mL/min |
| | 4 mg/mL | 250 mL | 1000 mg | 0.5 to 1.5 mL/min |

[1] All infusions should be made up to final volume with 5% dextrose injection, USP.
[2] The maintenance infusion rates are calculated to deliver 2 to 6 mg/min depending on body weight, renal elimination rate and steady-state plasma level needed to maintain control of the arrhythmia. The 4 mg/mL maintenance concentration may be preferred if total infused volume must be limited.

Cautiously administer the IV injection to avoid a possible hypotensive response. Initial arrhythmia control, under blood pressure and ECG monitoring, may usually be accomplished safely within 30 minutes by either of the 2 methods that follow:

1) Slowly direct injection into a vein or into tubing of an established infusion line at a rate not to exceed 50 mg/min. It is advisable to dilute the 500 mg/mL concentrations prior to IV injection to facilitate control of dosage rate. Doses of 100 mg may be administered every 5 minutes at this rate until the arrhythmia is suppressed or until 500 mg has been administered, after which it is advisable to wait 10 minutes or longer to allow for more distribution into tissues before resuming.

2) Alternatively, a loading infusion containing 20 mg/mL (1 g diluted to 50 mL with 5% dextrose injection, USP) may be administered at a constant rate of 1 mL/min for 25 to 30 minutes to deliver 500 to 600 mg. Some effects may be seen after infusion of the first 100 or 200 mg; it is unusual to require more than 600 mg to achieve satisfactory antiarrhythmic effects.

The maximum advisable dosage to be given either by repeated bolus injections or such loading infusion is 1 g.

To maintain therapeutic levels, a more dilute IV infusion at a concentration of 2 mg/mL is convenient (1 g in 500 mL 5% dextrose injection), and may be administered at 1 to 3 mL/min. If daily total fluid intake must be limited, a 4 mg/mL concentration (1 g in 250 mL of 5% dextrose injection) administered at 0.5 to 1.5 mL/min will deliver an equivalent 2 to 6 mg/min. Assess the amount needed in a given patient to maintain the therapeutic level principally from the clinical response. Adjust based on close observation. A maintenance infusion rate of 50 mcg/kg/min to a person with a normal renal procainamide elimination half-life of 3 hours should produce a plasma level of about 6.5 mcg/mL.

Terminate IV therapy if persistent conduction disturbances or hypotension develop. As soon as the patient's basic cardiac rhythm appears to be stabilized, oral antiarrhythmic maintenance therapy is preferable (if indicated and possible). A period of approximately 3 to 4 hours (one half-life for renal elimination, ordinarily) should elapse after the last IV dose before administering the first dose of oral procainamide.

*Children:* The following doses have been suggested.
 *Oral* – 15 to 50 mg/kg/day divided every 3 to 6 hours; maximum 4 g/day.
 *IM* – 20 to 30 mg/kg/day.
 *IV* – Loading dose: 3 to 6 mg/kg/dose over 5 minutes. Maintenance: 20 to 80 mcg/kg/min continuous infusion. Maximum 100 mg/dose or 2 g/day.

## Actions

*Pharmacology:* Procainamide, a class IA antiarrhythmic, increases the effective refractory period of the atria, and to a lesser extent the bundle of His-Purkinje system and ventricles of the heart.

*Electrophysiology* – The ECG may show slight sinus tachycardia and widened QRS complexes and, less regularly, prolonged QT and PR intervals, as well as some decrease in QRS and T-wave amplitude.

*Pharmacokinetics:*
 *Absorption/Distribution* – Oral procainamide is resistant to digestive hydrolysis, and the drug is well absorbed from the entire small intestinal surface, but individual patients vary in their completeness of absorption. Following oral use, plasma levels peak at approximately 45 to 120 minutes. Following IM injection, plasma levels peak in 15 to 60 minutes. IV use can produce therapeutic plasma levels within minutes. About 15% to 20% is reversibly bound to plasma proteins. The apparent volume of distribution eventually reaches approximately 2 L/kg with a half-life of approximately 5 minutes.

 *Metabolism/Excretion* – A significant fraction of the circulating procainamide may be metabolized in hepatocytes to N-acetylprocainamide (NAPA), ranging from 16% to 33% of an administered dose. NAPA also has significant antiarrhythmic activity and somewhat slower renal clearance than procainamide. The elimination half-life of procainamide is 3 to 4 hours in patients with normal renal function, but reduced creatinine clearance (Ccr) and advancing age each prolong the elimination half-life. Half-life and renal clearance are also reduced in infants. Thirty percent to 60% of the drug is excreted as unchanged procainamide, and 6% to 52% as the NAPA derivative. Both procainamide and NAPA are eliminated by active tubular secretion as well as by glomerular filtration.

### Contraindications

Complete heart block; idiosyncratic hypersensitivity; lupus erythematosus; torsades de pointes.

### Warnings

*Blood dyscrasias:* Agranulocytosis, bone marrow depression, neutropenia, hypoplastic anemia and thrombocytopenia in patients receiving procainamide have been reported at a rate of approximately 0.5%. Fatalities have occurred (with approximately 20% to 25% mortality in reported cases of agranulocytosis). Perform complete blood counts including white cell, differential, and platelet counts at weekly intervals for the first 3 months of therapy, and periodically thereafter. Perform complete blood counts promptly if the patient develops any signs of infection (eg, fever, chills, sore throat, stomatitis), bruising, or bleeding. If any of these hematologic disorders are identified, discontinue therapy. Blood counts usually return to normal within 1 month of discontinuation. Use caution in patients with preexisting marrow failure or cytopenia of any type.

*Mortality:* Considering the known proarrhythmic properties of procainamide and the lack of evidence of improved survival for any antiarrhythmic drug in patients without life-threatening arrhythmias, reserve the use of procainamide and other antiarrhythmic agents for patients with life-threatening ventricular arrhythmias.

*Complete heart block:* Do not administer to patients with complete heart block because of its effects in suppressing nodal or ventricular pacemakers and the hazard of asystole. If significant slowing of ventricular rate occurs during treatment without evidence of AV conduction appearing, stop procainamide. In cases of second-degree AV block or various types of hemiblock, avoid or discontinue procainamide because of the possibility of increased severity of block, unless the ventricular rate is controlled by an electrical pacemaker.

*Torsades de pointes:* Procainamide may aggravate this special type of ventricular extrasystole or tachycardia instead of suppressing it.

*Lupus erythematosus:* If the lupus erythematosus-like syndrome develops in a patient with recurrent life-threatening arrhythmias not controlled by other agents, corticosteroid suppressive therapy may be used concomitantly with procainamide. Because the procainamide-induced lupoid syndrome rarely includes the dangerous pathologic renal changes, therapy may not necessarily have to be stopped unless the symptoms of serositis and the possibility of further lupoid effects are of greater risk than the benefit of procainamide in controlling arrhythmias. Patients with rapid acetylation capability are less likely to develop the lupoid syndrome after prolonged therapy.

*Digitalis intoxication:* Exercise caution in the use of procainamide in arrhythmias associated with digitalis intoxication. Procainamide can suppress digitalis-induced arrhythmias; however, if there is concomitant marked disturbance of AV conduction, additional depression of conduction and ventricular asystole or fibrillation may result. Consider use of procainamide only if discontinuation of digitalis, and therapy with potassium, lidocaine, or phenytoin are ineffective.

*First-degree heart block:* Exercise caution if the patient exhibits or develops first-degree heart block while taking procainamide; dosage reduction is advised. If the block persists despite dosage reduction, evaluate the continuation of procainamide on the basis of current benefit vs risk of increased heart block.

*Predigitalization for atrial flutter or fibrillation:* Cardiovert or digitalize patients with atrial flutter or fibrillation prior to procainamide administration to avoid enhancement of AV conduction, which may result in ventricular rate acceleration beyond tolerable limits. Adequate digitalization reduces the possibility of sudden increase in ventricular rate.

*CHF:* Use with caution in patients with CHF and in those with acute ischemic heart disease or cardiomyopathy because even slight depression of myocardial contractility may further reduce cardiac output of the damaged heart.

*Concurrent antiarrhythmic agents:* Concurrent antiarrhythmic agents may produce enhanced prolongation of conduction or depression of contractility and hypotension, especially in patients with cardiac decompensation. Reserve concurrent use of procainamide with other Class IA antiarrhythmic agents (eg, quinidine, disopyramide) for patients with serious arrhythmias unresponsive to a single drug and use only if close observation is possible.

*Myasthenia gravis:* Procainamide administration in myasthenia gravis patients may be hazardous without optimal adjustment of anticholinesterase medications and other precautions. Immediately after initiation of therapy, closely observe patients for muscular weakness if myasthenia gravis is a possibility.

*Renal insufficiency:* Renal insufficiency may lead to accumulation of high plasma levels from conventional oral doses of procainamide, with effects similar to those of overdosage unless dosage is adjusted for the individual patient.

*Hypersensitivity reactions:* In patients sensitive to procaine or other ester-type local anesthetics, cross-sensitivity to procainamide is unlikely; however, consider the possibility. Do not use procainamide if it produces acute allergic dermatitis, asthma or anaphylactic symptoms.

*Pregnancy: Category C.*

*Lactation:* Both procainamide and NAPA are excreted in breast milk and absorbed by the nursing infant. Discontinue nursing or the drug, taking into account the importance of the drug to the mother.

*Children:* Safety and efficacy have not been established. However, see Administration and Dosage.

## Precautions

*Monitoring:* After achieving and maintaining therapeutic plasma concentrations and satisfactory ECG and clinical responses, continue frequent periodic monitoring of vital signs and ECG. If evidence of QRS widening of more than 25% or marked prolongation of the QT interval occurs, concern for overdosage is appropriate; reduction in dosage is advisable if a 50% increase occurs. Elevated serum creatinine or urea nitrogen, reduced Ccr or history of renal insufficiency, as well as use in older patients (older than 50 years of age), provide grounds to anticipate that less than the usual dosage and longer time intervals between doses may suffice. If facilities are available for measurement of plasma procainamide and NAPA levels or acetylation capability, individual dose adjustment for optimal therapeutic levels may be easier, but close observation of clinical effectiveness is the most important criterion.

*Embolization:* In conversion of atrial fibrillation to normal sinus rhythm by any means, dislodgment of mural thrombi may lead to embolization.

*Sulfite sensitivity:* Some of these products contain sulfites that may cause allergic-type reactions including anaphylactic symptoms and life-threatening or less severe asthmatic episodes. Sulfite sensitivity is seen more frequently in asthmatic or atopic nonasthmatic persons.

## Drug Interactions

Drugs that may affect procainamide include amiodarone, anticholinergics, antiarrhythmics, beta-blockers, ethanol, histamine $H_2$ antagonists, propranolol, quinidine, quinolones, thioridazine, trimethoprim, and ziprasidone. Drugs that may be affected by procainamide include neuromuscular blockers (succinylcholine). Tests that depend on fluorescence measurement may also be affected.

## Adverse Reactions

Significant adverse reactions include a lupus erythematosus-like syndrome of arthralgia, pleural or abdominal pain, and sometimes arthritis, pleural effusion, pericarditis, fever, chills, myalgia, and possibly related hematologic or skin lesions (after prolonged administration); neutropenia; thrombocytopenia; agranulocytosis (after repeated use; deaths have occurred); anorexia; nausea; vomiting; abdominal pain; bitter taste; diarrhea.

# DISOPYRAMIDE

| | |
|---|---|
| **Capsules:** 100 and 150 mg (Rx) | Various, *Norpace* (Searle) |
| **Capsules, extended-release:** 100 and 150 mg (Rx) | Various, *Norpace* CR (Searle) |

**Warning:**
In the National Heart, Lung, and Blood Institute's Cardiac Arrhythmia Suppression Trial (CAST), a long-term, multicenter, randomized, double-blind study in patients with asymptomatic non-life-threatening ventricular arrhythmias who had an MI more than 6 days but less than 2 years previously, an excessive mortality or nonfatal cardiac arrest rate (7.7%) was seen in patients treated with encainide or flecainide compared with that seen in patients assigned to carefully matched placebo-treated groups (3%). The average duration of treatment with encainide or flecainide in this study was 10 months.

The applicability of the CAST results to other populations (eg, those without recent MI) is uncertain. Considering the known proarrhythmic properties of disopyramide and the lack of evidence of improved survival for any antiarrhythmic drug in patients without life-threatening arrhythmias, the use of disopyramide as well as other antiarrhythmic agents should be reserved for patients with life-threatening ventricular arrhythmias.

### Indications
Treatment of documented ventricular arrhythmias (eg, sustained ventricular tachycardia) considered to be life-threatening.

### Administration and Dosage
Individualize dosage. Initiate treatment in the hospital.

*Adults:* 400 to 800 mg/day. The recommended dosage for most adults is 600 mg/day. For patients less than 50 kg (110 pounds), give 400 mg/day. Divide the total daily dose and administer every 6 hours in the immediate release form or every 12 hours in the controlled-release form.

In the event of increased anticholinergic side effects, plasma levels of disopyramide should be monitored and the dose of the drug adjusted accordingly. A reduction of the dose by one third, from the recommended 600 mg/day to 400 mg/day, would be reasonable, without changing the dosing interval.

*Children:* Divide daily dosage and administer equal doses every 6 hours or at intervals according to patient needs. Closely monitor plasma levels and therapeutic response. Hospitalize patients during initial treatment and start dose titration at the lower end of the ranges provided below:

| Suggested Total Daily Disopyramide Dosage in Children[1] | |
|---|---|
| Age (years) | Disopyramide (mg/kg/day) |
| < 1 | 10 to 30 |
| 1 to 4 | 10 to 20 |
| 4 to 12 | 10 to 15 |
| 12 to 18 | 6 to 15 |

[1] Prepare a 1 to 10 mg/mL suspension by adding contents of the immediate release capsule to cherry syrup, NF. The resulting suspension, when refrigerated, is stable for 1 month; shake thoroughly before measuring dose. Dispense in an amber glass bottle. Do not use the controlled-release form to prepare the solution.

*Initial loading dose:* For rapid control of ventricular arrhythmia, give an initial loading dose of 300 mg immediate release (200 mg for patients less than 50 kg [110 lbs]). Therapeutic effects are attained in 30 minutes to 3 hours. If there is no response or no evidence of toxicity within 6 hours of the loading dose, 200 mg every 6 hours may be administered instead of the usual 150 mg. If there is no response within 48 hours, discontinue the drug or carefully monitor subsequent doses of 250 or 300 mg every 6 hours.

Do not use the controlled-release form initially if rapid plasma levels are desired.

*Severe refractory ventricular tachycardia:* A limited number of patients have tolerated up to 1600 mg/day (400 mg every 6 hours), resulting in plasma levels up to 9 mcg/mL. Hospitalize patients for close evaluation and continuous monitoring.

*Cardiomyopathy or possible cardiac decompensation:* Do not administer a loading dose, and limit the initial dosage to 100 mg immediate release every 6 to 8 hours. Make subsequent dosage adjustments gradually.

*Renal/Hepatic function impairment:* For patients with moderate renal insufficiency (Ccr greater than 40 mL/min) or hepatic insufficiency, the recommended dosage is 400 mg/day given in divided doses (either 100 mg every 6 hours for immediate release or 200 mg every 12 hours for controlled release).

In severe renal insufficiency (Ccr up to 40 mL/min), the recommended dosage is 100 mg of the immediate release form given at the intervals shown in the table below, with or without an initial loading dose of 150 mg.

| Disopyramide Dosage in Renal Impairment | | | |
| --- | --- | --- | --- |
| Creatinine clearance (mL/min) | Loading dose (mg) | Dose (mg) | Dosage interval (h) |
| 30-40 | 150 | 100 | 8 |
| 15-30 | 150 | 100 | 12 |
| < 15 | 150 | 100 | 24 |

*Transfer to disopyramide:* Use the regular maintenance schedule, without a loading dose, 6 to 12 hours after the last dose of quinidine or 3 to 6 hours after the last dose of procainamide. Where withdrawal of quinidine or procainamide is likely to produce life-threatening arrhythmias, consider hospitalization.

When transferring from immediate to controlled release, start maintenance schedule of controlled release 6 hours after the last dose of immediate release.

**Actions**
*Pharmacology:*
*Mechanism of action* – Disopyramide is a class IA antiarrhythmic agent that decreases the rate of diastolic depolarization (phase 4), decreases the upstroke velocity (phase 0), increases the action potential duration of normal cardiac cells, and prolongs the refractory period (phases 2 and 3). It also decreases the disparity in refractoriness between infarcted and adjacent normally perfused myocardium and does not affect alpha- or beta-adrenergic receptors.

*Pharmacokinetics:*
*Absorption/Distribution* – Following oral administration of immediate-release disopyramide, the drug is rapidly and almost completely (approximately 90%) absorbed. Peak plasma levels usually occur within 2 hours. Therapeutic plasma levels of disopyramide are 2 to 4 mcg/mL. Protein binding is concentration-dependent and varies from 50% to 65%; it is difficult to predict the concentration of the free drug when total drug is measured.

*Metabolism/Excretion* – About 50% is excreted in the urine as the unchanged drug and 30% as metabolites (20% mono-N-dealkyldisopyramide [MND]). The plasma concentration of MND is approximately one-tenth that of disopyramide. The mean plasma half-life is 6.7 hours (range, 4 to 10 hours). In impaired renal function, half-life values ranged from 8 to 18 hours. Therefore, decrease the dose in renal failure to avoid drug accumulation.

*Immediate-release vs controlled-release* – Following multiple doses, steady-state plasma levels of between 2 and 4 mcg/mL were attained following either 150 mg every 6 hours (immediate release) or 300 mg every 12 hours (controlled release).

**Contraindications**

Cardiogenic shock; preexisting second- or third-degree AV block (if no pacemaker is present); congenital QT prolongation; sick sinus syndrome; hypersensitivity to disopyramide.

**Warnings**

*Proarrhythmic effects:* Because of the proarrhythmic effects, use with lesser arrhythmias is generally not recommended.

*Asymptomatic ventricular premature contractions:* Avoid treatment of patients with this condition.

*Survival:* Antiarrhythmic drugs have not been shown to enhance survival in patients with ventricular arrhythmias.

*Negative inotropic properties:*

*Heart failure/hypotension* – May cause or aggravate CHF or produce severe hypotension, especially in patients with depressed systolic function. Do not use in patients with uncompensated or marginally compensated CHF or hypotension unless secondary to cardiac arrhythmia. Treat patients with a history of heart failure with careful attention to the maintenance of cardiac function, including optimal digitalization. If hypotension occurs or CHF worsens, discontinue use; restart at a lower dosage after adequate cardiac compensation has been established.

Do not give a loading dose to patients with myocarditis or other cardiomyopathy; closely monitor initial dosage and subsequent adjustments.

*QRS widening* – QRS widening (greater than 25%), although unusual, may occur; discontinue use in such cases.

*$QT_c$ prolongation* – $QT_c$ prolongation and worsening of the arrhythmia, including ventricular tachycardia and fibrillation, may occur. Patients who have QT prolongation in response to quinidine may be at particular risk. Disopyramide has been associated with torsade de pointes. If QT prolongation greater than 25% is observed and if ectopy continues, monitor closely and consider discontinuing the drug.

*Atrial tachyarrhythmias:* Digitalize patients with atrial flutter or fibrillation prior to administration to ensure that enhancement of AV conduction does not increase ventricular rate beyond acceptable limits.

*Conduction abnormalities:* Use caution in patients with sick sinus syndrome, Wolff-Parkinson-White syndrome or bundle branch block.

*Heart block:* If first-degree heart block develops, reduce dosage. If the block persists, drug continuation must depend upon the benefit compared with the risk of higher degrees of heart block. Development of second- or third-degree AV block or unifascicular, bifascicular, or trifascicular block requires discontinuation of therapy, unless ventricular rate is controlled by a ventricular pacemaker.

*Concomitant antiarrhythmic therapy:* Reserve concomitant use of disopyramide with other class IA antiarrhythmics or propranolol for life-threatening arrhythmias unresponsive to a single agent. Such use may produce serious negative inotropic effects or may excessively prolong conduction, particularly with cardiac decompensation.

*Hypoglycemia:* Hypoglycemia has been reported in rare instances. Monitor blood glucose levels in patients with CHF, chronic malnutrition, hepatic disease, and in those taking drugs which could compromise normal glucoregulatory mechanisms in the absence of food.

*Anticholinergic activity:* Do not use in patients with urinary retention, glaucoma, or myasthenia gravis unless adequate overriding measures are taken. Males with benign prostatic hypertrophy are at particular risk of having urinary retention. In patients with a family history of glaucoma, measure intraocular pressure before initiating therapy.

*Renal function impairment:* Reduce dosage in impaired renal function. Carefully monitor ECG for signs of overdosage. The controlled-release form is not recommended for patients with severe renal insufficiency (Ccr up to 40 mL/min).

*Hepatic function impairment:* Impairment increases plasma half-life; reduce dosage in such patients. Carefully monitor the ECG. Patients with cardiac dysfunction have a higher potential for hepatic impairment.

*Pregnancy:* Category C.

*Lactation:* Disopyramide has been detected in breast milk.

### Precautions
*Potassium imbalance:* Disopyramide may be ineffective in *hypo*kalemia and its toxic effects may be enhanced in *hyper*kalemia. Correct any potassium deficit before instituting therapy.

### Drug Interactions
Drugs that may affect disopyramide include antiarrhythmics, beta blockers, cisapride, clarithromycin, erythromycin, fluoroquinolones, hydantoins, quinidine, thioridazine, rifampin, verapamil, and ziprasidone. Drugs that may be affected by disopyramide include quinidine, anticoagulants, and digoxin.

### Adverse Reactions
The most serious adverse reactions are hypotension and CHF. The most common reactions are anticholinergic and are dose-dependent. These may be transitory, but may be persistent or severe. Urinary retention is the most serious anticholinergic effect. Adverse reactions occurring in 3% or more of patients include urinary retention, frequency and urgency; dizziness; fatigue; headache; nausea; pain; bloating; gas; dry mouth; urinary hesitancy; constipation; blurred vision; dry nose; eyes and throat; muscle weakness; malaise; aches/pain.

# LIDOCAINE HCI

| | |
|---|---|
| **Injection**: (for IM administration) 300 mg/3 mL automatic injection device (*Rx*) | *LidoPen Auto-Injector* (Survival Technology) |
| (for direct IV administration) 1% (10 mg/mL), 2% (20 mg/mL) (*Rx*) | Various, *Xylocaine HCl IV for Cardiac Arrhythmias* (Astra) |
| (for IV admixtures) 10% (100 mg/mL) (*Rx*) | Various |
| (for IV admixtures) 4% (40 mg/mL), 20% (200 mg/mL) (*Rx*) | Various, *Xylocaine HCl IV for Cardiac Arrhythmias* (Astra) |
| (for IV infusion) 0.2% (2 mg/mL), 0.4% (4 mg/mL), 0.8% (8 mg/mL) (*Rx*) | Various |

### Indications
*IV:* Acute management of ventricular arrhythmias occurring during cardiac manipulation, such as cardiac surgery or in relation to acute myocardial infarction (MI).

*IM:* Single doses are justified in the following exceptional circumstances: When ECG equipment is not available to verify the diagnosis but the potential benefits outweigh the possible risks; when facilities for IV administration are not readily available; by the patient in the prehospital phase of suspected acute MI, directed by qualified medical personnel viewing the transmitted ECG.

*Unlabeled uses:* In pediatric patients with cardiac arrest, less than 10% develop ventricular fibrillation, and others develop ventricular tachycardia; the hemodynamically compromised child may develop ventricular couplets or frequent premature ventricular beats. In these cases, administer 1 mg/kg lidocaine by the IV, intraosseous, or endotracheal route. A second 1 mg/kg dose may be given in 10 to 15 minutes. Start a lidocaine infusion if the second dose is required; a third bolus may be needed in 10 to 15 minutes to maintain therapeutic levels.

### Administration and Dosage
*IM:* 300 mg. The deltoid muscle is preferred. Avoid intravascular injection. Use only the 10% solution for IM injection.

The *LidoPen Auto-Injector* unit is for self-administration into deltoid muscle or anterolateral aspect of thigh. Patient instructions are provided with product.

*Replacement therapy* – As soon as possible, change patient to IV lidocaine or to an oral antiarrhythmic preparation for maintenance therapy. However, if necessary, an additional IM injection may be administered after 60 to 90 minutes.

IV: Use only lidocaine injection without preservatives, clearly labeled for IV use. Monitor ECG constantly to avoid potential overdosage and toxicity.

*IV bolus* – IV bolus is used to establish rapid therapeutic blood levels. Continuous IV infusion is necessary to maintain antiarrhythmic effects. The usual dose is 50 to 100 mg, given at a rate of 25 to 50 mg/min. If the initial injection does not produce the desired clinical response, give a second bolus dose after 5 minutes. Give no more than 200 to 300 mg/hour.

*Reduce loading (bolus) doses* – Reduce loading (bolus) doses in patients with congestive heart failure (CHF) or reduced cardiac output and in the elderly. However, some investigators recommend the usual loading dose be administered and only the maintenance dosage be reduced.

*IV continuous infusion* – IV continuous infusion is used to maintain therapeutic plasma levels following loading doses in patients in whom arrhythmias tend to recur and who cannot receive oral antiarrhythmic drugs. Administer at a rate of 1 to 4 mg/min (20 to 50 mcg/kg/min). Reduce maintenance doses in patients with heart failure or liver disease, or who are also receiving other drugs known to decrease clearance of lidocaine or decrease liver blood flow and in patients older than 70 years of age. Reassess the rate of infusion as soon as the cardiac rhythm stabilizes or at the earliest signs of toxicity. Change patients to oral antiarrhythmic agents for maintenance therapy as soon as possible. It is rarely necessary to continue IV infusions for prolonged periods. Use a precision volume control IV set for continuous IV infusion.

*Children* – The American Heart Association's Standards and Guidelines recommend a bolus dose of 1 mg/kg, followed by an infusion of 30 mcg/kg/min. The following dosage has also been suggested:

*Loading dose* – Loading dose, 1 mg/kg/dose given IV or intratracheally every 5 to 10 min to desired effect, maximum total dose 5 mg/kg; Maintenance: 20 to 50 mcg/kg/min.

## Actions

*Pharmacology:* Therapeutic concentrations of lidocaine attenuate phase 4 diastolic depolarization, decrease automaticity and cause a decrease or no change in excitability and membrane responsiveness. Action potential duration and effective refractory period (ERP) of Purkinje fibers and ventricular muscle are decreased, while the ratio of ERP to action potential duration is increased. Lidocaine raises ventricular fibrillation threshold. AV nodal conduction time is unchanged or shortened. Lidocaine increases the electrical stimulation threshold of the ventricle during diastole.

*Pharmacokinetics:*

*Absorption/Distribution* – Lidocaine is ineffective orally; it is most commonly administered IV with an immediate onset (within minutes) and brief duration (10 to 20 minutes) of action following a bolus dose. Continuous IV infusion of lidocaine (1 to 4 mg/min) is necessary to maintain antiarrhythmic effects. Following IM administration, therapeutic serum levels are achieved in 5 to 15 minutes and may persist for up to 2 hours. Higher and more rapid serum levels are achieved by injection into the deltoid muscle. Therapeutic serum levels are 1.5 to 6 mcg/mL; serum levels greater than 6 to 10 mcg/mL are usually toxic. Lidocaine is approximately 50% protein bound (concentration-dependent).

*Metabolism/Excretion* – Extensive biotransformation in the liver (approximately 90%) results in at least 2 active metabolites, monoethylglycinexylidide and glycinexylidide. Lidocaine exhibits a biphasic half-life. The distribution phase is approximately 10 minutes. The elimination half-life is 1.5 to 2 hours; half-life may be 3 hours or more following infusions of more than 24 hours. Any condition that alters liver function, including changes in liver blood flow, which could result from severe CHF or shock, may alter lidocaine kinetics. Less than 10% of the parent drug is excreted unchanged in the urine. Renal elimination plays an important role in the elimination of the metabolites.

### Contraindications

Hypersensitivity to amide local anesthetics; Stokes-Adams syndrome; Wolff-Parkinson-White syndrome; severe degrees of sinoatrial, atrioventricular (AV), or intraventricular block in the absence of an artificial pacemaker.

### Warnings

*Survival:* Prophylactic single dose lidocaine administered in a monitored environment does not appear to affect mortality in the earliest phase of acute MI, and may harm some patients who are later shown not to have suffered an acute MI.

*Constant ECG monitoring:* Constant ECG monitoring is essential for proper administration. Have emergency resuscitative equipment and drugs immediately available.

*IV use:* Signs of excessive depression of cardiac conductivity should be followed by dosage reduction and, if necessary, prompt cessation of IV infusion.

*IM use:* May increase creatine phosphokinase levels. Use of the enzyme determination without isoenzyme separation, as a diagnostic test for acute MI, may be compromised.

*Cardiac effects:* Use with caution and in lower doses in patients with CHF, reduced cardiac output, digitalis toxicity accompanied by AV block and in the elderly.

In sinus bradycardia or incomplete heart block, lidocaine administration for the elimination of ventricular ectopy without prior acceleration in heart rate (eg, by atropine, isoproterenol or electric pacing) may promote more frequent and serious ventricular arrhythmias or complete heart block. Use with caution in patients with hypovolemia and shock, and all forms of heart block.

*Acceleration of ventricular rate* – Acceleration of ventricular rate may occur when administered to patients with atrial flutter or fibrillation.

*Hypersensitivity reactions:* Hypersensitivity reactions may occur. Refer to Management of Acute Hypersensitivity Reactions.

*Renal/Hepatic function impairment:* Use caution with repeated or prolonged use in liver or renal disease; possible toxic accumulation may occur.

*Pregnancy:* Category B.

*Lactation:* Exercise caution when administering to a nursing woman.

*Children:* Safety and efficacy have not been established; reduce dosage. The IM autoinjector device is not recommended in children less than 50 kg.

### Precautions

*Malignant hyperthermia:* Amide local anesthetic administration has been associated with acute onset of fulminant hypermetabolism of skeletal muscle known as malignant hyperthermic crisis. Recognition of early unexplained signs of tachycardia, tachypnea, labile blood pressure, and metabolic acidosis may precede temperature elevation. Successful outcome depends on early diagnosis, prompt discontinuance of the triggering agent and institution of treatment, including oxygen, supportive measures, and IV dantrolene sodium.

### Drug Interactions

Drugs that may affect lidocaine include beta-blockers, cimetidine, procainamide, tocainide, and succinylcholine.

### Adverse Reactions

Significant drug interactions include light-headedness; nervousness; drowsiness; dizziness; apprehension; confusion; mood changes; hallucinations; tremors; convulsions; unconsciousness; hypotension; bradycardia; cardiovascular collapse, which may lead to cardiac arrest; febrile response; soreness/infection at the injection site; venous thrombosis or phlebitis extending from the site of injection; extravasation; vomiting; respiratory depression/arrest.

# PROPAFENONE HCl

| | |
|---|---|
| **Tablets**: 150, 225, and 300 mg (*Rx*) | *Rythmol* (Various, eg Reliant) |
| **Capsules, extended-release**: 225, 325, and 425 mg (*Rx*) | *Rythmol SR* (Reliant) |

**Warning:**
In the National Heart, Lung, and Blood Institute's Cardiac Arrhythmia Suppression Trial (CAST), a long-term, multicenter, randomized, double-blind study in patients with asymptomatic non-life-threatening ventricular arrhythmias who had an MI more than 6 days but less than 2 years previously, an increased rate of death or reversed cardiac arrest rate (7.7%) was seen in patients treated with encainide or flecainide (Class 1C antiarrhythmics) compared with that seen in patients assigned to placebo (3%). The average duration of treatment with encainide or flecainide in this study was 10 months.

The applicability of the CAST results to other populations (eg, those without recent MI) or other antiarrhythmic drugs is uncertain, but at present, it is prudent to consider any 1C antiarrhythmic to have a significant risk in patients with structural heart disease. Given the lack of any evidence that these drugs improve survival, antiarrhythmic agents should generally be avoided in patients with nonlife-threatening ventricular arrhythmias, even if the patients are experiencing unpleasant, but not life-threatening symptoms or signs.

## Indications

Treatment of documented life-threatening ventricular arrhythmias, such as sustained ventricular tachycardia.

*Atrial fibrillation/flutter:*
    *Immediate-release (IR)* – To prolong the time to recurrence of paroxysmal atrial fibrillation/flutter associated with disabling symptoms in patients without structural heart disease.

    *Extended-release (ER)* – To prolong the time to recurrence of symptomatic atrial fibrillation in patients with structural heart disease.

Because of the proarrhythmic effects of propafenone, reserve its use for patients in whom the benefits of treatment outweigh the risks. The use of propafenone is not recommended in patients with less severe ventricular arrhythmias, even if the patients are symptomatic.

## Administration and Dosage

*IR*: Individually titrate on the basis of response and tolerance. Initiate with 150 mg every 8 hours (450 mg/day). Dosage may be increased at a minimum of 3 to 4 day intervals to 225 mg every 8 hours (675 mg/day) and, if necessary, to 300 mg every 8 hours (900 mg/day). The safety and efficacy of dosages exceeding 900 mg/day have not been established. In those patients in whom significant widening of the QRS complex or second- or third-degree AV block occurs, consider dose reduction.

    As with other antiarrhythmics, in the elderly or patients with marked previous myocardial damage, increase dose more gradually during initial treatment phase.

*SR*: Individually titrate on the basis of response and tolerance. Therapy should be initiated with 225 mg given every 12 hours. Dosage may be increased at a minimum of 5-day intervals to 325 mg given every 12 hours. If additional therapeutic effect is needed, the dose may be increased to 425 mg given every 12 hours.

    The SR capsules can be taken with or without food. Do not crush or further divide the contents of the capsule.

## Actions

*Pharmacology*: Propafenone is a Class IC antiarrhythmic with local anesthetic effects and direct stabilizing action on myocardial membranes.

*Pharmacokinetics:*
    *Absorption/Distribution* – Propafenone is nearly completely absorbed after oral administration with peak plasma levels occurring approximately 3.5 hours after adminis-

tration. It exhibits extensive first-pass metabolism resulting in a dose-dependent and dosage-form-dependent absolute bioavailability. Propafenone follows a nonlinear pharmacokinetic disposition presumably due to saturation of first-pass hepatic metabolism as the liver is exposed to higher concentrations of propafenone and shows a very high degree of interindividual variability.

*Metabolism/Excretion* – There are 2 genetically determined patterns of propafenone metabolism. In more than 90% of patients, the drug is rapidly and extensively metabolized with an elimination half-life of 2 to 10 hours. These patients metabolize propafenone into two active metabolites: 5-hydroxypropafenone and N-depropylpropafenone. They both are usually present in concentrations less than 20% of propafenone. The saturable hydroxylation pathway is responsible for the nonlinear pharmacokinetic disposition.

## Contraindications

Uncontrolled CHF; cardiogenic shock; sinoatrial, AV and intraventricular disorders of impulse generation or conduction (eg, sick sinus node syndrome, AV block) in the absence of an artificial pacemaker; bradycardia; marked hypotension; bronchospastic disorders; manifest electrolyte imbalance; hypersensitivity to the drug.

## Warnings

*Mortality:* An excessive mortality or nonfatal cardiac arrest rate was seen in patients treated with encainide or flecainide compared with that seen in patients assigned to carefully matched placebo-treated groups.

*Proarrhythmic effects:* Propafenone may cause new or worsened arrhythmias. Such proarrhythmic effects range from an increase in frequency of PVCs to the development of more severe ventricular tachycardia, ventricular fibrillation or torsade de pointes, which may lead to fatal consequences. It is essential that each patient be evaluated electrocardiographically and clinically prior to, and during therapy to determine whether response to propafenone supports continued use.

*Non-life-threatening arrhythmias:* Use of propafenone is not recommended in patients with less severe ventricular arrhythmias, even if the patients are symptomatic.

*Survival:* There is no evidence from controlled trials that the use of propafenone favorably affects survival or the incidence of sudden death.

*Nonallergic bronchospasm (eg, chronic bronchitis, emphysema):* In general, these patients should not receive propafenone or other agents with beta-adrenergic blocking activity.

*CHF:* New or worsened CHF has occurred in 3.7% of patients.

As propafenone exerts both beta blockade and a (dose-related) negative inotropic effect on cardiac muscle, fully compensate patients with CHF before receiving propafenone. If CHF worsens, discontinue propafenone unless CHF is due to the cardiac arrhythmia and, if indicated, restart at a lower dosage only after adequate cardiac compensation has been established.

*Conduction disturbances:* Propafenone causes first-degree AV block. Average PR interval prolongation and increases in QRS duration are closely correlated with dosage increases and concomitant increases in propafenone plasma concentrations. Development of second- or third-degree AV block requires a reduction in dosage or discontinuation of propafenone. Bundle branch block and intraventricular conduction delay have occurred. Bradycardia has also occurred. Patients with sick sinus node syndrome should not be treated with propafenone.

*Effects on pacemaker threshold:* Pacing and sensing thresholds of artificial pacemakers may be altered. Monitor and program pacemakers accordingly during therapy.

*Hematologic disturbances:* Agranulocytosis with fever and sepsis has occurred. Unexplained fever or decrease in white cell count, particularly during the first 3 months of therapy, warrants consideration of possible agranulocytosis/granulocytopenia.

*Renal function impairment:* A considerable percentage of propafenone metabolites are excreted in the urine. Administer cautiously in impaired renal function.

*Hepatic function impairment:* Propafenone is highly metabolized by the liver; administer cautiously to patients with impaired hepatic function. The clearance of propafenone is reduced and the elimination half-life increased in patients with significant hepatic dysfunction. The dose of propafenone should be approximately 20% to 30% of the dose given to patients with normal hepatic function.

*Elderly:* Because of the possible increased risk of impaired hepatic or renal function in this age group, use with caution. The effective dose may be lower in these patients.

*Pregnancy:* Category C.

*Lactation:* Propafenone is excreted in breast milk. Decide whether to discontinue nursing or to discontinue the drug, taking into account the importance of the drug to the mother.

*Children:* The safety and efficacy in children have not been established.

## Precautions

*Elevated ANA titers:* Positive ANA titers have occurred. They have been reversible upon cessation of treatment and may disappear even with continued therapy. Carefully evaluate patients who develop an abnormal ANA test and, if persistent or worsening elevation of ANA titers is detected, consider discontinuing therapy.

*Renal/Hepatic changes:* Renal changes have been observed in the rat following 6 months of oral administration of propafenone at doses of 180 and 360 mg/kg/day (2 to 4 times the maximum recommended human dose). Both inflammatory and noninflammatory changes in the renal tubules with accompanying interstitial nephritis were observed.

*Neuromuscular dysfunction:* Exacerbation of myasthenia gravis has been reported during propafenone therapy.

## Drug Interactions

Drugs that inhibit CYP2D6, CYP1A2, and CYP3A4 might lead to increased plasma levels of propafenone. Drugs that may affect propafenone include local anesthetics, cimetidine, quinidine, cisapride, rifampin, ritonavir, and SSRIs. Drugs that may be affected by propafenone include anticoagulants, beta blockers, cisapride, cyclosporine, desipramine, digoxin, mexiletine, and theophylline.

## Adverse Reactions

Adverse reactions occurring in at least 3% of patients include angina; first-degree AV block; CHF; intraventricular conduction delay; palpitations; proarrhythmia; ventricular tachycardia; dizziness; fatigue; headache; constipation; dyspepsia; nausea/vomiting; unusual taste; blurred vision; dyspnea. About 20% of patients discontinued treatment due to adverse reactions.

# MEXILETINE HYDROCHLORIDE

| **Capsules:** 150, 200, and 250 mg (*Rx*) | Various, *Mexitil* (Boehringer Ingelheim) |
|---|---|

**Warning:**
> *Mortality:* In the National Heart, Lung and Blood Institute's Cardiac Arrhythmia
> Suppression Trial (CAST), a long-term, multicentered, randomized, double-
> blind study in patients with asymptomatic non-life-threatening ventricular
> arrhythmias who had an MI more than 6 days but less than 2 years previously,
> an excessive mortality or nonfatal cardiac arrest rate was seen in patients
> treated with encainide or flecainide (7.7%) compared with that seen in patients
> assigned to matched placebo-treated groups (3%). The average duration of
> treatment with encainide or flecainide in this study was 10 months.
>
> The applicability of these results to other populations (eg, those without recent
> MI) is uncertain. Considering the known proarrhythmic properties of mexiletine
> and the lack of evidence of improved survival for any antiarrhythmic drug in
> patients without life-threatening arrhythmias, the use of mexiletine as well as
> other antiarrhythmic agents should be reserved for patients with life-threatening
> ventricular arrhythmia.

### Indications
Treatment of documented, life-threatening ventricular arrhythmias, such as sustained
ventricular tachycardia. Because of the proarrhythmic effects of mexiletine, use with
lesser arrhythmias is generally not recommended.

### Administration and Dosage
Individualize dosage. Administer with food or antacids.

Perform clinical and ECG evaluation as needed to determine whether the desired antiarrhythmic effect has been obtained and to guide titration and dose adjustment.

*Initial dose:* 200 mg every 8 hours when rapid control of arrhythmia is not essential,
with a minimum of 2 to 3 days between adjustments. Adjust dose in 50 or 100 mg
increments.

Control can be achieved in most patients with 200 to 300 mg given every 8 hours.
If satisfactory response is not achieved at 300 mg every 8 hours, and the patient tolerates mexiletine well, try 400 mg every 8 hours. The severity of CNS side effects
increases with total daily dose; do not exceed 1200 mg/day.

*Renal/hepatic function impairment:* In general, patients with renal failure will require the
usual doses of mexiletine. Patients with severe liver disease, however, may require
lower doses and must be monitored closely. Similarly, marked right-sided CHF can
reduce hepatic metabolism and reduce the dose needed.

*Loading dose:* When rapid control of ventricular arrhythmia is essential, administer an
initial loading dose of 400 mg, followed by a 200 mg dose in 8 hours. Onset of therapeutic effect is usually observed within 30 minutes to 2 hours.

*Twice-daily dosage:* If adequate suppression is achieved on a dose of 300 mg or less every
8 hours, the same total daily dose may be given in divided doses every 12 hours
with monitoring. The dose may be adjusted to a maximum of 450 mg every 12 hours.

*Transferring to mexiletine:* When transferring from other Class I oral antiarrhythmics to
mexiletine, based on theoretical considerations, initiate with a 200 mg dose, and
titrate to response as described above, 6 to 12 hours after the last dose of quinidine sulfate, 3 to 6 hours after the last dose of procainamide, 6 to 12 hours after
the last disopyramide dose or 8 to 12 hours after the last tocainide dose.

Hospitalize patients in whom withdrawal of the previous antiarrhythmic agent
is likely to produce life-threatening arrhythmias.

When transferring from lidocaine to mexiletine, stop the lidocaine infusion when
the first oral dose of mexiletine is administered. Maintain the IV line until suppres-

sion of the arrhythmia appears satisfactory. Consider the similarity of adverse effects of lidocaine and mexiletine and the additive potential.

## Actions

*Pharmacology:*

*Mechanism* – Structurally like lidocaine, mexiletine inhibits the inward sodium current, thus reducing the rate of rise of the action potential, Phase 0. Mexiletine decreases the effective refractory period (ERP) in Purkinje fibers. The decrease in ERP is of lesser magnitude than the decrease in action potential duration (APD), with a resulting increase in ERP/APD ratio.

*Hemodynamic effects* – Small decreases in cardiac output and increases in systemic vascular resistance have occurred, with no significant negative inotropic effect. Blood pressure and pulse rate remain essentially unchanged. Mild depression of myocardial function has been observed following IV mexiletine (dosage form not available in the US) in patients with cardiac disease.

*Electrophysiology* – Mexiletine is a local anesthetic and a Class IB antiarrhythmic compound with electrophysiologic properties similar to lidocaine.

*Pharmacokinetics:*

*Absorption/Distribution* – Mexiletine is well absorbed (approximately 90%) from the GI tract. The absorption rate is reduced in clinical situations (such as acute MI) in which gastric emptying time is increased.

Peak blood levels are reached in 2 to 3 hours. The therapeutic range is approximately 0.5 to 2 mcg/mL. An increase in the frequency of CNS adverse effects has been observed when plasma levels exceed 2 mcg/mL. It is 50% to 60% bound to plasma protein with a volume of distribution of 5 to 7 L/kg.

*Metabolism/Excretion* – Mexiletine is metabolized in the liver primarily by CYP2D6, although it is a substrate for CYP1A2. The most active minor metabolite is N-methylmexiletine, which is less than 20% as potent as mexiletine. Urinary excretion of N-methylmexiletine is less than 0.5%.

In healthy subjects, the elimination half-life is 10 to 12 hours. Hepatic impairment prolongs it to a mean of 25 hours. Little change in half-life occurs with reduced renal function. In eight patients with creatinine clearance less than 10 mL/min, the mean plasma elimination half-life was 15.7 hours; in seven patients with creatinine clearance between 11 and 40 mL/min, the mean half-life was 13.4 hours.

## Contraindications

Cardiogenic shock; preexisting second- or third-degree AV block (if no pacemaker).

## Warnings

*Proarrhythmia:* Mexiletine can worsen arrhythmias; it is uncommon in patients with less serious arrhythmias (frequent premature beats or nonsustained ventricular tachycardia) but is of greater concern in patients with life-threatening arrhythmias, such as sustained ventricular tachycardia.

*Survival:* Antiarrhythmic drugs have not been shown to enhance survival in patients with ventricular arrhythmias.

*Initial therapy:* As with other antiarrhythmics, initiate therapy in the hospital.

*Mortality:* Considering the known proarrhythmic properties of mexiletine and the lack of evidence of improved survival for any antiarrhythmic drug in patients without life-threatening arrhythmias, the use of mexiletine should be reserved for patients with life-threatening ventricular arrhythmia.

*Hepatic function impairment:* Since mexiletine is metabolized in the liver, and hepatic impairment prolongs the elimination half-life, carefully monitor patients with liver disease. Observe caution in patients with hepatic dysfunction secondary to CHF.

Abnormal liver function tests have been reported, some in the first few weeks of therapy with mexiletine. Most have occurred along with CHF or ischemia; their relationship to mexiletine has not been established.

*Pregnancy: Category C.*

*Lactation:* Mexiletine appears in breast milk in concentrations similar to those in plasma. If mexiletine is essential, consider alternative infant feeding.

*Children:* Safety and efficacy in children have not been established.

## Precautions

*Cardiovascular effects:* If a ventricular pacemaker is operative, patients with second- or third-degree heart block may be treated with mexiletine if continuously monitored. Exercise caution in such patients or in patients with preexisting sinus node dysfunction or intraventricular conduction abnormalities.

Use with caution in patients with hypotension and severe CHF.

*AST elevation and liver injury:* Elevations of AST more than 3 times the upper limit of normal occurred in about 1% of both mexiletine-treated and control patients.

Rare instances of severe liver injury, including hepatic necrosis, have been reported. Carefully evaluate patients in whom an abnormal liver test has occurred, or who have signs or symptoms suggesting liver dysfunction.

*Hematologic effects:* Marked leukopenia (neutrophils less than $1000/mm^3$) or agranulocytosis were seen in 0.06%; milder depressions of leukocytes were seen in 0.08% and thrombocytopenia was observed in 0.16%. Many of these patients were seriously ill and were receiving concomitant medications with known hematologic adverse effects. Rechallenge with mexiletine in several cases was negative. If significant hematologic changes are observed, carefully evaluate the patient and, if warranted, discontinue mexiletine. Blood counts usually return to normal within 1 month of discontinuation.

*CNS effects:* Convulsions occurred in about 2 of 1000 patients. Convulsions occurred in patients with and without a history of seizures. Use with caution in patients with a known seizure disorder.

*Urinary pH:* Avoid concurrent drugs or diets which may markedly alter urinary pH. Minor fluctuations in urinary pH associated with normal diet do not affect mexiletine excretion.

## Drug Interactions

Drugs that may affect mexiletine include aluminum-magnesium hydroxide, atropine, narcotics, cimetidine, fluvoxamine, hydantoins, metoclopramide, propafenone, rifampin, urinary acidifiers, and urinary alkalinizers.

Drugs that may be affected by mexiletine include cimetidine, caffeine, and theophylline.

*CYP450 system:* Because mexiletine is a substrate for CYP2D6 and CYP1A2, inhibition or induction of either of these enzymes would be expected to alter mexiletine concentrations.

## Adverse Reactions

The most frequent adverse reactions were upper GI distress, tremor, lightheadedness, and coordination difficulties. These reactions were generally not serious, dose-related, and reversible if the dosage was reduced, if the drug was taken with food or antacids or if it was discontinued.

Other adverse events occurring in at least 3% of patients include palpitations, chest pain, nervousness, changes in sleep habits, headache, blurred vision/visual disturbances, paresthesias/numbness, weakness, fatigue, diarrhea, constipation, rash, nonspecific edema, dyspnea/respiratory.

*Postmarketing:* There have been isolated, spontaneous reports of pulmonary changes including pulmonary infiltration and pulmonary fibrosis during mexiletine therapy with or without other drugs or diseases that are known to produce pulmonary toxicity.

# FLECAINIDE ACETATE

**Tablets:** 50, 100, and 150 mg *(Rx)*                    *Tambocor* (3M Pharm)

**Warning:**

*Mortality:* Flecainide was included in the National Heart Lung and Blood Institute's Cardiac Arrhythmia Suppression Trial (CAST), a long-term, multicenter, randomized, double-blind study in patients with asymptomatic non-life-threatening ventricular arrhythmias who had an MI more than 6 days but less than 2 years previously. An excessive mortality or nonfatal cardiac arrest rate was seen in patients treated with flecainide compared with that seen in patients assigned to a carefully matched placebo-treated group. This rate was 5.1% for flecainide and 2.3% for the matched placebo. The average duration of treatment with flecainide in this study was 10 months.

The applicability of the CAST results to other populations (eg, those without recent MI) is uncertain, but at present, it is prudent to consider the risks of Class IC agents (including flecainide), coupled with the lack of any evidence of improved survival, generally unacceptable in patients without life-threatening ventricular arrhythmias, even if the patients are experiencing unpleasant, but not life-threatening, symptoms or signs.

*Ventricular proarrhythmic effects in patients with atrial fibrillation/flutter:* A review of the world literature revealed reports of 568 patients treated with oral flecainide for paroxysmal atrial fibrillation/flutter (PAF). Ventricular tachycardia was experienced in 0.4% of these patients. Of 19 patients in the literature with chronic atrial fibrillation (CAF), 10.5% experienced ventricular tachycardia (VT) or ventricular fibrillation (VF). Flecainide is not recommended for use in patients with CAF. Case reports of ventricular proarrhythmic effects in patients treated with flecainide for atrial fibrillation/flutter have included increased premature ventricular contractions (PVCs), VT, VF, and death.

As with other Class I agents, patients treated with flecainide for atrial flutter have been reported with 1:1 atrioventricular conduction due to slowing the atrial rate. A paradoxical increase in the ventricular rate also may occur in patients with atrial fibrillation who receive flecainide. Concomitant negative chronotropic therapy such as digoxin or beta-blockers may lower the risk of this complication.

## Indications

*Atrial fibrillation:* For the prevention of paroxysmal atrial fibrillation/flutter (PAF) associated with disabling symptoms and paroxysmal supraventricular tachycardias (PSVT), including atrioventricular nodal reentrant tachycardia, atrioventricular reentrant tachycardia, and other supraventricular tachycardias of unspecified mechanism associated with disabling symptoms in patients without structural heart disease.

*Ventricular arrhythmias:* Prevention of documented life-threatening ventricular arrhythmias, such as sustained ventricular tachycardia.

Not recommended in patients with less severe ventricular arrhythmias even if the patients are symptomatic. Because of proarrhythmic effects of flecainide, reserve use for patients in whom benefits outweigh risks.

## Administration and Dosage

For patients with sustained ventricular tachycardia, initiate therapy in the hospital and monitor rhythm.

Do not increase dosage more frequently than once every 4 days, because optimal effect may not be achieved during the first 2 to 3 days of therapy.

An occasional patient not adequately controlled by (or intolerant of) a dose given at 12-hour intervals may be dosed at 8-hour intervals.

Once the arrhythmia is controlled, it may be possible to reduce the dose, as necessary, to minimize side effects or effects on conduction.

*PSVT and PAF:* The recommended starting dose is 50 mg every 12 hours. Doses may be increased in increments of 50 mg twice daily every 4 days until efficacy is achieved. For PAF patients, a substantial increase in efficacy without a substantial increase in discontinuation for adverse experiences may be achieved by increasing the flecainide dose from 50 to 100 mg twice/day. The maximum recommended dose for patients with paroxysmal supraventricular arrhythmias is 300 mg/day.

*Sustained ventricular tachycardia:*
Initial dose – 100 mg every 12 hours. Increase in 50 mg increments twice daily every 4 days until effective. Most patients do not require more than 150 mg every 12 hours (300 mg/day). Maximum dose is 400 mg/day.

Use of higher initial doses and more rapid dosage adjustments have resulted in an increased incidence of proarrhythmic events and CHF, particularly during the first few days of dosing. A loading dose is not recommended.

*CHF or MI* – Use cautiously in patients with a history of CHF or myocardial dysfunction (see Warnings).

*Renal function impairment:* In severe renal impairment (Ccr 35 mL/min/1.73 m$^2$ or less), the initial dosage is 100 mg once daily (or 50 mg twice/day). Frequent plasma level monitoring is required to guide dosage adjustments. In patients with less severe renal disease, initial dosage is 100 mg every 12 hours. Increase dosage cautiously at intervals greater than 4 days, observing the patient closely for signs of adverse cardiac effects or other toxicity. It may take more than 4 days before a new steady-state plasma level is reached following a dosage change. Monitor plasma levels to guide dosage adjustments.

*Transfer to flecainide:* Theoretically, when transferring patients from another antiarrhythmic to flecainide, allow at least 2 to 4 plasma half-lives to elapse for the drug being discontinued before starting flecainide at the usual dosage. Consider hospitalization of patients in whom withdrawal of a previous antiarrhythmic is likely to produce life-threatening arrhythmias.

*Administration with amiodarone:* When flecainide is given in the presence of amiodarone, reduce the usual flecainide dose by 50% and monitor the patient closely for adverse effects. Plasma level monitoring is strongly recommended to guide dosage with such combination therapy.

*Plasma level monitoring:* The majority of patients treated successfully had trough plasma levels between 0.2 and 1 mcg/mL. The probability of adverse experiences, especially cardiac, may increase with higher trough plasma levels, especially levels greater than 1 mcg/mL. Monitor trough plasma levels periodically, especially in patients with severe or moderate chronic renal failure or severe hepatic disease and CHF, as drug elimination may be slower.

### Actions
*Pharmacology:* Flecainide has local anesthetic activity and belongs to the membrane stabilizing (Class I) group of antiarrhythmic agents; it has electrophysiologic effects characteristic of the IC class of antiarrhythmics.

*Pharmacokinetics:*
*Absorption/Distribution* – Oral absorption is nearly complete. Peak plasma levels are attained at approximately 3 hours. The plasma half-life ranges from 12 to 27 hours after multiple oral doses. Steady-state levels are approached in 3 to 5 days; once at steady-state, no accumulation occurs during chronic therapy. Plasma levels are approximately proportional to dose. In patients with congestive heart failure (CHF; NYHA class III), the rate of flecainide elimination from plasma is moderately slower than for healthy subjects. Plasma protein binding is about 40% and is independent of plasma drug level over the range of 0.015 to about 3.4 mcg/mL.

*Metabolism/Excretion* – About 30% of a single oral dose (range, 10% to 50%) is excreted in urine unchanged. The two major urinary metabolites are meta-O-dealkylated flecainide (active, but about as potent) and the meta-O-dealkylated lactam (inactive). These two metabolites (primarily conjugated) account for most of the remaining portion of the dose. With increasing renal impairment, the extent of unchanged drug in urine is reduced and the half-life is prolonged. Hemodialysis removes only about 1% of an oral dose as unchanged flecainide.

**Contraindications**

Preexisting second- or third-degree AV block, right bundle branch block when associated with a left hemiblock (bifascicular block), unless a pacemaker is present to sustain the cardiac rhythm if complete heart block occurs; recent myocardial infarction (MI); presence of cardiogenic shock; hypersensitivity to the drug.

**Warnings**

*Mortality:* An excessive mortality or nonfatal cardiac arrest rate was seen in patients treated with flecainide compared with that seen in a carefully matched placebo-treated group.

*Ventricular proarrhythmic effects in patients with atrial fibrillation/flutter:* Flecainide is not recommended for use in patients with chronic atrial fibrillation. Case reports of ventricular proarrhythmic effects in patients treated with flecainide for atrial fibrillation/flutter have included increased premature ventricular contractions (PVCs), ventricular tachycardia (VT), ventricular fibrillation (VF), and death.

*Non-life-threatening ventricular arrhythmias:* It is prudent to consider the risks of Class IC agents, coupled with the lack of any evidence of improved survival, generally unacceptable in patients whose ventricular arrhythmias are not life-threatening, even if the patients are experiencing unpleasant but not life-threatening symptoms or signs.

*Proarrhythmic effects:* Flecainide can cause new or worsened arrhythmias. Such proarrhythmic effects range from an increase in frequency of PVCs to the development of more severe ventricular tachycardia.

*Sick sinus syndrome:* Use only with extreme caution; the drug may cause sinus bradycardia, sinus pause, or sinus arrest. The frequency probably increases with higher trough plasma levels.

*Heart failure:* Flecainide has a negative inotropic effect and may cause or worsen CHF, particularly in patients with cardiomyopathy, preexisting severe heart failure (NYHA functional class III or IV), or low ejection fractions (less than 30%). The initial dosage should be no more than 100 mg twice/day; monitor patients carefully. Give close attention to maintenance of cardiac function, including optimal digitalis, diuretic or other therapy. Where CHF has developed or worsened during treatment, the time of onset has ranged from a few hours to several months after starting therapy. Some patients who develop reduced myocardial function while on flecainide can continue with adjustment of digitalis or diuretics; others may require dosage reduction or discontinuation of flecainide. When feasible, monitor plasma flecainide levels. Keep trough plasma levels less than 1 mcg/mL.

*Cardiac conduction:* Flecainide slows cardiac conduction in most patients to produce dose-related increases in PR, QRS, and QT intervals. The degree of lengthening of PR and QRS intervals does not predict either efficacy or the development of cardiac adverse effects. Patients may develop new first-degree AV heart block. Use caution and consider dose reductions. The JT interval (QT minus QRS) only widens approximately 4% on the average. Rare cases of torsade de pointes-type arrhythmias have occurred.

If second- or third-degree AV block, or right bundle branch block associated with a left hemiblock occurs, discontinue therapy unless a ventricular pacemaker is in place to ensure an adequate ventricular rate.

*Electrolyte disturbance:* Hypokalemia or hyperkalemia may alter the effects of Class I antiarrhythmic drugs. Correct preexisting hypokalemia or hyperkalemia before administration.

*Effects on pacemaker thresholds:* Flecainide increases endocardial pacing thresholds and may suppress ventricular escape rhythms. These effects are reversible. Use with caution in patients with permanent pacemakers or temporary pacing electrodes. Do not administer to patients with existing poor thresholds or nonprogrammable pacemakers unless suitable pacing rescue is available.

*Urinary pH:* Flecainide elimination is altered by urinary pH; alkalinization decreases, and acidification increases flecainide renal excretion.

*Hepatic function impairment:* Because flecainide elimination from plasma can be markedly slower in patients with significant hepatic impairment, do not use in such patients unless the potential benefits outweigh the risks. If used, make dosage increases very cautiously when plasma levels have plateaued (after more than 4 days).

*Elderly:* Patients up to 80 years of age and above have been safely treated with usual doses.

*Pregnancy:* Category C.

*Lactation:* Flecainide is excreted in breast milk; determine whether to discontinue nursing or discontinue the drug, taking into account the importance of the drug to the mother.

*Children:* Safety and efficacy for use in children younger than 18 years of age have not been established.

Based on several studies flecainide appears to be beneficial in treating supraventricular and ventricular arrhythmias in children. Elimination half-life is shorter and volume of distribution is smaller.

### Drug Interactions

Drugs that may affect flecainide include amiodarone, cimetidine, cisapride, disopyramide, propranolol, ritonavir, urinary acidifiers/alkalinizers, and verapamil. Smoking may also have an effect. Drugs that may be affected by flecainide include cisapride, propranolol, and digoxin.

### Adverse Reactions

Adverse interactions occurring in at least 3% of patients include dizziness; dyspnea; headache; nausea; fatigue; palpitation; chest pain; asthenia; tremor; constipation; edema; abdominal pain; visual disturbances.

In post-MI patients with asymptomatic PVCs and nonsustained ventricular tachycardia, flecainide therapy was associated with a 5.1% rate of death and nonfatal cardiac arrest, compared with a 2.3% rate in a matched placebo group.

# BRETYLIUM TOSYLATE

| | |
|---|---|
| **Injection:** 50 mg/mL (*Rx*) | Various, *Bretylol* (DuPont Critical Care) |
| 2 mg/mL (500 mg/vial) in 5% dextrose, 4 mg/mL (1,000 mg/vial) in 5% dextrose (*Rx*) | Various |

### Indications

For prophylaxis and therapy of ventricular fibrillation.

In the treatment of life-threatening ventricular arrhythmias (ie, ventricular tachycardia) which have failed to respond to first-line antiarrhythmic agents (eg, lidocaine).

*Unlabeled uses:* Bretylium is a second-line agent following lidocaine in the protocol for advanced cardiac life support during CPR. For resistant VF and VT (after lidocaine, defibrillation, and procainamide failures), give bretylium 5 to 10 mg/kg IV; repeat as needed up to 30 mg/kg; use a bolus every 15 to 30 minutes, infusion 1 to 2 mg/min. For life-threatening arrhythmia use an undiluted infusion of 1 g/250 mL.

### Administration and Dosage

For short-term use only.

Keep patient supine during therapy or closely observe for postural hypotension. The optimal dose has not been determined. Dosages greater than 40 mg/kg/day have been used without apparent adverse effect. As soon as possible, and when indicated, change patient to an oral antiarrhythmic agent for maintenance therapy.

Immediate life-threatening ventricular arrhythmias (eg, ventricular fibrillation, hemo-dynamically unstable ventricular tachycardia): Administer undiluted, 5 mg/kg by rapid IV injection. If ventricular fibrillation persists, increase dosage to 10 mg/kg and repeat as necessary.

*Maintenance:* For continuous suppression, administer the diluted solution by continu-ous IV infusion at 1 to 2 mg/min. Alternatively, infuse the diluted solution at a dos-age of 5 to 10 mg/kg over more than 8 minutes, every 6 hours. More rapid infusion may cause nausea and vomiting.

*Other ventricular arrhythmias:*
     *IV* – Dilute before administration. Administer 5 to 10 mg/kg by IV infusion over more than 8 minutes. More rapid infusion may cause nausea and vomiting. Give subsequent doses at 1 to 2 hour intervals if the arrhythmia persists. For mainte-nance therapy, the same dosage may be administered every 6 hours, or a constant infusion of 1 to 2 mg/min may be given.
     *IM* – 5 to 10 mg/kg undiluted. Do not dilute prior to injection. Give subsequent doses at 1 to 2 hour intervals if the arrhythmia persists. Thereafter, maintain with same dosage every 6 to 8 hours.
          Do not give more than 5 mL in any one site. Do not inject into or near a major nerve; vary injection sites. Repeated injection into the same site may cause atro-phy and necrosis of muscle tissue, fibrosis, vascular degeneration, and inflammatory changes.

*Children:*  The following dosages have been suggested.
     *Acute ventricular fibrillation* – 5 mg/kg/dose IV, followed by 10 mg/kg at 15- to 30-minute intervals, maximum total dose 30 mg/kg. Maintenance: 5 to 10 mg/kg/dose every 6 hours.
     *Other ventricular arrhythmias* – 5 to 10 mg/kg/dose every 6 hours.

## Actions

*Pharmacology:* Bretylium tosylate inhibits norepinephrine release by depressing adrener-gic nerve terminal excitability, inducing a chemical sympathectomy-like state. Bretylium blocks the release of norepinephrine in response to neuron stimulation. Peripheral adrenergic blockade causes orthostatic hypotension but has less effect on supine blood pressure. It has a positive inotropic effect on the myocardium.

*Pharmacokinetics:* Peak plasma concentration and peak hypotensive effects are seen within 1 hour of IM administration. However, suppression of premature ventricu-lar beats is not maximal until 6 to 9 hours after dosing, when mean plasma concen-tration declines to less than 50% of peak level. Antifibrillatory effects occur within minutes of an IV injection. Suppression of ventricular tachycardia and other ven-tricular arrhythmias develops more slowly, usually 20 minutes to 2 hours after par-enteral administration.

The terminal half-life ranges from 6.9 to 8.1 hours. During dialysis, a 2-fold increase in clearance occurs. The drug is eliminated intact by the kidneys. Approxi-mately 70% to 80% of an IM dose is excreted in the urine during the first 24 hours, with an additional 10% excreted over the next 3 days.

## Warnings

*Hypotension:* Hypotension (postural) occurs regularly in about 50% of patients while they are supine, manifested by dizziness, light-headedness, vertigo, or faintness. Tolerance occurs unpredictably but may be present after several days. Hypotension with supine systolic pressure above 75 mm Hg need not be treated unless symp-tomatic. If supine systolic pressure falls below 75 mm Hg, infuse dopamine or nor-epinephrine to increase blood pressure; use dilute solution and monitor blood pressure closely because pressor effects are enhanced by bretylium. Perform volume expansion with blood or plasma and correct dehydration where appropriate.

*Transient hypertension and increased frequency of arrhythmias:* Transient hypertension and increased frequency of arrhythmias may occur due to initial release of norepin-ephrine from adrenergic postganglionic nerve terminals.

*Fixed cardiac output:* Avoid use with fixed cardiac output because severe hypotension may result from a fall in peripheral resistance without a compensatory increase in cardiac output. If survival is threatened by arrhythmia, the drug may be used, but give vasoconstrictive catecholamines promptly if severe hypotension occurs.

*Renal function impairment:* Because the drug is excreted principally via the kidney, increase the dosage interval in patients with impaired renal function.

*Pregnancy: Category* C. Reduced uterine blood flow with fetal hypoxia (bradycardia) is a potential risk. Give to a pregnant woman only if clearly needed.

*Children:* Safety and efficacy for use in children have not been established.

**Drug Interactions**
Drugs that may affect bretylium include catecholamines and digoxin.

**Adverse Reactions**
Adverse reactions occurring in at least 3% of patients include hypotension and postural hypotension; nausea and vomiting, primarily after rapid IV administration.

## AMIODARONE HCl

| **Tablets**: 200 and 400 mg (*Rx*) | Various, *Cordarone* (Wyeth-Ayerst), *Pacerone* (Upsher Smith) |
|---|---|
| **Injection**: 50 mg/mL (*Rx*) | *Cordarone* (Wyeth-Ayerst) |

**Indications**
*Ventricular arrhythmias:*
Oral – Only for treatment of the following documented life-threatening recurrent ventricular arrhythmias that do not respond to documented adequate doses of other antiarrhythmics or when alternative agents are not tolerated:
1.) Recurrent ventricular fibrillation (VF).
2.) Recurrent hemodynamically unstable ventricular tachycardia (VT).

*Parenteral* – Initiation of treatment and prophylaxis of frequently recurring VF and hemodynamically unstable VT in patients refractory to other therapy. It can also be used to treat patients with VT/VF for whom oral amiodarone is indicated, but who are unable to take oral medication.

During or after treatment with IV amiodarone, patients may be transferred to oral amiodarone therapy. Use IV amiodarone for acute treatment until the patient's ventricular arrhythmias are stabilized. Most patients require this therapy for 48 to 96 hours, but IV amiodarone may be given safely for longer periods if needed.

**Administration and Dosage**
In order to ensure that an antiarrhythmic effect will be observed without waiting several months, loading doses are required. Individual patient titration is suggested.

*Life-threatening ventricular arrhythmias (ventricular fibrillation or hemodynamically unstable ventricular tachycardia):* Administer the loading dose in a hospital. Loading doses of 800 to 1600 mg/day are required for 1 to 3 weeks (occasionally longer) until initial therapeutic response occurs. Administer in divided doses with meals for total daily doses of at least 1000 mg, or when GI intolerance occurs. If side effects become excessive, reduce the dose. Elimination of recurrence of ventricular fibrillation and tachycardia usually occurs within 1 to 3 weeks, along with reduction in complex and total ventricular ectopic beats.

When starting amiodarone therapy, attempt to gradually discontinue prior antiarrhythmic drugs. When adequate arrhythmia control is achieved, or if side effects become prominent, reduce dose to 600 to 800 mg/day for 1 month and then to the maintenance dose, usually 400 mg/day. Some patients may require larger maintenance doses, up to 600 mg/day, and some can be controlled on lower doses.

*Concurrent antiarrhythmic agents* – In general, reserve the combination of amiodarone with other antiarrhythmic therapy for patients with life-threatening arrhythmias who are incompletely responsive to a single agent or incompletely responsive to amiodarone. During transfer to amiodarone, reduce the dose levels of previously administered agents by 30% to 50% several days after the addition of amiodarone when arrhythmia suppression should be beginning. Review the continued need for the other antiarrhythmic agent after the effects of amiodarone have been established, and attempt discontinuation. If the treatment is continued, carefully monitor these patients for adverse effects, especially conduction disturbances and exacerbation of tachyarrhythmias, as amiodarone is continued. In amiodarone-treated patients who require additional antiarrhythmic therapy, the initial dose of such agents should be approximately 50% of the usual recommended dose.

*Parenteral:* Amiodarone shows considerable interindividual variation in response. Thus, although a starting dose adequate to suppress life-threatening arrhythmias is needed, close monitoring with adjustment of dose as needed is essential. The recommended starting dose of amiodarone IV is as follows.

| Amiodarone IV Dose Recommendations During the First 24 Hours | |
| --- | --- |
| Loading infusions | |
| *First* rapid | 150 mg over the *first* 10 minutes (15 mg/min). Add 3 mL amiodarone IV (150 mg) to 100 mL D5W (concentration, 1.5 mg/mL). Infuse 100 mL/10 min. |
| *Followed by* slow | 360 mg over the *next* 6 hours (1 mg/min). Add 18 mL amiodarone IV (900 mg) to 500 mL D5W (concentration, 1.8 mg/mL). |
| Maintenance infusion | 540 mg over the *remaining* 18 hours (0.5 mg/min). Decrease the rate of the slow loading infusion to 0.5 mg/min. |

After the first 24 hours, continue the maintenance infusion rate of 0.5 mg/min (720 mg/24 hours) utilizing a concentration of 1 to 6 mg/mL. In the event of breakthrough episodes of VF or hemodynamically unstable VT, 150 mg supplemental infusions of amiodarone IV mixed in 100 mL D5W may be given. Administer such infusions over 10 minutes to minimize the potential for hypotension. The rate of the maintenance infusion may be increased to achieve effective arrhythmia suppression.

The first 24-hour dose may be individualized for each patient; however, in controlled clinical trials, mean daily doses greater than 2100 mg were associated with an increased risk of hypotension. The initial infusion rate should not exceed 30 mg/min.

Based on the experience from clinical studies, a maintenance infusion of up to 0.5 mg/min can be cautiously continued for 2 to 3 weeks regardless of the patient's age, renal function, or left ventricular function. There has been limited experience in patients receiving amiodarone IV for more than 3 weeks.

The surface properties of solutions containing injectable amiodarone are altered such that the drop size may be reduced. This reduction may lead to underdosage of the patient by up to 30%. If drop counter infusion sets are used, amiodarone must be delivered by a volumetric infusion pump.

Amiodarone IV concentrations greater than 3 mg/mL in D5W have been associated with a high incidence of peripheral vein phlebitis; however, concentrations of 2.5 mg/mL or less appear to be less irritating. Therefore, for infusions more than 1 hour, amiodarone IV concentrations should not exceed 2 mg/mL unless a central venous catheter is used. Use an in-line filter during administration.

Amiodarone IV infusions exceeding 2 hours must be administered in glass or polyolefin bottles containing D5W.

Amiodarone adsorbs to polyvinyl chloride (PVC) tubing, and the clinical trial dose administration schedule was designed to account for this adsorption. Clinical trials were conducted using PVC tubing; therefore its use is recommended. The concentrations and rates of infusion provided in Administration and Dosage reflect doses identified in these studies. It is important that the recommended infusion regimen be followed closely.

Amiodarone IV has been found to leach out plasticizers, including DEHP (di-[2-ethylhexyl]phthalate) from IV tubing (including PVC tubing). The degree of leaching increases when infusing amiodarone IV at higher concentrations and lower flow rates than recommended.

*Admixture incompatibility:* Amiodarone IV in D5W, in a concentration of 4 mg/mL, forms a precipitate and is incompatible with the following drugs: Aminophylline, cefamandole, cefazolin, mezlocillin, heparin (no amiodarone concentration stated), and sodium bicarbonate (amiodarone concentration of 3 mg/mL).

*IV to oral transition:* During or after treatment with IV amiodarone, patients may be transferred to oral amiodarone therapy. Use IV amiodarone for acute treatment until the patient's ventricular arrhythmias are stabilized. Most patients require this therapy for 48 to 96 hours, but IV amiodarone may be given safely for longer periods if necessary. The optimal dose for changing from IV to oral administration will depend on the IV dose already administered, as well as the bioavailability of oral amiodarone.

The following table provides suggested doses of oral amiodarone to be initiated after varying durations of IV administration. These recommendations are made on the basis of a comparable total body amount of amiodarone delivered by the IV and oral routes, based on 50% bioavailability of oral amiodarone.

| Recommendations for Oral Amiodarone Dosage After IV Infusion | |
|---|---|
| Duration of amiodarone IV infusions[1] | Initial daily dose of oral amiodarone |
| < 1 week | 800 to 1600 mg |
| 1 to 3 weeks | 600 to 800 mg |
| > 3 weeks[2] | 400 mg |

[1] Assuming a 720 mg/day infusion (0.5 mg/min).
[2] Amiodarone IV is not intended for maintenance treatment.

## Actions

*Pharmacology:* Amiodarone possesses electrophysiologic characteristics of all 4 Vaughan Williams Classes but has predominantly Class III antiarrhythmic effects. The antiarrhythmic effect may be due to at least 2 major properties: Prolongation of the myocardial cell-action potential duration and refractory period, and noncompetitive α- and β-adrenergic inhibition.

*Pharmacokinetics:*

*Absorption* – Following oral administration, amiodarone is slowly and variably absorbed; bioavailability is approximately 50%. Maximum plasma concentrations are attained 3 to 7 hours after a single dose. Plasma concentrations with chronic dosing at 100 to 600 mg/day are approximately dose-proportional, with a mean 0.5 mg/L increase for each 100 mg/day.

Peak concentrations after 10-minute infusions of 150 mg in patients with VF or hemodynamically unstable VT range between 7 and 26 mg/L. Due to rapid distribution, serum concentrations decline to 10% of peak values within 30 to 45 minutes after the end of the infusion.

*Distribution* – Amiodarone has a very large but variable volume of distribution, averaging about 60 L/kg. One major metabolite, desethylamiodarone (DEA), accumulates to an even greater extent in almost all tissues. The drug is highly protein bound (approximately 96%).

*Metabolism* – Amiodarone is metabolized principally by CYP3A4 into DEA, the major active metabolite of amiodarone. DEA serum concentrations greater than 0.05 mg/L are not usually seen until after several days of continuous infusion but with prolonged therapy reach approximately the same concentration as amiodarone.

*Excretion* – Following discontinuation of chronic oral therapy, amiodarone has a biphasic elimination with an initial one-half reduction of plasma levels after 2.5 to 107 days. A much slower terminal plasma elimination phase shows a half-life of the parent compound of approximately 53 days. For the metabolite, mean plasma elimination half-life was approximately 61 days. Antiarrhythmic effects persist for weeks or months after the drug is discontinued.

The main route of elimination is via hepatic excretion into bile; some enterohepatic recirculation may occur. The drug has a very low plasma clearance with negligible renal excretion. Neither amiodarone nor its metabolite is dialyzable.

## Contraindications

Hypersensitivity to the drug or any of its components.

*Oral:* Severe sinus-node dysfunction, causing marked sinus bradycardia; second- and third-degree AV block; when episodes of bradycardia have caused syncope (except when used in conjunction with a pacemaker).

*Parenteral:* Marked sinus bradycardia; second- and third-degree AV block unless a functioning pacemaker is available; cardiogenic shock.

## Warnings

*Potentially fatal toxicities:* Potentially fatal toxicities with pulmonary toxicity have occurred with ventricular arrhythmias (at approximately 400 mg/day), and symptomless abnormal diffusion capacity has occurred in much higher percentages. Pulmonary toxicity has been fatal approximately 10% of the time. Hepatic injury is common, but usually mild, and evidenced by abnormal liver enzymes. Overt liver disease can occur and has been fatal. Amiodarone has made arrhythmia less well tolerated or more difficult to reverse. Significant heart block or sinus bradycardia has been seen. These events should be manageable in the proper clinical setting. Although such events do not appear more frequently with amiodarone than with other agents, effects are prolonged. In patients at high risk of arrhythmic death in whom amiodarone toxicity is an acceptable risk, amiodarone poses major management problems that could be life-threatening in a population at risk of sudden death so that every effort should be made to use alternative agents first.

Hospitalize patients while the loading dose is given. The time at which a life-threatening arrhythmia will recur after discontinuation or dose adjustment is unpredictable, ranging from weeks to months. The patient risk is greatest during this time. Substituting other antiarrhythmics when amiodarone must be stopped is made difficult by gradually, but unpredictably, changing amiodarone body stores. When amiodarone is ineffective, it still poses the risk of interacting with subsequent treatment.

*Life-threatening arrhythmias:* Use amiodarone only in patients with the indicated life-threatening arrhythmias because its use is accompanied by substantial toxicity.

*Survival* – There is no evidence that the use of amiodarone favorably affects survival.

*Ophthalmologic effects:* Optic neuropathy or neuritis may occur at any time following initiation of therapy, in some cases, visual impairment has progressed to permanent blindness. Corneal microdeposits appear in virtually all adults treated with amiodarone. They give rise to symptoms such as visual halos or blurred vision in as many as 10% of patients. Corneal microdeposits are reversible upon reduction of dose or drug discontinuation. Asymptomatic microdeposits are not a reason to reduce dose or stop treatment. Some patients develop photophobia and dry eyes. Vision is rarely affected and drug discontinuation is rarely needed.

*Pulmonary toxicity:*

*Oral* – Amiodarone may cause a clinical syndrome of cough and progressive dyspnea accompanied by functional, radiographic, gallium scan, and pathological data consistent with pulmonary toxicity. The frequency varies from 2% to 17%; fatalities occur in about 10% of cases. However, in patients with life-threatening arrhythmias, discontinuation of amiodarone therapy due to suspected drug-induced pulmonary toxicity should be undertaken with caution, as the most common cause of death in these patients is sudden cardiac death.

Any new respiratory symptom suggests pulmonary toxicity, therefore repeat and evaluate the history, physical exam, chest x-ray, gallium scan, and pulmonary function tests (with diffusion capacity). In some cases, rechallenge at a lower dose has not resulted in return of interstitial/alveolar pneumonitis.

Perform baseline chest x–rays and pulmonary function tests, including diffusion capacity before therapy initiation. A history and physical exam and chest x-ray should be repeated every 3 to 6 months. Patients with preexisting pulmonary disease have a poorer prognosis if pulmonary toxicity does develop.

*Hypersensitivity pneumonitis* – Hypersensitivity pneumonitis usually appears earlier in the course of therapy, and rechallenging these patients results in a more rapid recurrence of greater severity.

*Interstitial/alveolar pneumonitis* – Interstitial/alveolar pneumonitis is characterized by findings of diffuse alveolar damage, interstitial pneumonitis or fibrosis in lung biopsy specimens. A diagnosis of amiodarone-induced interstitial/alveolar pneumonitis should lead to dose reduction or to withdrawal of amiodarone to establish reversibility. With these measures, a reduction in symptoms of amiodarone-induced pulmonary toxicity was usually noted within the first week. In some cases, rechallenge with amiodarone at a lower dose has not resulted in return of toxicity. Recent reports suggest that lower loading and maintenance doses of amiodarone are associated with a decrease incidence of amiodarone-induced pulmonary toxicity.

If a diagnosis of amiodarone-induced hypersensitivity pneumonitis is made, discontinue amiodarone and institute steroid treatment. If a diagnosis of amiodarone-induced interstitial/alveolar pneumonitis is made, institute steroid therapy and discontinue amiodarone or, at a minimum, reduce dosage.

*Parenteral* –

ARDS: 2% of patients were reported to have adult respiratory distress syndrome (ARDS) during clinical studies.

*Pulmonary fibrosis:* Only 1 of more than 1000 patients treated with amiodarone IV in clinical studies developed pulmonary fibrosis.

**Cardiac effects:**

*Proarrhythmias* – Amiodarone can cause serious exacerbation of the presenting arrhythmia, a risk that may be enhanced by concomitant antiarrhythmics. In addition, amiodarone has caused symptomatic bradycardia, heart block, or sinus arrest with suppression of escape foci. Treat bradycardia by slowing the infusion rate or discontinuing amiodarone IV. In some patients, inserting a pacemaker is required. Cardiac conduction abnormalities are infrequent and reversible on discontinuation.

*Hypotension* – Hypotension is the most common adverse effect seen with amiodarone IV. Clinically significant hypotension during infusions was seen most often in the first several hours of treatment and appeared to be related to the rate of infusion. Hypotension necessitating alterations in therapy was reported in 3% of patients, with permanent discontinuation required in less than 2% of patients. Treat hypotension initially by slowing the infusion; additional standard therapy may be needed.

**Surgery:**

*Volatile anesthetic agents* – Close perioperative monitoring is recommended in patients undergoing general anesthesia who are on amiodarone therapy as they may be more sensitive to the myocardial depressant and conduction effects of halogenated inhalational anesthetics.

*Hypotension postbypass* – Rare occasions of hypotension upon discontinuation of cardiopulmonary bypass during open-heart surgery in patients receiving amiodarone have been reported.

**Hepatic effects:**

*Oral* – Elevated hepatic enzyme levels (AST and ALT) are frequent, and in most cases are asymptomatic. If the increase exceeds 3 times normal, or doubles in a patient with an elevated baseline, consider discontinuation or dosage reduction.

*Parenteral* – Elevations of blood hepatic enzyme values, ALT, AST, and GGT, are seen commonly in patients with immediately life-threatening VT/VF.

In patients with life-threatening arrhythmias, weigh the potential risk of hepatic injury against the potential benefit of therapy. Monitor carefully for evidence of progressive hepatic injury. Give consideration to reducing the rate of administration or withdrawing amiodarone IV in such cases.

**Elderly:** Healthy subjects older than 65 years of age show lower clearances of amiodarone than younger subjects and an increase in half-life.

**Pregnancy:** Category D.

*Lactation:* Amiodarone is excreted in breast milk. When amiodarone therapy is indicated, advise the mother to discontinue nursing.

*Children:* Safety and efficacy for use in children have not been established. Amiodarone is not recommended in children.

### Precautions

*Thyroid abnormalities:* Amiodarone inhibits peripheral conversion of thyroxine ($T_4$) to tri-iodothyronine ($T_3$), prompting increased $T_4$ levels, increased levels of inactive reverse $T_3$ and decreased levels of $T_3$. It is also a potential source of large amounts of inorganic iodine. It can cause hypothyroidism or hyperthyroidism. High plasma iodide levels, altered thyroid function, and abnormal thyroid function tests may persist for several weeks or even months following amiodarone withdrawal.

*Hypothyroidism* – Hypothyroidism is best managed by dose reduction or thyroid hormone supplement.

*Hyperthyroidism* – Hyperthyroidism usually poses a greater hazard to the patient than hypothyroidism because of the possibility of arrhythmia breakthrough or aggravation. If any new signs of arrhythmia appear, consider the possibility of hyperthyroidism. Aggressive medical treatment is indicated, including, dose reduction or withdrawal of amiodarone.

*Electrolyte disturbances:* Correct potassium or magnesium deficiency before therapy begins as these disorders can exaggerate the degree of QTc prolongation and increase the potential for torsades de pointes.

*Benzyl alcohol:* Benzyl alcohol, contained in some of these products as a preservative, has been associated with a fatal "gasping syndrome" in premature infants.

*Photosensitivity:* Amiodarone has induced photosensitization in about 10% of patients. During long-term treatment, a blue-gray discoloration of the exposed skin may occur; some protection may be afforded by sun barrier creams or protective clothing. This is slowly and occasionally incompletely reversible on discontinuation of drug.

### Drug Interactions

Drugs that may affect amiodarone include hydantoins, cholestyramine, fluoroquinolones, rifamycins, ritonavir, and cimetidine. Drugs that may be affected by amiodarone include anticoagulants, beta-blockers, calcium channel blockers, cyclosporine, dextromethorphan, digoxin, disopyramide, fentanyl, flecainide, hydantoins, lidocaine, methotrexate, procainamide, quinidine, and theophylline.

*Drug/Lab test interactions:* Amiodarone alters the results of thyroid function tests, causing an increase in serum $T_4$ and serum reverse $T_3$ levels and a decline in serum $T_3$ levels. Despite these biochemical changes, most patients remain clinically euthyroid.

*Drug/Food interactions:* Food increases the rate and extent of absorption.

### Adverse Reactions

*Oral* – Adverse reactions requiring discontinuation include: Pulmonary infiltrates or fibrosis; paroxysmal ventricular tachycardia; CHF; elevation of liver enzymes; visual disturbances; solar dermatitis; blue discoloration of skin; hyperthyroidism; hypothyroidism. Adverse reactions occurring in at least 3% of patients include CHF; GI complaints (nausea, vomiting, constipation, anorexia); dermatologic reactions (photosensitivity, solar dermatitis); neurologic problems (malaise, fatigue, tremor/abnormal involuntary movements, lack of coordination, abnormal gait/ataxia, dizziness, paresthesias); abnormal liver function tests.

*Parenteral* – The most important treatment-emergent adverse effects were hypotension, asystole/cardiac arrest/electromechanical dissociation (EMD), cardiogenic shock, CHF, bradycardia, liver function test abnormalities, VT, and AV block. The most common adverse effects leading to discontinuation of IV therapy were hypotension, asystole/cardiac arrest/EMD, VT, and cardiogenic shock. Adverse reactions occurring in at least 3% of patients include nausea.

# CALCIUM CHANNEL BLOCKING AGENTS

**AMLODIPINE**

**Tablets**: 2.5, 5, and 10 mg (*Rx*) — *Amvaz* (Reddy), *Norvasc* (Pfizer)

**DILTIAZEM HCl**

**Tablets**: 30, 60, 90, and 120 mg (*Rx*) — Various, *Cardizem* (Biovail)

**Tablets, extended-release**: 120, 180, 240, 300, 360, 420 mg — *Cardizem LA* (Biovail)

**Capsules, extended-release**: 60 and 90 mg (*Rx*) — Various

120, 180, and 240 mg (*Rx*) — Various, *Cardizem CD* (Biovail), *CartiaXT* (Andrx), *Dilacor XR* (Watson), *Diltia XT* (Andrx), *Tiazac* (Forest), *Taztia XT* (Andrx)

300 mg (*Rx*) — Various, *Cardizem CD* (Biovail), *CartiaXT* (Andrx), *Tiazac* (Forest), *Taztia XT* (Andrx)

360 mg (*Rx*) — Various, *Cardizem CD* (Biovail), *Tiazac* (Forest), *Taztia XT* (Andrx)

420 mg (*Rx*) — *Tiazac* (Forest)

**Injection**: 5 mg/mL (*Rx*) — Various, *Cardizem* (Biovail)

**FELODIPINE**

**Tablets, extended-release**: 2.5, 5, and 10 mg (*Rx*) — *Plendil* (AstraZeneca)

**ISRADIPINE**

**Tablets, controlled-release**: 5 and 10 mg (*Rx*) — *DynaCirc CR* (Reliant)

**Capsules**: 2.5 and 5 mg (*Rx*) — *DynaCirc* (Reliant)

**NICARDIPINE HCl**

**Capsules**: 20 and 30 mg (*Rx*) — Various, *Cardene* (Roche)

**Capsules, sustained-release**: 30, 45, and 60 mg (*Rx*) — *Cardene SR* (Roche)

**Injection**: 2.5 mg/mL (*Rx*) — *Cardene I.V.* (Wyeth-Ayerst)

**NIFEDIPINE**

**Tablets, extended-release**: 30, 60, and 90 mg (*Rx*) — Various, *Adalat CC* (Bayer), *Nifedical XL* (Teva), *Procardia XL* (Pfizer)

**Capsules**: 10 and 20 mg (*Rx*) — Various, *Procardia* (Pfizer), *Adalat* (Bayer)

**NIMODIPINE**

**Capsules, liquid-filled**: 30 mg (*Rx*) — *Nimotop* (Bayer)

**NISOLDIPINE**

**Tablets, extended-release**: 10, 20, 30, and 40 mg (*Rx*) — *Sular* (First Horizon)

**VERAPAMIL HCl**

**Tablets**: 40, 80, and 120 mg (*Rx*) — Various, *Calan* (Searle)

**Tablets, extended-release**: 120, 180, and 240 mg (*Rx*) — Various, *Covera-HS* (Searle)

**Tablets, sustained-release**: 120, 180, and 240 mg (*Rx*) — Various, *Calan SR* (Searle), *Isoptin SR* (Abbott)

**Capsules, extended-release**: 120, 180, and 240 mg (*Rx*) — Various

100, 200, and 300 mg (*Rx*) — *Verelan PM* (Schwarz Pharma)

**Capsules, sustained-release**: 120, 180, 240, and 360 mg (*Rx*) — *Verelan* (Schwarz Pharma)

**Injection**: 2.5 mg/mL (*Rx*) — Various

**Warning:**
**Bepridil** has Class I antiarrhythmic properties and, like other such drugs, can induce new arrhythmias, including ventricular tachycardia/ventricular fibrillation (VT/VF). In addition, because of its ability to prolong the QT interval, bepridil can cause torsades de pointes type VT. Because of these properties, reserve bepridil for patients in whom other antianginal agents do not offer a satisfactory effect (see Warnings).

### Indications

| Calcium Channel Blocking Agents – Summary of Indications[1] | | | | | | | | | | | | | | | | | |
| --- | --- | --- | --- | --- | --- | --- | --- | --- | --- | --- | --- | --- | --- | --- | --- | --- | --- |
| Indications | Amlodipine | Diltiazem | Diltiazem SR | Diltiazem ER | Diltiazem IV | Felodipine | Isradipine | Nicardipine | Nicardipine SR | Nicardipine IV | Nifedipine | Nifedipine ER | Nimodipine | Nisoldipine | Verapamil | Verapamil SR | Verapamil ER | Verapamil IV |
| Angina pectoris | | | | | | | | | | | | | | | | | | |
|   Vasospastic | ✔ | ✔ | | ✔ | | | | | | | ✔ | ✔[2] | | | ✔ | | ✔[3] | |
|   Chronic stable | ✔ | ✔ | | ✔ | | | ✔ | | | | ✔ | ✔[2] | | | ✔ | | ✔[3] | |
|   Unstable | | | | | | | | | | | | | | | ✔ | | ✔[3] | |
| Hypertension | ✔ | | ✔ | ✔ | | ✔ | ✔ | ✔ | ✔ | ✔ | | ✔ | | ✔ | ✔ | ✔ | ✔ | ✔ |
| Subarachnoid hemorrhage | | | | | | | | | | | | | ✔ | | | | | |
| Atrial fibrillation/flutter | | | | | ✔ | | | | | | | | | | | | | ✔ |
| Paroxysmal supraventricular tachycardia | | | | | ✔ | | | | | | | | | | | | ✔[4] | ✔ |

[1] For more detailed information, see the information below and individual drug monographs.
[2] Except *Adalat* CC.
[3] *Covera-HS* only.
[4] For prophylaxis of repetitive paroxysmal supraventricular tachycardia.

#### Administration and Dosage

Swallow extended-release tablets and sustained-release capsule forms whole; do not bite, open, chew, crush, or divide.

*AMLODIPINE:* May be taken without regard to meals.

*Hypertension* – Usual dose is 5 mg once daily. Maximum dose is 10 mg once daily. Small, fragile, or elderly patients or patients with hepatic insufficiency may be started on 2.5 mg once daily; this dose may also be used when adding amlodipine to other antihypertensive therapy. In general, titrate over 7 to 14 days; proceed more rapidly if clinically warranted with frequent assessment of the patient.

*Angina (chronic stable or vasospastic)* – 5 to 10 mg, using the lower dose for elderly and patients with hepatic insufficiency. Most patients require 10 mg.

*DILTIAZEM HCl:*
  Oral –
    *Tablets, immediate-release:* Start with 30 mg 4 times/day before meals and at bedtime; gradually increase dosage to 180 to 360 mg (given in divided doses 3 or 4 times/day) at 1- to 2-day intervals until optimum response is obtained. The average optimum dosage range appears to be 180 to 360 mg/day.

    *Tablets, extended-release:* Intended for once daily administration. Patients treated with diltiazem alone or in combination with other medications may be switched safely to once daily extended-release diltiazem tablets at the nearest equivalent total daily dose. Subsequent titration to higher or lower doses may be necessary and should be initiated as clinically warranted.

    Swallow tablets whole; do not crush or chew. Take tablets at about the same time once every day, either in the morning or at bedtime.

*Hypertension* – Starting dose usually is 180 to 240 mg once daily. Maximum antihypertensive effect usually is observed by 14 days of chronic therapy. May be titrated to a maximum dose of 540 mg daily.

*Angina* – Initial dose of 180 mg may be increased at intervals of 7 to 14 days if adequate response is not obtained. Doses above 360 mg appear not to confer any additional benefit.

*Extended-release capsules:*

*Hypertension* – Start with 60 to 120 mg twice daily or 180 to 240 mg once daily. Optimum dosage range is 240 to 360 mg/day. Individual patients may respond to higher doses of up to 480 mg once daily.

*Angina* – Start with 120 or 180 mg once daily. Individual patients may respond to higher doses of up to 480 mg once daily. When necessary, carry titration out over 7 to 14 days.

*Cardizem CD and Cartia XT* –

*Hypertension:* 180 to 240 mg once daily. Maximum antihypertensive effect is usually achieved by 14 days chronic therapy. Usual range is 240 to 360 mg once daily; experience with doses more than 360 mg is limited.

*Angina:* Start with 120 or 180 mg once daily. Some patients may respond to higher doses of up to 480 mg once daily. When necessary, titration may be carried out over a 7- to 14-day period.

*Dilacor XR and Diltia XT* –

*Hypertension:* 180 to 240 mg once daily. Individual patients, particularly those 60 years of age or older, may respond to a lower dose of 120 mg. Usual range is 180 to 480 mg once daily. Do not exceed 540 mg once daily.

*Angina:* Start with 120 mg once daily, which may be titrated to doses of up to 480 mg once daily. When necessary, titration may be carried out over a 7- to 14-day period.

Administration in the morning on an empty stomach is recommended.

*Tiazac* –

*Hypertension:* Usual starting doses are 120 to 240 mg once daily. Maximum antihypertensive effect is usually observed by 14 days of chronic therapy. The usual dosage range is 120 to 540 mg once daily.

*Angina:* Start with a dose of 120 to 180 mg once daily. Patients may respond to higher doses of up to 540 mg once daily. When necessary titration should be carried out over 7 to 14 days.

*Parenteral* –

*Direct IV single injections (bolus):* The initial dose is 0.25 mg/kg as a bolus administered over 2 minutes (20 mg is a reasonable dose for the average patient). If response is inadequate, a second dose may be administered after 15 minutes. The second bolus dose should be 0.35 mg/kg administered over 2 minutes (25 mg is a reasonable dose for the average patient). Individualize subsequent IV bolus doses. Dose patients with low body weights on a mg/kg basis. Some patients may respond to an initial dose of 0.15 mg/kg, although duration of action may be shorter.

*Continuous IV infusion:* For continued reduction of the heart rate (up to 24 hours) in patients with atrial fibrillation or atrial flutter, an IV infusion may be administered. Immediately following bolus administration of 20 mg (0.25 mg/kg) or 25 mg (0.35 mg/kg) and reduction of heart rate, begin an IV infusion. The recommended initial infusion rate is 10 mg/h. Some patients may maintain response to an initial rate of 5 mg/h. The infusion rate may be increased in 5 mg/h increments up to 15 mg/h as needed, if further reduction in heart rate is required. The infusion may be maintained for up to 24 hours. Therefore, infusion duration more than 24 hours and infusion rates more than 15 mg/h are not recommended.

*Concomitant therapy:* Concomitant therapy with β-blockers or digitalis is usually well tolerated, but the effects of coadministration cannot be predicted, especially in patients with left ventricular dysfunction or cardiac conduction abnormalities.

Use caution in titrating dosages for impaired renal or hepatic function patients, since dosage requirements are not available.

*FELODIPINE:* The recommended starting dose is 5 mg once daily. Depending on the patient's response the dosage can be decreased to 2.5 mg or increased to 10 mg once daily. These adjustments should occur generally at intervals of not less than 2 weeks. The recommended dosage range is 2.5 to 10 mg once daily. Closely monitor blood pressure in patients more than 65 years of age and in impaired hepatic function during dosage adjustment; generally, do not consider doses more than 10 mg.

*ISRADIPINE:*

*Capsules* – Recommended initial dose is 2.5 mg twice daily. Response usually occurs within 2 to 3 hours; maximal response may require 2 to 4 weeks. If a satisfactory response does not occur after this period, the dose may be adjusted in increments of 5 mg/day at 2 to 4 week intervals up to a maximum of 20 mg/day.

*Tablets, controlled-release* – Recommended initial dose is 5 mg once daily. Response usually occurs within 2 hours with the peak antihypertensive response occurring 8 to 10 hours postdose. If necessary, the dose may be adjusted in increments of 5 mg at 2- to 4-week intervals up to a maximum dose of 20 mg/day.

Swallow controlled-release tablets whole; do not bite or divide.

*NICARDIPINE HCl:*

*Oral –*

*Angina (immediate release only):* Usual initial dose is 20 mg 3 times/day (range, 20 to 40 mg 3 times/day). Allow at least 3 days before increasing dose.

*Hypertension (immediate release only):* Initial dose is 20 mg 3 times/day (range, 20 to 40 mg 3 times/day). The maximum BP-lowering effect occurs approximately 1 to 2 hours after dosing.

*Hypertension (sustained release):* Initial dose is 30 mg twice daily. Effective doses have ranged from 30 to 60 mg twice daily. The maximum BP lowering effect at steady-state is sustained from 2 to 6 hours after dosing.

Titrate patients currently receiving the immediate-release form with the sustained-release form starting at their current daily dose of immediate-release, then re-examine to assess adequacy of BP control.

*Renal impairment:* Titrate dose beginning with 20 mg 3 times/day (immediate-release) or 30 mg twice/day (sustained-release).

*Hepatic impairment:* Starting dose is 20 mg twice/day (immediate-release) with individual titration.

*Parenteral –*

*Dosage:*

*Substitute for oral nicardipine* – The IV infusion rate required to produce an average plasma concentration equivalent to a given oral dose at steady state is shown in the following table:

| Equivalent Nicardipine Doses: Oral vs IV Infusion | |
| --- | --- |
| Oral dose | Equivalent IV infusion rate |
| 20 mg every 8 h | 0.5 mg/h |
| 30 mg every 8 h | 1.2 mg/h |
| 40 mg every 8 h | 2.2 mg/h |

*Initiation in a drug free patient* – Administer by slow continuous infusion at a concentration of 0.1 mg/mL. With constant infusion, blood pressure begins to fall within minutes. It reaches about 50% of its ultimate decrease in about 45 minutes and does not reach final steady state for about 50 hours.

When treating acute hypertensive episodes in patients with chronic hypertension, discontinuation of infusion is followed by a 50% offset of action in 30 minutes but plasma levels of drug and gradually decreasing antihypertensive effects exist for about 50 hours.

*Titration* – For gradual reduction in blood pressure, initiate therapy at 50 mL/h (5 mg/h). If desired reduction is not achieved, the infusion rate may be increased by 25 mL/h (2.5 mg/h) every 15 minutes up to a maximum of 150 mL/h (15 mg/h) until desired reduction of blood pressure is achieved. For more rapid reduction of blood pressure, initiate at 50 mL/h. If desired reduction is not achieved, the infusion rate may be increased by 25 mL/h every 5 minutes up to a maximum of 150 mL/h until desired reduction of blood pressure is achieved. Following achievement of the blood pressure goal, decrease the infusion rate to 30 mL/h.

*Hypotension or tachycardia* – If there is concern of impending hypotension or tachycardia, discontinue the infusion. When blood pressure has stabilized, infusion may be restarted at low doses (eg, 30 to 50 mL/h) and adjusted to maintain desired blood pressure.

*Infusion site changes* – Change the infusion site every 12 hours if administered via peripheral vein.

*Transfer to oral antihypertensives* – If treatment includes transfer to an oral antihypertensive other than nicardipine, generally initiate therapy upon discontinuation of the infusion. If oral nicardipine is to be used, administer the first dose of a 3-times-daily regimen 1 hour prior to discontinuation of the infusion.

NIFEDIPINE: Individualize dosage. Excessive doses can result in hypotension.

*Initial dosage (capsule)* – 10 mg 3 times/day; swallow whole. Usual range is 10 to 20 mg 3 times/day. Some patients, especially those with coronary artery spasm, respond to 20 to 30 mg 3 or 4 times/day. Doses more than 120 mg/day are rarely necessary. More than 180 mg/day is not recommended.

Titrate throughout 7 to 14 days to assess response to each dose level; monitor blood pressure before proceeding to higher doses.

*Sustained release* –

*Procardia XL/Nifedical XL:* 30 or 60 mg once daily. Titrate over a 7- to 14-day period. Titration may proceed more rapidly if the patient is frequently assessed. Titration to doses more than 120 mg is not recommended.

Angina patients maintained on the nifedipine capsule formulation may be switched to the sustained release tablet at the nearest equivalent total daily dose. Experience with doses more than 90 mg in angina is limited.

*Adalat CC:* Administer once daily on an empty stomach. In general, titrate over a 7- to 14-day period starting with 30 mg once daily. Usual maintenance dose is 30 to 60 mg once daily. Titration to doses more than 90 mg daily is not recommended.

*Concomitant drug therapy* – Concomitant drug therapy with β-blockers may be beneficial in chronic stable angina; however, the effects of concurrent treatment cannot be predicted, especially in patients with compromised left ventricular function or cardiac conduction abnormalities.

NIMODIPINE: Commence therapy within 96 hours of the subarachnoid hemorrhage (SAH), using 60 mg every 4 hours for 21 consecutive days.

If the capsule cannot be swallowed (eg, time of surgery, unconscious patient), make a hole in both ends of the capsule with an 18 gauge needle and extract the contents into a syringe. Empty the contents into the patient's in situ nasogastric tube and wash down the tube with 30 mg normal saline.

NISOLDIPINE: Administer nisoldipine orally once daily. Avoid administration with a high fat meal. Avoid grapefruit products before and after dosing. Swallow whole; do not bite, divide, or crush.

Initiate therapy with 20 mg orally once daily, then increase by 10 mg/week, or longer intervals, to attain adequate control of blood pressure. The usual maintenance dosage is 20 to 40 mg once daily. BP response increases over the 10 to 60 mg/day dose range, but adverse event rates also increase. Doses more than 60 mg once daily are not recommended.

*Elderly/Hepatic function impairment* – In patients more than 65 years of age or patients with hepatic function impairment. A starting dose not exceeding 10 mg/day is recommended in patients older than 65 years of age or patients with hepatic function impairment.

VERAPAMIL HCl: Avoid verapamil in patients with severe left ventricular dysfunction (eg, ejection fractions less than 30%) or moderate to severe symptoms of cardiac failure and in patients with any degree of ventricular dysfunction if they are receiving a beta-adrenergic blocker.

Do not exceed 480 mg/day; safety and efficacy are not established.

Lower initial doses may be warranted in patients who may have an increased response to verapamil (eg, elderly people, those of small stature, impaired hepatic function). Base upward titration on therapeutic efficacy and safety evaluated approximately 24 hours after dosing. The antihypertensive effects of verapamil are evident within the first week of therapy.

*Immediate-release –*

*Angina:* Usual initial dose is 80 to 120 mg 3 times/day; 40 mg 3 times/day may be warranted if patients may have increased response to verapamil (eg, decreased hepatic function, elderly). Base upward titration of safety and efficacy evaluated about 8 hours after dosing. Increase dosage daily (eg, unstable angina) or weekly until optimum clinical response is obtained.

*Arrhythmias:* Dosage range in digitalized patients with chronic atrial fibrillation is 240 to 320 mg/day in divided doses 3 or 4 times/day. Dosage range for prophylaxis of paroxysmal supraventricular tachycardia (PSVT) (non-digitalized patients) is 240 to 480 mg/day in divided doses 3 or 4 times/day. In general, maximum effects will be apparent during the first 48 hours of therapy.

*Hypertension:* The usual initial monotherapy dose is 80 mg 3 times/day (240 mg/day). Daily dosages of 360 and 480 mg have been used, but there is no evidence that dosages more than 360 mg provide added effect.

*Extended-release –* When administered at bedtime, office evaluation of blood pressure (BP) during morning and early afternoon hours is essentially a measure of peak effect. The usual evaluation of trough effect would be just prior to bedtime. Swallow whole; do not chew, break, or crush the tablets.

*Capsules:* The usual daily dose is 240 mg once daily in the morning.

*Tablets:* Initiate therapy with 180 mg given in the morning.

*Covera-HS tablets:* Initiate therapy with 180 mg/day at bedtime. Clinical trials explored dose ranges between 180 and 540 mg given at bedtime and found effects to persist throughout the dosing interval.

*Verelan PM:* Usual daily dose is 200 mg/day at bedtime.

*Sustained-release –* When switching from the immediate-release formulation, total daily dose (in mg) may remain the same.

*Calan SR and Isoptin SR:* Initiate therapy with 180 mg given in the morning with food.

Sustained release characteristics are not altered when the tablet is divided in half.

*Verelan:* Usual daily dose is 240 mg once daily in the morning.

*Pellet-filled capsules:* Do not chew or crush the contents of the capsule. Pellet-filled capsules also may be administered by carefully opening the capsule and sprinkling the pellets on a spoonful of applesauce. Swallow the applesauce immediately without chewing and follow with a glass of cool water to ensure complete swallowing of the pellets. The applesauce used should not be hot, and it should be soft enough to be swallowed without chewing. Use any pellet/applesauce mixture immediately and do not store for future use. Subdividing the contents of the capsule is not recommended.

*Parenteral (supraventricular tachyarrhythmias) –* For IV use only. Give as slow IV injection over at least 2 minutes under continuous ECG and blood pressure monitoring. An IV infusion has been used (5 mg/hour); precede the infusion with an IV loading dose.

*Initial dose:* 5 to 10 mg (0.075 to 0.15 mg/kg) as IV bolus over 2 minutes.

*Repeat dose:* 10 mg (0.15 mg/kg) 30 minutes after the first dose if the initial response is not adequate.

*Older patients:* Give over at least 3 minutes to minimize risk of untoward drug effects.

*Children:*

*1 year of age or younger* – 0.1 to 0.2 mg/kg (usual single dose range, 0.75 to 2 mg) as an IV bolus over 2 minutes (under continuous ECG monitoring).

*1 to 15 years of age* – 0.1 to 0.3 mg/kg (usual single dose range, 2 to 5 mg) IV over 2 minutes. Do not exceed 5 mg.

*Repeat dose* – Repeat above dose 30 minutes after the first dose if the initial response is not adequate (under continuous ECG monitoring). Do not exceed a single dose of 10 mg in patients 1 to 15 years of age.

## Actions

*Pharmacology:* The calcium channel blockers share the ability to inhibit movement of calcium ions across the cell membrane. The effects on the cardiovascular system include depression of mechanical contraction of myocardial and smooth muscle and depression of both impulse formation (automaticity) and conduction velocity. **Bepridil** also inhibits fast sodium inward channels. Calcium channel blockers are classified by structure as follows: Diphenylalkylamines – verapamil; benzothiazepines – diltiazem; dihydropyridines – amlodipine, felodipine, isradipine, nicardipine, nifedipine, nimodipine, nisoldipine.

*Pharmacokinetics:*

### Calcium Channel Blocking Agents: Pharmacokinetics[*]

| Parameters | Amlodipine | Diltiazem | Felodipine | Isradipine | Nicardipine | Nifedipine | Nimodipine | Nisoldipine | Verapamil |
|---|---|---|---|---|---|---|---|---|---|
| Extent of absorption (oral) (%) | nd | nd | ≈ 100 | 90-95 | ≈ 100 | 100 | nd | nd | > 90 |
| Absolute bioavailability (oral) (%) | 64-90 | 40 | ≈ 20 | 15-24 | ≈ 35 | 45-75 (IR) 84-89 (ER) | ≈ 13 | ≈ 5 | 20-35 (IR) |
| Volume of distribution | nd | ≈ 305 L (IV) | 10 L/kg | 3 L/kg | 8.3 L/kg (IV) | nd | nd | nd | nd |
| $T_{max}$ (h) | 6-12 | 2-4 (IR) 10-14 (ER) 6-11 (SR) | 2.5-5 | 1.5 (IR) 7-18 (CR) | 0.5-2 (IR) 1-4 (SR) | 0.5 (IR) 6 (ER) | 1 | 6-12 | 1-2 (IR) ≈ 11 (ER) ≈ 7-9 (SR) |
| Protein binding (%) | 93 | 70-80 | > 99 | 95 | > 95 | 92-98 | > 95 | > 99 | ≈ 90 |
| Metabolism | Hepatic | Hepatic | Hepatic | Hepatic | Hepatic | Hepatic | Hepatic | Hepatic | Hepatic |
| Major metabolites | 90% converted to inactive | Desacetyl-diltiazem[2] | 6 inactive | Mono acids and cyclic lactone[3] | nd | Inactive | Numerous, inactive | 5 major urinary metabolites | Norverapamil[4] |
| Half-life, elimination (h) | 30-50 | 3-4.5 (IR) 4-9.5 (ER) 5-7 (SR) ≈ 3.4 (IV) | 11-16 | 8 | 2-4 | ≈ 2 (IR) ≈ 7 (ER) | ≈ 8-9[7] | 7-12 | 2.8-7.4[8] 4.5-12[9] ≈ 12 (SR) 2-5 (IV) |
| Clearance, systemic | nd | ≈ 65 L/h (IV) | ≈ 0.8 L/min | 1.4 L/min | 0.4 L/h•kg (IV) | nd | nd | nd | nd |
| Excreted unchanged in urine (%) | 10 | 2-4 | ± | 0 | < 1 | < 0.1 | < 1 | trace | 3-4 |
| Excreted in urine (%) | nd | nd | 70 | 60-65 | 60 (oral) 49 (IV) | 60-80 | nd | 60-80 | ≈ 70 |
| Excreted in feces (%) | nd | nd | 10 | 25-30 | 35 (oral) 43 (IV) | 15 | nd | nd | ≥ 16 |

| | Calcium Channel Blocking Agents: Pharmacokinetics[*] | | | | | | | | |
|---|---|---|---|---|---|---|---|---|---|
| Parameters | Amlodipine | Diltiazem | Felodipine | Isradipine | Nicardipine | Nifedipine | Nimodipine | Nisoldipine | Verapamil |
| **ECG Changes** Heart rate | ± | 0-↓ | ↑↑ | ↑ | ↑↑ | 0-↑ | na | ± | ± |
| QRS complex | 0 | nd | 0 | 0 | 0 | nd | | 0 | nd |
| PR interval | 0 | ↑ | 0 | 0 | 0 | nd | | 0 | ↑ |
| QT interval | 0 | nd | 0 | ↑ | ↑ | nd | | 0 | nd |
| **Hemodynamics** Myocardial contractility | 0-↓ | 0-↓ | 0-↓ | ↓ | 0-↓ | 0-↓ | | 0-↓ | ↓↓ |
| Cardiac output/index | ↑ | 0-↑ | nd | ↑ | ↑↑ | ↑ | | nd | ± |
| Peripheral vascular resistance | ↓↓ | ↓↓[10] | ↓↓[10] | ↓↓ | ↓↓↓ | ↓↓↓ | | ↓↓[10] | ↓↓ |

[*] ↑↑↑ or ↓↓↓ = pronounced effect; ↑↑ or ↓↓ = moderate effect; ↑ or ↓ = slight effect; ± = negligible amount or effect; nd = no data; na = not applicable.
[1] Activity of metabolites is unknown.
[2] 25% to 50% as potent a coronary vasodilator as diltiazem; plasma levels are 10% to 20% of the parent drug.
[3] Of 6 metabolites identified, accounting for more than 75%.
[4] Major metabolite; cardiovascular activity is approximately 20% that of verapamil.
[5] Following cessation of multiple dosing.
[6] During a given dosing interval.
[7] Earlier elimination rates are much more rapid, equivalent to a half-life of 1 to 2 hours.
[8] After single doses.
[9] After repetitive doses.
[10] Dose-related.

## Contraindications

Hypersensitivity to the drug; hypersensitivity to dihydropyridine calcium channel blockers (**nisodipine**); sick sinus syndrome or second- or third-degree AV block except with a functioning pacemaker, hypotension less than 90 mm Hg systolic (**diltiazem** and **verapamil**).

*Diltiazem:* Acute MI and pulmonary congestion.

> *Injectable* –
> - Sick sinus syndrome except in the presence of a functioning ventricular pacemaker.
> - Second- or third-degree AV block except in the presence of a functioning ventricular pacemaker.
> - Severe hypotension or cardiogenic shock.
> - Hypersensitivity to the drug.
> - IV diltiazem and IV beta-blockers should not be administered together or in close proximity (within a few hours).
> - Atrial fibrillation or atrial flutter associated with an accessory bypass tract such as in Wolff-Parkinson-White syndrome or short PR syndrome.
> - Initial use of injectable forms of diltiazem should be, if possible, in a setting where monitoring and resuscitation capabilities, including DC cardioversion/defibrillation, are present. Once familiarity of the patient's response is established, use in an office setting may be acceptable.
> - Ventricular tachycardia.
> - In newborns, because of the presence of benzyl alcohol (*Cardizem Lyo-Ject Syringe* only).

*Verapamil:* Severe left ventricular dysfunction; cardiogenic shock and severe CHF, unless secondary to a supraventricular tachycardia amenable to verapamil therapy and in patients with atrial flutter or atrial fibrillation and an accessory bypass tract.

> *Verapamil IV* – Do not administer concomitantly with IV β-adrenergic blocking agents (within a few hours), because both may depress myocardial contractility and AV conduction; ventricular tachycardia (VT), because use in patients with wide-complex VT (QRS 0.12 seconds or more) can result in marked hemodynamic dete-

rioration and ventricular fibrillation; atrial fibrillation or atrial flutter associated with an accessory bypass tract.

*Nicardipine:* Advanced aortic stenosis.

*Bepridil:* History of serious ventricular arrhythmias; uncompensated cardiac insufficiency; congenital QT interval prolongation; use with other drugs that prolong QT interval.

**Warnings**

*Induction of new serious arrhythmias (bepridil):* Bepridil has Class I antiarrhythmic properties and, like other such drugs, can induce new arrhythmias, including VT/VF. In addition, because of its ability to prolong the QT interval, bepridil can cause torsades de pointes-type VT. Because of these properties, reserve for patients in whom other antianginal agents do not offer a satisfactory effect.

While the safe upper limit of QT is not defined, it is suggested that the interval not be permitted to exceed 0.52 seconds during treatment. If dose reduction does not eliminate the excessive prolongation, stop the drug. If concomitant diuretics are needed, consider low doses and the addition or primary use of a potassium-sparing diuretic and monitor serum potassium.

*Hypotension:* Hypotension, usually modest and well tolerated, may occasionally occur during initial therapy or with dosage increases, and may be more likely in patients taking concomitant β-blockers.

*CHF:* CHF has developed rarely, usually in patients receiving a β-blocker, after beginning **nifedipine**.

**Oral verapamil** may precipitate heart failure. Control patients with milder ventricular dysfunction with digitalis or diuretics before verapamil, if possible.

Use **diltiazem, nicardipine, isradipine, felodipine,** and **amlodipine** with caution in CHF patients.

*Cardiac conduction:* **IV verapamil** slows AV nodal conduction and SA nodes; it rarely produces second- or third-degree AV block, bradycardia, and in extreme cases, asystole. This is more likely to occur in patients with sick sinus syndrome.

**Oral verapamil** – Oral verapamil may lead to first-degree AV block and transient bradycardia, sometimes accompanied by nodal escape rhythms.

**IV diltiazem** – If second- or third-degree AV block occurs in sinus rhythm, discontinue and institute appropriate supportive measures.

*Premature ventricular contractions (PVCs):* During conversion or marked reduction in ventricular rate, benign complexes of unusual appearance (sometimes resembling PVCs) may occur after **IV verapamil**.

*Hypertrophic cardiomyopathy (IHSS):* Serious adverse effects were seen in 120 patients with IHSS (especially with pulmonary artery wedge pressure more than 20 mm Hg and left ventricular outflow obstruction) who received oral **verapamil** at doses up to 720 mg/day. Sinus bradycardia occurred in 11%, second-degree AV block in 4% and sinus arrest in 2%.

*Withdrawal syndrome:* Abrupt withdrawal of calcium channel blockers may be associated with an exacerbation of angina. Gradually taper the dose.

*β-blocker withdrawal:* Patients recently withdrawn from β-blockers may develop a withdrawal syndrome with increased angina, probably related to increased sensitivity to catecholamines. Initiation of **nifedipine** will not prevent this occurrence and might exacerbate it by provoking reflex catecholamine release. Taper β-blockers rather than stopping them abruptly before beginning nifedipine.

Gradually reduce beta-blocker dose over 8 to 10 days with nicardipine administration.

*Hepatic function impairment:* The pharmacokinetics, bioavailability and patient response to **verapamil** and **nifedipine** may be significantly affected by hepatic cirrhosis.

Because **amlodipine, diltiazem, nicardipine, felodipine,** and **nimodipine** are extensively metabolized by liver, use with caution in impaired hepatic function or reduced hepatic blood flow.

*Renal function impairment:* The pharmacokinetics of **diltiazem** and **verapamil** in patients with impaired renal function are similar to the pharmacokinetic profile of patients with normal renal function. However, caution is still advised. **Nifedipine**'s plasma concentration is slightly increased in patients with renal impairment. **Nicardipine**'s mean plasma concentrations, AUC and maximum concentration were about 2-fold higher in patients with mild renal impairment.

*Increased angina:* Occasional patients have increased frequency, duration or severity of angina on starting **nifedipine** or **nicardipine** or at the time of dosage increases.

*Duchenne muscular dystrophy:* **Verapamil** may decrease neuromuscular transmission in patients with Duchenne muscular dystrophy and prolong recovery from the neuromuscular blocking agent vecuronium. Decrease in verapamil dosage may be necessary.

*Elderly:* **Verapamil, nifedipine,** and **felodipine** may cause a greater hypotensive effect than that seen in younger patients, probably due to age-related changes in drug disposition.

*Pregnancy:* Category C.

*Lactation:* Discontinue nursing while taking **amlodipine, diltiazem, nicardipine, verapamil,** or **nimodipine.** If using **felodipine, isradipine, nifedipine,** or **nisoldipine,** decide whether to discontinue nursing or discontinue the drug, taking into account the importance of the drug to the mother.

*Children:* Safety and efficacy of oral **verapamil, diltiazem, felodipine, amlodipine, nicardipine, nifedipine, nisoldipine,** and **isradipine** have not been established. Use of *Procardia* in the pediatric population is not recommended.

Controlled studies of **IV verapamil** have not been conducted in pediatric patients, but uncontrolled experience indicates that results of treatment are similar to those in adults. Patients less than 6 months of age may not respond to IV verapamil; this resistance may be related to a developmental difference of AV node responsiveness.

## Precautions

*Acute hepatic injury:* In rare instances, symptoms consistent with acute hepatic injury, as well as significant elevations in enzymes such as alkaline phosphatase, CPK, LDH, AST, and ALT have occurred with **diltiazem** and **nifedipine.**

Elevations of transaminases with and without concomitant elevations in alkaline phosphatase and bilirubin have occurred with **verapamil.**

Isolated cases of elevated LDH, alkaline phosphatase, and ALT levels have occurred rarely with **nimodipine.**

Clinically significant transaminase elevations have occurred in approximately 1% of patients receiving; however, no patient became clinically symptomatic or jaundiced, and values returned to normal when the drug was stopped.

*Edema:* Edema, mild to moderate, typically associated with arterial vasodilation and not due to left ventricular dysfunction, occurs in 10% to 30% of patients receiving **nifedipine.** It occurs primarily in the lower extremities and usually responds to diuretics. In patients with CHF, differentiate this peripheral edema from the effects of decreasing left ventricular function.

Peripheral edema, generally mild and not associated with generalized fluid retention, may occur with **felodipine** within 2 to 3 weeks of therapy initiation. The incidence is both age- and dose-dependent, with frequency ranging from 10% in patients less than 50 years of age taking 5 mg/day to 30% in patients more than 60 years of age taking 20 mg/day.

## Drug Interactions

Drugs that may affect calcium blockers include amiodarone, antineoplastics, azole antifungals, barbiturates, beta blockers, calcium salts, carbamazepine, oxcarbazepine, cisapride, cyclosporine, erythromycin, H$_2$ antagonists, hydantoins, melatonin, nafcillin, quinupristine/dalfopristin, moricizine, quinidine, rifampin, ritonavir, sparfloxacin, St. John's wort, valproic acid. Drugs that may be affected by calcium blockers include anesthetics, antiarrhythmic agents, antineoplastics, benzodiazepines, buspirone, carbamazepine, digoxin, dofetilide, ethanol, HMG-CoA reductase inhibitors, lovastatin, imipramine, lithium, methylprednisolone, moricizine, nondepolarizing muscle relaxants, prazosin, quinidine, sirolimus, tacrolimus, theophyllines, vincristine.

**Diltiazem** and **verapamil** inhibit other CYP3A4 substrates, whereas the dihydropyridines do not.

*Drug/Food interactions:* **Nifedipine, amlodipine**, and **verapamil** may be administered without regard to meals.

Bioavailability of **felodipine** is not affected by food, but increased more than 2-fold when taken with doubly concentrated grapefruit juice vs water or orange juice.

High-fat meals and grapefruit juice with **nisoldipine** should be avoided.

**Adverse Reactions**
Generally not serious; rarely requires discontinuation or dosage adjustment.

| Calcium Channel Blocker Adverse Reactions (%)[*] | | | | | | | | | |
|---|---|---|---|---|---|---|---|---|---|
| Adverse reactions | Amlodipine | Diltiazem Oral (IV)[1] | Felodipine | Isradipine[1] | Nicardipine Oral (IV)[1] | Nifedipine[1] | Nimodipine | Nisoldipine | Verapamil Oral (IV)[1] |
| **Cardiovascular** | | | | | | | | | |
| Angina increased | | | | | 5.6[2] | ≤ 1 | | | |
| AV block (1°, 2°, or 3°) | | ≤ 7.6 (< 1) | | | (†) | | | ≤ 1 | 0.8-1.7 |
| Bradycardia | ≤ 1 | ≤ 6 (< 1) | | | | < 1 | ≤ 1 | | 1.4 (1.2) |
| Edema | 1.8-14.6[4] | ≤ 6 (< 1) | | 3.5-35.9[2] | 0.6-1 | 10-30[2] | ≤ 1.2[2] | | 1.7-3 |
| ECG abnormalities | | ≤ 4.1 | | | 0.6 (1.4) | | ≤ 1.4 | | 2 |
| Hypotension | ≤ 1 | < 2 | 0.5-1.5 | ≤ 1 | † (5.6) | < 1 | ≤ 8.1[2] | ≤ 1 | 0.7-2.5 |
| Hypotension, symptomatic | | (3.2) | | | | | | | (1.5) |
| Palpitations | 0.7-4.5[2] | ≤ 2 | 0.4-2.5 | 1-5.1[2] | 2.8-4.1 | ≤ 7 | < 1 | 3 | ≤ 1 |
| Peripheral edema | | 2-15 (4.3) | 2-17.4 | | (†) | 7-29[2] | | 7-29[2] | 3.7 |
| Tachycardia | ≤ 1 | < 2 | 0.5-1.5 | ≤ 3.4 | 0.8-3.4 (3.5) | ≤ 1 | ≤ 1.4 | | |
| Vasodilation | | ≤ 3 | | | 4.7-5.5 (0.7) | | | 4 | |
| **CNS** | | | | | | | | | |
| Asthenia | 1-2 | ≤ 4 (< 1) | 2.2-3.9 | | 0.9-5.8 (0.7) | ≤ 4 | | | 2 |
| Dizziness/Lightheadedness | ≤ 3.4[2] | ≤ 10 (< 1) | 2.7-3.7 | 3.4-8 | 1.6-6.9 (1.4) | 4-27 | < 1 | 3-10[2] | 3-4.7 (1.2) |
| Drowsiness | | | | ≤ 1 | | | | | |
| Fatigue/Lethargy | 4.5[2] | | | ≤ 8.5[2] | | 4-5.9 | | | 1.7-4.5 |
| Headache | 7.3 | ≤ 12 (< 1) | 10.6-14.7 | 10.3-22 | 6.2-8.2 | 10-23 | ≤ 4.1[2] | 22 | 2.2-12.1 (1.2) |
| Nervousness | ≤ 1 | ≤ 2 | 0.5-1.5 | ≤ 1 | 0.6 | ≤ 7 | | ≤ 1 | |
| Tremor | ≤ 1 | < 2 | | | 0.6 | ≤ 8 | | ≤ 1 | |
| Weakness | | | | ≤ 1.2 | | 10-12 | | | |

## Calcium Channel Blocker Adverse Reactions (%)[*]

| | Adverse reactions | Amlodipine | Diltiazem Oral (IV)[1] | Felodipine | Isradipine[1] | Nicardipine Oral (IV)[1] | Nifedipine[1] | Nimodipine | Nisoldipine | Verapamil Oral (IV)[1] |
|---|---|---|---|---|---|---|---|---|---|---|
| GI | Abdominal discomfort | 1.6 | 1 | 0.5-1.5 | ≤ 5.1 | (0.7) | < 3 | | | (0.6) |
| | Anorexia | ≤ 1 | < 2 | | | | | | ≤ 1 | |
| | Constipation | ≤ 1 | ≤ 3.6 (< 1) | 0.3-1.5 | ≤ 3.8 | 0.6 | ≤ 3.3 | | | 3.9-11.7 |
| | Diarrhea | ≤ 1 | ≤ 2 | 0.5-1.5 | ≤ 3.4 | | < 3 | ≤ 4.2 | ≤ 1 | ≤ 2.4 |
| | Dry mouth | ≤ 1 | < 2 (< 1) | 0.5-1.5 | ≤ 1 | 0.4-1.4 | < 3 | | ≤ 1 | ≤ 1 |
| | Dyspepsia | 1-2 | ≤ 6 | 0.5-3.9 | | 0.8-1.5 (†) | < 3 | | ≤ 1 | 2.5-2.7 |
| | GI distress | | | | | | | | | ≤ 1 |
| | Nausea | 2.9[2] | ≤ 2.2 (< 1) | 1-1.7 | 1-5.1 | 1.9-2.2 (4.9) | 2-11 | 0.6-1.4 | 2 | 1.7-2.7 (0.9) |
| | Vomiting | ≤ 0.1 | ≤ 2 (< 1) | 0.5-1.5 | ≤ 1.3 | 0.4-0.6 (4.9) | ≤ 1 | < 1 | | |
| Respiratory | Cough | ≤ 0.1 | | 0.8-1.7 | ≤ 1 | | ≤ 6 | | | |
| | Dyspnea | 1-2 | ≤ 6 (< 1) | 0.5-1.5 | ≤ 3.4 | 0.6 (0.7) | ≤ 6 | ≤ 1.2 | ≤ 1 | 1.4 |
| | Nasal congestion | | < 2 | | | | ≤ 6 | | | |
| | Pharyngitis | | 1.4-6 | 0.5-1.5 | | | < 1 | | ≤ 5 | 3 |
| | Rhinitis | ≤ 0.1 | ≤ 9.6 | | | † | | | ≤ 1 | 2.7 |
| | Upper respiratory infection | | | 0.7-3.9 | | | ≤ 1 | | | 5.4 |
| | Wheezing | | | | | | 6 | < 1 | | |
| Miscellaneous | Flu-like illness/syndrome/symptoms | | ≤ 2.3 | 0.5-1.5 | | | | | ≤ 1 | 3.7 |
| | Flushing | 0.7-4.5[4] | ≤ 3 (1.7) | 3.9-6.9 | 1.2-5.1[2] | 5.6-9.7 | ≤ 25 | ≤ 2.1 | | 0.6-0.8 |
| | Injection site reactions | | (3.9) | | | (1.4) | | | | |
| | Infection | | ≤ 6 | | | † | | | | 12.1 |
| | Muscle cramps | 1-2 | < 2 | 0.5-1.5 | | | ≤ 8 | ≤ 1.4 | | ≤ 1 |
| | Pain | ≤ 1 | ≤ 6 | | | 0.6 | < 3 | | | |
| | Sore throat | | | | | † | 6 | | | |
| | Tinnitus | ≤ 1 | < 2 | | | † (†) | ≤ 1 | | ≤ 1 | ≤ 1 |
| | Urinary frequency | ≤ 1 | | 0.5-1.5 | 1.3-3.4 | ≤ 0.6 (†) | ≤ 3 | | ≤ 1 | ≤ 1 |

[*] Data are pooled from separate studies and are not necessarily comparable.
[1] Includes data for SR/ER form.
[2] Dose-related.
[3] Functional rhythm or isorhythmic dissociation.
[4] Dose-related and higher in females.
†Occurs, no incidence reported.

# VASOPRESSORS USED IN SHOCK

*Vasopressors:* Sympathomimetic agents are used in shock to treat hypoperfusion in normovolemic patients and in patients unresponsive to whole blood or plasma volume expanders. These agents increase myocardial contractility, constrict capacitance vessels, and dilate resistance vessels. In cardiogenic shock or advanced shock from other causes associated with a low cardiac output, they may be combined with vasodilators (eg, nitroprusside, nitroglycerin) to maintain blood pressure while the vasodilator improves myocardial performance. Nitroprusside is used to reduce preload and afterload and improve cardiac output. Nitroglycerin directly relaxes the venous vasculature and decreases preload.

*Pharmacology:* Sympathomimetic agents produce $\alpha$-adrenergic stimulation (vasoconstriction), $\beta_1$-adrenergic stimulation (increase myocardial contractility, heart rate, automaticity, and AV conduction), and $\beta_2$-adrenergic activity (peripheral vasodilation). Dopamine also causes vasodilation of the renal and mesenteric, cerebral, and coronary beds by dopaminergic receptor activation.

*Monitoring:* Monitoring shock patients and their response to drugs requires special vigilance. Monitor heart rate, blood pressure, and ECG continuously. Record urine output and fluid intake frequently. Due to rapid and life-threatening changes that can occur in the hemodynamically unstable patient, optimal drug selection, dose titration, and management is probably best achieved with the use of invasive hemodynamic monitoring.

*Administration:* Administration only should be via the IV route using a large-bore, free flowing IV in the antecubital vein, or a central vein due to unpredictable absorption. Small IVs in the extremities are both unreliable and unsafe for vasopressor administration. Frequent monitoring of the IV sites for extravasation injury is essential when vasopressor agents are being used.

*Prolonged, high-dose therapy:* Prolonged, high-dose therapy can produce cyanosis and tissue necrosis of distal extremities. The principle of using the lowest dose that produces an adequate response for the shortest period of time is very important when using these agents.

*Plasma volume depletion:* Prolonged use of vasopressors may result in plasma volume depletion; correct this by appropriate fluid and electrolyte replacement therapy. If plasma volumes are not corrected, hypotension may recur when these drugs are discontinued.

*Acidosis:* Acidosis lessens the response to vasopressors; therefore, correct acidosis if it exists or develops during the course of vasopressor therapy.

*Avoid continuous IV therapy:* Acute tolerance develops during continuous IV administration. High concentration/low volume (250 mL) vasopressor solutions administered with the aid of an infusion control device allows for maximum dosing flexibility because fluids and drugs can be regulated independently and the development of tolerance is minimized.

286  VASOPRESSORS USED IN SHOCK

| Effects of Vasopressors Used in Shock | | | | | | | | |
|---|---|---|---|---|---|---|---|---|
| | Sites of action | | | | Hemodynamic response | | | |
| | Heart | | Blood vessels | | | | | |
| +++ pronounced effect<br>++ moderate effect<br>+ slight effect<br>0 no effect<br>↑ increase<br>↓ decrease | Contractility (Inotropic) | SA Node Rate (Chronotropic) | Vasoconstriction | Vasodilatation | Renal Perfusion | Cardiac Output | Total Peripheral Resistance | Blood Pressure |
| | $\beta_1$ | $\beta_1$ | $\alpha$ | $\beta_2$ | | | | |
| **Inotropic** Isoproterenol | +++ | +++ | 0 | +++ | ↑[1] or ↓[2] | ↑ | ↓ | ↑[3]↓[4] |
| Dobutamine | +++ | 0 to +[5] | 0 to +[5] | + | 0 | ↑ | ↓ | ↑ |
| Dopamine | +++ | + to ++[5] | + to +++[5] | 0 to +[6] | ↑[5] | ↓ | ↓[5] or ↑ | 0 to ↑ |
| **Mixed** Epinephrine | +++ | +++ | +++[5] | ++[5] | ↓ | ↑ | ↓ | ↑[3]↓[4] |
| Norepinephrine | ++ | ++[7] | +++ | 0 | ↓ | 0 or ↓ | ↑ | ↑ |
| Ephedrine | ++ | ++ | + | 0 to + | ↓ | ↑ | ↑ or ↓ | ↑ |
| Mephentermine | + | + | + | ++ | ↑ or ↓ | ↑ | 0 to ↑ | ↑ |
| Metaraminol | + | + | ++ | 0 | ↓ | ↓ | ↑ | ↑ |
| **Pressors** Methoxamine | 0 | 0[7] | +++ | 0 | ↓ | 0 or ↓ | ↑ | ↑ |
| Phenylephrine | 0 | 0[7] | +++ | 0 | ↓ | ↓ | ↑ | ↑ |

[1] Cardiogenic or septicemic shock.
[2] Normotensive patient.
[3] Systolic effect.
[4] Diastolic effect.
[5] Effects are dose dependent.
[6] Dilates renal and splanchnic beds via dopaminergic effect at doses less than 10 mcg/kg/min.
[7] Decreased heart rate may result from reflex mechanisms.

| Common Dilutions and Infusion Rates for Selected Drugs Used in Shock | | |
|---|---|---|
| Drug | Usual Dilution for IV Infusion | Infusion Rate |
| Isoproterenol | 2 mg (10 mL) in 500 mL D5W (4 mcg/mL) or 1 mg (5 mL) in 250 mL D5W | 5 mcg/min |
| Dobutamine | 250 mg in 250 to 500 mL NS or D5W (500 to 1000 mcg/mL) | 2.5 to 15 mcg/kg/min |
| Dopamine | 200 to 800 mg in 250 to 500 mL NS or D5W (400 to 3200 mcg/mL) | Low dose – 2.5 to 10 mcg/kg/min<br>High dose – 20 to 50 mcg/kg/min |
| Norepinephrine | 4 mg in 250 mL of D5W (16 mcg/mL) | Initial: 8 to 12 mcg/min<br>Maintenance: 2 to 4 mcg/min |

# BETA-ADRENERGIC BLOCKING AGENTS

| | |
|---|---|
| **ACEBUTOLOL HCl** | |
| **Capsules**: 200 and 400 mg (*Rx*) | Various, *Sectral* (Wyeth-Ayerst) |
| **ATENOLOL** | |
| **Tablets**: 25, 50, and 100 mg (*Rx*) | Various, *Tenormin* (AstraZeneca) |
| **Injection**: 5 mg/10 mL (*Rx*) | *Tenormin* (AstraZeneca) |
| **BETAXOLOL HCl** | |
| **Tablets**: 10 and 20 mg (*Rx*) | *Kerlone* (Searle) |
| **BISOPROLOL FUMARATE** | |
| **Tablets**: 5 and 10 mg (*Rx*) | *Zebeta* (Lederle) |
| **CARTEOLOL HCl** | |
| **Tablets**: 2.5 and 5 mg (*Rx*) | *Cartrol* (Abbott) |
| **ESMOLOL HCl** | |
| **Injection**: 10 or 250 mg/mL (*Rx*) | *Brevibloc* (Baxter) |
| **METOPROLOL** | |
| **Tablets**: 50 and 100 mg (*Rx*) | *Lopressor* (Novartis) |
| **Tablets, extended-release**: 25, 50, 100, and 200 mg (*Rx*) | *Toprol XL* (AstraZeneca) |
| **Injection**: 1 mg/mL (*Rx*) | Various, *Lopressor* (Novartis) |
| **NADOLOL** | |
| **Tablets**: 20, 40, 80, 120, and 160 mg (*Rx*) | Various, *Corgard* (Bristol-Myers Squibb) |
| **PENBUTOLOL SULFATE** | |
| **Tablets**: 20 mg (*Rx*) | *Levatol* (Schwarz Pharma) |
| **PINDOLOL** | |
| **Tablets**: 5 and 10 mg (*Rx*) | Various, *Visken* (Novartis) |
| **PROPRANOLOL** | |
| **Tablets**: 10, 20, 40, 60, 80, and 90 mg (*Rx*) | Various, *Inderal* (Wyeth-Ayerst) |
| **Capsules, sustained-release**: 60, 80, 120, and 160 mg (*Rx*) | Various, *Inderal LA* (Wyeth-Ayerst), *InnoPran XL* (Reliant) |
| **Solution, oral**: 4 and 8 mg/mL (*Rx*) | Various |
| **Solution, concentrated oral**: 80 mg/mL (*Rx*) | *Propranolol Intensol* (Roxane) |
| **Injection**: 1 mg/mL (*Rx*) | Various, *Inderal* (Wyeth-Ayerst) |
| **SOTALOL HCl** | |
| **Tablets**: 80, 120, 160, and 240 mg (*Rx*) | Various, *Betapace* (Berlex) |
| 80, 120, 160 mg (*Rx*) | *Betapace AF* (Berlex) |
| **TIMOLOL MALEATE** | |
| **Tablets**: 5, 10, and 20 mg (*Rx*) | Various, *Blocadren* (Merck) |

**Warning:**

To minimize the risk of induced arrhythmia, patients initiated or reinitiated on *Betapace* or *Betapace AF* should be placed for a minimum of 3 days (on their maintenance dose) in a facility that can provide cardiac resuscitation, continuous electrocardiographic monitoring, and calculations of creatinine clearance. For detailed instructions regarding dose selection and special cautions for people with renal impairment, see Administration and Dosage.

Do not substitute *Betapace* for *Betapace AF* because of significant differences in labeling (eg, patient package insert, dosing administration, safety information).

## Indications

| Beta-Adrenergic Blocking Agents — Summary of Indications | | | | | | | | | | | | |
|---|---|---|---|---|---|---|---|---|---|---|---|---|
| Indications<br>✔ = labeled<br>x = unlabeled | Acebutolol | Atenolol | Betaxolol | Bisoprolol | Carteolol | Esmolol | Metoprolol | Nadolol | Penbutolol | Pindolol | Propranolol | Sotalol | Timolol |
| Hypertension | ✔ | ✔ | ✔ | ✔ | ✔ | | ✔ | ✔ | ✔ | ✔ | ✔ | | ✔ |
| Angina pectoris | | ✔ | | | | | ✔ | ✔ | | | ✔¹ | | |
| Cardiac arrhythmias | | | | | | | | | | | | | |
| Supraventricular arrhythmias/tachycardias | | | | | | ✔ | | | | | ✔² | | |
| Sinus tachycardia | | | | | | ✔ | | | | | | | |
| Intraoperative and postoperative tachycardia and hypertension | | | | | | ✔ | | | | | | | |
| Ventricular arrhythmias/tachycardias | | | | | | | | | | | ✔ | ✔³ | |
| Premature ventricular contractions (PVCs) | ✔ | | | | | | | | | | ✔ | | |
| Digitalis-induced tachyarrhythmias | | | | | | | | | | | ✔ | | |
| Resistant tachyarrhythmias (during anesthesia) | | | | | | | | | | | ✔ | | |
| Atrial ectopy | | | | | | x | | | | | | | |
| Maintenance of normal sinus rhythm | | | | | | | | | | | | ✔ | |
| MI | | ✔ | | | | | ✔ | | | | ✔² | | ✔ |
| CHF (stable)⁴ | | | | x | | | ✔⁵ | | | | | | |
| Pheochromocytoma | | | | | | | | | | | ✔² | | |
| Migraine prophylaxis | | x | | | | | x | x | | | ✔¹ | | ✔ |
| Hypertrophic subaortic stenosis | | | | | | | | | | | ✔¹ | | |
| Essential tremors | | | | | | | | | | | ✔² | | |
| Parkinsonian tremors | | | | | | | | x | | | x⁶ | | |
| Akathisia, antipsychotic-induced | | | | | | | x | | | | x | | |
| Variceal bleeding in portal hypertension | | x | | | | | x | x | | | x | | x |
| Atrial fibrillation | | | | | | | | | | | | | |
| Rapid heart rate control | | | | | | x | | | | | | | |
| Maintenance heart rate control | | | | | | x | | | | | | | |
| Generalized anxiety disorder | | | | | | | | | | | x | | |
| Angina | | | | | | | | | | | | | |
| Stable | x | | | x | | | | | | | | | |
| Unstable | | x | | | | x | x | | | | | | |

¹ Except *InnoPram XL*.
² Except extended-release.
³ Not *Betapace AF*.
⁴ See Precautions or Warnings.
⁵ *Toprol-XL* 25 mg only.
⁶ Sustained-release only.

### Administration and Dosage

ACEBUTOLOL HCl:

*Hypertension –*

*Initial dose:* 400 mg in uncomplicated mild to moderate hypertension. May be given as a single daily dose, but 200 mg twice/day may be required for adequate control. Optimal response usually occurs with 400 to 800 mg/day (range, 200 to 1200 mg/day given twice daily).

*Ventricular arrhythmia –*

*Initial dose:* 400 mg (200 mg twice/day). Increase dosage gradually until optimal response is obtained, usually 600 to 1200 mg/day.

*Elderly –* Because bioavailability increases about 2-fold, older patients may require lower maintenance doses. Avoid doses greater than 800 mg/day.

*Renal/Hepatic function impairment* – Reduce the daily dose by 50% when creatinine clearance is less than 50 mL/min/1.73$^2$. Reduce by 75% when it is less than 25 mL/min/1.73$^2$. Use cautiously in impaired hepatic function.

ATENOLOL:
*Hypertension (oral)* –
Initial dosage: 50 mg once daily, used alone or in combination with other antihypertensive agents. If an optimal response is not achieved, increase to 100 mg/day. Dosage greater than 100 mg/day is unlikely to produce any further benefit.

*Angina pectoris (oral)* –
Initial dosage: 50 mg/day. If an optimal response is not achieved within 1 week, increase to 100 mg/day. Some patients may require 200 mg/day for optimal effect.

With once-daily dosing, 24-hour control is achieved by giving doses larger than necessary to achieve an immediate maximum effect. The maximum early effect on exercise tolerance occurs with doses of 50 to 100 mg, but the effect at 24 hours is attenuated, averaging approximately 50% to 75% of that with once-daily doses of 200 mg.

*Acute MI* –
IV: Initiate treatment as soon as possible after the patient's arrival in the hospital and after eligibility is established. Begin treatment with 5 mg over 5 minutes followed by another 5 mg IV injection 10 minutes later. Dilutions in dextrose injection, sodium chloride injection, or sodium chloride and dextrose injection may be used. These admixtures are stable for 48 hours if not used immediately.

*Oral:* In patients who tolerate the full 10 mg IV dose, initiate 50 mg tablets 10 minutes after the last IV dose followed by another 50 mg dose 12 hours later. Thereafter, administer 100 mg once daily or 50 mg twice/day for a further 6 to 9 days or until discharge from the hospital.

If there is any question concerning the use of IV atenolol, eliminate the IV administration and use the tablets at a dosage of 100 mg once daily or 50 mg twice/day for 7 days or more.

*Renal function impairment* –

| Atenolol Dosage Adjustments in Severe Renal Impairment | | |
|---|---|---|
| Creatinine clearance (mL/min/1.73 m$^2$) | Elimination half-life (h) | Maximum dosage |
| 15 to 35 | 16 to 27 | 50 mg/day |
| < 15 | > 27 | 50 mg every other day |

*Hemodialysis* – Give 25 or 50 mg after each dialysis.

BETAXOLOL HCl:
*Initial dose* – 10 mg once daily, alone or added to diuretic therapy. If the desired response is not achieved the dose can be doubled. Increasing the dose to more than 20 mg has not produced a statistically significant additional hypertensive effect; however, the 40 mg dose is well tolerated.

*Elderly* – Consider reducing the starting dose to 5 mg.

*Renal function impairment* – In patients with renal impairment, clearance of betaxolol declines with decreasing renal function.

In patients with severe renal impairment and those undergoing dialysis, the initial dose is 5 mg once daily. If the desired response is not achieved, dosage may be increased by 5 mg/day increments every 2 weeks to a maximum dose of 20 mg/day.

BISOPROLOL FUMARATE: May be given without regard to meals.
*Initial dose* – 5 mg once daily. In some patients, 2.5 mg may be appropriate. If the antihypertensive effect of 5 mg is inadequate, the dose may be increased to 10 mg and then, if necessary, to 20 mg once daily.

*Renal/Hepatic function impairment* – In patients with renal dysfunction (Ccr less than 40 mL/min) or hepatic impairment (hepatitis or cirrhosis), use an initial daily dose of 2.5 mg and use caution in dose titration.

*Elderly* – Dose adjustment is not necessary.

CARTEOLOL HCl:
   Initial dose – 2.5 mg as a single daily dose, either alone or with a diuretic. If adequate response is not achieved, gradually increase to 5 and 10 mg as single daily doses. Doses greater than 10 mg/day are unlikely to produce further benefit, and may decrease response.
   Maintenance – 2.5 to 5 mg once daily.
   Renal function impairment –

| Carteolol Dosage in Renal Impairment | |
| --- | --- |
| Creatinine clearance (mL/min/1.73 m²) | Dosage interval (h) |
| > 60 | 24 |
| 20 to 60 | 48 |
| < 20 | 72 |

ESMOLOL HCl:
   Supraventricular tachycardia – 50 to 200 mcg/kg/min; average dose is 100 mcg/kg/min although dosages as low as 25 mcg/kg/min have been adequate. Dosages as high as 300 mcg/kg/min provide little added effect and an increased rate of adverse effects, and are not recommended.

| Dosage in Supraventricular Tachycardia | | | | |
| --- | --- | --- | --- | --- |
| Time | Loading dose (over 1 minute) | | Maintenance dose (over 4 minutes) | |
| (minutes) | mcg/kg/min | mg/kg/min | mcg/kg/min | mg/kg/min |
| 0 to 1 | 500 | 0.5 | | |
| 1 to 5 | | | 50 | 0.05 |
| 5 to 6 | 500 | 0.5 | | |
| 6 to 10 | | | 100 | 0.1 |
| 10 to 11 | 500 | 0.5 | | |
| 11 to 15 | | | 150 | 0.15 |
| 15 to 16 | — | — | | |
| 16 to 20 | | | 200[1] | 0.2[1] |
| 20 to (24 hours) | | | Maintenance dose titrated to heart rate or other clinical endpoint | |

[1] As the desired heart rate or endpoint is approached, the loading infusion may be omitted and the maintenance infusion titrated to 300 mcg/kg/min (0.3 mg/kg/min) or downward as appropriate. Maintenance dosages more than 200 mcg/kg/min (0.2 mg/kg/min) have not been shown to have significantly increased benefits. The interval between titration steps may be increased.

   If adequate therapeutic effect is not observed within 5 minutes, repeat loading dose and follow with maintenance infusion increased to 100 mcg/kg/min. Continue titration procedure, repeating loading infusion, increasing maintenance infusion by increments of 50 mcg/kg/min (for 4 minutes). As desired heart rate or a safety endpoint (eg, lowered blood pressure) is approached, omit loading infusion and titrate the maintenance dosage up or down to endpoint. Also, if desired, increase interval between titration steps from 5 to 10 minutes.
   This specific dosage regimen has not been intraoperatively studied. Because of the time required for titration, it may not be optimal for intraoperative use.
   The safety of dosages greater than 300 mcg/kg/min has not been studied.
   In the event of an adverse reaction, reduce dosage or discontinue the drug. If a local infusion site reaction develops, use an alternative site. Avoid butterfly needles.
   Transfer to alternative agents – After achieving adequate heart rate control and stable clinical status, transition to alternative antiarrhythmic agents may be accomplished.
   Reduce the dosage of esmolol as follows: 30 minutes after the first dose of the alternative agent, reduce esmolol infusion rate by 50%. Following the second dose of the alternative agent, monitor patient's response and, if satisfactory control is maintained for the first hour, discontinue esmolol infusion.

*Intraoperative and postoperative tachycardia and hypertension* – In the intraoperative and postoperative settings, it is not always advisable to slowly titrate the dose of esmolol to a therapeutic effect. Therefore, 2 dosing options are presented: Immediate control dosing and a gradual control when the physician has time to titrate.

*Immediate control:* For intraoperative treatment of tachycardia and hypertension, give an 80 mg (approximately 1 mg/kg) bolus dose over 30 seconds followed by a 150 mcg/kg/min infusion, if necessary. Adjust the infusion rate as required up to 300 mcg/kg/min to maintain desired heart rate or blood pressure.

*Gradual control:* For postoperative tachycardia and hypertension, the dosing schedule is the same as that used in supraventricular tachycardia. To initiate treatment, administer a loading dosage infusion of 500 mcg/kg/min for 1 minute followed by a 4-minute maintenance infusion of 50 mcg/kg/min. If an adequate therapeutic effect is not observed within 5 minutes, repeat the same loading dosage and follow with a maintenance infusion increased to 100 mcg/kg/min (see Supraventricular tachycardia).

*Withdrawal effects* – The use of esmolol infusions for up to 24 hours has been well documented. Limited data indicate that esmolol is well tolerated for up to 48 hours.

*Preparation of solution* –

*250 mg/mL ampule:* Aseptically prepare a 10 mg/mL infusion by adding two 2500 mg ampuls to a 500 mL container or one 2500 mg ampule to a 250 mL container of one of the IV fluids listed below (see Compatibility/Stability). This yields a final concentration of 10 mg/mL. The diluted solution is stable for 24 hours or more at room temperature. Esmolol has been well tolerated when administered via a central vein.

The 250 mg/mL strength is concentrated, and is not for direct IV injection; dilute prior to infusion. Do not mix with sodium bicarbonate. Do not mix with other drugs prior to dilution in a suitable IV fluid.

*10 mg/mL:* This dosage form is prediluted to provide a ready-to-use 10 mg/mL concentration. It may be used to administer an esmolol loading dose infusion by hand-held syringe while the maintenance infusion is being prepared.

*Compatibility/Stability* – Esmolol, at a final concentration of 10 mg/mL, is compatible with the following solutions and is stable for 24 hours or more at controlled room temperature or under refrigeration: 5% dextrose injection; 5% dextrose in Lactated Ringer's injection; 5% dextrose in Ringer's injection; 5% dextrose and 0.9% or 0.45% sodium chloride injection; Lactated Ringer's injection; potassium chloride (40 mEq/L) in 5% dextrose injection; 0.9% or 0.45% sodium chloride injection.

Esmolol is *not* compatible with 5% sodium bicarbonate injection.

METOPROLOL:

*Tablets (immediate-release) and injection* –

*Hypertension:*

*Initial dosage* – 100 mg/day in single or divided doses, used alone or added to a diuretic taken with or immediately after meals. The dosage may be increased at weekly (or longer) intervals until optimum blood pressure reduction is achieved.

*Maintenance dosage* – 100 to 450 mg/day. Dosages greater than 450 mg/day have not been studied. While once daily dosing is effective and can maintain a reduction in blood pressure throughout the day, lower doses (especially 100 mg) may not maintain a full effect at the end of the 24-hour period; larger or more frequent daily doses may be required.

*Angina pectoris:*

*Initial dosage* – 100 mg/day in 2 divided doses. Dosage may be gradually increased at weekly intervals until optimum clinical response is obtained or a pronounced slowing of heart rate occurs. Effective dosage range is 100 to 400 mg/day. Dosages above 400 mg/day have not been studied.

*MI:*

*Early treatment* – During the early phase of definite or suspected acute MI, initiate treatment as soon as possible. Administer 3 IV bolus injections of 5 mg each at approximately 2 minute intervals.

In patients who tolerate the full IV dose (15 mg), give 50 mg orally every 6 hours 15 minutes after the last IV dose and continue for 48 hours. Thereafter, administer a maintenance dosage of 100 mg twice daily.

In patients who do not tolerate the full IV dose, start with 25 or 50 mg orally every 6 hours (depending on the degree of intolerance) 15 minutes after the last IV dose or as soon as the clinical condition allows.

*Late treatment* – Patients with contraindications to early treatment, patients who do not tolerate the full early treatment, and patients in whom therapy is delayed for any other reason should be started at 100 mg orally, twice daily, as soon as their clinical condition allows. Continue for 3 months or more.

*Tablets, extended release* – The extended-release tablets are for once daily administration. When switching from immediate-release metoprolol tablets to extended-release, use the same daily dose.

*Hypertension:* The usual initial dosage is 50 to 100 mg/day in a single dose whether used alone or added to a diuretic. The dosage may be increased at weekly (or longer) intervals until optimum blood pressure reduction is achieved. Dosages greater than 400 mg/day have not been studied.

*Angina pectoris:* The usual initial dosage is 100 mg/day in a single dose. The dosage may be gradually increased at weekly intervals until optimum clinical response has been obtained or there is a pronounced slowing of the heart rate. Dosages greater than 400 mg/day have not been studied.

*CHF:* Dosage must be individualized and closely monitored during up-titration. Prior to initiation of therapy, stabilize the dosing of diuretics, ACE inhibitors, and digitalis (if used). The recommended starting dose is 25 mg once daily for 2 weeks in patients with NYHA Class II heart failure and 12.5 mg once daily in patients with more severe heart failure. Then double the dose every 2 weeks to the highest dosage level tolerated by the patient or up to 200 mg. If transient worsening of heart failure occurs, it may be treated with increased dose of diuretics, and it may be necessary to lower the dose of metoprolol or temporarily discontinue it. The dose should not be increased until symptoms of worsening heart failure have been stabilized; initial difficulty with titration should not preclude later attempts to introduce metoprolol. If heart failure patients experience symptomatic bradycardia, reduce the dose.

NADOLOL:

*Angina pectoris* –

*Initial dose:* 40 mg/day. Gradually increase dosage in 40 to 80 mg increments at 3- to 7-day intervals until optimum clinical response is obtained or there is pronounced slowing of the heart rate.

*Maintenance dosage:* Usual dose is 40 to 80 mg once daily. Up to 160 to 240 mg once daily may be needed. The safety and efficacy of dosages exceeding 240 mg/day have not been established.

*Hypertension* –

*Initial dose:* 40 mg once daily, alone or in addition to diuretic therapy. Gradually increase dosage in 40 to 80 mg increments until optimum blood pressure reduction is achieved.

*Maintenance dose:* Usual dose is 40 to 80 mg once daily. Up to 240 to 320 mg once daily may be needed.

*Renal function impairment* –

| Nadolol Dosage Adjustments in Renal Failure | |
| --- | --- |
| Creatinine clearance (mL/min/1.73$^2$) | Dosage interval (h) |
| > 50 | 24 |
| 31 to 50 | 24 to 36 |
| 10 to 30 | 24 to 48 |
| < 10 | 40 to 60 |

*PENBUTOLOL SULFATE:* Usual starting and maintenance dose is 20 mg once daily. Doses of 40 to 80 mg have been well tolerated but have not shown greater antihypertensive effect. A dose of 10 mg also lowers blood pressure, but the full effect is not seen for 4 to 6 weeks.

*PINDOLOL:*

*Initial dose* – 5 mg twice daily, alone or with other antihypertensive agents. If a satisfactory reduction in blood pressure does not occur within 3 to 4 weeks, adjust dose in increments of 10 mg/day at 3 to 4 week intervals, to a maximum of 60 mg/day.

*PROPRANOLOL HCl:*

| Propranolol Dosage Based on Indication |||||
|---|---|---|---|---|
| Indication | Initial dosage | Usual range | Maximum daily dosage |
| Arrhythmias | | 10-30 mg tid-qid (given ac and hs) | |
| Hypertension | 40 mg bid or 80 mg once daily (ER) | 120-240 mg/day (given bid or tid) or 80-160 mg once daily (ER) | 640 mg |
| Angina | 80 mg once daily (ER) | 80-320 mg bid, tid, qid or 160 mg once daily (ER) | 320 mg |
| MI | | 180-240 mg/day (given bid or tid) | 240 mg |
| IHSS | | 20-40 mg tid-qid (given ac and hs) or 8-160 mg once daily (ER) | |
| Pheochromocytoma | | 60 mg/day × 3 days preoperatively (in divided doses) | |
| Inoperable tumor | | 30 mg/day (in divided doses) | |
| Migraine | 80 mg/day once daily (ER) or in divided doses | 160-240 mg once daily (ER) or in divided doses | |
| Essential tremor | 40 mg bid | 120 mg/day | 320 mg |

*Extended-release capsules* – The extended-release capsule should be administered once daily. Administer *InnoPran XL* at bedtime (approximately 10 pm) consistently either on an empty stomach or with food. The starting dose is 80 mg but dosage should be individualized and titration may be needed to a dose of 120 mg or higher. Doses of *InnoPran XL* above 120 mg had no additional effects on blood pressure. The time needed for full antihypertensive response is variable, but is usually achieved within 2 to 3 weeks.

*Parenteral* –

*Usual dose:* 1 to 3 mg. Do not exceed 1 mg/min. If necessary, give a second dose after 2 minutes. Thereafter, do not give additional drug in under 4 hours. Transfer to oral therapy as soon as possible.

*Pediatrics* – IV use is not recommended; however, an unlabeled dose of 0.01 to 0.1 mg/kg/dose to a maximum of 1 mg/dose by slow infusion over 5 minutes has been used for arrhythmias.

Oral dosage for treating hypertension requires titration, beginning with a 1 mg/kg/day dosage regimen (eg, 0.5 mg/kg twice daily). May be increased at 3- to 5-day intervals to a maximum of 16 mg/kg/day.

The usual pediatric dosage range is 2 to 4 mg/kg/day in 2 equally divided doses (eg, 1 to 2 mg/kg twice daily). Dosage calculated by weight generally produces plasma levels in a therapeutic range similar to that in adults. Do not use doses more than 16 mg/kg/day.

*Concentrated oral solution* – Mix with liquid or semi-solid food such as water, juices, soda or soda-like beverages, applesauce, and puddings. Draw into the dropper the amount prescribed for a single dose. Then squeeze the dropper contents into a liquid or semi-solid food. Stir the liquid or food gently for a few seconds. The entire amount of the mixture, of drug and liquid or drug and food, should be consumed immediately. Do not store for future use.

SOTALOL HCl:

Betapace – The recommended initial dose is 80 mg twice daily. This dose may be increased if necessary, after appropriate evaluation, to 240 or 320 mg/day (120 to 160 mg bid). In most patients, a therapeutic response is obtained at a total daily dose of 160 to 320 mg/day, given in 2 or 3 divided doses. Some patients with life-threatening refractory ventricular arrhythmias may require doses as high as 480 to 640 mg/day.

Adjust dosage gradually, allowing 3 days between dosing increments to attain steady-state plasma concentrations and allow monitoring of QT intervals.

Renal function impairment:

| Sotalol Dosing Interval in Renal Impairment | |
|---|---|
| Creatinine clearance (mL/min) | Dosing interval (hours)[1] |
| ≥ 60 | 12 |
| 30 to 59 | 24 |
| 10 to 29 | 36 to 48 |
| < 10 | Individualize dosage |

[1] The initial dose of 80 mg and subsequent doses should be administered at these intervals. See following paragraph for dosage escalations.

Dose escalations in renal impairment should be done after administration of at least 5 to 6 doses at appropriate intervals (see above table).

Exercise extreme caution in the use of sotalol in patients with renal failure undergoing hemodialysis. The half-life of sotalol is prolonged (up to 69 hours) in anuric patients. However, sotalol can be partly removed by dialysis with subsequent partial rebound in concentrations when dialysis is completed. Safety (heart rate, QT interval) and efficacy (arrhythmia control) must be closely monitored.

Betapace AF – Therapy with Betapace AF must be initiated (and if necessary, titrated) in a setting that provides continuous ECG monitoring and in the presence of personnel trained in the management of serious ventricular arrhythmias. Continue to monitor patients in this way for a minimum of 3 days on the maintenance dose. In addition, do not discharge patients within 12 hours of electrical or pharmacological conversion to normal sinus rhythm.

The QT interval is used to determine patient eligibility for Betapace AF treatment and for monitoring safety during treatment. The baseline QT interval must be less than or equal to 450 msec in order for a patient to be started on Betapace AF therapy. During initiation and titration, monitor the QT interval 2 to 4 hours after each dose. If the QT interval prolongs to 500 msec or more, the dose must be reduced or the drug discontinued.

The dose of Betapace AF must be individualized according to creatinine clearance. Modify the dosing interval according to the following table.

| Betapace AF Dosing Interval in Renal Impairment | |
|---|---|
| Creatinine clearance (mL/min) | Dosing interval (hours) |
| > 60 | 12 |
| 40 to 60 | 24 |
| < 40 | Contraindicated |

The recommended initial dose of Betapace AF is 80 mg and is initiated as shown in the dosing algorithm described below. The 80 mg dose can be titrated upward to 120 mg during initial hospitalization or after discharge on 80 mg in the event of recurrence, by rehospitalization and repeating the same steps used during the initiation of therapy (see Upward Titration of Dose).

Anticoagulate patients with atrial fibrillation according to usual medical practice. Correct hypokalemia before initiation of Betapace AF therapy (see Warnings).

Patients to be discharged on Betapace AF therapy from an inpatient setting should have an adequate supply of Betapace AF to allow uninterrupted therapy until the patient can fill a Betapace AF prescription.

*Initiation of therapy:*

1.) Electrocardiographic assessment: Prior to administration of the first dose, the QT interval must be determined using an average of 5 beats. If the baseline QT is greater than 450 msec (JT 330 msec or more if QRS over 100 msec), *Betapace AF* is contraindicated.

2.) Starting dose: The starting dose of *Betapace AF* is 80 mg twice daily if the creatinine clearance is greater than 60 mL/min, and 80 mg once daily if the creatinine clearance is 40 to 60 mL/min. If the creatinine clearance is less than 40 mL/min, *Betapace AF* is contraindicated.

3.) Administer the appropriate daily dose of *Betapace AF* and begin continuous ECG monitoring with QT interval measurements 2 to 4 hours after each dose.

4.) If the 80 mg dose level is tolerated and the QT interval remains less than 500 msec after at least 3 days (after 5 or 6 doses if patient is receiving once daily dosing), the patient can be discharged. Alternatively, during hospitalization, the dose can be increased to 120 mg twice daily and the patient followed for 3 days on this dose (followed for 5 or 6 doses if the patient is receiving once daily doses).

*Upward titration of dose:* If the 80 mg dose level (given once or twice daily depending upon the creatinine clearance) does not reduce the frequency of relapses of AFIB/AFL and is tolerated without excessive QT interval prolongation (ie, 520 msec or more), the dose level may be increased to 120 mg (once or twice daily depending on the creatinine clearance). As proarrhythmic events can occur not only at initiation of therapy, but also with each upward dosage adjustment, steps 2 through 5 used during initiation of *Betapace AF* therapy should be followed when increasing the dose level. In a US multicenter dose-response study, a 120 mg dose (once or twice daily) was found to be the most effective in prolonging the time to ECG documented symptomatic recurrence of AFIB/AFL. If the 120 mg dose does not reduce the frequency of early relapse of AFIB/AFL and is tolerated without excessive QT interval prolongation (520 msec or more), an increase to 160 mg (once or twice daily depending on the creatinine clearance) can be considered. Steps 2 through 5 used during the initiation of therapy should be used again to introduce such an increase.

*Maintenance of Betapace AF therapy:* Regularly re-evaluate renal function and QT if medically warranted. If QT is at least 520 msec (JT 430 msec or greater if QRS is greater than 100 msec), reduce the dose of *Betapace AF* therapy and carefully monitor patients until QT returns to less 520 msec. If the QT interval is 520 msec or more while on the lowest maintenance dose level (80 mg), discontinue the drug. If renal function deteriorates, reduce the daily dose in half by administering the drug once daily as described in Initiation of Therapy, step 3.

*Special considerations:* The maximum recommended dose in patients with a calculated creatinine clearance greater than 60 mL/min is 160 mg twice/day, doses greater than 160 mg twice/day have been associated with an increased incidence of torsades de pointes and are not recommended.

A patient who misses a dose should not double the next dose. The next dose should be taken at the usual time.

*Transfer to sotalol from other antiarrhythmic therapy* – Before starting sotalol, generally withdraw previous antiarrhythmic therapy under careful monitoring for a minimum of 2 to 3 plasma half-lives if the patient's clinical condition permits. Treatment has been initiated in some patients receiving IV lidocaine without ill effect. After discontinuation of amiodarone, do not initiate sotalol until the QT interval is normalized.

*Transfer to Betapace AF from Betapace* – Patients with a history of symptomatic atrial fibrillation/atrial flutter (AFIB/AFL) who are currently receiving *Betapace* for the maintenance of normal sinus rhythm should be transferred to *Betapace AF* because of the significant differences in labeling (ie, patient package insert for *Betapace AF*, dosing, administration, and safety information).

*TIMOLOL MALEATE:*

*Hypertension –*

*Initial dosage:* 10 mg twice/day used alone or added to a diuretic.

*Maintenance dosage:* 20 to 40 mg/day. Titrate, depending on blood pressure and heart rate. Increases to a maximum of 60 mg/day divided into 2 doses may be necessary. There should be an interval of at least 7 days between dosage increases.

*MI (long-term prophylactic use in patients who have survived the acute phase of MI)* – 10 mg twice/day.

*Migraine* – Initial dosage is 10 mg twice/day. During maintenance therapy the 20 mg/day dosage may be given as a single dose. Total daily dosage may be increased to a maximum of 30 mg in divided doses or decreased to 10 mg once daily depending on clinical response and tolerability. Discontinue if a satisfactory response is not obtained after 6 to 8 weeks of the maximum daily dosage.

## Actions

*Pharmacology:*

| Pharmacologic/Pharmacokinetic Properties of Beta-Adrenergic Blocking Agents | | | | | | | | | |
|---|---|---|---|---|---|---|---|---|---|
| 0 – none<br>+ – low<br>++ – moderate<br>+++ – high<br>Drug | Adrenergic-receptor blocking activity | Membrane stabilizing activity | Intrinsic sympathomimetic activity | Lipid solubility | Extent of absorption (%) | Absolute oral bioavailability (%) | Half-life (h) | Protein binding (%) | Metabolism/Excretion |
| Acebutolol | $\beta_1$[1] | +[2] | + | Low | 90 | 20-60 | 3-4 | 26 | Hepatic; renal excretion 30% to 40%; nonrenal excretion 50% to 60% (bile; intestinal wall) |
| Atenolol | $\beta_1$[1] | 0 | 0 | Low | 50 | 50-60 | 6-7 | 6-16 | ≈ 50% excreted unchanged in feces |
| Betaxolol | $\beta_1$[1] | + | 0 | Low | ≈ 100 | 89 | 14-22 | ≈ 50 | Hepatic; > 80% recovered in urine, 15% unchanged |
| Bisoprolol | $\beta_1$[1] | 0 | 0 | Low | ≥ 90 | 80 | 9-12 | ≈ 30 | ≈ 50% excreted unchanged in urine, remainder as inactive metabolites; < 2% excreted in feces. |
| Esmolol | $\beta_1$[1] | 0 | 0 | Low | na[3] | na[3] | 0.15 | 55 | Rapid metabolism by esterases in cytosol of red blood cells |
| Metoprolol | $\beta_1$[1] | 0[2] | 0 | Moderate | ≈ 100 | 40-50 | 3-7 | 12 | Hepatic; renal excretion, < 5% unchanged |
| Metoprolol, long-acting | | | | | | 77[4] | | | |
| Carteolol | $\beta_1$  $\beta_2$ | 0 | ++ | Low | 85 | 85 | 6 | 23-30 | 50% to 70% excreted unchanged in urine |
| Nadolol | $\beta_1$  $\beta_2$ | 0 | 0 | Low | 30 | 30-50 | 20-24 | 30 | Urine, unchanged |
| Penbutolol | $\beta_1$  $\beta_2$ | 0 | + | High | ≈ 100 | ≈ 100 | ≈ 5 | 80-98 | Hepatic (conjugation, oxidation); renal excretion of metabolites (17% as conjugate) |
| Pindolol | $\beta_1$  $\beta_2$ | 0 | +++ | Low | > 95 | ≈ 100 | 3-4[5] | 40 | Urinary excretion of metabolites (60% to 65%) and unchanged drug (35% to 40%) |

| Pharmacologic/Pharmacokinetic Properties of Beta-Adrenergic Blocking Agents | | | | | | | | | |
|---|---|---|---|---|---|---|---|---|---|
| 0 – none<br>+ – low<br>++ – moderate<br>+++ – high<br>Drug | Adrenergic-receptor blocking activity | Membrane stabilizing activity | Intrinsic sympathomimetic activity | Lipid solubility | Extent of absorption (%) | Absolute oral bioavailability (%) | Half-life (h) | Protein binding (%) | Metabolism/Excretion |
| Propranolol | β₁  β₂ | ++ | 0 | High | < 90 | 30 | 3-5 | 90 | Hepatic; < 1% excreted unchanged in urine |
| Propranolol, long-acting | | | | | | 9-18 | 8-11 | | |
| Sotalol | β₁  β₂ | 0 | 0 | Low | nd⁶ | 90-100 | 12 | 0 | Not metabolized; excreted unchanged in urine |
| Timolol | β₁  β₂ | 0 | 0 | Low to moderate | 90 | 75 | 4 | < 10 | Hepatic; urinary excretion of metabolites and unchanged drug |

[1] Inhibits β₂ receptors (bronchial and vascular) at higher doses.
[2] Detectable only at doses much greater than required for beta blockade.
[3] Not applicable (available IV only).
[4] Average bioavailability; not absolute.
[5] In elderly hypertensive patients with normal renal function, t½ variable: 7 to 15 hours.
[6] No data.

## Contraindications

Sinus bradycardia; greater than first degree heart block; cardiogenic shock; congestive heart failure (CHF) unless secondary to a tachyarrhythmia treatable with β-blockers; overt cardiac failure; hypersensitivity to β-blocking agents.

*Acebutolol, carteolol:* Persistently severe bradycardia.

*Propranolol, nadolol, timolol, penbutolol, carteolol, sotalol, and pindolol:* Bronchial asthma or bronchospasm, including severe chronic obstructive pulmonary disease.

*Metoprolol:* Treatment of MI in patients with a heart rate less than 45 beats/min; significant heart block greater than first degree (PR interval 0.24 seconds or more); systolic blood pressure less than 100 mm Hg; moderate to severe cardiac failure.

*Sotalol:* Congenital or acquired long QT syndromes.

## Warnings

*Proarrhythmia:* Like other antiarrhythmic agents, **sotalol** can provoke new or worsened ventricular arrhythmias in some patients, including sustained ventricular tachycardia or ventricular fibrillation, with potentially fatal consequences. Because of its effect on cardiac repolarization, is the most common form of proarrhythmia associated with sotalol, occurring in approximately 4% of high-risk patients.

*Cardiac failure:* Sympathetic stimulation is a vital component supporting circulatory function in CHF, and β-blockade carries the potential hazard of further depressing myocardial contractility and precipitating more severe failure.

*Wolff-Parkinson-White syndrome:* In several cases, the tachycardia was replaced by a severe bradycardia requiring a demand pacemaker after **propranolol** administration with as little as 5 mg.

*Abrupt withdrawal:* The occurrence of a β-blocker withdrawal syndrome is controversial. However, hypersensitivity to catecholamines has been observed in patients withdrawn from β-blocker therapy. Exacerbation of angina, MI, ventricular arrhythmias, and death have occurred after abrupt discontinuation of therapy. Reduce dosage gradually over 1 to 2 weeks and carefully monitor the patient.

Because coronary artery disease may be unrecognized, do not discontinue therapy abruptly, even in patients treated only for hypertension, as abrupt withdrawal may result in transient symptoms.

*Peripheral vascular disease:* Treatment with β-antagonists reduces cardiac output and can precipitate or aggravate the symptoms of arterial insufficiency in patients with peripheral or mesenteric vascular disease.

*Nonallergic bronchospasm (eg, chronic bronchitis, emphysema):* In general, do not administer β-blockers to patients with bronchospastic diseases. Administer **nadolol, timolol, penbutolol, propranolol, sotalol,** and **pindolol** with caution, because they may block bronchodilation produced by endogenous or exogenous catecholamine stimulation of β_2 receptors.

Because of their relative β_1 selectivity, low doses of **metoprolol, acebutolol, bisoprolol,** and **atenolol** may be used with caution in patients with bronchospastic disease who do not respond to, or cannot tolerate, other antihypertensive treatment.

*Bradycardia:* **Metoprolol** produces a decrease in sinus heart rate in most patients; this decrease is greatest among patients with high initial heart rates and least among patients with low initial heart rates.

*Pheochromocytoma:* It is hazardous to use **propranolol** or **atenolol** unless α-adrenergic blocking drugs are already in use, because this would predispose to serious blood pressure elevation.

*Sinus bradycardia:* Sinus bradycardia (heart rate less than 50 beats/min) occurred in 13% of patients receiving **sotalol** in clinical trials, and led to discontinuation in about 3%. Bradycardia itself increases risk of torsade de pointes.

*Electrolyte disturbances:* Do not use **sotalol** in patients with hypokalemia or hypomagnesemia prior to correction of imbalance.

*Hypotension:* If hypotension (systolic blood pressure up to 90 mm Hg) occurs, discontinue drug and carefully assess patient's hemodynamic status and extent of myocardial damage.

*Anaphylaxis:* Anaphylaxis has occurred and may include symptoms such as profound hypotension, bradycardia with or without AV nodal block, severe sustained bronchospasm, hives, and angioedema. Deaths have occurred. Refer to Management of Acute Hypersensitivity Reactions.

*Anesthesia and major surgery:* Necessity, or desirability, of withdrawing β-blockers prior to major surgery is controversial. β-blockade impairs the heart's ability to respond to β-adrenergically mediated reflex stimuli. While this might help prevent arrhythmic response, risk of excessive myocardial depression during general anesthesia may be enhanced, and difficulty restarting and maintaining heart beat has occurred. If β-blockers are withdrawn, allow 48 hours between the last dose and anesthesia. Others may recommend withdrawal of β-blockers well before surgery takes place.

*AV block:* **Metoprolol** slows AV conduction and may produce significant first (PR interval 0.26 seconds or more), second; or third-degree heart block. Acute MI also produces heart block.

*Sick sinus syndrome:* Use **sotalol** only with extreme caution in patients with sick sinus syndrome associated with symptomatic arrhythmias, because it may cause sinus bradycardia, sinus pauses, or sinus arrest.

*Concomitant use of calcium channel blockers (atenolol):* Bradycardia and heart block can occur and the left ventricular end diastolic pressure can rise when beta-blockers are administered with verapamil or diltiazem. Patients with preexisting conduction abnormalities or left ventricular dysfunction are particularly susceptible.

*Recent acute MI (sotalol):* Sotalol can be used safely and effectively in the long-term treatment of life-threatening ventricular arrhythmias following an MI. However, experience in the use of sotalol to treat cardiac arrhythmias in the early phase of recovery from acute MI is limited and at least at high initial doses is not reassuring. In the first 2 weeks post-MI, caution is advised and careful dose titration is especially important, particularly in patients with markedly impaired ventricular function.

*Intraoperative and postoperative tachycardia and hypertension:* Do not use esmolol as the treatment for hypertension in patients in whom the increased blood pressure is primarily caused by the vasoconstriction associated with hypothermia.

*Renal/Hepatic function impairment:* Use with caution.

*Pregnancy: Category D* (**atenolol**).

*Category C* (**betaxolol, esmolol, metoprolol, nadolol, timolol, propranolol, penbutolol, carteolol, bisoprolol**).

*Category B* (**acebutolol, pindolol, sotalol**).

*Lactation:* In general, nursing should not be undertaken by mothers receiving these drugs.

*Children:* Safety and efficacy for use in children have not been established.

IV administration of **propranolol** is not recommended in children; however, oral propranolol has been used.

## Precautions

*Diabetes/Hypoglycemia:* β-adrenergic blockade may blunt premonitory signs and symptoms (eg, tachycardia, blood pressure changes) of acute hypoglycemia. Nonselective β-blockers may potentiate insulin-induced hypoglycemia.

*Thyrotoxicosis:* β-adrenergic blockers may mask clinical signs (eg, tachycardia) of developing or continuing hyperthyroidism. Abrupt withdrawal may exacerbate symptoms of hyperthyroidism, including thyroid storm.

In contrast, propranolol may be beneficial in reducing the symptoms of thyrotoxicosis.

*Serum lipid concentrations:* β-blockers may alter serum lipids including an increase in the concentration of total triglycerides, total cholesterol and LDL and VLDL cholesterol, and a decrease in the concentration of HDL cholesterol.

*Muscle weakness:* β-blockade has potentiated muscle weakness consistent with certain myasthenic symptoms (eg, diplopia, ptosis, generalized weakness).

## Drug Interactions

Drugs that may affect beta blockers include aluminum salts, barbiturates, calcium salts, cholestyramine, cimetidine, colestipol, diphenhydramine, hydroxychloroquine, NSAIDs, penicillins (ampicillin), rifampin, salicylates, SSRIs, sulfinpyrazole, calcium blockers, oral contraceptives, flecainide, haloperidol, hydralazine, loop diuretics, MAO inhibitors, phenothiazines, propafenone, quinidine, quinolones (ciprofloxacin), thioamines, and thyroid hormones.

Drugs that may be affected by beta blockers include flecainide, gabapentin, haloperidol, hydralazine, phenothiazines, anticoagulants, benzodiazepines, clonidine, disopyramide, epinephrine, ergot alkaloids, lidocaine, nondepolarizing muscle relaxants, prazosin, sulfonylureas, and theophylline.

*Drug/Lab test interactions:* These agents may produce hypoglycemia and interfere with glucose or insulin tolerance tests. **Propranolol** and **betaxolol** may interfere with the glaucoma screening test due to a reduction in intraocular pressure.

*Drug/Food interactions:* Food enhances the bioavailability of **metoprolol** and **propranolol**; this effect is not noted with **nadolol, bisoprolol,** or **pindolol**. The rate of **carteolol** and **penbutolol** absorption is slowed by the presence of food; however, extent of absorption is not appreciably affected. **Sotalol** absorption is reduced approximately 20% by a standard meal.

## Adverse Reactions

Most adverse effects are mild and transient and rarely require withdrawal of therapy.

*Cardiovascular:* Bradycardia; torsade de pointes and other serious new ventricular arrhythmias; chest pain; hypertension; hypotension; peripheral ischemia; pallor; flushing; worsening of angina and arterial insufficiency; shortness of breath; peripheral vascular insufficiency; CHF; edema; pulmonary edema; vasodilation; presyncope and syncope; tachycardia; palpitations; first-, second-, and third-degree heart block; abnormal ECG; supraventricular tachycardia.

*CNS:* Dizziness; vertigo; tiredness/fatigue; headache; mental depression; peripheral neuropathy; paresthesias; lethargy; anxiety; nervousness; diminished concentration/memory; somnolence; restlessness; insomnia; sleep disturbances; sedation; change in behavior; mood change; incoordination; hallucinations; acute mental changes in the elderly; increase in signs and symptoms of myasthenia gravis.

It has been suggested that the more lipophilic the β-blocker, the higher the CNS penetration and subsequent incidence of adverse CNS effects.

*Dermatologic:* Rash; pruritus; skin irritation; increased pigmentation; sweating/hyperhidrosis; alopecia; dry skin; psoriasis; acne; eczema; flushing; purpura; erythematous rash.

*Endocrine:* Hyperglycemia; hypoglycemia; unstable diabetes.

*GI:* Gastric/epigastric pain; flatulence; gastritis; constipation; nausea; diarrhea; dry mouth; vomiting; heartburn; appetite disorder; anorexia; bloating; abdominal discomfort/pain; dyspepsia; taste distortion.

*GU:* Sexual dysfunction; impotence or decreased libido; dysuria; nocturia; urinary retention or frequency.

*Hematologic:* Agranulocytosis; nonthrombocytopenic or thrombocytopenic purpura; bleeding; thrombocytopenia; eosinophilia; leukopenia; hyperlipidemia.

*Hypersensitivity:* Pharyngitis; photosensitivity reaction; erythematous rash; fever combined with aching and sore throat; laryngospasm; respiratory distress; angioedema; anaphylaxis.

*Musculoskeletal:* Joint pain; arthralgia; muscle cramps/pain; back/neck pain; arthritis; twitching/tremor; localized pain; extremity pain; myalgia.

*Ophthalmic:* Eye irritation/discomfort; dry/burning eyes; blurred vision; conjunctivitis; ocular pain/pressure; abnormal lacrimation.

*Respiratory:* Bronchospasm; dyspnea; cough; bronchial obstruction; wheezing; nasal stuffiness; pharyngitis; laryngospasm with respiratory distress; asthma; rhinitis; sinusitis.

*Miscellaneous:* Facial swelling; weight gain; weight loss; Raynaud's phenomenon; speech disorder; earache; asthenia; malaise; fever; death.

*Lab test abnormalities:* **Propranolol** may elevate blood urea levels in patients with severe heart disease. **Propranolol** and **metoprolol** may cause elevated serum transaminase, alkaline phosphatase and LDH.

Minor persistent elevations in AST and ALT have occurred in 7% of patients treated with **pindolol**. Elevations of AST and ALT of 1 to 2 times normal have occurred with **bisoprolol** (3.9% to 6.2%).

# LABETALOL HCl

| | |
|---|---|
| **Tablets**: 100, 200, and 300 mg (Rx) | Various, *Trandate* (Faro Pharmaceuticals) |
| **Injection**: 5 mg/mL (Rx) | Various, *Normodyne* (Key), *Trandate* (Faro Pharmaceuticals) |

### Indications
*Oral:* Hypertension, alone or with other agents, especially thiazide and loop diuretics.

*Parenteral:* For control of blood pressure in severe hypertension.

### Administration and Dosage
*Oral:*
    *Initial dose* – 100 mg twice/day, alone or added to a diuretic. After 2 or 3 days, using standing BP as an indicator, titrate dosage in increments of 100 mg twice/day, every 2 or 3 days.

    *Maintenance dose* – 200 to 400 mg twice/day. Patients with severe hypertension may require 1.2 to 2.4 g/day. Should side effects (principally nausea or dizziness) occur with twice daily dosing, the same total daily dose given 3 times/day may improve tolerability. Titration increments should not exceed 200 mg twice/day.

*Parenteral:*
    *Repeated IV injection* – Initially, 20 mg (0.25 mg/kg for an 80 kg patient) slowly over 2 minutes. Additional injections of 40 or 80 mg can be given at 10 minute intervals until a desired supine BP is achieved or a total of 300 mg has been injected. The maximum effect usually occurs within 5 minutes of each injection.

    *Slow continuous infusion* – Give at a rate of 3 mL/min (2 mg/min). Continue infusion until satisfactory response is obtained; then discontinue infusion and start oral labetalol. Effective IV dose range is 50 to 200 mg, up to 300 mg.

*Transfer to oral dosing (hospitalized patients):* Begin oral dosing when supine diastolic BP begins to rise. Recommended initial dose is 200 mg, then 200 or 400 mg, 6 to 12 hours later, depending on BP response. Thereafter, proceed as follows:

| Inpatient Titration Instructions | |
|---|---|
| IV regimen | Oral daily dose* |
| 200 mg twice a day | 400 mg |
| 400 mg twice a day | 800 mg |
| 800 mg twice a day | 1600 mg |
| 1200 mg twice a day | 2400 mg |

* Total daily dose may be given in 3 divided doses.

### Actions
*Pharmacology:* Labetalol combines both selective, competitive postsynaptic $\alpha_1$-adrenergic blocking, and nonselective, competitive β-adrenergic blocking activity. The α- and β-blocking actions decrease BP. Standing BP is lowered more than supine.

*Pharmacokinetics:*
    *Absorption/Distribution* – Oral labetalol is completely absorbed; peak plasma levels occur in 1 to 2 hours. Steady-state plasma levels during repetitive dosing are reached by about the third day. Due to an extensive first-pass effect, absolute bioavailability is 25%. Protein binding is approximately 50%.

    *Metabolism/Excretion* – Metabolism is mainly through conjugation to glucuronide metabolites, which are excreted in urine and in feces (via bile). Elimination half-life is 5.5 to 8 hours. About 55% to 60% of a dose appears in urine as conjugates or unchanged drug in the first 24 hours.

    *Onset/Peak/Duration* –
        *Oral:* The peak effects of single oral doses occur within 2 to 4 hours and lasts 8 to 12 hours. The maximum, steady-state BP response upon oral, twice-a-day dosing occurs within 24 to 72 hours.

        *IV:* The maximum effect of each IV injection of labetalol at each dose level occurs within 5 minutes. Following discontinuation of IV therapy, BP approaches pretreatment baseline values in 16 to 18 hours.

## Contraindications

Bronchial asthma; overt cardiac failure; greater than first-degree heart block; cardiogenic shock; severe bradycardia.

## Warnings

*Cardiac failure:* Avoid use in overt CHF; may be used with caution in patients with a history of heart failure who are well compensated. CHF has been observed in patients receiving labetalol.

*Patients without history of cardiac failure (latent cardiac insufficiency):* Continued depression of myocardium with β-blockers can lead to cardiac failure.

*Withdrawal:* Hypersensitivity to catecholamines has been seen in patients withdrawn from β-blockers. When discontinuing chronic labetalol, particularly in ischemic heart disease, gradually reduce dosage over 1 to 2 weeks and carefully monitor.

*Nonallergic bronchospasm (eg, chronic bronchitis, emphysema):* Patients with bronchospastic disease should, in general, not receive β-blockers.

*Diabetes mellitus and hypoglycemia:* β-blockade may prevent the appearance of premonitory signs and symptoms of acute hypoglycemia. β-blockade also reduces insulin release; it may be necessary to adjust antidiabetic drug dose.

*Major surgery:* Withdrawing β-blockers prior to major surgery is controversial. Protracted severe hypotension and difficulty restarting or maintaining heartbeat have been reported with beta blockers.

*Rapid decreases of BP:* Observe caution when reducing severely elevated BP. Achieve desired BP lowering over as long a time as possible.

*Hepatic function impairment:* Drug metabolism may be diminished.

*Jaundice or hepatic dysfunction* – Jaundice or hepatic dysfunction has rarely been associated with labetalol.

*Elderly:* Bioavailability is increased in elderly patients.

*Pregnancy:* Category C.

*Lactation:* Small amounts are excreted in breast milk.

*Children:* Safety and efficacy for use in children have not been established.

## Precautions

*Hypotension:* Symptomatic postural hypotension is most likely to occur 2 to 4 hours after a dose, especially following a large initial dose or upon large changes in dose. It is likely to occur if patients are tilted or allowed to assume the upright position 3 hours or less of receiving labetalol injection.

## Drug Interactions

Drugs that may interact with labetalol include beta-adrenergic agonists, cimetidine, glutethimide, halothane, and nitroglycerin.

*Drug/Lab test interactions:* A labetalol metabolite may falsely increase urinary catecholamine levels when measured by a nonspecific trihydroxyindole reaction.

*Drug/Food interactions:* Food may increase bioavailability of the drug.

## Adverse Reactions

Significant adverse reactions include fatigue; headache; drowsiness; paresthesias; difficulty in micturition; diarrhea; reversible increases in serum transaminases; dyspnea; bronchospasm; asthenia; muscle cramps; nausea; vomiting; fever with aching and sore throat; toxic myopathy; rashes; systemic lupus erythematosus; vision abnormality; hypoesthesia; ventricular arrhythmias; intensification of AV block; mental depression; scalp tingling.

# CARVEDILOL

**Tablets:** 3.125, 6.25, 12.5, and 25 mg *(Rx)*                    *Coreg* (GlaxoSmithKline)

## Indications

*Essential hypertension:* Management of essential hypertension. It can be used alone or in combination with other antihypertensive agents, especially thiazide-type diuretics.

*Congestive heart failure (CHF):* For the treatment of mild to severe heart failure of ischemic or cardiomyopathic origin, in conjunction with digitalis, diuretics, and ACE inhibitors, to reduce the progression of disease.

*Left ventricular dysfunction (LVD) following MI:* To reduce cardiovascular mortality in clinically stable patients who have survived the acute phase of a MI and have a left ventricular ejection fraction of 40% or less (with or without symptomatic heart failure).

*Unlabeled uses:* Carvedilol appears to be beneficial in the treatment of the following conditions: Angina pectoris (25 to 50 mg twice daily).

## Administration and Dosage

*Hypertension:* The recommended starting dose is 6.25 mg twice daily. If this dose is tolerated, using standing systolic pressure measured about 1 hour after dosing as a guide, maintain the dose for 7 to 14 days, and then increase to 12.5 mg twice daily, if needed, based on trough blood pressure, again using standing systolic pressure 1 hour after dosing as a guide for tolerance. This dose also should be maintained for 7 to 14 days and can then be adjusted upward to 25 mg twice/day if tolerated and needed. The full antihypertensive effect of carvedilol is seen within 7 to 14 days. Total daily dose should not exceed 50 mg. Carvedilol should be taken with food to slow the rate of absorption and reduce the incidence of orthostatic effects.

*CHF:* Dosage must be individualized and closely monitored during up-titration. Prior to initiation, it is recommended that fluid retention be minimized.

The recommended starting dose of carvedilol is 3.125 mg twice daily for 2 weeks. If this dose is tolerated, it can then be increased to 6.25, 12.5, and 25 mg twice daily over successive intervals of at least 2 weeks. Maintain patients on lower doses if higher doses are not tolerated. A maximum dose of 50 mg twice daily has been administered to patients weighing over 85 kg (187 lbs) with mild to moderate heart failure.

Advise patients that initiation of treatment and (to a lesser extent) dosage increases may be associated with transient symptoms of dizziness or lightheadedness (and rarely syncope) within the first hour after dosing. Thus, during these periods, avoid situations such as driving or hazardous tasks, where symptoms could result in injury. In addition, vasodilatory symptoms often do not require treatment, but it may be useful to separate the time of dosing of carvedilol from that of the ACE inhibitor or to temporarily reduce the dose of the ACE inhibitor. Do not increase the dose of carvedilol until symptoms of worsening heart failure or vasodilation have been established.

Treat fluid retention (with or without transient worsening heart failure symptoms) with an increase in the dose of diuretics.

Reduce the dose of carvedilol if patients experience bradycardia (heart rate less than 55 beats/minute).

Episodes of dizziness or fluid retention during initiation of carvedilol can generally be managed without discontinuation of treatment and do not preclude subsequent successful titration of, or a favorable response to, carvedilol.

*LVD following MI:* Dosage must be individualized and monitored during up-titration. Treatment with carvedilol may be started as an inpatient or outpatient and started after the patient is hemodynamically stable and fluid retention has been minimized. It is recommended that carvedilol be started at 6.25 mg twice daily and increased after 3 to 10 days, based on tolerability to 12.5 mg twice daily, then again to the target dose of 25 mg twice daily. A lower starting dose may be used (3.125 mg twice daily) and/or, the rate of up-titration may be slowed if clinically indicated (eg, because of low BP, heart rate, fluid retention). Maintain patients on lower doses if higher doses are not tolerated. The recommended dosing regimen need not be altered in patients who received treatment with an IV or oral β-blocker during the acute phase of the MI.

*Discontinuation:* Because carvedilol has β-blocking activity, do not discontinue abruptly. Severe exacerbation of angina and the occurrence of MI and ventricular arrhythmias have been reported. Instead, discontinue over 1 or 2 weeks.

## Actions

*Pharmacology:* Carvedilol, an antihypertensive agent, is a racemic mixture in which nonselective β-adrenoreceptor blocking activity is present in the S(-) enantiomer and α-adrenergic blocking activity is present in both R(+) and S(-) enantiomers at equal potency. Carvedilol has no intrinsic sympathomimetic activity.

Carvedilol (1) reduces cardiac output, (2) reduces exercise- or isoproterenol-induced tachycardia, and (3) reduces reflex orthostatic tachycardia. Significant β-blocking effect is usually seen within 1 hour of drug administration.

Carvedilol also (1) attenuates the pressor effects of phenylephrine, (2) causes vasodilation, and (3) reduces peripheral vascular resistance. These effects contribute to the reduction of blood pressure and usually are seen within 30 minutes of drug administration.

*Pharmacokinetics:*

*Absorption/Distribution* – Carvedilol is rapidly and extensively absorbed following oral administration, with absolute bioavailability of approximately 25% to 35% due to a significant degree of first-pass metabolism. Following oral administration, the apparent mean terminal elimination half-life generally ranges from 7 to 10 hours. Plasma concentrations achieved are proportional to the oral dose administered.

Carvedilol is more than 98% bound to plasma proteins (primarily albumin). It has a steady-state volume of distribution of approximately 115 L, indicating substantial distribution into extravascular tissues. Plasma clearance ranges from 500 to 700 mL/min.

*Metabolism/Excretion* – Carvedilol is extensively metabolized. Following oral administration in healthy volunteers, carvedilol accounted for only about 7% of the total in plasma as measured by area under the curve. Less than 2% of the dose was excreted unchanged in the urine. The metabolites of carvedilol are excreted primarily via the bile into the feces.

## Contraindications

Patients with decompensated cardiac failure requiring the use of IV inotropic therapy (such patients should first be weaned from IV therapy before initiating carvedilol); bronchial asthma (see Warnings) or related bronchospastic conditions; second- or third-degree AV block; sick sinus syndrome or severe bradycardia (unless a permanent pacemaker is in place); cardiogenic shock; clinically manifest hepatic impairment; hypersensitivity to the drug.

## Warnings

*Abrupt withdrawal:* Because carvedilol has β-blocking activity, do not discontinue abruptly. Severe exacerbation of angina and the occurrence of MI and ventricular arrhythmias have been reported. Instead, discontinue over 1 or 2 weeks.

*Bronchial asthma:* Two cases of death from status asthmaticus have occurred in patients receiving single doses of carvedilol.

*Bronchospasm, nonallergic (eg, chronic bronchitis, emphysema):* In general, do not give β-blockers to patients with bronchospastic disease. However, carvedilol may be used with caution in patients who do not respond to, or cannot tolerate, other antihypertensive agents. If carvedilol is used, it is prudent to use the smallest effective dose so that inhibition of endogenous or exogenous β-agonists is minimized.

*Cardiac failure:* Worsening cardiac failure or fluid retention may occur during up-titration of carvedilol. If such symptoms occur, increase diuretics and do not advance the carvedilol dose until clinical stability resumes. Occasionally, it is necessary to lower the carvedilol dose or temporarily discontinue it. Such episodes do not preclude subsequent successful titration of carvedilol.

*Peripheral vascular disease:* β-blockers can precipitate or aggravate symptoms of arterial insufficiency in patients with peripheral vascular disease. Exercise caution.

*Hypotension and postural hypotension:* Hypotension and postural hypotension occurred in 9.7% and syncope in 3.4% of CHF patients receiving carvedilol, compared with 3.6% and 2.5% of placebo patients, respectively. The risk for these events was highest during the first 30 days of dosing.

*Anesthesia and major surgery:* If carvedilol treatment is to be continued perioperatively, take particular care with anesthetic agents which depress myocardial function.

*Diabetes and hypoglycemia:* β-blockers may mask some of the manifestations of hypoglycemia, particularly tachycardia. Nonselective β-blockers may potentiate insulin-induced hypoglycemia and delay recovery of serum glucose levels. Caution patients subject to spontaneous hypoglycemia, or diabetic patients receiving insulin or oral hypoglycemic agents about these possibilities and use carvedilol with caution.

*Thyrotoxicosis:* β-adrenergic blockade may mask clinical signs of hyperthyroidism, such as tachycardia. Abrupt withdrawal of β-blockade may be followed by an exacerbation of the symptoms of hyperthyroidism or may precipitate thyroid storm.

*Pheochromocytoma:* In patients with pheochromocytoma, an α-blocking agent should be initiated prior to use of any β-blocking agent. Although carvedilol has both α- and β-blocking pharmacologic activities, there has been no experience with its use in this condition. Therefore, use caution in administering carvedilol.

*Prinzmetal variant angina:* Agents with nonselective β-blocking activity may provoke chest pain in patients with Prinzmetal variant angina. Although the α-blocking activity of carvedilol may prevent such symptoms, take caution with patients suspected of having Prinzmetal variant angina.

*Hypersensitivity reactions:* While taking β-blockers, patients with a history of severe anaphylactic reaction to a variety of allergens may be more reactive to repeated challenge, either accidental, diagnostic, or therapeutic. Such patients may be unresponsive to the usual doses of epinephrine used to treat allergic reaction.

*Renal/Hepatic function impairment:* Rarely, use of carvedilol in patients with CHF has resulted in deterioration of renal function. Patients at risk appear to be those with low blood pressure (systolic BP less than 100 mm Hg), ischemic heart disease, and diffuse vascular disease or underlying renal insufficiency. Renal function returned to baseline when carvedilol was stopped. Discontinue the drug or reduce dosage if worsening of renal function occurs.

Use of carvedilol in patients with clinically manifest hepatic impairment is not recommended. Mild hepatocellular injury, confirmed by rechallenge, has occurred rarely with carvedilol therapy.

*Elderly:* Plasma levels of carvedilol average about 50% higher in the elderly compared with young subjects. With the exception of dizziness (8.8% in the elderly vs 6% in younger patients), there were no events for which the incidence in the elderly exceeded that in the younger population by more than 2%.

*Pregnancy:* Category C.

*Lactation:* It is not known whether this drug is excreted in breast milk.

*Children:* Safety and efficacy in patients younger than 18 years of age have not been established.

## Precautions

*Monitoring:* At the first symptoms/sign of liver dysfunction (eg, pruritus, dark urine, persistent anorexia, jaundice, right upper quadrant tenderness, unexplained flu-like symptoms) perform laboratory testing. If the patient has laboratory evidence of liver injury of jaundice, stop therapy and do not restart.

*Cardiovascular effects:* Because carvedilol has β-blocking activity, it should not be discontinued abruptly, particularly in patients with ischemic heart disease. Instead, discontinue over 1 to 2 weeks.

In clinical trials, carvedilol caused bradycardia in about 2% of patients. If pulse rate drops below 55 beats/min, reduce the dosage.

*Photosensitivity:* Photosensitivity may occur; therefore, caution patients to take protective measures (ie, sunscreens, protective clothing) against exposure to ultraviolet light or sunlight until tolerance is determined.

## Drug Interactions

Drugs that may affect carvedilol include cimetidine, rifampin and SSRIs (eg, fluoxetine, paroxetine, diphenhydramine, hydroxychloroquine).

Drugs that may be affected by carvedilol include antidiabetic agents, calcium blockers, clonidine, cyclosporine, disopyramide, catecholamine depleting agents (eg, reserpine), and digoxin.

*Drug/Food interactions:* When taken with food, rate of absorption is slowed but extent of bioavailability is not affected. Taking with food minimizes the risk of orthostatic hypotension.

## Adverse Reactions

*CHF patients* – Reactions occurring in 3% or more of patients include dizziness; fatigue; upper respiratory tract infection; chest pain; diarrhea; hyperglycemia; pain; injury; generalized and dependent edema; abnormal vision; fever; bradycardia; hypotension; syncope; headache; nausea; abdominal pain; vomiting; weight increase; gout; BUN increase; NPN increase; hypercholesterolemia; back pain; arthralgia; myalgia; sinusitis; bronchitis; pharyngitis and urinary tract infection.

*Hypertensive patients* – Adverse reactions occurring in 3% or more of patients include dizziness and fatigue.

# ANTIHYPERTENSIVES

Agents used in hypertension therapy are listed in the following tables:

| **Pharmacological Effects of Antihypertensive Agents** | | | | | | | | | | | | | |
|---|---|---|---|---|---|---|---|---|---|---|---|---|---|
| ↑ = increase<br>⇧= slight increases<br>0 = no change<br>⇩= slight decrease<br>↓ = decrease | Onset (min) | Peak effect[1] (h) | Duration of action[2] (h) | Plasma volume | Plasma renin activity | RBF[3] GFR | Peripheral resistance | Cardiac output | Heart rate | LVH | Total cholesterol | HDL | LDL | Triglycerides |
| **Antiadrenergic Agents – Centrally Acting** | | | | | | | | | | | | | |
| Methyldopa | 120 | 2-6 | 12-24 | ↑ | ⇩/0 | ⇩/0 | ↓ | ⇩/0 | ⇩/0 | ↓ | 0 | 0 | 0 | 0 |
| Clonidine | 30-60 | 2-5 | 12-24 | ↑ | ⇩ | ⇩/0 | ↓ | ⇩/0 | ↓ | ↓ | 0 | 0 | 0 | 0 |
| Guanabenz | 60 | 2-4 | 6-12 | 0 | ↓ | 0 | ↓ | 0 | ↓ | ↓ | 0 | 0 | 0 | 0 |
| Guanfacine | | 1-4 | 24 | ⇩/0 | ↓ | | ↓ | 0 | ⇩ | ↓ | 0 | 0 | 0 | 0 |
| **Antiadrenergic Agents – Peripherally Acting** | | | | | | | | | | | | | |
| Reserpine | days | 6-12 | 6-24 | ↑ | ⇩/0 | ⇩/0 | ↑ | 0/↓ | ↑ | | | | | |
| Guanethidine | | 6-8 | 24-48 | ↑ | ⇩/0 | ⇩/0 | ↓ | 0/↓ | ↑ | | | | | |
| Guanadrel | 30-120 | 4-6 | 9-14 | ↑ | | 0 | ↑ | 0 | ↓ | | | | | |
| Doxazosin | | 2-3 | | | | | | | | ↓ | ↓ | ↑ | 0/↓ | ↓ |
| Prazosin | 120-130 | 1-3 | 6-12 | 0/⇧ | ⇩/0 | 0 | ↓ | 0/⇧ | 0/⇧ | ↓ | ↓ | ↑ | 0/↑ | ↓ |
| Terazosin | 15 | 1-2 | 12-24 | 0 | 0 | 0 | ↑ | ⇧ | ⇧ | ↓ | ↓ | ↑ | 0/↓ | ↓ |
| **Antiadrenergic Agents – Beta-Adrenergic Blockers** | | | | | | | | | | | | | |
| Acebutolol | | 3-8 | 24-30 | | | | ⇩ | ↓ | ↓ | 0/↓ | 0/↑ | ↓ | ↑ | 0/↑ |
| Atenolol | | 2-4 | 24 + | | ⇩/0 | ↓/0 | 0 | ↓ | ↓ | ↓ | 0/↑ | ↓ | ↑ | 0/↑ |
| Betaxolol | | | | | | | ↓ | ↓ | | | 0/↑ | ↓ | ↑ | 0/↑ |
| Bisoprolol | | | | | | | ↓ | ↓ | | | 0 | | | 0 |
| Carteolol | | 1-3 | 24 + | | | | ↓ | ↓ | | 0 | 0 | | | 0 |
| Metoprolol | | 1.5 | 13-19 | ⇩/0 | ↓ | ⇩/0 | 0/↓ | ↓ | ↓ | ↓ | 0/↑ | ↓ | ↑ | 0/↑ |
| Nadolol | | 3-4 | 17-24 | | ⇩/0 | 0 | 0 | ↓ | ↓ | ↓ | 0/↑ | ↓ | ↑ | 0/↑ |
| Penbutolol | | 1.5-3 | 20 + | | ↓ | ⇩ | 0 | ↓ | ↓ | | 0 | 0/↑ | 0 | ↑/↓ |
| Pindolol | | 1 | 24 + | | 0 | 0 | ↓ | ⇩ | ↓ | 0/↓ | 0 | 0/↑ | 0 | ↑/↓ |
| Propranolol | | 2-4 | 8-12 | ⇩/0 | ↓ | ↓ | ⇩/0 | ↓ | ↓ | ↓ | 0 | 0/↑ | 0 | ↑/↓ |
| Timolol | | 1-3 | 12 | ⇩/0 | ↓ | | 0 | ↓ | ↓ | ↓ | 0 | 0/↑ | 0 | ↑/↓ |
| **Antiadrenergic Agents – Alpha/Beta-Adrenergic Blocker** | | | | | | | | | | | | | |
| Labetalol | | 2-4 | 8-12 | ↑ | ↓ | 0/↑ | ↓ | 0 | ↓ | ↓ | | | | |
| Carvedilol | 30 | | | | | | ↓ | ↓ | ↓ | | | | | |
| **Angiotensin Converting Enzyme (ACE) Inhibitors** | | | | | | | | | | | | | |
| Benazepril | 60 | 0.5-1 | 24 | | ↑ | RBF ↑<br>GFR 0 | ↓ | 0/↑ | 0 | ↓ | 0 | 0 | 0 | 0 |
| Captopril | 15-30 | 0.5-1.5 | 6-12 | ⇧ | ↑ | RBF ↑<br>GFR 0 | ↓ | 0/↑ | 0 | ↓ | 0 | 0 | 0 | 0 |
| Enalapril | 60 | 4-6 | 24 | 0/⇧ | ↑ | RBF ↑<br>GFR 0 | ↓ | ↑ | 0 | ↓ | 0 | 0 | 0 | 0 |
| Enalaprilat | 15 | 3-4 | ≈ 6 | | ↑ | RBF ↑<br>GFR 0 | ↓ | ↑ | 0 | ↓ | 0 | 0 | 0 | 0 |
| Fosinopril | 60 | ≈ 3 | 24 | | ↑ | RBF ↑<br>GFR 0 | ↓ | 0/↑ | 0 | ↓ | 0 | 0 | 0 | 0 |
| Lisinopril | 60 | ≈ 7 | 24 | | ↑ | RBF ↑<br>GFR 0 | ↓ | 0 | 0 | ↓ | 0 | 0 | 0 | 0 |
| Quinapril | 60 | 1 | 24 | | ↑ | RBF ↑<br>GFR 0 | ↓ | 0/↑ | 0 | ↓ | 0 | 0 | 0 | 0 |
| Ramipril | 60-120 | 1 | 24 | | ↑ | RBF ↑<br>GFR 0 | ↓ | 0/↑ | 0 | ↓ | 0 | 0 | 0 | 0 |

## Pharmacological Effects of Antihypertensive Agents

↑ = increase
⇧ = slight increases
0 = no change
⇩ = slight decrease
↓ = decrease

| | Onset (min) | Peak effect[1] (h) | Duration of action[2] (h) | Plasma volume | Plasma renin activity | RBF GFR[3] | Peripheral resistance | Cardiac output | Heart rate | LVH | Total cholesterol | HDL | LDL | Triglycerides |
|---|---|---|---|---|---|---|---|---|---|---|---|---|---|---|
| **Calcium Channel Blocking Agents** | | | | | | | | | | | | | | |
| Amlodipine | gradual | 6-12 | > 24 | 0 | 0 | ↑ | ↓↓↓ | 0 | 0 | ↓ | 0 | 0 | 0 | 0 |
| Diltiazem SR | 30-60 | 6-11 | | | | | ↓ | 0-↑ | ↓-0 | ↓ | 0 | 0 | 0 | 0 |
| Felodipine | 120-300 | 2.5-5 | | | | | ↓↓↓ | ↑ | ↑ | ↓ | 0 | 0 | 0 | 0 |
| Isradipine | 120 | 1.5 | | | | | ↓↓↓ | ↑ | ↑/↓ | ↓ | 0 | 0 | 0 | 0 |
| Nicardipine | 20 | 0.5-2 | | | ⇧/↑ | ⇧ | ↓ | ↑ | ↑ | ↓ | 0 | 0/⇧ | 0 | 0 |
| Nifedipine SR | 20 | 6 | | | | | ↓↓↓ | ↑↑ | ↑ | ↓ | 0 | 0 | 0 | 0 |
| Verapamil | 30 | 1-2.2 | | | 0/⇧ | 0 | ↓ | ↑/↓ | ↑/↓ | ↓ | 0 | 0/⇧ | 0 | 0 |
| **Diuretics** | | | | | | | | | | | | | | |
| Thiazides & deriv. | 60-120 | 4-12 | 6-72 | ↓ | ↑ | ↓ | ↓ | ↓ | 0 | 0/↓ | ↑ | 0 | ↑ | ↑ |
| Loop diuretics | within 60 | 1-2 | 4-8 | ↓ | ↑ | ↓ | ↓ | ↓ | 0 | 0/↓ | ↑ | 0 | ↑ | ↑ |
| Amiloride | 120 | 6-10 | 24 | ↓ | ↑ | 0 | ↓ | ↓ | 0 | | | | | |
| Spironolactone | 24-48 h | 48-72 | 48-72 | ↓ | ↑ | 0 | ↓ | 0 | 0 | | | | | |
| Triamterene | 2-4 h | 6-8 | 12-16 | | | | | | | | | | | |
| **Vasodilators** | | | | | | | | | | | | | | |
| Hydralazine | 45 | 0.5-2 | 6-8 | ↑ | ↑ | ↑ | ↓ | ↑ | ↑ | ↑ | | | | |
| Minoxidil | 30 | 2-3 | 24-72 | ↑ | ↑ | 0 | ↓ | ↑ | ↑ | ↑ | | | | |
| **Agents For Pheochromocytoma** | | | | | | | | | | | | | | |
| Phentolamine | immed. | | 5-10 min | ⇧ | ↑ | ↑ | ↓ | 0/↑ | ↑ | | | | | |
| Phenoxy-benzamine | gradual | 2-3 | 24 + | ⇧ | ↑ | ↑ | ↓ | ↑ | ↓ | | | | | |
| Metyrosine | | 6 + | 2-3 days | | | | ↓ | | ↓ | | | | | |
| **Agents For Hypertensive Emergencies/Urgencies** | | | | | | | | | | | | | | |
| Nitroprusside | 0.5-1 | | 3-5 min | ↑ | ↑ | 0 | ↓ | ⇩ | ⇧ | NA[4] | | | | |
| Diazoxide | 1-2 | 5 min | < 12 | ↑ | ↑ | ↑ | ↓ | ↑ | ↑ | | | | | |
| Trimethaphan camsylate | 1-2 | | 10-15 min | ↑ | ↓ | 0 | ↓ | ↓ | ↓ | | | | | |
| Nitroglycerin (IV) | immed. | | transient | 0 | 0 | | ↓ | ↑ | ↑ | | | | | |
| Captopril[5] | | | | ⇧ | ↑ | RBF ↑ GFR 0 | ↓ | 0/↑ | 0 | | | | | |
| Enalaprilat[5] | | | | | ↑ | RBF ↑ GFR 0 | ↓ | ↑ | 0 | | | | | |
| Hydralazine[5] | 10-20 | | 3-6 | | | | | | | | | | | |
| Labetalol[5] | 5-10 | | 3-6 | ↑ | ↓ | 0/↑ | ↓ | 0 | ↓ | | | | | |
| Nicardipine[5] | 1-5 | | 3-6 | | ⇧/↑ | ⇧ | ↓ | ↑ | ↑ | | | | | |
| Nifedipine[5] | | | | | | | ↓↓↓ | ↑↑ | ↑ | | | | | |
| Phentolamine[5] | 1-2 | | 3-10 min | | | | | | | | | | | |
| **Miscellaneous Agents** | | | | | | | | | | | | | | |
| Mecamylamine | 30-120 | | 6-12+ | ↑ | ↓ | ↓ | ↓ | ↓ | ↑ | | | | | |
| Pargyline | | 4-21 days | 3 weeks | | | ↓ | ↓ | 0 | 0 | | | | | |
| Tolazoline | | | | | | | ↓ | | | | | | | |

[1] Peak clinical effect following a single oral dose, except where indicated.
[2] Duration of action is frequently dose-dependent.
[3] Renal blood flow and glomerular filtration rate.
[4] NA = Not applicable.
[5] Unlabeled use.

*Stepped-Care Antihypertensive Regimen†:*
   Experience in treating essential hypertension (systolic blood pressure [BP] 140 mm Hg or greater and/or diastolic BP 90 mm Hg or greater) demonstrates the benefits of pharmacotherapy. Reducing BP decreases cardiovascular mortality and morbidity in patients with hypertension. Antihypertensive therapy protects against stroke, left ventricular hypertrophy, CHF, and progression to more severe hypertension. In addition to drug therapy, life-style modifications of adjunctive value include weight reduction, sodium and alcohol restriction, smoking cessation, regular exercise, and a diet low in saturated fat.

| Hypertension Categories | | |
|---|---|---|
| Range (mm Hg) | | |
| Systolic | Diastolic | Category[1] |
| < 130 | < 85 | Normal BP |
| 130-139 | 85-89 | High normal BP |
| 140-159 | 90-99 | Stage 1 (mild) hypertension |
| 160-179 | 100-109 | Stage 2 (moderate) hypertension |
| 180-209 | 110-119 | Stage 3 (severe) hypertension |
| ≥ 210 | ≥ 120 | Stage 4 (very severe) hypertension |

[1] When systolic and diastolic BP fall into different categories, select the higher category to classify the patient's BP (eg, classify 165/95 mm Hg as Stage 2, 170/115 mm Hg as Stage 3). Isolated systolic hypertension is systolic BP 140 mm Hg or greater and diastolic BP less than 90 mm Hg (stage appropriately).

   For purposes of risk classification and management, specify presence or absence of target-organ disease and additional risk factors in addition to classifying hypertension stages. For example, classify a diabetic patient with Stage 3 hypertension and left ventricular hypertrophy as "Stage 3 hypertension with target-organ disease (left ventricular hypertrophy) and with one additional risk factor (diabetes)."
   The *stepped-care approach* begins with life-style modifications. If BP remains at least 140/90 mm Hg for 3 to 6 months, start antihypertensive therapy, especially in patients with target-organ disease or other risk factors for cardiovascular disease. Initiate therapy with one agent, increase the dosage gradually, then add or substitute agents with gradual increases in doses until the therapeutic goal is achieved, side effects become intolerable or maximum dosages are reached. Try life-style modifications first.

| Stepped-Care Approach | | |
|---|---|---|
| I. Life-style modifications | Weight reduction<br>Moderation of alcohol intake<br>Regular physical activity | Reduction of sodium intake<br>Smoking cessation |
| II. Inadequate response | Continue life-style modifications<br>Initial pharmacological selection[1]<br>1) Diuretics or beta blockers[2]<br>2) ACE inhibitors, calcium blockers, alpha₁ blockers, alpha-beta blocker[3] | |
| III. Inadequate response | 1) Increase drug dose, or;<br>2) Substitute another drug, or;<br>3) Add a second agent from a different class.[4] | |
| IV. Inadequate response | Add a second or third agent or diuretic if not already prescribed.[4] | |

[1] Initial drug therapy is monotherapy for Stage 1 and Stage 2 hypertension.
[2] Preferred because a reduction in morbidity and mortality has been demonstrated.
[3] Equally effective in reducing BP; however, these have not been tested in long-term controlled trials to demonstrate reduction of morbidity and mortality. Reserve for special indications or when preferred agents are unacceptable or ineffective.
[4] Supplemental antihypertensive agents, which include centrally acting alpha₂-agonists (clonidine, guanabenz, guanfacine, methyldopa), peripheral-acting adrenergic antagonists (guanadrel, guanethidine, rauwolfia alkaloids) and direct vasodilators (hydralazine, minoxidil), are not routinely well suited for initial monotherapy.

   *Diuretics* – Generally initiate therapy with a thiazide or other oral diuretic. Thiazide-type diuretics are drugs of choice; hydrochlorothiazide or chlorthalidone are

† The Fifth-Report of the Joint National Committee on Detection, Evaluation, and Treatment of High Blood Pressure. *Arch Intern Med* 1993;153:154-83.

generally preferred. Reserve loop diuretics for selected patients. This therapy alone may control many cases of mild hypertension. Consider treating diuretic-induced hypokalemia (less than 3.5 mEq/L) with potassium supplementation or by adding a potassium-sparing diuretic to therapy.

*Beta-adrenergic blocking agents* – Beta-adrenergic blocking agents also may be used as initial drug monotherapy. Beta blockers are effective in older patients, but less effective in black people. Beta-adrenergic blocking agents decrease cardiac output without effects on vascular resistance. In addition, they inhibit renin release.

*Calcium channel blockers, ACE inhibitors, labetalol, and alpha₁ blockers* – Calcium channel blockers, ACE inhibitors, labetalol, and alpha$_1$ blockers may be used as initial monotherapy, although they are not routinely preferred over diuretics and beta-blockers. Black people tend to respond better to calcium blockers than ACE inhibitors; labetalol may be more effective in black people than other beta-blockers.

*Antiadrenergic agents* – Antiadrenergic agents (central and peripheral adrenergic inhibitors) are considered supplemental agents and are used when the initial drug therapy fails to achieve the desired effect. Diuretics are usually continued to provide synergistic effects and to prevent secondary fluid accumulation that may occur with use of antiadrenergic agents alone. Combination therapy also may minimize untoward reactions, which are more common at the higher doses necessary when a single drug is used alone.

Decreased adrenergic tone results in reduced cardiac output or decreased peripheral vascular resistance. Methyldopa, guanabenz, guanfacine, and clonidine act mainly in the CNS. Although reserpine has been used for years, other agents are preferred. Guanadrel is a peripheral antiadrenergic similar to guanethidine.

*Vasodilators:* Vasodilators also are considered supplemental agents and are not suited for initial monotherapy. A 3 drug regimen should include agents acting by different mechanisms. Hydralazine and minoxidil have direct vasodilating actions. In order to prevent reflex tachycardia caused by decreased peripheral resistance, these agents are most effective when used with a diuretic and a β-blocker. Minoxidil's undesirable side effects limit its use to severely hypertensive patients who do not respond to minimum doses of a diuretic and 2 other agents.

*Antihypertensive drug withdrawal syndrome* – Antihypertensive drug withdrawal syndrome may occur after discontinuation of antihypertensives.

To circumvent problems, encourage patient compliance, avoid excessive doses, avoid combining sympatholytics and β-blockers, and maintain antihypertensive medication in surgical patients. When discontinuing medication, taper the dose slowly, one drug at a time; use special caution in patients with coronary artery or cerebrovascular disease.

Treatment generally includes reinstitution of therapy, bed rest/sedation and, perhaps, therapy similar to treatment of malignant hypertension.

*Step-down therapy* – Attempt to decrease the dosage or the number of antihypertensive agents in patients; have them maintain life-style modifications. It may be possible to accomplish this in a deliberate, slow, progressive manner if the patient has been effectively controlled for 1 year and at least 4 visits.

# METHYLDOPA AND METHYLDOPATE HCl

**Tablets**: 250 and 500 mg methyldopa (*Rx*)          Various
**Injection**: 50 mg methyldopate HCl/mL (*Rx*)

### Indications
Hypertension.

**Methyldopate HCl** may be used to initiate treatment of acute hypertensive crises; however, due to its slow onset of action, other agents may be preferred for rapid reduction of blood pressure.

### Administration and Dosage

*Oral:*

   *Adults –*

      *Initial therapy:* 250 mg, 2 or 3 times/day in the first 48 hours. Adjust dosage at intervals of not less than 2 days until adequate response is achieved. To minimize sedation, increase dosage in the evening. By adjustment of dosage, morning hypotension may be prevented without sacrificing control of afternoon blood pressure.

      *Maintenance therapy:* 500 mg to 3 g daily in 2 to 4 doses. Methyldopa is usually administered in 2 divided doses; some patients may be controlled with a single daily dose given at bedtime.

      *Concomitant drug therapy:* When methyldopa is given with antihypertensives other than thiazides, limit the initial dosage to 500 mg/day in divided doses; when added to a thiazide, the dosage of thiazide need not be changed.

      *Children –* Individualize dosage. Initial oral dosage is based on 10 mg/kg/day in 2 to 4 doses. The maximum daily dosage is 65 mg/kg or 3 g, whichever is less.

   *IV:* Add dose to 100 mL 5% dextrose or give in 5% dextrose in water in a concentration of 10 mg/mL. Administer over 30 to 60 minutes. When control has been obtained, substitute oral therapy starting with the same parenteral dosage schedule.

      *Adults –* 250 to 500 mg every 6 hours as required (maximum 1 g every 6 hours).

      *Children –* 20 to 40 mg/kg/day in divided doses every 6 hours. The maximum daily dosage is 65 mg/kg or 3 g, whichever is less.

*Tolerance:* Tolerance may occur, usually between the second and third month of therapy. Adding a diuretic or increasing the dosage of methyldopa frequently restores blood pressure control. A thiazide is recommended if therapy was not started with a thiazide or if effective control of blood pressure cannot be maintained on 2 g methyldopa daily.

*Discontinuation:* Methyldopa has a relatively short duration of action; therefore, withdrawal is followed by return of hypertension, usually within 48 hours. This is not complicated by an overshoot of blood pressure above pretreatment levels.

*Impaired renal function:* Methyldopa is largely excreted by the kidneys; patients with impaired renal function may respond to smaller doses.

### Actions

*Pharmacology:* The proposed mechanism of action of methyldopa is probably due to the drug's metabolism to alpha-methyl norepinephrine, which lowers arterial pressure by the stimulation of central inhibitory $\alpha$-adrenergic receptors, false neurotransmission or reduction of plasma renin activity.

*Pharmacokinetics:*

   *Absorption/Distribution –* Following oral administration, methyldopa is variably absorbed. The mean bioavailability is approximately 50%. Methyldopa crosses the blood-brain barrier and is converted in the CNS to active alpha-methylnoradrenaline. Methyldopa crosses the placental barrier and appears in cord blood and breast milk. A decrease in BP occurs within 4 to 6 hours following IV or oral administration and lasts 10 to 16 hours or 12 to 24 hours, respectively.

   *Metabolism/Excretion –* Methyldopa is extensively metabolized. Approximately 17% of a dose of methyldopate HCl appears in plasma as free methyldopa. The average $T_{max}$ is 2 hours. The total volume of distribution is about 0.6 L/kg. Approximately 70% (oral) and approximately 49% (IV) of the drug that is absorbed is excreted in the urine as methyldopa and its mono-O-sulfate conjugate. Methyldopa is less than 20% bound to plasma proteins. The drug is removed by dialysis.

### Contraindications

Active hepatic disease, such as acute hepatitis or active cirrhosis; if previous methyldopa therapy has been associated with liver disorders; coadministration with MAOIs; hypersensitivity to any component of these formulations, including sulfites.

### Warnings

*Positive Coombs' test/Hemolytic anemia:* With prolonged therapy, 10% to 20% of patients develop a positive direct Coombs' test, usually between 6 and 12 months of therapy.

This is associated rarely with hemolytic anemia, which could lead to potentially fatal complications and is difficult to predict. Perform baseline and periodic blood counts to detect hemolytic anemia. If Coombs'-positive hemolytic anemia occurs, discontinue methyldopa; anemia usually remits promptly.

*Blood transfusions:* Should the need for transfusion arise in a patient receiving methyldopa, perform both a direct and indirect Coombs' test.

*Edema/Weight gain:* Some patients taking methyldopa experience clinical edema or weight gain, which may be controlled by use of a diuretic. Do not continue methyldopa if edema progresses or signs of heart failure appear.

*Hepatotoxicity:* Fever has occasionally occurred within the first 3 weeks of therapy, sometimes associated with eosinophilia or abnormalities in 1 liver function test or more. Jaundice with or without fever may occur, usually within the first 2 to 3 months of therapy. Incidence of elevated serum transaminase levels and impaired hepatic function ranges from 1% to 27%.

Perform periodic determinations of hepatic function, particularly during the first 6 to 12 weeks of therapy or when an unexplained fever occurs.

*Hematologic disorders:* Rarely, a reversible reduction of the white blood cell (WBC) count with a primary effect on granulocytes has been seen.

*Renal function impairment:* The active metabolites of methyldopa accumulate in uremia. Use with caution in renal failure. Prolonged hypotension has been reported.

Hypertension has recurred occasionally after dialysis in patients given methyldopa because the drug is removed by this procedure.

*Hepatic function impairment:* Use with caution in patients with previous liver disease or dysfunction.

*Elderly:* Syncope in older patients may be related to an increased sensitivity and advanced arteriosclerotic vascular disease. May be avoided by lower doses.

*Pregnancy: Category B* (oral); *Category C* (IV).

*Lactation:* Methyldopa is excreted in breast milk.

### Precautions

*Monitoring:* Blood count, Coombs' tests, and liver function tests are recommended before initiating therapy and at periodic intervals. Perform periodic determinations of hepatic function, particularly during the first 6 to 12 weeks of therapy or when an unexplained fever occurs.

*Paradoxical pressor response:* Paradoxical pressor response has been reported with IV methyldopa.

*Involuntary choreoathetotic movements:* Involuntary choreoathetotic movements have been observed rarely in patients with severe bilateral cerebrovascular disease. Should these occur, discontinue methyldopa therapy.

*Sedation:* Usually transient, sedation may occur during initial therapy or whenever the dose is increased.

*Urine discoloration:* Rarely, when urine is exposed to air, it may darken because of breakdown of methyldopa or its metabolites.

*Sulfite sensitivity:* These products contain sulfites that may cause allergic-type reactions in certain susceptible people. Sulfite sensitivity is seen more frequently in asthmatic or atopic nonasthmatic people.

### Drug Interactions

Drugs that may affect methyldopa include levodopa, nonselective beta-blockers (eg, propranolol), and ferrous sulfate or gluconate.

Drugs that may be affected by methyldopa include haloperidol, levodopa, lithium, sympathomimetics, MAOIs, anesthetics, and phenothiazines.

*Drug/Lab test interactions:* Methyldopa may interfere with tests for: Urinary uric acid by phosphotungstate method; serum creatinine by alkaline picrate method; AST by colorimetric methods. Because methyldopa causes fluorescence in urine samples at the same wavelengths as catecholamines, falsely high levels of urinary catecholamines may occur and will interfere with the diagnosis of pheochromocytoma.

**Adverse Reactions**

Possible adverse reactions include fever; lupus-like syndrome; rise in BUN; myalgia; septic shock-like syndrome; headache; asthenia; weakness; dizziness; symptoms of cerebrovascular insufficiency; paresthesias; parkinsonism; Bell's palsy; decreased mental acuity; involuntary choreoathetotic movements; psychic disturbances; verbal memory impairment; bradycardia; prolonged carotid sinus hypersensitivity; aggravation of angina pectoris; pericarditis; myocarditis; orthostatic hypotension; edema/weight gain (usually relieved by a diuretic; discontinue methyldopa if edema progresses or signs of heart failure appear); nausea; vomiting; constipation; diarrhea; colitis; sore or "black" tongue; pancreatitis; liver disorders; positive Coombs' test, bone marrow depression; leukopenia; granulocytopenia; thrombocytopenia; positive tests for antinuclear antibody, LE cells and rheumatoid factor; rash; toxic epidermal necrolysis; gynecomastia; lactation; amenorrhea.

# CLONIDINE HCI

| | |
|---|---|
| **Tablets**: 0.1 mg, 0.2 mg, and 0.3 mg (*Rx*) | Various, *Catapres* (Boehringer-Ingelheim) |
| **Transdermal system**: 2.5 mg (release rate 0.1 mg/24 h) (*Rx*) | *Catapres-TTS-1* (Boehringer-Ingelheim) |
| 5 mg (release rate 0.2 mg/24 h) (*Rx*) | *Catapres-TTS-2* (Boehringer-Ingelheim) |
| 7.5 mg (release rate 0.2 mg/24 h) (*Rx*) | *Catapres-TTS-3* (Boehringer-Ingelheim) |

**Indications**

Hypertension.

*Unlabeled uses:* Clonidine has been evaluated for use in the following conditions:

| Clonidine Unlabeled Uses | |
|---|---|
| Use | Dosage[1] |
| Alcohol withdrawal | 0.3 to 0.6 mg every 6 hours |
| Constitutional growth delay in children | 0.0375 to 0.15 mg/m$^2$/day |
| Diabetic diarrhea | 0.15 to 1.2 mg/day or 0.3 mg/24-hour patch (1 to 2 patches/week) |
| Gilles de la Tourette syndrome | 0.15 to 0.2 mg/day |
| Hypertensive "urgencies" (diastolic> 120 mm Hg) | Initially 0.1 to 0.2 mg, followed by 0.05 to 0.1 mg every hour to a maximum of 0.8 mg |
| Menopausal flushing | 0.1 to 0.4 mg/day or 0.1 mg/24-hour patch |
| Methadone/opiate detoxification | 15 to 16 mcg/kg/day |
| Pheochromocytoma diagnosis (overnight clonidine suppression test) | 0.3 mg |
| Postherpetic neuralgia | 0.2 mg/day |
| Reduction of allergen-induced inflammatory reactions in patients with extrinsic asthma | 0.15 mg for 3 days |
| Smoking cessation facilitation | 0.15 to 0.4 mg/day or 0.2 mg/24-hour patch |
| Ulcerative colitis | 0.3 mg 3 times a day |

[1] Dosage given as oral unless otherwise specified.

**Administration and Dosage**

*Oral:* Individualize dosage.

*Initial dose* – 0.1 mg twice daily. The elderly may benefit from a lower initial dose.

*Maintenance dose* – Increments of 0.1 or 0.2 mg/day may be made until desired response is achieved; most common range is 0.2 to 0.8 mg/day given in divided doses. The maximum dose is 2.4 mg/day. Minimize sedative effects by slowly increasing the daily dosage and giving the majority of the daily dose at bedtime.

*Children* – 5 to 25 mcg/kg/day in divided doses every 6 hours; increase at 5- to 7-day intervals.

*Unlabeled route of administration* – Sublingual clonidine, using a dosage of 0.2 to 0.4 mg/day, may be effective in hypertensive patients unable to take oral medication. The onset occurs within 30 to 60 minutes and blood pressure appears to be maintained on a twice daily regimen.

*Renal Impairment* – Adjust dosage according to degree of renal impairment and carefully monitor patients. Because only a minimal amount of clonidine is removed during hemodialysis, there is no need to give supplemental clonidine following dialysis.

*Transdermal:* Apply to a hairless area of intact skin on upper arm or torso, once every 7 days. Use a different skin site from the previous application. If the system loosens during the 7-day wearing, apply the adhesive overlay directly over the system to ensure good adhesion.

For initial therapy, start with the 0.1 mg system. If, after 1 or 2 weeks, desired blood pressure reduction is not achieved, add another 0.1 mg system or use a larger system. Dosage greater than two 0.3 mg systems usually does not improve efficacy. Note that the antihypertensive effect of the system may not commence until 2 to 3 days after application. Therefore, when substituting the transdermal system in patients on prior antihypertensive therapy, a gradual reduction of prior drug dosage is advised. Previous antihypertensive treatment may have to be continued, particularly in patients with severe hypertension.

### Actions

*Pharmacology:* Initially, clonidine stimulates peripheral α-adrenergic receptors producing transient vasoconstriction. Stimulation of alpha-adrenergic in the brain stem results in reduced sympathetic outflow from the CNS and a decrease in peripheral resistance, renal vascular resistance, heart rate, and blood pressure.

*Pharmacokinetics:* Blood pressure declines within 30 to 60 minutes after an oral dose. The peak plasma level occurs in approximately 3 to 5 hours with a plasma half-life of 12 to 16 hours. About 50% of the absorbed dose is metabolized in the liver. In patients with impaired renal function, half-life increases to 30 to 40 hours. Clonidine and its metabolites are excreted mainly in the urine. About 40% to 60% of the absorbed dose is recovered in the urine as unchanged drug in 24 hours.

*Transdermal system* – The system, a 0.2 mm thick film with 4 layers, contains a drug reservoir of clonidine, released at an approximately constant rate for 7 days.

Therapeutic plasma levels, achieved 2 to 3 days after initial application, are lower than during oral therapy with equipotent doses. When system is removed, therapeutic plasma clonidine levels persist for approximately 8 hours and then decline slowly over several days; blood pressure returns gradually to pretreatment levels. Elimination half-life is approximately 19 hours.

### Contraindications

Hypersensitivity to clonidine or any component of adhesive layer of transdermal system.

### Warnings

Use with caution in patients with severe coronary insufficiency, recent MI, cerebrovascular disease, or chronic renal failure.

*Tolerance:* Tolerance may develop, necessitating a reevaluation of therapy.

*Pregnancy: Category* C.

*Lactation:* Clonidine is excreted in breast milk.

*Children:* Safety and efficacy for use in children have not been established.

### Precautions

*Rebound hypertension:* Do not discontinue therapy without consulting a physician. Discontinue therapy by reducing the dose gradually over 2 to 4 days to avoid a rapid rise in blood pressure.

If an excessive rise in blood pressure occurs, it can be reversed by resumption of therapy or by IV phentolamine, phenoxybenzamine, or prazosin. Direct vasodilators and captopril also have been used. If therapy is to be discontinued in patients receiving β-blockers and clonidine concurrently, discontinue β-blockers several days before the gradual withdrawal of clonidine.

Rebound hypertension also has occurred following discontinuation of the transdermal patch.

*Ophthalmologic effects:* Perform periodic eye examinations, because retinal degeneration has been noted in animal studies.

*Perioperative use:* Continue administration of clonidine to within 4 hours of surgery and resume as soon as possible thereafter. Carefully monitor blood pressure and institute appropriate measures to control it. If transdermal therapy is started during the perioperative period, note that therapeutic plasma levels are not achieved until 2 to 3 days after initial application.

*Sensitization to transdermal clonidine:* In patients who develop an allergic reaction to transdermal clonidine, oral clonidine HCl substitution may elicit a similar reaction.

### Drug Interactions
Drugs that may interact with clonidine include beta-adrenergic blocking agents and tricyclic antidepressants.

### Adverse Reactions
*Oral* – Adverse reactions may include dry mouth; drowsiness; dizziness; sedation; constipation; anorexia; malaise; nausea and vomiting; parotid pain; mild transient abnormalities in liver function tests; gynecomastia; CHF; orthostatic symptoms; palpitations, tachycardia and bradycardia; Raynaud's phenomenon; ECG abnormalities; conduction disturbances, arrhythmias, sinus bradycardia; dreams or nightmares; insomnia; hallucinations; delirium; nervousness; anxiety; depression; headache; rash, angioneurotic edema, hives, urticaria; hair thinning and alopecia; pruritus; impotence; decreased sexual activity; difficulty in micturition; weakness; muscle or joint pain; increased sensitivity to alcohol; dryness, itching or burning of the eyes; dryness of the nasal mucosa; pallor; fever; weakly positive Coombs' test.

*Transdermal system* – Adverse reactions may include dry mouth, drowsiness (the most frequent systemic reactions); constipation; nausea; change in taste; fatigue; headache; sedation; insomnia; nervousness; dizziness; impotence/sexual dysfunction; transient localized skin reactions; hyperpigmentation; edema; excoriation; burning; papules; throbbing; generalized macular rash.

## ALPHA-1-ADRENERGIC BLOCKERS

| | | |
|---|---|---|
| **ALFUZOSIN HCL** | | |
| **Tablets, extended-release:** 10 mg (*Rx*) | *Uroxatral* (Sanofi-Syntholabo) | |
| **DOXAZOSIN MESYLATE** | | |
| **Tablets:** 1, 2, 4, and 8 mg (*Rx*) | *Cardura* (Pfizer) | |
| **PRAZOSIN** | | |
| **Capsules:** 1, 2, and 5 mg (*Rx*) | Various, *Minipress* (Pfizer) | |
| **TAMSULOSIN HCL** | | |
| **Capsules:** 0.4 mg (*Rx*) | *Flomax* (Abbott) | |
| **TERAZOSIN** | | |
| **Capsules:** 1, 2, 5, and 10 mg (*Rx*) | *Hytrin* (Abbott) | |

### Indications
*Hypertension (doxazosin, prazosin, terazosin):* For the treatment of hypertension, alone or in combination with other antihypertensive agents.

*Alfuzosin, doxazosin mesylate, terazosin, and tamsulosin:* Treatment of symptomatic benign prostatic hyperplasia.

### Administration and Dosage

ALFUZOSIN:

*Benign prostatic hyperplasia* – 10 mg/day alfuzosin extended-release tablet taken immediately after the same meal each day. Do not chew or crush tablets.

DOXAZOSIN MESYLATE:

*Hypertension* –

*Initial dosage:* 1 mg once daily. Postural effects are most likely to occur between 2 and 6 hours after a dose.

*Maintenance dose:* Depending on the standing blood pressure response, dosage may be increased to 2 mg and, if necessary, to 4, 8 and 16 mg to achieve the desired reduction in blood pressure. Increases in dose beyond 4 mg increase the likelihood of excessive postural effects.

*BPH* – 1 to 8 mg once daily.

*Maintenance:* Depending on the urodynamics and BPH symptomatology, dosage may then be increased to 2 mg and thereafter to 4 and 8 mg once daily, the maximum recommended dose for BPH. The recommended titration interval is 1 to 2 weeks. Evaluate blood pressure routinely.

PRAZOSIN:

*Hypertension* –

*Initial dose:* 1 mg 2 or 3 times daily. When increasing dosages, give the first dose of each increment at bedtime to reduce syncopal episodes.

*Maintenance dose:* 6 to 15 mg/day in divided doses. Doses higher than 20 mg usually do not increase efficacy; however, a few patients may benefit from up to 40 mg/day. After initial adjustment, some patients can be maintained on a twice-daily regimen.

*Children* – A dose of 0.5 to 7 mg 3 times a day has been suggested.

*Concomitant therapy* – When adding a diuretic or other antihypertensive agent, reduce dosage to 1 or 2 mg 3 times a day and then retitrate.

TAMSULOSIN:

*Benign prostatic hyperplasia* – 0.4 mg once daily, administered approximately 30 minutes following the same meal each day. Do not crush, chew, or open capsules.

For those patients who fail to respond to the 0.4 mg dose after 2 to 4 weeks of dosing, the dose can be increased to 0.8 mg once daily. If administration is discontinued or interrupted for several days at either the 0.4 or 0.8 mg dose, start therapy again with the 0.4 mg once-daily dose.

TERAZOSIN:

*Hypertension* – Adjust dose and the dose interval (12 or 24 hours) individually.

*Initial dose:* 1 mg at bedtime for all patients. Do not exceed this dose. Strictly observe this initial dosing regimen to avoid severe hypotensive effects.

*Subsequent doses:* Slowly increase the dose to achieve the desired blood pressure response. The recommended dose range is 1 to 5 mg daily; however, some patients may benefit from doses as high as 20 mg/day. If response is substantially diminished at 24 hours, consider an increased dose or a twice-daily regimen.

*Benign prostatic hyperplasia* –

*Initial dose:* 1 mg at bedtime is the starting dose for all patients; do not exceed as an initial dose. Closely monitor patients to minimize the risk of severe hypotensive response.

*Subsequent doses:* Increase the dose in a stepwise fashion to 2, 5, or 10 mg daily to achieve desired improvement of symptoms or flow rates. Doses of 10 mg once daily are generally required for clinical response; therefore, treatment with 10 mg for a minimum of 4 to 6 weeks may be required to assess whether a beneficial response has been achieved. There is insufficient data to support the use of doses greater than 20 mg in patients who do not respond.

*Concomitant therapy* – Observe caution when terazosin is administered concomitantly with other antihypertensive agents (eg, calcium antagonists) to avoid the possibility of significant hypotension. When adding a diuretic or other antihypertensive agent, dosage reduction and retitration may be necessary.

## Actions

*Pharmacology:* **Prazosin, terazosin, alfuzosin, tamsulosin,** and **doxazosin** selectively block postsynaptic α-1-adrenergic receptors. These peripherally acting drugs dilate both resistance (arterioles) and capacitance (veins) vessels. Both supine and standing blood pressure are lowered. The effect is most pronounced on diastolic blood pressure.

In the treatment of benign prostatic hyperplasia (BPH), the reduction in symptoms and improvement in urine flow rates is related to relaxation of smooth muscle produced by blockade of alpha$_1$ adrenoceptors in the bladder neck and prostate.

*Pharmacokinetics:* **Prazosin** is extensively metabolized. The metabolites of prazosin are active. Duration of antihypertensive effect is 10 hours.

**Terazosin** undergoes minimal hepatic first-pass metabolism; nearly all of the circulating dose is in the form of parent drug.

**Alfuzosin, doxazosin, tamsulosin** is extensively metabolized in the liver.

| Pharmacokinetics of Alpha-1-Adrenergic Blockers | | | | | |
| --- | --- | --- | --- | --- | --- |
| Parameters | Alfuzosin | Doxazosin | Prazosin | Tamsulosin | Terazosin |
| Oral bioavailability | 49% | 65% | 48% to 68% | 90% | 90% |
| Affected by food | Yes | nd[1] | No | Yes | No |
| Peak plasma level, time | 8 h | 2 to 3 h | 1 to 3 h | 4 to 5 h | 1 to 2 h |
| Protein binding | 82% to 90% | 98% | 92% to 97% | 94% to 99% | 90% to 94% |
| Half-life | 10 h | 22 h | 2 to 3 h | 4 to 7 h | 9 to 12 h |
| Excretion: Bile/feces | 69% | 63% | < 90% | 76% | 60% |
| Excretion: Urine | 24% | 9% | < 10% | 21% | 40% |

[1] nd = no data

## Contraindications

Hypersensitivity to quinazolines (eg, doxazosin, prazosin, terazosin); moderate or severe hepatic insufficiency; coadministration with potent CYP3A4 inhibitors (eg, ketoconazole, itraconazole, ritonavir).

## Warnings

*"First-dose" effect:* **Prazosin, terazosin, doxazosin, alfuzosin,** and **tamsulosin,** like other α-adrenergic blocking agents, can cause marked hypotension (especially postural hypotension) and syncope with sudden loss of consciousness with the first few doses. Anticipate a similar effect if therapy is interrupted for more than a few doses, if dosage is increased rapidly, or if another antihypertensive drug is introduced.

The "first-dose" phenomenon may be minimized by limiting the initial dose to 1 mg of terazosin or prazosin (given at bedtime) or doxazosin.

*Renal function impairment:* Exercise caution when **alfuzosin** is administered in patients with severe renal insufficiency.

*Hepatic function impairment:* Administer **doxazosin** and **alfuzosin** with caution to patients with evidence of impaired hepatic function or to patients receiving drugs known to influence hepatic metabolism.

*Pregnancy:* Category C (**prazosin, terazosin**); Category B (**doxazosin, alfuzosin, tamsulosin**).

*Lactation:* Safety has not been established.

*Children:* Safety and efficacy for use in children have not been established.

## Precautions

*Weight gain:* There was a tendency for patients to gain weight during **terazosin** therapy.

*Cholesterol:* During controlled clinical studies **prazosin, terazosin,** and **doxazosin** were associated with small decreases in LDL and cholesterol.

*Prostatic carcinoma:* Examine patients prior to starting therapy with **alfuzosin** to rule out the presence of carcinoma of the prostate.

*Coronary insufficiency:* Discontinue **alfuzosin** if symptoms of angina pectoris should newly appear or worsen.

*Patients with congenital or acquired QT prolongation:* The QT effect of 40 mg **alfuzosin** did not appear as large as that of the active control moxifloxacin. This observation should be considered in clinical decisions to prescribe **alfuzosin** for patients with a known history of QT prolongation or patients who are taking medications known to prolong QT. There has been no signal of torsades de pointe in postmarketing experience with **alfuzosin** outside the United States.

### Drug Interactions

Drugs that interact may include beta blockers, indomethacin, verapamil, and clonidine.

*Alfuzosin:* Do not coadminister with potent inhibitors of CYP3A4 because exposure is increased, (eg, ketoconazole, itraconazole, or ritonavir). Diltiazem is an antihypertensive medication and the combination of diltiazem and alfuzosin and antihypertensive medications has the potential to cause hypotension in some patients. The combination of alfuzosin with atenolol caused significant reductions in mean blood pressure and in mean heart rate.

*Tamsulosin:* Exercise caution with coadministration of warfarin and tamsulosin.

Use caution when using tamsulosin in combination with cimetidine, particularly at doses higher than 0.4 mg.

*Drug/Lab test interactions:* False-positive results may occur in screening tests for pheochromocytoma in patients who are being treated with **prazosin**.

### Adverse Reactions

| Alpha-1-Adrenergic Blocker Adverse Reactions | | | | | | |
|---|---|---|---|---|---|---|
| | Hypertension | | | BPH | | |
| Adverse reaction | Doxazosin | Prazosin | Terazosin | Terazosin | Alfuzosin | Tamsulosin |
| *Cardiovascular* | | | | | | |
| Palpitations | 2% | 5.3% | 4.3% | 0.9% | | |
| Postural hypotension/ hypotension | 0.3% to 1% | ✔[1] | 1.3% | 0.6% to 3.9% | 0.4% | 0.2% |
| *CNS* | | | | | | |
| Dizziness | 19% | 10.3% | 19.3% | 9.1% | 5.7% | 10.1% |
| Somnolence | 5% | no report | 5.4% | 3.6% | | 1.6% |
| Asthenia | 1% to 12% | ≈ 7% | 11.3% | 7.4% | | |
| Drowsiness | ✔[1] | 7.6% | ✔[1] | | | |
| *GI* | | | | | | |
| Nausea | 3% | 4.9% | 4.4% | 1.7% | | 3.2% |
| *Musculoskeletal* | | | | | | |
| Shoulder/neck/back/ extremity pain | < 0.5% to 2% | no report | 1% to 3.5% | | | 5.5 |
| *Respiratory* | | | | | | |
| Dyspnea | 1% | ✔[1] | 3.1% | 1.7% | | |
| Nasal congestion | no report | ✔[1] | 5.9% | 1.9% | | |
| Pharyngitis/rhinitis | 3% | no report | 1% | 1.9% | | 4.7 to 8.3 |
| *Miscellaneous* | | | | | | |
| Headache | 14% | 7.8% | 16.2% | 4.9% | 3% | 20.1% |
| Edema | 4% | ✔[1] | < 1% | | | |
| Peripheral edema | no report | no report | 5.5% | 0.9% | | |

[1] Reactions associated with the drug; incidence unknown.

# HYDRALAZINE HCl

**Tablets:** 10, 25, 50, and 100 mg (*Rx*)          Various, *Apresoline* (Ciba)
**Injection:** 20 mg/mL (*Rx*)

### Indications
*Oral:* Essential hypertension, alone or in combination with other agents.

*Parenteral:* Severe essential hypertension when the drug cannot be given orally or when the need to lower blood pressure is urgent.

*Unlabeled uses:* Hydralazine in doses up to 800 mg 3 times/day has been effective in reducing afterload in the treatment of congestive heart failure (CHF), severe aortic insufficiency, and after valve replacement.

### Administration and Dosage
Bioavailability of hydralazine tablets is enhanced by the concurrent ingestion of food.

*Initiate therapy:* Initiate therapy in gradually increasing dosages; individualize dosage. Start with 10 mg 4 times daily for the first 2 to 4 days, increase to 25 mg 4 times daily for the balance of the first week.

*Second and subsequent weeks:* Increase dosage to 50 mg 4 times daily.

*Maintenance:* Adjust dosage to lowest effective level. Twice daily dosage may be adequate. In a few resistant patients, up to 300 mg/day may be required for a significant antihypertensive effect. In such cases, consider a lower dosage of hydralazine combined with a thiazide or reserpine or a beta-blocker. However, when combining therapy, individual titration is essential to ensure the lowest possible therapeutic dose of each drug.

    *Children –*
      *Initial:* 0.75 mg/kg/day in 4 divided doses. Dosage may be increased gradually over the next 3 to 4 weeks to a maximum of 7.5 mg/kg or 200 mg daily.

*Parenteral:* Therapy in the hospitalized patient may be initiated IV or IM. Use parenterally only when the drug cannot be given orally. Usual dose is 20 to 40 mg, repeated as necessary. Certain patients (especially those with marked renal damage) may require a lower dose. Check blood pressure frequently; it may begin to fall within a few minutes after injection; average maximal decrease occurs in 10 to 80 minutes. Where there is a previously existing increased intracranial pressure, lowering the blood pressure may increase cerebral ischemia. Most patients can transfer to the oral form in 24 to 48 hours.

    *Children –* 0.1 to 0.2 mg/kg/dose every 4 to 6 hours as needed.
    *Eclampsia –* A dose of 5 to 10 mg every 20 minutes as an IV bolus has been recommended. If there is no effect after 20 mg, try another agent.

*Stability:* Use hydralazine injection as quickly as possible after drawing through a needle into a syringe. Hydralazine changes color after contact with a metal filter.

### Actions
*Pharmacology:* Hydralazine exerts a peripheral vasodilating effect through a direct relaxation of vascular smooth muscle.

*Pharmacokinetics:* Hydralazine is rapidly absorbed after oral use. Half-life is 3 to 7 hours. Protein binding is 87%, and bioavailability is 30% to 50%. Plasma levels vary widely among individuals. Peak plasma concentrations occur 1 to 2 hours after ingestion; duration of action is 6 to 12 hours. Hypotensive effects are seen 10 to 20 minutes after parenteral use and last 2 to 4 hours. Slow acetylators generally have higher plasma levels of hydralazine and require lower doses to maintain control of blood pressure. Hydralazine undergoes extensive hepatic metabolism; it is excreted in the urine as active drug (12% to 14%) and metabolites.

### Contraindications
Hypersensitivity to hydralazine; coronary artery disease; mitral valvular rheumatic heart disease.

## Warnings

*Lupus erythematosus:* Hydralazine may produce a clinical picture simulating systemic lupus erythematosus including glomerulonephritis. Symptoms usually regress when the drug is discontinued, but residual effects have been detected years later. Long-term treatment with steroids may be necessary.

Perform complete blood counts and antinuclear antibody (ANA) titer determinations before and during prolonged therapy, even in the asymptomatic patient. These studies also are indicated if the patient develops arthralgia, fever, chest pain, continued malaise, or other unexplained signs or symptoms. If the ANA titer reaction is positive, carefully weigh benefits to be derived from hydralazine.

*Renal function impairment:* In hypertensive patients with normal kidneys who are treated with hydralazine, there is evidence of increased renal blood flow and a maintenance of glomerular filtration rate. Renal function may improve where control values were below normal prior to administration. Use with caution in patients with advanced renal damage.

*Pregnancy: Category* C.

*Lactation:* Hydralazine is excreted in breast milk.

*Children:* Safety and efficacy for use in children have not been established.

## Precautions

*Cardiovascular:* The "hyperdynamic" circulation caused by hydralazine may accentuate specific cardiovascular inadequacies. It may reduce the pressor responses to epinephrine. Postural hypotension may result from hydralazine. Use with caution in patients with cerebral vascular accidents.

*Coronary artery disease* – Myocardial stimulation produced by hydralazine can cause anginal attacks and ECG changes of myocardial ischemia. The drug has been implicated in the production of MI. Use with caution in patients with suspected coronary artery disease.

*Pulmonary hypertension* – Use hydralazine with caution in patients with pulmonary hypertension. Severe hypotension may result. Monitor carefully.

*Lipids* – Hydralazine may cause some decrease in total cholesterol.

*Peripheral neuritis:* Peripheral neuritis evidenced by paresthesias, numbness, and tingling, has been observed. Add pyridoxine to the regimen if symptoms develop.

*Hematologic effects:* Blood dyscrasias consisting of reduction in hemoglobin and red cell count, leukopenia, agranulocytosis, and purpura have been reported. If such abnormalities develop, discontinue therapy. Periodic blood counts are advised.

*Tartrazine sensitivity:* Some of these products contain tartrazine, which may cause allergic-type reactions in susceptible individuals. Tartrazine sensitivity is frequently seen in patients who also have aspirin hypersensitivity.

## Drug Interactions

Drugs that may interact with hydralazine include beta blockers (eg, metoprolol, propranolol) and indomethacin.

*Drug/Food interactions:* Taking with food results in higher plasma hydralazine levels.

## Adverse Reactions

Possible adverse reactions include headache; anorexia; nausea; vomiting; diarrhea; palpitations; tachycardia; angina pectoris; toxic reactions (particularly the LE cell syndrome); lacrimation; conjunctivitis; dizziness; tremors; psychotic reactions; rash; urticaria; pruritus; fever; chills; arthralgia; eosinophilia; constipation; paralytic ileus; lymphadenopathy; splenomegaly; nasal congestion; flushing; edema; muscle cramps; hypotension; paradoxical pressor response; dyspnea; urination difficulty; adverse reactions with hydralazine are usually reversible when dosage is reduced. However, it may be necessary to discontinue the drug.

# MINOXIDIL

**Tablets:** 2.5 and 10 mg (Rx)                    Various, *Loniten* (Upjohn)

---

**Warning:**

Minoxidil may produce serious adverse effects. It can cause pericardial effusion, occasionally progressing to tamponade; it can exacerbate angina pectoris. Reserve for hypertensive patients who do not respond adequately to maximum therapeutic doses of a diuretic and 2 other antihypertensive agents.

In experimental animals, minoxidil caused several kinds of myocardial lesions and other adverse cardiac effects (see Warnings).

Administer under close supervision, usually concomitantly with a beta-adrenergic blocking agent, to prevent tachycardia and increased myocardial workload. Usually, it must be given with a diuretic, frequently one acting on the ascending limb of the loop of Henle, to prevent serious fluid accumulation. When first administering minoxidil, hospitalize and monitor patients with malignant hypertension and those already receiving guanethidine to avoid too rapid or large orthostatic decreases in blood pressure.

---

### Indications

*Severe hypertension:* Severe hypertension that is symptomatic or associated with target organ damage, and is not manageable with maximum therapeutic doses of a diuretic plus two other antihypertensives.

Topical minoxidil is used for the treatment of male pattern baldness (alopecia androgenetica) of the vertex of the scalp. Use of the tablets, in any formulation, to promote hair growth is not an approved use.

### Administration and Dosage

*Adults and children (12 years of age or older):* Initial dosage is 5 mg/day as a single dose. Daily dosage can be increased to 10, 20, then 40 mg in single or divided doses if required. Effective range is usually 10 to 40 mg/day. Maximum dosage is 100 mg/day.

*Children:* Initial dosage is 0.2 mg/kg/day as a single dose. Dose may be increased in 50% to 100% increments until optimum BP control is achieved. Effective range is usually 0.25 to 1 mg/kg/day. Maximum dosage is 50 mg/day.

*Dose frequency:* If supine diastolic pressure has been reduced less than 30 mm Hg, administer the drug only once a day; if reduced more than 30 mm Hg, divide the daily dosage into 2 equal parts.

*Dosage adjustment intervals:* Dosage adjustment intervals, which must be carefully titrated, should be 3 or more days because the full response to a given dose is not obtained until then.

*Concomitant drug therapy:*

    *Diuretics* – Use minoxidil with a diuretic in patients relying on renal function for maintaining salt and water balance. Diuretics have been used at the following dosages when starting minoxidil therapy: hydrochlorothiazide (50 mg twice daily) or other thiazides at equally effective doses; chlorthalidone (50 to 100 mg/day); furosemide (40 mg twice daily). If excessive salt and water retention results in a weight gain of more than 2.3 kg (5 lb), change diuretic therapy to furosemide. In furosemide-treated patients, increase dosage in accordance with their needs.

    *Beta-blockers/Other sympathetic nervous system suppressants* – When beginning therapy, the β-blocker dosage should be equal to 80 to 160 mg/day propranolol in divided doses. If β-blockers are contraindicated, use methyldopa 250 to 750 mg twice daily; give for at least 24 hours before starting minoxidil due to delay in onset. Clonidine may also be used to prevent tachycardia induced by minoxidil; usual dosage is 0.1 to 0.2 mg twice daily.

## Actions

*Pharmacology:* Minoxidil is a direct-acting peripheral vasodilator. Minoxidil elicits a reduction of peripheral arteriolar resistance. The exact mechanism of action on the vascular smooth muscle is unknown.

*Pharmacokinetics:*

*Absorption/Distribution* – Minoxidil is at least 90% absorbed from the GI tract. Plasma levels of the parent drug reach a maximum within the first hour and decline rapidly thereafter. Minoxidil is not protein bound; it concentrates in arteriolar smooth muscle.

*Onset/Duration:* The extent and time course of BP reduction by minoxidil do not correspond closely to its plasma concentration. When minoxidil is administered chronically, once or twice a day, the time required to achieve maximum effect on BP is inversely related to the size of the dose. Thus, maximum effect is achieved on 10 mg/day within 7 days, on 20 mg/day within 5 days and on 40 mg/day within 3 days.

*Metabolism/Excretion* – 90% is metabolized, predominantly by conjugation with glucuronic acid. Average plasma half-life is 4.2 hours.

## Contraindications

Hypersensitivity to any component of the product; pheochromocytoma (because the drug may stimulate secretion of catecholamines from the tumor through its antihypertensive action); acute MI; dissecting aortic aneurysm.

## Warnings

*Mild hypertension:* Because of the potential for serious adverse effects, use in milder degrees of hypertension is not recommended.

*Cardiac lesions:* Autopsies did not reveal right atrial or other hemorrhage pathology of the kind seen in animals.

*ECG changes:* Rarely, a large negative amplitude of the T wave may encroach upon the ST segment, but the ST segment is not independently altered. These changes usually disappear with continuance of treatment and revert to the pretreatment state if therapy is discontinued.

*Fluid and electrolyte balance:* Monitor fluid and electrolyte balance and body weight. Give with a diuretic to prevent fluid retention and possible CHF; a loop diuretic is usually required. If used without a diuretic, retention of several hundred mEq salt and corresponding volumes of water can occur in a few days, leading to increased plasma and interstitial fluid volume and local or generalized edema.

Refractory fluid retention rarely may require discontinuation of minoxidil. Under close medical supervision, it may be possible to resolve refractory salt retention by discontinuing the drug for 1 or 2 days, and then resuming treatment in conjunction with vigorous diuretic therapy.

*Tachycardia/Angina:* Minoxidil increases heart rate; this can be prevented by coadministration of a β-adrenergic blocking drug or other sympathetic nervous system suppressants. In addition, angina may worsen or appear for the first time during treatment, probably because of the increased oxygen demands associated with increased heart rate and cardiac output. This can usually be prevented by sympathetic blockade.

*Pericardial effusion:* Pericardial effusion, occasionally with tamponade, has occurred in approximately 3% of treated patients not on dialysis, especially those with inadequate or compromised renal function. Many cases were associated with connective tissue disease, the uremic syndrome, CHF or fluid retention, but were instances in which these potential causes of effusion were not present. Observe patients closely for signs of pericardial disorder. Perform echocardiographic studies if suspicion arises. More vigorous diuretic therapy, dialysis, pericardiocentesis, or surgery may be required. If the effusion persists, consider drug withdrawal.

*Hazard of rapid control of BP:* In patients with very severe BP elevation, too rapid control of BP can precipitate syncope, cerebrovascular accidents, MI and ischemia of special sense organs with resulting decrease or loss of vision or hearing. Patients with compromised circulation or cryoglobulinemia also may suffer ischemic episodes of affected organs. Although such events have not been unequivocally associated with minoxidil use, experience is limited.

Hospitalize any patient with malignant hypertension during initial treatment to ensure that blood pressure is not falling more rapidly than intended.

*Hemodilution:* Hematocrit, hemoglobin, and erythrocyte count usually fall about 7% initially and then recover to pretreatment levels.

*Hypersensitivity reactions:* Manifested as a skin rash, hypersensitivity reactions occur in fewer than 1% of patients and rare reports of bullous eruptions and Stevens-Johnson syndrome.

*Renal function impairment:* Renal failure or dialysis patients may require smaller doses; closely supervise to prevent cardiac failure or exacerbation of renal failure.

*Carcinogenesis:* Dietary administration of minoxidil to mice for up to 2 years was associated with an increased incidence of malignant lymphomas in females at all dose levels (10, 25, and 63 mg/kg/day) and an increased incidence of hepatic nodules in males (63 mg/kg/day).

*Fertility impairment:* There was a dose-dependent reduction in conception rate.

*Pregnancy:* Category C.

*Lactation:* Minoxidil is excreted in breast milk; do not nurse while taking minoxidil.

*Children:* Use in children is limited, particularly in infants. The recommendations under Administration and Dosage are only a rough guide; careful titration is essential.

### Precautions

*Monitoring:* Monitor initially and periodically thereafter body weight, blood pressure, fluid, and electrolyte balance; signs and symptoms of pericardial effusion; ECG changes; CBC; alkaline phosphatase; renal function tests.

*Myocardial infarction:* Minoxidil has not been used in patients who have had an MI within the preceding month. A reduction in arterial pressure with the drug might further limit blood flow to the myocardium, although this might be compensated by decreased oxygen demand because of lower BP.

*Hypertrichosis:* Elongation, thickening, and enhanced pigmentation of fine body hair develops within 3 to 6 weeks after starting therapy in approximately 80% of patients. It is usually first noticed on the temples, between the eyebrows, between the hairline and the eyebrows, or in the sideburn area of the upper lateral cheek, later extending to the back, arms, legs, and scalp. After discontinuation, 1 to 6 months may be required for restoration to pretreatment appearance. No endocrine abnormalities have been found to explain the abnormal hair growth; thus, it is hypertrichosis without virilism.

*Lab test abnormalities:* Repeat tests that are abnormal at initiation of minoxidil therapy to ascertain whether improvement or deterioration is occurring under therapy. Initially, perform such tests frequently, at 1 to 3 month intervals, and as stabilization occurs, at 6 to 12 month intervals.

### Drug Interactions
Drugs that may interact with minoxidil include guanethidine.

### Adverse Reactions
Adverse reactions may include Stevens-Johnson syndrome; pericardial effusion; T-wave changes; rebound hypertension (following gradual withdrawal in children); decreased initial hematocrit, hemoglobin and erythrocyte counts; nausea; vomiting; temporary edema; alkaline phosphatase/serum creatinine/BUN increase, hypertrichosis.

# ACE INHIBITORS

| | |
|---|---|
| **BENAZEPRIL HCl** | |
| **Tablets:** 5, 10, 20, and 40 mg (*Rx*) | *Lotensin* (Novartis) |
| **CAPTOPRIL** | |
| **Tablets:** 12.5, 25, 50, and 100 mg (*Rx*) | Various, *Capoten* (Par) |
| **ENALAPRIL** | |
| **Tablets:** 2.5, 5, 10, and 20 mg (*Rx*) | *Vasotec* (Merck) |
| **Injection:** 1.25 mg enalaprilat/mL (*Rx*) | *Vasotec I.V.* (Merck) |
| **FOSINOPRIL SODIUM** | |
| **Tablets:** 10, 20, and 40 mg (*Rx*) | *Monopril* (Bristol-Myers Squibb) |
| **LISINOPRIL** | |
| **Tablets:** 2.5, 5, 10, 20, and 40 mg (*Rx*) | *Prinivil* (Merck), *Zestril* (Zeneca) |
| **MOEXIPRIL HCl** | |
| **Tablets:** 7.5 and 15 mg (*Rx*) | *Univasc* (Schwarz Pharma) |
| **PERINDOPRIL ERBUMINE** | |
| **Tablets:** 2, 4, and 8 mg (*Rx*) | *Aceon* (Solvay Pharm.) |
| **QUINAPRIL HCl** | |
| **Tablets:** 5, 10, 20, and 40 mg (*Rx*) | *Accupril* (Parke-Davis) |
| **RAMIPRIL** | |
| **Capsules:** 1.25, 2.5, 5, and 10 mg (*Rx*) | *Altace* (Monarch) |
| **TRANDOLAPRIL** | |
| **Tablets:** 1, 2, and 4 mg (*Rx*) | *Mavik* (Knoll) |

> **Warning:**
> *Pregnancy:* When used in pregnancy during the second and third trimesters, ACEIs can cause injury and even death to the developing fetus. When pregnancy is detected, discontinue the ACEI as soon as possible.

## Indications

*Hypertension:* The ACEIs are effective alone and in combination with other antihypertensive agents, especially thiazide-type diuretics. Blood pressure (BP)-lowering effects of ACEIs and thiazides are approximately additive.

*Heart failure:* Some ACEIs are effective in the management of CHF, usually as adjunctive therapy and in patients who demonstrate clinical signs of CHF or have evidence of left ventricular systolic dysfunction within the first few days after an acute myocardial infarction (MI).

*MI:*
    *Lisinopril* – Treatment of hemodynamically stable patients within 24 hours of acute MI, to improve survival. Patients should receive, as appropriate, the standard recommended treatments such as thrombolytics, aspirin and beta-blockers.

*Left ventricular dysfunction (LVD):* Various ACEIs have demonstrated improved survival and decreased rates of development of overt heart failure in patients with varying degrees of LVD (from modest, asymptomatic to severe with CHF).

*Diabetic nephropathy:*
    *Captopril* – Treatment of diabetic nephropathy (proteinuria greater than 500 mg/day) in patients with type 1 insulin-dependent diabetes mellitus and retinopathy.

*Heart failure post-MI/left-ventricular dysfunction post-MI (trandolapril, ramipril):* For stable patients who have evidence of left-ventricular systolic dysfunction (identified by wall motion abnormalities) or who are symptomatic from CHF within the first few days after sustaining acute MI. Administration to white patients decreases the risk of death (principally cardiovascular death) and decreases risk of heart failure-related hospitalization.

*Perindopril:*
    *Essential hypertension* – For the treatment of patients with essential hypertension. It may be used alone or given with other classes of antihypertensives, especially thiazide diuretics.

*Ramipril:*

*Reduction in risk of MI, stroke, and death from cardiovascular causes* – In patients 55 years of age or older at high risk of developing a major cardiovascular event because of a history of coronary artery disease, stroke, peripheral vascular disease, or diabetes that is accompanied by at least 1 other cardiovascular risk factor (eg, hypertension, elevated total cholesterol levels, low HDL levels, cigarette smoking, documented microalbuminuria).

*Unlabeled uses:*

*Captopril* – Management of hypertensive crises (25 mg initially, 100 mg 90 to 120 minutes later, 200 to 300 mg/day for 2 to 5 days, then adjusted). Sublingual captopril 25 mg has also been used effectively.

Severe childhood hypertension (0.3 mg/kg initial dose, titrated 6 mg/day or less given in 2 or 3 divided doses).

Rheumatoid arthritis (75 to 150 mg/day in divided doses).

Raynaud syndrome (symptomatic relief) (37.5 mg/day).

*Enalaprilat* – May be used for hypertensive emergencies (1.25 to 5 mg every 6 hours), but the effects are often variable.

## Administration and Dosage
BENAZEPRIL HCl:

*Initial dose* – 10 mg once daily for patients not receiving a diuretic.

*Maintenance dosage* – 20 to 40 mg/day as a single dose or 2 divided doses. A dose of 80 mg gives an increased response, but experience is limited.

*Renal function impairment* – 5 mg once daily in patients with Ccr of less than 30 mL/min/1.73 $m^2$ (serum creatinine greater than 3 mg/dL). Dosage may be titrated upward until BP is controlled or to a maximum of 40 mg/day.

CAPTOPRIL: Administer 1 hour before meals.

*Hypertension* –

*Initial:* 25 mg 2 or 3 times/day. If satisfactory BP reduction is not achieved after 1 or 2 weeks, increase to 50 mg 2 or 3 times/day. If BP is not controlled after 1 or 2 weeks at this dose (and patient is not already on a diuretic), add a modest dose of a thiazide diuretic.

If further BP reduction is required, increase to 100 mg captopril 2 or 3 times/day and then, if necessary, to 150 mg 2 or 3 times/day (while continuing diuretic). Usual dose is 25 to 150 mg 2 or 3 times/day. Do not exceed daily dose of 450 mg.

*Accelerated or malignant hypertension:* Promptly initiate captopril at 25 mg 2 or 3 times daily under close supervision. Increase dose every 24 hours or less until a satisfactory response is obtained or the maximum dose is reached.

*Heart failure* – Usual initial dosage is 25 mg 3 times daily. After 50 mg 3 times daily is reached, delay further dosage increases, where possible, for at least 2 weeks to determine if a satisfactory response occurs. Most patients have had a satisfactory clinical improvement at 50 or 100 mg 3 times daily. Do not exceed a daily dose of 450 mg. Captopril should generally be used in conjunction with a diuretic and digitalis.

*LVD after MI* – 50 mg 3 times daily is the target maintenance dose. Therapy may be initiated as early as 3 days following an MI. After a single 6.25 mg dose, initiate at 12.5 mg 3 times daily, then increase to 25 mg 3 times daily during the next several days and to a target of 50 mg 3 times daily over the next several weeks as tolerated.

*Diabetic nephropathy* – Recommended dose for long-term use is 25 mg 3 times daily.

*Renal impairment* – Reduce initial dosage and use smaller increments for titration, which should be quite slow (1- to 2-week intervals). After the desired therapeutic effect is achieved, slowly back-titrate to the minimal effective dose.

ENALAPRIL:

*Oral* –

*Hypertension:*

*Patients taking diuretics* – Discontinue the diuretic, if possible, for 2 to 3 days before beginning therapy with enalapril to reduce the likelihood of hypotension. If the diuretic cannot be discontinued, use an initial dose of 2.5 mg under medical supervision for at least 2 hours and until BP has stabilized for at least an additional hour.

*Patients not taking diuretics* – Initial dose is 5 mg once a day. The usual dosage range is 10 to 40 mg/day as a single dose or in 2 divided doses.

*Impaired renal function* – Titrate the dosage upward until BP is controlled or until a maximum dose of 40 mg/day is reached. Use initial dose of 5 mg/day in normal renal function and mild impairment (Ccr 30 to 80 mL/min, serum creatinine 3 mg/dL or less); 2.5 mg/day in moderate to severe renal impairment (Ccr 30 mL/min or less, serum creatinine 3 mg/dL or more) and in dialysis patients on dialysis days.

*Heart failure:* As adjunctive therapy with diuretics and digitalis, the recommended starting dose is 2.5 mg twice daily. The usual therapeutic dosing range for the treatment of heart failure is 2.5 to 20 mg/day given in 2 divided doses. The maximum daily dose is 40 mg.

*Renal impairment or hyponatremia* –

*Serum sodium less than 130 mEq/L or with serum creatinine greater than 1.6 mg/dL:* Initiate at 2.5 mg/day under close medical supervision. The dose may be increased to 2.5 mg twice daily, then 5 mg twice daily and higher as needed, usually at intervals of 4 days or more. The maximum daily dose is 40 mg.

*Asymptomatic left ventricular dysfunction:* 2.5 mg twice daily, titrated as tolerated to the targeted daily dose of 20 mg in divided doses.

*Parenteral (enalaprilat)* – For IV administration only.

*Hypertension:* 1.25 mg every 6 hours IV over 5 minutes.

The dose for patients being converted to IV from oral therapy is 1.25 mg every 6 hours. For conversion from IV to oral therapy, the recommended initial dose of tablets is 5 mg/day for patients with Ccr greater than 30 mL/min and 2.5 mg/day for patients with Ccr 30 mL/min or less. Adjust dosage according to BP response.

*Patients taking diuretics:* Starting dose for hypertension is 0.625 mg IV over 5 minutes. If there is inadequate clinical response after 1 hour, repeat the 0.625 dose. Give additional doses of 1.25 mg at 6-hour intervals.

For conversion from IV to oral therapy, the recommended initial dose of enalapril maleate tablets for patients who have responded to 0.625 mg enalaprilat every 6 hours is 2.5 mg once a day with subsequent dosage adjustment as needed.

*High-risk patients:* Hypertensive patients at risk of excessive hypotension include those with the following concurrent conditions or characteristics: Heart failure, hyponatremia, high-dose diuretic therapy, recent intensive diureses or increase in diuretic dose, renal dialysis, or severe volume or salt depletion of any etiology. Single doses of enalaprilat as low as 0.2 mg have produced excessive hypotension in normotensive patients with these diagnoses. Because of the potential for an extreme hypotensive response in these patients, initiate therapy under very close medical supervision. The starting dose should be no more than 0.625 mg administered IV over a period of at least 5 minutes and preferably longer (up to 1 hour).

*Renal function impairment:* Administer 1.25 mg every 6 hours for patients with Ccr greater than 30 mL/min. For Ccr 30 mL/min or less, initial dose is 0.625 mg. If there is inadequate clinical response after 1 hour, the 0.625 mg dose may be repeated. May give additional 1.25 mg doses at 6-hour intervals. For dialysis patients, initial dose is 0.625 mg or less administered over 5 minutes or more, preferably longer (no more than 1 hour).

For conversion from IV to oral therapy, the recommended initial dose is 5 mg once a day for patients with Ccr greater than 30 mL/min and 2.5 mg once daily for patients with Ccr 30 mL/min or less.

*FOSINOPRIL SODIUM:*
  *Initial dose* – 10 mg once daily.

*Maintenance dosage* – Usual range needed to maintain a response is 20 to 40 mg/day but some patients appear to have a further response to 80 mg. If trough response is inadequate, consider dividing the daily dose.

LISINOPRIL:

*Hypertension –*

*Initial therapy:* 10 mg once/day in patients with uncomplicated essential hypertension not on diuretic therapy. The usual dosage range is 20 to 40 mg/day as a single daily dose.

*Diuretic-treated patients:* Discontinue the diuretic, if possible, for 2 to 3 days before beginning therapy with lisinopril to reduce the likelihood of hypotension. If the diuretic cannot be discontinued, use an initial dose of 5 mg under medical supervision for at least 2 hours and until BP has stabilized for at least an additional hour.

*CHF –*

*Initial dose:* 5 mg once daily with diuretics and digitalis. Usual effective dosage range is 5 to 20 mg/day as a single dose. In patients with hyponatremia (serum sodium less than 130 mEq/L), initiate dose at 2.5 mg once daily. If used with diuretics, initial dose is 5 mg/day.

*Elderly* – Make dosage adjustments with particular caution.

*Renal function impairment* – For hypertension, titrate dosage upward until BP is controlled or to a maximum of 40 mg daily.

In acute MI, initiate lisinopril with caution in patients with evidence of renal dysfunction (serum creatinine concentration exceeding 2 mg/dL).

| Lisinopril Dosage in Renal Impairment | | | |
|---|---|---|---|
| Renal status | Ccr (mL/min) | Serum creatinine (mg/dL) | Initial dose (mg/day) |
| Normal function to mild impairment | > 30 | ≤ 3 | 10 |
| Moderate to severe impairment | ≥ 10 to ≤ 30 | ≥ 3 | 5 |
| Dialysis patients | < 10 | — | 2.5[1] |

[1] Adjust dosage or dosing interval depending on the BP response.

*Acute MI* – In hemodynamically stable patients within 24 hours of the onset of symptoms of acute MI, the first dose is 5 mg, followed by 5 mg after 24 hours, 10 mg after 48 hours and then 10 mg once daily. Continue dosing for 6 weeks. Patients with a low systolic BP (120 mm Hg or less) when treatment is started or during the first 3 days after the infarct should be given a lower 2.5 mg dose. If hypotension occurs (systolic BP 100 mm Hg or less), a daily maintenance dose of 5 mg may be given with temporary reductions to 2.5 mg if needed. If prolonged hypotension occurs (systolic BP less than 90 mm Hg for more than 1 hour), withdraw lisinopril.

MOEXIPRIL HCl:

*Initial dose* – In patients not receiving diuretics, 7.5 mg 1 hour prior to meals once daily. If control is not adequate, increase the dose or divide the dosing.

*Maintenance dose* – 7.5 to 30 mg daily in 1 or 2 divided doses 1 hour before meals.

*Renal function impairment* – Cautiously use 3.75 mg once daily in patients with Ccr of 40 mL/min/1.73 m$^2$ or less. Dosage may be titrated upward to a maximum of 15 mg/day.

PERINDOPRIL:

*Use in uncomplicated hypertensive patients* – In patients with essential hypertension, the recommended initial dose is 4 mg once a day. The dosage may be titrated upward until BP, when measured just before the next dose, is controlled or to a maximum of 16 mg/day. The usual maintenance dose range is 4 to 8 mg administered as a single daily dose. It also may be administered in 2 divided doses. When once-daily dosing was compared to twice-daily dosing in clinical studies, the twice-daily regimen was generally slightly superior, but not by more than approximately 0.5 to 1 mm Hg.

*Use in elderly patients* – As in younger patients, the recommended initial dosages for the elderly (older than 65 years of age) is 4 mg daily in 1 or 2 divided doses. The daily dosage may be titrated upward until BP, when measured just before the next dose, is controlled, but experience with perindopril is limited in the elderly at doses greater than 8 mg. Administer dosages greater than 8 mg cautiously and under close medical supervision.

*Use in concomitant diuretics* – If BP is not adequately controlled with perindopril alone, a diuretic may be added. In patients currently being treated with a diuretic, symptomatic hypotension occasionally can occur following the initial dose of perindopril. To reduce likelihood of such reaction, the diuretic should, if possible, be discontinued 2 to 3 days prior to beginning perindopril therapy. Then, if BP is not controlled with perindopril alone, resume the diuretic.

If the diuretic cannot be discontinued, use an initial dose of 2 to 4 mg daily in 1 or 2 divided doses with careful medical supervision for several hours and until BP has stabilized. Titrate the dosage as described above.

*Use in patients with impaired renal function* – Perindoprilat elimination is decreased in renally impaired patients, with a marked increase in accumulation when Ccr drops below 30 mL/min. In patients with Ccr less than 30 mL/min, safety and efficacy have not been established. For patients with lesser degrees of impairment (Ccr more than 30 mL/min), the initial dosage should be 2 mg/day, and dosage should not exceed 8 mg/day because of limited clinical experience. During dialysis, perindopril is removed with the same clearance as in patients with normal renal function.

QUINAPRIL HCl:
   *Hypertension* –
   *Initial dose:* 10 or 20 mg once daily for patients not on diuretics.
   *Elderly (65 years of age or older):* 10 mg once daily followed by titration to the optimal response.
   *Renal function impairment:* Initial dose is 10 mg with Ccr greater than 60 mL/min, 5 mg with Ccr 30 to 60 mL/min and 2.5 mg with Ccr 10 to 30 mL/min.
   *CHF* – The recommended starting dose is 5 mg twice/day. If the initial dose is well tolerated, titrate patients at weekly intervals until an effective dose, usually 20 to 40 mg/day given in 2 equally divided doses, is reached or undesirable hypotension, orthostasis, or azotemia prohibit reaching this dose.
   *Renal impairment or hyponatremia:* In patients with heart failure and renal impairment, the recommended initial dose is 5 mg with Ccr greater than 30 mL/min and 2.5 mg with Ccr 10 to 30 mL/min. There is insufficient data for dosage recommendation in patients with Ccr less than 10 mL/min.

RAMIPRIL:
   *Reduction in risk of MI, stroke, and death from cardiovascular causes* –
   *Initial dose:* 2.5 mg once daily for 1 week, 5 mg once daily for the next 3 weeks, and then increased as tolerated to maintenance dose.
   *Maintenance dosage:* 10 mg once daily. If the patient is hypertensive or recently post-MI, it can also be given as a divided dose.
   *Renal function impairment:* In patients with Ccr of less than 40 mL/min/1.73 m$^2$ (serum creatinine approximately greater than 2.5 mg/dL) doses only 25% of those normally used should be expected to induce full therapeutic levels of ramiprilat.
   *Hypertension* –
   *Initial dose:* 2.5 mg once daily in patients not receiving a diuretic.
   *Maintenance dosage:* 2.5 to 20 mg/day as a single dose or in two equally divided doses. If BP is not controlled with ramipril alone, a diuretic can be added.
   *Renal function impairment:* 1.25 mg once daily in patients with Ccr of less than 40 mL/min/1.73 m$^2$ (serum creatinine approximately greater than 2.5 mg/dL). Dosage may be titrated upward until BP is controlled or to a maximum of 5 mg/day.
   *Heart failure post-MI* – Starting dose is 2.5 mg twice daily. A patient who becomes hypotensive at this dose may be switched to 1.25 mg twice daily, but all patients should then be titrated (as tolerated) toward a target dose of 5 mg twice daily, with dosage increases being approximately 3 weeks apart. After the initial dose, observe for at least 2 hours and until BP has stabilized for at least an additional hour. If possible, reduce the dose of any concomitant diuretic.
   *Renal function impairment:* 1.25 mg once daily in patients with Ccr of less than 40 mL/min/1.73 m$^2$ (serum creatinine approximately greater than 2.5 mg/dL). Dos-

age may be increased to 1.25 mg twice daily up to a maximum dose of 2.5 mg twice daily depending on clinical response and tolerability.

*Alternative route of administration* – Ramipril capsules are usually swallowed whole. However, the capsules may be opened and the contents sprinkled on a small amount of approximately 4 oz applesauce or mixed in apple juice or water.

TRANDOLAPRIL:
  Hypertension –
    *Initial dose:* The recommended initial dosage of trandolapril for patients not receiving a diuretic is 1 mg/day (2 mg in black patients). Adjust dosage according to the BP response. Make dosage adjustments at intervals of 1 week or more. Most patients have required dosages of 2 to 4 mg/day. There is little clinical experience with doses greater than 8 mg.

    *Maintenance* – Patients inadequately treated with once daily dosing at 4 mg may be treated with twice-daily dosing. If BP is not adequately controlled with trandolapril monotherapy, a diuretic may be added.

    *Concomitant diuretic* – In patients being treated with a diuretic, symptomatic hypotension can occasionally occur following the initial dose of trandolapril. To reduce the likelihood of hypotension, if possible, discontinue the diuretic 2 to 3 days prior to beginning therapy with trandolapril. If BP is not controlled with trandolapril alone, resume diuretic therapy. If the diuretic cannot be discontinued, give an initial dose of 0.5 mg trandolapril with careful medical supervision for several hours until BP has stabilized. Titrate dosage as described above to the optimal response.

  Heart failure post-MI or LVD post-MI –
    *Initial dose:* 1 mg/day
    *Maintenance dosage:* Titrate to greatest tolerated dose.
    *Target dose:* 4 mg/day.

  *Renal/Hepatic function impairment* – For patients with a Ccr less than 30 mL/min or with hepatic cirrhosis, the recommended starting dose, based on clinical and pharmacokinetic data, is 0.5 mg/day. Titrate as described above to the optimal response.

## Actions

*Pharmacology:* The angiotensin-converting enzyme inhibitors (ACEIs) appear to act primarily through suppression of the renin-angiotensin-aldosterone system; however, no consistent correlation has been described between renin levels and drug response.

Synthesized by the kidneys, renin is released into the circulation where it acts on a plasma globulin substrate to produce angiotensin I. Angiotensin I is then converted by angiotensin converting enzyme (ACE) to angiotensin II. These agents prevent the conversion of angiotensin I to angiotensin II by inhibiting ACE. ACEIs may also inhibit local angiotensin II at vascular and renal sites and attenuate the release of catecholamines from adrenergic nerve endings.

Increased prostaglandin synthesis may also play a role in the antihypertensive action of captopril.

Some ACEIs have demonstrated a beneficial effect on the severity of heart failure and an improvement in maximal exercise tolerance in patients with heart failure. In these patients, ACEIs significantly decrease peripheral (systemic vascular) resistance, BP (afterload), pulmonary capillary wedge pressure (preload), pulmonary vascular resistance and heart size and increase cardiac output and exercise tolerance time.

*Pharmacokinetics:*

| Pharmacokinetics of the Active Moieties of ACEIs | | | | | | | | |
|---|---|---|---|---|---|---|---|---|
| | | | | | Half-life | | Elimination (24 h) | |
| ACEI | Onset/ Duration (h) | Protein binding | Effect of food on absorption | Active metabolite | Normal renal function | Impaired renal function | Total | Un-changed |
| Benazepril | 1/24 | ≈ 96.7% (≈ 95.3%)[1] | slightly reduced | benazeprilat | 10-11 h[1] | prolonged | 11-12% bile[1] | trace |

| Pharmacokinetics of the Active Moieties of ACEIs | | | | | | | | |
|---|---|---|---|---|---|---|---|---|
| | | | | | Half-life | | Elimination (24 h) | |
| ACEI | Onset/ Duration (h) | Protein binding | Effect of food on absorption | Active metabolite | Normal renal function | Impaired renal function | Total | Un-changed |
| Captopril | nd[2]/ dose-related | ≈ 25%-30% | reduced | | < 2 h | prolonged | > 95% urine | 40%-50% in urine |
| Enalapril | 1/24 | nd[2] | none | enalaprilat | 1.3 h (11 h)[1] | nd[2] | 94% urine and feces | 54% in urine (40%)[1] |
| Enalapri-lat | 0.25/≈6 | na[3] | na[4] | | 11 h | prolonged | nd[2] | > 90% in urine |
| Fosinopril | 1/24 | ≈ 99.4% | slightly reduced | fosinoprilat | ≈ 12 h[1] | prolonged negligible clinical effect | 50% urine, 50% feces | negli-gible |
| Lisinopril | 1/24 | na[3] | none | - | 12 h | prolonged | nd[2] | 100% in urine |
| Moexipril | 1.5/24 | ≈ 50% | markedly reduced | moexiprilat | 2-9 h[1] | prolonged | 13% urine, 53% feces | 1% in urine, 1% in feces |
| Quinapril | 1/24 | ≈ 97% | reduced | quinaprilat | 2 h[1] | prolonged | ≈60% urine, ≈37% feces | trace |
| Ramipril | 1-2/24 | ≈ 73% (≈ 56%)[1] | slightly reduced | ramiprilat | 13-17 h[1] | prolonged | ≈ 60% urine, ≈ 40% feces | < 2% |
| Trandol-april | 4/24 | ≈ 80% | reduced | trandolapri-lat | ≈ 5 h (≈ 10 h)[1] | prolonged | 33% urine, 56% feces | nd[2] |

[1] Of active metabolite.
[2] nd – No data.
[3] na – Not applicable.
[4] na – Not applicable; available IV only.

### Contraindications
Hypersensitivity to these products.

### Warnings
*Neutropenia/Agranulocytosis:* Neutropenia (less than 1000/mm$^3$) with myeloid hypoplasia resulted from **captopril** use. About half of the neutropenic patients developed systemic or oral cavity infections or other features of agranulocytosis. Neutropenia/ agranulocytosis has occurred rarely with **enalapril** or **lisinopril** and in 1 patient on **quinapril**. Data are insufficient to show that **moexipril, ramipril, quinapril, benazepril, trandolapril,** or **fosinopril** do not cause agranulocytosis at similar rates. Periodically monitor WBC counts.

*Angioedema:* Angioedema has occurred. It may occur at any time during treatment, especially following the first dose of **enalapril** (0.2%), **captopril, lisinopril, trandolapril** (0.13%), **benazepril** (approximately 0.5%), **quinapril** (0.1%), or **moexipril** (less than 0.5%). Angioedema associated with laryngeal edema may be fatal. Black patients receiving ACE inhibitor monotherapy have been reported to have a higher incidence of angioedema compared with non-blacks.

*Proteinuria:* Total urinary proteins more than 1 g/day were seen in 0.7% of **captopril** patients. Nephrotic syndrome occurred in approximately 20% of these cases.

*Hypotension:*
    *First-dose effect* – ACEIs may cause a profound fall in BP following the first dose.
    *Heart failure* – In heart failure, where the BP was either normal or low, transient decreases in mean BP greater than 20% occurred in approximately 50% of the patients.

*Renal function impairment:* Some hypertensive patients with renal disease, particularly those with severe renal artery stenosis, have developed increases in BUN and serum creatinine after reduction of BP.

In patients with severe CHF whose renal function may depend on the activity of the renin-angiotensin-aldosterone system, treatment with ACEIs may be associated with oliguria or progressive azotemia and, rarely, with acute renal failure or death.

Impaired renal function decreases **lisinopril** elimination. The elimination half-life of quinaprilat increases as Ccr decreases. Dosage adjustment may be necessary for **quinapril, benazepril, ramipril,** and **lisinopril.** Impaired renal function decreases total clearance of fosinoprilat and approximately doubles the AUC.

*Hepatic function impairment:* Patients with impaired liver function could develop markedly elevated plasma levels of unchanged **fosinopril** or **ramipril.** In patients with alcoholic or biliary cirrhosis, the rate, but not extent of fosinopril hydrolysis was reduced. Quinaprilat concentrations are reduced in alcoholic cirrhosis.

*Elderly:* Elderly patients may have higher blood levels and AUC of **lisinopril, ramiprilat, quinaprilat,** and **moexiprilat.** This may relate to decreased renal function rather than to age itself.

*Pregnancy: Category C* (first trimester); *Category D* (second and third trimesters). See Warning Box.

*Lactation:* Several ACEIs have been detected in breast milk. Do not administer **trandolapril** or **ramipril** to nursing mothers. It is not known whether **lisinopril, moexipril,** or **ramipril** is excreted in breast milk. Discontinue nursing or the drug.

*Children:* Safety and efficacy have not been established. Use **captopril** in children only when other measures for controlling BP have not been effective.

## Precautions

*Hyperkalemia:* Elevated serum potassium (at least 0.5 mEq/L greater than the upper limit of normal) was observed in 0.4% of hypertensive patients given **trandolapril,** approximately 1% of hypertensive patients given **benazepril, enalapril, ramipril,** or **moexipril;** approximately 2% of patients receiving **quinapril** or **lisinopril,** approximately 2.6% of hypertensive patients given **fosinopril,** and approximately 4.8% of CHF patients given lisinopril. Hyperkalemia also occurred with **captopril.**

*Valvular stenosis:* Theoretically, patients with aortic stenosis might be at risk of decreased coronary perfusion when treated with vasodilators, because they do not develop as much afterload reduction as others.

*Surgery/Anesthesia:* In patients undergoing major surgery or during anesthesia with agents that produce hypotension, ACEIs will block angiotensin II formation secondary to compensatory renin release.

*Cough:* Chronic cough has occurred with the use of all ACEIs. Characteristically, the cough is nonproductive, persistent and resolves within 1 to 4 days after therapy discontinuation.

The incidence of cough, although still reported as 0.5% to 3% by some manufacturers, appears to range from 5% to 25% and has been reported to be as high as 39%, resulting in discontinuation rates as high as 15%.

## Drug Interactions

Drugs that may affect ACEIs may include antacids, capsaicin, indomethacin, phenothiazines, probenecid, and rifampin. Drugs that may be affected by ACEIs include allopurinol, digoxin, lithium, potassium preparations/potassium-sparing diuretics, and tetracycline.

*Drug/Lab test interactions:* Captopril may cause a false-positive test for urine acetone.

Fosinopril may cause a false low measurement of serum digoxin levels with the *Digi-Tab RIA Kit for Digoxin* other kits such as the *Coat-A-Count RIA Kit,* may be used.

*Drug/Food interactions:* Food significantly reduces the bioavailability of **captopril** by 30% to 40%. Administer captopril 1 hour before meals. The rate and extent of **quina-**

**pril** absorption are diminished moderately (25% to 30%) when administered during a high-fat meal. The rate, but not extent, of **ramipril** and **fosinopril** absorption is reduced by food. Food does not reduce the GI absorption of **benazepril**, **enalapril**, and **lisinopril**.

### Adverse Reactions
Adverse reactions may include chest pain, hypotension, headache, dizziness, fatigue, diarrhea, dysgeusia, cough, rash, dyspepsia, syncope, myalgia.

# ANGIOTENSIN II RECEPTOR ANTAGONISTS

| | |
|---|---|
| **CANDESARTAN CILEXETIL** | |
| **Tablets**: 4, 8, 16, and 32 mg (*Rx*) | *Atacand* (AstraZeneca) |
| **EPROSARTAN MESYLATE** | |
| **Tablets**: 600 mg (*Rx*) | *Teveten* (Biovail) |
| **IRBESARTAN** | |
| **Tablets**: 75, 150, and 300 mg (*Rx*) | *Avapro* (Bristol-Myers Squibb/Sanofi-Synthelabo) |
| **LOSARTAN POTASSIUM** | |
| **Tablets**: 25, 50, and 100 mg (*Rx*) | *Cozaar* (Merck) |
| **OLMESARTAN MEDOXOMIL** | |
| **Tablets**: 5, 20, and 40 mg (*Rx*) | *Benicar* (Sankyo Pharma) |
| **TELMISARTAN** | |
| **Tablets**: 20, 40, and 80 mg (*Rx*) | *Micardis* (Boehringer Ingelheim) |
| **VALSARTAN** | |
| **Capsules**: 40, 80, 160, and 320 mg (*Rx*) | *Diovan* (Novartis) |

**Warning:**
> *Pregnancy:* When used in pregnancy during the second and third trimesters, drugs that act directly on the renin-angiotensin system can cause injury and even death to the developing fetus. When pregnancy is detected, discontinue angiotensin II receptor antagonists as soon as possible.

### Indications
*Hypertension:* Treatment of hypertension alone or in combination with other antihypertensive agents.

*Nephropathy in type 2 diabetes (losartan and irbesartan):* Treatment of diabetic nephropathy with an elevated serum creatinine and proteinuria (urinary albumin to creatinine ratio greater than or equal to 300 mg/g) in patients with type 2 diabetes and a history of hypertension.

*Heart failure (valsartan):* Treatment of heart failure (NYHA class II to IV) in patients who are intolerant of angiotensin-converting enzyme (ACE) inhibitors.

*Hypertensive patients with left ventricular hypertrophy (losartan):* Used to reduce the risk of stroke in patients with hypertension and left ventricular hypertrophy, but there is evidence that this benefit does not apply to black patients.

### Administration and Dosage
CANDESARTAN:

*Hypertension* – Administer with or without food. The usual recommended starting dose is 16 mg once daily when used as monotherapy in patients who are not volume-depleted. Candesartan can be administered once or twice daily with total daily doses ranging from 8 to 32 mg. Most of the antihypertensive effect is present within 2 weeks; maximal blood pressure reduction generally is obtained within 4 to 6 weeks of treatment.

For patients with possible intravascular volume depletion (eg, patients treated with diuretics, particularly those with impaired renal function), initiate candesartan under close medical supervision and consider administering a lower dose.

EPROSARTAN:

*Hypertension* – The usual recommended starting dosage is 600 mg once daily when used as monotherapy in patients who are not volume-depleted. Eprosartan can also be administered once or twice daily with total daily doses ranging from 400 to 800 mg. There is limited experience with doses more than 800 mg/day.

If the antihypertensive effect using once-daily dosing is inadequate, a twice-a-day regimen at the same total daily dose or an increase in dose may give a more satisfactory response. Achievement of maximum blood pressure (BP) reduction in most patients may take 2 to 3 weeks.

Discontinuation of treatment with eprosartan does not lead to a rapid rebound increase in blood pressure.

*Elderly and Hepatic/Renal function impairment* – No initial dosing adjustment is generally necessary in patients with moderate and severe renal impairment, with maximum dose not exceeding 600 mg/day.

IRBESARTAN:

*Hypertension* – The recommended initial dosage of irbesartan is 150 mg once daily with or without food. Patients may be titrated to 300 mg once daily.

Patients not adequately treated by the maximum dose of 300 mg once daily are unlikely to derive additional benefit from a higher dose or twice-daily dosing.

*Nephropathy in type 2 diabetes* – The recommended target maintenance dose is 300 mg once daily.

*Children 6 to 12 years of age* – An initial dose of 75 mg once daily is reasonable. Titrate patients requiring further reduction in blood pressure to 150 mg once daily.

*Adolescents 13 to 16 years of age* – An initial dose of 150 mg once daily is reasonable. Titrate patients requiring further reduction in blood pressure to 300 mg once daily. Higher doses are not recommended.

*Volume- and salt-depleted patients* – A lower initial dose of 75 mg is recommended in patients with depletion of intravascular volume or salt (eg, patients treated vigorously with diuretics or on hemodialysis).

LOSARTAN POTASSIUM:

*Hypertension* – The usual starting dose is 50 mg once daily with 25 mg used in patients with possible depletion of intravascular volume (eg, patients treated with diuretics) and patients with a history of hepatic impairment. Losartan can be administered with or without food once or twice daily with total daily doses ranging from 25 to 100 mg.

If the antihypertensive effect using once-daily dosing is inadequate, a twice-daily regimen at the same total daily dose or an increase in dose may give a more satisfactory response.

Losartan may be administered with other antihypertensive agents. If blood pressure is not controlled by losartan alone, a low dose of a diuretic may be added. Hydrochlorothiazide has an additive effect.

*Hypertensive patients with left ventricular hypertrophy* – The usual starting dose is 50 mg of losartan once daily. Add hydrochlorothiazide 12.5 mg/day and/or increase the dose of losartan to 100 mg once daily followed by an increase in hydrochlorothiazide to 25 mg once daily based on blood pressure response.

*Nephropathy in type 2 diabetes* – The usual starting dose is 50 mg once daily. Increase the dose to 100 mg once daily based on blood pressure response. Losartan may be administered with insulin and other commonly used hypoglycemic agents (eg, sulfonylureas, glitazones, glucosidase inhibitors).

OLMESARTAN:

*Hypertension* – Dosage must be individualized. The usual recommended starting dose is 20 mg once daily with or without food when used as monotherapy in patients who are not volume-contracted. For patients requiring further reduction in blood pressure after 2 weeks of therapy, the dose may be increased to 40 mg. Doses above 40 mg do not appear to have greater effect. Twice-daily dosing offers no advantage over the same total dose given once daily.

If blood pressure is not controlled by olmesartan alone, a diuretic may be added. Olmesartan may be administered with other antihypertensive agents.

For patients with possible depletion of intravascular volume (eg, patients treated with diuretics, particularly those with impaired renal function), initiate olmesartan under close medical supervision and consider using a lower starting dose.

TELMISARTAN:

*Hypertension* – The usual starting dose is 40 mg/day. BP response is dose-related over the range of 20 to 80 mg. May be administered with or without food.

*Special risk patients:* Patients on dialysis may develop orthostatic hypotension; monitor blood pressure closely. Initiate treatment under close medical supervision for patients with biliary obstructive disorders or hepatic insufficiency. Correct the condition of patients with depletion of intravascular volume before initiating therapy and monitor closely.

VALSARTAN:

*Hypertension* – The recommended starting dose is 80 mg/day, with or without food, when used as monotherapy in patients who are not volume-depleted. Valsartan may be used over a dose range of 80 to 320 mg once daily. The full antihypertensive effect of this dose usually is seen in 2 to 4 weeks.

If additional antihypertensive effect is required, the dosage may be increased to 160 or 320 mg or a diuretic may be added.

*Heart failure* – The recommended starting dose is 40 mg twice daily. Up-titrate to 80 and 160 mg twice daily to the highest dose, as tolerated. Consider reducing the dose of concomitant diuretics. The maximum daily dose in clinical trials was 320 mg in divided doses. Concomitant use with an ACE inhibitor and a beta-blocker is not recommended.

*Hepatic/Renal function impairment* – Exercise care when dosing patients with severe hepatic or renal function impairment.

## Actions

*Pharmacology:* **Losartan, candesartan, irbesartan, olmesartan, telmisartan, eprosartan,** and **valsartan** are angiotensin II receptor (type $AT_1$) antagonists. Angiotensin II receptor antagonists (AIIRAs) block the vasoconstrictor and aldosterone-secreting effects of angiotensin II by selectively blocking the binding of angiotensin II to the $AT_1$ receptor found in many tissues.

AIIRAs do not inhibit ACE (kininase II, the enzyme that converts angiotensin I to angiotensin II and degrades bradykinin), nor do they bind to or block other hormone receptors or ion channels known to be important in cardiovascular regulation.

*Pharmacokinetics:*

| Angiotensin II Antagonist Pharmacokinetics | | | | | | | |
|---|---|---|---|---|---|---|---|
| Parameters | Cande-sartan | Eprosartan | Irbe-sartan | Losartan (metabolite)[1] | Olme-sartan | Telmi-sartan | Valsartan |
| Bioavail-ability | ≈ 15% | ≈ 13% | 60% to 80% | ≈ 33% | ≈ 26% | 42%/58% (40 mg/ 160 mg) | ≈ 25% |
| Food effect ($AUC/C_{max}$) | no effect | ↓< 25% | no effect | ↓10%/↓14% | no effect | ↓6%/↓20% (40 mg AUC/ 160 mg AUC) | ↓4C%/↓50% |
| Plasma bound | > 99% | ≈ 98% | 90% | 98.7% (99.8%) | 99% | > 99.5% | 95% |
| $T_{max}$ | 3 to 4 h | 1 to 2 h | 1.5 to 2 h | 1 h (3 to 4 h) | 1 to 2 h | 0.5 to 1 h | 2 to 4 h |
| Volume of dis-tribution | 0.13 L/kg | 308 L | 53 to 93 L | ≈ 34 L (≈ 12 L) | ≈ 17 L | ≈ 500 L | 17 L[2] |
| Converted to metabolites | minor | minor | < 20% | ≈ 14% | none | ≈ 11% | ≈ 20% |
| Metabolism | O-deethy-lation | glucuroni-dation | CYP2C9 | CYP2C9; CYP3A4 | none | conjugation | unknown |
| Terminal half-life | ≈ 9 h | 5 to 9 h | 11 to 15 h | ≈ 2 h (6 to 9 h) | ≈ 13 h | ≈ 24 h | ≈ 6 h[2] |
| Total plasma clearance | 0.37 mL/ min/kg | ≈ 130 mL/min[2] | 157 to 176 mL/min | ≈ 600 mL/min (≈ 50 mL/min) | 1.3 L/h | > 800 mL/min | ≈ 2 L/h[2] |

| Angiotensin II Antagonist Pharmacokinetics | | | | | | |
|---|---|---|---|---|---|---|
| Parameters | Cande-sartan | Eprosartan | Irbe-sartan | Losartan (metabolite)[1] | Olme-sartan | Telmi-sartan | Valsartan |
| Renal clearance | 0.19 mL/min/kg | ≈30 to 40 mL/min | 3 to 3.5 mL/min | ≈ 75 mL/min (≈ 25 mL/min) | 0.6 L/h | nd[3] | ≈ 0.62 L/h[2] |
| Recovered in the urine | ≈ 33% | ≈ 7% | ≈ 20% | ≈ 45/≈ 35% (IV/oral) | 35% to 50% | 0.91%/0.49% (IV/oral) | ≈ 13% |
| Recovered in the feces | ≈ 67% | ≈ 90% | ≈ 80% | ≈ 50/≈ 60% (IV/oral) | 50% to 65% | > 97% | ≈ 83% |

[1] Active.
[2] IV dosing.
[3] nd = no data

### Contraindications
Hypersensitivity to any component of these products.

### Warnings
*Hypotension/Volume- or salt-depleted patients:* In patients who are intravascularly volume-depleted (eg, those treated with diuretics), symptomatic hypotension may occur. Correct these conditions prior to administration.

*Race:* **Losartan** was effective in reducing blood pressure regardless of race, although the effect was somewhat less in black patients (usually a low-renin population). In healthy black subjects, **irbesartan** AUC values were approximately 25% greater than in whites.

*Cough:* In trials where **valsartan** was compared with an ACE inhibitor with or without placebo, the incidence of dry cough was significantly greater in the ACE inhibitor group (7.9%) than in the groups who received valsartan (2.6%) or placebo (1.5%). In patients who had dry cough when previously receiving ACE inhibitors, the incidences of cough in patients who received AIIRAs, HCTZ, or lisinopril were about 22.5%, about 18%, and 69%, respectively.

There was no significant difference in the incidence of cough between **losartan**, **olmesartan**, **eprosartan**, or **telmisartan** and placebo. **Irbesartan** use was not associated with an increased incidence of dry cough, as is typically associated with ACE inhibitor use.

*Renal function impairment:* In patients whose renal function may depend on the activity of the renin-angiotensin-aldosterone system (eg, patients with severe CHF), treatment with ACE inhibitors and angiotensin receptor antagonists has been associated with oliguria or progressive azotemia and with acute renal failure or death (rarely). No dosage adjustment is necessary for patients with renal impairment unless they are volume-depleted. AIIRAs are not dialyzable.

*Hepatic function impairment:*
Losartan – Compared with healthy subjects, the total plasma clearance in patients with hepatic insufficiency was about 50% lower and the oral bioavailability was about 2 times higher. A lower starting dose is recommended.

Valsartan – On average, patients with mild to moderate chronic liver disease have twice the exposure to valsartan of healthy volunteers. In general, no dosage adjustment is needed in patients with mild to moderate liver disease. However, exercise care in this patient population.

Olmesartan – Increases in $AUC_{0-\infty}$ and $C_{max}$ were observed in patients with moderate hepatic impairment compared with those in matched controls, with an increase in AUC of about 60%.

Telmisartan – As the majority of telmisartan is eliminated by biliary excretion, patients with biliary obstructive disorders or hepatic insufficiency can be expected to have reduced clearance. Use telmisartan with caution in these patients.

*Elderly:* No dosage adjustment is necessary when initiating AIIRAs in the elderly.

*Pregnancy:* Category C (first trimester); Category D (second and third trimesters).

*Lactation:* It is not known if AIIRAs are excreted in human breast milk.

*Children:* Safety and efficacy have not been established in children younger than 6 years of age.

**Precautions**

*Potassium supplements:* Tell patients receiving **losartan** not to use potassium supplements or salt substitutes containing potassium without consulting the prescribing physician.

*Lab test abnormalities:*

*Liver function tests* – Occasional elevations of liver enzymes or serum bilirubin have occurred.

*Creatinine/Blood urea nitrogen (BUN)* – Minor increases in BUN or serum creatinine were observed with **candesartan, losartan, valsartan, irbesartan,** and **eprosartan.** A rise of 0.5 mg/dL or more in creatinine was observed in 0.4% **telmisartan** patients compared with 0.3% placebo patients.

*Hemoglobin and hematocrit* – A decrease of more than 2 g/dL in hemoglobin was observed in 0.8% **telmisartan** patients compared with 0.3% placebo patients. No patients discontinued therapy because of anemia.

Small decreases in hemoglobin and hematocrit occurred frequently in patients treated with **losartan** alone but were rarely of clinical importance. Decreases of more than 20% in hemoglobin and hematocrit were observed in 0.4% and 0.8%, respectively, of **valsartan** patients, vs 0.1% and 0.1% with placebo.

Mean decreases in hemoglobin of 0.2 g/dL were observed in 0.2% of patients receiving **irbesartan.** Neutropenia (less than 1000 cells/mm$^3$) occurred at similar frequencies (0.3%).

Small decreases in hemoglobin and hematocrit (mean decreases of approximately 0.2 g/dL and 0.5 volume percent, respectively) were observed in patients treated with **candesartan** alone but were rarely of clinical importance.

*Serum potassium* – Increases of greater than 20% in serum potassium were observed in 4.4% of **valsartan**-treated patients vs 2.9% of placebo-treated patients.

A small increase (mean increase of 0.1 mEq/L) was observed in patients treated with **candesartan** alone but was rarely of clinical importance. One patient from a CHF trial was withdrawn for hyperkalemia (serum potassium, 7.5 mEq/L). This patient was also receiving spironolactone.

A potassium value of at least 5.6 mmol/L occurred in 0.9% of patients taking **eprosartan** and 0.3% of patients given placebo in controlled clinical trials.

*Hyperuricemia* – Hyperuricemia was rarely found (0.6% with **candesartan** vs 0.5% with placebo.)

**Drug Interactions**

Drugs that may interact with **losartan** include cimetidine, phenobarbital, fluconazole, indomethacin, and rifamycins.

Drugs that may interact with **telmisartan** include digoxin and warfarin.

In vitro studies show significant inhibition of the formation of oxidized **irbesartan** metabolites with the known cytochrome CYP2C9 substrates/inhibitors, tolbutamide, and nifedipine. However, clinical consequences were negligible.

*CYP450:* In vitro studies show significant inhibition of the formation of the active metabolite of **losartan** by inhibitors of cytochrome P450 3A4 (eg, ketoconazole, troleandomycin) or P450 2C9 (sulfaphenazole). The consequences of concomitant use of losartan and these inhibitors have not been examined.

*Potassium:* Concomitant use of potassium-sparing diuretics, potassium supplements, or salt substitutes containing potassium and AIIRAs may lead to increases in serum potassium.

**Adverse Reactions**

Adverse reactions occurring in at least 3% of patients include dizziness, upper respiratory tract infection, cough, viral infection, fatigue, diarrhea, pain, sinusitis, pharyngitis, rhinitis.

# EPLERENONE

**Tablets**: 25 and 50 mg (*Rx*)                    *Inspra* (Searle)

### Indications
*Congestive heart failure (CHF) post-myocardial infarction (MI)*: To improve survival of stable patients with left ventricular systolic dysfunction (ejection fraction 40% or less) and clinical evidence of CHF after an acute MI.

*Hypertension*: Treatment of hypertension alone or in combination with other antihypertensive agents.

### Administration and Dosage
The recommended starting dose is 50 mg administered once daily. The full therapeutic effect is apparent within 4 weeks. For patients with an inadequate response to 50 mg once daily, increase the dosage to 50 mg twice daily. Higher dosages are not recommended.

*CHF post-MI*: 50 mg once daily. Initiate treatment at 25 mg once daily and titrate to the target dose of 50 mg once daily, preferably within 4 weeks as tolerated by the patient.

| Eplerenone Dose Adjustment in CHF | | |
|---|---|---|
| Serum potassium (mEq/L) | Action | Dose adjustment |
| < 5 | Increase | 25 mg every other day to 25 mg every day<br>25 mg every day to 50 mg every day |
| 5 to 5.4 | Maintain | No adjustment |
| 5.5 to 5.9 | Decrease | 50 mg every day to 25 mg every day<br>25 mg every day to 25 mg every other day<br>25 mg every other day to withhold |
| ≥ 6 | Withhold | — |

Eplerenone can be restarted at a dose of 25 mg every other day when serum potassium levels have fallen below 5.5 mEq/L. Measure serum potassium before initiating eplerenone therapy, within the first week, and at 1 month after the start of treatment or dose adjustment. Periodically assess serum potassium thereafter. Factors such as patient characteristics and serum potassium levels may indicate that additional monitoring is appropriate.

For patients receiving weak CYP3A4 inhibitors (eg, erythromycin, saquinavir, verapamil, fluconazole), reduce the starting dose to 25 mg once daily.

### Actions
*Pharmacology*: Eplerenone blocks the binding of aldosterone, a component of the renin-angiotensin-aldosterone system (RAAS).

*Pharmacokinetics*:
   *Absorption* – Mean peak plasma concentrations are reached approximately 1.5 hours following oral administration. Steady state is reached within 2 days. Absorption is not affected by food.

   *Distribution* – The plasma protein binding of eplerenone is about 50%. The apparent volume of distribution at steady state ranged from 43 to 90 L. Eplerenone does not preferentially bind to red blood cells.

   *Metabolism* – Eplerenone is primarily metabolized via CYP3A4. Inhibitors of CYP3A4 increase blood levels of eplerenone.

   *Excretion* – The elimination half-life of eplerenone is approximately 4 to 6 hours. The apparent plasma clearance is approximately 10 L/h.

   *Special populations* –
      *Age and race*: At steady state, elderly subjects had increases in $C_{max}$ (22%) and AUC (45%) compared with younger subjects. At steady state, $C_{max}$ was 19% lower and AUC was 26% lower in blacks.

### Contraindications

All patients with the following conditions: Serum potassium greater than 5.5 mEq/L at initiation; Ccr 30 mL/min or less; concomitant use with the following potent CYP3A4 inhibitors: Ketoconazole, itraconazole, nefazodone, troleandomycin, clarithromycin, ritonavir, and nelfinavir.

Also contraindicated for the treatment of hypertension in patients with the following conditions: Type 2 diabetes with microalbuminuria; serum creatinine greater than 2 mg/dL in males or greater than 1.8 mg/dL in females; Ccr less than 50 mL/min; concomitant use of potassium supplements or potassium-sparing diuretics (amiloride, spironolactone, or triamterene).

### Warnings

*Hyperkalemia:* The principal risk of eplerenone is hyperkalemia. Hyperkalemia can cause serious, sometimes fatal arrhythmias. This risk can be minimized by patient selection, avoidance of certain concomitant treatments, dose reduction of eplerenone, and monitoring. The rates of hyperkalemia increase with declining renal function. Treat patients with CHF post-MI who have serum creatinine levels greater than 2 mg/dL (males) or greater than 1.8 mg/dL (females), patients who have Ccr 50 mL/min or less, and diabetic patients with CHF post-MI, including those with proteinuria, with caution.

*Renal function impairment:* No correlation was observed between plasma clearance of eplerenone and creatinine clearance. Eplerenone is not removed by hemodialysis.

*Hepatic function impairment:* In 16 subjects with mild to moderate hepatic impairment who received 400 mg of eplerenone, no elevations of serum potassium above 5.5 mEq/L were observed. The mean increase in serum potassium was 0.12 mEq/L in patients with hepatic impairment and 0.13 mEq/L in normal controls. The use of eplerenone in patients with severe hepatic impairment has not been evaluated.

*Pregnancy: Category B.*

*Lactation:* The concentration of eplerenone in human breast milk after oral administration is unknown.

*Children:* Safety and efficacy have not been established in pediatric patients.

### Drug Interactions

Drugs that may affect eplerenone include ACE inhibitors, angiotensin II antagonists, CYP3A4 inhibitors, NSAIDs, and St. John's wort. Drugs that may be affected by eplerenone include lithium.

### Adverse Reactions

Adverse reactions occurring in at least 3% of patients include hyperkalemia and dizziness, increased creatinine (more than 0.5 mg/dL).

# ANTIHYPERLIPIDEMIC AGENTS

Lowering cholesterol levels can arrest or reverse atherosclerosis in all vascular beds and can significantly decrease the morbidity and mortality associated with atherosclerosis. Each 10% reduction in cholesterol levels is associated with an approximately 20% to 30% reduction in the incidence of coronary heart disease. Hyperlipidemia, particularly elevated serum cholesterol and low density lipoprotein (LDL) levels, is a risk factor in the development of atherosclerotic cardiovascular disease.

Treatment of hyperlipidemia is based on the assumption that lowering serum lipids decreases morbidity and mortality of atherosclerotic cardiovascular disease.

The cornerstone of treatment in primary hyperlipidemia is diet restriction and weight reduction. Limit or eliminate alcohol intake. Use drug therapy in conjunction with diet, and after maximal efforts to control serum lipids by diet alone prove unsatisfactory, when tolerance to or compliance with diet is poor or when hyperlipidemia is severe and risk of complications is high. Treat contributory diseases such as hypothyroidism or diabetes mellitus.

Positive risk factors for CHD (other than high LDL) include: Age (men 45 years of age or older; women 55 years of age or older or women who go through premature menopause without estrogen replacement therapy); family history of premature CHD; smoking; hypertension (greater than 140/90 mm Hg); low HDL cholesterol (less than 35 mg/dL); obesity (more than 30% overweight); and diabetes mellitus. Physical inactivity is not listed but should also be considered.

Negative risk factors include: High HDL cholesterol (60 mg/dL or more); subtract one risk factor if the patient's HDL is at this level.

All Americans (except children younger than 2 years of age) should adopt a diet that reduces total dietary fat, decreases intake of saturated fat, increases intake of polyunsaturated fat, and reduces daily cholesterol intake to no more than 250 to 300 mg.

The following treatments guidelines are provided by the National Cholesterol Education Program Expert Panel on Detection, Evaluation and Treatment of High Blood Cholesterol in Adults 20 years of age and older.

| Classification of Total and HDL Cholesterol Levels | |
| --- | --- |
| Level (mg/dL) | Classification |
| < 200 (5.2 mmol/L) | desirable |
| 200 to 239 (5.2 to 6.2 mmol/L) | borderline-high |
| ≥ 240 (6.2 mmol/L) | high |
| HDL < 35 (0.9 mmol/L) | low |

1.) Total blood cholesterol less than 200 mg/dL: HDL 35 mg/dL or more, repeat total cholesterol and HDL measurements within 5 years or with physical exam; provide education on general population eating pattern, physical activity, and risk factor education. HDL less than 35 mg/dL, do lipoprotein analysis; base further action on LDL levels.

2.) Total blood cholesterol 200 to 239 mg/dL: HDL 35 mg/dL or more and less than 2 risk factors, provide information on dietary modification, physical activity, and risk factor reduction; reevaluate in 1 to 2 years, repeat total and HDL cholesterol measurements, and reinforce nutrition and physical activity education. HDL less than 35 mg/dL or at least 2 risk factors, analyze lipoprotein; base further action on LDL levels.

3.) Total blood cholesterol 240 mg/dL or more: Analyze lipoprotein; base further action on LDL levels.

| Classification of LDL- Cholesterol Levels | |
| --- | --- |
| Level (mg/dL) | Classification |
| < 130 (3.4 mmol/L) | desirable |
| 130 to 159 (3.4 to 4.1 mmol/L) | borderline-high |
| ≥ 160 (4.1 mmol/L) | high |

4.) LDL 160 mg/dL or more without CHD and with less than 2 risk factors: Dietary treatment.
5.) LDL 130 mg/dL or more without CHD and with at least 2 risk factors: Dietary treatment.
6.) LDL 190 mg/dL or more without CHD and with less than 2 other risk factors, or LDL 160 mg/dL or more without CHD and with at least 2 other risk factors: Drug treatment.

Elevations and treatment associated with each type of hyperlipidemia follow:

**Hyperlipidemias and Their Treatment[1]**

| | Hyperlipidemia type | | | | | |
|---|---|---|---|---|---|---|
| | I | IIa | IIb | III | IV | V |
| **Lipids** | | | | | | |
| Cholesterol | N-⇧ | ↑ | ↑ | N-↑ | N-⇧ | N-↑ |
| Triglycerides | ↑ | N | ↑ | N-↑ | ↑ | ↑ |
| **Lipoproteins** | | | | | | |
| Chylomicrons | ↑ | N | N | N | N | ↑ |
| VLDL (pre-β) | N-⇧ | N-↓ | ↑ | N-⇧ | ↑ | ↑ |
| ILDL (broad-β)[2] | | | | ↑ | | |
| LDL (β) | ↓ | ↑ | ↑ | ↑ | N-⇩ | ↓ |
| HDL (α) | ↓ | N | N | N | N-⇩ | ↓ |
| **Treatment** | Diet | Diet<br>Bile acid sequestrants<br>Dextrothyroxine<br>Nicotinic acid<br>Probucol<br>HMG-CoA reductase inhibitors | Diet<br>Bile acid sequestrants[3]<br>Clofibrate[4]<br>Gemfibrozil[5]<br>Nicotinic acid<br>HMG-CoA reductase inhibitors | Diet<br>Clofibrate<br>Gemfibrozil<br>Nicotinic acid | Diet<br>Clofibrate<br>Gemfibrozil<br>Nicotinic acid<br>Fenofibrate | Diet<br>Clofibrate<br>Gemfibrozil<br>Nicotinic acid<br>Fenofibrate |

[1] N = normal  ↑ = increase  ↓ = decrease  ⇧ = slight increase  ⇩ = slight decrease
[2] An abnormal lipoprotein.
[3] Particularly useful if hypercholesterolemia predominates.
[4] With high serum triglyceride levels and moderately elevated cholesterol.
[5] In patients with inadequate response to weight loss, bile acid sequestrants, and nicotinic acid.

**Antihyperlipidemic Drug Effects[1]**

| | Lipids | | Lipoproteins | | |
|---|---|---|---|---|---|
| Drug | Cholesterol | Triglycerides | VLDL (pre-β) | LDL (β) | HDL |
| Atorvastatin | ↓ | ↓ | ↓ | ↓ | ↑ |
| Cerivastatin | ↓ | ↓ | ↓ | ↓ | ↑ |
| Cholestyramine | ↓ | →↑ | →↑ | ↓ | →↑ |
| Clofibrate[2] | ↓ | ↓ | ↓ | →↓ | →↑ |
| Colestipol | ↓ | →↑ | ↑ | ↓ | →↑ |
| Dextrothyroxine[2] | ↓ | → | → | ↓ | → |
| Fenofibrate | ↓ | ↓ | ↓ | ↑ | ↑ |
| Fluvastatin | ↓ | ↓ | ↓ | ↓ | ↑ |
| Gemfibrozil | ↓ | ↓ | ↓ | →↓ | ↑ |
| Lovastatin | ↓ | ↓ | ↓ | ↓ | ↑ |
| Nicotinic Acid | ↓ | ↓ | ↓ | ↓ | ↑ |
| Pravastatin | ↓ | ↓ | ↓ | ↓ | ↑ |
| Simvastatin | ↓ | ↓ | ↓ | ↓ | ↑ |

[1] ↓ = decrease  ↑ = increase  → = unchanged.
[2] These agents are no longer commonly used as antihyperlipidemics.

# BILE ACID SEQUESTRANTS

## CHOLESTYRAMINE

| | |
|---|---|
| **Powder**: 4 g anhydrous cholestyramine resin/9 g powder (*Rx*) | Various, *LoCHOLEST* (Warner Chilcott), *Questran* (Bristol-Myers Squibb) |
| 4 g anhydrous cholestyramine resin/dose (*Rx*) | Various, *Cholestyramine Light* (Eon, Novopharm) |
| 4 g anhydrous cholestyramine resin/5.7 g powder (*Rx*) | *LoCHOLEST Light* (Warner Chilcott) |
| 4 g anhydrous cholestyramine resin/5.5 g powder (*Rx*) | *Prevalite* (Upsher Smith) |
| 4 g anhydrous cholestyramine resin/6.4 g powder (*Rx*) | *Questran Light* (Bristol-Myers Squibb) |

## COLESEVELAM HCl

| | |
|---|---|
| **Tablets**: 625 mg (*Rx*) | *Welchol* (Sankyo Parke Davis) |

## COLESTIPOL HCl

| | |
|---|---|
| **Tablets**: 1 g (*Rx*) | *Colestid* (Pharmacia) |
| **Granules**: 5 g colestipol HCl/dose, 5 g colestipol HCl/7.5 g powder (*Rx*) | |

### Indications

*Hyperlipoproteinemia:* Adjunctive therapy for the reduction of elevated serum cholesterol in patients with primary hypercholesterolemia (elevated LDL) who do not respond adequately to diet.

*Biliary obstruction (cholestyramine only):* Relief of pruritus associated with partial biliary obstruction.

### Administration and Dosage

Although generally given 3 to 4 times daily, there appears to be no advantage to dosing more frequently than twice daily.

CHOLESTYRAMINE:

> Powder –

> > *Adults:* 4 g 1 to 2 times daily.

> > *Maintenance dose:* 8 to 16 g/day divided into 2 doses. Use gradual increases in dose with periodic assessment of lipid/lipoprotein levels at intervals of at least 4 weeks. Maximum recommended daily dose is 24 g.

> > Suggested time of administration is at mealtime but may be modified to avoid interference with absorption of other medications. Although the recommended dosing schedule is twice daily, it may be given in 1 to 6 doses per day.

> > *Preparation:* Mix the contents of 1 powder packet or 1 level scoopful with 60 to 180 mL (2 to 6 fl oz) water or noncarbonated beverage. Do not take in dry form. Always mix with water or other fluids, highly fluid soups, or pulpy fruits, such as applesauce or crushed pineapple.

COLESEVELAM: Take with liquid.

> *Monotherapy* – The recommended starting dose is 3 tablets taken twice daily with meals or 6 tablets once daily with a meal. The dose can be increased to 7 tablets depending on desired therapeutic effect.

> *Combination therapy* – For maximal therapeutic effect in combination with an HMG-CoA reductase inhibitor, the recommended dose of colesevelam is 3 tablets taken twice daily with meals or 6 tablets taken once daily with a meal. Doses of 4 to 6 tablets/day have been shown to be safe and effective when coadministered with an HMG-CoA reductase inhibitor or when the 2 drugs are dosed apart.

COLESTIPOL HCl:

> Granules –

> > *Adults:* 5 to 30 g colestipol per day given once or in divided doses. The starting dose should be 5 g once or twice daily with a daily increment of 5 g at 1- or 2-month intervals.

> > *Preparation:* Mix in liquids, soups, cereals, or pulpy fruits. Do not take dry. Add the prescribed amount to a glassful (at least 90 mL) of liquid; stir until completely mixed. Colestipol will not dissolve. May also mix with carbonated beverages slowly stirred in a large glass. Rinse glass with a small amount of additional beverage to ensure that all the medication is taken.

*Tablets* – 2 to 16 g/day given once or in divided doses. The starting dose should be 2 g once or twice daily. Dosage increases of 2 g, once or twice daily, should occur at 1 or 2 month intervals.

Swallow tablets whole; do not cut, chew, or crush.

## Actions

*Pharmacology:* Bile acid sequestering resins bind bile acids in the intestine to form an insoluble complex, which is excreted in the feces. This results in a partial removal of bile acids from the enterohepatic circulation, preventing their absorption. The lipid-lowering effect of 4 g cholestyramine equals 5 g colestipol.

## Contraindications

Hypersensitivity to bile acid sequestering resins or any components of the products; complete biliary obstruction.

## Warnings

*Powder:* To avoid accidental inhalation or esophageal distress, do not take powder or granules dry. Mix with fluids.

*Pregnancy:* These agents are not absorbed systemically and are not expected to cause fetal harm when given during pregnancy in recommended doses.

*Lactation:* Exercise caution when administering to a nursing woman. The possible lack of proper vitamin absorption may have an effect on nursing infants.

*Children:* Dosage schedules have not been established.

## Precautions

*Malabsorption:* Because they sequester bile acids, these resins may interfere with normal fat absorption and digestion and may prevent absorption of fat-soluble vitamins such as A, D, E, and K.

Chronic use of resins may be associated with increased bleeding tendency due to hypoprothrombinemia associated with vitamin K deficiency.

*Reduced folate:* Reduction of serum or red cell folate has been reported over long-term administration of cholestyramine. Consider supplementation with folic acid.

*Hyperchloremic acidosis:* Prolonged use may cause hyperchloremic acidosis, especially in younger and smaller patients where relative dosage may be higher.

*Constipation:* These agents may produce or severely worsen preexisting constipation. Fecal impaction may occur and hemorrhoids may be aggravated.

## Drug Interactions

These resins may delay or reduce the absorption of concomitant oral medication by binding the drugs in the gut. Take other drugs at least 1 hour before or 4 to 6 hours after these agents.

Drugs that may be affected by bile acid sequestrants include anticoagulants, aspirin, clindamycin, clofibrate, diclofenac, digitalis glycosides, furosemide, gemfibrozil, glipizide, hydrocortisone, imipramine, iopanoic acid, methyldopa, mycophenolate, nicotinic acid (niacin), penicillin G, phenytoin, phosphate supplements, piroxicam, propranolol, tetracyclines, thiazide diuretics, thyroid hormones, tolbutamide, ursodiol, and vitamins A, D, E, and K.

## Adverse Reactions

*GI:*

*Most common* – Constipation; infection; flatulence.

*Less frequent* – Abdominal pain/distention/cramping; GI bleeding; belching; bloating; nausea; vomiting; diarrhea; loose stools; indigestion; dyspepsia; heartburn; anorexia; steatorrhea; rhinitis; pharyngitis.

*Miscellaneous:* Transient and modest elevations of AST, ALT, and alkaline phosphatase (colestipol); liver function abnormalities (cholestyramine); pain, flu syndrome, accidental injury, asthenia (colesevelam); headache (including migraine and sinus); anxiety; vertigo; dizziness; light-headedness; insomnia; fatigue; tinnitus; syncope; drowsiness; urticaria; dermatitis; asthma; wheezing; rash; backache; muscle/joint pains; hematuria; dysuria; burnt odor to urine; diuresis; uveitis; anorexia; weight loss/ gain; increased libido; swollen glands; edema; weakness; shortness of breath; swelling of hands/feet.

# HMG-CoA REDUCTASE INHIBITORS

| | |
|---|---|
| **ATORVASTATIN CALCIUM** | |
| **Tablets**: 10, 20, 40, and 80 mg (as base) (*Rx*) | *Lipitor* (Pfizer) |
| **FLUVASTATIN** | |
| **Capsules**: 20 and 40 mg (as base) (*Rx*) | *Lescol* (Novartis) |
| **Tablets, extended-release**: 80 mg (as base) (*Rx*) | *Lescol XL* (Novartis) |
| **LOVASTATIN** | |
| **Tablets**: 10, 20, and 40 mg (*Rx*) | Various, *Mevacor* (Merck) |
| **Tablets, extended-release**: 10, 20, 40, and 60 mg (*Rx*) | *Altocor* (Andrx) |
| **PRAVASTATIN SODIUM** | |
| **Tablets**: 10, 20, 40, and 80 mg (*Rx*) | *Pravachol* (Bristol-Myers Squibb) |
| **ROSUVASTATIN CALCIUM** | |
| **Tablets**: 5, 10, 20, and 40 mg (*Rx*) | *Crestor* (AstraZeneca) |
| **SIMVASTATIN** | |
| **Tablets**: 5, 10, 20, 40, and 80 mg (*Rx*) | *Zocor* (Merck) |

### Indications

*Antihyperlipidemics:* Use HMG-CoA reductase inhibitors in addition to a diet restricted in saturated fat and cholesterol when diet and other nonpharmacological therapies alone have produced inadequate responses. Refer to individual product monographs.

| HMG-CoA Reductase Inhibitor Indications | | | | | | |
|---|---|---|---|---|---|---|
| Indication | Atorvastatin | Fluvastatin | Lovastatin | Pravastatin | Rosuvastatin | Simvastatin |
| Primary hyper-cholesterolemia | ✔[1] | ✔[1] | ✔[1,5] | ✔[1] | ✔[1] | ✔[1] |
| Mixed dyslipidemia | ✔[2] | ✔[2] | | ✔[2] | ✔[2] | ✔[2] |
| Hypertriglyceridemia | ✔[3] | | | ✔[3] | ✔[3] | ✔[3] |
| Primary dysbetalipo-proteinemia | ✔[4] | | | ✔[4] | | ✔[4] |
| Homozygous familial hyperlipidemia | ✔ | | | | ✔ | ✔ |
| Primary prevention coronary events | ✔ | | ✔ | ✔ | | |
| Secondary prevention cardiovascular event(s) | ✔ | ✔ | ✔ | ✔ | | ✔ |
| Heterozygous familial hypercholesterolemia in adolescents | ✔ | | ✔[5,6] | ✔ | | ✔ |
| Hyperlipidemia | | | ✔[7] | | | |

[1] Includes heterozygous familial and nonfamilial hypercholesterolemia.
[2] Includes Fredrickson types IIa and IIb.
[3] Includes Fredrickson type IV.
[4] Includes Fredrickson type III.
[5] Immediate-release only.
[6] Adolescents 10 to 17 years of age.
[7] Extended-release only.

### Administration and Dosage

Place the patient on a standard cholesterol-lowering diet before receiving HMG-CoA reductase inhibitors, and continue on this diet during treatment.

ATORVASTATIN CALCIUM:

*Hypercholesterolemia (heterozygous familial and nonfamilial), mixed dyslipidemia (Fredrickson type IIa and IIb), and prevention of cardiovascular disease* – The recommended starting dose is 10 to 20 mg once/day. Patients who require a large reduction in LDL cholesterol (more than 45%) may be started at 40 mg once/day. Dosage range is 10 to 80 mg once/day, at any time of the day, with or without food. Individualize therapy according to goal of therapy and response. After initiation and/or upon titration of atorvastatin, analyze lipid levels within 2 to 4 weeks and adjust dosing accordingly. Because the goal of treatment is to decrease LDL cholesterol, the NCEP recommends that LDL cholesterol levels be used to initiate and assess treatment response. Use total cholesterol to monitor therapy only if LDL cholesterol levels are not available.

*Heterozygous familial hypercholesterolemia in pediatric patients 10 to 17 years of age* – Recommended starting dose is 10 mg/day; the maximum recommended dose is 20 mg/day. Individualize doses according to recommended goal of therapy. Make adjustments at intervals of 4 weeks or more.

*Homozygous familial hypercholesterolemia* – 10 to 80 mg/day. Use atorvastatin as an adjunct to other lipid-lowering treatments (eg, LDL apheresis) in these patients or if such treatments are unavailable.

*Concomitant lipid-lowering therapy* – Atorvastatin may be used in combination with a bile-acid-binding resin for additive effect. Generally, avoid the combination of HMG-CoA reductase inhibitors and fibrates.

FLUVASTATIN:

*Dose* – For patients requiring LDL cholesterol reduction to a goal of 25% or more, the recommended starting dose is 40 mg as 1 capsule, 80 mg as 1 tablet administered as a single dose in the evening, or 80 mg in divided doses of the 40 mg capsule given twice daily. For patients requiring LDL cholesterol reduction to a goal of less than 25%, a starting dose of 20 mg may be used. The recommended dosing range is 20 to 80 mg/day. Because the maximal reductions in LDL cholesterol of a given dose are seen within 4 weeks, perform periodic lipid determinations and adjust dosage according to the patient's response to therapy and established treatment guidelines. The therapeutic effect of fluvastatin is maintained with prolonged administration.

*Concomitant lipid-lowering therapy* – When administering a bile acid resin and fluvastatin, administer fluvastatin at bedtime, at least 2 hours following the resin.

*Renal function impairment* – Dose adjustments for mild to moderate renal impairment are not necessary. Fluvastatin has not been studied at doses greater than 40 mg in patients with severe renal impairment; exercise caution when treating such patients at higher doses.

LOVASTATIN: Give immediate-release tablets once/day with evening meal and give extended-release tablets once/day in evening at bedtime.

*Adults* –

*Immediate-release:* Usual recommended starting dose is 20 mg once/day with the evening meal. Recommended dosage range is 10 to 80 mg/day in a single or 2 divided doses. Individualize dose according to the recommended goal of therapy. Start patients requiring reductions in LDL cholesterol of 20% or more on 20 mg/day. Consider a starting dose of 10 mg for patients requiring smaller reductions. Adjust at intervals of 4 weeks or more. Maximum dose is 80 mg/day.

*Extended-release:* Usual recommended starting dose is 20, 40, or 60 mg once/day given in the evening at bedtime. The recommended dosing range is 10 to 60 mg/day in single doses. A starting dose of 10 mg may be considered for patients requiring smaller reductions. Adjust at intervals of 4 weeks or more. Swallow whole; do not chew or crush.

*Adolescents 10 to 17 years of age with heterozygous familial hypercholesterolemia (immediate-release only)* – The recommended dosing range is 10 to 40 mg/day; the maximum recommended dose is 40 mg/day. Start patients requiring reductions in LDL cholesterol of 20% or more on 20 mg/day. Consider a starting dose of 10 mg for patients requiring smaller reductions. Adjust at intervals of 4 weeks or more.

*Concomitant lipid-lowering therapy* – Generally avoid use of lovastatin with fibrates or niacin. If lovastatin is used in combination with gemfibrozil, other fibrates, or lipid-lowering doses (1 g/day or more) of niacin, the dose of lovastatin should not exceed 20 mg/day.

*Concomitant cyclosporine* – Initiate lovastatin at 10 mg/day in patients taking cyclosporine. Maximum dose is 20 mg/day.

*Concomitant amiodarone or verapamil (immediate-release only)* – In patients taking amiodarone or verapamil concomitantly with lovastatin, the dose should not exceed 40 mg/day.

*Renal function impairment* – In patients with severe renal insufficiency (Ccr less than 30 mL/min), carefully consider dosage increases above 20 mg/day.

PRAVASTATIN SODIUM: Pravastatin can be administered as a single dose at any time of the day, with or without food. Because the maximal effect of a given dose is seen within 4 weeks, perform periodic lipid determinations at this time and adjust dosage according to the patient's response to therapy and established treatment guidelines.

*Adults* – The recommended starting dose is 40 mg once/day. If a daily dose of 40 mg does not achieve desired cholesterol levels, 80 mg once/day is recommended.

*Pediatric patients* –

*Children 8 to 13 years of age (inclusive):* The recommended dose is 20 mg once daily. Doses greater than 20 mg have not been studied in this patient population.

*Adolescents 14 to 18 years of age:* The recommended starting dose is 40 mg once daily. Doses greater than 40 mg have not been studied in this patient population.

Reevaluate children and adolescents treated with pravastatin in adulthood and make appropriate changes to their cholesterol-lowering regimen to achieve adult goals for LDL-C.

*Concomitant immunosuppressants* – In patients taking immunosuppressive drugs such as cyclosporine concomitantly with pravastatin, begin therapy with pravastatin 10 mg once/day at bedtime and titrate to higher doses with caution. Most patients treated with this combination received a maximum pravastatin dose of 20 mg/day.

*Concomitant lipid-lowering therapy* – The lipid-lowering effects of pravastatin on total and LDL cholesterol are enhanced when combined with a bile acid binding resin. When administering a bile acid binding resin (eg, cholestyramine, colestipol) and pravastatin, give pravastatin either 1 hour or more before or at least 4 hours following the resin.

*Renal/Hepatic function impairment* – Use a starting dose of 10 mg/day in significant renal or hepatic function impairment.

ROSUVASTATIN CALCIUM:

*Hypercholesterolemia (heterozygous familial and nonfamilial) and mixed dyslipidemia (Fredrickson type IIa and IIb)* – The dose range for rosuvastatin is 5 to 40 mg once daily. Individualize rosuvastatin therapy according to goal of therapy and response. The usual recommended starting dose of rosuvastatin is 10 mg once daily. Initiation of therapy with 5 mg once daily may be considered for patients requiring less aggressive LDL-C reductions or who have predisposing factors for myopathy. For patients with marked hypercholesterolemia (LDL-C greater than 190 mg/dL) and aggressive lipid targets, consider a 20 mg starting dose. Reserve the 40 mg dose of rosuvastatin for those patients who have not achieved goal LDL-C at 20 mg. After initiation or upon titration of rosuvastatin, analyze lipid levels within 2 to 4 weeks and adjust dosage accordingly.

*Homozygous FH* – The recommended starting dose of rosuvastatin is 20 mg once daily in patients with homozygous FH. The maximum recommended daily dose is 40 mg. Rosuvastatin should be used in these patients as an adjunct to other lipid-lowering treatments (eg, LDL apheresis) or if such treatments are unavailable. Estimate response to therapy from pre-apheresis LDL-C levels.

*Dosage in patients taking cyclosporine* – In patients taking cyclosporine, limit therapy to rosuvastatin 5 mg once daily.

*Concomitant lipid-lowering therapy* – The effect of rosuvastatin on LDL-C and total-C may be enhanced when used in combination with a bile acid-binding resin. If rosuvastatin is used in combination with gemfibrozil, limit the dose of rosuvastatin to 10 mg once daily.

*Renal insufficiency* – No modification of dosage is necessary for patients with mild to moderate renal insufficiency. For patients with severe renal impairment (Ccr less than 30 mL/min/1.73 m$^2$) not on hemodialysis, start dosing at 5 mg once daily. Do not exceed 10 mg once daily.

SIMVASTATIN:

*Dose* – The recommended usual starting dose is 20 to 40 mg once/day in the evening. Patients who require a large reduction in LDL cholesterol (more than 45%) may be started at 40 mg/day in the evening. Dosage range is 5 to 80 mg/day. Individualize dosage according to baseline LDL cholesterol level, the recommended goal of therapy, and patient response. Adjust dose at intervals of 4 weeks or more.

*Homozygous familial hypercholesterolemia* – The recommended dosage is 40 mg/day in the evening or 80 mg/day in 3 divided doses of 20 mg, 20 mg, and an evening dose of 40 mg. Use simvastatin as an adjunct to other lipid-lowering treatments (eg, LDL apheresis) in these patients or if such treatments are unavailable.

*Adolescents 10 to 17 years of age with heterozygous familial hypercholesterolemia* – Usual recommended starting dose is 10 mg once a day in the evening. The recommended dosing range is 10 to 40 mg/day; maximum dose is 40 mg/day. Individualize dose according to recommended goal of therapy. Adjust at intervals of 4 weeks or more.

*Concomitant cyclosporine* – In patients taking cyclosporine concomitantly with simvastatin, begin therapy with 5 mg/day; do not exceed 10 mg/day.

*Concomitant amiodarone or verapamil* – In patients taking amiodarone or verapamil concomitantly with simvastatin, the dose should not exceed 20 mg/day.

*Concomitant lipid-lowering therapy* – Simvastatin is effective alone or when used concomitantly with bile acid sequestrants. The combined use of simvastatin with gemfibrozil, other fibrates, or lipid-lowering doses (1 g/day or more) of niacin should be avoided unless the benefit of further alteration in lipid levels is likely to outweigh the increased risk of this drug combination. However, if simvastatin is used in combination with fibrates or niacin, the dose of simvastatin generally should not exceed 10 mg/day.

*Renal function impairment* – Exercise caution when simvastatin is administered to patients with severe renal insufficiency. Initiate therapy in such patients with 5 mg/day and monitor closely.

## Actions

*Pharmacology:* These agents specifically competitively inhibit 3-hydroxy-3-methylglutaryl-coenzyme A (HMG-CoA) reductase, the enzyme which catalyzes the early rate-limiting step in cholesterol biosynthesis, conversion of HMG-CoA to mevalonate.

*Pharmacokinetics:*

| Pharmacokinetics of HMG-CoA Reductase Inhibitors | | | | | | |
|---|---|---|---|---|---|---|
| | Bioavailability | Excretion | t½ (h) | Major metabolites | Protein binding | Effects of renal/hepatic impairment |
| Atorvastatin | ≈ 14% absolute bioavailability; first-pass metabolism (CYP3A4) | < 2% (urine) | ≈ 14[1] | Metabolized to ortho- and parahydroxylated derivatives (active) | ≥ 98% | Plasma levels not affected by renal disease; markedly increased with chronic alcoholic liver disease. |

| Pharmacokinetics of HMG-CoA Reductase Inhibitors | | | | | | |
| --- | --- | --- | --- | --- | --- | --- |
| | Bioavailability | Excretion | t½ (h) | Major metabolites | Protein binding | Effects of renal/hepatic impairment |
| Fluvastatin | 98% absorbed; absolute bioavailability 24%; extensive first-pass metabolism (CYP2C9); mean relative bioavailability is ≈ 29% for XR compared with IR | ≈ 5% (urine) ≈ 90% (feces) | < 3 (IR) ≈ 9 (XR) | Hydroxylated metabolites (active, do not circulate systemically) | 98% | Potential drug accumulation with hepatic insufficiency. |
| Lovastatin | ≈ 30% absorbed; extensive first-pass metabolism (CYP3A4); < 5% of oral dose reaches general circulation as active inhibitors; bioavailability for XR was 190% compared with IR | 10% (urine) 83% (feces) | 3-4 | Beta-hydroxyacid; 6'-hydroxyderivative; 2 additional metabolites | > 95% | Increased plasma concentration with severe renal disease. |
| Pravastatin | 34% absorbed; absolute bioavailability 17%; extensive first-pass metabolism; plasma levels may not correlate with efficacy | ≈ 20% (urine) 70% (feces) | 77 | Major degradation product: 3α-hydroxy isomeric metabolite | ≈ 50% | Potential drug accumulation with renal or hepatic insufficiency. Mean AUC varied 18-fold in cirrhotic patients and peak values varied 47-fold. |
| Rosuvastatin | absolute bioavailability ≈ 20%; not extensively metabolized (≈ 10%; CYP2C9) | 90% (feces) | 19 | N-desmethyl rosuvastatin (≈ ⅙ to ½ activity of parent) | 88% | Increased plasma concentrations with severe renal impairment and hepatic disease. |
| Simvastatin | ≈ 85% absorbed; extensive first-pass metabolism (CYP3A4); < 5% of oral dose reaches general circulation | 13% (urine) 60% (feces) | — | Beta-hydroxyacid; 6'-hydroxy, 6'-hydroxymethyl, 6'-exomethylene derivatives | ≈ 95% | Higher systemic exposure may occur in hepatic and severe renal insufficiency. |

[1] For unmetabolized atorvastatin only. The t½ is 20 to 30 hours for the active metabolites.

## Contraindications

Hypersensitivity to any component of these products; active liver disease or unexplained persistent elevated liver function tests; pregnancy; lactation.

## Warnings

*Liver dysfunction:* Use with caution in patients who consume substantial quantities of alcohol or who have a history of liver disease.

**Pravastatin** and **fluvastatin** plasma clearance is decreased but no dose adjustment is needed.

*Skeletal muscle effects:* All statins have been associated with myalgia, myopathy (ie, muscle pain, tenderness, or weakness with creatine phosphokinase [CPK] values above 10 times the ULN), and rhabdomyolysis. Factors that may predispose patients to myopathy with HMG-CoA reductase inhibitors include advanced age (65 years of age or older), hypothyroidism, and renal insufficiency. The risk of myopathy/rhabdomyolysis is dose-related and also increases when statins are given concomitantly with other drugs that inhibit their metabolism (eg, cyclosporine, erythromycin, or azole antifungals) or other drugs that can cause myopathy when given alone (eg, fibrates or lipid-lowering doses of niacin).

Consider myopathy in any patient with diffuse myalgias, muscle tenderness or weakness, or marked elevation of CPK. Advise patients to report promptly muscle pain, tenderness or weakness, particularly with malaise or fever. Discontinue the drug if markedly elevated CPK levels occur or if myopathy is diagnosed or suspected.

*Endocrine effects:* Statins interfere with cholesterol synthesis and lower circulating cholesterol levels and, as such, might theoretically blunt adrenal or gonadal steroid hormone production. Small declines in total testosterone with no commensurate elevation in LH have been noted with the use of **fluvastatin**. **Pravastatin** showed inconsistent results with regard to possible effects on basal steroid hormone levels; **atorvastatin, lovastatin, rosuvastatin,** and **simvastatin** did not reduce basal plasma cortisol concentration or basal plasma testosterone concentration or impair adrenal reserve. Appropriately evaluate patients who display clinical evidence of endocrine dysfunction. Exercise caution when administering HMG-CoA reductase inhibitors with drugs that affect steroid levels or activity, such as ketoconazole, spironolactone, and cimetidine.

*Hyperlipidemia, secondary causes:* Prior to initiating therapy, exclude secondary causes of hyperlipidemia (eg, poorly controlled diabetes mellitus, hypothyroidism, nephrotic syndrome, dysproteinemias, obstructive liver disease, other drug therapy, alcoholism) and measure total-C, HDL-C, and triglycerides.

*Hypersensitivity reactions:* An apparent hypersensitivity syndrome has occurred. Refer to Management of Acute Hypersensitivity Reactions.

*Renal function impairment:* Closely monitor patients with renal impairment. Higher systemic exposure of **simvastatin** may occur in severe renal insufficiency. Plasma concentrations after a single dose of **lovastatin** were approximately 2-fold higher in patients with severe renal insufficiency. Plasma concentrations of **rosuvastatin** increased to a clinically significant extent (about 3-fold) in patients with severe renal impairment.

*Hepatic function impairment:* Marked persistent increases (greater than 3 times ULN) in serum transaminases occurred in patients treated with all agents ranging in frequency from less than 1% to 1.9%. When the drug was interrupted or discontinued or the dosage was reduced, transaminase levels usually fell slowly to pretreatment levels.

*Elderly:* In patients older than 70 years of age, the AUC of **lovastatin, pravastatin,** and **simvastatin** is increased. **Pravastatin** does not need dosage adjustment. The safety and efficacy of **atorvastatin, rosuvastatin,** and **lovastatin** extended-release in patients 70 years of age and older were similar to those of patients younger than 70 years of age. Elderly patients (65 years of age and older) demonstrated a greater treatment response in respect to LDL-C, total-C and LDL/HDL ratio than patients younger than 65 years of age.

*Pregnancy: Category X.*

*Lactation:* **Lovastatin** and **atorvastatin** are excreted in the milk of rats; atorvastatin is likely to be excreted in breast milk; it is not known whether **lovastatin, rosuvastatin,** and **simvastatin** are excreted in breast milk; a small amount of **pravastatin** is excreted in breast milk; **fluvastatin** is present in breast milk in a 2:1 ratio (milk:plasma).

*Children:* **Atorvastatin, simvastatin,** and **lovastatin** are indicated for treatment of patients 10 to 17 years of age with heterozygous familial hypercholesterolemia. **Pravastatin** is indicated for the treatment of patients 8 to 18 years of age with heterozygous familial hypercholesterolemia. Safety and efficacy have not been established for atorvastatin, simvastatin, and lovastatin in prepubertal patients and patients younger than 10 years of age. Safety and efficacy have not been established in patients younger than 8 years of age for pravastatin. Safety and efficacy have not been established in patients younger than 18 years of age for **fluvastatin**. Safety and efficacy of **rosuvastatin** have not been established in pediatric patients.

**Precautions**

*Monitoring:* For **lovastatin**, perform LFTs before initiating therapy, at 6 and 12 weeks after initiation of therapy or after dose elevation, and periodically thereafter (approximately 6-month intervals). For **rosuvastatin, fluvastatin,** and **atorvastatin,** it is recommended that LFTs be performed prior to and at 12 weeks following both the initiation of therapy and any elevation in dose, and periodically (eg, semiannually) thereafter. For **pravastatin** and **simvastatin**, perform LFTs prior to the initiation of therapy, prior to elevation of dose, and when otherwise clinically indicated. For patients titrated to the 80 mg dose of simvastatin, perform LFTs prior to titration, 3 months after titration to the 80 mg dose, and periodically thereafter (eg, semiannually) for the first year of treatment. Pay special attention to patients who develop elevated serum transaminase levels. If transaminase levels progress, particularly if they rise to 3 times the ULN and are persistent, discontinue the drug.

Because HMG-CoA reductase inhibitors may increase CPK and transaminase levels, consider this in the differential diagnosis of chest pain in patients treated with these agents.

*Diet:* Before instituting therapy, attempt to control hypercholesterolemia with diet, exercise, and weight reduction in obese patients.

*Homozygous familial hypercholesterolemia:* HMG-CoA reductase inhibitors are less effective in patients with the rare homozygous familial hypercholesterolemia, possibly because they have no functional LDL receptors.

*Ophthalmic effects:* There was a high prevalence of baseline lenticular opacities in the patient population included in the early clinical trials with **lovastatin**.

*Sleep disturbance:* **Lovastatin** and **simvastatin** may interfere with sleep, causing insomnia, whereas **pravastatin** does not appear to disturb sleep.

*Photosensitivity:* Photosensitization (photoallergy or phototoxicity) may occur.

### Drug Interactions

Drugs that may affect HMG-CoA reductase inhibitors include alcohol, amiodarone, antacids, azole antifungals, bile acid sequestrants, cimetidine, cyclosporine, diltiazem, erythromycin, gemfibrozil, isradipine, nefazodone, niacin, nicotinic acid, omeprazole, phenytoin, propranolol, protease inhibitors, ranitidine, rifampin, St. John's wort, and verapamil.

Drugs that may be affected by HMG-CoA reductase inhibitors include oral contraceptives, diclofenac, digoxin, glyburide, phenytoin, and warfarin.

**Atorvastatin**, **lovastatin**, and **simvastatin** are primarily metabolized by CYP3A4; they may interact with CYP3A4 inhibitors.

**Fluvastatin** is primarily metabolized by CYP2C9; it may interact with CYP2C9 inhibitors. Data indicate that **pravastatin** and **rosuvastatin** are not metabolized by CYP3A4 to a clinically significant extent.

### Adverse Reactions

| HMG-CoA Reductase Inhibitor Adverse Reactions (≥ 3%)[1] | | | | | | |
|---|---|---|---|---|---|---|
| Adverse reaction | Atorvastatin | Fluvastatin (n = 2326) | Lovastatin | Pravastatin (n = 900) | Rosuvastatin (n = 900) | Simvastatin (n = 1583) |
| *CNS* | | | | | | |
| Asthenia | 2.2-3.8 | ˅ | ˅ | ˅ | 2.7 | 1.6 |
| Dizziness | ≥ 2 | 2.2 | 0.7-2 | 3.3 | ≥ 2 | ˅ |
| Headache | 2.5-16.7 | 8.9 | 2.6-9.3 | 6.2 | 5.5 | 3.5 |
| *GI* | | | | | | |
| Abdominal pain/cramps | 2.1-3.8 | 4.9 | 2-5.7 | 5.4 | ≥ 2 | 3.2 |
| Constipation | 1.1-2.5 | 3.1 | 2-4.9 | 4 | ≥ 2 | 2.3 |
| Diarrhea | 2.7-5.3 | 4.9 | 2.6-5.5 | 6.2 | 3.4 | 1.9 |
| Dyspepsia | 1.3-2.8 | 7.9 | 1.3-3.9 | ˅ | 3.4 | 1.1 |
| Flatulence | 1.1-2.8 | 2.6 | 3.7-6.4 | 3.3 | ≥ 1 | 1.9 |
| Nausea/Vomiting | ≥ 2/< 2 | 3.2 | 1.9-4.7 | 7.3 | 3.4/≥ 1 | 1.3 |
| *Musculoskeletal* | | | | | | |
| Arthralgia | 2-5.1 | 4 | 0.5-1 | ˅ | ≥ 2 | ˅ |
| Arthritis | ≥ 2 | 2.1 | ˅ | ˅ | ≥ 2 | ˅ |
| Back pain | 1.1-3.8 | 5.7 | ˅ | ˅ | 2.6 | ˅ |
| Localized pain | ˅ | ˅ | 0.5-1 | 10 | ˅ | ˅ |

| | HMG-CoA Reductase Inhibitor Adverse Reactions (≥ 3%)[1] | | | | | |
|---|---|---|---|---|---|---|
| Adverse reaction | Atorvastatin | Fluvastatin (n = 2326) | Lovastatin | Pravastatin (n = 900) | Rosuvastatin (n = 900) | Simvastatin (n = 1583) |
| Myalgia | 1.3-5.6 | 5 | 2.4-2.6 | 2.7 | 2.8 | - |
| *Respiratory* | | | | | | |
| Bronchitis | ≥ 2 | - | - | - | ≥ 2 | - |
| Common cold | - | - | - | 7 | - | - |
| Pharyngitis | 1.3-2.5 | 3.8 | - | - | - | - |
| Rhinitis | ≥ 2 | 4.7 | - | 4 | 2.2 | - |
| Sinusitis | 2.5-6.4 | 2.6 | - | - | 2 | - |
| Upper respiratory tract infection | - | 16.2 | - | - | - | 2.1 |
| *Miscellaneous* | | | | | | |
| Accidental trauma | 1.3-4.2 | 5.2 | - | - | ≥ 2 | - |
| Cardiac chest pain | - | - | - | 4 | - | - |
| Chest pain | ≥ 2 | - | 0.5-1 | 3.7 | ≥ 2 | - |
| Fatigue | - | 2.7 | - | 3.8 | - | - |
| Infection | 2.8-10.3 | - | - | - | ≥ 2 | - |
| Influenza | 2.2-3.2 | 5.1 | - | 2.4 | - | - |
| Peripheral edema | ≥ 2 | - | - | - | ≥ 2 | - |
| Rash/Pruritus | 1.1-3.9/< 2 | 2.3 | 0.8 - 5.2 | 4 | ≥ 2/≥ 1 | - |

[1] All events. Data are pooled from separate studies and are not necessarily comparable.

# GEMFIBROZIL

**Tablets**: 600 mg (*Rx*)  
**Capsules**: 300 mg (*Rx*)

*Gemcor* (Upsher-Smith), *Lopid* (Parke-Davis)  
Various

## Indications

*Hypertriglyceridemia:* Hypertriglyceridemia in adult patients (Types IV and V hyperlipidemia) who present a risk of pancreatitis and who do not respond to diet. Consider therapy for those with triglyceride elevations between 1000 and 2000 mg/dL, and who have a history of pancreatitis or of recurrent abdominal pain typical of pancreatitis.

*Reducing coronary heart disease risk:* Consider gemfibrozil therapy in those Type IIb patients who have low HDL-cholesterol levels in addition to elevated LDL-cholesterol and triglycerides and who have not responded to weight loss, dietary therapy, exercise, and other pharmacologic agents.

Gemfibrozil is not useful for the hypertriglyceridemia of Type I hyperlipidemia.

## Administration and Dosage

*Adults:* 1200 mg/daily in 2 divided doses, 30 minutes before the morning and evening meals.

## Actions

*Pharmacology:* Gemfibrozil is a lipid-regulating agent that decreases serum triglycerides and very low density lipoprotein (VLDL) cholesterol, and increases high density lipoprotein (HDL) cholesterol. While modest decreases in total and low density lipoprotein (LDL) cholesterol may be observed with gemfibrozil therapy, treatment of patients with elevated triglycerides due to Type IV hyperlipoproteinemia often results in a rise in LDL-cholesterol. Gemfibrozil usually raises HDL-cholesterol significantly in Type IIb patients with elevations of both serum LDL-cholesterol and triglycerides.

*Pharmacokinetics:*

*Absorption/Distribution* – Gemfibrozil is well absorbed from the GI tract. Peak plasma levels occur in 1 to 2 hours.

*Metabolism/Excretion* – Gemfibrozil mainly undergoes oxidation to form a hydroxymethyl and a carboxyl metabolite. It has a plasma half-life of 1.5 hours following multiple doses. Biological half-life is considerably longer, as some of the drug undergoes enterohepatic circulation and is reabsorbed in the GI tract. Approximately 70% is excreted in the urine, mostly as the glucuronide conjugate.

### Contraindications

Hepatic or severe renal dysfunction, including primary biliary cirrhosis; preexisting gallbladder disease; hypersensitivity to gemfibrozil.

### Warnings

*Cholelithiasis:* If cholelithiasis is suspected, perform gallbladder studies. Discontinue therapy if gallstones are found.

*Concomitant therapy:* Concomitant therapy with gemfibrozil and lovastatin has been associated with rhabdomyolysis, markedly elevated creatine kinase (CK) levels and myoglobinuria, leading in a high proportion of cases to acute renal failure. In most subjects who have had an unsatisfactory lipid response to either drug alone, the possible benefit of combined therapy does not outweigh the risks. The use of gemfibrozil may occasionally be associated with myositis. If myositis is suspected or diagnosed, withdraw therapy.

*Renal function impairment:* There have been reports of worsening renal insufficiency upon the addition of gemfibrozil therapy in individuals with baseline plasma creatinine greater than 2 mg/dL. In such patients, consider the use of alternative therapy against the risks and benefits of a lower dose of gemfibrozil.

*Pregnancy:* Category C.

*Lactation:* Decide whether to discontinue nursing or discontinue the drug, taking into account the importance of the drug to the mother.

*Children:* Safety and efficacy in children have not been established.

### Precautions

*Estrogen therapy:* Estrogen therapy is sometimes associated with massive rises in plasma triglycerides, especially in subjects with familial hypertriglyceridemia.

*Contributory diseases:* Contributory diseases such as hypothyroidism or diabetes mellitus should be adequately treated.

*Monitoring therapy:* Perform adequate pretreatment laboratory studies. Obtain periodic determinations of serum lipids during administration. Withdraw the drug after 3 months if response is inadequate.

*Hematologic* – Mild hemoglobin, hematocrit and white blood cell decreases have been observed. Perform periodic blood counts during the first 12 months of administration.

*Liver function* – Abnormal elevations of AST, ALT, LDH, bilirubin, and alkaline phosphatase have occurred, and are usually reversible on drug discontinuation. Perform periodic liver function studies and terminate therapy if abnormalities persist.

*Blood glucose* – Gemfibrozil has a moderate hyperglycemic effect; carefully monitor blood glucose levels during therapy.

*Hazardous tasks:* May produce drowsiness (dizziness or blurred vision); patients should observe caution while driving or performing other tasks requiring alertness, coordination and physical dexterity.

### Drug Interactions

Drugs that may interact with gemfibrozil include oral anticoagulants and lovastatin.

### Adverse Reactions

Adverse reactions occurring in at least 3% of patients include dyspepsia; abdominal pain; diarrhea; fatigue.

# FENOFIBRATE

| **Tablets**: 54 and 160 mg (Rx) | _Tricor_ (Abbott) |
|---|---|

### Indications

Hypercholesterolemia: Adjunctive therapy to diet for the reduction of LDL-C, total-C, triglycerides, and apolipoprotein B (apo B) and to increase HDL-C in adult patients with primary hypercholesterolemia or mixed dyslipidemia (Fredrickson Types IIa and IIb).

### Administration and Dosage

Place patients on an appropriate lipid-lowering diet before receiving fenofibrate and continue this diet during treatment. Give with meals, thereby optimizing the bioavailability of the medication.

_Primary hypercholesterolemia/mixed hyperlipidemia:_ For the treatment of adult patients with primary hypercholesterolemia or mixed hyperlipidemia, the initial dose of fenofibrate is 160 mg/day.

_Hypertriglyceridemia:_ For adult patients with hypertriglyceridemia, the initial dose is 54 to 160 mg/day. Individualize dosage according to patient response and adjust if necessary following repeat lipid determinations at 4- to 8-week intervals. The maximum dose is 160 mg/day.

Monitor lipid levels periodically and give consideration to reducing the dosage if lipid levels fall significantly below the targeted range.

_Renal function impairment:_ Initiate treatment with fenofibrate at a dose of 54 mg/day in patients with impaired renal function, and increase only after evaluation of the effects on renal function and lipid levels at this dose.

_Elderly:_ In the elderly, limit the initial dose to 54 mg/day.

### Actions

_Pharmacology:_ Fenofibric acid, the active metabolite of fenofibrate, produces reductions in total cholesterol, LDL cholesterol, apo B, total triglycerides, and triglyceride rich lipoprotein (VLDL) in treated patients. In addition, treatment with fenofibrate results in increases in high-density lipoprotein (HDL) and apoproteins apoAI and apoAII.

_Pharmacokinetics:_

_Absorption/Distribution_ – Fenofibrate is well absorbed from the GI tract. Peak plasma levels of fenofibric acid occur within 6 to 8 hours after administration. Serum protein binding is approximately 99%.

_Metabolism_ – Fenofibrate is rapidly hydrolyzed by esterases to the active metabolite, fenofibric acid; no unchanged fenofibrate is detected in plasma. Fenofibric acid is primarily conjugated with glucuronic acid.

_Excretion_ – Fenofibrate is eliminated with a half-life of 20 hours. It is mainly excreted in urine in the form of metabolites, primarily fenofibric acid and fenofibric acid glucuronide; approximately 60% of the dose appears in urine and 25% in feces.

### Contraindications

Hepatic or severe renal dysfunction, including primary biliary cirrhosis, and patients with unexplained persistent liver function abnormality; preexisting gallbladder disease; hypersensitivity to fenofibrate.

### Warnings

_Pancreatitis:_ This has been reported in patients taking fenofibrate, gemfibrozil, and clofibrate. This occurrence may represent a failure of efficacy in patients with severe hypertriglyceridemia, a direct drug effect, or a secondary phenomenon mediated through biliary tract stone or sludge formation and obstruction of the common bile duct.

_Cholelithiasis:_ Fenofibrate, like clofibrate and gemfibrozil, may increase cholesterol excretion into the bile, leading to cholelithiasis. If cholelithiasis is suspected, gallbladder studies are indicated. Discontinue therapy if gallstones are found.

*Skeletal muscle effects:* The use of fibrates alone, including fenofibrate, may occasionally be associated with myopathy. Treatment with drugs of the fibrate class has been associated on rare occasions with rhabdomyolysis, usually in patients with impaired renal function. Consider myopathy in any patient with diffuse myalgias, muscle tenderness or weakness, or marked elevations of creatine phosphokinase levels.

*Hypersensitivity reactions:* Acute hypersensitivity reactions have occurred.

*Renal function impairment:* Minimize the dosage in patients who have Ccr less than 50 mL/min.

*Hepatic function impairment:* Fenofibrate is associated with significant increases in serum transaminases (AST or ALT). Increases to more than 3 times the upper limit of normal (ULN) occurred. Hepatocellular, chronic active and cholestatic hepatitis associated with fenofibrate therapy have been reported after exposures of weeks to several years.

*Pregnancy:* Category C.

*Lactation:* Fenofibrate should not be used in nursing mothers.

*Children:* Safety and efficacy in children have not been established.

**Precautions**

*Monitoring:* Obtain periodic determination of serum lipids during initial therapy in order to establish the lowest effective dose of fenofibrate. Withdraw therapy in patients who do not have an adequate response after 2 months of treatment with the maximum recommended dose of 160 mg/day. Also, perform liver function tests regularly.

*Initial therapy:* Ascertain that lipid levels are consistently abnormal before instituting fenofibrate therapy. Make every attempt to control serum lipids with appropriate diet, exercise, weight loss in obese patients, and control of any medical problems (eg, diabetes mellitus, hypothyroidism) that are contributing to the lipid abnormalities. If possible, discontinue or change medications known to exacerbate hypertriglyceridemia (eg, beta-blockers, thiazides, estrogens) prior to consideration of triglyceride-lowering drug therapy.

*Hematologic changes:* Mild to moderate hemoglobin, hematocrit, and white blood cell decreases have been observed in patients following initiation of fenofibrate therapy. However, these levels stabilize during long-term administration. Extremely rare spontaneous reports of thrombocytopenia and agranulocytosis have been received during postmarketing surveillance outside of the US. Periodic blood counts are recommended during the first 12 months of fenofibrate administration.

**Drug Interactions**

Drugs that may affect fenofibrate include bile acid sequestrants.

Drugs that may be affected by fenofibrate include anticoagulants, cyclosporine, and HMG-CoA reductase inhibitors.

*Drug/Food interactions:* The absorption of fenofibrate is increased by approximately 35% when administered with food.

**Adverse Reactions**

Adverse events occurring in at least 3% include abnormal liver function tests, increased ALT and AST, increased creatine phosphokinase, respiratory disorder, abdominal pain, back pain, headache.

# NIACIN

| | |
|---|---|
| **Tablets**: 500 mg (*Rx*) | *Niacor* (Upsher-Smith) |
| **Tablets, extended-release**: 500, 750, and 1,000 mg (*Rx*) | *Niaspan* (Kos Pharmaceuticals) |

## Indications

*Hyperlipidemia*: Adjunctive therapy for treatment in adult patients with very high serum triglyceride levels (Types IV and V hyperlipidemia) who present a risk of pancreatitis and who do not respond adequately to dietary control.

## Administration and Dosage

*Extended-release*: 500 mg at bedtime for 1 to 4 weeks, then 1000 mg at bedtime during weeks 5 to 8. After week 8, titrate to patient response and tolerance. If response to 1000 mg/day is inadequate, increase dose to 1500 mg/day; may subsequently increase dose to 2000 mg/day. Do not increase daily dose more than 500 mg in a 4-week period. Doses exceeding 2000 mg/day are not recommended.

*Immediate-release*: Adult dosage is 1 to 2 g given 2 to 3 times/day. Individualize the dose according to patient response. Initiate therapy at 250 mg as a single dose following the evening meal. The frequency of dosing and total daily dose may be increased every 4 to 7 days until the desired LDL or triglyceride level is achieved or the first-level therapeutic dose of 1.5 to 2 g/day is reached. If hyperlipidemia is not adequately controlled after 2 months at this level, increase dosage at 2- to 4-week intervals to 3 g/day (1 g 3 times/day). Do not exceed 6 g/day.

## Actions

*Pharmacology*: Nicotinic acid (but not nicotinamide) in gram doses produces an average 10% to 20% reduction in total and LDL cholesterol, a 30% to 70% reduction in triglycerides, and an average 20% to 35% increase in HDL cholesterol. Nicotinic acid also decreases serum levels of apolipoprotein B-100, the major component of VLDL and LDL fractions. The mechanism by which nicotinic acid exerts these effects is not entirely understood but may involve several actions, including a decrease in esterification of hepatic triglycerides.

*Pharmacokinetics*: The drug is rapidly absorbed from the GI tract. At a 1 g dose, peak plasma concentrations of 15 to 30 mcg/mL are reached within 30 to 60 minutes. About 88% of the immediate-release nicotinic acid oral dose is eliminated by the kidneys as unchanged drug and nicotinuric acid. Approximately 60% to 76% of the niacin dose administered as extended-release niacin (nicotinic acid) was recovered in urine as niacin and metabolites. The elimination half-life ranges from 20 to 45 minutes.

## Contraindications

Hepatic dysfunction; active peptic ulcer; arterial bleeding; hypersensitivity to niacin.

## Warnings

*Skeletal muscle effects*: Rare cases of rhabdomyolysis have been associated with coadministration of lipid-altering doses (1 g/day or greater) of nicotinic acid and HMG-CoA reductase inhibitors. Consider periodic serum creatine phosphokinase (CPK) and potassium determinations in such situations, although there is no assurance that such monitoring will prevent the occurrence of severe myopathy.

*Flushing*: When flushing is distressing or persistent, 325 mg aspirin given 30 minutes before each scheduled dose of nicotinic acid or slow upward dose adjustment may help ameliorate this reaction. Do not drink hot liquids with or immediately after administration; this increases flushing.

*Hepatic function impairment*: Cases of severe hepatic toxicity, including fulminant hepatic necrosis have occurred in patients who have substituted sustained-release (modified-release, timed-release) nicotinic acid products for immediate-release (crystalline) nicotinic acid at equivalent doses.

Perform liver function tests on all patients during therapy with nicotinic acid. Monitor serum transaminase levels, including ALT and AST, before treatment begins, every 6 to 12 weeks for the first year, and periodically thereafter (at approximately 6-month intervals). Discontinue the drug if the transaminase levels show evidence of progression, particularly if they rise to 3 times the upper limit of normal and are persistent or if they are associated with symptoms of nausea, fever, or malaise. Consider liver biopsy if elevations persist beyond discontinuation.

# EZETIMIBE

| Tablets: 10 mg (Rx) | Zetia (Merck/Schering-Plough) |
| --- | --- |

## Indications
*Primary hypercholesterolemia:*
    *Monotherapy* – Administered alone as adjunctive therapy to diet for the reduction of elevated total cholesterol (total-C), low density lipoprotein cholesterol (LDL-C), and apolipoprotein B (Apo B) in patients with primary (heterozygous familial and nonfamilial) hypercholesterolemia.
    *Combination therapy with HMG-CoA reductase inhibitors* – In combination with an HMG-CoA reductase inhibitor as adjunctive therapy to diet for the reduction of elevated total-C, LDL-C, and Apo B in patients with primary (heterozygous familial and nonfamilial) hypercholesterolemia.

*Homozygous familial hypercholesterolemia (HoFH):* With atorvastatin or simvastatin for the reduction of elevated total-C and LDL-C levels in patients with HoFH as an adjunct to other lipid-lowering treatments (eg, LDL apheresis) or if such treatments are unavailable.

*Homozygous sitosterolemia:* As adjunctive therapy to diet for the reduction of elevated sitosterol and campesterol levels in patients with homozygous familial sitosterolemia.

## Administration and Dosage
*Dose:* The recommended dose of ezetimibe is 10 mg once daily. Ezetimibe can be administered with or without food.

*Coadministration with HMG-CoA reductase inhibitors:* Ezetimibe may be administered with an HMG-CoA reductase inhibitor for incremental effect. For convenience, the daily dose of ezetimibe may be taken at the same time as the HMG-CoA reductase inhibitor, according to the dosing recommendations for the HMG-CoA reductase inhibitor.

*Coadministration with bile acid sequestrants:* Dosing of ezetimibe should occur at least 2 hours before or at least 4 hours after administration of a bile acid sequestrant.

## Actions
*Pharmacology:* Ezetimibe reduces total-C, LDL-C, Apo B, and triglycerides (TG), and increases HDL-C in patients with hypercholesterolemia. Ezetimibe reduces blood cholesterol by inhibiting the absorption of cholesterol by the small intestine.
    Ezetimibe has a mechanism of action that differs from those of other classes of cholesterol-reducing compounds. Ezetimibe does not inhibit cholesterol synthesis in the liver or increase bile acid excretion.

*Pharmacokinetics:*
    *Absorption* – After oral administration, ezetimibe is absorbed and extensively conjugated to a pharmacologically active phenolic glucuronide (ezetimibe-glucuronide). After a single 10 mg dose of ezetimibe to fasted adults, mean ezetimibe peak plasma concentrations ($C_{max}$) of 3.4 to 5.5 ng/mL were attained within 4 to 12 hours ($T_{max}$). The absolute bioavailability of ezetimibe cannot be determined, as the compound is virtually insoluble in aqueous media suitable for injection. Ezetimibe has variable bioavailability; the coefficient of variation, based on intersubject variability, was 35% to 60% for area under the curve (AUC) values.
    *Distribution* – Ezetimibe and ezetimibe-glucuronide are highly bound (greater than 90%) to human plasma proteins.
    *Metabolism/Excretion* – Ezetimibe is primarily metabolized in the small intestine and liver via glucuronide conjugation (a phase II reaction) with subsequent biliary and renal excretion.

*Special populations –*
  *Gender:* Plasma concentrations for total ezetimibe were slightly higher (less than 20%) in women than in men.

## Contraindications
Hypersensitivity to any component of the medication.

The combination of ezetimibe with an HMG-CoA reductase inhibitor is contraindicated in patients with active liver disease or unexplained persistent elevations in serum transaminases.

All HMG-CoA reductase inhibitors are contraindicated in pregnant and nursing women. When ezetimibe is administered with an HMG-CoA reductase inhibitor in a woman of childbearing potential, refer to the pregnancy category and product labeling for the HMG-CoA reductase inhibitor.

## Warnings
*Hyperlipidemia, secondary causes:* Prior to initiating therapy with ezetimibe, exclude or, if appropriate, treat secondary causes for dyslipidemia. Perform a lipid profile to measure total-C, LDL-C, HDL-C, and TG. For TG levels greater than 400 mg/dL (greater than 4.5 mmol/L), determine LDL-C concentrations by ultracentrifugation.

*Renal function impairment:* In patients with severe renal disease (mean Ccr less than or equal to 30 mL/min/1.73 $m^2$), the mean AUC values for total ezetimibe, ezetimibe-glucuronide, and ezetimibe were increased.

*Hepatic function impairment:* Because of the unknown effects of the increased exposure to ezetimibe in patients with moderate or severe hepatic insufficiency, ezetimibe is not recommended in these patients.

*Elderly:* Plasma concentrations for total ezetimibe were about 2-fold higher in older (65 years of age and older) healthy subjects compared with younger subjects.

*Pregnancy:* Category C.

*Lactation:* It is not known whether ezetimibe is excreted in human breast milk.

*Children:* Treatment with ezetimibe in children (younger than 10 years of age) is not recommended.

## Precautions
*Monitoring:* When ezetimibe is coadministered with an HMG-CoA reductase inhibitor, perform liver function tests at initiation of therapy and according to the recommendations of the HMG-CoA reductase inhibitor. At the time of hospitalization for an acute coronary event, take lipid measures on admission or within 24 hours.

*Liver enzymes:* When ezetimibe is coadministered with an HMG-CoA reductase inhibitor, perform liver function tests at initiation of therapy and according to the recommendations of the HMG-CoA reductase inhibitor.

*Skeletal muscle effects:* In clinical trials, there was no excess of myopathy or rhabdomyolysis associated with ezetimibe compared with the relevant control arm (placebo or HMG-CoA reductase inhibitor alone). However, myopathy and rhabdomyolysis are known adverse reactions to HMG-CoA reductase inhibitors and other lipid-lowering drugs.

## Drug Interactions
Drugs that may affect ezetimibe include antacids, cholestyramine, fibric acid derivatives, and cyclosporine.

*Drug/Food interactions:* Ezetimibe may be administered with or without food.

## Adverse Reactions
Adverse reactions occurring in at least 3% of patients include diarrhea, abdominal pain, back pain, arthralgia, sinusitis. In combination with HMG-CoA reductase inhibitors reactions included headache, myalgia, pharyngitis, URI, chest pain.

# ANTIHYPERLIPIDEMIC COMBINATIONS

## AMLODIPINE BESYLATE/ATORVASTATIN CALCIUM

**Tablets:** 5 mg amlodipine besylate/10 mg atorvastatin calcium (as base), 5 mg amlodipine besylate/20 mg atorvastatin calcium (as base), 5 mg amlodipine besylate/40 mg atorvastatin calcium (as base), 5 mg amlodipine besylate/80 mg atorvastatin calcium (as base), 10 mg amlodipine besylate/10 mg atorvastatin calcium (as base), 10 mg amlodipine besylate/20 mg atorvastatin calcium (as base), 10 mg amlodipine besylate/40 mg atorvastatin calcium (as base), 10 mg amlodipine besylate/80 mg atorvastatin calcium (as base) (Rx)

*Caduet* (Pfizer)

## ASPIRIN/PRAVASTATIN

**Tablets:** 81 mg aspirin (buffered)/20 mg pravastatin, 81 mg aspirin (buffered)/40 mg pravastatin, 81 mg aspirin (buffered)/80 mg pravastatin, 325 mg aspirin (buffered)/20 mg pravastatin, 325 mg aspirin (buffered)/40 mg pravastatin, 325 mg aspirin (buffered)/80 mg pravastatin (Rx)

*Pravigard PAC* (Bristol-Myers Squibb)

## NIACIN (EXTENDED-RELEASE)/LOVASTATIN

**Tablets:** 500 mg niacin/20 mg lovastatin and 1,000 mg niacin/20 mg lovastatin (Rx)

*Advicor* (Kos)

### Indications

*Primary hypercholesterolemia/mixed dyslipidemia:* For the treatment of primary hypercholesterolemia (heterozygous familial and nonfamilial) and mixed dyslipidemia (Frederickson Types IIa and IIb) in the following: Patients treated with lovastatin who require further TG-lowering or HDL-raising who may benefit from having niacin added to their regimen; patients treated with niacin who require further LDL-lowering who may benefit from having lovastatin added to their regimen.

### Administration and Dosage

The usual recommended starting dose for extended-release niacin tablets is 500 mg at bedtime. Niacin extended-release tablets must be titrated and the dose should not be increased by more than 500 mg every 4 weeks up to a maximum dose of 2000 mg/day, to reduce the incidence and severity of side effects. Patients already receiving a stable dose of niacin extended-release tablets may be switched directly to a niacin-equivalent dose of niacin extended-release/lovastatin tablets.

The usual recommended starting dose of lovastatin is 20 mg once/day. Make dose adjustments at intervals of 4 weeks or more. Patients already receiving a stable dose of lovastatin may receive concomitant dosage titration with niacin extended-release tablets, and switch to niacin extended-release/lovastatin tablets once a stable dose of niacin extended-release tablets has been reached.

Take niacin extended-release/lovastatin tablets at bedtime, with a low-fat snack, and individualize dose according to patient response.

Take whole; do not break, chew, or crush before swallowing. Do not increase the dose by more than 500 mg/day (based on the niacin extended release component) every 4 weeks. The lowest dose of niacin extended-release/lovastatin tablets is 500/20 mg. Doses greater than 2000/40 mg/day are not recommended. If therapy is discontinued for an extended period (greater than 7 days), begin reinstitution of therapy with the lowest dose.

# EZETIMIBE/SIMVASTATIN

**Tablets**: 10 mg ezetimibe/10 mg simvastatin, 10 mg ezeti-   *Vytorin* (Merck/Schering-Plough)
mibe/20 mg simvastatin, 10 mg ezetimibe/40 mg simvastatin,
10 mg ezetimibe/80 mg simvastatin (*Rx*)

See individual drug monographs for more information.

### Indications

*Primary hypercholesterolemia:* Adjunctive therapy to diet for reducing elevated total-C, LDL-C, Apo B, TG, and non-HDL-C, and increasing HDL-C in patients with primary (heterozygous familial and nonfamilial) hypercholesterolemia or mixed hyperlipidemia.

*Homozygous familial hypercholesterolemia:* For reducing elevated total-C and LDL-C in patients with homozygous familial hypercholesterolemia, as an adjunct to other lipid-lowering treatments (eg, LDL apheresis) or if such treatments are unavailable.

### Administration and Dosage

The patient should be placed on a standard cholesterol-lowering diet before receiving ezetimibe/simvastatin and should continue on this diet during treatment. Individualize the dosage according to the baseline LDL-C level, the recommended goal of therapy, and the patient's response. Take ezetimibe/simvastatin as a single daily dose in the evening, with or without food.

*Dose:* The recommended usual starting dose is 10 mg ezetimibe/20 mg simvastatin daily. Initiation of therapy with 10 mg ezetimibe/10 mg simvastatin daily may be considered for patients requiring less aggressive LDL-C reductions. Patients who require a larger reduction in LDL-C (more than 55%) may be started at 10 mg ezetimibe/40 mg simvastatin daily. After initiation or titration of ezetimibe/simvastatin, lipid levels may be analyzed after 2 or more weeks and dosage adjusted, if needed.

*Homozygous familial hypercholesterolemia:* The recommended dosage for patients with homozygous familial hypercholesterolemia is 10 mg ezetimibe/40 mg simvastatin daily or 10 mg ezetimibe/80 mg simvastatin daily in the evening. Use ezetimibe/simvastatin as an adjunct to other lipid-lowering treatments (eg, LDL apheresis) in these patients or if such treatments are unavailable.

*Hepatic function impairment:* Use is not recommended in patients with moderate or severe hepatic insufficiency.

*Renal function impairment:* For patients with severe renal insufficiency, do not start ezetimibe/simvastatin unless the patient has already tolerated treatment with simvastatin at a dose of 5 mg or higher. Exercise caution when ezetimibe/simvastatin is administered to these patients, and monitor them closely.

*Concomitant bile acid sequestrants:* Give ezetimibe/simvastatin either 2 hours or more before or 4 hours or more after administration of a bile acid sequestrant.

*Concomitant cyclosporine:* Exercise caution when initiating ezetimibe/simvastatin in the setting of cyclosporine. In patients taking cyclosporine, do not start ezetimibe/simvastatin unless the patient has already tolerated treatment with simvastatin at a dose of 5 mg or higher. Do not exceed 10 mg ezetimibe/10 mg simvastatin daily.

*Concomitant amiodarone or verapamil:* In patients taking amiodarone or verapamil concomitantly with ezetimibe/simvastatin, do not exceed 10 mg ezetimibe/20 mg simvastatin daily.

# Chapter 5

# RENAL & GENITOURINARY AGENTS

# ALPROSTADIL (Prostaglandin E₁; PGE₁)

| | |
|---|---|
| **Injection, aqueous:** 10, 20, and 40 mcg/mL (*Rx*) | *Caverject* (Pharmacia & Upjohn) |
| **Powder for injection, lyophilized:** 5, 10, 20, and 40 mcg/mL (after reconstitution) (*Rx*) | |
| **Powder for injection, lyophilized:** 10 mcg/0.5 mL, 20 mcg/ 0.5 mL (after reconstitution) (*Rx*) | *Caverject Impulse* (Pharmacia & Upjohn) |
| 5, 10, 20, and 40 mcg/mL (after reconstitution) (*Rx*) | *Edex* (Schwarz Pharma) |
| **Pellet:** 125, 250, 500, or 1000 mcg (*Rx*) | *Muse* (Vivus) |

### Indications

*Erectile dysfunction:* Treatment of erectile dysfunction caused by neurogenic, vasculogenic, psychogenic, or mixed etiology.

Intracavernosal alprostadil may be a useful adjunct to other diagnostic tests in the diagnosis of erectile dysfunction (*Caverject* only).

### Administration and Dosage

*Intercavernosal:* The first alprostadil injections must be done at the physician's office by medically trained personnel. The injection site is usually along the dorsolateral aspect of the proximal third of the penis. Avoid visible veins. Alternate the side of the penis that is injected and the site of injection.

The dose of alprostadil that is selected for self-injection treatment should provide the patient with an erection that is satisfactory for sexual intercourse and that is maintained for no longer than 1 hour. If the duration of erection is more than 1 hour, reduce the dose.

*Initial titration* – The patient must stay in the physician's office until complete detumescence occurs. If there is no response, then the next higher dose may be given within 1 hour. If there is a response, then wait at least 1 day before the next dose is given.

*Erectile dysfunction of vasculogenic, psychogenic, or mixed etiology* – Do not give more than 2 doses within a 24-hour period during initial titration. If there is no response to the initial 2.5 mcg dose, the second dose may be increased to 7.5 mcg within 1 hour. If additional titration is required, doses in increments of 5 to 10 mcg may be given at least 24 hours apart.

*Erectile dysfunction of pure neurogenic etiology (spinal cord injury)* – Initiate dosage titration at 1.25 mcg. The dose may be increased by 1.25 mcg to a dose of 2.5 mcg within 1 hour. Do not give more than 2 doses within a 24-hour period during initial titration. If additional titration is required, a dose of 5 mcg may be given during the next 24 hours. Doses in increments of 5 mcg may be given at least 24 hours apart until the dose that produces an erection suitable for intercourse and does not exceed a duration of 1 hour is reached.

*Adjunct to the diagnosis of erectile dysfunction (Caverject only)* – Patients are monitored for the occurrence of an erection after an intracavernosal injection of alprostadil. Use a single dose of alprostadil that induces a rigid erection.

*Maintenance therapy* – The first injections of alprostadil must be done at the physician's office by medically trained personnel. The recommended frequency of injection is 3 times/week or less, with at least 24 hours between each dose.

*Intraurethral:* Administer as needed to achieve an erection. The onset of effect is within 5 to 10 minutes after administration. The duration of effect is approximately 30 to 60 minutes. A medical professional should instruct each patient on proper technique for administering alprostadil prior to self-administration. The maximum frequency of use is no more than 2 systems per 24-hour period.

*Initiation of therapy* – Titrate dose under the supervision of a physician to test a patient's response to alprostadil, to demonstrate proper administration technique and to monitor for evidence of hypotension. Individually titrate patients to the lowest dose that is sufficient for sexual intercourse. If necessary, increase the dose (or decrease) on separate occasions in a stepwise manner until the patient achieves an erection that is sufficient for sexual intercourse.

## Actions

*Pharmacology:* Alprostadil induces erection by relaxation of trabecular smooth muscle and by dilation of cavernosal arteries.

*Pharmacokinetics:*

*Absorption* – For treatment of erectile dysfunction, alprostadil is administered by injection into the corpora cavernosa or inserted intraurethrally.

*Intracavernosal:* Following intracavernosal injection of 20 mcg, mean peripheral plasma concentrations at 30 to 60 minutes after injection (89 to 102 pcg/mL, respectively) were not significantly greater than baseline levels of endogenous alprostadil (96 pcg/mL).

*Intraurethral:* The transurethral absorption of alprostadil is rapid, with approximately 80% of an administered dose absorbed within 10 minutes. The mean time to the maximum plasma PGE₁ concentration after a 1000 mcg intraurethral dose is approximately 16 minutes.

*Distribution* –

*Intracavernosal:* Alprostadil is bound in plasma primarily to albumin (81% bound).

*Intraurethral:* The half-life is short, varying between 30 seconds and 10 minutes.

*Metabolism* – Following IV administration, 80% of circulating alprostadil is metabolized in one pass through the lungs, primarily by beta- and omega-oxidation. The near-complete pulmonary first-pass metabolism of PGE₁ is the primary factor influencing the systemic pharmacokinetics of alprostadil and is a reason that peripheral venous plasma levels of PGE₁ are low or undetectable (less than 2 pg/mL) following alprostadil administration. The enzyme catalyzing this process has been isolated from many tissues in the lower GU tract including the urethra, prostate, and corpus cavernosum.

*Excretion* – The metabolites of alprostadil are excreted primarily by the kidney, with almost 90% of an administered IV dose excreted in urine within 24 hours postdose. The remainder of the dose is excreted in the feces.

## Contraindications

Hypersensitivity to the drug; conditions that might predispose patients to priapism (eg, sickle cell anemia or trait, multiple myeloma, leukemia); patients with anatomical deformation of the penis; patients with penile implants (intracavernosal); use in women, children, or newborns; use in men for whom sexual activity is inadvisable or contraindicated; for sexual intercourse with a pregnant woman unless the couple uses a condom barrier.

*Intraurethral:* Urethral stricture; balanitis; severe hypospadias; patients with acute or chronic urethritis; thrombocythemia; polycythemia.

## Warnings

*Priapism:* Prolonged erection (lasting more than 4 to 6 or fewer hours) and priapism (erection lasting more than 6 hours) have occurred in patients using alprostadil. To minimize the chances of prolonged erection or priapism, titrate slowly to the lowest effective dose.

*Penile fibrosis:* Regular follow-up of patients, with careful examination of the penis, is strongly recommended to detect signs of penile fibrosis.

*Penile pain:* Penile pain after intracavernosal administration was reported. In the majority of the cases, penile pain was rated mild or moderate in intensity.

*Hematoma/Ecchymosis:* In most cases, hematoma/ecchymosis was judged to be a complication of a faulty injection technique.

*Hemodynamic changes:* Hemodynamic changes, manifested as decreases in blood pressure and increases in pulse rate, principally at doses more than 20 mcg, were observed during clinical studies, and appeared to be dose-dependent.

*Erectile dysfunction:* Diagnose and treat underlying treatable medical causes of erectile dysfunction prior to initiation of therapy.

*Pulmonary disease:* The pulmonary extraction of alprostadil following intravascular administration was reduced by 15% in patients with acute respiratory distress syndrome (ARDS).

*Pregnancy: Category* C. Do not use for sexual intercourse with a pregnant woman unless the couple uses a condom barrier.

*Children: Caverject* is not indicated for use in newborns or children. However, alprostadil (*Prostin VR Pediatric*) is used in newborns to maintain the patency of the ductus arteriosus in neonates with congenital heart defects.

### Drug Interactions
Drugs that may interact with alprostadil include anticoagulants and vasoactive agents.

### Adverse Reactions
Adverse reactions occurring in at least 3% of patients receiving alprostadil by intracavernosal administration include bleeding, ecchymosis, hematoma, penile angulation, penis disorder, penile fibrosis, penile pain, and prolonged erection.

Adverse reactions in at least 3% of patients receiving alprostadil by intraurethral administration include accidental injury, dizziness, flu syndrome, headache, hypotension, pain, penile pain, testicular pain, urethral bleeding/spotting, urethral burning, urethral pain, and URI.

The most common drug-related adverse event reported by female partners during clinical studies was vaginal burning/itching (5.8%).

## PHOSPHODIESTERASE TYPE 5 INHIBITORS

| | |
|---|---|
| **SILDENAFIL CITRATE** | |
| **Tablets**: 25, 50, and 100 mg (*Rx*) | *Viagra* (Pfizer) |
| **TADALAFIL** | |
| **Tablets**: 5, 10, and 20 mg (*Rx*) | *Cialis* (Lilly) |
| **VARDENAFIL HCL** | |
| **Tablets**: 2.5, 5, 10, and 25 mg (*Rx*) | *Levitra* (Bayer) |

### Indications
*Erectile dysfunction:* Treatment of erectile dysfunction.

### Administration and Dosage
*SILDENAFIL:* 50 mg taken as needed approximately 1 hour before sexual activity. However, sildenafil may be taken anywhere from 4 hours to 30 minutes before sexual activity. Based on effectiveness and tolerance, the dose may be increased to a maximum recommended dose of 100 mg or decreased to 25 mg. The maximum recommended dosing frequency is once per day.

*Dosage adjustment* – Consider a starting dose of 25 mg in the following patients: Older than 65 years of age, hepatic impairment, severe renal impairment, and concomitant use of potent cytochrome P450 3A4 inhibitors (eg, erythromycin, ketoconazole, itraconazole, saquinavir).

*Concomitant use with protease inhibitors:* Do not exceed a maximum single dose of 25 mg of sildenafil within a 48-hour period.

*Concomitant use with alpha-blockers:* Do not take 50 or 100 mg doses of sildenafil within 4 hours of alpha-blocker administration. A 25 mg dose of sildenafil may be taken at any time.

*TADALAFIL:* 10 mg taken prior to anticipated sexual activity. The dose may be increased to 20 mg or decreased to 5 mg, based on individual efficacy and tolerability. The maximum recommended dosing frequency is once daily in most patients. Tadalafil may be taken without regard to food.

Tadalafil was shown to improve erectile function compared with placebo up to 36 hours following dosing. Therefore, take this into consideration when advising patients on optimal use of tadalafil.

*Renal function impairment* – For patients with moderate (Ccr 31 to 50 mL/min) renal insufficiency, a starting dose of 5 mg not more than once daily is recommended, and the maximum dose is limited to 10 mg not more than once every 48 hours. For patients with severe (Ccr less than 30 mL/min) renal insufficiency on hemodialysis, the maximum recommended dose is 5 mg.

*Hepatic function impairment* – In mild or moderate hepatic impairment (Child-Pugh class A or B), do not exceed 10 mg once daily. In severe hepatic impairment (Child-Pugh class C), the use of tadalafil is not recommended.

*Concomitant medications* – For patients taking concomitant potent inhibitors of CYP3A4 (eg, ketoconazole, ritonavir), the maximum recommended dose of tadalafil is 10 mg, not to exceed once every 72 hours.

Concomitant use of nitrates in any form and alpha-adrenergic blockers (other than 0.4 mg once-daily tamsulosin) is contraindicated.

VARDENAFIL HCL: 10 mg taken orally approximately 60 minutes before sexual activity. The dose may be increased to a maximum recommended dose of 20 mg or decreased to 5 mg based on efficacy and side effects. The maximum recommended dosing frequency is once daily. Vardenafil can be taken with or without food.

*Elderly* – Consider a starting dose of 5 mg in patients 65 years of age and older.

*Hepatic function impairment* – A starting dose of 5 mg is recommended in patients with moderate hepatic impairment (Child-Pugh B). The maximum dose should not exceed 10 mg. Vardenafil has not been evaluated in patients with severe hepatic impairment (Child-Pugh C).

*Concomitant medications* – The dosage of vardenafil may require adjustment in patients receiving certain CYP3A4 inhibitors. For ritonavir, do not exceed a single dose of 2.5 mg vardenafil in a 72-hour period. For indinavir, ketoconazole 400 mg/day, and itraconazole 400 mg/day, do not exceed a single dose of 2.5 mg vardenafil in a 24-hour period. For ketoconazole 200 mg/day, itraconazole 200 mg/day, and erythromycin, do not exceed a single dose of 5 mg vardenafil in a 24-hour period.

**Actions**

*Pharmacology:* **Sildenafil**, **tadalafil**, and **vardenafil** are selective inhibitors of phosphodiesterase type 5 (PDE5).

*Pharmacokinetics:*

*Absorption/Distribution –*

| Phosphodiesterase Type 5 Inhibitors Pharmacokinetics | | | |
|---|---|---|---|
| Parameters | Sildenafil | Tadalafil | Vardenafil |
| Bioavailability | ≈ 40% | Not determined | ≈ 15% |
| $T_{max}$ | 0.5 to 2 h (median, 1 h)[a] | 0.5 to 6 h (median, 2 h)[b] | 0.5 to 2 h (median, 1 h)[c] |
| Effect of food (high-fat meal) | $C_{max}$ reduced by 29% $T_{max}$ increased by 1 h | No effect | $C_{max}$ reduced by 18% to 50% |
| Onset of action | ≈ 30 min | ≈ 30 min | ≈ 20 min[d] |
| Maximum effect | no data | no data | 45 to 90 min[d] |
| Duration of action | ≥ 4 h | 36 h | < 5 h |
| Volume of distribution[e] | 105 L | ≈ 63 L | 208 L |
| Protein binding[f] | ≈ 96% | 94% | ≈ 95% |
| Metabolism | CYP3A4 (major) CYP2C9 (minor) | CYP3A4 | CYP3A4 (major) CYP3A5, CYP2C isoforms (minor) |
| Active metabolite | Yes[g] | No | Yes[h] |
| Terminal half-life | ≈ 4 h | 17.5 h | 4 to 5 h |
| Excretion | Feces (≈ 80%) Urine (≈ 13%) | Feces (≈ 61%) Urine (≈ 36%) | Feces (≈ 91% to 95%) Urine (≈ 2% to 6%) |
| Clearance | no data | 2.5 L/h | 56 L/h |

[a] Oral dosing in the fasted state.
[b] Single oral dose.
[c] Single oral dose of 20 mg; fasted state.
[d] Based on animal studies.
[e] At steady state.
[f] For parent drug and major circulating metabolite.
[g] Accounts for approximately 20% of sildenafil's pharmacologic activity.
[h] Accounts for approximately 7% of vardenafil's pharmacologic activity.

*Metabolism/Excretion* – **Sildenafil, tadalafil,** and **vardenafil** are cleared predominantly by the CYP3A4 (major route), 3A5 (major route; vardenafil), and CYP2C9 (minor route) hepatic isoenzymes.

## Contraindications

Hypersensitivity to any component of the tablet; administration with nitrates (either regularly and/or intermittently) and nitric oxide donors because of the potentiation of hypotension (see Drug Interactions); coadministration with alpha-blockers (**vardenafil** only); coadministration with alpha-blockers other than 0.4 mg/day tamsulosin (**tadalafil** only).

## Warnings

*Priapism:* Prolonged erections more than 4 hours and priapism (painful erections more than 6 hours in duration) have been infrequently reported. In the event of an erection that persists more than 4 hours, advise the patient to seek immediate medical assistance.

*Cardiovascular effects:* Treatments for erectile dysfunction, including these agents, generally should not be used in men for whom sexual activity is inadvisable because of their underlying cardiovascular status.

Patients with the following underlying conditions can be particularly sensitive to the actions of vasodilators, including **sildenafil, tadalafil,** and **vardenafil:** Those with left ventricular outflow obstruction (eg, aortic stenosis, idiopathic hypertrophic subaortic stenosis) and those with severely impaired autonomic control of blood pressure.

The following groups of patients with cardiovascular disease were not included in clinical safety and efficacy trials for tadalafil, and, therefore, the use of tadalafil is not recommended in these groups until further information is available:

- Patients with an MI within the last 90 days
- patients with unstable angina or angina occurring during sexual intercourse
- patients with New York Heart Association Class 2 or greater heart failure in the last 6 months
- patients with uncontrolled arrhythmias, hypotension (BP less than 90/50 mm Hg), or uncontrolled hypertension (BP greater than 170/100 mm Hg)
- patients with a stroke within the last 6 months.

*Sildenafil* – Serious cardiovascular, cerebrovascular, and vascular events, including MI, sudden cardiac death, ventricular arrhythmia, cerebrovascular hemorrhage, transient ischemic attack, hypertension subarachnoid and intracerebral hemorrhages, and pulmonary hemorrhage have been reported postmarketing in temporal association with sildenafil.

*Vardenafil* –

*Congenital or acquired QT prolongation:* Patients with congenital QT prolongation and those taking Class IA (eg, quinidine, procainamide) or Class III (eg, amiodarone, sotalol) antiarrhythmic medications should avoid using vardenafil.

*Renal function impairment:* In volunteers with severe renal impairment (Ccr 30 mL/min or less), **sildenafil** clearance was reduced. Consider an initial sildenafil dose of 25 mg in these patients. There is no clinical data on the safety or efficacy of **vardenafil** in patients with end-stage renal disease requiring dialysis.

Limit **tadalafil** to 5 mg not more than once daily in patients with severe renal insufficiency or end-stage renal disease. The starting dose in patients with a moderate degree of renal insufficiency should be 5 mg not more than once daily, and the maximum dose should be limited to 10 mg not more than once in every 48 hours. No dose adjustment is required in patients with mild renal insufficiency.

In patients with moderate (Ccr 30 to 50 mL/min) to severe (Ccr less than 30 mL/min) renal impairment, the AUC of vardenafil was 20% to 30% higher. No dosage adjustment for vardenafil is required.

*Hepatic function impairment:* In volunteers with hepatic cirrhosis, **sildenafil** clearance was reduced. Consider an initial sildenafil dose of 25 mg in these patients. In patients with mild or moderate hepatic impairment, do not exceed a 10 mg dose of **tadalafil**. Because of insufficient information in patients with severe hepatic impairment, use in these patients is not recommended. In volunteers with mild and moderate hepatic impairment (Child-Pugh A), the $C_{max}$ and AUC following a 10 mg **vardenafil** dose were increased. Consequently, a starting dose of 5 mg is recommended for patients with moderate hepatic impairment, and the maximum dose should not exceed 10 mg. Vardenafil is not recommended in patients with severe (Child-Pugh C) hepatic impairment.

*Elderly:* Consider an initial **sildenafil** dose of 25 mg in these patients. Consider a lower starting dose of **vardenafil** (5 mg) in patients 65 years of age and older.

*Pregnancy: Category B.* These agents are not indicated for use in women.

*Lactation:* These agents are not indicated for use in women.

*Children:* These agents are not indicated for use in newborns and children.

### Precautions

*Erectile dysfunction:* Undertake thorough medical history and physical examination to diagnose erectile dysfunction, determine potential underlying causes, and identify appropriate treatment.

The safety and efficacy of combinations of **sildenafil** or **vardenafil** with other treatments for erectile dysfunction have not been studied. Therefore, the use of such combinations is not recommended.

*Deformation of penis:* Use agents for the treatment of erectile dysfunction with caution in patients with anatomical deformation of the penis or in patients who have conditions that may predispose them to priapism.

*Bleeding disorders:* **Sildenafil, tadalafil,** and **vardenafil** have no effect on bleeding time when taken alone or with aspirin.

*Visual disturbances:* Single oral doses of phosphodiesterase inhibitors have demonstrated transient, dose-related impairment of color discrimination (blue/green), with peak effects near the time of peak plasma levels. The findings were most evident 1 hour after administration, diminishing but still present 6 hours after administration.

*Retinitis pigmentosa:* There is no safety information on the administration of **sildenafil** or **vardenafil** to patients with known hereditary degenerative retinal disorders, including retinitis pigmentosa. Therefore, administer with caution to these patients.

### Drug Interactions

*CYP450 system:* PDE5 inhibitors are metabolized principally by the cytochrome P450 (CYP) isoforms 3A4 (major route), 3A5 (major route; **vardenafil**), and 2C9 (minor route; **sildenafil**, vardenafil). Therefore, inhibitors of these isoenzymes may increase PDE5 inhibitor concentrations and inducers of these isoenzymes may decrease PDE5 inhibitor concentrations. See the Administration and Dosage sections of the individual monographs for dosing recommendations.

Drugs that affect all phosphodiesterase type 5 inhibitors include the following: alcohol, amlodipine, angiotensin II receptor blockers, antacids, bendroflumethiazide, beta blockers, cimetidine, diuretics, enalapril, metoprolol, nifedipine, rifampin, tacrolimus.

Drugs that may be affected by PDE5 inhibitors include: alpha-blockers, amlodipine, angiotensin II receptor blockers, bendroflumethiazide, enalapril, metoprolol, nifedipine, nitrates, protease inhibitors.

*Drug/Food interactions:* When taken with a high-fat meal, the rate of **sildenafil** absorption is reduced, with a mean delay in $T_{max}$ of 60 minutes and a mean reduction in $C_{max}$ of 29%. High-fat meals caused a reduction in $C_{max}$ of **vardenafil** by 18% to 50%.

### Adverse Reactions

Adverse reactions occurring in 3% or more of patients receiving these agents during clinical trials included abnormal vision (mild and transient, predominantly color tinge to vision but also increased sensitivity to light or blurred vision), accidental injury, back pain, diarrhea, dyspepsia, flushing, flu syndrome, headache, limb pain, myalgia, nasal congestion, rhinitis, sinusitis, urinary tract infection.

# PENICILLAMINE

| | |
|---|---|
| **Capsules**: 125 and 250 mg (*Rx*) | *Cuprimine* (Merck) |
| **Tablets, titratable**: 250 mg (*Rx*) | *Depen* (Wallace) |

### Indications
Rheumatoid arthritis.

Wilson's disease (hepatolenticular degeneration).

Cystinuria.

### Administration and Dosage
Give penicillamine on an empty stomach at least 1 hour before meals or 2 hours after meals and at least 1 hour apart from any other drug, food, or milk.

*Wilson's disease:* Initial dosage is 1 g/day for children or adults. This may be increased, as indicated by the urinary copper analyses, but it is seldom necessary to exceed 2 g/day. In patients who cannot tolerate 1 g/day initially, initiating dosage with 250 mg/day and increasing gradually allows closer control of the drug. Give on an empty stomach in 4 divided doses, 30 minutes to 1 hour before meals and at bedtime ( 2 hours or more after the evening meal).

*Cystinuria:*
   Adult dosage – 2 g/day (range, 1 to 4 g/day) in 4 divided doses.
   *Pediatric dosage* – 30 mg/kg/day in 4 divided doses. If 4 equal doses are not feasible, give the larger portion at bedtime. Initiating dosage with 250 mg/day, and increasing gradually, allows closer control of the drug and may reduce the incidence of adverse reactions.

   Patients should drink about a pint of fluid at bedtime and another pint once during the night when urine is more concentrated and more acid than during the day. The greater the fluid intake, the lower the dosage of penicillamine required.

*Rheumatoid arthritis:* Administer on an empty stomach at least 1 hour before meals and at least 1 hour apart from any other drug, food, or milk.

*Initial therapy:* A single daily dose of 125 or 250 mg. Thereafter, increase dose at 1- to 3-month intervals by 125 or 250 mg/day as patient response and tolerance indicate. If satisfactory remission is achieved, continue the dose. If there is no improvement and if there are no signs of potentially serious toxicity after 2 to 3 months with doses of 500 to 750 mg/day, continue increases of 250 mg/day at 2- to 3-month intervals until satisfactory remission occurs or toxicity develops. If there is no discernible improvement after 3 to 4 months of treatment with 1 to 1.5 g/day, assume the patient will not respond and discontinue the drug.

*Maintenance therapy:* Many patients respond to less than or equal to 500 to 750 mg/day. In patients who respond but who evidence incomplete disease suppression after the first 6 to 9 months of treatment, increase daily dosage by 125 or 250 mg/day at 3-month intervals. Dosage more than 1 g/day is unusual, but 1.5 g/day or less has been required.

*Dosage frequency:* Dosages 500 mg/day or less can be given as a single daily dose. Administer dosages greater than 500 mg/day in divided doses.

### Actions
*Pharmacology:*
   *Rheumatoid arthritis* – The mechanism of action of penicillamine in rheumatoid arthritis is unknown. The onset of therapeutic response may not be seen for 2 or 3 months in those patients who respond.

   *Wilson's disease* – Penicillamine is a chelating agent that removes excess copper in patients with Wilson's disease. Noticeable improvement may not occur for 1 to 3 months.

   *Poisoning* – Penicillamine also forms soluble complexes with iron, mercury, lead, and arsenic, which are readily excreted by the kidneys. The drug may be used to treat poisoning by these metals.

   *Cystinuria* – Penicillamine reduces excess cystine excretion in cystinuria. Penicillamine with conventional therapy decreases crystalluria and stone formation and may decrease the size of or dissolve existing stones. This is done, at least in part, by disulfide interchange between penicillamine and cystine, resulting in a substance more soluble than cystine and readily excreted.

*Pharmacokinetics:* It is well absorbed from the GI tract after oral administration (40% to 70%); peak plasma levels occur in 1 to 3 hours. Most (80%) of the plasma penicillamine is protein bound, primarily to albumin. Penicillamine is rapidly excreted in the urine; 50% is excreted in the feces. Metabolites may be detected in the urine for up to 3 months after stopping the drug. Half-life ranges are 1.7 to 3.2 hours.

## Contraindications

History of penicillamine-related aplastic anemia or agranulocytosis; rheumatoid arthritis patients with a history or other evidence of renal insufficiency; pregnancy; breast-feeding.

## Warnings

*Fatalities:* Penicillamine has been associated with fatalities due to aplastic anemia, agranulocytosis, thrombocytopenia, Goodpasture's syndrome, and myasthenia gravis.

*Hematologic:* Leukopenia (2%) and thrombocytopenia (4%) have occurred. A reduction in WBC below 3500, neutrophils less than 2000/mm$^3$, or monocytes greater than 500/mm$^3$ mandate permanent withdrawal of therapy.

*Hepatotoxicity:* Penicillamine has been associated with a mild elevation of hepatic enzymes that usually returns to normal even with continuation of the drug.

*Autoimmune syndromes:* Autoimmune syndromes that may be caused by penicillamine include polymyositis, diffuse alveolitis and dermatomyositis, Goodpasture's syndrome, myasthenic syndrome, pemphigus, and obliterative bronchiolitis.

*Pemphigoid-type:* Pemphigoid-type reactions characterized by bullous lesions have required discontinuation of penicillamine and treatment with corticosteroids.

*Lupus erythematosus:* Certain patients will develop a positive antinuclear antibody (ANA) test and some may show a lupus erythematosus-like syndrome similar to other drug-induced lupus, but it is not associated with hypocomplementemia and may be present without nephropathy. A positive ANA test does not mandate drug discontinuance; however, a lupus erythematosus-like syndrome may develop later.

*Sensitivity reactions:* Once instituted for Wilson's disease or cystinuria, continue treatment with penicillamine on a daily basis. Interruptions for even a few days have been followed by sensitivity reactions after reinstitution of therapy.

*Hypersensitivity reactions:* Allergic reactions occur in approximately 33% of patients. They are more common at the start of treatment, and occur as generalized rashes or drug fever. Discontinue treatment and reinstitute at a low dosage such as 250 mg/day, with gradual increases. Administering prednisolone 20 mg/day for the first few weeks of penicillamine therapy reduces the severity of these reactions. Antihistamines may control pruritus.

*Renal function impairment:* Proteinuria and hematuria may develop and may be a warning sign of membranous glomerulopathy, which can progress to a nephrotic syndrome.

*Pregnancy:* Category D.

*Lactation:* Safety has not been established.

*Children:* The efficacy of penicillamine in juvenile rheumatoid arthritis has not been established.

## Precautions

*Monitoring:* When indicated, monitor drug toxicity or efficacy through urinalysis. In rheumatoid arthritis patients, discontinue the drug if unexplained gross hematuria or persistent microscopic hematuria develops. Perform liver function tests and an annual x–ray for renal stones.

Monitor white and differential blood cell count, hemoglobin determination, and direct platelet count every 2 weeks for the first 6 months of penicillamine therapy and monthly thereafter.

*Drug fever:* Drug fever may appear in some patients, usually in the second to third week of therapy; it is sometimes accompanied by a macular cutaneous eruption.

*Dermatologic:* Skin rashes are the most frequent (44% to 50%) adverse reactions. Early rash occurs during the first few months of treatment and is more common.

*A late rash:* A late rash is less commonly seen, usually after 6 months or more of treatment, and requires drug discontinuation. It usually appears on the trunk, is accompanied by intense pruritus, and is usually unresponsive to topical corticosteroids.

*Pemphigoid rash:* Pemphigoid rash, the most serious dermatologic reaction occurs most often after 6 to 9 months of penicillamine.

*Oral ulcerations:* Oral ulcerations may develop that may have the appearance of aphthous stomatitis. Although rare, cheilosis, glossitis, and gingivostomatitis have been reported.

*Hypogeusia:* Hypogeusia occurs in 25% to 33% of patients, except for a lesser incidence in Wilson's disease (4%).

*Dietary supplementation:* Because of their dietary restriction, give patients with Wilson's disease, cystinuria, and rheumatoid arthritis whose nutrition is impaired 25 mg/day of pyridoxine during therapy, because penicillamine increases the requirement for this vitamin.

Iron deficiency may develop, especially in children and in menstruating women. This may be caused by diet. If necessary, give iron in short courses. A period of 2 hours should elapse between administration of penicillamine and iron, because orally administered iron reduces the effects of penicillamine.

*Effects of penicillamine on collagen and elastin:* Effects of penicillamine on collagen and elastin make it advisable to consider a reduction in dosage to 250 mg/day when surgery is contemplated.

Penicillamine may cause increased skin friability at sites subject to pressure or trauma, such as shoulders, elbows, knees, toes, and buttocks.

### Drug Interactions
Drugs that may affect penicillamine include gold therapy, antimalarial or cytotoxic drugs, iron salts, antacids, and food.

Drugs that may be affected by penicillamine include digoxin.

### Adverse Reactions
Penicillamine has a high incidence (greater than 50%) of untoward reactions, some of which are potentially fatal.

Adverse reactions that may occur in 3% or more of patients include anorexia; epigastric pain; nausea; vomiting; diarrhea; blunting/diminution/total loss of taste; taste perversion; thrombocytopenia; generalized pruritus; early and late rashes; proteinuria.

# FLAVOXATE

| | |
|---|---|
| **Tablets:** 100 mg (*Rx*) | *Urispas* (ALZA) |

### Indications
For the symptomatic relief of dysuria, urgency, nocturia, suprapubic pain, frequency, and incontinence as may occur in cystitis, prostatitis, urethritis, urethrocystitis/urethrotrigonitis.

Not indicated for definitive treatment but is compatible with drugs used to treat urinary tract infections.

### Administration and Dosage
*Adults and children older than 12 years of age:* 100 or 200 mg 3 or 4 times/day. Reduce the dose when symptoms improve.

### Actions
*Pharmacology:* Counteracts smooth muscle spasm of the urinary tract and exerts its effect directly on the muscle.

### Contraindications
Pyloric or duodenal obstruction; obstructive intestinal lesions or ileus; achalasia; GI hemorrhage; obstructive uropathies of the lower urinary tract.

### Warnings
*Glaucoma:* Give cautiously in patients with suspected glaucoma.

*Pregnancy:* Category B.

*Lactation:* It is not known whether this drug is excreted in breast milk. Use caution when flavoxate is administered to a nursing woman.

*Children:* Safety and efficacy in children younger than 12 years of age have not been established.

### Adverse Reactions
Nausea; vomiting; dry mouth; nervousness; vertigo; headache; drowsiness; mental confusion (especially in the elderly patient); hyperpyrexia; blurred vision; increased ocular tension; disturbance in eye accommodation; urticaria and other dermatoses; dysuria; tachycardia; palpitations; eosinophilia; leukopenia.

# OXYBUTYNIN CHLORIDE

| | |
|---|---|
| **Tablets:** 5 mg (*Rx*) | Various, *Ditropan* (ALZA) |
| **Tablets, extended-release:** 5, 10, 15 mg (*Rx*) | *Ditropan XL* (ALZA) |
| **Syrup:** 5 mg/5 mL (*Rx*) | Various, *Ditropan* (ALZA) |
| **Transdermal system:** 36 mg delivering 3.9 mg oxybutynin per day. (*Rx*) | *Oxytrol* (Watson) |

### Indications
*Bladder instability/Overactive bladder:* For the relief of symptoms of bladder instability/treatment of overactive bladder associated with voiding in patients with uninhibited and reflex neurogenic bladder (eg, urgency, frequency, urinary leakage, urge incontinence, dysuria).

### Administration and Dosage
*Oxybutynin immediate-release tablets:*

*Adults* – 5 mg (tablets or syrup) 2 or 3 times/day. Maximum dose is 5 mg 4 times/day.

*Children (older than 5 years of age)* – 5 mg (tablets or syrup) 2 times/day. Maximum dose is 5 mg 3 times/day.

*Oxybutynin ER tablets:* 5 mg once daily. Dosage may be adjusted in 5 mg increments to achieve a balance of efficacy and tolerability (up to a maximum of 30 mg/day). Dosage adjustments may proceed at approximately weekly intervals.

The ER tablets may be administered with or without food and must be swallowed whole with the aid of liquids, and not be chewed, divided, or crushed.

*Transdermal system:* Apply system to dry, intact skin on the abdomen, hip, or buttock. Select a new application site with each new system to avoid reapplication to the same site within 7 days.

The dose is one 3.9 mg/day system applied twice weekly (every 3 to 4 days).

## Actions

*Pharmacology:* Oxybutynin exerts direct antispasmodic effect on smooth muscle and inhibits the muscarinic action of acetylcholine on smooth muscle.

In patients with conditions characterized by involuntary bladder contractions, oxybutynin increases vesical capacity, diminishes frequency of uninhibited contractions of the detrusor muscle, and delays initial desire to void. Oxybutynin thus decreases urgency and the frequency of incontinent episodes and voluntary urination.

Oxybutynin is well tolerated in patients administered the drug from 30 days to 2 years.

*Pharmacokinetics:*

ER tablets – Following the first dose of oxybutynin ER tablets, oxybutynin plasma concentrations rise for 4 to 6 hours; thereafter, steady concentrations are maintained for up to 24 hours, minimizing fluctuations between peak and trough concentrations associated with oxybutynin.

Steady-state oxybutynin plasma concentrations are achieved by day 3 of repeated oxybutynin ER dosing, with no observed drug accumulation or change in oxybutynin and desethyloxybutynin pharmacokinetic parameters.

*Transdermal system* – Following application of the first 3.9 mg/day transdermal system, oxybutynin plasma concentration increases for approximately 24 to 48 hours, reaching average maximum concentrations of 3 to 4 ng/mL. Thereafter, steady concentrations are maintained for up to 96 hours. Absorption of oxybutynin is bioequivalent when oxybutynin transdermal system is applied to the abdomen, buttocks, or hip.

## Contraindications

Untreated angle-closure glaucoma; untreated narrow anterior chamber angles; GI obstruction; paralytic ileus; intestinal atony in the elderly or debilitated; megacolon; toxic megacolon complicating ulcerative colitis; severe colitis; myasthenia gravis; obstructive uropathy; unstable cardiovascular status in acute hemorrhage; hypersensitivity to the drug or any component of the product.

## Warnings

*Heat prostration:* When administered in the presence of high environmental temperature, heat prostration (fever and heat stroke) may occur because of decreased sweating.

*Diarrhea:* Diarrhea may be an early symptom of incomplete intestinal obstruction, especially in patients with ileostomy or colostomy; discontinue treatment.

*GI disorders:* Doses administered to patients with ulcerative colitis may suppress GI motility and produce paralytic ileus and precipitate or aggravate toxic megacolon.

Administer ER tablets with caution to patients with GI obstructive disorders because of the risk of gastric retention.

The ER tablets and transdermal system, like other anticholinergic drugs, may decrease GI motility and should be used with caution in patients with conditions such as ulcerative colitis, intestinal atony, and myasthenia gravis.

Use the ER tablets and transdermal system with caution in patients who have gastroesophageal reflux or who are concurrently taking drugs (such as bisphosphonates) that can cause or exacerbate esophagitis.

As with other nondeformable material, use caution when administering the ER tablets to patients with preexisting severe GI narrowing (pathologic or iatrogenic). There have been rare reports of obstructive symptoms in patients with known strictures in association with the ingestion of other drugs in nondeformable controlled-release formulations.

*Urinary retention:* Administer ER tablets with caution to patients with clinically significant bladder outflow obstruction because of the risk of urinary retention.

*Renal/Hepatic function impairment:* Use ER tablets with caution in patients with hepatic or renal impairment.

*Pregnancy: Category B.*

*Lactation:* It is not known whether this drug is excreted in breast milk. Exercise caution when administering to a nursing woman.

*Children:* Safety and efficacy in children (younger than 5 years of age for immediate-release tablets) have not been established.

### Precautions
*Use with caution:* Use with caution in the elderly and patients with autonomic neuropathy and hepatic or renal disease.

*Cardiac and other effects:* Symptoms of hyperthyroidism, coronary heart disease, CHF, cardiac arrhythmias, tachycardia, hypertension, hiatal hernia, and prostatic hypertrophy may be aggravated.

*Hazardous tasks:* Patients should use caution while driving or performing other tasks requiring alertness, coordination, or physical dexterity.

### Drug Interactions
Drugs that interact with oxybutynin include atenolol, digoxin, haloperidol, phenothiazines, amantadine, and anticholinergic agents.

### Adverse Reactions
*Adverse reactions occurring in 3% or more of patients* – Palpitations; vasodilation; dizziness; insomnia; rash; constipation; dry mouth; nausea; urinary hesitance and retention.

*Immediate-release tablets:* Tachycardia; drowsiness; hallucinations; restlessness; decreased sweating; decreased GI motility; amblyopia; cycloplegia; decreased lacrimation; mydriasis; asthenia; impotence; suppression of lactation.

*Extended-release tablets:* Somnolence; headache; diarrhea; dyspepsia; blurred vision; dry eyes; asthenia; pain; rhinitis; urinary tract infection; hypertension; nervousness; confusion; dry skin; flatulence; gastroesophageal reflux; increased post-void residual volume; cystitis; upper respiratory tract infection; cough; sinusitis; bronchitis; dry nasal and sinus mucous membranes; pharyngitis; abdominal pain; accidental injury; back pain; flu syndrome; arthritis.

# TOLTERODINE TARTRATE

| | |
|---|---|
| **Tablets:** 1 and 2 mg (*Rx*) | *Detrol* (Pharmacia) |
| **Capsules, extended-release:** 2 and 4 mg (*Rx*) | *Detrol LA* (Pharmacia) |

### Indications
*Overactive bladder:* Treatment of patients with an overactive bladder with symptoms of urinary frequency, urgency, or urge incontinence.

### Administration and Dosage
*Immediate-release:* The initial recommended dose is 2 mg twice/day. The dose may be lowered to 1 mg twice/day based on individual response and tolerability. For patients with significantly reduced hepatic function or who are currently taking drugs that are inhibitors of cytochrome P450 3A4, the recommended dose is 1 mg twice/day.

*Extended-release (ER):* The recommended dose is 4 mg once daily taken with liquids and swallowed whole. The dose may be lowered to 2 mg/day based on individual response and tolerability; however, limited efficacy data is available for the 2 mg capsules.

For patients with significantly reduced hepatic or renal function or who are currently taking drugs that are potent inhibitors of CYP3A4, the recommended dose of the ER capsules is 2 mg/day.

#### Actions

*Pharmacology:* Tolterodine is a competitive muscarinic receptor antagonist for overactive bladder. Urinary bladder contraction and salivation are mediated via cholinergic muscarinic receptors.

After oral administration, tolterodine is metabolized in the liver, resulting in the formation of the 5-hydroxymethyl derivative, a major active metabolite. The 5-hydroxymethyl metabolite, which exhibits antimuscarinic activity similar to that of tolterodine, contributes significantly to the therapeutic effect.

Tolterodine has a pronounced effect on bladder function in healthy volunteers. The main effects following a 6.4 mg single dose of tolterodine were an increase in residual urine, reflecting an incomplete emptying of the bladder, and a decrease in detrusor pressure.

*Pharmacokinetics:*

*Absorption* – Tolterodine is rapidly absorbed; 77% or more is absorbed, but absolute bioavailability is highly variable (10% to 74%). Maximum steady-state serum concentrations ($C_{max}$) typically occur within 1 to 2 hours. The pharmacokinetics of tolterodine are dose-proportional over the range of 1 to 4 mg.

*Distribution* – Tolterodine is highly bound to plasma proteins, primarily $\alpha_1$-acid glycoprotein. The 5-hydroxymethyl metabolite is not extensively protein bound, with unbound fraction concentrations averaging approximately 36%.

*Metabolism* – Tolterodine undergoes extensive and variable first-pass hepatic metabolism following oral dosing. The primary metabolic route involves the oxidation of the 5-methyl group mediated by the cytochrome P450 2D6 leading to the formation of an active 5-hydroxymethyl metabolite. Further metabolism leads to formation of the 5-carboxylic acid and N-dealkylated 5-carboxylic acid metabolites, which account for approximately 51% and approximately 29% of the metabolites recovered in the urine, respectively.

*Variability in metabolism:* A subset (approximately 7%) of the population is devoid of CYP2D6, the enzyme responsible for the formation of the 5-hydroxymethyl metabolite of tolterodine. The identified pathway of metabolism for these individuals ("poor metabolizers") is by dealkylation via cytochrome P450 3A4 (CYP3A4) to N-dealkylated tolterodine. The remainder of the population is referred to as "extensive metabolizers." Pharmacokinetic studies revealed that tolterodine is metabolized at a slower rate in poor metabolizers than in extensive metabolizers; this results in significantly higher serum concentrations of tolterodine and in negligible concentrations of the 5-hydroxymethyl metabolite.

*Excretion* – Following a 5 mg oral dose in healthy volunteers, 77% was recovered in urine and 17% was recovered in feces. Less than 1% (less than 2.5% in poor metabolizers) of the dose was recovered as intact tolterodine, and 5% to 14% (less than 1% in poor metabolizers) was recovered as the active 5-hydroxymethyl metabolite.

*Special populations* –

*Renal insufficiency:* Exposure levels of other metabolites of tolterodine were significantly higher (10- to 30-fold) in renally impaired patients.

*Hepatic function impairment:* The elimination half-life of tolterodine was longer in cirrhotic patients (mean, 8.7 hours) than in healthy, young, and elderly volunteers (mean, 2 to 4 hours). The clearance of oral tolterodine was substantially lower in cirrhotic patients (approximately 1.1 L/h/kg) than in the healthy volunteers (approximately 5.7 L/h/kg).

#### Contraindications

Urinary retention; gastric retention; uncontrolled narrow-angle glaucoma; hypersensitivity to the drug or its ingredients.

#### Warnings

*Renal/Hepatic function impairment:* Patients with significantly reduced hepatic function should not receive doses greater than 1 mg twice/day (greater than 2 mg/day for ER capsules). Treat patients with renal impairment with caution.

*Pregnancy: Category* C.

*Lactation:* It is not known whether tolterodine is excreted in human breast milk; therefore, discontinue administration during nursing.

*Children:* Safety and efficacy have not been established.

**Precautions**

*Urinary/Gastric retention:* Administer with caution to patients with clinically significant bladder outflow obstruction because of the risk of urinary retention and to patients with GI obstructive disorders, such as pyloric stenosis, because of the risk of gastric retention.

*Controlled narrow-angle glaucoma:* Use with caution in patients being treated for narrow-angle glaucoma.

**Drug Interactions**

*Fluoxetine:* Fluoxetine is a potent inhibitor of cytochrome P450 2D6 activity. No dose adjustment is required when tolterodine and fluoxetine are coadministered.

*Cytochrome P450:*

*3A4 inhibitors* – Patients receiving cytochrome P450 3A4 inhibitors, such as macrolide antibiotics (erythromycin and clarithromycin), antifungal agents (ketoconazole, itraconazole, and miconazole), or cyclosporine or vinblastine should not receive doses of tolterodine greater than 1 mg twice/day (greater than 2 mg/day for ER capsules).

*2D6* – Tolterodine is not expected to influence the pharmacokinetics of drugs that are metabolized by cytochrome P450 2D6, such as flecainide, vinblastine, carbamazepine, and tricyclic antidepressants.

*Drug/Food interactions:* Food intake increases the bioavailability of tolterodine (average increase 53%). This change is not expected to be a safety concern and adjustment of dose is not needed.

**Adverse Reactions**

Adverse reactions occurring in 3% or more of patients include the following: Dry mouth, headache, dizziness, somnolence, abdominal pain, constipation, dyspepsia, xerophthalmia (extended- and immediate-release); diarrhea, fatigue, flu-like syndrome (immediate-release).

# TROSPIUM CHLORIDE

| **Tablets:** 20 mg *(Rx)* | *Sanctura* (Odyssey, Indevus) |

**Indications**

*Overactive bladder:* For the treatment of overactive bladder with symptoms of urge urinary incontinence, urgency, and urinary frequency.

**Administration and Dosage**

*TROSPIUM CHLORIDE:* The recommended dose is 20 mg twice daily. Dose at least 1 hour before meals or give on an empty stomach.

*Renal function impairment* – For patients with severe renal impairment (creatinine clearance [Ccr] less than 30 mL/min), the recommended dose is 20 mg once daily at bedtime.

*Elderly* – In elderly patients, 75 years of age and older, dose may be titrated down to 20 mg once daily based upon tolerability.

**Actions**

*Pharmacology:* Trospium is an antispasmodic, antimuscarinic agent. Trospium antagonizes the effect of acetylcholine on muscarinic receptors in cholinergically innervated organs. Its parasympatholytic action reduces the tonus of smooth muscle in the bladder. Trospium increases maximum cystometric bladder capacity and volume at first detrusor contraction.

*Pharmacokinetics:*

*Absorption* – After oral administration, less than 10% of the dose is absorbed. Mean absolute bioavailability of a 20 mg dose is 9.6% (range, 4% to 16.1%). Peak plasma concentrations ($C_{max}$) occur between 5 to 6 hours postdose. Mean $C_{max}$ increases greater than dose-proportionally; a 3-fold and 4-fold increase in $C_{max}$ was observed for dose increases from 20 to 40 mg and from 20 to 60 mg, respectively.

*Distribution* – Protein binding ranged from 50% to 85% when therapeutic concentration levels (0.5 to 50 ng/mL) were incubated with human serum in vitro. The majority of trospium is distributed in plasma. The apparent volume of distribution for a 20 mg oral dose is 395 ($\pm$ 140) L.

*Metabolism* – The metabolic pathway of trospium in humans has not been fully defined. Of the 10% of the dose absorbed, metabolites account for approximately 40% of the excreted dose following oral administration. The major metabolic pathway is hypothesized as ester hydrolysis with subsequent conjugation of benzylic acid to form azoniaspironortropanol with glucuronic acid. Cytochrome P450 is not expected to contribute significantly to the elimination of trospium.

*Excretion* – The plasma half-life for trospium following oral administration is approximately 20 hours. After administration of oral trospium, the majority of the dose (85.2%) was recovered in feces and a smaller amount (5.8%) was recovered in urine; 60% of the radioactivity excreted in urine was unchanged trospium. The mean renal clearance for trospium (29.07 L/h) is 4-fold higher than average glomerular filtration rate, indicating that active tubular secretion is a major route of elimination for trospium. There may be competition for elimination with other compounds that also are renally eliminated.

*Special populations* –

Gender: Studies comparing the pharmacokinetics in different genders had conflicting results. When a single 40 mg trospium dose was administered to 16 elderly subjects, exposure was 45% lower in elderly females compared with elderly males. When 20 mg trospium was dosed twice daily for 4 days to 6 elderly males and 6 elderly females (60 to 75 years of age), AUC and $C_{max}$ were 26% and 68% higher, respectively, in females without hormone replacement therapy than in males.

*Renal function impairment:* Severe renal impairment significantly altered the disposition of trospium. A 4.5-fold and 2-fold increase in mean $AUC_{0-\infty}$ and $C_{max}$, respectively, and the appearance of an additional elimination phase with a long half-life (approximately 33 hours) was detected in patients with severe renal insufficiency (Ccr less than 30 mL/min) compared with healthy, nearly age-matched subjects. The different pharmacokinetic behavior of trospium in patients with severe renal insufficiency necessitates adjustment of dosage frequency. The pharmacokinetics of trospium have not been studied in people with mild or moderate renal impairment (Ccr from 30 to 80 mL/min).

*Hepatic function impairment:* $C_{max}$ increased 12% and 63% in subjects with mild and moderate hepatic impairment, respectively, compared with healthy subjects. AUC was similar. Use caution when administering trospium to patients with moderate and severe hepatic dysfunction.

## Contraindications

Patients with urinary retention, gastric retention, or uncontrolled narrow-angle glaucoma and patients at risk for these conditions; hypersensitivity to the drug or its ingredients.

## Warnings

*Renal function impairment:* Dose modification is recommended in patients with severe renal insufficiency (Ccr less than 30 mL/min). In such patients, administer trospium as 20 mg once daily at bedtime.

*Hepatic function impairment:* Use caution when administering trospium in patients with moderate or severe hepatic dysfunction.

*Elderly:* In 2 studies, the incidence of commonly reported anticholinergic adverse events in patients treated with trospium (including dry mouth, constipation, dyspepsia, UTI, and urinary retention) was higher in patients 75 years of age and older as compared with younger patients. This effect may be related to an enhanced sensitivity to anticholinergic agents in this patient population.

*Pregnancy: Category C.*

*Lactation:* Trospium (2 mg/kg orally and 50 mcg/kg IV) was excreted, to a limited extent (less than 1%), into the milk of lactating rats. It is not known whether this drug is excreted in human milk. Exercise caution when administering trospium to a nursing mother. Use during lactation only if the potential benefit justifies the potential risk to the newborn.

*Children:* Safety and efficacy in pediatric patients have not been established.

## Precautions

*Cardiac effects:* Asymptomatic, nonspecific T-wave inversions were observed in 1 study more often in subjects receiving trospium than in subjects receiving moxifloxacin or placebo following 5 days of treatment. This finding was not observed during routine safety monitoring in 2 other placebo-controlled clinical trials in 591 trospium-treated overactive bladder patients. The clinical significance of T-wave inversion in this study is unknown.

*Decreased GI motility:* Use caution in patients with conditions such as ulcerative colitis, intestinal atony, and myasthenia gravis.

*Narrow-angle glaucoma:* In patients being treated for narrow-angle glaucoma, only use trospium if the potential benefits outweigh the risks and, in that circumstance, only with careful monitoring.

*Risk of urinary retention:* Administer trospium with caution to patients with clinically significant bladder outflow obstruction because of the risk of urinary retention.

## Drug Interactions

Drugs that may affect trospium include other anticholinergic agents; drugs eliminated by active tubular secretion.

Drugs that may be affected by trospium include those eliminated by active tubular secretion (eg, digoxin, procainamide, pancuronium, morphine, vancomycin, metformin, and tenofovir).

*Drug/Food interactions:* It is recommended that trospium be taken at least 1 hour prior to meals or on an empty stomach.

## Adverse Reactions

The three most common adverse events reported by patients receiving 20 mg trospium twice daily were dry mouth, constipation, and headache.

# THIAZIDES AND RELATED DIURETICS

| | |
|---|---|
| **BENDROFLUMETHIAZIDE** | |
| **Tablets:** 5 and 10 mg (*Rx*) | *Naturetin* (Princeton) |
| **CHLOROTHIAZIDE** | |
| **Tablets:** 250 and 500 mg (*Rx*) | Various, *Diuril* (Merck), *Diurigen* (Goldline) |
| **Suspension:** 250 mg/5 mL (*Rx*) | *Diuril* (Merck) |
| **Powder for injection, lyophilized:** 500 mg (as sodium) (*Rx*) | *Sodium Diuril* (Merck) |
| **CHLORTHALIDONE** | |
| **Tablets:** 15, 25, 50, and 100 mg (*Rx*) | Various, *Hygroton* (Rhone-Poulenc Rorer), *Thalitone* (Horus Therapeutics) |
| **HYDROCHLOROTHIAZIDE** | |
| **Tablets:** 25, 50, and 100 mg (*Rx*) | Various, *Esidrix* (Ciba), *Ezide* (Econo Med), *HydroDIURIL* (Merck), *Hydro-Par* (Parmed), *Oretic* (Abbott) |
| **Solution:** 50 mg/5 mL (*Rx*) | *Hydrochlorothiazide* (Roxane) |
| **INDAPAMIDE** | |
| **Tablets:** 1.25 and 2.5 mg (*Rx*) | Various, *Lozol* (Rhone-Poulenc Rorer) |
| **METHYCLOTHIAZIDE** | |
| **Tablets:** 2.5 and 5 mg (*Rx*) | Various, *Aquatensen* (Wallace), *Enduron* (Abbott) |
| **METOLAZONE** | |
| **Tablets:** 2.5, 5 and 10 mg (*Rx*) | *Zaroxolyn* (Fisons) |
| **0.5 mg** (*Rx*) | *Mykrox* (Fisons) |
| **QUINETHAZONE** | |
| **Tablets:** 50 mg (*Rx*) | *Hydromox* (Lederle) |
| **TRICHLORMETHIAZIDE** | |
| **Tablets:** 2 and 4 mg | Various, *Diurese* (American Urologicals), *Metahydrin* (Marion Merrell Dow), *Naqua* (Schering) |

### Indications

*Edema:* Adjunctive therapy in edema associated with congestive heart failure (CHF), hepatic cirrhosis, and corticosteroid and estrogen therapy. Useful in edema due to renal dysfunction (eg, nephrotic syndrome, acute glomerulonephritis, chronic renal failure).

*Indapamide* – Indapamide alone is indicated for edema associated with CHF.

*Metolazone* – Metolazone, rapidly acting (*Mykrox*), has not been evaluated for the treatment of CHF or fluid retention due to renal or hepatic disease, and the correct dosage for these conditions and other edematous states has not been established.

*Hypertension:* As the sole therapeutic agent or to enhance other antihypertensive drugs in more severe forms of hypertension.

### Administration and Dosage

BENDROFLUMETHIAZIDE:

*Edema* – 5 mg once daily, preferably in the morning.

*Initial:* Up to 20 mg once daily or divided into 2 doses.

*Maintenance:* 2.5 to 5 mg/day.

*Hypertension* –

*Initial:* 5 to 20 mg/day.

*Maintenance:* 2.5 to 15 mg/day.

CHLOROTHIAZIDE:

*Adults* –

*Edema:* 0.5 to 1 g once or twice/day, orally or IV. Reserve IV route for patients unable to take oral medication or for emergency situations.

*Hypertension (oral forms only):* Starting dose is 0.5 to 1 g/day as a single or divided dose. Rarely, some patients may require up to 2 g/day in divided doses.

*Infants and children* –

*Oral:* 22 mg/kg/day (10 mg/lb/day) in 2 doses. Infants younger than 6 months of age may require up to 33 mg/kg/day (15 mg/lb/day) in 2 doses.

On this basis, infants up to 2 years of age may be given 125 to 375 mg/day in 2 doses. Children from 2 to 12 years of age may be given 375 mg to 1 g/day in 2 doses.

IV use is not generally recommended.

CHLORTHALIDONE: Give as a single dose with food in the morning. Maintenance doses may be lower than initial doses.

*Edema* – Initiate therapy with 50 to 100 mg (*Thalitone*, 30 to 60 mg) daily, or 100 mg (*Thalitone*, 60 mg) on alternate days. Some patients may require 150 or 200 mg (*Thalitone*, 90 to 120 mg) at these intervals, or 120 mg *Thalitone* daily. However, dosages above this level do not usually create a greater response.

*Hypertension* – Initiate therapy with a single dose of 25 mg/day (*Thalitone*, 15 mg). If response is insufficient after a suitable trial, increase to 50 mg (*Thalitone*, increase from 30 to 50 mg). For additional control, increase dosage to 100 mg once daily (except *Thalitone*), or add a second antihypertensive.

*Note:* Doses greater than 25 mg/day are likely to potentiate potassium excretion but provide no further benefit in sodium excretion or blood pressure reduction.

HYDROCHLOROTHIAZIDE:
    *Adults* –
        *Edema:*
            *Initial* – 25 to 200 mg/day for several days, or until dry weight is attained.
            *Maintenance* – 25 to 100 mg/day or intermittently. Refractory patients may require up to 200 mg/day.
        *Hypertension* –
            *Initial:* 50 mg/day as a single or 2 divided doses. Doses greater than 50 mg are often associated with marked reductions in serum potassium. Patients usually do not require doses greater than 50 mg/day when combined with other antihypertensives.

        *Infants and children:* Usual dosage is 2.2 mg/kg (1 mg/lb) daily in 2 doses. Pediatric patients with hypertension only rarely will benefit from doses greater than 50 mg/day.

            *Infants (younger than 6 months of age)* – Up to 3.3 mg/kg (1.5 mg/lb) daily in 2 doses.

            *Infants (6 months to 2 years of age)* – 12.5 to 37.5 mg/day in 2 doses. Base dosage on body weight.

            *Children (2 to 12 years of age)* – 37.5 to 100 mg/day in 2 doses. Base dosage on body weight.

INDAPAMIDE:
    *Edema of congestive heart failure* –
        *Adults:* 2.5 mg as a single daily dose in the morning. If response is not satisfactory after 1 week, increase to 5 mg once daily.
    *Hypertension* –
        *Adults:* 1.25 mg as a single daily dose taken in the morning. If the response to 1.25 mg is not satisfactory after 4 weeks, increase the daily dose to 2.5 mg taken once daily. If the response to 2.5 mg is not satisfactory after 4 weeks, the daily dose may be increased to 5 mg taken once daily, but consider adding another antihypertensive.

METHYCLOTHIAZIDE:
    *Edema* –
        *Adults:* 2.5 to 10 mg once daily. Maximum effective single dose is 10 mg.
    *Hypertension* –
        *Adults:* 2.5 to 5 mg once daily. If blood pressure control is not satisfactory after 8 to 12 weeks with 5 mg once daily, add another antihypertensive.

METOLAZONE: Individualize dosage.
    *Zaroxolyn* –
        *Mild to moderate essential hypertension:* 2.5 to 5 mg once daily.
        *Edema of renal disease/cardiac failure:* 5 to 20 mg once daily.

Mykrox –

*Mild to moderate hypertension:* 0.5 mg as a single daily dose taken in the morning. If response is inadequate, increase the dose to 1 mg daily. Do not increase dosage if blood pressure is not controlled with 1 mg. Rather, add another antihypertensive agent with a different mechanism of action.

*Brand interchange* – The metolazone formulations are not bioequivalent or therapeutically equivalent at the same doses. Mykrox is more rapidly and completely bioavailable. Do not interchange brands.

QUINETHAZONE:

*Adults* – 50 to 100 mg once daily. Occasionally, 50 mg twice daily; 150 to 200 mg/day may be necessary infrequently.

TRICHLORMETHIAZIDE:

*Edema* – 2 to 4 mg once daily.

*Hypertension* – 2 to 4 mg once daily. In initiating therapy, doses may be given twice daily.

## Actions

*Pharmacology:* Thiazide diuretics increase the urinary excretion of sodium and chloride in approximately equivalent amounts. They inhibit reabsorption of sodium and chloride in the cortical thick ascending limb of the loop of Henle and the early distal tubules. Other common actions include: Increased potassium and bicarbonate excretion, decreased calcium excretion and uric acid retention. At maximal therapeutic dosages all thiazides are approximately equal in diuretic efficacy.

The antihypertensive action requires several days to produce effects. Administration for less than or equal to 2 to 4 weeks is usually required for optimal therapeutic effect. The duration of the antihypertensive effect of the thiazides is sufficiently long to adequately control blood pressure with a single daily dose.

*Pharmacokinetics:*

| Pharmacokinetics of Thiazides and Related Diuretics | | | | | | |
|---|---|---|---|---|---|---|
| Diuretic | Onset (hours) | Peak (hours) | Duration (hours) | Equivalent dose (mg) | Percent absorbed | Half-life (hours) |
| Bendroflumethiazide | 2 | 4 | 16 to 12 | 5 | $\approx$ 100 | 3 to 3.9 |
| Chlorothiazide | 2[2] | 4[2] | 16 to 12 | 500 | 10 to 21[3] | 0.75 to 2 |
| Chlorthalidone | 2 to 3 | 2 to 6 | 24 to 72 | 50 | 64[3] | 40 |
| Hydrochlorothiazide | 2 | 4 to 6 | 16 to 12 | 50 | 65 to 75 | 5.6 to 14.8 |
| Indapamide | 1 to 2 | $\leq$ 2 | up to 36 | 2.5 | 93 | $\approx$ 14 |
| Methyclothiazide | 2 | 6 | 24 | 5 | nd[1] | nd[1] |
| Metolazone[4] | 1 | 2 | 12 to 24 | 5 | 65 | nd[1] |
| Quinethazone | 2 | 6 | 18 to 24 | 50 | nd[1] | nd[1] |
| Trichlormethiazide | 2 | 6 | 24 | 2 | nd[1] | 2.3 to 7.3 |

[1] nd = No data.
[2] Following IV use, onset of action is 15 minutes; peak occurs in 30 minutes.
[3] Bioavailability may be dose-dependent.
[4] Mykrox only: Peak plasma concentrations reached in 2 to 4 h, t½ approximately 14 h.

## Contraindications

Anuria; renal decompensation; hypersensitivity to thiazides or related diuretics or sulfonamide-derived drugs; hepatic coma or precoma (**metolazone**).

## Warnings

*Parenteral use:* Use IV **chlorothiazide** only when patients are unable to take oral medication or in an emergency. In infants and children, IV use is not recommended.

*Lupus erythematosus:* Lupus erythematosus exacerbation or activation has occurred.

*Hypersensitivity reactions:* Hypersensitivity reactions may occur in patients with or without a history of allergy or bronchial asthma; cross-sensitivity with sulfonamides may also occur. Refer to Management of Acute Hypersensitivity Reactions.

*Renal function impairment:* Use with caution in severe renal disease because these agents may precipitate azotemia. Cumulative effects of the drug may develop in patients with impaired renal function. Monitor renal function periodically. **Metolazone** is the only thiazide-like diuretic that may produce diuresis in patients with GFR less than 20 mL/min. Indapamide may also be useful in patients with impaired renal function.

*Pregnancy: Category B* (chlorothiazide, chlorthalidone, hydrochlorothiazide, indapamide, metolazone); *Category C* (bendroflumethiazide, methyclothiazide, trichlormethiazide). Routine use during normal pregnancy is inappropriate.

*Lactation:* Thiazides may appear in breast milk. Discontinue nursing or the drug.

*Children:* Bendroflumethiazide, chlorthalidone, hydrochlorothiazide, methyclothiazide, metolazone, trichlormethiazide – Safety and efficacy have not been established. Metolazone is not recommended for use in children. In infants and children, IV use of chlorothiazide has been limited and is generally not recommended.

## Precautions

*Fluid/Electrolyte balance:* Perform initial and periodic determinations of serum electrolytes, BUN, uric acid and glucose. Observe patients for clinical signs of fluid or electrolyte imbalance (eg, hyponatremia, hypochloremic alkalosis, hypokalemia, changes in serum and urinary calcium).

*Hypokalemia* – Hypokalemia may develop during concomitant corticosteroids, ACTH, and especially with brisk diuresis, with severe liver disease or cirrhosis, vomiting or diarrhea, or after prolonged therapy.

*Hyponatremia/Hypochloremia* – A chloride deficit is generally mild and usually does not require specific treatment, except in extraordinary circumstances (as in liver or renal disease). Thiazide-induced hyponatremia has been associated with death and neurologic damage in elderly patients.

*Hypomagnesemia* – Thiazide diuretics have been shown to increase urinary excretion of magnesium, resulting in hypomagnesemia.

*Hypercalcemia* – Calcium excretion may be decreased by thiazide diuretics.

*Hyperuricemia* – Hyperuricemia may occur or acute gout may be precipitated in certain patients receiving thiazides, even in those patients without a history of gouty attacks.

*Glucose tolerance* – Hyperglycemia may occur with thiazide diuretics.

*Lipids:* Thiazides may cause increased concentrations of total serum cholesterol, total triglycerides and LDL (but not HDL) in some patients, although these appear to return to pretreatment levels with long-term therapy.

*Photosensitivity:* Photosensitization may occur.

## Drug Interactions

Drugs that may be affected by thiazides include the following: Allopurinol; anesthetics; anticoagulants; antigout agents; antineoplastics; calcium salts; diazoxide; digitalis glycosides; insulin; lithium; loop diuretics; methyldopa; nondepolarizing muscle relaxants; sulfonylureas; vitamin D. Drugs that may affect thiazides include: Amphotericin B; anticholinergics; bile acid sequestrants; corticosteroids; methenamines; NSAIDs.

*Drug/Lab test interactions:* Thiazides may decrease serum PBI levels without signs of thyroid disturbance. Thiazides also may cause diagnostic interference of serum electrolyte, blood, and urine glucose levels (usually only in patients with a predisposition to glucose intolerance), serum bilirubin levels, and serum uric acid levels. In uremic patients, serum magnesium levels may be increased. **Bendroflumethiazide** and **trichlormethiazide** may interfere with the phenolsulfonphthalein test due to decreased excretion. In the phentolamine and tyramine tests, bendroflumethiazide may produce false-negative and trichlormethiazide may produce false-positive results.

## Adverse Reactions

| Adverse reaction | Bendroflumethiazide | Chlorothiazide | Chlorthalidone | Hydrochlorothiazide | Indapamide | Methyclothiazide | Metolazone | Quinethazone | Trichlormethiazide |
|---|---|---|---|---|---|---|---|---|---|
| *Cardiovascular* | | | | | | | | | |
| Orthostatic hypotension | ✔ | ✔ | | ✔ | <5% | ✔ | <2%[1] | ✔ | ✔ |
| Palpitations | | | | | <5% | | <2%[2] | | ✔ |
| *CNS* | | | | | | | | | |
| Dizziness/Lightheadedness | ✔ | ✔ | ✔ | ✔ | ≥5% | ✔ | 10%[2] | ✔ | ✔ |
| Vertigo | ✔ | ✔ | ✔ | ✔ | <5% | ✔ | ✔[3] | ✔ | ✔ |
| Headache | ✔ | ✔ | ✔ | ✔ | ≥5% | ✔ | 9%[2] | ✔ | ✔ |
| Paresthesias | ✔ | ✔ | ✔ | ✔ | | ✔ | ✔[3] | ✔ | ✔ |
| Xanthopsia | ✔ | ✔ | ✔ | ✔ | | ✔ | | ✔ | ✔ |
| Weakness | ✔ | ✔ | ✔ | ✔ | ≥5% | ✔ | <2%[4] | ✔ | ✔ |
| Restlessness/Insomnia | ✔ | ✔ | ✔ | ✔ | <5% | ✔ | ✔[3] | ✔ | ✔ |
| Drowsiness | | | | | <5% | | ✔[3] | | ✔ |
| Fatigue/Lethargy/Malaise/Lassitude | | | | | ≥5% | | 4%[2] | | ✔ |
| Anxiety | | | | | ≥5% | | <2%[3] | | |
| Depression | | | | | <5% | | <2%[2] | | ✔ |
| Nervousness | | | | | ≥5% | | <2%[3] | | |
| Blurred vision (may be transient) | ✔ | ✔ | | ✔ | <5% | | ✔[3] | | |
| *GI* | | | | | | | | | |
| Anorexia | ✔ | ✔ | ✔ | ✔ | <5% | ✔ | ✔[3] | ✔ | ✔ |
| Gastric irritation/epigastric distress | ✔ | ✔ | ✔ | ✔ | <5% | ✔ | | ✔ | ✔ |
| Nausea | ✔ | ✔ | ✔ | ✔ | <5% | ✔ | <2%[2] | ✔ | ✔ |
| Vomiting | ✔ | ✔ | ✔ | ✔ | <5% | ✔ | <2%[4] | ✔ | ✔ |
| Abdominal pain/cramping/bloating | ✔ | ✔ | ✔ | ✔ | <5% | ✔ | <2%[2] | ✔ | ✔ |
| Diarrhea | ✔ | ✔ | ✔ | ✔ | <5% | ✔ | <2%[2] | ✔ | ✔ |
| Constipation | ✔ | ✔ | ✔ | ✔ | <5% | ✔ | <2%[2] | ✔ | ✔ |
| Jaundice (intrahepatic/cholestatic) | ✔ | ✔ | ✔ | ✔ | | ✔ | ✔[3] | ✔ | ✔ |
| Pancreatitis | ✔ | ✔ | ✔ | ✔ | | ✔ | ✔[3] | ✔ | ✔ |
| Dry mouth | | | | | <5% | | <2%[1] | | ✔ |
| *GU* | | | | | | | | | |
| Nocturia | | | | | <5% | | <2%[1] | | |
| Impotence/Reduced libido | ✔ | ✔ | ✔ | ✔ | <5% | ✔ | <2%[2] | ✔ | ✔ |
| *Hematologic* | | | | | | | | | |
| Leukopenia | ✔ | ✔ | ✔ | ✔ | | ✔ | ✔[3] | ✔ | ✔ |
| Thrombocytopenia | ✔ | ✔ | ✔ | ✔ | | ✔ | | ✔ | ✔ |
| Agranulocytosis | ✔ | ✔ | ✔ | ✔ | | ✔ | ✔[3] | ✔ | ✔ |
| Aplastic/Hypoplastic anemia | ✔ | ✔ | ✔ | ✔ | | ✔ | ✔[3] | ✔ | ✔ |
| *Dermatologic* | | | | | | | | | |
| Purpura | ✔ | ✔ | ✔ | ✔ | | ✔ | ✔[3] | ✔ | ✔ |
| Photosensitivity/Photosensitivity dermatitis | ✔ | ✔ | ✔ | ✔ | | ✔ | ✔[3] | ✔ | ✔ |
| Rash | ✔ | ✔ | ✔ | ✔ | <5% | ✔ | <2%[2] | ✔ | ✔ |
| Urticaria | ✔ | ✔ | ✔ | ✔ | | | ✔[3] | ✔ | ✔ |
| Necrotizing angiitis, vasculitis, cutaneous vasculitis | ✔ | ✔ | ✔ | ✔ | <5% | ✔ | ✔[2] | ✔ | ✔ |
| Pruritus | ✔ | | | | <5% | | <2%[1] | | |

## Adverse Reactions of Thiazides and Related Diuretics

| Adverse reaction | Bendroflumethiazide | Chlorothiazide | Chlorthalidone | Hydrochlorothiazide | Indapamide | Methyclothiazide | Metolazone | Quinethazone | Trichlormethiazide |
|---|---|---|---|---|---|---|---|---|---|
| *Metabolic* | | | | | | | | | |
| Hyperglycemia | ✔ | ✔ | ✔ | ✔ | <5% | ✔ | ✔[3] | ✔ | ✔ |
| Glycosuria | ✔ | ✔ | ✔ | ✔ | <5% | ✔ | ✔[3] | ✔ | ✔ |
| Hyperuricemia | ✔ | ✔ | ✔ | ✔ | <5% | ✔ | | | ✔ |
| *Miscellaneous* | | | | | | | | | |
| Muscle cramp/spasm | ✔ | ✔ | ✔ | ✔ | ≥5% | ✔ | 6%[2] | ✔ | ✔ |

[1] Percentage of occurrence refers to rapidly acting doseform; however this adverse reaction also occurred with the slow acting doseform.
[2] IV doseform.
[3] Possibly with life-threatening anaphylactic shock.
[4] Slow acting doseform only.

# LOOP DIURETICS

| | |
|---|---|
| **BUMETANIDE** | |
| **Tablets**: 0.5, 1, and 2 mg (*Rx*) | Various, *Bumex* (Roche) |
| **Injection**: 0.25 mg/mL (*Rx*) | |
| **ETHACRYNIC ACID** | |
| **Tablets**: 25 and 50 mg (*Rx*) | *Edecrin* (Merck) |
| **Powder for Injection**: 50 mg (as ethacrynate sodium) per vial (*Rx*) | *Edecrin Sodium* (Merck) |
| **FUROSEMIDE** | |
| **Tablets**: 20, 40, and 80 mg (*Rx*) | Various, *Lasix* (Hoechst-Roussel) |
| **Oral Solution**: 10 mg/mL (*Rx*) | |
| **Injection**: 10 mg/mL (*Rx*) | |
| **TORSEMIDE** | |
| **Tablets**: 5, 10, 20, and 100 mg (*Rx*) | *Demadex* (Boehringer Mannheim) |
| **Injection**: 10 mg/mL (*Rx*) | |

> **Warning:**
> These agents are potent diuretics; excess amounts can lead to a profound diuresis with water and electrolyte depletion.

### Indications

*Edema:* Edema associated with CHF, hepatic cirrhosis, and renal disease, including the nephrotic syndrome. Particularly useful when greater diuretic potential is desired.

Parenteral administration is indicated when a rapid onset of diuresis is desired (eg, acute pulmonary edema), when GI absorption is impaired or when oral use is not practical for any reason. As soon as it is practical, replace with oral therapy.

*Hypertension (furosemide, oral; torsemide, oral):* Alone or in combination with other antihypertensive drugs.

*Ethacrynic acid:*

*Ascites* – Short-term management of ascites due to malignancy, idiopathic edema, and lymphedema.

*Congenital heart disease, nephrotic syndrome* – Short-term management of hospitalized pediatric patients, other than infants.

*Pulmonary edema, acute* – Adjunctive therapy.

### Administration and Dosage

BUMETANIDE:

*Oral* – 0.5 to 2 mg/day, given as a single dose. If diuretic response is not adequate, give a second or third dose at 4- to 5-hour intervals, up to a maximum daily dose of 10 mg. An intermittent dose schedule, given on alternate days or for 3 to 4 days with rest periods of 1 to 2 days in between, is the safest and most effective method for the continued control of edema. In patients with hepatic failure, keep the dose to a minimum, and if necessary, increase the dose carefully.

*Parenteral* – Initially, 0.5 to 1 mg IV or IM. Administer IV over a period of 1 to 2 minutes. If the initial response is insufficient, give a second or third dose at intervals of 2 to 3 hours; do not exceed a daily dosage of 10 mg. End parenteral treatment and start oral treatment as soon as possible.

*Renal function impairment* – In patients with severe chronic renal insufficiency, a continuous infusion of bumetanide (12 mg over 12 hours) may be more effective and less toxic than intermittent bolus therapy.

ETHACRYNIC ACID:

*Oral* –

*Initial therapy:* Give minimally effective dose (usually, 50 to 200 mg/day) on a continuous or intermittent dosage schedule to produce gradual weight loss of 2.2 to 4.4 kg/day (1 to 2 lb/day). Adjust dose in 25 to 50 mg increments. Higher doses, up to 200 mg twice daily, achieved gradually, are most often required in patients with severe, refractory edema.

*Children:* Initial dose is 25 mg. Make careful increments of 25 mg to achieve maintenance. Dosage for infants has not been established.

*Maintenance therapy:* Administer intermittently after an effective diuresis is obtained using an alternate daily schedule or more prolonged periods of diuretic therapy interspersed with rest periods.

*Parenteral* – Do not give subcutaneously or IM because of local pain and irritation. The usual IV dose for the average adult is 50 mg, or 0.5 to 1 mg/kg. Give slowly through the tubing of a running infusion or by direct IV injection over several minutes. Usually, only 1 dose is necessary; occasionally, a second dose may be required; use a new injection site to avoid thrombophlebitis. A single IV dose, not exceeding 100 mg, has been used. Insufficient pediatric experience precludes recommendation for this age group.

FUROSEMIDE:
Oral –

*Edema:* 20 to 80 mg/day as a single dose. Depending on response, administer a second dose 6 to 8 hours later. If response is not satisfactory, increase by increments of 20 or 40 mg, no sooner than 6 to 8 hours after previous dose, until desired diuresis occurs. This dose should then be given once or twice daily (eg, at 8 am and 2 pm). Dosage may be titrated up to 600 mg/day in patients with severe edema.

Mobilization of edema may be most efficiently and safely accomplished with an intermittent dosage schedule; the drug is given 2 to 4 consecutive days each week. With doses greater than 80 mg/day, clinical and laboratory observations are advisable.

*Hypertension:* 40 mg twice a day; adjust according to response. If the patient does not respond, add other antihypertensive agents. Reduce dosage of other agents by at least 50% as soon as furosemide is added to prevent excessive drop in blood pressure.

*Infants and children:* 2 mg/kg. If diuresis is unsatisfactory, increase by 1 or 2 mg/kg, no sooner than 6 to 8 hours after previous dose. Doses greater than 6 mg/kg are not recommended. For maintenance therapy, adjust dose to the minimum effective level. A dose range of 0.5 to 2 mg/kg twice daily has also been recommended.

*CHF and chronic renal failure:* It has been suggested that doses as high as 2 to 2.5 g/day or more are well tolerated and effective in these patients.

Parenteral –

*Edema:* Initial dose: 20 to 40 mg IM or IV. Give the IV injection slowly (1 to 2 minutes). If needed, another dose may be given in the same manner 2 hours later. The dose may be raised by 20 mg and given no sooner than 2 hours after previous dose, until desired diuretic effect is obtained. This dose should then be given once or twice daily. Administer high-dose parenteral therapy as a controlled infusion at a rate 4 mg/min or less.

*Acute pulmonary edema:* The usual initial dose is 40 mg IV (over 1 to 2 minutes). If response is not satisfactory within 1 hour, increase to 80 mg IV (over 1 to 2 minutes).

*Infants and children:* 1 mg/kg IV or IM given slowly under close supervision. If diuretic response after the initial dose is not satisfactory, increase the dosage by 1 mg/kg, no sooner than 2 hours after previous dose, until desired effect is obtained. Doses greater than 6 mg/kg are not recommended.

*CHF and chronic renal failure:* It has been suggested that doses as high as 2 to 2.5 g/day or more are well tolerated and effective in these patients. For IV bolus injections, the maximum should not exceed 1 g/day given over 30 minutes.

TORSEMIDE: Torsemide may be given at any time in relation to a meal.

Because of high bioavailability, oral and IV doses are therapeutically equivalent, so patients may be switched to and from the IV form with no change in dose. Administer the IV injection slowly over a period of 2 minutes.

*Congestive heart failure/chronic renal failure* – The usual initial dose is 10 or 20 mg once daily oral or IV. If the diuretic response is inadequate, titrate the dose upward by approximately doubling until the desired diuretic response is obtained. Single doses greater than 200 mg have not been adequately studied.

*Hepatic cirrhosis* – The usual initial dose is 5 or 10 mg once daily oral or IV, administered together with an aldosterone antagonist or a potassium-sparing diuretic. If the diuretic response is inadequate, titrate the dose upward by approximately doubling until the desired diuretic response is obtained. Single doses greater than 40 mg have not been adequately studied.

*Hypertension* – The usual initial dose is 5 mg once daily. If the 5 mg dose does not provide adequate reduction in blood pressure within 4 to 6 weeks, the dose may be increased to 10 mg once daily.

### Actions

*Pharmacology:* Furosemide and ethacrynic acid inhibit primarily reabsorption of sodium and chloride, not only in proximal and distal tubules, but also the loop of Henle. In contrast, bumetanide is more chloruretic than natriuretic and may have an additional action in the proximal tubule; it does not appear to act on the distal tubule. Torsemide acts from within the lumen of the thick ascending portion of the loop of Henle, where it inhibits the $Na^+/K^+/2Cl^-$-carrier system.

*Pharmacokinetics:* These agents are metabolized and excreted primarily through the urine. Protein binding of these agents exceeds 90%. Furosemide is metabolized approximately 30% to 40%, and its urinary excretion is 60% to 70%. Oral administration of bumetanide revealed that 81% was excreted in urine, 45% of it as unchanged drug. Torsemide is cleared from the circulation by both hepatic metabolism (approximately 80% of total clearance) and excretion into the urine (approximately 20% of total clearance).

| Pharmacokinetic Parameters of the Loop Diuretics | | | | | | | | |
|---|---|---|---|---|---|---|---|---|
| Diuretic | Bioavail-ability (%) | Half-life (min) | Onset of action (min) | Peak (min) | Duration (h) | Dosage (mg) | Relative potency | Doses/day |
| Bumetanide | | | | | | | | |
| Oral | 72-96 | 60-90[5] | 30-60 | 60-120 | 4-6 | 0.5-2 | ≈ 40 | 1 |
| IV | | | within minutes | 15-30 | 0.5-1 | 0.5-1 | ≈ 40 | 1-3 |
| Ethacrynic acid | | | | | | | | |
| Oral | ≈100 | 60 | ≤ 30 | 120 | 6-8 | 50-100 | 0.6-0.8 | 1-2 |
| IV | | | ≤ 5 | 15-30 | 2 | 50 | 0.6-0.8 | 1-2 |
| Furosemide | | | | | | | | |
| Oral | 60-64[1] | ≈ 120[2] | ≤ 60 | 60-120[3] | 6-8 | 20-80 | 1 | 1-2 |
| IV or IM | | | ≤ 5[4] | 30 | 2 | 20-40 | 1 | |
| Torsemide | | | | | | | | |
| Oral | ≈ 80 | 210 | ≤ 60 | 60-120 | 6-8 | 5-20 | 2-4 | 1 |
| IV | | | ≤ 10 | ≤ 60 | 6-8 | 5-20 | 2-4 | 1 |

[1] Decreased in uremia and nephrosis.
[2] Prolonged in renal failure, uremia and in neonates.
[3] Decreased in CHF.
[4] Somewhat delayed after IM administration.
[5] Prolonged in renal disease.

### Contraindications

Anuria; hypersensitivity to these compounds or to sulfonylureas; infants (ethacrynic acid); patients with hepatic coma or in states of severe electrolyte depletion until the condition is improved or corrected (bumetanide).

### Warnings

*Dehydration:* Excessive diuresis may result in dehydration and reduction in blood volume with circulatory collapse and the possibility of vascular thrombosis and embolism, particularly in elderly patients.

*Hepatic cirrhosis and ascites:* In these patients, sudden alterations of electrolyte balance may precipitate hepatic encephalopathy and coma. Do not institute therapy until the basic condition is improved.

*Ototoxicity:* Tinnitus, reversible and irreversible hearing impairment, deafness, and vertigo with a sense of fullness in the ears have been reported. Deafness is usually reversible and of short duration (1 to 24 hours); however, irreversible hearing impairment has occurred. Usually, ototoxicity is associated with rapid injection, with severe renal impairment, with doses several times the usual dose, and with concurrent use with other ototoxic drugs.

*Systemic lupus erythematosus:* Systemic lupus erythematosus may be exacerbated or activated.

*Thrombocytopenia:* Because there have been rare spontaneous reports of thrombocytopenia with **bumetanide,** observe regularly for possible occurrence.

*Hypersensitivity reactions:* Patients with known sulfonamide sensitivity may show allergic reactions to **furosemide, torsemide,** or **bumetanide.** Bumetanide use following instances of allergic reactions to furosemide suggests a lack of cross-sensitivity. Refer to Management of Acute Hypersensitivity Reactions.

*Renal function impairment:* If increasing azotemia, oliguria, or reversible increases in BUN or creatinine occur during treatment of severe progressive renal disease, discontinue therapy.

*Pregnancy:* Category B (ethacrynic acid, torsemide); Category C (furosemide, bumetanide). Since furosemide may increase the incidence of patent ductus arteriosus in preterm infants with respiratory-distress syndrome, use caution when administering before delivery.

*Lactation:* **Furosemide** appears in breast milk.

*Children:* Safety and efficacy for use of **torsemide** in children, **bumetanide** in children younger than 18 years of age, and **ethacrynic acid** in infants (oral) and children (IV) have not been established.

*Furosemide* – Furosemide stimulates renal synthesis of prostaglandin $E_2$ and may increase the incidence of patent ductus arteriosus when given in the first few weeks of life, to premature infants with respiratory-distress syndrome.

## Precautions

*Monitoring:* Observe for blood dyscrasias, liver or kidney damage, or idiosyncratic reactions. Perform frequent serum electrolyte, calcium, glucose, uric acid, $CO_2$, creatinine, and BUN determinations during the first few months of therapy and periodically thereafter.

*Cardiovascular effects:* Too vigorous a diuresis, as evidenced by rapid and excessive weight loss, may induce an acute hypotensive episode. In elderly cardiac patients, avoid rapid contraction of plasma volume and the resultant hemoconcentration to prevent thromboembolic episodes, such as cerebral vascular thromboses and pulmonary emboli.

*Electrolyte imbalance:* Electrolyte imbalance may occur, especially in patients receiving high doses with restricted salt intake. Perform periodic determinations of serum electrolytes.

*Hypokalemia:* Hypokalemia prevention requires particular attention to the following: Patients receiving digitalis and diuretics for CHF, hepatic cirrhosis, and ascites; in aldosterone excess with normal renal function; potassium-losing nephropathy; certain diarrheal states; or where hypokalemia is an added risk to the patient (eg, history of ventricular arrhythmias).

*Hypomagnesemia:* Loop diuretics increase the urinary excretion of magnesium.

*Hypocalcemia:* Serum calcium levels may be lowered (rare cases of tetany have occurred).

*Hyperuricemia:* Asymptomatic hyperuricemia can occur, and rarely, gout may be precipitated.

*Glucose:* Increases in blood glucose and alterations in glucose tolerance tests (fasting and 2 hour postprandial sugar) have been observed.

*Lipids:* Increases in LDL and total cholesterol and triglycerides with minor decreases in HDL cholesterol may occur.

*Photosensitivity:* Photosensitization (photoallergy or phototoxicity) may occur.

### Drug Interactions

Loop diuretics may affect the following drugs: Aminoglycosides; anticoagulants; chloral hydrate; digitalis glycosides; lithium; nondepolarizing neuromuscular blockers; propranolol; sulfonylureas; theophyllines. Loop diuretics may be affected by the following drugs: Charcoal; cisplatin; clofibrate; hydantoins; NSAIDs; probenecid; salicylates; thiazide diuretics.

*Drug/Food interactions:* The bioavailability of **furosemide** is decreased and its degree of diuresis reduced when administered with food. Simultaneous food intake with **torsemide** delays the time to $C_{max}$ by about 30 minutes, but overall bioavailability and diuretic activity are unchanged.

### Adverse Reactions

Adverse reactions associated with loop diuretics include nausea; vomiting; diarrhea; gastric irritation; headache; fatigue; dizziness; thrombocytopenia; rash; orthostatic hypotension; hyperuricemia; hyperglycemia; electrolyte imbalance (decreased chloride, potassium and sodium); dehydration.

*Bumetanide:* Adverse reactions may include impaired hearing, ear discomfort, dry mouth, pain, renal failure, weakness, arthritic pain, muscle cramps, ECG changes, chest pain, hives, pruritus, itching, sweating, hyperventilation.

*Ethacrynic acid:* Adverse reactions may include anorexia, pain, GI bleeding, severe neutropenia, agranulocytosis, fever, chills, confusion, fatigue, malaise, sense of fullness in the ears, blurred vision, tinnitus, hearing loss (irreversible), rash.

*Furosemide:* Adverse reactions may include anorexia, cramping, constipation, blurred vision, hearing loss, restlessness, fever, anemia, purpura, thrombocytopenia, agranulocytosis, photosensitivity, urticaria, pruritus, thrombophlebitis, muscle spasm, weakness.

*Torsemide:* Adverse reactions may include excessive urination.

# POTASSIUM-SPARING DIURETICS

### Actions

*Pharmacology:* In the kidney, potassium is filtered at the glomerulus and then absorbed parallel to sodium throughout the proximal tubule and thick ascending limb of the loop of Henle, so that only minor amounts reach the distal convoluted tubule. As a result, potassium appearing in urine is secreted at the distal tubule and collecting duct. The potassium-sparing diuretics interfere with sodium reabsorption at the distal tubule, thus decreasing potassium secretion. They exert a weak diuretic and antihypertensive effect when used alone. Their major use is to enhance the action and counteract the kaliuretic effect of thiazide and loop diuretics.

*Spironolactone* – Spironolactone, a competitive inhibitor of aldosterone, binds to aldosterone receptors of the distal tubule and prevents the formation of a protein important in sodium transport. It is effective in primary and secondary hyperaldosteronism. Spironolactone is effective in lowering systolic and diastolic blood pressure in primary hyperaldosteronism and essential hypertension, although aldosterone secretion may be normal in benign essential hypertension.

*Amiloride and triamterene* – **Amiloride** and **triamterene** not only inhibit sodium reabsorption induced by aldosterone, but they also inhibit basal sodium reabsorption. They are not aldosterone antagonists, but act directly on the renal distal tubule, cortical collecting tubule and collecting duct. They induce a reversal of polarity of the transtubular electrical-potential difference and inhibit active transport of sodium and potassium. Amiloride may inhibit sodium, potassium-ATPase.

| Potassium-Sparing Diuretics: Pharmacological and Pharmacokinetic Properties | | | |
|---|---|---|---|
| Parameters | Amiloride | Spironolactone | Triamterene |
| *Pharmacology* | | | |
| Tubular site of action | Proximal = distal | Distal | Distal |
| Mechanism of action | $Na^+$, $K^+$–ATPase inhibition; $Na^+/H^+$ exchange mechanism inhibition (proximal tubule) | Aldosterone antagonism | Membrane effect |
| Action: | | | |
| Onset (hours) | 2 | 24 to 48 | 2 to 4 |
| Peak (hours) | 6 to 10 | 48 to 72 | 6 to 8 |
| Duration (hours) | 24 | 48 to 72 | 12 to 16 |
| *Pharmacokinetics* | | | |
| Bioavailability | 15% to 25% | > 90% | 30% to 70% |
| Protein binding | 23% | ≥ 98%[1] | 50% to 67% |
| Half-life (hours) | 6 to 9 | 20[2] | 3 |
| Active metabolites | none | canrenone | hydroxytriamterene sulfate |
| Peak plasma levels (hours) | 3 to 4 | canrenone: 2 to 4 | 3 |
| Excreted unchanged in urine | ≈ 50%[3] | †[4] | ≈ 21% |
| *Dosage* | | | |
| Daily dose (mg) | 5 to 20 | 25 to 400 | 200 to 300 |

[1] Canrenone > 98%.
[2] 10 to 35 hours for canrenone.
[3] 40% excreted in stool within 72 hours.
[4] Metabolites primarily excreted in urine, but also in bile.

# AMILORIDE HCl

| Tablets: 5 mg (Rx) | Midamor (Merck) |
|---|---|

### Indications
Adjunctive treatment with thiazide or loop diuretics in CHF or hypertension to: Help restore normal serum potassium in patients who develop hypokalemia on the kaliuretic diuretic; prevent hypokalemia in patients who would be at particular risk if hypokalemia were to develop (eg, digitalized patients or patients with significant cardiac arrhythmias).

*Unlabeled uses:* Amiloride (10 to 20 mg/day) may be useful in reducing lithium-induced polyuria without increasing lithium levels as is seen with thiazide diuretics.

### Administration and Dosage
Administer with food.

*Concomitant therapy:* Add amiloride 5 mg/day to the usual antihypertensive or diuretic dosage of a kaliuretic diuretic. Increase dosage to 10 mg/day, if necessary; doses > 10 mg are usually not needed. If persistent hypokalemia is documented with 10 mg, increase the dose to 15 mg, then 20 mg, with careful titration of the dose and careful monitoring of electrolytes.

In patients with CHF, potassium loss may decrease after an initial diuresis; reevaluate the need or dosage for amiloride. Maintenance therapy may be intermittent.

*Single drug therapy:* The starting dose is 5 mg/day. Increase to 10 mg/day, if necessary; doses greater than 10 mg are usually not needed. If persistent hypokalemia is documented with 10 mg, increase the dose to 15 mg, then 20 mg, with careful monitoring of electrolytes.

### Contraindications
Hypersensitivity to amiloride; serum potassium greater than 5.5 mEq/L; antikaliuretic therapy or potassium supplementation; renal function impairment patients receiving spironolactone or triamaterene.

### Warnings
*Hyperkalemia:* Amiloride may cause hyperkalemia (serum potassium greater than 5.5 mEq/L) that, if uncorrected, is potentially fatal. Monitor serum potassium carefully. Symptoms of hyperkalemia include paresthesias, muscular weakness, fatigue, flaccid paralysis of the extremities, bradycardia, shock, and ECG abnormalities.

*Diabetes mellitus:* Avoid use of amiloride in diabetic patients. If it is used, monitor serum electrolytes and renal function frequently. Discontinue use 3 days or more before glucose tolerance testing.

*Metabolic or respiratory acidosis:* Cautiously institute amiloride in severely ill patients in whom respiratory or metabolic acidosis may occur, such as patients with cardiopulmonary disease or poorly controlled diabetes. Monitor acid-base balance frequently. Shifts in acid-base balance alter the ratio of extracellular/intracellular potassium; the development of acidosis may be associated with rapid increases in serum potassium.

*Renal function impairment:* Anuria, acute or chronic renal insufficiency and evidence of diabetic nephropathy are contraindications because potassium retention is accentuated and may result in the rapid development of hyperkalemia. Do not give to patients with evidence of renal impairment (BUN greater than 30 mg/dL or serum creatinine greater than 1.5 mg/dL) or diabetes mellitus without continuous monitoring of serum electrolytes, creatinine, and BUN levels.

*Hepatic function impairment:* In patients with preexisting severe liver disease, hepatic encephalopathy (manifested by tremors, confusion, and coma, and increased jaundice) may occur. Because amiloride is not metabolized by the liver, drug accumulation is not anticipated in patients with hepatic dysfunction, but accumulation can occur if hepatorenal syndrome develops.

*Pregnancy: Category B.*

*Lactation:* It is not known whether amiloride is excreted in breast milk.

*Children:* Safety and efficacy for use in children have not been established.

**Precautions**

*Electrolyte imbalance and BUN increases:* Hyponatremia and hypochloremia may occur when amiloride is used with other diuretics. Increases in BUN levels usually accompany vigorous fluid elimination, especially when diuretic therapy is used in seriously ill patients, such as those who have hepatic cirrhosis with ascites and metabolic alkalosis, or those with resistant edema.

**Drug Interactions**

Drugs that may interact include digoxin, potassium preparations, ACE inhibitors, and NSAIDs.

**Adverse Reactions**

Possible adverse reactions include headache, nausea, anorexia, diarrhea, vomiting.

# SPIRONOLACTONE

| **Tablets:** 25, 50, and 100 mg *(Rx)* | Various, *Aldactone* (Searle) |
| --- | --- |

**Indications**

*Primary hyperaldosteronism:* Diagnosis of primary hyperaldosteronism.

Short-term preoperative treatment of patients with primary hyperaldosteronism.

Long-term maintenance therapy for patients with discrete aldosterone-producing adrenal adenomas who are poor operative risks, or who decline surgery.

Long-term maintenance therapy for patients with bilateral micronodular or macronodular adrenal hyperplasia (idiopathic hyperaldosteronism).

*Edematous conditions when other therapies are inappropriate or inadequate:*

CHF – Management of edema and sodium retention; also indicated with digitalis.

*Cirrhosis of the liver accompanied by edema or ascites* – For maintenance therapy in conjunction with bed rest and the restriction of fluid and sodium.

*Nephrotic syndrome.*

*Essential hypertension:* Usually in combination with other drugs.

*Hypokalemia:* Hypokalemia and the prophylaxis of hypokalemia in patients taking digitalis.

*Unlabeled uses:* Spironolactone has been used in the treatment of hirsutism (50 to 200 mg/day) due to its antiandrogenic properties. One study suggested that a lower dosage (50 mg twice/day on days 4 through 21 of the menstrual cycle) may help minimize the risk of metrorrhagia that occurs with higher doses.

Symptoms of premenstrual syndrome (PMS) have been relieved at a dosage of 25 mg 4 times daily beginning on day 14 of the menstrual cycle.

The combination of spironolactone (2 mg/kg/day) and testolactone (20 to 40 mg/kg/day) for 6 months or more may be effective for short-term treatment of familial male precocious puberty.

Spironolactone 100 mg/day appears effective in short-term treatment of acne vulgaris.

**Administration and Dosage**

Spironolactone may be administered in single or divided doses.

*Diagnosis of primary hyperaldosteronism:* As initial diagnostic measure to provide presumptive evidence of primary hyperaldosteronism in patients on normal diets, as follows:

*Long test* – 400 mg/day for 3 to 4 weeks. Correction of hypokalemia and hypertension provides presumptive evidence for diagnosis of primary hyperaldosteronism.

*Short test* – 400 mg/day for 4 days. If serum potassium increases but decreases when spironolactone is discontinued, consider a presumptive diagnosis of primary hyperaldosteronism.

*Maintenance therapy for hyperaldosteronism:* 100 to 400 mg/day in preparation for surgery. For patients unsuitable for surgery, employ the drug for long-term maintenance therapy at lowest possible dose.

*Edema:*

*Adults (CHF, hepatic cirrhosis, nephrotic syndrome)* – Initially, 100 mg/day (range, 25 to 200 mg/day). When given as the sole diuretic agent, continue for ≥ 5 days at the initial dosage level, then adjust to the optimal level. If after 5 days an adequate diuretic response has not occurred, add a second diuretic, which acts more proximally in the renal tubule. Because of the additive effect of spironolactone with such diuretics, an enhanced diuresis usually begins on the first day of combined treatment; combined therapy is indicated when more rapid diuresis is desired. Spironolactone dosage should remain unchanged when other diuretic therapy is added.

*Children* – 3.3 mg/kg/day (1.5 mg/lb/day) administered in single or divided doses.

*Essential hypertension:*

*Adults* – Initially, 50 to 100 mg/day in single or divided doses. May also be combined with diuretics, which act more proximally, and with other antihypertensive agents. Continue treatment for 2 weeks or more because the maximal response may not occur sooner. Individualize dosage.

*Children* – A dose of 1 to 2 mg/kg twice/day has been recommended.

*Hypokalemia:* 25 to 100 mg/day. Useful in treating diuretic-induced hypokalemia when oral potassium supplements or other potassium-sparing regimens are considered inappropriate.

## Contraindications

Anuria; acute renal insufficiency; significant impairment of renal function; hyperkalemia; patients receiving amiloride or triamterene.

## Warnings

*Hyperkalemia:* Carefully evaluate patients for possible fluid and electrolyte balance disturbances. Hyperkalemia may occur with impaired renal function or excessive potassium intake and can cause cardiac irregularities that may be fatal. Ordinarily, do not give potassium supplements with spironolactone.

*Renal function impairment:* Use of spironolactone may cause a transient elevation of BUN, especially in patients with preexisting renal impairment. The drug may cause mild acidosis.

*Carcinogenesis:* Spironolactone was a tumorigen in chronic toxicity studies in rats.

*Pregnancy:* Spironolactone or its metabolites may cross the placental barrier.

*Lactation:* Canrenone, a metabolite of spironolactone, appears in breast milk. The labeling suggests that an alternative method of infant feeding be instituted when using spironolactone; however, the American Academy of Pediatrics considers the drug to be compatible with breastfeeding.

## Precautions

*Hyponatremia:* Hyponatremia may be caused or aggravated by spironolactone, especially in combination with other diuretics. Symptoms include dry mouth, thirst, lethargy, drowsiness.

*Gynecomastia:* Gynecomastia may develop and appears to be related to dosage and duration of therapy. It is normally reversible when therapy is discontinued.

*Reversible hyperchloremic metabolic acidosis:* Reversible hyperchloremic metabolic acidosis, usually in association with hyperkalemia, occurs in some patients with decompensated hepatic cirrhosis, even in the presence of normal renal function.

## Drug Interactions

Drugs that may affect spironolactone include ACE inhibitors, salicylates, and food. Drugs that may be affected by spironolactone include anticoagulants, digitalis glycosides, mitotane, digoxin, and potassium preparations.

## Adverse Reactions

Adverse reactions are usually reversible upon discontinuation of the drug.

Possible adverse reactions include cramping; diarrhea; gastric bleeding; ulceration; gastritis; vomiting; drowsiness; lethargy; headache; mental confusion; ataxia; irregular menses; carcinoma of the breast.

# TRIAMTERENE

**Capsules**: 50 and 100 mg (*Rx*)                    *Dyrenium* (Wellspring Pharmaceuticals)

### Indications
*Edema*: Edema associated with CHF, hepatic cirrhosis, and the nephrotic syndrome; steroid-induced edema, idiopathic edema, and edema due to secondary hyperaldosteronism.

May be used alone or with other diuretics, either for additive diuretic effect or antikaliuretic (potassium-sparing) effect. It promotes increased diuresis in patients resistant or only partially responsive to other diuretics because of secondary hyperaldosteronism.

### Administration and Dosage
Individualize dosage.

When used alone, the usual starting dose is 100 mg twice/daily after meals. When combined with other diuretics or antihypertensives, decrease the total daily dosage of each agent initially, and then adjust to the patient's needs. Do not exceed 300 mg/day.

### Contraindications
Patients receiving spironolactone or amiloride; anuria; severe hepatic disease; hyperkalemia; hypersensitivity to triamterene; severe or progressive kidney disease or dysfunction, with the possible exception of nephrosis; preexisting elevated serum potassium (impaired renal function, azotemia) or patients who develop hyperkalemia while on triamterene.

### Warnings
*Hyperkalemia*: Abnormal elevation of serum potassium levels (5.5 mEq/L or more) can occur. Hyperkalemia is more likely to occur in patients with renal impairment and diabetes (even without evidence of renal impairment), and in the elderly or severely ill. Because uncorrected hyperkalemia may be fatal, serum potassium levels must be monitored at frequent intervals, especially when dosages are changed or with any illness that may influence renal function.

When triamterene is added to other diuretic therapy, or when patients are switched to triamterene from other diuretics, discontinue potassium supplementation.

*Hypersensitivity reactions:* Monitor patients regularly for blood dyscrasias, liver damage, or other idiosyncratic reactions.

*Renal function impairment:* Perform periodic BUN and serum potassium determinations to check kidney function, especially in patients with suspected or confirmed renal insufficiency and in elderly or diabetic patients; diabetic patients with nephropathy are especially prone to develop hyperkalemia.

*Hepatic function impairment:* Triamterene is extensively metabolized in the liver. The overall diuretic response may not be affected.

*Pregnancy: Category B.*

*Lactation:* If the drug is essential, the patient should stop nursing.

*Children:* Safety and efficacy have not been established.

### Precautions
*Electrolyte imbalance:* In CHF, renal disease, or cirrhosis, electrolyte imbalance may be aggravated or caused by diuretics. The use of full doses of a diuretic when salt intake is restricted can result in a low salt syndrome.

*Renal stones:* Triamterene has been found in renal stones with other usual calculus components. Use cautiously in patients with histories of stone formation.

*Hematologic effects:* Triamterene is a weak folic acid antagonist. Because cirrhotics with splenomegaly may have marked variations in hematological status, it may contribute to the appearance of megaloblastosis in cases where folic acid stores have been depleted. Perform periodic blood studies in these patients.

*Metabolic acidosis:* Triamterene may cause decreasing alkali reserve with a possibility of metabolic acidosis.

*Diabetes mellitus:* Triamterene may raise blood glucose levels for adult-onset diabetes; dosage adjustments of hypoglycemic agents may be necessary. Concurrent use with chlorpropamide may increase the risk of severe hyponatremia.

*Photosensitivity:* Photosensitization is likely to occur; avoid prolonged exposure to sunlight.

### Drug Interactions
Drugs that may affect triamterene include ACE inhibitors, cimetidine, and indomethacin. Drugs that may be affected by triamterene include amantadine and potassium preparations. Triamterene will interfere with the fluorescent measurement of quinidine serum levels.

### Adverse Reactions
Diarrhea; nausea; vomiting; jaundice; liver enzyme abnormalities. Azotemia; elevated BUN/creatinine; increased serum uric acid levels (in patients predisposed to gouty arthritis); thrombocytopenia; megaloblastic anemia; weakness; dizziness; hypokalemia; headache; dry mouth; anaphylaxis.

# CARBONIC ANHYDRASE INHIBITORS

| | |
|---|---|
| **ACETAZOLAMIDE** | |
| **Tablets:** 125 and 250 mg (*Rx*) | Various, *Diamox* (Lederle) |
| **Capsules, sustained-release:** 500 mg (*Rx*) | *Diamox Sequels* (Lederle) |
| **METHAZOLAMIDE** | |
| **Tablets:** 25 and 50 mg (*Rx*) | Various, *Neptazane* (Lederle) |

### Indications

*Glaucoma:* For adjunctive treatment of chronic simple (open-angle) glaucoma and secondary glaucoma; preoperatively in acute angle-closure glaucoma when delay of surgery is desired to lower intraocular pressure (IOP).

*Acetazolamide:*

*Tablets, sustained-release capsules, and injection* – For the prevention or amelioration of symptoms associated with acute mountain sickness in climbers attempting rapid ascent and in those who are susceptible to acute mountain sickness despite gradual ascent.

*Tablets and injection only* – For adjunctive treatment of edema due to CHF, drug-induced edema, and centrencephalic epilepsy (petit mal, unlocalized seizures).

### Administration and Dosage

ACETAZOLAMIDE:

*Chronic simple (open-angle) glaucoma* –

Adults: 250 mg to 1 g/day, usually in divided doses for amounts greater than 250 mg. Dosage greater than 1 g/day does not usually increase the effect.

*Secondary glaucoma and preoperative treatment of acute congestive (closed-angle) glaucoma* –

Adults:

Short-term therapy – 250 mg every 4 hours or 250 mg twice/day.

Acute cases – 500 mg followed by 125 or 250 mg every 4 hours.

IV therapy may be used for rapid relief of increased intraocular pressure. A complementary effect occurs when used with miotics or mydriatics.

Children:

Parenteral – 5 to 10 mg/kg/dose, IM or IV, every 6 hours.

Oral – 10 to 15 mg/kg/day in divided doses, every 6 to 8 hours.

*Diuresis in congestive heart failure* –

Adults: Initially, 250 to 375 mg (5 mg/kg) once daily in the morning. If, after an initial response, the patient stops losing edema fluid, do not increase the dose; allow for kidney recovery by skipping medication for a day. Best diuretic results occur when given on alternate days, or for 2 days alternating with a day of rest. Failures in therapy may result from overdosage or from too frequent dosages.

*Drug-induced edema* – Most effective if given every other day or for 2 days alternating with a day of rest.

Adults: 250 to 375 mg once daily for 1 or 2 days.

Children: 5 mg/kg/dose, oral or IV, once daily in the morning.

*Epilepsy* –

Adults and children: 8 to 30 mg/kg/day in divided doses. The optimum range is 375 to 1000 mg/day. When given in combination with other anticonvulsants, the starting dose is 250 mg once daily.

*Acute mountain sickness* – 500 to 1000 mg/day, in divided doses of tablets or sustained release capsules. For rapid ascent (ie, in rescue or military operations), use the higher dose (1000 mg). If possible, initiate dosing 24 to 48 hours before ascent and continue for 48 hours while at high altitude, or longer as needed to control symptoms.

*Sustained release* – May be used twice daily, but is only indicated for use in glaucoma and acute mountain sickness.

*Parenteral* – Direct IV administration is preferred; IM administration is painful because of the alkaline pH of the solution.

METHAZOLAMIDE:

*Glaucoma* – 50 to 100 mg 2 or 3 times/day. May be used with miotic and osmotic agents.

## Actions

*Pharmacology:* These agents are nonbacteriostatic sulfonamides that inhibit the enzyme carbonic anhydrase. This action reduces the rate of aqueous humor formation, resulting in decreased IOP.

*Pharmacokinetics:*

| Pharmacokinetics of Carbonic Anhydrase Inhibitors | | | | |
|---|---|---|---|---|
| Carbonic anhydrase inhibitor | IOP Lowering Effects | | | Relative inhibitor potency |
| | Onset (h) | Peak effect (h) | Duration (h) | |
| Acetazolamide | | | | |
| Tablets | 1 to 1.5 | 1 to 4 | 8 to 12 | 1 |
| Sustained release capsules | 2 | 3 to 6 | 18 to 24 | |
| Injection (IV) | 2 min | 15 min | 4 to 5 | |
| Methazolamide | 2 to 4 | 6 to 8 | 10 to 18 | †[1] |

[1] † Quantitative data not available; reported to be more active than acetazolamide.

## Contraindications

Hypersensitivity to these agents; depressed sodium or potassium serum levels; marked kidney and liver disease or dysfunction; suprarenal gland failure; hyperchloremic acidosis; adrenocortical insufficiency; severe pulmonary obstruction with inability to increase alveolar ventilation since acidosis may be increased (dichlorphenamide); cirrhosis (acetazolamide, methazolamide); long-term use in chronic noncongestive angle-closure glaucoma.

## Warnings

*Hepatic function impairment:* Use of **methazolamide** in this condition could precipitate hepatic coma.

*Pregnancy:* Category C.

*Lactation:* Safety has not been established.

*Children:* Safety and efficacy for use in children have not been established.

## Precautions

*Monitoring:* Monitor for hematologic reactions common to sulfonamides. Obtain baseline CBC and platelet counts before therapy and at regular intervals during therapy.

> *Hypokalemia* – Hypokalemia may develop when severe cirrhosis is present, during concomitant use of steroids or ACTH, and with interference with adequate oral electrolyte intake.

*Dose increases:* Increasing the dose of **acetazolamide** does not increase diuresis and may increase drowsiness or paresthesia; it often results in decreased diuresis. However, very large doses have been given with other diuretics to promote diuresis in complete refractory failure.

*Pulmonary conditions:* These drugs may precipitate or aggravate acidosis. Use with caution in patients with pulmonary obstruction or emphysema when alveolar ventilation may be impaired.

*Cross-sensitivity:* Cross-sensitivity between antibacterial sulfonamides and sulfonamide derivative diuretics, including acetazolamide and various thiazides, has been reported.

## Drug Interactions

Drugs that may interact with carbonic anhydrase inhibitors include cyclosporine, primidone, salicylates, and diflunisal.

## Adverse Reactions

Sulfonamide-type adverse reactions may occur.

*CNS:* Convulsions; weakness; malaise; fatigue; nervousness; drowsiness; depression; dizziness; disorientation; confusion; ataxia; tremor; tinnitus; headache.

*Dermatologic:* Urticaria; pruritus; skin eruptions; rash (including erythema multiforme, Stevens-Johnson syndrome, toxic epidermal necrolysis); photosensitivity.

*GI:* Melena; anorexia; nausea; vomiting; constipation; taste alteration; diarrhea.

*Hematologic:* Bone marrow depression; thrombocytopenia; thrombocytopenic purpura; hemolytic anemia; leukopenia; pancytopenia; agranulocytosis.

*Renal:* Hematuria; glycosuria; urinary frequency.

*Miscellaneous:* Weight loss; fever; decreased/absent libido; impotence; electrolyte imbalance; hepatic insufficiency.

# Chapter 6
# RESPIRATORY AGENTS

# SYMPATHOMIMETICS

**ALBUTEROL**

| | |
|---|---|
| **Tablets**: 2 and 4 mg (as sulfate) (*Rx*) | Various, *Proventil* (Schering) |
| **Syrup**: 2 mg (as sulfate)/5 mL (*Rx*) | Various, *Proventil* (Schering) |
| **Aerosol**: Delivers 90 mcg/actuation (*Rx*) | Various, *Proventil* (Schering) |
| Delivers 90 mcg (as sulfate)/actuation (*Rx*) | *Proventil HFA* (Key), *Ventolin HFA* (GlaxoSmith-Kline) |
| **Solution for inhalation**: 0.083% and 0.5% (as sulfate) (*Rx*) | Various, *Proventil* (Schering) |
| 0.63 mg (as sulfate)/3 mL, 1.25 mg/3 mL (*Rx*) | *AccuNeb* (Dey) |

**BITOLTEROL**

| | |
|---|---|
| **Solution for inhalation**: 0.2% (*Rx*) | *Tornalate* (Elan) |

**EPHEDRINE SULFATE**

| | |
|---|---|
| **Capsules**: 25 mg (*otc*) | *Ephedrine Sulfate* (West-Ward) |
| **Injection**: 50 mg/mL (*Rx*) | Various |

**EPINEPHRINE**

| | |
|---|---|
| **Solution for inhalation**: 1:100 (10 mg/mL as hydrochloride) (*Rx*) | *Adrenalin Chloride Solution* (Monarch) |
| 2.25% racepinephrine hydrochloride (1.125% epinephrine base) (*otc*) | *microNefrin* (Bird), *Nephron* (Nephron), *S2* (Nephron) |
| **Topical solution**: 1:1000 (1 mg/mL as hydrochloride) (*Rx*) | *Adrenalin Chloride Solution* (Monarch) |
| **Aerosol**: 0.22 mg epinephrine/spray (*otc*) | Various, *Primatene Mist* (Whitehall Robins) |
| **Injection**: 1:1000 (1 mg/mL as hydrochloride) solution (*Rx*) | Various, *Adrenalin Chloride Solution* (Monarch) |
| 1:10,000 (0.1 mg/mL) solution (*Rx*) | *Epinephrine* (Abbott) |

**FORMOTEROL FUMARATE**

| | |
|---|---|
| **Inhalation powder in capsules**: 12 mcg | *Foradil Aerolizer* (Schering) |

**ISOETHARINE HYDROCHLORIDE**

| | |
|---|---|
| **Solution for inhalation**: 1% (*Rx*) | *Isoetharine Hydrochloride* (Roxane) |

**ISOPROTERENOL HYDROCHLORIDE**

| | |
|---|---|
| **Injection**: (1:5000 solution) 0.2 mg/mL (*Rx*) | *Isoproterenol Hydrochloride* (ESI Lederle), *Isuprel* (Abbott) |
| (1:50,000 solution) 0.02 mg/mL (*Rx*) | *Isoproterenol Hydrochloride* (Abbott) |

**LEVALBUTEROL HYDROCHLORIDE**

| | |
|---|---|
| **Solution for inhalation**: 0.31 mg/3 mL (as base), 0.63 mg/3 mL (as base), 1.25 mg/3 mL (as base) (*Rx*) | *Xopenex* (Sepracor) |

**METAPROTERENOL SULFATE**

| | |
|---|---|
| **Aerosol**: Delivers 0.65 mg/actuation (*Rx*) | *Alupent* (Boehringer Ingelheim) |
| **Solution for inhalation**: 0.4%, 0.6%, and 5% (*Rx*) | Various, *Alupent* (Boehringer Ingelheim) |

**PIRBUTEROL ACETATE**

| | |
|---|---|
| **Aerosol**: Delivers 0.2 mg (as acetate)/actuation (*Rx*) | *Maxair Autohaler* (3M Pharm) |

**SALMETEROL XINAFOATE**

| | |
|---|---|
| **Powder for inhalation**: 50 mcg (as base) (*Rx*) | *Serevent Diskus* (GlaxoSmithKline) |

**TERBUTALINE SULFATE**

| | |
|---|---|
| **Tablets**: 2.5 and 5 mg (*Rx*) | *Terbutaline Sulfate* (Global), *Brethine* (aaiPharma) |
| **Injection**: 1 mg/mL (*Rx*) | *Brethine* (aaiPharma) |

## Indications

*Sympathomimetics:* According to the National Asthma Education and Prevention Program's Expert Panel Report II, long-acting $\beta_2$-agonists (eg, **salmeterol**) are used concomitantly with anti-inflammatory medications for long-term control of symptoms, especially nocturnal symptoms. They also prevent exercise-induced bronchospasm (EIB). Short-acting $\beta_2$-agonists (eg, **albuterol**, **bitolterol**, **pirbuterol**, **terbutaline**) are the therapy of choice for relief of acute symptoms and prevention of EIB.

*Albuterol:* Relief and prevention of bronchospasm in patients with reversible obstructive airway disease; prevention of EIB.

*Bitolterol:* Prophylaxis and treatment of bronchial asthma and reversible bronchospasm. May be used with or without concurrent theophylline or steroid therapy.

*Ephedrine sulfate:*
　　*Asthma* – Ephedrine sulfate injection is indicated in the treatment of allergic disorders, such as bronchial asthma. Oral ephedrine is indicated for temporary relief of shortness of breath, tightness of chest, and wheezing caused by bronchial asthma. Eases breathing for asthma patients by reducing spasms of bronchial muscles.

*Epinephrine:*
　　*Inhalation* – For temporary relief of acute paroxysms (eg, shortness of breath, tightness of chest, wheezing) of bronchial asthma; postintubation and infectious croup.

　　*MicroNefrin:* Chronic obstructive lung disease, chronic bronchitis, bronchiolitis, bronchial asthma, and other peripheral airway diseases; croup (postintubation and infectious).

　　*Injection* – To relieve respiratory distress in bronchial asthma or during acute asthma attacks and for reversible bronchospasm in patients with chronic bronchitis, emphysema, and other obstructive pulmonary diseases; severe acute anaphylactic reactions, including anaphylactic shock and cardiac arrest; to restore cardiac rhythm.

　　Allergic reactions (eg, bronchospasm, urticaria, pruritus, angioneurotic edema, or swelling of the lips, eyelids, tongue, and nasal mucosa) due to anaphylactic shock caused by stinging insects (primarily of the order Hymenoptera, that includes bees, wasps, hornets, yellow jackets, bumble bees, and fire ants); severe allergic or anaphylactoid reactions caused by allergy injections; exposures to pollens, dusts, molds, foods, drugs, and exercise or unknown substances (so-called idiopathic anaphylaxis); severe, life-threatening asthma attacks characterized by wheezing, dyspnea, and inability to breathe.

*Formoterol fumarate:*
　　*Asthma* – For long-term, twice-daily (morning and evening) administration in the maintenance treatment of asthma and in the prevention of bronchospasm in adults and children 5 years of age and older with reversible obstructive airways disease, including patients with symptoms of nocturnal asthma, who require regular treatment with inhaled, short-acting, $\beta_2$-agonists.

　　*EIB* – For the acute prevention of EIB in adults and children 12 years of age and older when administered on an occasional, as-needed basis.

　　*Concomitant therapy* – Can be used concomitantly with short-acting $\beta_2$-agonists, inhaled or systemic corticosteroids, and theophylline therapy. A satisfactory clinical response to formoterol does not eliminate the need for continued treatment with an anti-inflammatory.

　　Formoterol is not a substitute for inhaled or oral corticosteroids. Do not stop or reduce corticosteroids at the time formoterol is initiated.

　　*Chronic obstructive pulmonary disease (COPD)* – For long-term, twice daily (morning and evening) administration in the maintenance of bronchoconstriction in patients with COPD including chronic bronchitis and emphysema.

*Isoetharine:* For bronchial asthma and reversible bronchospasm that occurs with bronchitis and emphysema.

*Isoproterenol:*
　　*Injection* – Management of bronchospasm during anesthesia.

*Isoproterenol and phenylephrine bitartrate:* Treatment of bronchospasm associated with acute and chronic asthma; reversible bronchospasm that may be associated with emphysema or chronic bronchitis.

*Levalbuterol:* For the treatment or prevention of bronchospasm in adults, adolescents, and children 6 years of age and older with reversible obstructive airway disease.

*Metaproterenol:* For bronchial asthma and reversible bronchospasm; treatment of acute asthmatic attacks in children 6 years of age and older (5% solution for inhalation only).

*Pirbuterol:* Prevention and reversal of bronchospasm in patients with reversible bronchospasm including asthma. Use with or without concurrent theophylline or steroid therapy.

*Salmeterol:*

*Asthma/Bronchospasm* – Long-term, twice-daily (morning and evening) administration in the maintenance treatment of asthma and in the prevention of bronchospasm in patients 4 years of age and older with reversible obstructive airway disease, including patients with symptoms of nocturnal asthma, who require regular treatment with inhaled, short-acting $\beta_2$-agonists. It should not be used in patients whose asthma can be managed by occasional use of short-acting, inhaled $\beta_2$-agonists. Salmeterol may be used with or without concurrent inhaled or systemic corticosteroid therapy.

*EIB* – Prevention of EIB in patients 4 years of age and older.

*COPD* – Maintenance treatment of bronchospasm associated with COPD (including emphysema and chronic bronchitis).

*Terbutaline:* A bronchodilator for bronchial asthma and for reversible bronchospasm that may occur with bronchitis and emphysema.

## Administration and Dosage
ALBUTEROL:

*Inhalation aerosol* –

*Adults and children 4 years of age and older (12 years of age and older for Proventil):* 2 inhalations every 4 to 6 hours. In some patients, 1 inhalation every 4 hours may be sufficient. More frequent administration or a larger number of inhalations is not recommended. If previously effective dosage fails to provide relief, this may be a marker of destabilization of asthma and requires re-evaluation of the patient and treatment regimen.

*Maintenance therapy (Proventil only):* For maintenance therapy or to prevent exacerbation of bronchospasm, 2 inhalations 4 times/day should be sufficient.

*Prevention of EIB:*

*Adults and children 4 years of age and older (12 years of age and older for Proventil)* – 2 inhalations 15 minutes prior to exercise.

*Inhalation solution* –

*Adults and children 12 years of age and older:* 2.5 mg 3 to 4 times/day by nebulization. Dilute 0.5 mL of the 0.5% solution with 2.5 mL sterile normal saline. Deliver over approximately 5 to 15 minutes.

*Children 2 to 12 years of age (15 kg or more):* 2.5 mg (1 UD vial) 3 to 4 times/day by nebulization. Children weighing less than 15 kg who require less than 2.5 mg/dose (ie, less than a full UD vial) should use the 0.5% inhalation solution. Deliver over approximately 5 to 15 minutes.

*AccuNeb:* The usual starting dosage for patients 2 to 12 years of age is 1.25 or 0.63 mg administered 3 or 4 times/day, as needed, by nebulization. More frequent administration is not recommended. Deliver over 5 to 15 minutes. *AccuNeb* has not been studied in the setting of acute attacks of bronchospasm.

*Tablets* –

*Adults and children 12 years of age and older:* Usual starting dosage is 2 or 4 mg 3 or 4 times/day. Do not exceed a total daily dose of 32 mg. Use doses greater than 4 mg 4 times/day only when the patient fails to respond. If a favorable response does not occur, cautiously increase stepwise, up to a maximum of 8 mg 4 times/day, as tolerated.

*Children 6 to 12 years of age:* Usual starting dosage is 2 mg 3 to 4 times/day. For those who fail to respond to the initial starting dosage, cautiously increase stepwise, but do not exceed 24 mg/day in divided doses.

*Elderly patients and those sensitive to $\beta$-adrenergic stimulants:* Start with 2 mg 3 or 4 times/day. If adequate bronchodilation is not obtained, increase dosage gradually to as much as 8 mg 3 or 4 times/day.

*Tablets, extended release* –

*Adults and children older than 12 years of age:* Usual recommended dose is 8 mg every 12 hours; in some patients, 4 mg every 12 hours may be sufficient. In unusual circumstances (eg, low adult body weight), initial doses may be 4 mg every 12 hours and progress to 8 mg every 12 hours according to response. The dose may be cautiously increased stepwise under physician supervision to a maximum of 32 mg/day in divided doses (eg, every 12 hours) if symptoms are not controlled.

*Children 6 to 12 years of age:* Usual recommended dose is 4 mg every 12 hours. The dose may be cautiously increased stepwise under physician supervision to a maximum of 24 mg/day in divided doses (eg, every 12 hours) if symptoms are not controlled.

*Switching to extended-release tablets:* Patients maintained on regular-release albuterol tablets or syrup can be switched to extended-release tablets. A 4 mg extended-release tablet every 12 hours is equivalent to a regular 2 mg tablet every 6 hours. Multiples of this regimen up to the maximum recommended dose also apply.

*Syrup –*

*Adults and children older than 12 years of age:* Usual dose is 2 or 4 mg 3 or 4 times/day. Give doses greater than 4 mg 4 times/day only when patient fails to respond. If a favorable response does not occur, cautiously increase, but do not exceed 8 mg 4 times/day.

*Children 6 to 12 years of age:* Usual starting dose is 2 mg 3 or 4 times/day. If patient does not respond to 2 mg 4 times/day, cautiously increase stepwise. Do not exceed 24 mg/day in divided doses.

*Children 2 to 6 years of age:* Initiate at 0.1 mg/kg 3 times/day. Do not exceed 2 mg 3 times/day. If the patient does not respond to the initial dose, increase stepwise to 0.2 mg/kg 3 times/day. Do not exceed 4 mg 3 times/day.

*Elderly patients and those sensitive to β-adrenergic stimulation –* Restrict initial dose to 2 mg 3 or 4 times/day. Individualize dosage thereafter.

BITOLTEROL:
*Bronchospasm –*

*Adults and children older than 12 years of age:* 2 inhalations at an interval of at least 1 to 3 minutes, followed by a third inhalation if needed.

*Solution for inhalation:* Administer during a 10- to 15-minute period.

| Dosing Regimens for Bitolterol Solution for Inhalation 0.2% | | | | |
|---|---|---|---|---|
| | Continuous flow nebulization | | Intermittent flow nebulization | |
| Doses | Volume (mL) | Bitolterol (mg) | Volume (mL) | Bitolterol (mg) |
| Usual dose | 1.25 | 2.5 | 0.5 | 1 |
| Decreased dose | 0.75 | 1.5 | 0.25 | 0.5 |
| Increased dose | 1.75 | 3.5 | 0.75 | 1.5 |

Up to 1 mL solution for inhalation, 0.2% (2 mg) can be administered with the intermittent flow system to severely obstructed patients.

The usual frequency of treatments is 3 times/day. Treatments may be increased up to 4 times/day; however, the interval between treatments should be at least 4 hours. For some patients, 2 treatments a day may be adequate. Seek medical advice immediately if the previously effective dosage regimen fails to provide the usual relief, as this is often a sign of seriously worsening asthma that would require reassessment of therapy.

Do not exceed the maximum daily dose of 8 mg with an intermittent flow nebulization system or 14 mg with a continuous flow nebulization system.

EPHEDRINE SULFATE: Ephedrine sulfate is a sympathomimetic alkaloid that stimulates alpha and beta receptors as well as the CNS. It is effective orally and parenterally. It is less potent than epinephrine.

*Adults and children 12 years of age and older –* Oral dosage is 12.5 to 25 mg every 4 hours, not to exceed 150 mg in 24 hours.

*Adults –* The usual parenteral dose is 25 to 50 mg administered subcutaneously or IM, or 5 to 25 mg administered slowly IV repeated every 5 to 10 minutes, if necessary.

*Children –*

*Capsules:* For use in children younger than 12 years of age, consult a physician.

*Injection:* The usual subcutaneous, IV, or IM dose is 0.5 to 0.75 mg/kg or 16.7 to 25 mg/m$^2$ every 4 to 6 hours.

*EPINEPHRINE:* Refer to specific product labeling for detailed administration and dosage information.

*Inhalation aerosol* – Start treatment at the first symptoms of bronchospasm. Individualize dosage.

*Adults and children 4 years of age and older:* Start with 1 inhalation, then wait at least 1 minute. If not relieved, use once more. Do not use again for 3 hours or more.

*Nebulization –*

*Adults and children 4 years of age and older:*

*Hand pump nebulizer* – Place 0.5 mL (10 drops) epinephrine into the nebulizer reservoir. Place the nebulizer nozzle into the partially opened mouth. Squeeze the bulb 1 to 3 times. Inhale deeply. Do not administer more than every 3 hours. Supervise children during use.

*Aerosol-nebulizer* – Add 0.5 mL (approximately 10 drops) racemic epinephrine to 3 mL diluent or 0.2 to 0.4 mL (approximately 4 to 8 drops) *MicroNefrin* to 4.6 to 4.8 mL water. Administer for 15 minutes every 3 to 4 hours. Supervise children during use.

*Children younger than 4 years of age:* Consult a physician.

*Topical solution* – Apply locally as drops or spray, or with a sterile swab, as required. See product labeling for dilution instructions.

*Injection –*

*Solution (1:1000):*

*Initial adult dose* – 0.2 to 1 mL (0.2 to 1 mg) subcutaneously (preferred) or IM; repeat every 4 hours.

*For infants and children* – Give 0.01 mL/kg or 0.3 mL/m$^2$ (0.01 mg/kg or 0.3 mg/m$^2$) subcutaneously. Do not exceed 0.5 mL (0.5 mg) in a single pediatric dose. Repeat every 4 hours if necessary.

*Solution (1:10,000):* The adult IV dose for hypersensitivity reactions or to relieve bronchospasm usually ranges from 0.1 to 0.25 mg (1 to 2.5 mL of 1:10,000 solution) injected slowly. Neonates may be given a dose of 0.01 mg/kg; for the infant, 0.05 mg is an adequate initial dose, and this may be repeated at 20- to 30-minute intervals in the management of asthma attacks.

Alternatively, if the patient has been intubated, epinephrine can be injected via the endotracheal tube directly into the bronchial tree at the same dosage for IV injection. It is rapidly absorbed through the lung capillary bed.

*FORMOTEROL:* Administer formoterol capsules only by the oral inhalation route and only using the *Aerolizer Inhaler.* Do not ingest formoterol (ie, swallowed) orally. Always store capsules in the blister, and only remove immediately before use.

When beginning treatment with formoterol, instruct patients who have been taking inhaled, short-acting $\beta_2$-agonists on a regular basis (eg, 4 times/day) to discontinue the regular use of these drugs and use them only for symptomatic relief of acute asthma symptoms.

*Asthma/Bronchospasm* – For adults and children 5 years of age and older, the usual dosage is the inhalation of the contents of one 12 mcg formoterol capsule every 12 hours using the *Aerolizer Inhaler.* The patient must not exhale into the device. The total daily dose of formoterol should not exceed 1 capsule twice daily (24 mcg total daily dose). If symptoms arise between doses, take an inhaled short-acting $\beta_2$-agonist for immediate relief.

*Prevention of EIB* – For adults and adolescents 12 years of age and older, the usual dosage is the inhalation of the contents of one 12 mcg formoterol capsule at least 15 minutes before exercise administered on an occasional as-needed basis.

*Maintenance treatment of COPD* – The usual dosage is the inhalation of the contents of one 12 mcg formoterol capsule every 12 hours using the *Aerolizer Inhaler.*

*ISOETHARINE HYDROCHLORIDE:*

| Isoetharine Doses (Volume) Based on Strength of Solution | | |
|---|---|---|
| Method of administration | Usual dose | Range of dose of 1:3 dilution[a] |
| Hand bulb nebulizer | 4 inhalations | 3 to 7 inhalations undiluted |
| Oxygen aerosolization[b] | 0.5 mL | 1 to 2 mL |
| IPPB[c] | 0.5 mL | 1 to 4 mL |

[a] Dilution of 1 part isoetharine plus 3 parts of normal saline solution.
[b] Administered with oxygen flow adjusted to 4 to 6 L/min over 15 to 20 minutes.
[c] Usually an inspiratory flow rate of 15 L/min at a cycling pressure of 15 cm $H_2O$ is recommended. It may be necessary, according to patient and type of IPPB apparatus, to adjust flow rate to 6 to 30 L/min, cycling pressure to 10 to 15 cm $H_2O$, and further dilution according to the needs of the patient.

*ISOPROTERENOL:*

*Injection* – For the management of bronchospasm during anesthesia, dilute 1 mL (0.2 mg) of a 1:5000 solution to 10 mL with sodium chloride injection or 5% dextrose injection. Administer an initial dose of 0.01 to 0.02 mg (0.5 to 1 mL of diluted solution) IV; repeat when necessary; or use a 1:50,000 undiluted solution and administer an initial dose of 0.01 to 0.02 mg (0.5 to 1 mL).

*LEVALBUTEROL:*

*Children 6 to 11 years of age* – The recommended dosage is 0.31 mg administered 3 times/day by nebulization. Do not exceed routine dosing of 0.63 mg 3 times/day.

*Adults and children 12 years of age and older* – 0.63 mg administered 3 times/day, every 6 to 8 hours, by nebulization. May increase to 1.25 mg 3 times/day. Closely monitor patients receiving the higher dose for adverse systemic effect, and balance the risks of such effects against the potential for improved efficacy.

*METAPROTERENOL:*

*Metered dose inhaler* – 2 to 3 inhalations every 3 to 4 hours. Do not exceed 12 inhalations/day. Not recommended for children younger than 12 years of age.

*Inhalant solutions* – Usually, treatment need not be repeated more often than every 4 hours to relieve acute bronchospasm attacks. In chronic bronchospastic pulmonary diseases, give 3 to 4 times/day. A single dose of nebulized metaproterenol in the treatment of an acute attack of asthma may not completely abort an attack. Not recommended for children younger than 12 years of age.

| Dosage and Dilution for Metaproterenol Inhalant Solutions | | | |
|---|---|---|---|
| Administration | Usual dose | Range | Dilution |
| Adults and children ≥ 12 years of age | | | |
| Hand bulb nebulizer | 10 inhalations | 5 to 15 inhalations | No dilution |
| IPPB[a] | 0.3 mL | 0.2 to 0.3 mL | In ≈ 2.5 mL saline or other diluent |
| Children 6 to 12 years of age | | | |
| Nebulizer | 0.1 mL | 0.1 to 0.2 mL | In saline to a total volume of 3 mL |

[a] IPPB = intermittent positive pressure breathing

*PIRBUTEROL:*

*Adults and children 12 years of age and older* – 2 inhalations (0.4 mg) repeated every 4 to 6 hours. One inhalation (0.2 mg) may be sufficient for some patients.

Do not exceed a total daily dose of 12 inhalations.

If previously effective dosage regimen fails to provide the usual relief, seek medical advice immediately, as this is often a sign of seriously worsening asthma that would require reassessment of therapy.

*SALMETEROL:*

*Asthma/Bronchospasm* – For asthma/bronchospasm in children 4 years of age and older, use 1 inhalation/disk (50 mcg) twice daily (12 hours apart). Adverse effects are more likely to occur with higher doses of salmeterol, and more frequent administration or administration of a larger number of inhalations is not recommended.

To gain full therapeutic benefit, administer twice daily (morning and evening) in the treatment of reversible airway obstruction.

*Prevention of EIB* – 1 inhalation at least 30 minutes before exercise protects patients against EIB. When used intermittently as needed for prevention of EIB, this protection may last up to 9 hours in adolescents and adults and up to 12 hours in patients 4 to 11 years of age. Do not use additional doses of salmeterol for 12 hours after administration of this drug. In patients who are receiving salmeterol twice daily (morning and evening), do not use additional salmeterol for prevention of EIB. If this dose is not effective, consider other appropriate therapy for EIB.

*COPD* – For maintenance treatment of bronchospasm associated with COPD (including chronic bronchitis and emphysema), the usual dosage for adults is 1 powder inhalation (50 mcg) twice daily (morning and evening, approximately 12 hours apart).

*TERBUTALINE:*
Oral –

*Adults and children older than 15 years of age:* 5 mg, given at 6-hour intervals, 3 times/ day during waking hours. If side effects are pronounced, dose may be reduced to 2.5 mg 3 times/day. Do not exceed 15 mg in 24 hours.

*Children 12 to 15 years of age:* 2.5 mg 3 times/day. Do not exceed 7.5 mg in 24 hours. Not recommended for children younger than 12 years of age.

*Parenteral* – Usual dose is 0.25 mg subcutaneously into the lateral deltoid area. If significant improvement does not occur in 15 to 30 minutes, administer a second 0.25 mg dose. Do not exceed a total dose of 0.5 mg in 4 hours. If a patient fails to respond to a second 0.25 mg dose within 15 to 30 minutes, consider other therapeutic measures.

## Actions

*Pharmacology:* These agents are used to produce bronchodilation. They relieve reversible bronchospasm by relaxing the smooth muscles of the bronchioles in conditions associated with asthma, bronchitis, emphysema, or bronchiectasis. Bronchodilation may additionally facilitate expectoration.

The pharmacologic actions of these agents include: Alpha-adrenergic stimulation (vasoconstriction, nasal decongestion, pressor effects); $\beta_1$-adrenergic stimulation (increased myocardial contractility and conduction); and $\beta_2$-adrenergic stimulation (bronchial dilation and vasodilation, enhancement of mucociliary clearance, inhibition of cholinergic neurotransmission).

The relative selectivity of action of sympathomimetic agents is the primary determinant of clinical usefulness; it can predict the most likely side effects. The $\beta_2$ selective agents provide the greatest benefit with minimal side effects. Direct administration via inhalation provides prompt effects and minimizes systemic activity.

| Sympathomimetic Bronchodilators: Pharmacologic Effects and Pharmacokinetic Properties | | | | | |
|---|---|---|---|---|---|
| Sympathomimetic | Adrenergic receptor activity | $\beta_2$ potency[a] | Route | Onset (min) | Duration (h) |
| Albuterol[b] | $\beta_1 < \beta_2$ | 2 | PO | within 30 | 4 to 8 |
| | | | Inh[c] | within 5 | 3 to 6 |
| Bitolterol[b] | $\beta_1 < \beta_2$ | 5 | Inh | 2 to 4 | 5 ≥ 8 |
| Ephedrine | $\alpha$  $\beta_1$  $\beta_2$ | — | PO | 15 to 60 | 3 to 5 |
| | | | SC | > 20 | ≤ 1 |
| | | | IM | 10 to 20 | ≤ 1 |
| | | | IV | immediate | |
| Epinephrine | $\alpha$  $\beta_1$  $\beta_2$ | — | SC | 5 to 10 | 4 to 6 |
| | | | IM | — | 1 to 4 |
| | | | Inh[c] | 1 to 5 | 1 to 3 |

| Sympathomimetic Bronchodilators: Pharmacologic Effects and Pharmacokinetic Properties | | | | | |
|---|---|---|---|---|---|
| Sympathomimetic | Adrenergic receptor activity | $\beta_2$ potency[a] | Route | Onset (min) | Duration (h) |
| Isoetharine[b] | $\beta_1 < \beta_2$ | 6 | Inh[c] | within 5 | 2 to 3 |
| Isoproterenol | $\beta_1 \quad \beta_2$ | 1 | IV | immediate | < 1 |
| | | | Inh[c] | 2 to 5 | 1 to 3 |
| Metaproterenol[b] | $\beta_1 < \beta_2$ | 15 | PO | ≈ 30 | 4 |
| | | | Inh[c] | 5 to 30 | 1 to 6 |
| Salmeterol[b] | $\beta_1 < \beta_2$ | 0.5 | Inh | within 20 | 12 |
| Pirbuterol[b] | $\beta_1 < \beta_2$ | 5 | Inh | within 5 | 5 |
| Terbutaline[b] | $\beta_1 < \beta_2$ | 4 | PO | 30 | 4 to 8 |
| | | | SC | 5 to 15 | 1.5 to 4 |
| | | | Inh | 5 to 30 | 3 to 6 |

[a] Relative molar potency: 1 = most potent.
[b] These agents all have minor $\beta_1$ activity.
[c] May be administered via aerosol or bulb nebulizer or IPPB administration.

## Contraindications

Hypersensitivity to any component (allergic reactions are rare); cardiac arrhythmias associated with tachycardia; angina, preexisting cardiac arrhythmias associated with tachycardia, known hypersensitivity to sympathomimetic amines, and ventricular arrhythmias requiring inotropic therapy, tachycardia or heart block caused by digitalis intoxication (**isoproterenol**); patients with organic brain damage, local anesthesia of certain areas (eg, fingers, toes) because of the risk of tissue sloughing, labor, cardiac dilatation, coronary insufficiency, cerebral arteriosclerosis, organic heart disease (**epinephrine**); in those cases where vasopressors may be contraindicated; narrow-angle glaucoma, nonanaphylactic shock during general anesthesia with halogenated hydrocarbons or cyclopropane (**epinephrine, ephedrine**).

## Warnings

*Special risk patients:* Administer with caution to patients with diabetes mellitus, hyperthyroidism, prostatic hypertrophy (**ephedrine**) or history of seizures; elderly; psychoneurotic individuals, patients with long-standing bronchial asthma and emphysema who have developed degenerative heart disease (**epinephrine**).

In patients with status asthmaticus and abnormal blood gas tensions, improvement in vital capacity and blood gas tensions may not accompany apparent relief of bronchospasm following **isoproterenol**.

*Diabetes* – Large doses of IV **albuterol** and IV **terbutaline** may aggravate preexisting diabetes mellitus and ketoacidosis. Relevance to the use of oral or inhaled albuterol and oral terbutaline is unknown. Diabetic patients receiving any of these agents may require an increase in dosage of insulin or oral hypoglycemic agents.

*Cardiovascular effects:* Use with caution in patients with cardiovascular disorders including coronary insufficiency, ischemic heart disease, history of stroke, coronary artery disease, cardiac arrhythmias, CHF, and hypertension.

Closely monitor patients receiving **epinephrine**. Inadvertently induced high arterial blood pressure may result in angina pectoris, aortic rupture, or cerebral hemorrhage. Cardiac arrhythmias develop in some individuals even after therapeutic doses.

Beta-adrenergic agonists can produce significant cardiovascular effects measured by pulse rate, blood pressure, symptoms, or ECG changes (eg, flattening of T-waves, prolongation of the QTc interval, and ST-segment depression).

**Isoproterenol** doses sufficient to increase the heart rate more than 130 bpm may increase the likelihood of inducing ventricular arrhythmias.

**Ephedrine** may cause hypertension resulting in intracranial hemorrhage. It may induce anginal pain in patients with coronary insufficiency or ischemic heart disease.

Large doses of inhaled or oral **salmeterol** (12 to 20 times the recommended dose) have been associated with clinically significant prolongation of the QTc interval, which has the potential for producing ventricular arrhythmias.

*Paradoxical bronchospasm:* Occasionally patients have developed severe paradoxical airway resistance with repeated, excessive use of inhalation preparations; the cause is unknown. Discontinue the drug immediately and institute alternative therapy.

*Usual dose response:* Advise patients to contact a physician if they do not respond to their usual dose of a sympathomimetic amine.

Further therapy with **isoproterenol** aerosol alone is inadvisable when 3 to 5 treatments within 6 to 12 hours produce minimal or no relief.

Reduce **epinephrine** dose if bronchial irritation, nervousness, restlessness, or sleeplessness occurs. Do not continue to use epinephrine, but seek medical assistance immediately if symptoms are not relieved within 20 minutes or become worse.

*CNS effects:* Sympathomimetics may produce CNS stimulation.

*Long-term use:* Prolonged use of **ephedrine** may produce a syndrome resembling an anxiety state; many patients develop nervousness; a sedative may be needed.

*Acute symptoms:* Do not use **salmeterol** to relieve acute asthma symptoms. If the patient's short-acting, inhaled $\beta_2$-agonist becomes less effective (eg, the patient needs more inhalations than usual), medical evaluation must be obtained immediately.

*Excessive use of inhalants* – Deaths have been reported; the exact cause is unknown, but cardiac arrest following an unexpected severe acute asthmatic crisis and subsequent hypoxia is suspected.

*Morbidity/Mortality* – Regularly scheduled, daily use of beta agonists is not recommended.

*Use with short-acting $\beta_2$-agonists* – When patients begin treatment with salmeterol, advise those who have been taking short-acting, inhaled $\beta_2$-agonists on a regular daily basis to discontinue their regular daily-dosing regimen and clearly instruct them to use short-acting, inhaled $\beta_2$-agonists only for symptomatic relief if they develop asthma symptoms while taking salmeterol.

*Overdosage or inadvertent IV injection:* Overdosage or inadvertent IV injection of conventional subcutaneous **epinephrine** doses may cause severe or fatal hypertension or cerebrovascular hemorrhage resulting from the sharp rise in blood pressure. Fatalities may also occur from pulmonary edema resulting from peripheral constriction and cardiac stimulation.

*Hypersensitivity reactions:* Hypersensitivity reactions can occur after administration of **bitolterol, albuterol, metaproterenol, terbutaline, ephedrine, salmeterol,** and possibly other bronchodilators.

*Elderly:* Lower doses may be required due to increased sympathomimetic sensitivity.

*Pregnancy: Category* B (terbutaline). *Category* C (**albuterol, bitolterol, ephedrine, epinephrine, isoetharine, isoproterenol, metaproterenol, salmeterol, pirbuterol**).

*Labor and delivery* – Use of $\beta_2$ active sympathomimetics inhibits uterine contractions. Other reactions include increased heart rate, transient hyperglycemia, hypokalemia, cardiac arrhythmias, pulmonary edema, cerebral and myocardial ischemia, and increased fetal heart rate and hypoglycemia in the neonate. Although these effects are unlikely with aerosol use, consider the potential for untoward effects.

Do not use parenteral **ephedrine** in obstetrics when maternal blood pressure exceeds 130/80.

*Lactation:* **Terbutaline, ephedrine,** and **epinephrine** are excreted in breast milk. It is not known whether other agents are excreted in breast milk.

*Children:*

*Inhalation* – Safety and efficacy for use of **bitolterol, pirbuterol, isoetharine, salmeterol,** and **terbutaline** in children 12 years of age and younger have not been established. **Albuterol** aerosol in children younger than 4 years of age and **albuterol** solution for inhalation in children younger than 2 years of age have not been established. **Metaproterenol** may be used in children 6 years of age and older.

*Injection* – Parenteral **terbutaline** is not recommended for use in children younger than 12 years of age. Administer **epinephrine** with caution to infants and children. Syncope has occurred following administration to asthmatic children.

*Oral* – **Terbutaline** is not recommended for use in children younger than 12 years of age. Safety and efficacy of **albuterol** have not been established for children younger than 2 years (syrup), 6 years (tablets) and 12 years (tablets, extended release) of age.

In children, **ephedrine** is effective in the oral therapy of asthma. Because of its CNS-stimulating effect, it is rarely used alone. This effect is usually countered by an appropriate sedative; however, its rationale has been questioned.

### Precautions

*Tolerance:* Tolerance may occur with prolonged use of sympathomimetic agents, but temporary cessation of the drug restores its original effectiveness.

*Hypokalemia:* Decreases in serum potassium levels have occurred, possibly through intracellular shunting, which can produce adverse cardiovascular effects.

*Hyperglycemia:* **Isoproterenol** causes less hyperglycemia than does **epinephrine**.

*Parkinson disease:* Epinephrine may temporarily increase rigidity and tremor.

*Parenteral use:* Administer **epinephrine** with great caution and in carefully circumscribed quantities in areas of the body served by end arteries or with otherwise limited blood supply (eg, fingers, toes, nose, ears, genitals) or if peripheral vascular disease is present to avoid vasoconstriction-induced tissue sloughing.

*Combined therapy:* Concomitant use with other sympathomimetic agents is not recommended, as it may lead to deleterious cardiovascular effects. This does not preclude the judicious use of an adrenergic stimulant aerosol bronchodilator in patients receiving tablets. Do not give on a routine basis. If regular coadministration is required, consider alternative therapy.

Do not use 2 or more β-adrenergic aerosol bronchodilators simultaneously because of the potential of additive effects.

Patients must be warned not to stop or reduce corticosteroid therapy without medical advice, even if they feel better when they are being treated with $\beta_2$-agonists. These agents are not to be used as a substitute for oral or inhaled corticosteroids.

*Drug abuse and dependence:* Prolonged abuse of **ephedrine** can lead to symptoms of paranoid schizophrenia. Patients exhibit such signs as tachycardia, poor nutrition and hygiene, fever, cold sweat, and dilated pupils. Some measure of tolerance develops, but addiction does not occur.

### Drug Interactions

Most interactions listed apply to sympathomimetics when used as vasopressors; however, consider the interaction when using the bronchodilator sympathomimetics. Drugs that may interact include antihistamines, alpha-adrenergic blockers, beta-blockers, cardiac glycosides, diuretics, ergot alkaloids, furazolidone, general anesthetics, guanethidine, levothyroxine, methyldopa, MAO inhibitors, nitrates, oxytocic drugs, phenothiazines, rauwolfia alkaloids, tricyclic antidepressants, digoxin, theophylline, insulin, or oral hypoglycemic agents.

*Drug/Lab test interactions:* **Isoproterenol** causes false elevations of bilirubin as measured in vitro by a sequential multiple analyzer. Isoproterenol inhalation may result in enough absorption of the drug to produce elevated urinary epinephrine values. Although small with standard doses, the effect is likely to increase with larger doses.

**Adverse Reactions**

| | Adverse reaction | Albuterol | Bitolterol | Ephedrine | Epinephrine | Isoetharine | Isoproterenol | Metaproterenol | Pirbuterol | Salmeterol | Terbutaline |
|---|---|---|---|---|---|---|---|---|---|---|---|
| | **Sympathomimetic Bronchodilator Adverse Reactions (≥ 3%)[a]** | | | | | | | | | | |
| Cardiovascular | Palpitations | < 1-10 | 1.5-3 | ✔ | 7.8-30 | ✔[b] | < 5-22 | 0.3-4 | 1.3-1.7 | 1-3 | ≤ 23 |
| | Tachycardia | 1-10 | < 3.7 | ✔ | ≤ 2.6 | ✔ | 2-12 | < 17 | 1.2-1.3 | 1-3 | 1.3-3 |
| | Blood pressure changes/hypertension | 1-5 | < 1 | | ✔ | ✔ | 2-5 | 0.3 | | | < 1 |
| | Chest tightness/pain/ discomfort, angina | < 3 | ≤ 1.5 | | ≤ 2.6 | | ✔ | 0.2 | < 1.3 | | 1.3-1.5 |
| | PVCs, arrhythmias, skipped beats | | 0.5 | ✔ | ✔ | | < 1-3 | | < 1 | | ≈ 4 |
| CNS | Tremor | < 1-24.2 | 9-26.6 | | 16-18 | ✔ | < 15 | 1-33 | 1.3-6 | 4 | < 5-38 |
| | Dizziness/vertigo | < 1-7 | 1-4 | ✔ | 3.3-7.8 | ✔ | 1.5-5 | 1-4 | 0.6-1.2 | ≥ 3 | 1.3-10 |
| | Shakiness/nervous-ness/tension | 1-20 | 1.5-11.1 | ✔ | 8.5-31 | ✔ | < 15 | 2.6-14 | 4.5-7 | 1-3 | < 5-31 |
| | Drowsiness | < 1 | | | 8.2-14 | | < 5 | 0.7 | | | < 5-11.7 |
| | Hyperactivity/Hyper-kinesia, excitement | 1-20 | < 1 | | | ✔ | ✔ | | < 1 | | |
| | Headache | 2-22 | ≤ 8.4 | ✔ | 3.3-10 | ✔ | 1.5-10 | ≤ 4 | 1.3-2 | 28 | 7.8-10 |
| | Insomnia | 1-11 | < 1 | ✔ | ✔ | ✔ | 1.5 | 1.8 | < 1 | | ✔ |
| GI | Nausea/Vomiting | 2-15 | ≤ 3 | ✔ | 1-11.5 | ✔ | < 15 | < 14 | ≤ 1.7 | 1-3 | 1.3-10 |
| | Heartburn/GI distress/ disorder | ≤ 5 | | | | | ≤ 5-10 | ≤ 4 | | 1-3 | < 10 |
| | Diarrhea | 1 | | | | | | 0.7 | < 1.3 | 1-3 | |
| Respiratory | Cough | < 1-5 | ≤ 4.1 | | | | 1-5 | ≤ 4 | 1.2 | 7 | |
| | Bronchospasm | 1-15.4 | ≤ 1.5 | | | | ≤ 18 | | | | |
| | Throat dryness/irrita-tion, pharyngitis | ≤ 6 | 2.5-5 | | | | 3.1 | ≤ 4 | < 1 | ≥ 3 | ✔ |

[a] Data pooled for all routes of administration, all age groups, from separate studies, and are not necessarily comparable.
[b] ✔ = Reported; no incidence given.

Adverse reactions are generally transient, and no cumulative effects have been reported. It is usually not necessary to discontinue treatment; however, in selected cases temporarily reduce dosage.

*Albuterol:*
　*Respiratory* – Bronchitis (1.5% to 4%); epistaxis (1% to 3%).
　*Miscellaneous* – Increased appetite, stomachache (3%); muscle cramps (1% to 3%).
*Bitolterol:* Light-headedness (6.8%). The overall incidence of cardiovascular effects was approximately 5%.

*Isoproterenol:* Bronchitis (5%).

*Metaproterenol:* Asthma exacerbation (1% to 4%).

*Salmeterol:*
　*Musculoskeletal* – Joint/back pain, muscle cramp/contraction, myalgia/myositis, muscular soreness (1% to 3%).
　*Respiratory* – Upper respiratory tract infection, nasopharyngitis (14%); nasal cavity/ sinus disease (6%); sinus headache, lower respiratory tract infection (4%); allergic rhinitis (more than 3%); rhinitis, laryngitis, tracheitis/bronchitis (1% to 3%).
　*Miscellaneous* – Giddiness, influenza (more than 3%); viral gastroenteritis, urticaria, dental pain, malaise/fatigue, rash/skin eruption, dysmenorrhea (1% to 3%).

# XANTHINE DERIVATIVES

### AMINOPHYLLINE

| | |
|---|---|
| **Tablets:** 100 mg (equiv. to 79 mg theophylline), 200 mg (equiv. to 158 mg theophylline) (*Rx*) | Various |
| **Tablets, controlled-release (12 hours):** 225 mg (equiv. to 178 mg theophylline) (*Rx*) | *Phyllocontin* (Purdue Frederick) |
| **Oral liquid:** 105 mg (equiv. to 90 mg theophylline) per 5 mL (*Rx*) | Various |
| **Injection:** 250 mg (equiv. to 197 mg theophylline) per 10 mL (*Rx*) For IV use. | Various |
| **Suppositories:** 250 mg (equiv. to 197.5 mg theophylline) and 500 mg (equiv. to 395 mg theophylline) (*Rx*) | Various, *Truphylline* (G & W) |

### DYPHYLLINE

| | |
|---|---|
| **Tablets:** 200 or 400 mg (*Rx*) | Various, *Dilor* (Savage) |
| **Elixir:** 100 or 160 mg/15 mL (33.3 or mg/5 mL) (*Rx*) | *Lufyllin* (Medpointe), *Dilor* (Savage) |
| **Injection:** 250 mg/mL (*Rx*) | *Lufyllin* (Medpointe) |

### OXTRIPHYLLINE

| | |
|---|---|
| **Tablets:** 100 mg (equiv. to 64 mg theophylline) and 200 mg (equiv. to 127 mg theophylline) (*Rx*) | Various, *Choledyl* (Parke-Davis) |
| **Syrup, pediatric:** 50 mg (equiv. to 32 mg theophylline) per 5 mL (*Rx*) | Various, *Choledyl* (Parke-Davis) |
| **Elixir:** 100 mg (equiv. to 64 mg theophylline) per 5 mL (*Rx*) | Various, *Choledyl* (Parke-Davis) |

### THEOPHYLLINE

| | |
|---|---|
| **Tablets:** 100, 125, 200, 250, and 300 mg (*Rx*) | Various, *Slo-Phyllin* (Rhone-Poulenc Rorer), *Quibron-T Dividose* (Bristol Labs) |
| **Capsules:** 100 and 200 mg (*Rx*) | *Bronkodyl* (Winthrop), |
| **Syrup:** 80 mg and 150 mg/15 mL (26.7 or 50 mg/5 mL) (*Rx*) | *Accurbron* (Marion Merrell Dow) |
| **Elixir:** 80 mg/15 mL (26.7 mg/5 mL) (*Rx*) | Various, *Asmalix* (Century), *Elixomin* (Cenci), *Elixophyllin* (Forest), *Lanophyllin* (Lannett) |
| **Solution:** 80 mg/15 mL (26.7 mg/5 mL) (*Rx*) | Various |
| **Capsules, timed-release (8 to 12 hours):** 50, 60, 65, 75, 100, 125, 130, 200, 250, 260, and 300 mg (sustained-release) (*Rx*) | *Aerolate* (Fleming), *Slo-bid Gyrocaps* (Rhone-Poulenc Rorer), |
| **Capsules, timed-release (24 hours):** 100, 200, and 300 mg (*Rx*) | *Theo-24* (Whitby) |
| **Capsules, extended-release:** 100, 125, 200, and 300 mg (*Rx*) | Various |
| **Tablets, timed-release (12 to 24 hours):** 100, 200, 300, and 450 mg (*Rx*) | Various |
| **Tablets, extended-release:** 450 mg (*Rx*) | Various |
| **Tablets, extended-release (12 to 24 hours):** 100, 200, and 300 mg (*Rx*) | *Theochron* (Various) |
| **Tablets, timed-release (8 to 12 hours):** 200, 250, 300, and 500 mg (*Rx*) | *Theolair-SR* (3M Pharm), *Quibron-T/SR* (Roberts), *Respbid* (Boehringer Ingelheim) |
| **Tablets, controlled-release (12 to 24 hours):** 100, 200, and 300 mg (*Rx*) | Various |
| **Tablets, timed-release (24 hours):** 400 mg (*Rx*) | *Uniphyl* (Purdue Frederick) |

### THEOPHYLLINE AND DEXTROSE

| | |
|---|---|
| **Injection:** 200, 400, and 800 mg/container (*Rx*) | Various |

### Indications

Symptomatic relief or prevention of bronchial asthma and reversible bronchospasm associated with chronic bronchitis and emphysema.

*Unlabeled uses:* Theophylline 10 mg/kg/day may significantly improve pulmonary function and dyspnea in patients with chronic obstructive pulmonary disease.

### Administration and Dosage

AMINOPHYLLINE:

*IV* – The loading dose may be infused into 100 to 200 mL of 5% Dextrose Injection or 0.9% Sodium Chloride Injection. Do not exceed 25 mg/min infusion rate.

*Parenteral administration* – Inject aminophylline slowly, up to 25 mg/min, when given IV. Substitute oral therapy for IV aminophylline as soon as adequate improvement is achieved.

*Loading dose:*

In patients currently not receiving theophylline products – 6 mg/kg.

In patients currently receiving theophylline products – Each 0.5 mg/kg theophylline (0.6 mg/kg aminophylline) will increase the serum theophylline concentration by approximately 1 mcg/mL. When respiratory distress warrants a small risk, 2.5 mg/kg theophylline (3.1 mg aminophylline IV) increases serum concentration by ≈ 5 mcg/mL. If the patient is not experiencing theophylline toxicity, this is unlikely to result in dangerous side effects.

*Maintenance infusions* – Administer by a large volume infusion to deliver the desired amount of drug each hour.

| Aminophylline Maintenance Infusion Rates (mg/kg/h) | | |
| --- | --- | --- |
| Patient group | First 12 hours | > 12 hours |
| Neonates to infants < 6 months of age | Not recommended | |
| Children 6 months to 9 years of age | 1.2 | 1 |
| Children 9 to 16 years of age and young adult smokers | 1 | 0.8 |
| Otherwise healthy nonsmoking adults | 0.7 | 0.5 |
| Older patients and those with cor pulmonale | 0.6 | 0.3 |
| Patients with CHF, liver disease | 0.5 | 0.1-0.2 |

*DYPHYLLINE:* Dyphylline is a derivative of theophylline; it is not a theophylline salt, and is not metabolized to theophylline in vivo. Although dyphylline is 70% theophylline by molecular weight ratio, the amount of dyphylline equivalent to a given amount of theophylline is not known. Specific dyphylline serum levels may be used to monitor therapy; serum theophylline levels will not measure dyphylline. The minimal effective therapeutic concentration is 12 mcg/mL.

*Oral* –

*Adults:* Up to 15 mg/kg every 6 hours.

*IM* – (Not for IV administration.)

*Adults:* 250 to 500 mg injected slowly every 6 hours. Do not exceed 15 mg/kg every 6 hours.

*Children:* Safety and efficacy have not been established.

*OXTRIPHYLLINE:*

*Adults* – 4.7 mg/kg every 8 hours.

*Children (9 to 16 years of age) and adult smokers* – 4.7 mg/kg every 6 hours.

*Children (1 to 9 years of age)* – 6.2 mg/kg every 6 hours.

*Sustained action* – If total daily maintenance dosage is established at approximately 800 or 1200 mg, 1 sustained-action tablet every 12 hours may be substituted.

*THEOPHYLLINE:* Individualize dosage. Base dosage adjustments on clinical response and improvement in pulmonary function with careful monitoring of serum levels. If possible, monitor serum levels to maintain levels in the therapeutic range of 10 to 20 mcg/mL. Levels greater than 20 mcg/mL may produce toxicity, and it may even occur with levels between 15 to 20 mcg/mL, particularly when factors known to reduce theophylline clearance are present. Once stabilized on a dosage, serum levels tend to remain constant.

Calculate dosages on the basis of lean body weight, because theophylline does not distribute into fatty tissue. Regardless of salt used, dosages should be equivalent based on anhydrous theophylline content.

*Individualize frequency of dosing* – Individualize frequency of dosing. With immediate release products, dosing every 6 hours is generally required, especially in children; intervals 8 hours or less may be satisfactory in adults. Some children and adults requiring higher than average doses (those having rapid rates of clearance; eg, half-lives less than 6 hours) may be more effectively controlled during chronic therapy with sustained-release products. Determine dosage intervals to produce minimal fluctuations between peak and trough serum theophylline concentrations. Consider the absorption profile and the elimination rate. When converting from an immediate-release to a sustained-release product, the total daily dose should remain the same, and only the dosing interval adjusted.

*Acute symptoms requiring rapid theophyllinization in patients not receiving theophylline* – To achieve a rapid effect, an initial loading dose is required. Dosage recommendations are for theophylline anhydrous.

| Dosage Guidelines for Rapid Theophyllinization | | |
|---|---|---|
| Patient Group | Oral loading | Maintenance |
| Children 1 to 9 years of age | 5 mg/kg | 4 mg/kg q 6 h |
| Children 9 to 16 years of age and young adult smokers | 5 mg/kg | 3 mg/kg q 6 h |
| Otherwise healthy nonsmoking adults | 5 mg/kg | 3 mg/kg q 8 h |
| Older patients, patients with cor pulmonale | 5 mg/kg | 2 mg/kg q 8 h |
| Patients with CHF | 5 mg/kg | 1-2 mg/kg q 12 h |

*Infants (preterm to younger than 1 year)* –

| Theophylline Dosage Guidelines for Infants | |
|---|---|
| Age | Initial maintenance dose |
| *Premature infants* | |
| ≤ 24 days postnatal | 1 mg/kg q 12 h |
| > 24 days postnatal | 1.5 mg/kg q 12 h |
| *Infants (6 to 52 weeks)* | $[(0.2 \times$ age in weeks$) = 5] \times$ kg = 24 h dose in mg |
| Up to 26 weeks | Divide into q 8 h dosing |
| 26 to 52 weeks | Divide into q 6 h dosing |

*Acute symptoms requiring rapid theophyllinization in patients receiving theophylline* – Each 0.5 mg/kg theophylline administered as a loading dose will increase the serum theophylline concentration by approximately 1 mcg/mL. Ideally, defer the loading dose if a serum theophylline concentration can be obtained rapidly.

If this is not possible, exercise clinical judgment. When there is sufficient respiratory distress to warrant a small risk, then 2.5 mg/kg of theophylline administered in rapidly absorbed form is likely to increase serum concentration by approximately 5 mcg/mL. If the patient is not experiencing theophylline toxicity, this is unlikely to result in dangerous adverse effects.

*Chronic therapy* – Slow clinical titration is generally preferred.

*Initial dose:* 16 mg/kg/24 hours or 400 mg/24 hours, whichever is less, of anhydrous theophylline in divided doses at 6- or 8-hour intervals.

*Increasing dose:* The above dosage may be increased in approximately 25% increments at 3-day intervals so long as the drug is tolerated or until the maximum dose (indicated below) is reached.

*Maximum dose (where the serum concentration is not measured)* – Do not attempt to maintain any dose that is not tolerated.

| Maximum Daily Theophylline Dose Based on Age | |
|---|---|
| Age | Maximum daily dose[1] |
| 1 to 9 years | 24 mg/kg/day |
| 9 to 12 years | 20 mg/kg/day |
| 12 to 16 years | 18 mg/kg/day |
| > 16 years | 13 mg/kg/day |

[1] Not to exceed listed dose or 900 mg, whichever is less.

Exercise caution in younger children who cannot complain of minor side effects. Older adults and those with cor pulmonale, CHF, or liver disease may have unusually low dosage requirements; they may experience toxicity at the maximal dosages recommended.

*Measurement of serum theophylline concentrations during chronic therapy* – The table below provides guidance to dosage adjustments based on serum theophylline level determinations:

| Dosage Adjustment After Serum Theophylline Measurement | | |
|---|---|---|
| If serum theophylline is: | | Directions |
| Too low | 5 to 10 mcg/mL | Increase dose by about 25% at 3-day intervals until either the desired clinical response or serum concentration is achieved.[1] |
| Within desired range | 10 to 20 mcg/mL | Maintain dosage if tolerated. Recheck serum theophylline concentration at 6- to 12-month intervals.[2] |
| Too high | 20 to 25 mcg/mL | Decrease doses by ≈ 10%. Recheck serum theophylline concentration after 3 days.[2] |
| | 25 to 30 mcg/mL | Skip next dose and decrease subsequent doses by 25%. Recheck serum theophylline after 3 days. |
| | > 30 mcg/mL | Skip next 2 doses and decrease subsequent doses by 50%. Recheck serum theophylline after 3 days. |

[1] The total daily dose may need to be administered at more frequent intervals if asthma symptoms occur repeatedly at the end of a dosing interval.
[2] Finer adjustments in dosage may be needed for some patients.

*Timed-release capsules* – These dosage forms gradually release the active medication so that the total daily dosage may be administered in 1 to 3 doses divided by 8 to 24 hours, depending on the patient's pharmacokinetic profile, thus reducing the number of daily doses required. These products are not necessarily interchangeable. If patients are switched from one brand to another, closely monitor their theophylline serum levels; serum concentrations may vary greatly following brand interchange.

THEOPHYLLINE and DEXTROSE: Substitute oral therapy for IV theophylline as soon as adequate improvement is achieved.

*Children (younger than 6 months of age)* – Due to marked variation in theophylline metabolism, use this drug only if clearly needed in infants.

### Actions

*Pharmacology:* The methylxanthines (theophylline, its soluble salts and derivatives) directly relax the smooth muscle of the bronchi and pulmonary blood vessels, stimulate the CNS, induce diuresis, increase gastric acid secretion, reduce lower esophageal sphincter pressure, and inhibit uterine contractions. Theophylline is also a central respiratory stimulant. Aminophylline has a potent effect on diaphragmatic contractility in healthy people and may then be capable of reducing fatigability and thereby improve contractility in patients with chronic obstructive airways disease.

*Pharmacokinetics:*

*Absorption* – Theophylline is well absorbed from oral liquids and uncoated plain tablets; maximal plasma concentrations are reached in 2 hours. Rectal absorption from suppositories is slow and erratic, the oral route is generally preferred. Enteric-coated tablets and some sustained-release dosage forms may be unreliably absorbed.

*Distribution* – Average volume of distribution is 0.45 L/kg (range, 0.3 to 0.7 L/kg). Theophylline does not distribute into fatty tissue. Approximately 40% is bound to plasma protein. Therapeutic serum levels generally range from 10 to 20 mcg/mL. Although some bronchodilatory effect occurs at lower concentrations, stabilization of hyperreactive airways is most evident at levels greater than 10 mcg/mL, and adverse effects are uncommon at levels less than 20 mcg/mL.

*Metabolism/Excretion* – Xanthines are biotransformed in the liver (85% to 90%) to 1, 3-dimethyluric acid, 3-methylxanthine and 1-methyluric acid; 3-methylxanthine accumulates in concentrations approximately 50% of those of theophylline.

Excretion is by the kidneys; less than 15% of the drug is excreted unchanged. Elimination kinetics vary greatly. Plasma elimination half-life averages about 3 to 15 hours in adult nonsmokers, 4 to 5 hours in adult smokers (1 to 2 packs per day), 1 to 9 hours in children, and 20 to 30 hours for premature neonates. In the neonate, theophylline is metabolized partially to caffeine. The premature neonate excretes approximately 50% unchanged theophylline and may accumulate the caffeine metabolite.

*Equivalent dose* – Because of differing theophylline content, the various salts and derivatives are not equivalent on a weight basis.

| Theophylline Content and Equivalent Dose of Various Theophylline Salts | | |
| --- | --- | --- |
| Theophylline salts | Theophylline % | Equivalent dose |
| Theophylline anhydrous | 100 | 100 mg |
| Theophylline monohydrate | 91 | 110 mg |
| Aminophylline anhydrous | 86 | 116 mg |
| Aminophylline dihydrate | 79 | 127 mg |
| Oxtriphylline | 64 | 156 mg |

*Dyphylline* – Dyphylline, a chemical derivative of theophylline, is not a theophylline salt as are the other agents. It is about one-tenth as potent as theophylline. Following oral administration, dyphylline is 68% to 82% bioavailable. Peak plasma concentrations are reached within 1 hour, and its half-life is 2 hours. The minimal effective therapeutic concentration is 12 mcg/mL. It is not metabolized to theophylline and 83% ± 5% is excreted unchanged in the urine.

## Contraindications
Hypersensitivity to any xanthine; peptic ulcer; underlying seizure disorders (unless receiving appropriate anticonvulsant medication).

*Aminophylline:* Hypersensitivity to ethylenediamine.

*Aminophylline rectal suppositories:* Irritation or infection of rectum or lower colon.

## Warnings
*Status asthmaticus:* Status asthmaticus is a medical emergency and is not rapidly responsive to usual doses of conventional bronchodilators. Oral theophylline products alone are not appropriate for status asthmaticus.

*Toxicity:* Excessive doses may cause severe toxicity; monitor serum levels to ensure maximum benefit with minimum risk.

Serious side effects such as ventricular arrhythmias, convulsions, or even death may appear as the first sign of toxicity without any previous warning. Less serious signs of toxicity (eg, nausea, restlessness) may occur frequently when initiating therapy, but are usually transient; when such signs are persistent during maintenance therapy, they are often associated with serum concentrations greater than 20 mcg/mL. Serious toxicity is not reliably preceded by less severe side effects.

*Cardiac effects:* Theophylline may cause dysrhythmias or worsen pre-existing arrhythmias.

*Pregnancy: Category* C.

*Lactation:* Theophylline distributes readily into breast milk.

*Children:* Sufficient numbers of infants younger than 1 year of age have not been studied in clinical trials to support use in this age group; however, there is evidence that the use of dosage recommendations for older infants and young children may result in the development of toxic serum levels.

## Precautions
*Use with caution:* Cardiac disease; hypoxemia; hepatic disease; hypertension; CHF; alcoholism; elderly (particularly males); and neonates.

*GI effects:* Use cautiously in peptic ulcer. Local irritation may occur.

## Drug Interactions
Agents that may decrease theophylline levels include aminoglutethimide, barbiturates, charcoal, hydantoins, ketoconazole, rifampin, smoking (cigarettes and marijuana), sulfinpyrazone, sympathomimetics (β-agonists), thioamines, carbamazepine, isoniazid, and loop diuretics.

Agents that may increase theophylline levels include allopurinol, beta blockers (nonselective), calcium channel blockers, cimetidine, oral contraceptives, corticosteroids, disulfiram, ephedrine, influenza virus vaccine, interferon, macrolides, mexiletine, quinolones, thiabendazole, thyroid hormones, carbamazepine, isoniazid, and loop diuretics.

The following agents may be affected by theophylline: Benzodiazepines, halothane, ketamine, lithium, nondepolarizing muscle relaxants, and propofol. Probenecid may increase the effects of dyphylline.

*Drug/Food interactions:* Theophylline elimination is increased (half-life shortened) by a low carbohydrate, high protein diet, and charcoal broiled beef (due to a high polycyclic carbon content). Conversely, elimination is decreased (prolonged half-life) by a high carbohydrate low protein diet. Food may alter the bioavailability and absorption pattern of certain sustained-release preparations. Some sustained-release preparations may be subject to rapid release of their contents when taken with food, resulting in toxicity. It appears that consistent administration in the fasting state allows predictability of effects.

### Adverse Reactions

Adverse reactions/toxicity are uncommon at serum theophylline levels less than 20 mcg/mL.

*Levels greater than 20 mcg/mL* – 75% of patients experience adverse reactions (eg, nausea, vomiting, diarrhea, headache, insomnia, irritability).

*Levels greater than 35 mcg/mL* – Hyperglycemia; hypotension; cardiac arrhythmias; tachycardia (greater than 10 mcg/mL in premature newborns); seizures; brain damage; death.

*Other* – Fever; flushing; hyperglycemia; inappropriate antidiuretic hormone syndrome; rash; alopecia. Ethylenediamine in aminophylline can cause sensitivity reactions, including exfoliative dermatitis and urticaria.

*Cardiovascular:* Palpitations; tachycardia; extrasystoles; hypotension; circulatory failure; life-threatening ventricular arrhythmias.

*CNS:* Irritability; restlessness; headache; insomnia; reflex hyperexcitability; muscle twitching; convulsions.

*GI:* Nausea; vomiting; epigastric pain; hematemesis; diarrhea; rectal irritation or bleeding (aminophylline suppositories). Therapeutic doses of theophylline may induce gastroesophageal reflux during sleep or while recumbent, increasing the potential for aspiration, which can aggravate bronchospasm.

*Renal:* Proteinuria; potentiation of diuresis.

*Respiratory:* Tachypnea; respiratory arrest.

# CORTICOSTEROIDS

| | |
|---|---|
| **BECLOMETHASONE** | |
| **Aerosol:** 40 and 80 mcg/actuation (*Rx*) | *QVAR* (IVAX) |
| **BUDESONIDE** | |
| **Powder:** Each actuation delivers ≈ 160 mcg (*Rx*) | *Pulmicort Turbuhaler* (AstraZeneca) |
| **Inhalation suspension:** 0.25 mg/2 mL, 0.5 mg/2 mL (*Rx*) | *Pulmicort Respules* (AstraZeneca) |
| **FLUNISOLIDE** | |
| **Aerosol:** Each actuation delivers ≈ 250 mcg (*Rx*) | *AeroBid* (Forest), *AeroBid-M* (Forest) |
| **FLUTICASONE** | |
| **Aerosol:** 44, 110, and 220 mcg (*Rx*) | *Flovent* (GlaxoSmithKline) |
| **Powder:** 50, 100, and 250 mcg (*Rx*) | *Flovent Rotadisk* (GlaxoSmithKline), *Flovent Diskus* (GlaxoSmithKline) |
| **TRIAMCINOLONE** | |
| **Aerosol:** Each actuation delivers ≈ 100 mcg. Contains 60 mg triamcinolone acetonide (*Rx*) | *Azmacort* (Aventis) |

**Warning:**

   Particular care is needed in patients who are transferred from systemically active corticosteroids to flunisolide inhaler because deaths because of adrenal insufficiency have occurred in asthmatic patients during and after transfer from systemic corticosteroids to aerosol corticosteroids. After withdrawal from systemic corticosteroids, a number of months are required for recovery of hypothalamic-pituitary-adrenal (HPA) function. During this period of HPA suppression, patients may exhibit signs and symptoms of adrenal insufficiency when exposed to trauma, surgery, or infections, particularly gastroenteritis. Although flunisolide inhaler may provide control of asthmatic symptoms during these episodes, it does not provide the systemic steroid that is necessary for coping with these emergencies. During periods of stress or a severe asthmatic attack, instruct patients who have been withdrawn from systemic corticosteroids to resume systemic steroids (in large doses) immediately and to contact their physician for further instruction. Also instruct these patients to carry a warning card indicating that they may need supplementary systemic steroids during periods of stress or a severe asthma attack. To assess the risk of adrenal insufficiency in emergency situations, periodically perform routine tests of adrenal cortical function, including measurement of early morning resting cortisol levels, in all patients. An early morning resting cortisol level may be accepted as normal if it falls at or near the normal mean level.

## Indications

   *Asthma, chronic:* Maintenance and prophylactic treatment of asthma; includes patients who require systemic corticosteroids and those who may benefit from systemic dose reduction/elimination; for the maintenance treatment of asthma and as prophylactic therapy in children 12 months to 8 years of age (budesonide respules).

   Not indicated for relief of asthma that can be controlled by bronchodilators and other nonsteroid medications, in patients who require systemic corticosteroid treatment infrequently, or in the treatment of nonasthmatic bronchitis.

## Administration and Dosage

| Estimated Comparative Daily Dosages for Inhaled Corticosteroids (Adults)[1] | | | |
|---|---|---|---|
| Drug | Low dose | Medium dose | High dose |
| Beclomethasone dipropionate | 168 to 504 mcg | 504 to 840 mcg | > 840 mcg |
| 42 mcg/puff | 4 to 12 puffs | 12 to 20 puffs | > 20 puffs |
| 84 mcg/puff | 2 to 6 puffs | 6 to 10 puffs | > 10 puffs |
| Budesonide *Turbuhaler* | 200 to 400 mcg | 400 to 600 mcg | > 600 mcg |
| 200 mcg/dose | 1 to 2 inhalations | 2 to 3 inhalations | > 3 inhalations |

### Estimated Comparative Daily Dosages for Inhaled Corticosteroids (Adults)[1]

| Drug | Low dose | Medium dose | High dose |
|---|---|---|---|
| Flunisolide<br>250 mcg/puff | 500 to 1000 mcg<br>2 to 4 puffs | 1000 to 2000 mcg<br>4 to 8 puffs | > 2000 mcg<br>> 8 puffs |
| Fluticasone<br>MDI:[2] 44, 110,<br>220 mcg/puff | 88 to 264 mcg<br>2 to 6 puffs (44 mcg)<br>or 2 puffs (110 mcg) | 264 to 660 mcg<br>2 to 6 puffs (110 mcg) | > 660 mcg<br>> 6 puffs<br>(110 mcg)<br>or > 3 puffs<br>(220 mcg) |
| DPI:[3] 50, 100, 250 mcg/puff | 2 to 6 inhalations<br>(50 mcg) | 3 to 6 inhalations<br>(100 mcg) | > 6 inhalations<br>(100 mcg) or<br>> 2 inhalations<br>(250 mcg) |
| Triamcinolone acetonide<br>100 mcg/puff | 400 to 1000 mcg<br>4 to 10 puffs | 1000 to 2000 mcg<br>10 to 20 puffs | > 2000 mcg<br>> 20 puffs |

[1] Guidelines for the Diagnosis and Management of Asthma. Expert Panel Report 2. National Institutes of Health. National Heart, Lung, and Blood Institute. February 1997. http://www.lungusa.org/asthma/astnhlbi.html
[2] MDI = Metered dose inhaler.
[3] DPI = Dry powder inhaler.

### Estimated Comparative Daily Dosages for Inhaled Corticosteroids (Children)[1]

| Drug | Low dose | Medium dose | High dose |
|---|---|---|---|
| Beclomethasone dipropionate<br>(6 to 12 years of age)<br>42 mcg/puff<br>84 mcg/puff | 84 to 336 mcg<br>2 to 8 puffs<br>1 to 4 puffs | 336 to 672 mcg<br>8 to 16 puffs<br>4 to 8 puffs | > 672 mcg<br>> 16 puffs<br>> 8 puffs |
| Budesonide Turbuhaler<br>(≥ 6 years of age)<br>200 mcg/dose | 100 to 200 mcg | 200 to 400 mcg<br>1 to 2 inhalations | > 400 mcg<br>> 2 inhalations |
| Flunisolide<br>(6 to 15 years of age)<br>250 mcg/puff | 500 to 750 mcg<br>2 to 3 puffs | 1000 to 1250 mcg<br>4 to 5 puffs | > 1250 mcg<br>> 5 puffs |
| Fluticasone<br>(≥ 12 years of age)<br>MDI:[2] 44, 110 mcg/puff | 88 to 176 mcg<br>2 to 4 puffs<br>(44 mcg) | 176 to 440 mcg<br>4 to 10 puffs<br>(44 mcg) or<br>2 to 4 puffs<br>(110 mcg) | > 440 mcg<br>> 4 puffs (110 mcg) |
| DPI:[3] 50, 100, 250 mcg/dose | 2 to 4 inhalations<br>(50 mcg) | 2 to 4 inhalations<br>(100 mcg) | > 4 inhalations<br>(100 mcg) or<br>> 2 inhalations<br>(250 mcg) |
| Triamcinolone acetonide<br>(6 to 12 years of age)<br>100 mcg/puff | 400 to 800 mcg<br>4 to 8 puffs | 800 to 1200 mcg<br>8 to 12 puffs | > 1200 mcg<br>> 12 puffs |

[1] Guidelines for the Diagnosis and Management of Asthma. Expert Panel Report 2. National Institutes of Health. National Heart, Lung, and Blood Institute. February 1997. http://www.lungusa.org/asthma/astnhlbi.html
[2] MDI = Metered dose inhaler.
[3] DPI = Dry powder inhaler.

*Patients receiving concomitant systemic steroids:* Slowly wean patients from systemic corticosteroids after transferring to steroid inhalers. Monitor lung function ($FEV_1$ or AM PEFR), beta-agonist use, and asthma symptoms during withdrawal of oral corticosteroids. Transfer to steroid inhalant and subsequent management may be more difficult because of slow HPA function recovery that may last up to 12 months. These agents may be effective and may permit replacement or significant reduction in corticosteroid dosage.

Stabilize the patient's asthma before treatment is started. Initially, use aerosol concurrently with usual maintenance dose of systemic steroid. After approximately 1 week, start gradual withdrawal of the systemic steroid by reducing the daily or alternate daily dose. Make the next reduction after 1 to 2 weeks, depending on response. Generally, these decrements should not exceed 25% of the prednisone dose or its equivalent. A slow rate of withdrawal cannot be overemphasized.

During withdrawal, some patients may experience symptoms of steroid withdrawal (eg, joint or muscular pain, lassitude, depression) despite maintenance or even improvement of respiratory function. Encourage continuance with the inhaler, but observe for objective signs of adrenal insufficiency (eg, fatigue, lassitude, weakness, nausea and vomiting, hypotension). If adrenal insufficiency occurs, increase the systemic steroid dose temporarily and continue further withdrawal more slowly.

During periods of stress or severe asthma attack, transfer patients will require supplementary systemic steroids.

BECLOMETHASONE: Test aerosol by spraying 2 times into the air before first use and in cases where the product has not been used for over 10 days. Rinse mouth after inhalation.

The safety and efficacy in children less than 5 years of age have not been established.

The onset and degree of symptom relief will vary in individual patients. Improvement in asthma symptoms should be expected within the first or second week of starting treatment, but maximum benefit should not be expected until 3 to 4 weeks of therapy. For patients who do not respond adequately to the starting dose after 3 to 4 weeks of therapy, higher doses may provide additional asthma control. The safety and efficacy of beclomethasone when administered in excess of recommended doses have not been established.

The aerosol solution does not require shaking. Two actuations of the 40 mcg strength should provide a dose comparable to 1 actuation of the 80 mcg strength. The recommended dosage relative to CFC-based beclomethasone dipropionate (CFC-BDP) inhalation aerosols is lower because of differences in delivery characteristics between the products.

| Recommended Doses in Patients ≥ 5 Years of Age | | |
| --- | --- | --- |
| Previous therapy | Recommended starting dose | Highest recommended dose |
| Adults and adolescents | | |
| Bronchodilators alone | 40 to 80 mcg twice daily | 320 mcg twice daily |
| Inhaled corticosteroids | 40 to 160 mcg twice daily | 320 mcg twice daily |
| Children 5 to 11 years of age | | |
| Bronchodilators alone | 40 mcg twice daily | 80 mcg twice daily |
| Inhaled corticosteroids | 40 mcg twice daily | 80 mcg twice daily |

Titrate the dose downward over time to the lowest level that maintains proper asthma control. The aerosol may have a different taste and inhalation sensation than that of an inhaler containing CFC propellant.

*Patients not receiving systemic corticosteroids* – Follow the doses recommended above. In patients who respond to beclomethasone, improvement in pulmonary function is usually apparent within 1 to 4 weeks after the start of therapy. Once the desired effect is achieved, consider tapering to the lowest effective dose.

*Concomitant systemic corticosteroid therapy* – See Administration in group monograph.

BUDESONIDE:

| Budesonide Recommended Starting Dose and Highest Recommended Dose | | |
| --- | --- | --- |
| Previous therapy | Recommended starting dose[1] | Highest recommended dose |
| *Turbuhaler* | | |
| *Adults* | | |
| Bronchodilators alone | 200-400 mcg twice/day | 400 mcg twice/day |
| Inhaled corticosteroids[2] | 200-400 mcg twice/day | 800 mcg twice/day |
| Oral corticosteroids | 400-800 mcg twice/day | 800 mcg twice/day |

| Budesonide Recommended Starting Dose and Highest Recommended Dose | | |
|---|---|---|
| Previous therapy | Recommended starting dose[1] | Highest recommended dose |
| *Children ≥ 6 years of age*[3] | | |
| Bronchodilators alone | 200 mcg twice/day | 400 mcg twice/day |
| Inhaled corticosteroids[2] | 200 mcg twice/day | 400 mcg twice/day |
| Oral corticosteroids | The highest recommended dose in children is 400 mcg twice/day. | |
| *Respules* | | |
| *Children 12 months to 8 years of age* | | |
| Bronchodilators alone | 0.5 mg total daily dose administered either once or twice daily in divided doses | 0.5 mg total daily dose |
| Inhaled corticosteroids | 0.5 mg total daily dose administered either once or twice daily in divided doses | 1 mg total daily dose |
| Oral corticosteroids | 1 mg total daily dose administered either as 0.5 mg twice/day or 1 mg once daily | 1 mg total daily dose |

[1] 200 mcg released with each actuation delivers ≈ 160 mcg to the patient (*Turbuhaler*).
[2] In patients with mild to moderate asthma who are well controlled on inhaled corticosteroids, dosing budesonide 200 mcg or 400 mcg once daily may be considered. Administer budesonide once daily either in the morning or evening.
[3] Insufficient information is available to warrant use in children < 6 years of age.

*Budesonide turbuhaler* – In all patients, it is desirable to titrate to the lowest effective dose once asthma stability is achieved.

Each actuation delivers ≈ 160 mcg budesonide.

Improvement in asthma control following inhaled administration of budesonide can occur within 24 hours of treatment initiation, although maximum benefit may not be achieved for 1 to 2 weeks or more.

*Budesonide respules* – Administer by the inhaled route via jet nebulizer connected to an air compressor in asthmatic patients 12 months to 8 years of age. Improvement in asthma control following inhaled administration of budesonide can occur within 2 to 8 days of initiation of treatment, although maximum benefit may not be achieved for 4 to 6 weeks. It is desirable to downward-titrate to the lowest effective dose once asthma stability is achieved. In symptomatic children not responding to nonsteroidal therapy and in patients who require maintenance therapy of their asthma, a starting dose of 0.25 mg once daily may also be considered.

If once-daily treatment with budesonide does not provide adequate control of asthma symptoms, increase the total daily dose or administer as a divided dose.

Ultrasonic nebulizers are not suitable for the adequate administration of budesonide respules and therefore, are not recommended. The effects of mixing budesonide respules with other nebulizable medications has not been adequately assessed; administer separately in the nebulizer.

*Patients maintained on chronic oral corticosteroids* – Initially use concurrently with the patient's usual maintenance dose of systemic corticosteroid. Initiate at 1 mg/day.

FLUNISOLIDE: Each actuation delivers approximately 250 mcg flunisolide.

*Adults* – 2 inhalations (500 mcg) twice daily, morning and evening (total daily dose 1000 mcg). Do not exceed 4 inhalations twice daily (2000 mcg).

*Children 6 to 15 years of age* – 2 inhalations twice daily, morning and evening (total daily dose 1000 mcg). Higher doses have not been studied. Safety and efficacy for use in children younger than 6 years of age have not been established. With chronic use, monitor children for growth as well as for effects on the HPA axis. Insufficient information is available to warrant use in children younger than 6 years of age.

*Patients not receiving systemic steroids* – In responsive patients, pulmonary function usually improves within 1 to 4 weeks.

FLUTICASONE:
*Fluticasone aerosol (12 years of age or older)* –

| Recommended Doses for Fluticasone Aerosol | | |
|---|---|---|
| Previous therapy | Recommended starting dose | Highest recommended dose |
| Bronchodilators alone | 88 mcg twice/day | 440 mcg twice/day |
| Inhaled corticosteroids | 88-220 mcg twice/day[1] | 440 mcg twice/day |
| Oral corticosteroids | 880 mcg twice/day | 880 mcg twice/day |

[1] Starting doses > 88 mcg twice/day may be considered for patients with poorer asthma control or those who have previously required doses of inhaled corticosteroids that are in the higher range for that specific agent.

*Fluticasone powder (4 years of age and older)* –

| Recommended Doses for Fluticasone Powder | | |
|---|---|---|
| Previous therapy | Recommended starting dose | Highest recommended dose |
| *Adults and adolescents* | | |
| Bronchodilators alone | 100 mcg twice/day | 500 mcg twice/day |
| Inhaled corticosteroids | 100-250 mcg twice/day[1] | 500 mcg twice/day |
| Oral corticosteroids | 1000 mcg twice/day | 1000 mcg twice/day |
| *Children 4 to 11 years of age* | | |
| Bronchodilators alone | 50 mcg twice/day | 100 mcg twice/day |
| Inhaled corticosteroids | 50 mcg twice/day | 100 mcg twice/day |

[1] Starting doses > 100 mcg twice/day for adults and adolescents and 50 mcg twice daily for children 4 to 11 years of age may be considered for patients with poorer asthma control or those who have previously required doses of inhaled corticosteroids that are in the higher range for that specific agent.

TRIAMCINOLONE: 200 mcg released with each actuation delivers approximately 100 mcg.

*Adults* – The usual dosage is 2 inhalations (approximately 200 mcg) 3 to 4 times/day or 4 inhalations (400 mcg) twice daily. Do not exceed a maximum daily intake of 16 inhalations (1600 mcg). Higher initial doses (12 to 16 inhalations/day) may be advisable in patients with more severe asthma.

*Children 6 to 12 years of age* – The usual dosage is 1 or 2 inhalations (100 to 200 mcg) 3 to 4 times/day or 2 to 4 inhalations (200 to 400 mcg) twice daily. Do not exceed a maximum daily intake of 12 inhalations (1200 mcg). Clinical data are insufficient with respect to use in children younger than 6 years of age. Maximum benefit may not be achieved for 2 weeks or more.

*Patients not receiving systemic steroids* – Follow above directions. In responsive patients, an improvement in pulmonary function is usually apparent within 1 to 2 weeks but maximum benefit may not be achieved for 2 weeks or more.

### Actions

*Pharmacology:* These agents are synthetic adrenocortical steroids with basic glucocorticoid actions and effects. Glucocorticoids may decrease number and activity of inflammatory cells, enhance effect of beta-adrenergic drugs on cyclic AMP production, inhibit bronchoconstrictor mechanisms, or produce direct smooth muscle relaxation. Inhaler use provides effective local steroid activity with minimal systemic effect.

*Pharmacokinetics:*

| Pharmacokinetics of Inhaled Corticosteroids | | | | | |
|---|---|---|---|---|---|
| | Corticosteroids | | | | |
| Parameters | Beclomethasone | Budesonide | Flunisolide | Fluticasone | Triamcinolone |
| Absorption<br>Systemic bioavaila-<br>bility from lungs | ≈ 20% | 25% | 40% | 20 | 21.5% |
| Distribution<br>Vd (L/kg)<br>Protein binding | NA<br>87% | 4.3<br>85% to 90% | 1.8<br>NA | 3.5<br>91% | 1.4<br>≈ 68% |
| Metabolism<br>Site | liver (CYP3A) | liver (CYP3A) | liver | liver (CYP3A4) | mostly from<br>liver, less<br>extensively<br>from the<br>kidneys |
| Metabolites<br>(Activity) | beclomethasone<br>17-mono-pro-<br>pionate (active),<br>free beclome-<br>thasone (very<br>weak anti-in-<br>flammatory<br>effects) | 16α-hydroxy-<br>prednisolone<br>and 6β-hydroxy-<br>budesonide<br>(< 1% of parent) | 6β-OH (low<br>corticosteroid<br>potency) | 17β-carboxylic<br>acid (negli-<br>gible in ani-<br>mal studies) | 6β-hydroxy-<br>triamcinolone<br>acetonide, 21-<br>carboxy-triam-<br>cinolone aceto-<br>nide, and 21-<br>carboxy-6β-<br>hydroxytriam-<br>cinolone ace-<br>tonide (less<br>active than<br>parent) |
| Excretion<br>Site<br><br>$T_{1/2}$ | feces, urine<br>(< 10%)<br>2.8 h | urine<br>(≈ 60%), feces<br>2.8 h | renal (50%),<br>feces (40%)<br>≈ 1.8 h | feces, urine<br>(< 0.02%)<br>3.1 h | urine (≈ 40%),<br>feces (≈ 60%)<br>1.5 h |

**Contraindications**

Relief of acute bronchospasm; primary treatment of status asthmaticus or other acute episodes of asthma when intensive measures are required; hypersensitivity to any ingredient; systemic fungal infections; persistently positive sputum cultures for *Candida albicans*.

*Vanceril:* Relief of asthma that can be controlled by bronchodilators and other nonsteroid medications; in patients who require systemic corticosteroid treatment infrequently; treatment of nonasthmatic bronchitis.

**Warnings**

*Infections:* Localized fungal infections with *Candida albicans* or *Aspergillus niger* have occurred in the mouth, pharynx, and occasionally in the larynx. The incidence of clinically apparent infection is low, and may require treatment with appropriate antifungal therapy or discontinuance of aerosol steroid treatment. Use inhaled corticosteroids with caution, if at all, in patients with active or quiescent tuberculous infection of the respiratory tract, untreated systemic fungal, bacterial, parasitic or viral infection, or ocular herpes simplex.

*Acute asthma:* These products are not bronchodilators and are not for rapid relief of bronchospasm. See Black Box Warning.

*Bronchospasm:* Bronchospasm may occur with an immediate increase in wheezing following dosing; treat immediately with a fast-acting inhaled bronchodilator. See Black Box Warning.

*Combination with prednisone:* Combination therapy of inhaled corticosteroids with systemic corticosteroids may increase the risk of HPA suppression compared with a therapeutic dose of either one alone. Use inhaled corticosteroids with caution in patients already receiving prednisone.

*Replacement therapy:* Transfer from systemic steroid therapy may unmask allergic conditions previously suppressed. During withdrawal from oral steroids, some patients may experience withdrawal symptoms despite maintenance or improvement of respiratory function.

*Pregnancy:* Category C; Category B (budesonide only).

*Lactation:* Glucocorticoids are excreted in breast milk. It is not known whether inhaled corticosteroids are excreted in breast milk, but it is likely.

*Children:* Insufficient information is available to warrant use in children younger than 6 years of age or younger than 12 years of age with **fluticasone** and **beclomethasone**. Monitor growth in children and adolescents because there is evidence that oral corticosteroids may suppress growth in a dose-related fashion, particularly in higher doses for extended periods.

### Precautions

*Steroid withdrawal:* During withdrawal from oral steroids, some patients may experience symptoms of systemically active steroid withdrawal (eg, joint or muscular pain, lassitude, depression), despite maintenance or even improvement of respiratory function. Although steroid withdrawal effects are usually transient and not severe, severe and even fatal exacerbation of asthma can occur if the previous daily oral corticosteroid requirement had significantly exceeded 10 mg/day of prednisone or equivalent.

*HPA suppression:* In responsive patients, inhaled corticosteroids may permit control of asthmatic symptoms with less HPA suppression. Because these agents are absorbed and can be systemically active, the beneficial effects in minimizing or preventing HPA dysfunction may be expected only when recommended dosages are not exceeded. Take particular care in observing patients postoperatively or during periods of stress for evidence of a decrease in adrenal function.

*Flunisolide* – Because of the possibility of higher systemic absorption, monitor patients using **flunisolide** for any evidence of systemic corticosteroid effect. If such changes occur, discontinue slowly, consistent with accepted procedures for discontinuing oral corticosteroids. When flunisolide is used chronically at 2 mg/day, monitor patients periodically for effects on the HPA axis.

*Glaucoma:* Rare instances of glaucoma, increased intraocular pressure, and cataracts have been reported following the inhaled administration of corticosteroids.

*Long-term effects:* The effects of long-term glucocorticoid inhalation are unknown. Although there is no clinical evidence of adverse effects, the local and systemic effects on developmental or immunologic processes in the mouth, pharynx, trachea, and lung are unknown.

There is no information about effects on acute, recurrent, or chronic pulmonary infection (including active or quiescent tuberculosis) or effects of long-term use on lung or other tissues. Use with caution (see Warnings).

*Pulmonary infiltrates:* Pulmonary infiltrates with eosinophilia may occur with beclomethasone or flunisolide.

*Reduction in growth velocity:* Closely follow the growth of adolescents taking corticosteroids, and weigh the benefits of corticosteroid therapy and asthma control against the possibility of growth suppression.

### Drug Interactions

*Ketoconazole:* A potent inhibitor of cytochrome P450 3A4 may increase plasma levels of **budesonide** and **fluticasone** during concomitant dosing. The clinical significance is unknown. Use caution.

### Adverse Reactions

*Local:* Throat irritation; hoarseness/dysphonia, coughing; dry mouth; rash; wheezing; facial edema; flu syndrome.

*Systemic:* Suppression of HPA function has occurred. Deaths caused by adrenal insufficiency have occurred during and after transfer from systemic to aerosol corticosteroids.

*Beclomethasone* – Adverse reactions occurring in 3% or more of patients include headache; nasal congestion; dysmenorrhea; dyspepsia; rhinitis; pharyngitis; coughing; upper respiratory tract infection; viral infections; sinusitis.

*Budesonide* – Adverse reactions occurring in 3% or more of patients include pain; fever; back pain; upper respiratory tract infection; sinusitis; pharyngitis; coughing; conjunctivitis; headache; rhinitis; epistaxis; otitis media; ear infection; viral infections; flu syndrome; voice alteration.

*Flunisolide* – Adverse reactions occurring in 3% or more of patients include palpitations; chest pain; dizziness; irritability; nervousness; shakiness; nausea; vomiting; abdominal pain; anorexia; heartburn; upper respiratory tract infection; nasal and sinus congestion; unpleasant taste; loss of smell or taste; edema; fever; menstrual disturbance; eczema; itching/pruritus, rash; sore throat; diarrhea; upset stomach; general flu; oral candidiasis; headache; rhinitis; sinusitis; cold symptoms; runny nose; sinus drainage/infection; hoarseness; sputum; wheezing; chest congestion; coughing; sneezing; ear infection.

*Fluticasone* – Adverse reactions occurring in 3% or more of patients include headache; pharyngitis; nasal congestion; sinusitis; rhinitis; upper respiratory tract infection; influenza; oral candidiasis; diarrhea; dysphonia; menstrual disturbance; nasal discharge; allergic rhinitis; fever.

*Triamcinolone* – Adverse reactions occurring in 3% or more of patients include pharyngitis; sinusitis; flu syndrome; headache; back pain.

# ACETYLCYSTEINE (N-Acetylcysteine)

**Solution:** 10% and 20% (*Rx*)        Various, *Mucomyst* (Apothecon)

### Indications
*Mucolytic:* Adjuvant therapy for abnormal, viscid, or inspissated mucus secretions in chronic bronchopulmonary disease (chronic emphysema, emphysema with bronchitis, chronic asthmatic bronchitis, tuberculosis, bronchiectasis, primary amyloidosis of lung).

Acute bronchopulmonary disease (pneumonia, bronchitis, tracheobronchitis).

Pulmonary complications of cystic fibrosis.

Tracheostomy care.

Pulmonary complications associated with surgery.

Use during anesthesia.

Posttraumatic chest conditions.

Atelectasis due to mucus obstruction.

Diagnostic bronchial studies (bronchograms, bronchospirometry, bronchial wedge catheterization).

*Antidote:* To prevent or lessen hepatic injury that may occur following ingestion of a potentially hepatotoxic quantity of acetaminophen.

### Administration and Dosage
*Nebulization (face mask, mouth piece, tracheostomy):* 1 to 10 mL of the 20% solution or 2 to 20 mL of the 10% solution every 2 to 6 hours; the dose for most patients is 3 to 5 mL of the 20% solution or 6 to 10 mL of the 10% solution 3 to 4 times/day.

*Nebulization (tent, croupette):* Very large volumes are required, occasionally up to 300 mL during a treatment period. The dose is the volume of solution that will maintain a very heavy mist in the tent or croupette for the desired period. Administration for intermittent or continuous prolonged periods, including overnight, may be desirable.

*Instillation:*
    *Direct* – 1 to 2 mL of a 10% to 20% solution as often as every hour.

    *Tracheostomy* – 1 to 2 mL of a 10% to 20% solution every 1 to 4 hours by instillation into the tracheostomy.

May be introduced directly into a particular segment of the bronchopulmonary tree by inserting (under local anesthesia and direct vision) a plastic catheter into the trachea. Instill 2 to 5 mL of the 20% solution by a syringe connected to the catheter.

*Percutaneous intratracheal catheter* – 1 to 2 mL of the 20% solution or 2 to 4 mL of the 10% solution every 1 to 4 hours by a syringe attached to the catheter.

*Diagnostic bronchograms:* 2 or 3 administrations of 1 to 2 mL of the 20% solution or 2 to 4 mL of the 10% solution by nebulization or by instillation intratracheally, prior to the procedure.

*Equipment compatibility:* Certain materials in nebulization equipment react with acetylcysteine, especially certain metals (notably iron and copper) and rubber. Where materials may come into contact with acetylcysteine solution, use parts made of the following materials: Glass, plastic, aluminum, anodized aluminum, chromed metal, tantalum, sterling silver, or stainless steel. Silver may become tarnished after exposure, but this is not harmful to the drug action or to the patient.

*Admixture incompatibility:* Tetracycline, chlortetracycline, oxytetracycline, erythromycin lactobionate, amphotericin B, and sodium ampicillin are incompatible when mixed in the same solution with acetylcysteine. Administer from separate solutions. Iodized oil, chymotrypsin, trypsin, and hydrogen peroxide are also incompatible.

## Actions

*Pharmacology:* The mucolytic action of acetylcysteine is related to the sulfhydryl group in the molecule, which acts directly to split disulfide linkages between mucoprotein molecular complexes, resulting in depolymerization and a decrease in mucus viscosity. The mucolytic activity of acetylcysteine increases with increasing pH.

Acetylcysteine also reduces the extent of liver injury following acetaminophen overdose. It is thought that acetylcysteine protects the liver by maintaining or restoring glutathione levels, or by acting as an alternate substrate for conjugation with, and thus, detoxification of, the reactive metabolite of acetaminophen.

*Pharmacokinetics:* Following a 200 to 400 mg oral dose, peak plasma concentrations of 0.35 to 4 mg/L are achieved within 1 to 2 hours. Protein binding is approximately 50% 4 hours postdose. Volume of distribution is 0.33 to 0.47 L/kg. The terminal half-life of reduced acetylcysteine is 6.25 hours. Approximately 70% of total body clearance is nonrenal.

## Contraindications

Hypersensitivity to acetylcysteine. As an antidote, there are no contraindications.

## Warnings

*Bronchial secretions:* An increased volume of liquefied bronchial secretions may occur; when cough is inadequate, maintain an open airway by mechanical suction if necessary. When there is a large mechanical block due to a foreign body or local accumulation, clear the airway by endotracheal aspiration, with or without bronchoscopy.

*Asthmatics:* Carefully observe asthmatics under treatment with acetylcysteine. If bronchospasm progresses, discontinue medication immediately.

*Antidotal use:*

*Allergic effects* – Generalized urticaria has been observed rarely. If this or other allergic symptoms appear, discontinue treatment unless it is deemed essential and the allergic symptoms can be otherwise controlled.

*Hepatic effects* – If encephalopathy due to hepatic failure occurs, discontinue treatment to avoid further administration of nitrogenous substances.

*Vomiting* – Vomiting, occasionally severe and persistent, occurs as a symptom of acute acetaminophen overdose. Treatment with oral acetylcysteine may aggravate vomiting. Evaluate patients at risk of gastric hemorrhage concerning the risk of upper GI hemorrhage vs the risk of developing hepatic toxicity. Diluting acetylcysteine minimizes its propensity to aggravate vomiting.

*Pregnancy: Category B.*

*Lactation:* It is not known whether this drug is excreted in breast milk.

**Precautions**

*Disagreeable odor:* Administration may initially produce a slight disagreeable odor which soon disappears.

*Face mask use:* A face mask may cause stickiness on the face after nebulization; remove with water.

*Solution color:* Solution color may change in the opened bottle, but does not significantly impair the drug's safety or efficacy.

*Continued nebulization:* Continued nebulization of acetylcysteine with a dry gas results in concentration of drug in the nebulizer due to evaporation. Extreme concentration may impede nebulization and drug delivery. Dilute with Sterile Water for Injection as concentration occurs.

**Adverse Reactions**

Adverse reactions may include stomatitis; nausea; vomiting; fever; rhinorrhea; drowsiness; clamminess; chest tightness; bronchoconstriction; bronchospasm; irritation to the tracheal and bronchial tracts.

*Antidotal use* – Large doses of oral acetylcysteine may result in nausea, vomiting, and other GI symptoms. Rash (with or without mild fever), pruritus, angioedema, bronchospasm, tachycardia, hypotension, and hypertension have occurred.

# IPRATROPIUM BROMIDE

**Aerosol:** Each actuation delivers 18 mcg (*Rx*)
**Solution for Inhalation:** 0.02% (500 mcg/vial) (*Rx*)
**Nasal spray:** 0.03% (21 mcg/spray) and
0.06% (42 mcg/spray) (Rx)

*Atrovent* (Boehringer Ingelheim)
Various, *Atrovent* (Boehringer Ingelheim)
*Atrovent* (Boehringer Ingelheim)

**Indications**

*Bronchospasm (solution and aerosol):* Used alone or in combination with other bronchodilators (especially beta-adrenergics) as a bronchodilator for maintenance treatment of bronchospasm associated with chronic obstructive pulmonary disease (COPD), including chronic bronchitis and emphysema. Ipratropium is not indicated for the initial treatment of acute episodes of bronchospasms.

*Rhinorrhea:*

*Perennial rhinitis (0.03% nasal spray)* – Symptomatic relief of rhinorrhea associated with allergic and nonallergic perennial rhinitis in patients 6 years of age or older.

*Common cold (0.06% nasal spray)* – Symptomatic relief of rhinorrhea associated with the common cold in patients 5 years of age or older.

**Administration and Dosage**

*Aerosol:* The usual dose is 2 inhalations (36 mcg) 4 times/day. Patients may take additional inhalations as required; however, do not exceed 12 inhalations in 24 hours.

*Solution:* The usual dose is 500 mcg (1 unit dose vial) administered 3 to 4 times/day by oral nebulization, with doses 6 to 8 hours apart. The solution can be mixed in the nebulizer with albuterol if used within 1 hour.

*Nasal spray:*

*0.03% (patients 6 years of age or older)* – The usual dose is 2 sprays (42 mcg) per nostril 2 or 3 times/day (total dose, 168 to 252 mcg/day). Optimum dosage varies.

*0.06% (patients 5 years of age or older)* – Recommended dose is 2 sprays (84 mcg) per nostril 3 or 4 times/day (total dose, 504 to 672 mcg/day). Optimum dosage varies.

*Children 5 to 11 years of age:* Recommended dose is 2 sprays (84 mcg) per nostril 3 times/day (total dose, 504 mcg/day).

The safety and efficacy of use for more than 4 days in patients with the common cold have not been established.

**Actions**

*Pharmacology:* Ipratropium for oral inhalation is a synthetic quaternary anticholinergic (parasympatholytic) ammonium compound chemically related to atropine. It appears to inhibit vagally mediated reflexes by antagonizing the action of acetylcholine. The bronchodilation following inhalation is primarily a local, site-specific effect, not a systemic one.

*Pharmacokinetics:* Much of an inhaled dose is swallowed as shown by fecal excretion studies. Ipratropium is not readily absorbed into the systemic circulation either from the surface of the lung or from the GI tract as confirmed by blood levels and renal excretion studies. The elimination half-life is approximately 1.6 hours.

**Contraindications**

Hypersensitivity to ipratropium, atropine, or its derivatives; a history of hypersensitivity to soya lecithin or related food products such as soy bean or peanut (inhalation aerosol).

**Warnings**

*Acute bronchospasm:* Ipratropium is not indicated as a single agent for relief of bronchospasm in acute COPD exacerbation.

*Special risk patients:* Use with caution in patients with narrow-angle glaucoma, prostatic hypertrophy, or bladder neck obstruction.

*Pregnancy:* Category B.

*Lactation:* It is not known whether this drug is excreted in breast milk.

*Children:* Safety and efficacy in children younger than 12 years of age (aerosol and solution), younger than 6 years of age (0.03% nasal spray), and younger than 5 years of age (0.06% nasal spray) have not been established.

**Drug Interactions**

Ipratropium has been used concomitantly with other drugs, including sympathomimetic bronchodilators, methylxanthines, steroids, and cromolyn sodium, commonly used in the treatment of chronic obstructive pulmonary disease, without adverse drug reactions.

**Adverse Reactions**

Adverse reactions from **inhalational products** may include nervousness, cough, dryness of the oropharynx, irritation from aerosol, exacerbation of symptoms, dizziness, headache, GI distress, dry mouth, influenza-like symptoms, back or chest pain, nausea, dyspnea, bronchitis, upper respiratory tract infection, epistaxis, pharyngitis, nasal dryness, and miscellaneous nasal symptoms.

Adverse reactions from **nasal spray** may include epistaxis, nasal dryness, headache, and upper respiratory tract infection.

# TIOTROPIUM BROMIDE

**Powder for inhalation:** 18 mcg (as base) (*Rx*)                    *Spiriva* (Boehringer Ingelheim)

**Indications**

*Chronic obstructive pulmonary disease (COPD):* For the long-term, once-daily, maintenance treatment of bronchospasm associated with COPD, including chronic bronchitis and emphysema.

**Administration and Dosage**

*Dose:* Inhalation of the contents of 1 capsule, once daily, with the *HandiHaler* inhalation device.

*Administration:* Tiotropium capsules are for inhalation only; do not swallow.

1.) Immediately before using the tiotropium dose, peel back the aluminum foil using the tab until 1 capsule is fully visible. Peel back the foil lidding only as far as the "STOP" line printed on the blister foil to prevent exposure of more than 1 capsule. Immediately use the drug after opening the packaging over an individual capsule or its efficacy may be reduced.

2.) Open the dust cap of the *HandiHaler* by pulling it upwards, then open the mouthpiece.

3.) Place the capsule in the center chamber. It does not matter which end of the capsule is placed in the chamber.

4.) Firmly close the mouthpiece until a click is heard, leaving the dust cap open.

5.) Hold the *HandiHaler* device with the mouthpiece upwards, press the piercing button completely in once, and release. This makes holes in the capsule and allows the medication to be released.

6.) Breathe out completely. Do not breathe into the mouthpiece at any time.

7.) Raise the *HandiHaler* device to mouth and close lips tightly around the mouthpiece.

8.) Keep head in an upright position, and breathe in slowly and deeply but at a rate sufficient to hear the capsule vibrate. Breathe in until lungs are full, then hold breath as long as is comfortable. At the same time, take the *Handi-Haler* device out of mouth. Resume normal breathing.

9.) To ensure getting the full dose of tiotropium, repeat this once again.

10.) After finishing taking the daily dose of tiotropium, open the mouthpiece again. Tip out the used capsule and dispose. Close the mouthpiece and dust cap for storage.

### Actions

*Pharmacology:* Tiotropium is a long-acting, antimuscarinic agent, which is often referred to as an anticholinergic. In the airways, it exhibits pharmacological effects through inhibition of $M_3$-receptors at the smooth muscle, leading to bronchodilation. The bronchodilation following inhalation of tiotropium is predominantly a site-specific effect.

*Pharmacokinetics:*

*Absorption* – The majority of a delivered dose is deposited in the GI tract and, to a lesser extent, in the lung, the intended organ. The absolute bioavailability of 19.5% suggests that the fraction reaching the lung is highly bioavailable. Maximum tiotropium plasma concentrations were observed 5 minutes after inhalation.

*Distribution* – Tiotropium shows a volume of distribution of 32 L/kg, indicating that the drug binds extensively to tissues. The drug is bound 72% to plasma proteins. At steady state, peak plasma levels in COPD patients were 17 to 19 pg/mL when measured 5 minutes after an 18 mcg dry powder inhalation dose and decreased rapidly in a multicompartmental manner. Steady-state trough plasma concentrations were 3 to 4 pg/mL.

*Metabolism* – The extent of biotransformation appears to be small. In vitro experiments with human liver microsomes and human hepatocytes suggest that a fraction of the administered dose (74% of an IV dose is excreted unchanged in the urine, leaving 25% for metabolism) is metabolized by cytochrome P450-dependent oxidation and subsequent glutathione conjugation to a variety of phase 2 metabolites. This enzymatic pathway can be inhibited by CYP450 2D6 and 3A4 inhibitors (eg, quinidine, ketoconazole, and gestodene).

*Excretion* – The terminal elimination half-life is between 5 and 6 days following inhalation. After dry powder inhalation, urinary excretion is 14% of the dose, the remainder being mainly nonabsorbed drug in the gut, which is eliminated via the feces. The renal clearance of tiotropium exceeds the Ccr, indicating active secretion into the urine. After chronic, once-daily inhalation by COPD patients, pharmacokinetic steady state was reached after 2 to 3 weeks with no accumulation thereafter.

### Contraindications

History of hypersensitivity to atropine or its derivatives, including ipratropium, or to any component of the product.

### Warnings

*Bronchospasm:* Tiotropium is not indicated for the initial treatment of acute episodes of bronchospasm (ie, rescue therapy). Inhaled medicines, including tiotropium, may cause paradoxical bronchospasm. If this occurs, stop treatment with tiotropium and consider other treatments.

*QT prolongation:* In a multicenter, randomized, double-blind trial that enrolled 198 patients with COPD, the number of subjects with changes from baseline-corrected QT interval of 30 to 60 msec was higher in the tiotropium group as compared with placebo. No patients in either group had QT of more than 500 msec.

*Hypersensitivity reactions:* Immediate hypersensitivity reactions, including angioedema, may occur after administration of tiotropium. If such a reaction occurs, stop therapy at once and consider alternative treatment.

*Renal function impairment:* Renal impairment was associated with increased plasma drug concentrations and reduced drug clearance after IV infusion and dry powder inhalation. Mild renal impairment (Ccr 50 to 80 mL/min) increased tiotropium plasma concentrations (39% increase in $AUC_{0-4}$ after IV infusion). In COPD patients with moderate to severe renal impairment (Ccr less than 50 mL/min), the IV administration of tiotropium resulted in doubling of the plasma concentrations (82% increase in $AUC_{0-4}$), which was confirmed by plasma concentrations after dry powder inhalation. Because tiotropium is a predominantly renally excreted drug, closely monitor patients with moderate to severe renal impairment (Ccr 50 mL/min or less).

*Elderly:* Advanced age was associated with a decrease of tiotropium renal clearance, which may be explained by decreased renal function. In the placebo-controlled studies, a higher frequency of dry mouth, constipation, and urinary tract infections was observed with increasing age in the tiotropium group.

*Pregnancy: Category C.*

*Lactation:* It is not known whether tiotropium is excreted in human milk. Exercise caution if administering to a nursing woman.

*Children:* Safety and efficacy have not been established.

**Precautions**

*Special risk:* As an anticholinergic drug, tiotropium potentially may worsen signs and symptoms associated with narrow-angle glaucoma, prostatic hyperplasia, or bladder-neck obstruction; use with caution in patients with any of these conditions.

**Drug Interactions**

*Anticholinergic agents:* The coadministration of tiotropium with other anticholinergic-containing drugs (eg, ipratropium) has not been studied and, therefore, is not recommended.

**Adverse Reactions**

Adverse reactions occurring in 3% or more of patients include abdominal pain, accidents, chest pain (nonspecific), constipation, dry mouth, dyspepsia, edema (dependent), epistaxis, infection, moniliasis, myalgia, pharyngitis, rash, rhinitis, sinusitis, upper respiratory tract infection, urinary tract infection, vomiting.

# IPRATROPIUM BROMIDE AND ALBUTEROL SULFATE

| | |
|---|---|
| **Aerosol**: Each actuation delivers 18 mcg ipratropium bromide and 103 mcg albuterol sulfate (*Rx*) | *Combivent* (Boehringer Ingelheim) |
| **Inhalation solution**: 0.5 mg ipratropium bromide and 3 mg albuterol sulfate (equiv. to 2.5 mg albuterol base) | *DuoNeb* (Dey) |

**Indications**

*Bronchospasm:* Use in patients with chronic obstructive pulmonary disease (COPD) on a regular aerosol bronchodilator who continue to have evidence of bronchospasm and require a second bronchodilator.

**Administration and Dosage**

*Combivent:* Shake well before using.

The recommended dose is 2 inhalations 4 times/day. Patients may take additional inhalations as required; however, advise the patient not to exceed 12 in 24 hours. It is recommended to "test spray" 3 times before using the first time and in cases where the aerosol has not be used for more than 24 hours.

*DuoNeb:* The recommended dose is one 3 mL vial administered 4 times/day via nebulization with up to 2 additional 3 mL doses allowed per day, if needed. Administer via jet nebulizer connected to an air compressor with an adequate air flow, equipped with mouthpiece or suitable face mask.

The use of these agents can be continued as medically indicated to control recurring bouts of bronchospasm. If a previously effective regimen fails to provide the usual relief, medical advice should be sought immediately, as this is often a sign of worsening COPD, which would require reassessment of therapy.

# CROMOLYN SODIUM (Disodium Cromoglycate)

| | |
|---|---|
| **Inhalation (for nebulization)**: 20 mg/2 mL (*Rx*) | Various |
| **Solution (for nebulizer only)**: 20 mg/amp (*Rx*) | *Intal* (King) |
| **Aerosol spray**: Each actuation delivers 800 mcg (*Rx*) | |
| **Nasal Solution**: 40 mg/mL | *Nasalcrom* (Pharmacia) |
| Each actuation delivers 5.2 mg (*otc*) | |
| **Oral concentrate**: 5 mL/100 mg (*Rx*) | *Gastrocrom* (Celltech) |

### Indications
*Bronchial asthma (inhalation solution, aerosol):* As prophylactic management of bronchial asthma. Cromolyn is given on a regular, daily basis in patients with frequent symptomatology requiring a continuous medication regimen.

*Prevention of bronchospasm (inhalation solution, aerosol):* To prevent acute bronchospasm induced by exercise, toluene diisocyanate, environmental pollutants, and known antigens.

*Allergic rhinitis (nasal solution):* To prevent and treat allergic rhinitis caused by airborne pollens from trees, grasses, or ragweed, and by mold, animals, and dust. To prevent and relieve the following nasal symptoms: Runny/itchy nose, sneezing, and allergic stuffy nose.

*Mastocytosis (oral):* Improves diarrhea, flushing, headaches, vomiting, urticaria, abdominal pain, nausea and itching in some patients.

*Unlabeled uses:* Cromolyn has been used as an alternative therapy in refractory forms of chronic urticaria/angioedema. Oral cromolyn has been used for the treatment of food allergies and mucosal and serosal eosinophilic gastroenteritis.

### Administration and Dosage
*Nebulizer solution:*
 *Adults and children 2 or more years of age* – Initially, 20 mg inhaled 4 times/day at regular intervals. The effectiveness of therapy depends upon administration at regular intervals.

 Administer solution from a power operated nebulizer having an adequate flow rate and equipped with a suitable face mask or mouthpiece. *Hand operated nebulizers are not suitable.*

 Introduce cromolyn into the patient's therapeutic regimen when the acute episode has been controlled, the airway has been cleared, and the patient is able to inhale adequately.

 Improvement ordinarily occurs within the first 4 weeks of administration, although some patients may demonstrate an immediate response. Efficacy is manifested by a decrease in the severity of clinical symptoms, or the need for concomitant therapy, or both.

*Prevention of acute bronchospasm:* Inhale 20 mg (1 amp/vial) administered by nebulization shortly before exposure to the precipitating factor.

*Aerosol:* For management of bronchial asthma in adults and children 5 or more years of age, the usual starting dose is two metered sprays inhaled 4 times/day at regular intervals. Do not exceed this dose. Not all patients will respond to the recommended dose, and a lower dose may provide efficacy in younger patients.

Advise patients with chronic asthma that the effect of therapy is dependent upon its administration at regular intervals, as directed. Introduce therapy into the patient's therapeutic regimen when the acute episode has been controlled, the airway has been cleared and the patient is able to inhale adequately.

*Prevention of acute bronchospasm* – The usual dose is inhalation of 2 metered dose sprays shortly (ie, 10 to 15 minutes but not more than 60 minutes) before exposure to the precipitating factor.

Nasal solution:

*Adults and children 2 or more years of age* – One spray in each nostril 3 to 6 times/day at regular intervals every 4 to 6 hours. Maximum effects may not be seen for 1 to 2 weeks. Clear the nasal passages before administering the spray and inhale through the nose during administration.

Oral:

*Adults (13 or more years of age)* – Two ampules 4 times/day, 30 minutes before meals and at bedtime.

*Children 2 to 12 years of age* – One ampule 4 times/day 30 minutes before meals and bedtime.

If satisfactory control of symptoms is not achieved within 2 to 3 weeks, the dosage may be increased but should not exceed 40 mg/kg/day.

The effect of therapy is dependent upon its administration at regular intervals as directed. Not for inhalation or injection.

*Maintenance* – Once a therapeutic response has been achieved the dose may be reduced to the minimum required to maintain the patient with a lower degree of symptomatology. To prevent relapses, maintain the dosage.

Administer as a solution in water 30 or more minutes before meals after preparation according to the following directions.

1.) Break open and squeeze liquid contents of ampule(s) into a glass of water.
2.) Stir solution.
3.) Drink all of the liquid.

*Concomitant corticosteroid treatment:* Continue concomitant corticosteroid treatment and bronchodilators following the introduction of cromolyn. If the patient improves, attempt to decrease corticosteroid dosage. Even if the steroid-dependent patient fails to improve following cromolyn use, attempt gradual tapering of steroid dosage while maintaining close patient supervision. Consider reinstituting steroid therapy for a patient subjected to significant stress while being treated or within 1 year (occasionally up to 2 years) after steroid treatment has been terminated, in case of adrenocortical insufficiency. When the inhalation of cromolyn is impaired, a temporary increase in the amount of steroids or other agents may be required.

Cautiously withdraw cromolyn in cases where its use has permitted a reduction in the maintenance dose of steroids as there may be a sudden reappearance of asthma that will require immediate therapy and possible reintroduction of corticosteroids.

*Nonsteroidal agents:* Add cromolyn (inhalation solution and aerosol) to the patient's existing treatment regimen (eg, bronchodilators). Concomitant medications may be decreased gradually when a clinical response to cromolyn is evident (approximately 2 to 4 weeks) and asthma is under good control. Titrate the frequency of cromolyn administration downward to the lowest effective level if concomitant medications are discontinued or required on no more than an as-needed basis. The usual decrease is from 4 to 3 ampules/vials per day for the nebulizer solution, or from 2 metered inhalations 4 times/day to 3 times/day to twice daily for the inhalation aerosol. Gradually reduce dosage to avoid asthma exacerbations. Clinical deterioration in these patients whose dosage has been decreased to less than 4 ampules/vials or 4 inhalations per day may require an increase in cromolyn dosage and the introduction of, or increase in, symptomatic medications.

*Compatibility:* Cromolyn **nebulizer solution** is compatible with metaproterenol sulfate, ipratropium bromide, isoproterenol HCl, isoetharine HCl, epinephrine HCl, terbutaline sulfate, and 20% acetylcysteine solution for 1 hour or more after their admixture. It also was compatible with 0.6% and 5% metaproterenol sulfate, 0.2% atropine sulfate, 0.5% albuterol sulfate, and 0.9% sodium chloride solution for at least 90 minutes after their admixture.

### Actions

*Pharmacology:* Cromolyn is an anti-inflammatory agent. It has no intrinsic bronchodilator, antihistaminic, anticholinergic, vasoconstrictor, or glucocorticoid activity. The drug inhibits the release of mediators, histamine, and SRS-A (the slow-reacting substance of anaphylaxis, a leukotriene) from the mast cell. Cromolyn acts locally on the lung to which it is directly applied.

*Pharmacokinetics:* After inhalation, approximately 8% is absorbed from the lung and is rapidly excreted unchanged in bile and urine. The remainder is either exhaled, or deposited in the oropharynx, swallowed and excreted via the alimentary tract.

Cromolyn is poorly absorbed from the GI tract. No more than 1% of an administered dose is absorbed after oral administration, the remainder excreted in the feces.

### Contraindications

Hypersensitivity to cromolyn or to any ingredient contained in these products.

### Warnings

*Acute asthma:* Cromolyn has no role in the treatment of acute asthma, especially status asthmaticus; it is a prophylactic drug with no benefit for acute situations.

*Hypersensitivity reactions:* Severe anaphylactic reactions may occur rarely.

*Renal/Hepatic function impairment:* Decrease the dose or discontinue the drug in these patients.

*Pregnancy:* Category B.

*Lactation:* Safety for use in the nursing mother has not been established.

*Children:*

*Aerosol* – Safety and efficacy in children younger than 2 years of age are not established.

*Nebulizer solution* – Safety and efficacy in children younger than 2 years of age not established.

*Nasal solution* – Safety and efficacy in children younger than 2 years of age are not established.

*Oral* – In term infants up to 6 months of age, data suggest the dose not exceed 20 mg/kg/day. Reserve use in children younger than 2 years of age for patients with severe disease in which potential benefits clearly outweigh risks.

### Precautions

*Bronchospasm/cough:* Occasionally, patients experience cough or bronchospasm following inhalation.

*Asthma:* Asthma may recur if drug is reduced below recommended dosage or discontinued.

*Eosinophilic pneumonia:* Pulmonary infiltrates with eosinophilia. If this occurs during the course of therapy, discontinue the drug.

*Aerosol:* Because of the propellants in this preparation, use with caution in patients with coronary artery disease or cardiac arrhythmias.

### Adverse Reactions

The most frequently reported adverse reactions attributed to cromolyn sodium (on the basis of recurrence following readministration) involve the respiratory tract and include bronchospasm (sometimes severe, associated with a precipitous fall in pulmonary function [$FEV_1$]), cough, laryngeal edema (rare), nasal congestion (sometimes severe), pharyngeal irritation, and wheezing.

Adverse reactions associated with *aerosol* may include throat irritation or dryness, bad taste, cough, wheeze, and nausea.

Reactions from the **nebulizer solution** may include cough, nasal congestion, wheezing, sneezing, nasal itching, epistaxis, nose burning, serum sickness, and stomach ache.

Adverse events associated with the **nasal solution** may include sneezing, nasal stinging, and nasal irritation.

Adverse reactions from oral concentrate may include headache and diarrhea.

# NEDOCROMIL SODIUM

| | |
|---|---|
| Aerosol: 1.75 mg/actuation (*Rx*) | *Tilade* (Monarch) |

### Indications
*Asthma:* Maintenance therapy in the management of adult and pediatric patients 6 years of age and older with mild to moderate asthma.

### Administration and Dosage
Two inhalations 4 times/day at regular intervals to provide 14 mg/day. In patients under good control on 4 times/day dosing (ie, patients whose only medication need is occasional [not more than twice a week] inhaled or oral beta-agonists, and who have no serious exacerbations with respiratory infections), a lower dose can be tried.

Add nedocromil to the patient's existing treatment regimen (eg, bronchodilators). When a clinical response to nedocromil is evident and if the asthma is under good control, an attempt may be made to decrease concomitant medication usage gradually.

Advise patients that the optimal effect of nedocromil therapy depends on its administration at regular intervals, even during symptom-free periods.

Each nedocromil inhaler canister must be primed with 3 actuations prior to the first use. If a canister remains unused for more than 7 days, then it should be reprimed with 3 actuations.

### Actions
*Pharmacology:* Nedocromil is an inhaled anti-inflammatory agent for the preventive management of asthma. It inhibits the in vitro activation of, and mediator release from, a variety of inflammatory cell types associated with asthma, including eosinophils, neutrophils, macrophages, mast cells, monocytes and platelets. Nedocromil inhibits the development of early and late bronchoconstriction responses to inhaled antigen.

*Pharmacokinetics:* Systemic bioavailability is low.

The mean 24 hour urinary excretion after either single- or multiple-dose administration represented approximately 5% of the administered dose.

Nedocromil is approximately 89% bound to plasma protein over a concentration range of 0.5 to 50 mcg/mL. This binding is reversible. It is not metabolized after IV administration and is excreted unchanged.

### Contraindications
Hypersensitivity to nedocromil or other ingredients in the preparation.

### Warnings
*Acute bronchospasm:* Nedocromil is not a bronchodilator and, therefore, should not be used for the reversal of acute bronchospasm, particularly status asthmaticus.

*Pregnancy:* Category B.

*Lactation:* It is not known whether this drug is excreted in breast milk.

*Children:* Safety and efficacy in children younger than 6 years of age have not been established.

### Precautions
*Coughing/Bronchospasm:* Inhaled medications can cause coughing and bronchospasm in some patients.

*Corticosteroids:* If systemic or inhaled steroid therapy is at all reduced, monitor patients carefully.

### Adverse Reactions
Adverse reactions associated with nedocromil may include coughing, pharyngitis, rhinitis, upper respiratory tract infection, bronchospasm, nausea, headache, chest pain, and unpleasant taste.

# NASAL DECONGESTANTS

**EPHEDRINE SULFATE**
**Solution:** 0.25% (*otc*)
  *Pretz-D* (Parnell)

**EPINEPHRINE HCl**
**Solution:** 1 mg/mL (*Rx*)
  *Adrenalin Chloride*[1] (Monarch)

**NAPHAZOLINE HCl**
**Solution:** 0.05% (*otc*)
  *Privine* (Ciba Consumer)

**OXYMETAZOLINE HCl**
**Solution:** 0.05% (*otc*)
  Various, *Afrin 12-Hour, Afrin Severe Congestion, Afrin No-Drip, Afrin Sinus, Duration* (Schering-Plough Healthcare), *Genasal* (Goldline), *Twice-A-Day 12-Hour Nasal* (Major), *Dristan 12-Hr Nasal* (Whitehall-Robins), *Duramist Plus 12-Hr Decongestant* (Pfeiffer), *Neo-Synephrine* (Bayer Corp.), *Nōstrilla 12-Hour* (Heritage), *Vicks Sinex 12-Hour* (Proctor & Gamble)

**PHENYLEPHRINE HCl**
**Tablets, chewable:** 10 mg (*otc*)
  *AH-chew D* (WE Pharm)
**Solution:** 0.125% (*otc*)
  *Little Noses Gentle Formula, Infants & Children* (Vetco)

0.25% (*otc*)
  *Afrin Children's Pump Mist* (Schering-Plough Healthcare), *Neo-Synephrine 4-Hour Mild Formula* (Bayer Corp.), *Little Colds For Infants and Children* (Vetco), *Rhinall*[1] (Scherer)

0.5% (*otc*)
  *Neo-Synephrine 4-Hour Regular Strength* (Bayer Corp.), *Vicks Sinex Ultra Fine Mist* (Proctor & Gamble)

1% (*otc*)
  Various, *4-Way Fast Acting* (Bristol-Myers), *Neo-Synephrine 4-Hour Extra Strength* (Bayer Corp.)

**PSEUDOEPHEDRINE HCl**
**Tablets:** 30 mg (*otc*)
  Various, *Genaphed* (Goldline), *Sudafed Non-Drowsy, Maximum Strength* (Warner-Lambert Consumer), *Medi-First Sinus Decongestant, Sudodrin* (Textilease Medique), *Simply Stuffy* (McNeil Consumer)

60 mg (*otc*)
  Various, *Cenafed* (Century)
**Tablets, chewable:** 15 mg (*otc*)
  *Sudafed, Children's Non-Drowsy* (Warner-Lambert Consumer), *Triaminic Allergy Congestion Softchews* (Novartis Consumer)

**Tablets, extended-release:** 120 mg (*otc*)
  *Sudafed Non-Drowsy 12 Hour Long Acting* (Warner Lambert Consumer), *Dimetapp, Maximum Strength 12-Hour Non-Drowsy Extentabs* (Whitehall-Robins)

**Tablets, controlled-release:** 240 mg (*otc*)
  *Efidac/24* (Ciba), *Sudafed Non-Drowsy 24 hour Long-Acting* (Warner-Lambert Consumer)

**Capsules:** 60 mg (*otc*)
  *Sinustop* (Nature's Way)
**Capsules, softgel:** 30 mg (*otc*)
  *Dimetapp, Maximum Strength, Non-Drowsy Liqui-Gels* (Whitehall-Robins)

**Liquid:** 15 mg/5 mL (*otc*)
  Various, *Triaminic Allergy Congestion* (Novartis Consumer), *Sudafed, Children's Non-Drowsy* (Warner-Lambert Consumer)

30 mg/5 mL (*otc*)
  Various, *Cenafed Syrup* (Century), *Silfedrine, Children's* (Silarx)
**Drops:** 7.5 mg/0.8 mL (*otc*)
  Various, *Dimetapp Decongestant Pediatric* (Whitehall-Robins), *Kid Kare* (Rugby), *PediaCare Infants' Decongestant* (Pharmacia Consumer)

**PSEUDOEPHEDRINE SULFATE**
**Tablets, extended-release:** 120 mg (*otc*)
  *Drixoral 12 Hour Non-Drowsy Formula* (Schering-Plough Healthcare)

**TETRAHYDROZOLINE HCl**
**Solution:** 0.05% (*Rx*)
  *Tyzine Pediatric* (Kenwood)
0.1% (*Rx*)
  *Tyzine* (Kenwood)

### XYLOMETAZOLINE HCl

**Solution**: 0.05% *(otc)*

Otrivin Pediatric Nasal (Novartis Consumer), Natru-Vent (Boehringer Ingelheim Consumer Health)

0.1% *(otc)*

Otrivin (Novartis Consumer), Natru-Vent (Boehringer Ingelheim Consumer Health)

### NASAL DECONGESTANT COMBINATIONS

**Solution**: 0.5% phenylephrine HCl and 0.2% pheniramine maleate *(otc)*

Dristan Fast Acting Formula (Whitehall-Robins)

### NASAL DECONGESTANT INHALERS

**Inhaler**: 250 mg propylhexedrine *(otc)*

Benzedrex (B.F. Ascher)

50 mg l-desoxyephedrine *(otc)*

Vicks Vapor Inhaler (Proctor & Gamble Consumer)

### NASAL PRODUCTS

**Solution**: Sodium chloride

Various, Pretz Moisturizing, Pretz Irrigation (Parnell), Afrin Saline (Schering-Plough Healthcare), Simply Saline (Blairex)

0.4% Sodium chloride

SalineX (Muro)

0.65% Sodium chloride

Ayr Saline (B.F. Ascher), Breathe Free (Thompson Medical), HuMist Moisturizing Mist (Scherer), NaSal (Bayer Corp.), Nasal Moist (Blairex), Ocean (Fleming and Co.), Mycinaire Saline Mist (Pfeiffer)

15% polyethylene glycol/5% propylene glycol, 15% polyethylene glycol/20% propylene glycol *(otc)*

Rhinaris Lubricating Mist (Pharmascience)

Zinc acetate, zinc gluconate

Nasal•Ease with Zinc, Nasal•Ease with Zinc Gluconate (Health Care Products)

[1] Contains sodium bisulfite.

#### Indications

*Oral:* For temporary relief of nasal congestion due to the common cold, hay fever, or other upper respiratory allergies, and nasal congestion associated with sinusitis; to promote nasal or sinus drainage.

*Topical:* Symptomatic relief of nasal and nasopharyngeal mucosal congestion due to the common cold, sinusitis, hay fever, or other upper respiratory allergies.

#### Administration and Dosage

| | Recommended Dosage Guidelines for Oral and Topical Nasal Decongestants (Dosage Maximum/24 h)[1] | | |
|---|---|---|---|
| Drug and route | Adults ≥ 12 years of age | Children 6 to < 12 years of age | Children 2 to < 6 years of age |
| *Ephedrine sulfate* Topical Sprays | 0.25%: 2 or 3 sprays in each nostril no more than q 4 h (6 doses/24 h) | 0.25%: 1 or 2 sprays in each nostril no more than q 4 h (6 doses/24 h) | not recommended |
| *Epinephrine HCl* Topical | 0.1%: Apply as drops or spray or with sterile swab as required | same as adults | not recommended |
| *Naphazoline* Topical Sprays | 0.05%: 1 or 2 sprays in each nostril no more than q 6 h (4 doses/24 h) | not recommended | not recommended |
| Drops | 0.05%: 1 or 2 drops in each nostril no more than q 6 h (4 doses/24 h) | not recommended | not recommended |

| Recommended Dosage Guidelines for Oral and Topical Nasal Decongestants (Dosage Maximum/24 h)[1] | | |
|---|---|---|
| Drug and route | Adults ≥ 12 years of age | Children 6 to < 12 years of age | Children 2 to < 6 years of age |
| **Oxymetazoline HCl**<br>Topical<br>Sprays | 0.05%: 2 or 3 sprays in each nostril q 10 to 12 h (2 doses/24 h) | same as adults | not recommended |
| **Phenylephrine HCl**<br>Oral | 10-20 mg q 4 h (120 mg/24 h) | 10 mg q 4 h (60 mg/24 h) | 0.25% drops: 1 mL q 4 h (6 doses/24 h); (15 mg/24 h) |
| Topical<br>Sprays | 0.25%, 0.5%, 1%: 2 to 3 sprays in each nostril no more than q 4 h (6 doses/24 h) | 0.25%: 2 to 3 sprays in each nostril no more than q 4 h (6 doses/24 h) | not recommended |
| Drops | 0.25%, 0.5%, 1%: 2 to 3 drops in each nostril no more than q 4 h (6 doses/24 h) | | 0.125%: 2 to 3 drops in each nostril no more than q 4 h (6 doses/24 h) |
| **Pseudoephedrine HCl**<br>Oral | 60 mg q 4 to 6 h (240 mg/24 h) | 30 mg q 4 to 6 h (120 mg/24 h) | 15 mg q 4 to 6 h (60 mg/24 h) |
| Oral SR, CR | 120 mg SR q 12 h or 240 mg CR q 24 h (240 mg/24 h) | not recommended | not recommended |
| **Pseudoephedrine sulfate**<br>Oral ER | 120 mg ER q 12 h (240 mg/24 h) | not recommended | not recommended |
| **Tetrahydrozoline HCl**<br>Topical<br>Sprays | 0.1%: 3 to 4 sprays in each nostril prn, no more than q 3 h (8 doses/24 h) | same as adults | not recommended |
| Drops | 0.1%: 2 to 4 drops in each nostril prn, no more than q 3 h (8 doses/24 h) | same as adults | 0.05%: 2 to 3 drops in each nostril prn no more than q 3 h (8 doses/24 h) |
| **Xylometazoline HCl**<br>Topical<br>Sprays | 0.1%: 1 to 3 sprays in each nostril q 8 to 10 h (3 doses/24 h) | 0.05%: 1 spray in each nostril q 8 to 10 h (3 doses/24 h) | same dose for 2 to 12 years of age |
| Drops | 0.1%: 2 to 3 drops in each nostril q 8 to 10 h (3 doses/24 h) | 0.05%: 2 to 3 drops in each nostril q 8 to 10 h (3 doses/24 h) | same dose for 2 to 12 years of age |

[1] Refer to manufacturer's directions.
SR = sustained release; CR = controlled release; ER = extended release

## Actions

*Pharmacology:* Decongestants act on the adrenergic receptors in the nasal mucosa by affecting the blood vessels' sympathetic tone and provoking vasoconstriction.

Decongestants improve nasal ventilation by shrinking swollen nasal mucosa. Constriction in the mucous membranes results in their shrinkage; this promotes drainage, thus improving ventilation and the stuffy feeling.

Oral agents are not as effective as topical products, especially on an immediate basis, but generally have a longer duration of action, cause less local irritation and are not associated with rebound congestion (rhinitis medicamentosa).

## Contraindications

Monoamine oxidase inhibitor (MAOI) therapy; hypersensitivity.

*Oral:*
*Sustained-release pseudoephedrine* – Children younger than 12 years of age.

*Oral:*
*Sustained release pseudoephedrine and naphazoline* – Children younger than 12 years of age.

*Topical:*
*Tetrahydrozoline* – 0.1% solution in children younger than 6 years of age; 0.05% solution in infants younger than 2 years of age.

## Warnings

*Special risk patients:* Administer with caution to patients with thyroid disease, diabetes mellitus, cardiovascular disease, coronary artery disease, hypertension, peripheral vascular disease, heart disease, ischemic heart disease, increased intraocular pressure, or prostatic hypertrophy.

*Oral* – Rarely, some tablets may cause bowel obstruction or blockage, usually in people with severe narrowing of the bowel, esophagus, stomach, or intestine. If a patient has had obstruction or narrowing of the bowel, have him or her consult a physician before taking oral tablet products. Advise patients to contact their physician if they experience persistent abdominal pain or vomiting.

*Hypertension:* Hypertensive patients should use these products only with medical advice, as they may experience a change in blood pressure because of the added vasoconstriction. Studies suggest pseudoephedrine is the drug of choice. Sustained-action preparations may affect the cardiovascular system to a lesser degree.

*Excessive use:* Do not exceed recommended dosage. If nervousness, dizziness, or sleeplessness occur, discontinue use and have the patient consult a physician. Do not take topical products for more than 3 days or oral products for more than 7 days. If symptoms do not improve or are accompanied by a fever, the patient should consult a physician.

*Rebound congestion (rhinitis medicamentosa):* May occur following topical application after the vasoconstriction subsides. Patients may increase the amount of drug and frequency of use, producing toxicity and perpetuating the rebound congestion.

*Treatment* – A simple but uncomfortable solution is to completely withdraw the topical medication. A more acceptable method is to gradually withdraw therapy by initially discontinuing the medication in one nostril, followed by total withdrawal. Substituting an oral decongestant for a topical one may also be useful.

*Elderly:* Patients 60 years of age and older are more likely to experience adverse reactions to sympathomimetics. Overdosage may cause hallucinations, convulsions, CNS depression, and death.

*Pregnancy:* Category C.

*Lactation:*
*Oral preparations* – Consult a physician before using.
*Topical* – It is not known if these agents are excreted in breast milk.

*Children:* Use in children is product specific.

## Precautions

*Acute use:* Use topical decongestants only in acute states and not longer than 3 to 5 days. Use sparingly (especially the imidazolines) in all patients, particularly infants, children, and patients with cardiovascular disease.

*Stinging sensation:* Some individuals may experience a mild, transient stinging sensation after topical application.

*Sulfite sensitivity:* Some of the nasal decongestant products contain sulfites that may cause allergic-type reactions including anaphylactic symptoms and life-threatening or less severe asthmatic episodes in certain susceptible people. Products containing sulfites are identified in the product listings.

### Drug Interactions

Most interactions listed apply to sympathomimetics when used as vasopressors; however, consider the interaction when using the nasal decongestants.

Drugs that may affect nasal decongestants include beta blockers, furazolidone, guanethidine, methyldopa, MAO inhibitors, rauwolfia alkaloids, tricyclic antidepressants, urinary acidifiers, and urinary alkalinizers.

Drugs that may be affected by nasal decongestants include guanethidine.

### Adverse Reactions

Arrhythmias; palpitations; tachycardia; transient hypertension; bradycardia; headache; lightheadedness; dizziness; drowsiness; tremor; insomnia; nervousness; restlessness; giddiness; psychological disturbances; prolonged psychosis; weakness; nausea; gastric irritation; hypersensitivity reactions such as rash, urticaria, leukopenia, agranulocytosis, and thrombocytopenia; orofacial dystonia; sweating; blepharospasm; urinary retention may occur in patients with prostatic hypertrophy.

*Topical use* – Burning; stinging; sneezing; dryness; local irritation; rebound congestion.

# INTRANASAL STEROIDS

| | |
|---|---|
| **BECLOMETHASONE DIPROPIONATE** | |
| **Spray:** 42 mcg/actuation (*Rx*) | *Beconase AQ* (GlaxoSmithKline) |
| **BUDESONIDE** | |
| **Spray:** 32 mcg/actuation (*Rx*) | *Rhinocort Aqua* (AstraZeneca) |
| **FLUNISOLIDE** | |
| **Solution:** 25 mcg/actuation (*Rx*) | *Flunisolide* (Bausch & Lomb) |
| **Spray:** 29 mcg/actuation (*Rx*) | *Nasarel* (Ivax) |
| **FLUTICASONE PROPIONATE** | |
| **Spray:** 50 mcg/actuation (*Rx*) | *Flonase* (GlaxoSmithKline) |
| **MOMETASONE FUROATE MONOHYDRATE** | |
| **Spray:** 50 mcg/actuation (*Rx*) | *Nasonex* (Schering) |
| **TRIAMCINOLONE ACETONIDE** | |
| **Spray:** 55 mcg/actuation (*Rx*) | *Nasacort AQ* (Aventis) |
| **Aerosol:** 55 mcg/actuation (*Rx*) | *Nasacort HFA* (Aventis) |

**Indications**

| Intranasal Steroids Indications | | | | | | |
|---|---|---|---|---|---|---|
| | Beclomethasone | Budesonide | Flunisolide | Fluticasone | Mometasone | Triamcinolone |
| Nasal polyps | ✔[a] | X[b] | | X | | |
| Nonallergic (vasomotor) rhinitis | ✔ | | | ✔ | | |
| Perennial allergic rhinitis | ✔ | ✔ | ✔ | ✔ | ✔ | ✔ |
| Seasonal allergic rhinitis | ✔ | ✔ | ✔ | ✔ | ✔[c] | ✔ |
| Recurrent chronic sinusitis[d] | | X | | X | X | |

[a] ✔ = Approved uses.
[b] X = Unlabeled uses.
[c] Treatment and prophylaxis.
[d] As adjunctive therapy with an antibiotic and/or decongestant.

**Administration and Dosage**

Improvement in symptoms usually becomes apparent within a few days. However, relief may not occur in some patients for as long as 2 weeks. Do not continue beyond 3 weeks in absence of significant symptomatic improvement.

BECLOMETHASONE DIPROPIONATE:

*Adults and children 12 years of age and older* – 1 or 2 nasal inhalations (42 to 84 mcg) in each nostril twice daily (total dose, 168 to 336 mcg/day).

*Children 6 to 11 years of age* – Start with 1 nasal inhalation in each nostril twice daily (168 mcg). Patients not adequately responding or those with more severe symptoms may use 2 sprays in each nostril twice daily (336 mcg/day).

*Maximum dosage* – 2 sprays in each nostril twice daily (336 mcg/day).

*Maintenance dose* – Once adequate control is achieved, decrease the dosage to 1 spray in each nostril twice daily.

*Nasal polyps* – Treatment of symptoms associated with nasal polyps may have to be continued for several weeks or more before a therapeutic result can be fully assessed. Recurrence of symptoms caused by polyps can occur after stopping treatment, depending on the severity of the disease.

BUDESONIDE:

*Adults and children 6 years of age and older* – 1 spray in each nostril once daily (64 mcg/day). Some patients who do not achieve symptom control at the recommended starting dose may benefit from an increased dose.

*Maximum dose* –

*Adults 12 years of age and older:* 4 sprays in each nostril once daily (256 mcg/day).

*Children 6 through 11 years of age:* 2 sprays in each nostril once daily (128 mcg/day).

*Maintenance dose* – After the desired clinical effect is obtained, reduce the maintenance dose to the smallest amount necessary to control symptoms.

FLUNISOLIDE:

*Adults* – Starting dose is 2 sprays (50 mcg) in each nostril 2 times/day (total dose 200 mcg/day). May increase to 2 sprays in each nostril 3 times/day (total dose 300 mcg/day). Maximum daily dose is 8 sprays in each nostril (400 mcg/day).

*Children (6 to 14 years of age)* – Starting dose is 1 spray (25 mcg) in each nostril 3 times/day or 2 sprays (50 mcg) in each nostril 2 times/day (total dose 150 to 200 mcg/day). Maximum daily dose is 4 sprays in each nostril (200 mcg/day).

*Maintenance dose* – After desired clinical effect is obtained, reduce maintenance dose to smallest amount necessary to control symptoms. Some patients with perennial rhinitis may be maintained on 1 spray in each nostril/day.

FLUTICASONE:

*Adults* – Recommended starting dose is 2 sprays (50 mcg each) per nostril once daily (total daily dose, 200 mcg). The same dosage divided into 100 mcg given twice daily (eg, 8:00 am and 8:00 pm) is also effective. After the first few days, dosage may be reduced to 100 mcg (1 spray per nostril) once daily for maintenance therapy. Maximum total daily dosage should not exceed 200 mcg/day.

*Adolescents 4 years of age and older* – Start most adolescents with 100 mcg (1 spray/nostril/day). Patients not adequately responding to 100 mcg may use 200 mcg (2 sprays/nostril). Depending on response, dosage may be decreased to 100 mcg daily. Total daily dosage should not exceed 200 mcg/day.

*Children younger than 4 years of age* – Use not recommended.

MOMETASONE FUROATE MONOHYDRATE:

*Adults and children 12 years of age and older* – 2 sprays (50 mcg) in each nostril once daily (total daily dose, 200 mcg).

In patients with a known seasonal allergen that precipitates nasal symptoms of seasonal allergic rhinitis, prophylaxis with mometasone (200 mcg/day) is recommended 2 to 4 weeks prior to the anticipated start of the pollen season.

*Children 2 to 11 years of age* – 1 spray (50 mcg) in each nostril once daily (total daily dose, 100 mcg).

TRIAMCINOLONE:

*Adults and children 12 years of age and older* – 2 sprays in each nostril once daily (220 mcg/day).

*Children 6 to 11 years of age* –

Nasacort AQ: 1 spray in each nostril once daily (110 mcg/day).

Nasacort HFA: 2 sprays in each nostril once daily (220 mcg/day).

*Maximum adult dose* –

Nasacort AQ: 2 sprays in each nostril once daily (220 mcg/day).

Nasacort HFA: 4 sprays in each nostril once daily (440 mcg/day).

*Maintenance dose* – When the maximum benefit has been achieved and symptoms have been controlled, titrate to the lowest effective dose (eg, 110 mcg/day). Use the minimum effective dose to ensure continued control of symptoms. Greater symptom control may be achieved with regular scheduled use.

*Duration* – Improvement in symptoms may be seen within the first day of treatment; generally, it takes 1 week of treatment to reach maximum benefit. Do not use for more than 3 weeks in the absence of significant symptomatic improvement.

*Priming* –

Nasacort AQ: Before use, prime the nasal spray by pushing down on the actuator until a fine spray appears (5 pumps). If the pump has not been used for more than 14 days, the spray must be reprimed with 1 spray.

Nasacort HFA: The canister must be primed with 3 actuations prior to the first use or after 3 days of nonuse.

## Actions

*Pharmacology:* These drugs have potent glucocorticoid and weak mineralocorticoid activity. The mechanisms responsible for the anti-inflammatory action of corticosteroids on the nasal mucosa are unknown. However, glucocorticoids have a wide range of inhibitory activities against multiple cell types and mediators involved in allergic and nonallergic/irritant-mediated inflammation. These agents, when administered topically in recommended doses, exert direct local anti-inflammatory effects with minimal systemic effects.

*Pharmacokinetics:* The amount of an intranasal dose that reaches systemic circulation is generally low, and metabolism is rapid.

## Contraindications

Untreated localized infections involving the nasal mucosa; hypersensitivity to the drug or any component of the product.

## Warnings

*Systemic corticosteroids:* The combined administration of alternate-day systemic prednisone with these products may increase the likelihood of HPA suppression.

*Excessive doses/sensitivity:* If recommended doses of intranasal **beclomethasone** are exceeded or if individuals are particularly sensitive or predisposed by virtue of recent systemic steroid therapy, symptoms of hypercorticism may occur, including, very rarely, menstrual irregularities, acneiform lesions, and cushingoid features.

*Hypersensitivity reactions:* Rare cases of immediate and delayed hypersensitivity reactions, including angioedema, urticaria, rash, and bronchospasm, have occurred.

*Pregnancy:* Category C.

Carefully observe infants born of mothers who have received substantial doses of corticosteroids during pregnancy for signs of adrenal insufficiency.

*Lactation:* Advise mothers taking pharmacologic doses not to nurse.

Beclomethasone, budesonide, flunisolide, triamcinolone – It is not known whether these drugs are excreted in breast milk.

*Children:* Safety and efficacy for use in children younger than 6 years of age (4 years of age or younger for **fluticasone**; younger than 2 years of age for **mometasone**) have not been established. Use in children younger than 6 years of age is not recommended; carefully follow growth and development if prolonged therapy is used.

## Precautions

*Infections:* Localized infections of the nose and pharynx with *Candida albicans* have developed only rarely.

Use with caution in patients with active or quiescent tuberculosis infections of the respiratory tract, or in untreated fungal, bacterial, or systemic viral infections, or ocular herpes simplex.

Individuals receiving immunosuppressant agents are more susceptible to infections than healthy individuals. Avoid exposure to chicken pox or measles.

*Wound healing:* Because of the inhibitory effect of corticosteroids on wound healing in patients who have experienced recent nasal septal ulcers, recurrent epistaxis, nasal surgery, or trauma, use nasal steroids with caution until healing has occurred.

*Vasoconstrictors:* In the presence of excessive nasal mucosa secretion or edema of the nasal mucosa, the drug may fail to reach the site of intended action. In such cases, use a nasal vasoconstrictor during the first 2 to 3 days of therapy.

*Systemic effects:* Although systemic absorption is low when used in recommended dosage, HPA suppression and other systemic effects may occur, especially with excessive doses.

*Long-term treatment:* Examine patients periodically over several months or longer for possible changes in the nasal mucosa.

## Drug Interactions

Use caution when coadministering high and prolonged doses of **fluticasone** with ketoconazole and other known cytochrome P450 inhibitors.

## Adverse Reactions

Adverse reactions associated with intranasal steroids include mild nasopharyngeal irritation, nasal irritation, burning, stinging, dryness, and headache.

Those associated with **budesonide** in particular include epistaxis, increased cough, and pharyngitis.

# ANTIHISTAMINES

**AZELASTINE HYDROCHLORIDE**
| | |
|---|---|
| **Nasal spray**: 137 mcg/spray (*Rx*) | *Astelin* (Medpointe) |

**BROMPHENIRAMINE TANNATE**
| | |
|---|---|
| **Tablets, chewable**: 12 mg (*Rx*) | *BröveX CT* (Athlon) |
| **Tablets, extended release**: 6 mg (*Rx*) | *Bidhist* (PharmaFab), *LoHist 12 Hour* (Larken) |
| **Capsules, extended release**: 12 mg (*Rx*) | *Lodrane 24* (ECR Pharmaceuticals) |
| **Liquid**: 2 mg/5 mL (*Rx*) | *VaZol* (WraSer) |
| **Oral suspension**: 8 mg/5 mL, 12 mg/5 mL (*Rx*) | *BröveX* (Athlon), *Lodrane XR* (ECR Pharmaceuticals) |

**CARBINOXAMINE MALEATE**
| | |
|---|---|
| **Tablets**: 4 mg (*Rx*) | *Palgic* (Pamlab) |
| **Tablets, timed release**: 8 mg (*Rx*) | *Histex CT* (Teamm Pharm) |
| **Capsules, extended release**: 10 mg (*Rx*) | *Histex I/E*[a] (Teamm Pharm) |
| **Liquid**: 1.5 mg/5 mL (*Rx*) | *Pediatex* (Zyber Pharmaceuticals) |
| **Liquid**: 4 mg/5 mL (*Rx*) | *Histex Pd* (Teamm Pharm), *Palgic* (Pamlab) |
| **Oral suspension**: 3.6 mg/5 mL (*Rx*) | *Pediatex 12* (Zyber) |

**CETIRIZINE HYDROCHLORIDE**
| | |
|---|---|
| **Tablets**: 5 and 10 mg (*Rx*) | *Zyrtec* (Pfizer) |
| **Tablets, chewable**: 5 and 10 mg (*Rx*) | |
| **Syrup**: 5 mg/5 mL (*Rx*) | |

**CHLORPHENIRAMINE MALEATE**
| | |
|---|---|
| **Tablets**: 4 mg (*otc*) | Various |
| **Tablets, chewable**: 2 mg (*otc*) | *Chlo-Amine* (Hollister-Stier) |
| **Tablets, extended release**: 8 mg (*otc*) | *Chlor-Trimeton Allergy 8 Hour* (Schering-Plough Healthcare) |
| 12 mg (*otc*) | *Chlor-Trimeton Allergy 12 Hour* (Schering-Plough Healthcare) |
| 16 mg (*otc*) | *Efidac 24*[b] (Hogil) |
| **Capsules, sustained release**: 8 and 12 mg (*Rx*) | Various |
| **Syrup**: 2 mg/5 mL (*otc*) | *Aller-Chlor* (Rugby) |

**CLEMASTINE FUMARATE**
| | |
|---|---|
| **Tablets**: 1.34 mg as fumarate (equiv. to 1 mg clemastine) (*otc*) | Various, *Dayhist-1* (Major), *Tavist Allergy* (Novartis Consumer Health) |
| 2.68 mg (equiv. to 2 mg clemastine) (*Rx*) | Various |
| **Syrup**: 0.67 mg (equiv. to 0.5 mg clemastine)/5 mL (*Rx*) | Various |

**CYPROHEPTADINE HYDROCHLORIDE**
| | |
|---|---|
| **Tablets**: 4 mg (*Rx*) | Various |
| **Syrup**: 2 mg/5 mL (*Rx*) | Various |

**DESLORATADINE**
| | |
|---|---|
| **Tablets**: 5 mg (*Rx*) | *Clarinex* (Schering) |
| **Tablets, rapidly disintegrating**: 5 mg (*Rx*) | *Clarinex RediTabs* (Schering) |
| **Syrup**: 2.5 mg/5 mL (*Rx*) | *Clarinex* (Schering) |

**DEXCHLORPHENIRAMINE MALEATE**
| | |
|---|---|
| **Tablets, extended release**: 4 and 6 mg (*Rx*) | Various |
| **Syrup**: 2 mg/5 mL (*Rx*) | (Morton Grove) |

**DIPHENHYDRAMINE HYDROCHLORIDE**
| | |
|---|---|
| **Tablets**: 25 mg (*otc*) | Various |
| 50 mg (*otc*) | *AllerMax Caplets, Maximum Strength* (Pfeiffer) |
| **Tablets, chewable**: 12.5 mg (*otc*) | *Benadryl Allergy* (Pfizer) |
| **Tablets, orally disintegrating**: 12.5 mg (*otc*) | *Children's Benadryl Allergy Fastmelt* (Pfizer) |
| **Capsules**: 25 mg (*otc/Rx*) | Various |
| 50 mg (*otc/Rx*) | Various |
| **Liquid**: 12.5 mg/5 mL (*otc*) | *AllerMax* (Pfeiffer), *Benadryl Children's Allergy* (Pfizer), *Benadryl Children's Dye-Free Allergy* (Pfizer), *Diphen AF* (Morton Grove), *Genahist* (Goldline), *Scot-Tussin Allergy Relief Formula Clear* (Scot-Tussin) |
| **Oral solution**: 12.5 mg/5 mL (*otc*) | *Diphenhist* (Rugby) |
| **Elixir**: 12.5 mg/5 mL (*otc*) | *Banophen Allergy* (Major), *Siladryl* (Silarx) |

| | |
|---|---|
| **Syrup**: 12.5 mg/5 mL (*Rx*) | *Tusstat* (Century) |
| **Injection**: 50 mg/mL (*Rx*) | Various, *Benadryl* (Parke-Davis) |
| **FEXOFENADINE HYDROCHLORIDE** | |
| **Tablets**: 30, 60, and 180 mg (*Rx*) | *Allegra* (Aventis) |
| **Capsules**: 60 mg (*Rx*) | |
| **HYDROXYZINE** | |
| **Tablets** (as hydrochloride): 10, 25, and 50 mg (*Rx*) | Various |
| **Capsules** (as pamoate): 25, 50, and 100 mg (*Rx*) | Various, *Vistaril* (Pfizer) |
| **Syrup** (as hydrochloride): 10 mg/5 mL (*Rx*) | Various |
| **Oral suspension** (as pamoate): 25 mg/5 mL (*Rx*) | *Vistaril* (Pfizer) |
| **Injection** (as hydrochloride): 25 and 50 mg/mL (*Rx*) | Various |
| **LORATADINE** | |
| **Tablets**: 10 mg (*otc*) | Various |
| **Tablets, orally disintegrating**: 10 mg (*otc*) | *Alavert* (Wyeth Consumer), *Triaminic Allerchews* (Novartis), *Dimetapp Children's ND Non-Drowsy Allergy* (Wyeth) |
| **Tablets, rapidly disintegrating**: 10 mg (*otc*) | *Claritin RediTabs* (Schering) |
| **Syrup**: 5 mg/5 mL (*otc*) | *Claritin* (Schering), *Dimetapp Children's ND Non-Drowsy Allergy* (Wyeth), *Alavert Children's* (Wyeth) |
| **PHENINDAMINE TARTRATE** | |
| **Tablets**: 25 mg (*otc*) | *Nolahist* (Amarin) |
| **PROMETHAZINE HYDROCHLORIDE** | |
| **Tablets**: 25 and 50 mg (*Rx*) | Various, *Phenergan* (Wyeth Labs) |
| **Syrup**: 6.25 mg/5 mL (*Rx*) | Various |
| **Suppositories**: 12.5 mg (*Rx*) | *Phenadoz* (Paddock), *Phenergan* (Wyeth Labs) |
| 25 mg (*Rx*) | *Promethazine Hydrochloride* (Alpharma) |
| 50 mg (*Rx*) | Various, *Phenergan* (Wyeth Labs) |
| **Injection**: 25 and 50 mg/mL (*Rx*) | Various, *Phenergan* (Wyeth Labs) |
| **TRIPROLIDINE HYDROCHLORIDE** | |
| **Liquid**: 1.25 mg/5 mL (*Rx*) | *Zymine* (Vindex Pharmaceuticals) |
| **ANTIHISTAMINE COMBINATIONS** | |
| **Elixir**: 4 mg phenyltoloxamine citrate, 4 mg pyrilamine maleate, 4 mg pheniramine maleate/5 mL (*Rx*) | *Poly-Histine* (Sanofi-Synthelabo) |

[a] 2 mg immediate-release and 8 mg extended-release.
[b] 4 mg immediate-release and 12 mg controlled-release.

### Indications

*Oral:* Relief of symptoms associated with the following: Perennial and seasonal allergic rhinitis; vasomotor rhinitis; allergic conjunctivitis (eg, caused by inhalant allergens or food); temporary relief of sneezing, itchy or watery eyes, itchy nose or throat, and runny nose caused by hay fever (allergic rhinitis), or other respiratory allergies and the common cold; allergic and nonallergic pruritic symptoms; mild, uncomplicated, allergic skin manifestations of urticaria and angioedema; amelioration of allergic reactions to blood or plasma; dermatographism; adjunctive therapy in anaphylactic reactions; lacrimation.

*Parenteral:* When oral therapy is not possible or contraindicated.

*Brompheniramine: VaZol* also is indicated for the temporary relief of runny nose and sneezing caused by the common cold; treatment of allergic and nonallergic pruritic symptoms; temporary relief of mild, uncomplicated urticaria and angioedema; amelioration of allergic reactions to blood or plasma; adjunctive therapy in anaphylactic reactions.

*Cetirizine, desloratadine, fexofenadine:* Cetirizine, desloratadine, and fexofenadine also are indicated for chronic idiopathic urticaria.

*Cyproheptadine:* Cold urticaria.

*Diphenhydramine:* Diphenhydramine also is indicated for active treatment of motion sickness (injection only); for parkinsonism in the elderly intolerant of more potent agents, for mild cases in other age groups, and in combination with centrally acting anticholinergics; as a cough suppressant (syrup only).

*Hydroxyzine:* Hydroxyzine also is indicated for sedation (oral only); analgesia, adjunctive therapy (parenteral only); antiemetic (parenteral only); as adjunctive therapy in allergic conditions with strong emotional overlay, such as asthma, chronic urticaria, and pruritus (parenteral only).

Also indicated for management of anxiety, tension, and psychomotor agitation in conditions of emotional stress.

*Promethazine:* Promethazine also is indicated for preoperative, postoperative, or obstetric sedation; prevention and control of nausea and vomiting associated with certain types of anesthesia and surgery; an adjunct to analgesics for control of postoperative pain; sedation and relief of apprehension, and to produce light sleep; antiemetic effect in postoperative patients; active and prophylactic treatment of motion sickness (oral and rectal only).

### Administration and Dosage

AZELASTINE: Before initial use, prime the delivery system with 4 sprays or until a fine mist appears. When at least 3 days have elapsed since last use, reprime the pump with 2 sprays or until a fine mist appears.

*Seasonal allergic rhinitis –*

*Adults and children 12 years of age and older:* 2 sprays per nostril twice daily.

*Children 5 to 11 years of age:* 1 spray per nostril twice daily.

*Vasomotor rhinitis –*

*Adults and children 12 years of age and older:* 2 sprays per nostril twice daily.

BROMPHENIRAMINE TANNATE:

*Tablets, extended release –* Take with food, water, or milk to minimize gastric irritation. Swallow whole; do not crush tablets.

*Adults and children older than 12 years of age:* 1 or 2 tablets (6 to 12 mg) every 12 hours.

*Children 6 to 12 years of age:* 1 tablet (6 mg) every 12 hours.

*Tablets, chewable –*

*Adults and children 12 years of age and older:* 1 or 2 tablets (12 to 24 mg) every 12 hours, up to 4 tablets (48 mg) in 24 hours.

*Children 6 to younger than 12 years of age:* ½ to 1 tablet (6 to 12 mg) every 12 hours, up to 2 tablets (24 mg) in 24 hours.

*Children 2 to younger than 6 years of age:* ½ tablet (6 mg) every 12 hours, up to 1 tablet (12 mg) in 24 hours.

*Capsules, extended release –* Take with food, water or milk to minimize gastric irritation. Swallow whole; do not crush capsules.

*Adults and children 12 years of age and older:* 1 or 2 capsules (12 to 24 mg) once daily.

*Children 6 to younger than 12 years of age:* 1 capsule (12 mg) once daily.

*Oral suspension –* Shake well before use.

*Adults and children 12 years of age and older:* 5 to 10 mL (12 to 24 mg) every 12 hours, up to 20 mL (48 mg) in 24 hours.

*Children 6 to younger than 12 years of age:* 5 mL (12 mg) every 12 hours, up to 10 mL (24 mg) in 24 hours.

*Children 2 to younger than 6 years of age:* 2.5 mL (6 mg) every 12 hours, up to 5 mL (12 mg) in 24 hours.

*Children 12 months to 2 years of age:* 1.25 mL (3 mg) every 12 hours, up to 2.5 mL (6 mg) in 24 hours.

*Oral liquid –*

*Adults and children older than 12 years of age:* 10 mL (4 mg) 4 times daily.

*Children 6 to 12 years of age:* 5 mL (2 mg) 4 times daily.

*Children 2 to 6 years of age:* 2.5 mL (1 mg) 4 times daily

*Children younger than 2 years of age:* Titrate dosage individually based on 0.5 mg/kg/day in equally divided doses, 4 times daily.

*Lodrane XR –*

*Adults and children older than 12 years of age:* 5 mL every 12 hours, not to exceed 2 doses in 24 hours.

*Children 6 to 12 years of age:* 2.5 mL every 12 hours, not to exceed 2 doses in 24 hours.

*Children 2 to 6 years of age:* 1.25 mL every 12 hours, not to exceed 2 doses in 24 hours.

*Children younger than 2 years of age:* As recommended by a physician.

CARBINOXAMINE MALEATE:

*Tablets –*

*Histex CT:* Histex CT tablets are not recommended for children younger than 6 years of age. Tablets may be broken in half for ease of administration, but should not be crushed or chewed.

*Adults and children 12 years of age and older* – 1 tablet (8 mg) twice daily (every 12 hours).

*Children 6 to 12 years of age* – ½ tablet twice daily (every 12 hours).

*Palgic:*

*Adults* – 1 or 2 tablets (4 to 8 mg) 3 to 4 times daily.

*Children 6 years of age and older* – 1 to 1½ tablets (4 to 6 mg) 3 or 4 times daily.

*Children 3 to 6 years of age* – ½ to 1 tablet (2 to 4 mg) 3 or 4 times daily.

*Children 1 to 3 years of age* – ½ tablet (2 mg) 3 or 4 times daily.

*Capsules –*

*Adults and children 12 years of age and older:* 1 capsule every 12 hours, up to 2 a day.

*Liquids –*

*Histex Pd:*

*Adults and children 6 years of age and older* – 5 mL 4 times/day.

*Children –*

*18 months to 6 years of age:* 2.5 mL 4 times/day.

*9 to 18 months of age:* 1.25 to 2.5 mL 4 times/day.

*Palgic:*

*Adults* – 5 or 10 mL 3 to 4 times/day.

*Children –*

*Older than 6 years of age:* 5 to 7.5 mL 3 or 4 times/day.

*3 to 6 years of age:* 2.5 to 5 mL 3 or 4 times/day.

*1 to 3 years of age:* 2.5 mL 3 or 4 times/day.

*Pediatex:*

*Adults and children 6 years of age and older* – 10 mL 4 times/day.

*Children –*

*18 months to 6 years of age:* 5 mL 4 times/day.

*9 to 18 months of age:* 3.75 to 5 mL 4 times/day.

*6 to 9 months of age:* 3.75 mL 4 times/day.

*3 to 6 months of age:* 2.5 mL 4 times/day.

*1 to 3 months of age:* 1.25 mL 4 times/day.

*Oral suspension –*

*Adults and children 12 years of age and older:* 2 to 4 teaspoonsful every 12 hours.

*Children 6 to 12 years of age:* 1 to 2 teaspoonsful every 12 hours.

*Children 2 to 6 years of age:* ½ to 1 teaspoonful every 12 hours.

CETIRIZINE HYDROCHLORIDE: May be given with or without food.

*Adults and children 12 years of age and older* – 5 or 10 mg once daily depending on symptom severity.

*Children –*

*6 to 11 years of age:* 5 or 10 mg once daily depending on symptom severity.

*2 to 5 years of age:* 2.5 mg once daily. May increase to a maximum dose of 5 mg/day as 5 mg once daily or as 2.5 mg given every 12 hours.

*6 months up to 2 years of age:* 2.5 mg once daily. The dose in children 12 to 23 months of age can be increased to a maximum dose of 5 mg/day given as 2.5 mg every 12 hours.

*Elderly (77 years of age and older)* – 5 mg once daily as recommended.

*Renal/Hepatic function impairment* – In patients 12 years of age and older with decreased renal function (Ccr 11 to 31 mL/min), hemodialysis patients (Ccr less than 7 mL/min), and in hepatically impaired patients, 5 mg once daily is recommended.

CHLORPHENIRAMINE MALEATE: Individualize dosage.

*Tablets or syrup –*

*Adults and children 12 years of age and older:* 4 mg every 4 to 6 hours. Do not exceed 24 mg in 24 hours.

*Children:*

6 to 12 years of age – 2 mg every 4 to 6 hours. Do not exceed 12 mg in 24 hours.

*Younger than 6 years of age* – Consult a doctor.

*Extended-release tablets –*

*Adults and children 12 years of age and older:* 8 mg every 8 to 12 hours or 12 mg every 12 hours. Do not exceed 24 mg in 24 hours.

*Efidac:*

*Adults and children 12 years of age and older* – 16 mg with liquid every 24 hours. Do not exceed 16 mg in 24 hours. Swallow each tablet whole; do not divide, crush, chew, or dissolve.

*Sustained-release capsules –*

*Adults and children 12 years of age and older:* 8 or 12 mg every 12 hours, up to 16 to 24 mg/day.

*Children 6 to 12 years of age:* 8 mg at bedtime or during the day as indicated.

CLEMASTINE FUMARATE:

*Allergic rhinitis –*

*Adults:* 1.34 mg every 12 hours or twice daily. Do not exceed 8.04 mg for the syrup or 2.68 mg for the tablets in 24 hours.

*Children 6 to 12 years of age (syrup only):* 0.67 mg twice daily. Single doses of up to 2.25 mg have been well tolerated. Do not exceed 4.02 mg/day.

*Urticaria/Angioedema –*

*Adults:* 2.68 mg twice daily, not to exceed 8.04 mg/day.

*Children 6 to 12 years of age (syrup only):* 1.34 mg twice daily, not to exceed 4.02 mg/day.

CYPROHEPTADINE HYDROCHLORIDE:

*Adults* – 4 to 20 mg/day. Initiate therapy with 4 mg 3 times/day. Most patients require 12 to 16 mg/day and occasionally as much as 32 mg/day. Do not exceed 0.5 mg/kg/day.

*Children* – Calculate total daily dosage as approximately 0.25 mg/kg or 8 mg/m$^2$.

*7 to 14 years of age:* 4 mg 2 or 3 times/day. Do not exceed 16 mg/day.

*2 to 6 years of age:* 2 mg 2 or 3 times/day. Do not exceed 12 mg/day.

DESLORATADINE: Fexofenadine should not be taken closely in time with aluminum- and magnesium-containing antacids.

*Adults and children 12 years of age and older* – 5 mg once daily. In patients with liver or renal impairment, a starting dose of 5 mg every other day is recommended.

Place rapidly disintegrating tablets on the tongue immediately after opening the blister. Administer with or without water.

*Children 6 to 11 years of age* – 2.5 mg once daily.

*Children 12 months to 5 years of age* – 1.25 mg once daily.

*Children 6 to 11 months of age* – 1 mg once daily.

*Renal/Hepatic function impairment* – In adults, a starting dose of one 5 mg tablet every other day is recommended.

DEXCHLORPHENIRAMINE MALEATE:

*Adults 12 years of age and older* – 4 to 6 mg at bedtime, or every 8 to 10 hours.

*Children 6 to 12 years of age* – 4 mg/day, preferably at bedtime.

DIPHENHYDRAMINE HYDROCHLORIDE: Individualize dosage.

*Hypersensitivity reactions, type I/Antiparkinsonism/Motion sickness –*

*Oral:*

*Adults* – 25 to 50 mg, every 4 to 6 hours, not to exceed 300 mg/day.

*Children 6 to younger 12 years of age* – 12.5 to 25 mg, every 4 to 6 hours, not to exceed 150 mg/day.

*Parenteral:* Administer IV or deeply IM.

*Adults* – 10 to 50 mg administered IV at a rate generally not exceeding 25 mg/min, or deep IM; 100 mg if required. Maximum daily dosage is 400 mg.

Children – 5 mg/kg/day or 150 mg/m²/day. Maximum daily dosage is 300 mg divided into 4 doses administered IV at a rate generally not exceeding 25 mg/min, or deep IM.

*Antitussive (syrup only)* –

*Adults:* 25 mg every 4 hours, not to exceed 150 mg in 24 hours.

*Children:*

6 to 12 years of age – 12.5 mg every 4 hours, not to exceed 75 mg in 24 hours.

2 to 6 years of age – 6.25 mg every 4 hours, not to exceed 25 mg in 24 hours.

FEXOFENADINE:

*Seasonal allergic rhinitis* –

*Adults and children 12 years of age and older:* 60 mg twice/day or 180 mg once daily.

*Children 6 to 11 years of age:* 30 mg twice/day.

*Chronic idiopathic urticaria* –

*Adults and children 12 years of age and older:* 60 mg twice/day.

*Children 6 to 11 years of age:* 30 mg twice/day.

*Renal function impairment* –

*Adults and children 12 years of age and older:* 60 mg once daily as a starting dose.

*Children 6 to 11 years of age:* 30 mg once daily as a starting dose.

HYDROXYZINE: Administer by deep IM only; may be given without further dilution. Avoid IV, subcutaneous, or intra-arterial administration. Do not administer IM injections into the lower and mid-third of the upper arm.

*Pruritus* –

Oral:

*Adults* – 25 mg 3 or 4 times/day.

*Children* –

6 years of age: 50 to 100 mg/day in divided doses.

Younger than 6 years of age: 50 mg/day in divided doses.

*Parenteral:*

*Adults* – 25 mg 3 to 4 times/day.

*Sedation (oral only)* –

*Adults:* 50 to 100 mg. Hydroxyzine may potentiate concomitant narcotics and barbiturates; reduce dosages accordingly. Atropine and other belladonna alkaloids may be given as appropriate.

*Children:* 0.6 mg/kg.

*Antiemetic/Analgesia, adjunctive therapy (parenteral only)* –

*Adults:* 25 to 100 mg IM. Reduce dosage of concomitant CNS depressants and narcotics by as much as 50%.

*Children:* 0.5 mg/lb IM. Reduce dosage of concomitant CNS depressants and narcotics by as much as 50%.

LORATADINE:

*Adults and children 6 years of age and older* – 10 mg once daily.

*Children 2 to 5 years of age* – 5 mg (5 mL) syrup once daily.

*Hepatic/Renal function impairment (GFR less than 30 mL/min)* –

*Adults and children 6 years of age and older:* 10 mg every other day as starting dose.

*Children 2 to 5 years of age:* 5 mg every other day as starting dose.

*Rapidly disintegrating tablets* – Place tablets on the tongue. Administer with or without water. Use within 6 months of opening laminated foil pouch and immediately upon opening individual tablet blister.

PHENINDAMINE TARTRATE:

*Adults and children 12 years of age and older* – 25 mg every 4 to 6 hours. Do not exceed 150 mg in 24 hours.

*Children 6 to under 12 years of age* – 12.5 mg (½ tablet) every 4 to 6 hours. Do not exceed 75 mg in 24 hours.

PROMETHAZINE HYDROCHLORIDE: The preferred parenteral route of administration is deep IM injection; properly administered IV doses are well tolerated, but this method is associated with increased hazard. IV administration should not exceed 25 mg/mL at a rate no more than 25 mg/min. Avoid subcutaneous and intra-arterial injection.

*Hypersensitivity reactions, Type 1 –*

*Adults and children older than 2 years of age:* Usual dose is 25 mg at bedtime; 12.5 mg before meals and at bedtime may be given, if necessary. Single 25 mg doses at bedtime or 6.25 to 12.5 mg taken 3 times daily will usually suffice. Doses of 25 mg will control minor transfusion reactions of an allergic nature.

*Parenteral:*

*Adults* – 25 mg; may repeat dose within 2 hours if needed.

*Children 2 years of age and older* – Dose should not exceed half the adult dose.

*Sedation –*

*Oral/Rectal:* If used for preoperative sedation, administer the night before surgery to relieve apprehension and produce quiet sleep.

*Adults* – 25 to 50 mg at bedtime.

*Children older than 2 years of age* – 12.5 to 25 mg at bedtime.

*Parenteral:*

*Adults* – 25 to 50 mg at bedtime for nighttime sedation. Doses of 50 mg provide sedation and relieve apprehension during early stages of labor. When labor is definitely established, 25 to 75 mg may be given IM or IV with an appropriately reduced dose of any desired narcotic. If necessary, promethazine injection with a reduced dose of analgesic may be repeated once or twice at 4-hour intervals. Do not exceed 100 mg/24 hours for patients in labor.

*Children 2 to 12 years of age* – Do not exceed half the adult dose.

*Antiemetic –*

*Oral/Rectal:*

*Adults* – Usual dose is 25 mg; doses of 12.5 to 25 mg may be repeated every 4 to 6 hours as needed.

*Children more than 2 years of age* – Usual dose is 25 mg or 0.5 mg/lb; doses of 12.5 to 25 mg may be repeated every 4 to 6 hours as needed.

Antiemetics are not recommended for treatment of uncomplicated vomiting in children; limit use to prolonged vomiting of known etiology.

*Parenteral:*

*Adults* – Usual dose is 12.5 to 25 mg, may repeat every 4 hours as needed. If used postoperatively, reduce doses of concomitant analgesics or barbiturates accordingly.

*Children 2 to 12 years of age* – Do not exceed half the adult dose. Do not use when etiology of vomiting is unknown.

*Motion sickness (oral and rectal only) –*

*Adults:* Usual dose is 25 mg twice/day; take first dose 30 to 60 minutes before anticipated travel; repeat 8 to 12 hours later if needed. On successive travel days, take 25 mg upon rising and again before the evening meal.

*Children older than 2 years of age:* 12.5 to 25 mg twice/day.

*Pre- and postoperative use –*

*Oral/Rectal:*

*Adults* – For preoperative use, 25 to 50 mg administered with an appropriately reduced dose of narcotic or barbiturate and the required amount of a belladonna alkaloid. For postoperative use, 25 to 50 mg doses in adults.

*Children older than 2 years of age* – For preoperative use, 0.5 mg/lb in combination with an appropriately reduced dose of narcotic or barbiturate and the appropriate dose of an atropine-like drug. For postoperative use, 12.5 to 25 mg in children.

*Parenteral:*

*Adults* – 25 to 50 mg in combination with appropriately reduced doses of analgesics, hypnotics, and atropine-like drugs as appropriate.

*Children 2 to 12 years of age* – 0.5 mg/lb in combination with an appropriately reduced dose of narcotic or barbiturate and the appropriate dose of an atropine-like drug.

*Use in children* – Exercise caution when administering to children 2 years of age and older because of the potential for fatal respiratory depression. The extrapyramidal symptoms that can occur secondary to promethazine administration may be confused with the CNS signs of undiagnosed primary disease (eg, encephalopathy,

Reye syndrome). Avoid use in children whose signs and symptoms may suggest Reye syndrome or other hepatic diseases.

*TRIPROLIDINE HYDROCHLORIDE:*

*Adults and children (12 years of age and older)* – 10 mL every 4 to 6 hours, not to exceed 40 mL in 24 hours.

*Children –*

*6 to 12 years of age:* 5 mL every 4 to 6 hours, not to exceed 20 mL in 24 hours.

*4 to 6 years of age:* 3.75 mL every 4 to 6 hours, not to exceed 15 mL in 24 hours.

*2 to 4 years of age:* 2.5 mL every 4 to 6 hours, not to exceed 10 mL in 24 hours.

*4 months to 2 years of age:* 1.25 mL every 4 to 6 hours, not to exceed 5 mL in 24 hours.

*ANTIHISTAMINE COMBINATION:*

*Adults 12 years of age and older* – 10 mL every 4 hours.

*Children –*

*6 to 12 years of age:* 5 mL every 4 hours.

*2 to 6 years of age:* 2.5 mL every 4 hours.

*Younger than 2 years of age:* Use only as directed by the physician.

## Actions

*Pharmacology:*

| Antihistamines: Dosage and Effects | | | | |
|---|---|---|---|---|
| Antihistamine | Sedative effects | Antihistaminic activity | Anticholinergic activity | Antiemetic effects |
| First-Generation (nonselective) | | | | |
| *Alkylamines* | | | | |
| Brompheniramine | + | +++ | ++ | — |
| Chlorpheniramine | + | ++ | ++ | — |
| Dexchlorpheniramine | + | +++ | ++ | — |
| Pheniramine | ++ | — | — | — |
| Triprolidine | + | — | — | — |
| *Ethanolamines* | | | | |
| Carbinoxamine | +++ | — | +++ | — |
| Clemastine | ++ | + to ++ | +++ | ++ to +++ |
| Diphenhydramine | +++ | + to ++ | +++ | ++ to +++ |
| *Ethylenediamine* | | | | |
| Pyrilamine | + | — | ± | — |
| *Phenothiazines* | | | | |
| Promethazine | +++ | +++ | +++ | ++++ |
| *Piperazines* | | | | |
| Hydroxyzine | +++ | ++ to +++ | ++ | +++ |
| *Piperidines* | | | | |
| Azatadine | ++ | ++ | ++ | — |
| Cyproheptadine | + | ++ | ++ | — |
| Phenindamine | ± | ++ | ++ | — |
| Second-Generation (peripherally selective) | | | | |
| *Phthalazinone* | | | | |
| Azelastine[c] | ± | ++ to +++ | ± | — |
| *Piperazine* | | | | |
| Cetirizine | + | ++ to +++ | ± | — |

| Antihistamines: Dosage and Effects | | | | |
|---|---|---|---|---|
| Antihistamine | Sedative effects | Antihistaminic activity | Anticholinergic activity | Antiemetic effects |
| *Piperidines* | | | | |
| Desloratadine | ± | — | ± | — |
| Fexofenadine | ± | — | ± | — |
| Loratadine | ± | ++ to +++ | ± | — |

* ++++ = very high, +++ = high, ++ = moderate, + = low, ± = low to none.
a Usual single adult dose.
b For conventional dosage forms.
c Some effects may be enhanced or reduced as a result of administration via the nasal route.

Antihistamines are reversible, competitive $H_1$ receptor antagonists that reduce or prevent most of the physiologic effects that histamine normally induces at the $H_1$ receptor site. First-generation antihistamines bind nonselectively to central and peripheral $H_1$ receptors and can result in CNS stimulation or depression. Second-generation antihistamines are selective for peripheral $H_1$ receptors and, as a group, are less sedating. First-generation agents with strong anticholinergic properties bind to central muscarinic receptors and produce antiemetic effects.

*Pharmacokinetics:*

*Pharmacokinetics* – Pharmacokinetics of first-generation agents have not been extensively studied. These agents are generally well absorbed following oral administration, have an onset of action within 15 to 30 minutes, are maximal within 1 to 2 hours, and have a duration of approximately 4 to 6 hours, although some are longer acting. Most are metabolized by liver. Antihistamine metabolites and small amounts of unchanged drug are excreted in urine.

*Second-generation agents* – Intranasal administration of **azelastine** yields peak levels in 2 to 3 hours, with an elimination half-life of 22 hours. Metabolism by the P450 system results in steady-state peak levels of a major active metabolite (desmethylazelastine), which are 20% to 50% of azelastine levels. The elimination half-life of the metabolite is predicted to be 54 hours. The major route of excretion is via feces.

| Pharmacokinetics of Peripherally Selective $H_1$ Antagonists (Oral) | | | | |
|---|---|---|---|---|
| | Onset of action | $T_{max}$ (h) | Elimination $t\frac{1}{2}$ (h) | Protein binding (%) |
| Cetirizine | rapid | 1 | 8.3 | 93 |
| Fexofenadine | rapid | 2.6 | 14.4 | 60 to 70 |
| Loratadine | rapid | 1.3 to 2.5[a] | 8.4 to 28[b] | 97 (75)[b] |

↑ = High ↓ = Low ↓↓ = Very low
a All active constituents (parent drug and active metabolites)
b Active metabolite

## Contraindications

*First-generation antihistamines:* Hypersensitivity to specific or structurally related antihistamines; newborns or premature infants; nursing mothers; monoamine oxidase (MAO) therapy; pregnancy (**hydroxyzine**); angle-closure glaucoma, stenosing peptic ulcer, symptomatic prostatic hypertrophy, bladder neck obstruction, pyloroduodenal obstruction, elderly, debilitated patients (**cyproheptadine**).

*Second-generation antihistamines:* Hypersensitivity to specific or structurally related antihistamines. **Desloratadine** is contraindicated in those who are hypersensitive to **loratadine**. **Cetirizine** is contraindicated in those who are hypersensitive to **hydroxyzine**.

## Warnings

*Neuroleptic malignant syndrome (NMS):* A potentially fatal symptom complex sometimes referred to as NMS has been reported in association with **promethazine** alone or in combination with antipsychotic drugs. Clinical manifestations of NMS are hyperpyrexia, muscle rigidity, altered mental status, and evidence of autonomic instability (eg, irregular pulse or blood pressure, tachycardia, diaphoresis, cardiac dysrhythmias).

*CNS depression:* Antihistamines may impair the mental and/or physical abilities required for the performance of potentially hazardous tasks, such as driving a vehicle or operating machinery. The impairment may be amplified by concomitant use of other CNS depressants such as alcohol, sedatives/hypnotics (including barbiturates), narcotics, narcotic analgesics, general anesthetics, tricyclic antidepressants, and tranquilizers. Therefore, such agents either should be eliminated or given in reduced dosage in the presence of certain antihistamines with strong CNS depressant effects.

When given concomitantly with **promethazine**, reduce the dose of barbiturates by at least one half, and reduce the dose of the narcotics by one quarter to one half. Individualize dosage. Excessive amounts of promethazine relative to a narcotic may lead to restlessness and motor hyperactivity in the patient with pain.

*Special risk patients:* Use antihistamines with caution in patients with narrow-angle glaucoma, stenosing peptic ulcer, pyloroduodenal obstruction, symptomatic prostatic hypertrophy, bladder neck obstruction, bronchial asthma, increased intraocular pressure, hyperthyroidism, cardiovascular disease, and hypertension.

*Respiratory depression:* Avoid sedatives and CNS depressants in patients with compromised respiratory function (eg, chronic obstructive pulmonary disease [COPD], sleep apnea).

*Respiratory disease:* In general, antihistamines are not recommended to treat lower respiratory tract symptoms, because their anticholinergic effects may cause thickening of secretions and impair expectoration. However, several reports indicate antihistamines can be safely used in asthmatic patients with severe perennial allergic rhinitis.

*Seizure threshold:* **Promethazine** may lower the seizure threshold; consider this when giving to people with known seizure disorders or when giving in combination with narcotics or local anesthetics that also may affect seizure threshold.

*Hypersensitivity reactions:* Hypersensitivity reactions may occur, and any of the usual manifestations of drug allergy may develop.

*Renal/Hepatic function impairment:* Use a lower initial dose of **loratadine, desloratadine,** and **cetirizine** in patients with renal or hepatic impairment.

*Elderly:* Antihistamines are more likely to cause dizziness, excessive sedation, syncope, toxic confusional states, and hypotension in elderly patients. Dosage reduction may be required. Phenothiazine side effects (extrapyramidal signs, especially parkinsonism, akathisia, and persistent dyskinesia) are more prone to develop in the elderly.

*Pregnancy:* Category B – **azatadine, cetirizine, chlorpheniramine, clemastine, cyproheptadine, dexchlorpheniramine, diphenhydramine, loratadine.** Category C – **azelastine, brompheniramine, carbinoxamine, desloratadine, fexofenadine, hydroxyzine, pheniramine, phenytoloxamine, promethazine, pyrilamine, triprolidine.**

*Lactation:* Antihistamine therapy is contraindicated in nursing mothers.

*Children:* Antihistamines may diminish mental alertness; conversely, they may occasionally produce excitation, particularly in the young child.

Promethazine is not recommended in children younger than 2 years of age. Exercise caution when administering promethazine to children because of the potential for fatal respiratory depression. Limit antiemetics to prolonged vomiting of known etiology. Avoid use in children whose signs and symptoms may suggest Reye syndrome or other hepatic diseases. In children with dehydration, there is an increased susceptibility to dystonias with the use of promethazine.

### Precautions

*Hematologic:* Use **promethazine** with caution in bone marrow depression. Leukopenia and agranulocytosis have been reported, usually when used with other toxic agents.

*Anticholinergic effects:* Antihistamines have varying degrees of atropine-like actions; use with caution in patients with a predisposition to urinary retention, history of bronchial asthma, increased intraocular pressure, hyperthyroidism, cardiovascular disease, or hypertension.

*Phenothiazines:* Use phenothiazines with caution in patients with cardiovascular disease, liver dysfunction, or ulcer disease. Promethazine has been associated with cholestatic jaundice.

Use cautiously in people with acute or chronic respiratory impairment, particularly children, because phenothiazines may suppress the cough reflex. If hypotension occurs, epinephrine is not recommended because phenothiazines may reverse its usual pressor effect and cause a paradoxical further lowering of blood pressure. Because these drugs have an antiemetic action, they may obscure signs of intestinal obstruction, brain tumor, or overdosage of toxic drugs.

Phenothiazines elevate prolactin levels.

*Phenylketonurics:* Inform phenylketonuric patients that some of these products contain phenylalanine.

*Tartrazine sensitivity:* Some of these products contain tartrazine (FD&C yellow #5), which may cause allergic-type reactions (including bronchial asthma) in susceptible individuals. Although the incidence of sensitivity is low, it is frequently seen in patients who also have aspirin hypersensitivity. Specific products containing tartrazine are identified in the product listings.

*Hazardous tasks:* May cause drowsiness and reduce mental alertness; patients should not drive or perform tasks requiring alertness, coordination, or physical dexterity.

*Photosensitivity:* Photosensitization may occur.

**Drug Interactions**

Drugs that may affect antihistamines include aluminum/magnesium-containing acids, cimetidine, erythromycin , ketoconazole, MAO inhibitors, and rifamycins (eg, rifampin). Drugs that may be affected by antihistamines include alcohol and CNS depressants, beta-blockers, MAO inhibitors, metyrapone, nefazodone, selective serotonin reuptake inhibitors (SSRIs), and venlafaxine.

See the Antipsychotic Agents monograph for drug interactions that relate to **promethazine**.

*Drug/Lab test interactions:* Diagnostic pregnancy tests based on hCG may result in false-negative or false-positive interpretations in patients on promethazine. Increased blood glucose has occurred in **promethazine** patients.

Phenothiazines may increase serum cholesterol, spinal fluid protein, and urinary urobilinogen levels; decrease protein bound iodine; yield false-positive urine bilirubin tests; interfere with urinary ketone and steroid determinations.

Discontinue antihistamines approximately 4 days prior to skin testing procedures; these drugs may prevent or diminish otherwise positive reactions to dermal reactivity indicators.

*Drug/Food interactions:* Food increased the AUC of **loratadine** by approximately 40% and the metabolite by approximately 15%; absorption was delayed by 1 hour. Although not expected to be clinically important, take on an empty stomach.

Certain fruit juices (ie, apple, orange, grapefruit) administered with **fexofenadine** significantly reduced the AUC and $C_{max}$ of fexofenadine. Therefore, fexofenadine's clinical effect may be decreased. It would be prudent for patients to take fexofenadine with a liquid other than these juices.

**Adverse Reactions**

Adverse reactions may include the following: acute labyrinthitis; agranulocytosis; anaphylactic shock; anemias; anorexia; aplastic anemiahemolytic anemia; asthma; blurred vision; bradycardia; cardiac arrest; catatonic-like states; chest tightness; chills; confusion; constipation; convulsions; dermatitis; diarrhea; diplopia; disorientation; disturbed coordination; disturbing dreams/nightmares; dizziness; drowsiness (often transient); drug rash; dry mouth, nose, and throat; dysuria; early menses; ECG changes, including blunting of T-waves and prolongation of the QT interval; elevated spinal fluid proteins; elevation of plasma cholesterol levels; epigastric distress, especially ethylenediamines; erythema; euphoria; excessive perspiration; excitation; extrasystoles; faintness; fatigue; grand mal seizures; glycosuria; gynecomastia; hallucinations; headache; high or prolonged glucose tolerance curves; hypertension; hypoplastic anemia; hypotension; hysteria; increased appetite and weight gain; increases and decreases in blood pressure; induced lactation; inhibition of ejaculation; insomnia; lassitude; leukopenia; lupus erythematosus-like syndrome; nasal stuffiness; nausea; neuritis; obstructive jaundice (usually reversible upon discontinuation); oculogyric crisis; palpitations; pancytopenia; paresthesias; peripheral, angioneurotic, and laryngeal edema; pharyngitis; photosensitivity; postural hypotension; pseudoschizophrenia; reflex tachycardia; respiratory depression; restlessness; sedation; sore throat; stomatitis; tachycardia; thickening of bronchial secretions; thrombocytopenia; thrombocytopenic purpura; tingling, heaviness, and weakness of the hands; tinnitus; tissue necrosis following subcutaneous administration of IV **promethazine**; tongue protrusion (usually in association with IV administration or excessive dosage); torticollis; tremor; urinary frequency; urinary retention; urticaria; venous thrombosis at injection site (IV **promethazine**); vertigo; vomiting; weakness; wheezing.

Extrapyramidal reactions may occur with high doses; these reactions usually respond to dose reduction.

*Nasal spray:* Bitter taste; conjunctivitis; epistaxis; eye abnormality; eye pain; glossitis; increased ALT; nasal burning; rhinitis; paroxysmal sneezing; taste loss; temporomandibular dislocation; ulcerative and aphthous stomatitis; watery eyes.

These antihistamines infrequently cause typical phenothiazine adverse effects. See the Antipsychotic Agents monograph for a complete discussion.

## Patient Information

Instruct patients to inform a physician of a history of glaucoma, peptic ulcer, urinary retention, or pregnancy before starting antihistamine therapy.

Some antihistamines may cause nervousness, insomnia, and dry mouth.

Some antihistamines may cause drowsiness or dizziness; advise patients to observe caution while driving or performing other tasks requiring alertness, coordination, or physical dexterity and to avoid alcohol and other CNS depressants (eg, sedatives, hypnotics, tranquilizers, antianxiety agents).

Some antihistamines may cause GI upset; instruct patients to take with food.

Advise patients to avoid prolonged exposure to sunlight; some agents may cause photosensitivity.

Instruct patients not to crush or chew sustained-release preparations.

Fexofenadine should not be taken closely in time with aluminum- and magnesium-containing antacids.

*Phenothiazines:* Advise patients to report any involuntary muscle movements or unusual sensitivity to sunlight.

# DEXTROMETHORPHAN HBr

**Gelcaps**: 30 mg (*otc*)
**Lozenges**: 5 mg (*otc*)

7.5 mg (*otc*)
**Liquid**: 7.5 mg/5 mL (*otc*)
10 mg/15 mL (3.33 mg/5 mL) (*otc*)
15 mg/5 mL (*otc*)

30 mg/5 mL (*otc*)
**Syrup**: 7.5 mg/5 mL
10 mg/5 mL
**Liquid, sustained action**: Dextromethorphan polistirex equivalent to 30 mg dextromethorphan HBr/5 mL (*otc*)

*DexAlone* (DexGen)
*Hold DM* (B.F. Ascher), *Scot-Tussin DM Cough Chasers* (Scot-Tussin)
*Trocal* (Textilease)
*Benylin Pediatric* (Pfizer)
*Creo-Terpin* (Lee)
*Benylin Adult* (Pfizer), *Robitussin Maximum Strength Cough* (Whitehall-Robins)
*Vicks 44 Cough Relief* (Proctor and Gamble)
*Robitussin Pediatric Cough* (Whitehall-Robins)
*Silphen DM* (Silarx)
*Delsym* (Celltech)

### Indications

Temporarily relieves cough caused by minor throat and bronchial irritation as may occur with the common cold or inhaled irritants.

### Administration and Dosage

*Gelcaps:*
    *Adults and children 12 years of age and older* – 30 mg every 6 to 8 hours. Do not exceed 120 mg in 24 hours.

*Lozenges:*
    *Adults and children 12 years of age and older* – 5 to 15 mg every 1 to 4 hours up to 120 mg/day.
    *Children 6 to under 12 years of age* – 5 to 10 mg every 1 to 4 hours up to 60 mg/day.
    Do not give to children under 6 years of age unless directed by a physician.

*Liquid and syrup:*
    *Adults and children 12 years of age and older* – 10 to 20 mg every 4 hours or 30 mg every 6 to 8 hours up to 120 mg/day.
    *Children* –
        *6 to under 12 years of age:* 15 mg every 6 to 8 hours up to 60 mg/day.
        *2 to under 6 years of age:* 7.5 mg every 6 to 8 hours up to 30 mg/day.

*Extended-release suspension:*
    *Adults and children 12 years of age and older* – 60 mg every 12 hours up to 120 mg/day.
    *Children* –
        *6 to under 12 years of age:* 30 mg every 12 hours up to 60 mg/day.
        *2 to under 6 years of age:* 15 mg every 12 hours up to 30 mg/day.

### Actions

*Pharmacology:* Dextromethorphan is the d-isomer of the codeine analog of levorphanol. Its cough suppressant action is due to a central action on the cough center in the medulla. Dextromethorphan 15 to 30 mg equals 8 to 15 mg codeine as an antitussive.

*Pharmacokinetics:* Dextromethorphan is rapidly absorbed from the GI tract. It undergoes metabolism in the liver and is then excreted in the urine as unchanged drug and demethylated metabolites.

### Contraindications

Hypersensitivity to any component.

### Warnings

*Use:* For persistent or chronic cough or cough accompanied by excessive secretions, consult a doctor before use.

*Pregnancy: Category C.*

*Lactation:* It is not known if dextromethorphan is excreted in breast milk.

### Precautions

Anecdotal reports of abuse of dextromethorphan-containing cough/cold products has increased, especially among teenagers.

### Drug Interactions

Drugs that may interact with dextromethorphan include MAO inhibitors, quinidine, and sibutramine.

### Adverse Reactions

Adverse reactions may include dizziness, drowsiness, and GI disturbances.

# DIPHENHYDRAMINE HCI

| | |
|---|---|
| **Liquid:** 12.5 mg/5 mL (*otc*) | *AllerMax* (Pfeiffer) |
| **Syrup:** 12.5 mg/5 mL (*otc*)[1] | Various, *Silphen Cough* (Silarx), *Tusstat* (Century) |

[1] Products available *otc* or *Rx* depending on product labeling.

### Indications

For the control of cough due to colds, allergy, or bronchial irritation.

### Administration and Dosage

*Adults:* 25 mg every 4 hours, not to exceed 150 mg in 24 hours.

*Children (6 to 12 years of age):* 12.5 mg every 4 hours, not to exceed 75 mg in 24 hours.

*Children (2 to 6 years of age):* 6.25 mg every 4 hours, not to exceed 25 mg in 24 hours.

# BENZONATATE

| | |
|---|---|
| **Capsules:** 100 and 200 mg (*Rx*) | Various, *Tessalon Perles* (Forest) |

### Indications

Symptomatic relief of cough.

### Administration and Dosage

*Adults and children (older than 10 years of age):* 100 to 200 mg 3 times/day, up to 600 mg/day.

### Actions

*Pharmacology:* Benzonatate anesthetizes stretch receptors in respiratory passages, lungs, and pleura, dampening their activity, and reducing the cough reflex. It has no inhibitory effect on the respiratory center in recommended dosage. Onset of action is 15 to 20 minutes; effects last 3 to 8 hours.

### Contraindications

Hypersensitivity to benzonatate or related compounds (eg, tetracaine).

### Warnings

*Behavior changes:* Isolated instances of bizarre behavior, including mental confusion and visual hallucinations, have been reported in patients taking benzonatate in combination with other prescribed drugs.

*Hypersensitivity reactions:* Severe hypersensitivity reactions (eg, bronchospasm, laryngospasm, cardiovascular collapse) have been reported that may be related to local anesthesia from sucking or chewing the capsule instead of swallowing it. Severe reactions have required intervention with vasopressor agents and supportive measures.

*Pregnancy:* Category C.

*Lactation:* It is not known whether this drug is excreted in breast milk.

### Precautions

*CNS effects:* Benzonatate has been associated with adverse CNS effects possibly related to a prior sensitivity to similar agents or interaction with concomitant medication.

*Local anesthesia:* Release of benzonatate in the mouth can produce a temporary local anesthesia of the oral mucosa. Swallow the capsules without chewing.

**Adverse Reactions**

Sedation; headache; dizziness; mental confusion; visual hallucinations; constipation; nausea; GI upset; pruritus; skin eruptions; nasal congestion; sensation of burning in the eyes; a vague "chilly" sensation; chest numbness; hypersensitivity.

# DEXTROMETHORPHAN HBr and BENZOCAINE

| | |
|---|---|
| **Lozenges**: 5 mg dextromethorphan and 2 mg benzocaine (*otc*) | *Cough* X (B.F. Ascher) |
| 10 mg dextromethorphan HBr and 15 mg benzocaine (*otc*) | *Tetra-Formula* (Reese Pharm.) |

**Indications**

Temporarily suppresses cough caused by minor throat and bronchial irritants that may occur with the common cold. Also for the temporary relief of occasional minor irritation and sore throat.

**Administration and Dosage**

Do not use for more than 2 days for sore throat or for more than 7 days for cough unless directed by a doctor. Do not use for persistent or chronic cough such as occurs with smoking, asthma, emphysema, or if cough is accompanied by excessive phlegm unless directed by a doctor. Allow lozenge to dissolve slowly in the mouth.

*Cough-X:*

   *Adults and children 6 years of age and older* – One lozenge every 2 hours as needed, not to exceed 12 lozenges in 24 hours or as directed by a physician.

   *Children 2 to 6 years of age* – One lozenge every 4 hours not to exceed 6 lozenges in 24 hours, or as directed by a physician.

   In children, take care to prevent choking on lozenge.

*Tetra-Formula:*

   *Adults and children 6 years of age and older* – Dissolve 1 lozenge slowly in the mouth; do not chew. May be repeated every 4 hours or as directed by a physician.

   *Children under 6 years of age* – Consult a physician.

# ZAFIRLUKAST

**Tablets:** 10 and 20 mg *(Rx)*                     *Accolate* (AstraZeneca)

### Indications
*Asthma:* Prophylaxis and chronic treatment of asthma in adults and children 5 years of age and older.

### Administration and Dosage
Because food reduces bioavailability of zafirlukast, take at least 1 hour before or 2 hours after meals.

*Adults and children 12 years of age and older:* The recommended dose of zafirlukast is 20 mg twice daily.

*Children 5 to 11 years of age:* The recommended dose of zafirlukast is 10 mg twice daily.

### Actions
*Pharmacology:* Zafirlukast is a selective and competitive leukotreine receptor antagonist (LTRA) of leukotreine $D_4$ and $E_4$, components of slow-reacting substance of anaphylaxis (SRSA). Leukotriene production and receptor occupation have been correlated with airway edema, smooth muscle constriction and altered cellular activity associated with the inflammatory process, which contribute to the signs and symptoms of asthma.

*Pharmacokinetics:* Oral zafirlukast is rapidly absorbed. Peak plasma concentrations are achieved 3 hours after dosing. The mean terminal elimination half-life is about 10 hours. Zafirlukast is more than 99% bound to plasma proteins, predominantly albumin.

Zafirlukast is extensively metabolized. Urinary excretion accounts for about 10% of the dose and the remainder is excreted in the feces. Liver microsomes that hydroxylate metabolites of zafirlukast are formed through the cytochrome P450 2C9 (CYP2C9) enzyme pathway.

Additional studies show that zafirlukast inhibits the CYP3A4 and CYP2C9 isoenzymes.

### Contraindications
Hypersensitivity to zafirlukast or any of its inactive ingredients.

### Warnings
*Acute asthma attacks:* Zafirlukast is not indicated for use in the reversal of bronchospasm in acute asthma attacks, including status asthmaticus. Continue zafirlukast during acute exacerbations of asthma.

*Infection:* An increased proportion of zafirlukast patients older than 55 years of age reported infections as compared to placebo-treated patients.

*Hypersensitivity reactions:* Hypersensitivity reactions, including urticaria, angioedema, and rashes, with or without blistering have been reported with zafirlukast therapy.

*Hepatic function impairment:* The clearance of zafirlukast is reduced in patients with hepatic impairment.

*Elderly:* The clearance of zafirlukast is reduced in elderly patients (65 years of age or older), such that $C_{max}$ and AUC are approximately twice those of younger adults.

*Pregnancy:* Category B.

*Lactation:* Zafirlukast is excreted in breast milk.

*Children:* The safety and effectiveness of zafirlukast in patients less than 5 years of age have not been established.

### Precautions
*Hepatotoxicity:* Rarely, elevations of 1 or more liver enzymes have occurred in patients receiving zafirlukast. Most of these have been observed at doses 4 times higher than the recommended dose. The following hepatic events predominantly in females) have been reported in patients who have received the recommended dose of zafirlukast (40 mg/day): Cases of symptomatic hepatitis without other attributable cause; and, rarely, hyperbilirubinemia without other elevated liver function tests. In

most, symptoms abated and the liver enzymes returned to healthy or near healthy after stopping zafirlukast. If liver dysfunction is suspected, discontinue zafirlukast.

*Eosinophilia:* Physicians should be alert to eosinophilia, vasculitic rash, worsening pulmonary symptoms, cardiac complications, or neuropathy presenting in their patients. In rare cases, patients on zafirlukast therapy may present with systemic eosinophilia. These events usually, but not always, have been associated with the reduction of oral steroid therapy.

### Drug Interactions

Due to zafirlukast's inhibition of cytochrome P450 2C9 and 3A4 isoenzymes, use caution with coadministration of drugs known to be metabolized by these isoenzymes.

Drugs that may affect zafirlukast include aspirin, erythromycin, and theophylline.

Drugs that may be affected by zafirlukast include warfarin.

*Drug/Food interactions:* The bioavailability of zafirlukast may be decreased when taken with food. Take zafirlukast at least 1 hour before or 2 hours after meals.

### Adverse Reactions

Adverse reactions occurring in 3% or more of patients include headache, nausea, infection.

# MONTELUKAST SODIUM

**Tablets**: 10 mg (as base) *(Rx)*
**Tablets, chewable**: 4 and 5 mg (as base) *(Rx)*
**Granules**: 4 mg/packet *(Rx)*

*Singulair* (Merck)

### Indications

*Asthma:* Prophylaxis and chronic treatment of asthma in adults and pediatric patients 12 months of age and older.

*Seasonal allergic rhinitis:* Relief of symptoms of seasonal allergic rhinitis in adults and pediatric patients 2 years of age and older.

### Administration and Dosage

*Adults and adolescents 15 years of age and older:* One 10 mg tablet daily, taken in the evening.

*Children 6 to 14 years of age:* One 5 mg chewable tablet daily, taken in the evening.

*Children 2 to 5 years of age:* One 4 mg chewable tablet daily, taken in the evening.

*Children 12 to 23 months of age:* One packet of 4 mg granules daily taken in the evening.

Safety and effectiveness in pediatric patients below 12 months of age have not been established.

*Administration of oral granules:* Montelukast 4 mg oral granules can be administered directly in the mouth or mixed with a spoonful of cold or room temperature soft foods; based on stability studies, use only applesauce, carrots, rice, or ice cream. Do not open the packet until ready to use. After opening the packet, the full dose (with or without mixing with food) must be administered within 15 minutes. If mixed with food, the oral granules must not be stored for future use. Discard any unused portion. Montelukast oral granules are not intended to be dissolved in liquid for administration. However, liquids may be taken subsequent to administration. The granules can be administered without regard to the time of meals.

### Actions

*Pharmacology:* Montelukast is a selective and orally active leukotriene receptor antagonist that inhibits the cysteinyl leukotrine ($CysLT_1$) receptor.

Leukotrienes are products of arachidonic acid metabolism and are released from mast cells and eosinophils. Leukotrienes and leukotriene receptor occupation have been correlated with airway edema, smooth muscle contraction, and altered cellular activity associated with the inflammatory process, which contribute to the signs and symptoms of asthma.

*Pharmacokinetics:* Montelukast is rapidly absorbed following oral administration. The mean peak plasma concentration ($C_{max}$) is achieved in 3 to 4 hours ($T_{max}$). The mean oral bioavailability is 64%. Montelukast is more than 99% bound to plasma proteins and is extensively metabolized by the cytochrome P4503A4 and 2C9 pathways. The plasma clearance of montelukast averages 45 mL/min in healthy adults. Montelukast and its metabolites are excreted almost exclusively via the bile. The mean plasma half-life ranged from 2.7 to 5.5 hours in healthy young adults.

## Contraindications

Hypersensitivity to any component of this product.

## Warnings

*Acute asthma attacks:* Montelukast is not indicated for use in acute asthma attacks, including status asthmaticus. Advise patients to have appropriate rescue medication available. Montelukast therapy can be continued during acute exacerbations of asthma.

*Elderly:* Plasma half-life is slightly longer in the elderly. No dosage adjustment is required.

*Pregnancy: Category B.*

Merck maintains a registry to monitor the pregnancy outcomes of pregnant women exposed to montelukast. Health care providers are encouraged to report any prenatal exposure to montelukast by calling the Pregnancy Registry at (800) 986-8999.

*Lactation:* It is not known if montelukast is excreted in human breast milk.

*Children:* Safety and efficacy in children less than 12 months of age have not been established.

## Precautions

*Exercise-induced bronchoconstriction:* Do not use montelukast as monotherapy. Patients should continue to use their usual regimen of inhaled beta-agonists as prophylaxis and have a short-acting inhaled beta-agonist available for rescue.

*Concurrent corticosteroids:* While the dose of inhaled corticosteroid may be reduced gradually under medical supervision, montelukast should not be abruptly substituted for inhaled or oral corticosteroids.

*Eosinophilia:* Physicians should be alert to eosinophilia, vasculitic rash, worsening pulmonary symptoms, cardiac complications, or neuropathy in their patients. In rare cases, patients on therapy with montelukast may present with systemic eosinophilia. These events usually, but not always, have been associated with the reduction of oral corticosteroid therapy.

*Aspirin sensitivity:* Patients with known aspirin sensitivity should continue avoidance of aspirin and nonsteroidal anti-inflammatory agents while taking montelukast.

*Phenylketonurics:* Inform phenylketonuric patients that the 4 and 5 mg chewable tablets contain phenylalanine.

## Drug Interactions

Drugs that may interact with montelukast include phenobarbital and rifampin.

## Adverse Reactions

Adverse reactions occurring in more than 3% of patients include headache and influenza. In children 6 to 14 years of age, the following events occurred with a frequency of 2%: Diarrhea, laryngitis, pharyngitis, nausea, otitis, sinusitis, viral infections. In children 2 to 5 years of age the following events occurred with a frequency of 2%: Rhinorrhea, otitis, ear pain, bronchitis, leg pain, thirst, sneezing, rash, and urticaria. In children 12 to 23 months of age, the following events occurred with a frequency of 2% or more: Upper respiratory infection; wheezing; otitis media; pharyngitis; tonsillitis; cough; rhinitis.

# ZILEUTON

**Tablets:** 600 mg (*Rx*)           Zyflo (Abbott)

### Indications
*Asthma:* The prophylaxis and chronic treatment of asthma in adults and children 12 years of age or older.

### Administration and Dosage
The recommended dosage of zileuton for the symptomatic treatment of patients with asthma is 600 mg 4 times/day for a total daily dose of 2400 mg. For ease of administration, zileuton may be taken with meals and at bedtime.

### Actions
*Pharmacology:* Zileuton is a specific inhibitor of 5-lipoxygenase and thus inhibits leukotriene ($LTB_1$, $LTC_1$, $LTD_1$, $LTe_1$) formation.

Zileuton inhibits leukotriene-dependent smooth muscle contractions. Pretreatment with zileuton attenuated bronchoconstriction caused by cold air challenge in patients with asthma.

*Pharmacokinetics:*

*Absorption* – Zileuton is rapidly absorbed upon oral administration with a mean time to peak plasma concentration ($T_{max}$) of 1.7 hours and a mean peak level ($C_{max}$) of 4.98 mcg/mL. Plasma concentrations of zileuton are proportional to dose.

*Distribution* – The apparent volume of distribution of zileuton is approximately 1.2 L/kg. Zileuton is 93% bound to plasma proteins, primarily to albumin, with minor binding to alpha-acid glycoprotein.

*Metabolism* – Several zileuton metabolites have been identified in plasma and urine. These include two diastereomeric O-glucuronide conjugates (major metabolites) and an N-dehydroxylated metabolite and unchanged zileuton each accounted for less than 0.5% of the dose. Liver microsomes have shown that zileuton and its N-dehydroxylated metabolite can be oxidatively metabolized by the cytochrome P450 isoenzymes 1A2, 2C9, and 3A4 (CYP1A2, CYP2C9, and CYP3A4).

*Excretion* – Elimination of zileuton is predominantly via metabolism with a mean terminal half-life of 2.5 hours. Zileuton activity is primarily because of the parent drug. Orally administered zileuton is well absorbed into the systemic circulation with 94.5% and 2.2% of the dose recovered in urine and feces, respectively.

### Contraindications
Active liver disease or transaminase elevations 3 times or more the upper limit of normal, hypersensitivity to zileuton or any of its inactive ingredients.

### Warnings
*Hepatotoxicity:* Elevations of 1 or more liver function tests may occur during zileuton therapy. These laboratory abnormalities may progress, remain unchanged or resolve with continued therapy.

*Acute asthma attacks:* Zileuton is not indicated for use in the reversal of bronchospasm in acute asthma attacks, including status asthmaticus.

*Hematologic:* Occurrences of low white blood cell count (up to $2.8 \times 10^9/L$) were observed in 1% of 1678 patients taking zileuton and 0.6% of 1056 patients taking placebo.

*Hepatic function impairment:* Use with caution in patients who consume substantial quantities of alcohol or have a history of liver disease.

*Pregnancy: Category C.*

*Lactation:* Zileuton and its metabolites are excreted in rat milk. It is not known if zileuton is excreted in breast milk.

*Children:* The safety and effectiveness of zileuton in pediatric patients younger than 12 years of age have not been established.

### Precautions
*Monitoring:* Evaluate hepatic transaminases at initiation of and during therapy with zileuton. Monitor serum ALT before treatment begins, once-a-month for the first

3 months, every 2 to 3 months for the remainder of the first year and periodically thereafter for patients receiving long-term zileuton therapy. If symptoms of liver dysfunction develop or transaminase elevations greater than 5 times the ULN occur, discontinue therapy and follow transaminase levels until normal.

### Drug Interactions

Liver microsomes have shown that zileuton and its N-dehydroxylated metabolite can be oxidatively metabolized by the cytochrome P450 isoenzymes 1A2, 2C9, and 3A4. Use caution when prescribing a medication that inhibits any of these enzymes.

Drugs that may be affected by zileuton include propranolol, terfenadine, theophylline, and warfarin.

Drugs that may affect zileuton include digoxin, oral contraceptives, phenytoin, and prednisone.

### Adverse Reactions

Adverse reactions occurring 3% or more of patients include headache; pain; abdominal pain; asthenia; accidental injury; dyspepsia; nausea; ALT elevation; myalgia.

# FLUTICASONE PROPIONATE/SALMETEROL

**Powder for inhalation:** 100 mcg fluticasone propionate/ 50 mcg salmeterol, 250 mcg fluticasone propionate/50 mcg salmeterol, 500 mcg fluticasone propionate/50 mcg salmeterol (*Rx*)

*Advair Diskus* (GlaxoSmithKline)

**Warning:**
Data from a large, placebo-controlled US study that compared the safety of salmeterol or placebo added to usual asthma therapy showed a small but significant increase in asthma-related deaths in patients receiving salmeterol (13 deaths out of 13,174 patients treated for 28 weeks) vs those on placebo (4 of 13,179). Subgroup analyses suggest the risk may be greater in blacks compared with whites.

## Indications

*Asthma, chronic:* For the long-term, twice-daily maintenance treatment of asthma in patients 4 years of age and older.

Not indicated for the relief of acute bronchospasm.

*Chronic obstructive pulmonary disease (COPD) associated with chronic bronchitis:* For the twice-daily maintenance treatment of airflow obstruction in patients with COPD associated with chronic bronchitis. Fluticasone propionate/salmeterol 250 mcg/50 mcg twice daily is the only approved dosage for the treatment of COPD associated with chronic bronchitis. Higher doses, including fluticasone propionate/salmeterol 500 mcg/50 mcg, are not recommended.

## Administration and Dosage

Administer by the orally inhaled route only. The maximum recommended dose of fluticasone propionate/salmeterol is 500 mcg/50 mcg twice/day.

*Asthma, chronic:*

*Adults and children 12 years of age and older –* 1 inhalation twice/day (morning and evening, approximately 12 hours apart).

More frequent administration or a higher number of inhalations of the prescribed strength is not recommended, as some patients are more likely to experience adverse effects with higher doses of salmeterol.

For all patients, titrate to the lowest effective strength after adequate asthma stability is achieved.

If symptoms arise in the period between doses, administer an inhaled, short-acting $\beta_2$-agonist for immediate relief.

Patients receiving fluticasone propionate/salmeterol twice daily should not use salmeterol or other inhaled, long-acting $\beta_2$-agonists (eg, formoterol) for prevention of exercise-induced bronchospasm, or for any other reason.

Improvement in asthma control following inhaled administration of fluticasone propionate/salmeterol can occur within 30 minutes of beginning treatment, although maximum benefit may not be achieved for at least 1 week. Individual patients will experience a variable time to onset and degree of symptom relief.

Replacing the current strength of fluticasone propionate/salmeterol with a higher strength may provide additional asthma control for patients who do not respond adequately to the starting dose after 2 weeks of therapy.

If a previously effective dosage regimen fails to provide adequate asthma control, reevaluate the therapeutic regimen and consider additional therapeutic options, such as replacing the current strength of fluticasone propionate/salmeterol with a higher strength, adding additional inhaled corticosteroid, or initiating oral corticosteroids.

Advise patients to rinse mouth after inhalation without swallowing.

*Patients not currently on an inhaled corticosteroid –* A starting dose of fluticasone propionate/salmeterol 100 mcg/50 mcg twice/day is recommended for patients who are not currently on an inhaled corticosteroid and whose disease severity warrants treatment with 2 maintenance therapies, including patients on noncorticosteroid maintenance therapy.

*Patients currently on an inhaled corticosteroid* – The following table provides the recommended starting dose for patients currently on an inhaled corticosteroid.

| Recommended Starting Doses of Fluticasone Propionate/Salmeterol for Asthma Patients (Age ≥ 12) Taking Inhaled Corticosteroids | | |
|---|---|---|
| Current daily dose of inhaled corticosteroid | | Recommended strength and dosing schedule of fluticasone propionate/salmeterol |
| Beclomethasone dipropionate | ≤ 420 mcg | 100 mcg/50 mcg twice/day |
| | 462 to 840 mcg | 250 mcg/50 mcg twice/day |
| Budesonide | ≤ 400 mcg | 100 mcg/50 mcg twice/day |
| | 800 to 1,200 mcg | 250 mcg/50 mcg twice/day |
| | 1,600 mcg[a] | 500 mcg/50 mcg twice/day |
| Flunisolide | ≤ 1,000 mcg | 100 mcg/50 mcg twice/day |
| | 1,250 to 2,000 mcg | 250 mcg/50 mcg twice/day |
| Fluticasone propionate inhalation aerosol | ≤ 176 mcg | 100 mcg/50 mcg twice/day |
| | 440 mcg | 250 mcg/50 mcg twice/day |
| | 660 to 880 mcg[a] | 500 mcg/50 mcg twice/day |
| Fluticasone propionate inhalation powder | ≤ 200 mcg | 100 mcg/50 mcg twice/day |
| | 500 mcg | 250 mcg/50 mcg twice/day |
| | 1,000 mcg[a] | 500 mcg/50 mcg twice/day |
| Triamcinolone acetonide | ≤ 1000 mcg | 100 mcg/50 mcg twice/day |
| | 1,100 to 1,600 mcg | 250 mcg/50 mcg twice/day |

[a] Do not use fluticasone propionate/salmeterol for transferring patients from systemic corticosteroid therapy.

*Children 4 to 11 years of age* – For patients 4 to 11 years of age who are symptomatic on an inhaled corticosteroid, the dosage is 1 inhalation of fluticasone propionate/salmeterol 100 mcg/50 mcg twice/day (morning and evening, approximately 12 hours apart).

*COPD associated with chronic bronchitis:* The dosage for adults is 1 inhalation (250 mcg/50 mcg) twice/day (morning and evening, approximately 12 hours apart). Higher doses are not recommended because no additional improvement in lung function was observed in clinical trials and higher doses of corticosteroids increase the risk of systemic effects. The benefit of treating patients with COPD associated with chronic bronchitis with fluticasone propionate/salmeterol 250 mcg/50 mcg for periods longer than 6 months has not been evaluated. Periodically reevaluate patients treated with fluticasone propionate/salmeterol 250 mcg/50 mcg for COPD associated with chronic bronchitis for periods longer than 6 months to assess the continuing benefits and potential risks of treatment.

If shortness of breath occurs in the period between doses, administer an inhaled, short-acting $\beta_2$-agonist for immediate relief.

Patients receiving fluticasone propionate/salmeterol twice daily should not use additional salmeterol or other inhaled, long-acting $\beta_2$-agonists (eg, formoterol) for the maintenance treatment of COPD, or for any other reason.

# Chapter 7

# CENTRAL NERVOUS SYSTEM AGENTS

# AMPHETAMINES

**DEXTROAMPHETAMINE SULFATE**

**Tablets:** 5 mg (c-ıı) — Various, *Dexedrine* (GlaxoSmithKline), *Dextrostat* (Shire Richwood)

**Tablets:** 10 mg (c-ıı) — Various, *Dextrostat* (Shire Richwood)

**Capsules, sustained-release:** 5, 10, and 15 mg (c-ıı) — Various, *Dexedrine Spansules* (GlaxoSmithKline)

**METHAMPHETAMINE HCl (Desoxyephedrine HCl)**

**Tablets:** 5 mg (c-ıı) — *Desoxyn* (Abbott)

**AMPHETAMINE MIXTURES**

**Tablets:** 5, 7.5, 10, 12.5, 15, 20, and 30 mg mixed salts of a single entity amphetamine product (c-ıı) — *Adderall* (Shire Richwood)

**Capsules:** 10, 20, and 30 mg mixed salts of a single entity amphetamine product (c-ıı) — *Adderall XR* (Shire)

**Warning:**
> *Drug dependence:* Amphetamines have a high potential for abuse. Use in weight reduction programs only when alternative therapy has been ineffective. Administration for prolonged periods may lead to drug dependence and must be avoided. Pay particular attention to the possibility of subjects obtaining amphetamines for nontherapeutic use or distribution to others. Prescribe or dispense sparingly.

## Indications

*Narcolepsy:* To improve wakefulness in patients with excessive daytime sleepiness associated with narcolepsy.

*Attention deficit disorder with hyperactivity (ADHD):* Indicated as an integral part of a total treatment program that includes other remedial measures (psychological, educational, social) for a stabilizing effect in children 3 to 16 years of age with a behavioral syndrome characterized by moderate to severe distractibility, short attention span, hyperactivity, emotional lability, and impulsivity. Do not diagnose this syndrome with finality when these symptoms are only of comparatively recent origin. Nonlocalizing (soft) neurological signs, learning disability, and abnormal EEG may be present and a diagnosis of CNS dysfunction may be warranted.

*Exogenous obesity (methamphetamine only):* As a short-term adjunct in a regimen of weight reduction based on caloric restriction, for patients refractory to alternative therapy (eg, repeated diets, group programs, other drugs). Weigh the limited usefulness against the possible risks inherent in use.

## Administration and Dosage

Administer at the lowest effective dosage and adjust individually. Avoid late evening doses, particularly with the long-acting form, because of the resulting insomnia.

*Attention deficit disorder (ADD):* When treating ADD in children, occasionally interrupt drug administration to determine if there is a recurrence of behavioral symptoms sufficient to require continued therapy.

DEXTROAMPHETAMINE SULFATE:
*Narcolepsy* – 5 to 60 mg/day in divided doses.

*Children (6 to 12 years of age):* Initial dose is 5 mg/day; increase in increments of 5 mg at weekly intervals until optimal response is obtained (maximum 60 mg/day).

*Adults (12 years of age or older):* Start with 10 mg/day; raise in increments of 10 mg/day at weekly intervals. If adverse reactions appear (eg, insomnia, anorexia), reduce dose. Long-acting forms may be used for once/day dosage. With tablets, give first dose on awakening; additional doses at intervals of 4 to 6 hours.

*ADHD* – Not recommended for children under 3 years of age.

*Children (3 to 5 years of age):* 2.5 mg/day; increase in increments of 2.5 mg/day at weekly intervals until optimal response is obtained.

*Children (6 years of age or older):* 5 mg once or twice/day; increase in increments of 5 mg/day at weekly intervals until optimal response is obtained. Dosage rarely will exceed 40 mg/day.

Long-acting forms may be used for once/day dosage. With tablets, give first dose on awakening; additional doses may be given at intervals of 4 to 6 hours.

METHAMPHETAMINE HCl:

*ADHD* – Initially, 5 mg once or twice/day; increase in increments of 5 mg/day at weekly intervals until an optimum response is achieved. Usual effective dose is 20 to 25 mg/day.

Total daily dose may be given in 2 divided doses. Where possible, interrupt drug administration to determine if there is a recurrence of behavioral symptoms sufficient to require continued therapy.

*Obesity* – 5 mg, 30 minutes before each meal.

Treatment duration should not exceed a few weeks. Do not use in children under 12 years of age.

AMPHETAMINE MIXTURES: These mixtures contain various salts of amphetamine and dextroamphetamine. Refer to Administration and Dosage for Dextroamphetamine for information about immediate-release tablets.

*Extended-release capsules* – In children with ADHD who are at least 6 years of age and are starting treatment for the first time or switching from another medication, start with 10 mg once daily in the morning; daily dosage may be raised in increments of 10 mg at weekly intervals. Administer amphetamines at the lowest effective dosage. The maximum recommended dose is 30 mg/day; doses larger than 30 mg/day of extended-release amphetamine mixture capsules have not been studied.

Extended-release amphetamine mixture capsules may be taken whole, or the capsule may be opened and the entire contents sprinkled on applesauce. If the patient is using the sprinkle administration method, the sprinkled applesauce should be consumed immediately. Patients should take the applesauce with sprinkled beads in its entirety without chewing.

Give extended-release amphetamine mixture capsules upon awakening. Avoid afternoon doses because of the potential for insomnia.

## Actions

*Pharmacology:* Amphetamines are sympathomimetic amines with CNS stimulant activity. CNS effects are mediated by release of norepinephrine from central noradrenergic neurons. Peripheral activities include elevation of systolic and diastolic blood pressures and weak bronchodilator and respiratory stimulant action.

*Pharmacokinetics:*

*Dextroamphetamine* – Following administration of 15 mg, maximum plasma dextroamphetamine concentrations were reached in approximately 3 hours (tablets) and 8 hours (extended-release capsules). The average plasma half-life was similar, approximately 12 hours.

*Methamphetamine* – Methamphetamine is rapidly absorbed from the GI tract. The primary site of metabolism is in the liver. The biological half-life is in the range of 4 to 5 hours. Excretion occurs in the urine and is dependent on urine pH. Alkaline urine increases the drug half-life.

*Amphetamine mixture* – Peak plasma concentrations occur in about 3 hours (*Adderall*) and 7 hours (*Adderall XR*). Elimination half-life is 10 to 13 hours in adults and 9 to 11 hours in children. Extended-release amphetamine mixture capsules demonstrate linear pharmacokinetics. There is no unexpected accumulation at steady state. Food does not affect the extent of absorption of extended-release amphetamine mixture capsules, but prolongs $T_{max}$ by 2.5 hours.

*Special populations:*

*Children* – Children eliminated amphetamine faster than adults.

## Contraindications

Advanced arteriosclerosis; symptomatic cardiovascular disease; moderate to severe hypertension; hyperthyroidism; hypersensitivity or idiosyncrasy to the sympathomimetic amines; glaucoma; agitated states; history of drug abuse; during or within 14 days following administration of monoamine oxidase (MAO) inhibitors (hypertensive crises may result).

### Warnings

*Tolerance:* When tolerance to the anorectic effect develops, do not exceed recommended dose in an attempt to increase the effect; rather, discontinue the drug.

*Drug dependence:* Amphetamines have been extensively abused. Tolerance, extreme psychological dependence, and severe social disability have occurred. Patients may increase the dosage to many times that recommended. Abrupt cessation following prolonged high dosage results in extreme fatigue, mental depression, and changes on the sleep EEG.

*Manifestations of chronic intoxication* – Severe dermatoses, marked insomnia, irritability, hyperactivity, and personality changes have occurred. Disorganization of thoughts, poor concentration, visual hallucinations, and compulsive behavior often occur. The most severe manifestation of chronic intoxication is psychosis, often clinically indistinguishable from paranoid schizophrenia. This is rare with oral amphetamines.

*Growth inhibition:* Decrements in the predicted growth (ie, weight gain or height) rate have been reported with the long-term use of stimulants in children.

*Pregnancy: Category C.*

*Lactation:* Amphetamines are excreted in breast milk.

*Children:* Safety and efficacy have not been established for the use of amphetamines as anorectic agents in children under 12 years of age.

Extended-release amphetamine mixture capsules are indicated for children 6 years of age and older. Effects in children 3 to 5 years of age have not been studied.

### Precautions

*Hypertension:* Use cautiously even in mild hypertension.

*Prescribe or dispense:* Prescribe or dispense the least amount feasible at one time to minimize the possibility of overdosage.

*Potentially hazardous tasks:* Amphetamines may impair the ability of the patient to engage in potentially hazardous activities such as operating machinery or vehicles; caution the patient accordingly.

*ADD:* Drug treatment is not indicated in all cases.

*Fatigue:* Do not use **methamphetamine** to combat fatigue or replace rest in normal people.

*Tartrazine sensitivity:* Some of these products contain tartrazine, which may cause allergic-type reactions (including bronchial asthma) in susceptible individuals.

### Drug Interactions

Drugs that may affect amphetamines include furazolidone, MAO inhibitors, SSRIs, urinary acidifiers, and urinary alkalinizers. Drugs that may be affected by amphetamines include guanethidine.

Insulin requirements in diabetes mellitus may be altered in association with the use of **methamphetamine** and the concomitant dietary regimen.

*Drug/Lab test interactions:* Plasma **corticosteroid** levels may be increased. **Urinary steroid** determinations may be altered by amphetamines.

### Adverse Reactions

Adverse reactions may include palpitations; tachycardia; elevation of blood pressure; reflex decrease in heart rate; arrhythmias (at larger doses); overstimulation; restlessness; dizziness; insomnia; dyskinesia; euphoria; dysphoria; tremor; headache; changes in libido; dry mouth; unpleasant taste; diarrhea; constipation; urticaria; impotence.

# ANOREXIANTS

| | |
|---|---|
| **BENZPHETAMINE HCL** | |
| **Tablets**: 50 mg (c-III) | Didrex (Pharmacia) |
| **DIETHYLPROPION HCl** | |
| **Tablets**: 25 mg (c-IV) | Various, Tenuate (Aventis) |
| **Tablets, sustained-release**: 75 mg (c-IV) | Various, Tenuate Dospan (Aventis) |
| **PHENDIMETRAZINE TARTRATE** | |
| **Tablets**: 35 mg (c-III) | Various, Bontril PDM (Amerin) |
| **Capsules, sustained-release**: 105 mg (c-III) | Prelu-2 (Roxane), Melfiat-105 Unicelles (Numark), Bontril Slow-Release (Amerin) |
| **PHENTERMINE HCl** | |
| **Tablets**: 8 and 37.5 mg (c-IV) | Various, Zantryl (Ion), Adipex-P (Gate), Pro-Fast SA (American Pharm.) |
| **Capsules**: 15, 18.75, 30, and 37.5 mg (c-IV) | Various, Adipex-P (Gate), Ionamin (Celltech), Pro-Fast HS (American Pharm.), Pro-Fast SR (American Pharm.) |
| **SIBUTRAMINE** | |
| **Capsules**: 5, 10, and 15 mg (c-IV) | Meridia (Knoll) |

### Indications
*Exogenous obesity:* As a short-term (8 to 12 weeks) adjunct in a regimen of weight reduction based on caloric restriction. Measure the limited usefulness of these agents against their inherent risks.

*Sibutramine:*
> *Obesity treatment* – Management of obesity, including weight loss and maintenance of weight loss, in conjunction with a reduced calorie diet.

### Administration and Dosage
Intermittent or interrupted courses of therapy may be useful in the treatment of obesity. A 3- to 6-week course of therapy followed by a discontinuation period of half the original treatment length has been suggested.

*BENZPHETAMINE HCl:* Initiate dosage with 25 to 50 mg once/day; increase according to response. Dosage ranges from 25 to 50 mg, 1 to 3 times/day.

*DIETHYLPROPION HCl:*
> *Tablets* – 25 mg 3 times/day, 1 hour before meals and in mid-evening if needed to overcome night hunger.
> *Sustained release tablets* – 75 mg once/day, in mid-morning.

*PHENDIMETRAZINE TARTRATE:*
> *Tablets and capsules* – 35 mg 2 or 3 times/day, 1 hour before meals.
> *Sustained-release capsules* – 105 mg once/day in the morning 30 to 60 minutes before breakfast.

*PHENTERMINE HCl:* Take 8 mg 3 times/day, 30 minutes before meals, or 15 to 37.5 mg as a single daily dose before breakfast or 10 to 14 hours before retiring.
> Take *Pro-Fast HS* and *Pro-Fast SR* capsules approximately 2 hours after breakfast for appetite control. Take *Adipex-P* capsules and tablets before breakfast or 1 to 2 hours after breakfast; the tablet dosage may be adjusted to the patient's need (ie, ½ tablet [18.75 mg] daily or 18.75 mg 2 times/day may be adequate).
> Swallow *Ionamin* capsules whole.
> Avoid late-evening medication because of the possibility of resulting insomnia.

*SIBUTRAMINE:* The recommended starting dose is 10 mg administered once/day with or without food. If there is inadequate weight loss, the dose may be titrated after 4 weeks to a total of 15 mg once/day. Reserve the 5 mg dose for patients who do not tolerate the 10 mg dose. Blood pressure and heart rate changes should be taken into account when making decisions regarding dose titration.
> Doses more than 15 mg/day are not recommended. In most of the clinical trials, sibutramine was given in the morning.
> The safety and efficacy of sibutramine when taken for more than 2 years have not been determined at this time.

### Actions

*Pharmacology:* Adrenergic agents (eg, **diethylpropion, benzphetamine, phendimetra-zine, phentermine**) act by modulating central norepinephrine and dopamine receptors through the promotion of catecholamine release. Aside from phenter-mine, other adrenergic agents are infrequently used, perhaps because of the lack of long-term, well-controlled data or the fear of their potential abuse. Older adren-ergic weight-loss drugs (eg, amphetamine, methamphetamine, phenmetrazine), which strongly engage in dopamine pathways, are no longer recommended because of the risk of their abuse.

*Pharmacokinetics:*

*Absorption* – **Diethylpropion** is rapidly absorbed from the GI tract after oral admin-istration and is extensively metabolized through a complex pathway of biotransfor-mation involving N-dealkylation and reduction. Many of these metabolites are biologically active and may participate in the therapeutic action of diethylpropion.

Sibutramine is rapidly absorbed from the GI tract ($T_{max}$ 1.2 hours) following oral administration.

*Metabolism* – Sibutramine is metabolized in the liver principally by the cytochrome P450 ($3A_4$) isoenzyme.

*Excretion* – Most of the drug and metabolites are excreted via the kidneys.

### Contraindications

Advanced arteriosclerosis; symptomatic cardiovascular disease; moderate to severe hypertension; hyperthyroidism; known hypersensitivity or idiosyncrasy to sym-pathomimetic amines; glaucoma; agitated states; history of drug abuse; during or up to 14 days following the administration of MAO inhibitors (hypertensive crises may result); coadministration with other CNS stimulants; pregnancy (benzphet-amine HCl); patients with anorexia nervosa, patients taking other centrally acting appetite-suppressant drugs (sibutramine).

### Warnings

*Blood pressure and pulse:* Sibutramine substantially increases blood pressure in some patients.

*Concurrent monoamine oxidase inhibitors:* Do not use sibutramine concomitantly with MAOIs. There should be at least a 2-week interval after starting or stopping MAOIs before starting treatment with sibutramine.

*Serotonin syndrome (sibutramine):* The rare, but serious, constellation of symptoms also has been reported with the concomitant use of selective serotonin reuptake inhibitors and agents for migraine therapy (eg, sumatriptan, dihydroergotamine), certain opioids (eg, dextromethorphan, meperidine, pentazocine, fentanyl), lithium, or tryp-tophan. Because sibutramine inhibits serotonin reuptake, it should not be admin-istered with other serotonergic agents.

*Concomitant cardiovascular disease:* Do not use sibutramine in patients with a history of coronary artery disease, CHF, arrhythmias, or stroke.

*Glaucoma:* Because sibutramine can cause mydriasis, use with caution in patients with narrow-angle glaucoma.

*Tolerance:* Tolerance to the anorectic effects may develop within a few weeks. If toler-ance to the anorectic effect develops, do not exceed the recommended dose in an attempt to increase the effect; rather, discontinue the drug.

*Other drugs:* These agents should not be used in combination with other anorectic agents, including prescribed drugs (eg, SSRIs [eg, fluoxetine, sertraline, fluvox-amine, paroxetine]), otc preparations, and herbal products. When using CNS-ac-tive agents, consider the possibility of adverse interactions with alcohol.

*Primary pulmonary hypertension (PPH):* PPH, a rare, frequently fatal disease of the lungs, has been reported to occur in patients receiving certain anorectic agents. The ini-tial symptom of PPH is usually dyspnea. Other initial symptoms include the fol-lowing: Angina pectoris, syncope, or lower extremity edema. Advise patients to report immediately any deterioration in exercise tolerance. Discontinue treatment in patients who develop new, unexplained symptoms of dyspnea, angina pectoris, syncope, or lower extremity edema.

*Valvular heart disease:* Serious regurgitant cardiac valvular disease, primarily affecting the mitral, aortic, or tricuspid valves, has been reported in otherwise healthy people who had taken certain anorectic agents in combination for weight loss. The etiology of these valvulopathies has not been established and their course in individuals after the drugs are stopped is not known.

*Pregnancy:* (*Category* X – benzphetamine HCl; *category* C – sibutramine, phentermine, phendimetrazine; *category* B – diethylpropion).

*Lactation:* Safety for use in the nursing mother has not been established.

*Children:* Not recommended for use in children younger than 12 years of age. The safety and efficacy of sibutramine in pediatric patients younger than 16 years of age have not been established.

### Precautions

*Psychological disturbances:* Psychological disturbances occurred in patients who received an anorectic agent together with a restrictive diet.

*Cardiovascular disease:* Use with caution and monitor blood pressure in patients with mild hypertension. Not recommended for patients with symptomatic cardiovascular disease, including arrhythmias.

*Convulsions:* Convulsions may increase in some epileptics receiving **diethylpropion**.

*Seizures:* Use **sibutramine** cautiously in patients with a history of seizures; discontinue in any patient who develops seizures.

*Diabetes:* Insulin requirements in diabetes mellitus may be altered in association with the use of anorexigenic drugs and the concomitant dietary restrictions.

*PPH (sibutramine):* Certain centrally acting weight loss agents that cause release of serotonin from nerve terminals have been associated with PPH.

*Drug abuse and dependence:* These drugs are chemically and pharmacologically related to the amphetamines and have abuse potential. Intense psychological or physical dependence and severe social dysfunction may be associated with long-term therapy or abuse. If this occurs, gradually reduce the dosage to avoid withdrawal symptoms.

*Hazardous tasks:* May produce dizziness, extreme fatigue, and depression after abrupt cessation of prolonged high dosage therapy; patients should observe caution while driving or performing other tasks requiring alertness.

### Drug Interactions

Drugs that may affect anorexiants include MAO inhibitors, furazolidone, and SSRIs. Drugs that may be affected by anorexiants include guanethidine and TCAs. Drugs that may affect **sibutramine** include alcohol, cimetidine, erythromycin, ketoconazole, and other CYP3A inhibitors. Sibutramine may affect agents that may raise blood pressure or heart rate, CNS-active drugs, MAOIs, SSRIs, ergot alkaloids, lithium, certain opioids, $5HT_1$ receptor antagonists, and tryptophan.

### Adverse Reactions

Adverse reactions may include the following: Palpitations; tachycardia; arrhythmias; hypertension or hypotension; fainting; overstimulation; nervousness; restlessness; dizziness; insomnia; weakness or fatigue; malaise; anxiety; tension; euphoria; elevated mood; drowsiness; depression; agitation; dysphoria; tremor; dyskinesia; dysarthria; confusion; incoordination; tremor; headache; change in libido; dry mouth; unpleasant taste; nausea; vomiting; abdominal discomfort; diarrhea; constipation; stomach pain; anorexia; increased appetite; dyspepsia; urticaria; rash; erythema; burning sensation; mydriasis; eye irritation; blurred vision; dysuria; polyuria; urinary frequency; impotence; menstrual upset; bone marrow depression; agranulocytosis; leukopenia; hair loss; ecchymosis; muscle pain; chest pain; excessive sweating; clamminess; chills; flushing; fever; myalgia; gynecomastia; back pain; flu syndrome; injury accident; asthenia; dysmenorrhea; arthralgia; rhinitis; pharyngitis; sinusitis; cough increase.

# NARCOTIC AGONIST ANALGESICS

**ALFENTANIL HCL**
Injection: 500 mcg (as HCl)/mL (c-II) | Alfenta (Janssen)

**CODEINE**
Tablets: 15, 30, and 60 mg (as sulfate) (c-II) | Various
Tablets, soluble: 30 and 60 mg (as sulfate) (c-II) | Various
Solution, oral: 15 mg/5 mL (as phosphate) (c-II) | Various
Injection: 30 and 60 mg (as phosphate) (c-II) | Various

**FENTANYL**
Injection: 0.05 mg base (as citrate)/mL (c-II) | Various, Sublimaze (Taylor)

**FENTANYL TRANSDERMAL SYSTEM**
Patch: 25 mcg/h, 50 mcg/h, 75 mcg/h, and 100 mcg/h (c-II) | Duragesic-25, Duragesic-50[1], Duragesic-75[1], Duragesic-100[1] (Janssen)

**FENTANYL TRANSMUCOSAL SYSTEM**
Lozenges: 100, 200, 300, and 400 mcg (c-II) | Fentanyl Oralet (Abbott)
Lozenge on a stick: 200, 400, 600, 800, 1200, and 1600 mcg (c-II) | Actiq (Abbott)

**HYDROMORPHONE HCl**
Tablets: 1, 2, 3, 4, and 8 mg (c-II) | Various, Dilaudid (Knoll)
Liquid: 5 mg/5 mL (c-II) | Various, Dilaudid (Knoll)
Suppositories: 3 mg (c-II) | Various, Dilaudid (Knoll)
Injection: 1 mg/mL, 2 mg/mL, 4 mg/mL, and 10 mg/mL (c-II) | Various, Dilaudid (Knoll), Dilaudid-HP (Knoll)
Powder for injection, lyophilized: 250 mg (10 mg/mL after reconstitution) | Dilaudid-HP (Knoll)

**LEVORPHANOL TARTRATE**
Tablets: 2 mg (c-II) | Levo-Dromoran (ICN), Levorphanol Tartrate (Roxane)

**MEPERIDINE HCl**
Tablets: 50 and 100 mg (c-II) | Various, Demerol (Sanofi-Synthelabo, Abbott)
Syrup: 50 mg/5 mL (c-II)
Injection: 25 mg/mL, 50 mg/mL, 75 mg/mL, and 100 mg/mL (c-II)
Injection: 50 mg/mL, 75 mg/mL, and 100 mg/mL (c-II)

**METHADONE HCl**
Tablets: 5 and 10 mg (c-II) | Methadone HCl (Roxane), Methadose (Mallinckrodt)
Dispersible Tablets: 40 mg (c-II) | Methadone HCl Diskets[2] (Eli Lilly), Methadose[2] (Mallinckrodt)
Oral Solution: 5 mg/5 mL and 10 mg/5 mL (c-II) | Various, Methadone HCl (Roxane)
Oral Concentrate: 10 mg/mL (c-II) | Various, Methadone HCl[2] (UDL), Methadone HCl Intensol (Roxane), Methadose[2] (Mallinckrodt)
Injection: 10 mg/mL (c-II) | Dolophine HCl (Roxane)
Powder: 50, 100, and 500 g | Various, Methadose[2] (Mallinckrodt)

**MORPHINE SULFATE**
Soluble Tablets: 10, 15, and 30 mg (c-II) | Various
Tablets: 15 and 30 mg (c-II) | Various, MSIR (Purdue Frederick)
Tablets, controlled-release: 15, 30, 60, 100, and 200 mg (c-II) | MS Contin (Purdue Frederick), Oramorph SR (Roxane)
Capsules, sustained-release: 20, 30, 50, 60, 100 mg (c-II) | Kadian (AstraZeneca)
Solution: 10 mg/5 mL, 20 mg/5 mL, 20 mg/mL, and 100 mg/5 mL (c-II) | Various, MSIR (Purdue Frederick), Roxanol (Roxane), Roxanol 100 (Roxane), Roxanol T (Roxane)
Rectal Suppositories: 5, 10, 20, and 30 mg (c-II) | Various, RMS (Upsher-Smith)
Injection: 0.5, 1, 2, 4, 5, 8, 10, 15, 25, and 50 mg/mL (c-II) | Various, Astramorph PF (AstraZeneca), Duramorph (Baxter), Infumorph 200 (ESI Lederle)
Compounding powder | Morphine Sulfate (Paddock)

**OPIUM**
Liquid: 10% (c-II) | Opium Tincture, Deodorized (Ranbaxy)
Liquid (camphorated tincture of opium): 2 mg morphine equiv./5 mL (c-III) | Paregoric (Various)

| | |
|---|---|
| **OXYCODONE HCl** | |
| **Tablets**: 5 mg (c-II) | Various, *Endocodone* (Endo), *M-oxy* (Mallinckrodt), *Percolone* (Endo Labs), *Roxicodone* (Roxane) |
| **Tablets, controlled-release**: 10, 20, 40, 80, 160 mg² (c-II) | *OxyContin* (Purdue Pharma LP) |
| **Tablets, immediate-release**: 15 and 30 mg (c-II) | *Roxicodone* (Roxane) |
| **Capsules, immediate release**: 5 mg (c-II) | Various, *OxyIR* (Purdue Pharma LP) |
| **Oral solution**: 5 mg/5 mL (c-II) | *Roxicodone* (Roxane) |
| **Solution, concentrate**: 20 mg/mL (c-II) | *OxyFAST* (Purdue Pharma LP), *Roxicodone Intensol* (Roxane), *Oxydose* (Ethex) |
| **OXYMORPHONE HCl** | |
| **Injection**: 1 mg/mL and 1.5 mg/mL (c-II) | *Numorphan* (Endo Labs) |
| **Suppositories**: 5 mg (c-II) | *Numorphan* (Endo Labs) |
| **PROPOXYPHENE HCl** | |
| **Capsules**: 65 mg (as HCl) (c-IV) | Various, *Darvon Pulvules* (Eli Lilly) |
| **PROPOXYPHENE NAPSYLATE** | |
| **Tablets**: 100 mg (c-IV) | *Darvon-N* (Eli Lilly) |
| **REMIFENTANIL HCl** | |
| **Powder for injection, lyophilized**: 1 mg/mL (as HCl; after reconstitution) (c-II) | *Ultiva* (Abbott) |
| **SUFENTANIL CITRATE** | |
| **Injection**: 50 mcg (as citrate)/mL (c-II) | Various, *Sufenta* (Taylor) |

[1] For use in opioid-tolerant patients only.
[2] For detoxification and maintenance only.

### Indications

ALFENTANIL HCl: As an analgesic adjunct given in incremental doses in the maintenance of anesthesia with barbiturate/nitrous oxide/oxygen.

As an analgesic administered by continuous infusion with nitrous oxide/oxygen in the maintenance of general anesthesia.

As a primary anesthetic for induction of anesthesia in general surgery when endotracheal intubation and mechanical ventilation are required.

Analgesic component for monitored anesthesia care (MAC).

CODEINE: Relief of mild to moderate pain and for coughing induced by chemical or mechanical irritation of the respiratory system.

FENTANYL:

Pain – For analgesic action of short duration during anesthesia (premediaction, induction, maintenance) and in the immediate postoperative period (recovery room) as needed.

For use as a narcotic analgesic supplement in general or regional anesthesia.

For administration with a neuroleptic such as droperidol as an anesthetic premedication, for induction of anesthesia and as an adjunct in maintenance of general and regional anesthesia.

For use as an anesthetic agent with oxygen in selected high-risk patients (open heart surgery or certain complicated neurological or orthopedic procedures.

FENTANYL TRANSDERMAL SYSTEM:

Pain – Management of chronic pain in patients requiring opioid analgesia.

FENTANYL TRANSMUCOSAL SYSTEM:

Anesthesia (Fentanyl Oralet only) – Only indicated for use in a hospital setting 1) as an anesthetic premedication in the operating room setting or 2) to induce conscious sedation prior to a diagnostic or therapeutic procedure in other monitored anesthesia care settings in the hospital.

Breakthrough cancer pain (Actiq only) – Only indicated for the management of breakthrough cancer pain in patients with malignancies who are already receiving and are tolerant to opioid therapy for their underlying persistent cancer pain. Patients considered opioid-tolerant are those who are taking 60 mg or more morphine/day, 50 mcg transdermal fentanyl/hour, or an equianalgesic dose of another opioid for 1 week or more.

HYDROMORPHONE HCl: Relief of moderate to severe pain.

*LEVORPHANOL TARTRATE:*
  *Pain (Levorphanol Tartrate only)* – Management of pain where an opioid analgesic is appropriate.
  *Pain/Preoperative medication (Levo-Dromoran only)* – Management of moderate to severe pain or as a preoperative medication where an opioid analgesic is appropriate.

*MEPERIDINE HCl:*
  *Oral and parenteral* – Relief of moderate to severe pain.
  *Parenteral* – For preoperative medication, support of anesthesia and obstetrical analgesia.

*METHADONE HCl:* For relief of severe pain; detoxification and temporary maintenance treatment of narcotic addiction. Methadone is ineffective for the relief of general anxiety.

*MORPHINE SULFATE:*
  *Oral* –
    *Immediate-release tablets/solution:* Relief of moderate to severe pain.
    *Controlled/Extended/Sustained-release tablets:* Relief of moderate to severe pain in those who require opioid analgesics for more than a few days.
  *Parenteral* –
    *IV:* Relief of severe pain; pain of MI; used preoperatively to sedate the patient and allay apprehension, facilitate anesthesia induction, and reduce anesthetic dosage; control postoperative pain; relieve anxiety and reduce left ventricular work by reducing preload pressure; treatment of dyspnea associated with acute left ventricular failure and pulmonary edema; produce anesthesia for open-heart surgery.
    *subcutaneous/IM:* Relief of severe pain; relieve preoperative apprehension; preoperative sedation; control postoperative pain; supplement to anesthesia; analgesia during labor; acute pulmonary edema; allay anxiety.
    *IV/Epidural/Intrathecal:* Management of pain not responsive to nonnarcotic analgesics (*Duramorph, Astramorph PF; Infumorph* for continuous epidural/intrathecal use only).
  *Rectal* – Severe acute and chronic pain.

*OPIUM:*
  *Diarrhea* – For treatment of diarrhea.
  *Unlabeled uses* –
    *Neonatal abstinence syndrome:* Treatment of opioid-related drug withdrawal (neonates). Diluted opium tincture is the preferred treatment for neonatal withdrawal in newborns. Paregoric contains benzoic acid (an oxidative product of benzyl alcohol), usually camphor, and other ingredients that may have potential toxic effects.
    *Management of short bowel syndrome:* Used to slow gastric emptying and delay bowel transit time in short bowel syndrome.

*OXYCODONE HCl:*
  *Pain* – Relief of moderate to severe pain.
    *Immediate-release tablets:* Management of moderate to severe pain where use of an opioid analgesic is appropriate.
    *Controlled-release tablets:* Management of moderate to severe pain when a continuous, around-the-clock analgesic is needed for an extended period of time. Not intended for use as a prn analgesic.
      Not indicated for pain in the immediate postoperative period (the first 12 to 24 hours following surgery), or if the pain is mild or not expected to persist for an extended period of time. Oxycodone controlled-release tablets are only indicated for postoperative use if the patient is already receiving the drug prior to surgery or if the postoperative pain is expected to be moderate to severe and persist for an extended period of time. Individualize treatment, moving from parenteral to oral analgesics as appropriate.
    *Unlabeled uses* – Postherpetic neuralgia (controlled-release).

*OXYMORPHONE HCl:* Relief of moderate to severe pain.

Parenterally for preoperative medication, support of anesthesia, obstetrical analgesia, and for relief of anxiety in patients with dyspnea associated with acute left ventricular failure and pulmonary edema.

*PROPOXYPHENE (Dextropropoxyphene):* Relief of mild to moderate pain.

*REMIFENTANIL HCl:*

*General anesthesia* – An analgesic agent for use during the induction and maintenance of general anesthesia for inpatient and outpatient procedures and for continuation as an analgesic into the immediate postoperative period under the direct supervision of an anesthesia practitioner in a postoperative anesthesia care unit or intensive care setting.

*Monitored anesthesia care* – An analgesic component of monitored anesthesia care.

*SUFENTANIL CITRATE:* Analgesic adjunct at dosages up to 8 mcg/kg to maintain balanced general anesthesia.

A primary anesthetic agent at dosages 8 mcg/kg or more to induce and maintain anesthesia with 100% oxygen in patients undergoing major surgical procedures, such as cardiovascular surgery or neurosurgical procedures in the sitting position, to provide favorable myocardial and cerebral oxygen balance or when extended postoperative ventilation is anticipated.

*Pain* – For analgesic action of short duration during anesthesia (premedication, induction, maintenance), and in the immediate postoperative period (recovery room) as needed.

For use as a narcotic analgesic supplement in general or regional anesthesia.

For administration with a neuroleptic such as droperidol as an anesthetic premedication, for induction of anesthesia and as an adjunct in maintenance of general and regional anesthesia.

For use as an anesthetic agent with oxygen in selected high-risk patients (open heart surgery or certain complicated neurological or orthopedic procedures).

### Administration and Dosage

In obese patients (more than 20% above ideal total body weight), determine dosage on the basis of lean body weight. Reduce dose in elderly or debilitated patients.

The most important factor to be considered in determining the appropriate dose is the extent of pre-existing opioid tolerance. Reduce initial doses in elderly or debilitated patients.

*ALFENTANIL HCl:*

*Children younger than 12 years of age* – Use is not recommended.

| Alfentanil Dosage Range for Use During General Anesthesia | | | | |
|---|---|---|---|---|
| Clinical status | ≈ Duration of anesthesia | Induction (Initial dose) | Maintenance (Increments/ Infusion) | Total dose |
| Spontaneously breathing/ Assisted ventilation | ≤ 30 min | 8-20 mcg/kg | 3-5 mcg/kg every 5-20 min or 0.5-1 mcg/kg/min | 8-40 mcg/kg |
| Assisted or controlled ventilation | | | | |
| Incremental injection (to attenuate response to laryngoscopy and intubation) | 30-60 min | 20-50 mcg/kg | 5-15 mcg/kg every 5-20 min | ≤ 75 mcg/kg |
| Continuous infusion[1] (to provide attenuation of response to intubation and incision) | > 45 min | 50-75 mcg/kg | 0.5-3 mcg/kg/min. Average infusion rate 1-1.5 mcg/kg/min | dependent on duration of procedure |
| Anesthetic induction (give slowly [over 3 min]). Reduce concentration of inhalation agents by 30%-50% for initial hour) | > 45 min | 130-245 mcg/kg | 0.5-1.5 mcg/kg/min or general anesthetic | dependent on duration of procedure |
| MAC (for sedated and responsive spontaneously breathing patients) | ≤ 30 min | 3-8 mcg/kg | 3-5 mcg/kg every 5-20 min or 0.25 to 1 mcg/kg/min | 3-40 mcg/kg |

[1] 0.5 to 3 mcg/kg/min with nitrous oxide/oxygen in general surgery. Following anesthetic induction dose, reduce infusion rate requirements by 30% to 50% for the first hour of maintenance. Vital sign changes that indicate response to surgical stress or lightening of anesthesia may be controlled by increasing rate to a max of 4 mcg/kg/min or administering bolus doses of 7 mcg/kg. If changes are not controlled after 3 bolus doses given over 5 minutes, use a barbiturate, vasodilator, or inhalation agent. Always adjust infusion rates downward in the absence of these signs until there is some response to surgical stimulation. Rather than an increase in infusion rate, administer 7 mcg/kg bolus doses of alfentanil or a potent inhalation agent in response to signs of lightening of anesthesia within the last 15 minutes of surgery. Discontinue infusion ≥ 10 to 15 minutes prior to the end of surgery.

CODEINE:
  *Analgesic* –
      *Adults:* 15 to 60 mg every 4 to 6 hours, orally, IM, IV or subcutaneously. Usual dose is 30 mg. Do not exceed 360 mg in 24 hours.
      *Children (1 year of age or older):* 0.5 mg/kg or 15 m$^2$ of body surface every 4 to 6 hours subcutaneously, IM or orally. Do not use IV in children
      *Antitussive* – (See also Respiratories chapter).
      *Adults:* 10 to 20 mg every 4 to 6 hours. Do not exceed 120 mg in 24 hours.
      *Children (6 to 12 years of age):* 5 to 10 mg orally every 4 to 6 hours. Do not exceed 60 mg in 24 hours.
      *(2 to 6 years of age)* – 2.5 to 5 mg orally every 4 to 6 hours. Do not exceed 30 mg in 24 hours.

FENTANYL:
  *Premedication* – 0.05 to 0.1 mg IM, 30 to 60 minutes prior to surgery.
  *Adjunct to general anesthesia* –
      *Total low dosage:* 0.002 mg/kg in small doses for minor, painful surgical procedures and postoperative pain relief; *maintenance low dosage:* Infrequently needed.
      *Total low dosage:* 0.002 to 0.02 mg/kg.
      *Maintenance moderate dosage:* 0.025 to 0.1 IV or IM when movement or changes in vital signs indicate surgical stress or lightening of analgesia.
      *Total high dosage:* 0.02 to 0.05 mg/kg. For "stress free" anesthesia. Use during open heart surgery and complicated neurosurgical and orthopedic procedures where surgery is prolonged and the stress response is detrimental.
      *Maintenance high dosage:* Ranging from 0.025 mg to half the initial loading dose.
      *Adjunct to regional anesthesia* – 0.05 to 0.1 mg IM or slowly IV over 1 to 2 minutes as required.
      *Postoperatively (recovery room)* – 0.05 to 0.1 mg IM for the control of pain, tachypnea, and emergence delirium; repeat dose in 1 to 2 hours as needed.
      *Children (2 to 12 years)* – For induction and maintenance, a reduced dose as low as 2 to 3 mcg/kg is recommended. Safety and efficacy in children younger than 2 years of age have not been established.
      *General anesthetic:* 0.05 to 0.1 mg/kg with oxygen and a muscle relaxant when attenuation of the responses to surgical stress is especially important. Up to 0.15 mg/kg may be necessary.

FENTANYL TRANSDERMAL SYSTEM:
  *Application* – Each system may be worn continuously for 72 hours. If analgesia for longer than 72 hours is required, apply a new system to a different skin site after removal of the previous transdermal system.
  *Dose selection* – Maintain each patient at the lowest dose providing acceptable pain control. Unless the patient has pre-existing opioid tolerance, use the lowest dose, 25 mcg/h, as the initial dose.
      Upwards titration may be done no more frequently than 3 days after the initial dose; thereafter, it may be done no more frequently than every 6 days. For delivery rates in excess of 100 mcg/h, multiple systems may be used.

| Fentanyl Transdermal Dose Based on Daily Morphine Equivalence Dose[1] | | |
|---|---|---|
| Oral 24 hour morphine (mg/day) | IM 24 hour morphine (mg/day) | Fentanyl transdermal (mcg/h) |
| 45-134 | 8-22 | 25 |
| 135-224 | 23-37 | 50 |
| 225-314 | 38-52 | 75 |

| Fentanyl Transdermal Dose Based on Daily Morphine Equivalence Dose[1] | | |
|---|---|---|
| Oral 24 hour morphine (mg/day) | IM 24 hour morphine (mg/day) | Fentanyl transdermal (mcg/h) |
| 315-404 | 53-67 | 100 |
| 405-494 | 68-82 | 125 |
| 495-584 | 83-97 | 150 |
| 585-674 | 98-112 | 175 |
| 675-764 | 113-127 | 200 |
| 765-854 | 128-142 | 225 |
| 855-944 | 143-157 | 250 |
| 945-1034 | 158-172 | 275 |
| 1035-1124 | 173-187 | 300 |

[1] A 10 mg IM or 60 mg oral dose of morphine every 4 hours for 24 hours for 24 hours (total of 60 mg/day IM or 360 mg/day IM or 360 mg/day oral) was considered approximately equivalent to fentanyl transdermal 100 mcg/h.

The majority of patients are adequately maintained with transdermal fentanyl administered every 72 hours. A small number of patients may require systems to be applied every 48 hours.

During the initial application, patients should use short-acting analgesics for the first 24 hours as needed until analgesic efficacy with the transdermal system is attained. Thereafter, some patients still may require periodic supplemental doses of other short-acting analgesics for breakthrough pain.

*Dose titration* – Base appropriate dosage increments on the daily dose of supplementary opioids, using the ratio of 90 mg/24 hours of oral morphine to a 25 mcg/h increase in transdermal fentanyl dose.

*Discontinuation* – Upon system removal, it takes 17 hours or more for the fentanyl serum concentration to fall by 50% after system removal. Titrate the dose of the new analgesic based on the patient's report of pain until adequate analgesia has been attained. For patients requiring discontinuation of opioids, a gradual downward titration is recommended because it is not known at what dose level the opioid may be discontinued without producing the signs and symptoms of abrupt withdrawal.

*FENTANYL TRANSMUCOSAL SYSTEM:*

*Fentanyl Oralet* – Fentanyl transmucosal doses of 5 mcg/kg provide effects similar to usual doses of fentanyl given IM (0.75 to 1.25 mcg/kg). Larger doses have not been shown to increase efficacy. Adults should not receive doses more than 5 mcg/kg (400 mcg), and most children not apprehensive at onset may be managed with the same 5 mcg/kg dose. Children apprehensive at onset and some younger children may need doses of 5 to 15 mcg/kg with an attendant increased risk of hypoventilation.

*Children:* Because of the excessive frequency of significant hypoventilation at higher doses, doses more than 15 mcg/kg (maximum, 400 mcg) are contraindicated in children.

*Adults:* Because of the excessive frequency of significant hypoventilation at higher doses, doses more than 5 mcg/kg (maximum, 400 mcg) are contraindicated in adults.

*Vulnerable patients:* Consider selection of a lower dose for vulnerable patients (eg, patients with head injury, cardiovascular or pulmonary disease, hepatic disease, liver dysfunction). If signs of excessive opioid effects appear before the unit is consumed, remove the dosage unit from the patient's mouth immediately.

*Elderly:* If fentanyl transmucosal is to be used in patients older than 65 years of age, reduce the dose to 2.5 to 5 mcg/kg.

*Administration:* Begin administration of the unit 20 to 40 minutes prior to the anticipated need of desired effect. Patients typically take 10 to 20 minutes for complete consumption. Peak effect occurs approximately 20 to 30 minutes after the start of administration.

*Actiq* – Use has not been established with opioid-tolerant children younger than 16 years of age. Keep out of the reach of children.

Open the foil package immediately prior to product use. Place the unit in the patient's mouth between the cheek and lower gum, moving it from one side to the other using the handle. Instruct the patient to suck, not chew, the lozenge. A unit dose, if chewed and swallowed, might result in lower peak concentrations and lower bioavailability.

Instruct the patient to consume the lozenge over a 15-minute period. Longer or shorter consumption times may produce less efficacy than reported in clinical trials. If signs of excessive opioid effects appear before the unit is consumed, remove the drug matrix from the patient's mouth immediately and decrease future doses.

*Dose titration:* Initial dose to treat episodes of breakthrough cancer pain should be 200 mcg.

*Redosing within a single episode* – Redosing may start 15 minutes after the previous unit has been completed (30 minutes after the start of the previous unit). Do not give more than 2 units for each individual breakthrough cancer pain episode while patients are in the titration phase and consuming units which individually may be subtherapeutic.

*Increasing the dose* – Evaluate each new dose used over several episodes of breakthrough cancer pain (generally 1 to 2 days) to determine whether it provides adequate efficacy with acceptable side effects.

*Daily limit* – Once a successful dose has been found, instruct patients to limit consumption to 4 units/day or less. If consumption increases to more than 4 units/day, reevaluate the dose of the long-acting opioid for persistent cancer pain.

*Discontinuation* – Recommend a gradual downward titration for discontinuation because it is not known at what dose level the opioid may be discontinued without producing the signs and symptoms of abrupt withdrawal.

*Safety and handling* – *Actiq* is supplied in individually sealed child-resistant foil pouches.

*Disposal* – Dispose all units remaining from a prescription as soon as they are no longer needed. Dispose all units immediately after use.

*Storage/Stability* – Protect from freezing and moisture. Do not store *Fentanyl Oralet* above 30°C (86°F) or *Actiq* above 25°C (77°F).

HYDROMORPHONE HCl:
> *Oral* –
> > *Tablet:* 2 to 4 mg every 4 to 6 hours; 4 mg or more every 4 to 6 hours for more severe pain.
> > *Liquid:* 2.5 to 10 mg every 4 to 6 hours.
> > *Parenteral* – 1 to 2 mg subcutaneously or IM every 4 to 6 hours as needed. For severe pain, administer 3 to 4 mg every 4 to 6 hours as needed. May be given by slow IV injection over 2 to 5 minutes.
> > *Rectal* – 3 mg every 6 to 8 hours.
> > *Children* – Safety and efficacy have not been established.

LEVORPHANOL TARTRATE:
> *Oral* – Recommended starting dose is 2 mg. Repeat in 6 to 8 hours (*Levo-Dromoran*) or 3 to 6 hours (*Levorphanol Tartrate*) as needed, provided the patient is assessed for signs of hypoventilation and excessive sedation.

> > *Levo-Dromoran:* If necessary, increase the dose to up to 3 mg every 6 to 8 hours, after adequate evaluation of the patient's response. Higher doses may be appropriate in opioid-tolerant patients. Adjust dosage according to the severity of the pain; the patient's age, weight, physical status, and underlying diseases; use of concomitant medications; and other factors.

The effective daily dosage range, depending on the severity of the pain, is 8 to 16 mg in 24 hours in the nontolerant patient. Total oral daily doses of more than 6 to 12 mg in 24 hours are generally not recommended as starting doses in non-opioid-tolerant patients; lower total daily doses may be appropriate.

*Levorphanol Tartrate:* The effective daily dosage range, depending on the severity of the pain, is 8 to 16 mg in 24 hours in the nontolerant patient. Total oral daily doses of more than 16 mg in 24 hours are generally not recommended as starting doses in non-opioid-tolerant patients.

*Chronic pain* – Individualize dosage. Because there is incomplete cross-tolerance among opioids, when converting a patient from morphine to levorphanol, begin the total daily dose of oral levorphanol at approximately $\frac{1}{15}$ to $\frac{1}{12}$ of the total daily dose of oral morphine that such patients had previously required, and then adjust the dose to the patient's clinical response. If a patient is to be placed on fixed-schedule dosing (round-the-clock) with this drug, take care to allow adequate time after each dose change (approximately 72 hours) for the patient to reach a new steady state before a subsequent dose adjustment to avoid excessive sedation because of drug accumulation.

*Perioperative period (Levo-Dromoran)* – Levorphanol has been used for analgesic action during premedication and the postoperative period. Factors to be considered in determining the dosage include age, body weight, physical status, underlying pathological condition, use of other drugs, type of anesthesia used, the surgical procedure involved, and the severity of pain.

*Premedication (Levo-Dromoran)* – Individualize the preoperative medication dose. Two mg levorphanol is approximately equivalent to 10 to 15 mg of morphine or 100 mg of meperidine.

*MEPERIDINE HCl:*

*Relief of pain* – While subcutaneous administration is suitable for occasional use, IM administration is preferred for repeated doses. If IV administration is required, decrease dosage and inject very slowly, preferably using a diluted solution. Meperidine is less effective when administered orally than when given parenterally. Reduce proportionately (usually by 25% to 50%) when administering concomitantly with phenothiazines and other tranquilizers.

*Adults:* 50 to 150 mg IM, subcutaneously, or orally every 3 to 4 hours, as necessary.

*Children:* 1.1 to 1.75 mg/kg (0.5 to 0.8 mg/lb) IM, subcutaneously, or orally up to adult dose, every 3 or 4 hours, as necessary.

*Preoperative medication* –

*Adults:* 50 to 100 mg IM or subcutaneously, 30 to 90 minutes before beginning anesthesia.

*Children:* 1.1 to 2.2 mg/kg (0.5 to 1 mg/lb) IM or subcutaneously, up to adult dose, 30 to 90 minutes before beginning anesthesia.

*Support of anesthesia* – Meperidine may be administered in repeated doses diluted to 10 mg/mL by slow IV injection, or by continuous IV infusion of solution diluted to 1 mg/mL.

*Obstetrical analgesia* – When pains become regular, administer 50 to 100 mg IM or subcutaneously; repeat at 1- to 3-hour intervals.

*METHADONE HCl:*

*Warning* – To treat narcotic addiction in detoxification or maintenance programs, methadone may be dispensed only by pharmacies and maintenance programs approved by the FDA and designated state authorities. Approved maintenance programs shall dispense and use methadone in oral form only and according to treatment requirements stipulated in Federal Methadone Regulations (21 CFR 291.505). Failure to abide by the requirements in these regulations may result in criminal prosecution, seizure of drug supply, revocation of program approval, and injunction precluding program operation.

Methadone, used as an analgesic, may be dispensed in any licensed pharmacy.

*Note* – If used to treat heroin dependence for longer than 3 weeks, the procedure passes from treatment of acute withdrawal syndrome (detoxification) to maintenance therapy. Maintenance may be undertaken only by approved methadone programs. This does not preclude maintenance addicts hospitalized for other conditions and who require temporary maintenance during the critical period of their stays or whose enrollment has been verified in a program approved for maintenance treatment with methadone.

Oral methadone is approximately ½ as potent as parenteral. Oral administration results in a delay of onset, a lower peak, and an increased duration of analgesic effect. Duration of effect increases with repeated use because of cumulative effects.

*Pain* –

*Adults:* 2.5 to 10 mg IM, subcutaneously, or orally every 3 or 4 hours as necessary. Adjust dosage according to the severity of pain and patient response. For exceptionally severe pain, or in those tolerant of narcotic analgesia, it may be necessary to exceed the usual recommended dosage. Injection IM is preferred for repeated doses; subcutaneously use may cause local irritation.

*Children:* Not for analgesic use because of insufficient documentation.

*Detoxification treatment* – Detoxification treatment should not exceed 21 days and may not be repeated earlier than 4 weeks after completion of the preceding course.

Initially, 15 to 20 mg will often suppress withdrawal symptoms. When patients are physically dependent on high doses, 40 mg/day in single or divided doses is usually an adequate stabilizing dose. Continue stabilization for 2 to 3 days, then gradually decrease the dose on a daily basis or at 2-day intervals.

*Maintenance treatment* – Initial dosage should control abstinence symptoms following narcotic withdrawal, but should not cause sedation, respiratory depression, or other effects of acute intoxication. Adjust dosage as tolerated and required, up to 120 mg/day.

*For a complete description of detoxification and maintenance regulations and dosage protocols, consult a local approved methadone program.*

MORPHINE SULFATE: Morphine may suppress respiration in the elderly, those taking other CNS depressants, the very ill, and those patients with respiratory problems; therefore, lower doses may be required.

*Oral* –

*Immediate-release:* 5 to 30 mg (solution or tablets) every 4 hours or as directed by physician.

*Controlled/Extended/Sustained-release:* Swallow whole; do not break, chew, or crush. See below for sustained-release capsule administration.

*Initial therapy* – There has been no evaluation of controlled/extended/sustained-release morphine as an initial opioid analgesic in the management of pain. Because it may be more difficult to titrate a patient to adequate analgesia using a controlled/extended/sustained-release morphine, it is ordinarily advisable to begin treatment using an immediate-release morphine formulation.

The MS *Contin* 200 mg tablet is for use only in opioid-tolerant patients requiring daily morphine-equivalent dosages of 400 mg or more. Reserve this strength for patients who have already been titrated to a stable analgesic regimen using lower strengths of MS *Contin* or other opioids. If *Kadian* is chosen, start with 20 mg in those who do not have a proven tolerance to opioids. Increase at a rate up to 20 mg every other day. Individualize dosage.

*Conversion from conventional immediate-release oral morphine to controlled/extended/sustained-release oral morphine* – Give ½ the total daily oral morphine dose every 12 hours; ⅓ the total daily oral morphine requirement every 8 hours (MS *Contin* and extended-release tablets only); or the full daily morphine dose every 24 hours (*Kadian* only). Use the 15 mg tablet for initial conversion for patients whose total daily requirement is expected to be less than 60 mg. The 30 mg tablet strength is recommended for patients with a daily morphine requirement of 60 to 120 mg. When the total daily dose is expected to be more than 120 mg, the appropriate combination of tablet strengths should be employed.

*Conversion from parenteral morphine or other opioids (parenteral or oral) to controlled/extended/sustained-release* – Exercise particular care in the conversion process. Because of uncertainty about, and intersubject variation in, relative estimates of opioid potency and cross-tolerance, initial dosing regimens should be conservative; that is, an underestimation of the 24-hour oral morphine requirement is preferred to an overestimate. To this end, estimate initial individual doses conservatively. In patients whose daily morphine requirements are expected to be 120 mg/day or less, the 30 mg tablet strength is recommended for the initial titration period. Once a stable dose regimen is reached, the patient can be converted to the 60 or 100 mg tablet strength, or appropriate combination of tablet strengths, if desired.

*Conversion from controlled/extended/sustained-release oral morphine to parenteral opioids* – It is best to assume that the parenteral-to-oral potency is high. For example, to estimate the required 24-hour dose of morphine for IM use, one could employ a conversion of 1 mg morphine IM for every 6 mg of morphine as controlled-release tablet. Of course, the IM 24-hour dose would have to be divided by 6 and administered every 4 hours. This approach is recommended because it is least likely to cause overdose. For *Kadian*, initiate treatment at half the calculated equivalent parenteral dose. For example, to estimate the 24-hour dose of parenteral morphine for a patient taking *Kadian*, one would take the 24-hour *Kadian* dose, divide by an oral-to-parenteral conversion ratio of 3, divide the estimated 24-hour parenteral dose into 6 divided doses (for a 4-hour dosing interval), then halve this dose as an initial trial.

*Conversion of sustained-release (Kadian) to other controlled-release oral forms* – *Kadian* is not bioequivalent to other controlled-release formulations. Conversion from *Kadian* to the same total daily dose may lead to either excessive sedation at peak or inadequate analgesia at trough; observe closely and adjust dosage as appropriate.

*Dosing adjustments* – If signs of excessive opioid effects are observed early in a dosing interval, reduce the next dose. If this adjustment leads to inadequate analgesia (ie, "breakthrough" pain occurs late in the dosing interval), the dosing interval may be shortened. Alternatively, a supplemental dose of a short-acting analgesic may be given. As experience is gained, adjustments can be made to obtain an appropriate balance between pain relief, opioid side effects, and the convenience of the dosing schedule. It is recommended that the dosing interval never be extended beyond 12 hours because the administration of very large single doses may lead to acute overdose.

*Sustained-release (Kadian):* Capsules may be opened and the entire contents sprinkled on a small amount of applesauce immediately prior to ingestion. The pellets in the capsules should not be chewed, crushed, or dissolved because of risk of overdose.

Open the capsule and sprinkle entire contents over approximately 10 mL of water and flush with swirling through a prewetted 16 French gastrostomy tube fitted with funnel at the port end. Additional aliquots of water are used to transfer all pellets and to flush the tube. Do not attempt the administration of pellets through a nasogastric tube.

May be given once or twice/day.

*Subcutaneously/IM* – Prepare soluble tablets in sterile water and filter through a 0.22 micron membrane filter.

*Adults:* 10 mg (range, 5 to 20 mg)/70 kg every 4 hours as needed.

*Children:* 0.05 to 0.2 mg/kg every 4 hours as needed. Do not exceed 10 to 15 mg/dose.

*IV –*

*Adults:* 2 to 10 mg/70 kg of body weight. A strength of 2.5 to 15 mg of morphine may be diluted in 4 to 5 mL of Water for Injection. Administer slowly over 4 to 5 minutes. Rapid IV use increases the incidence of adverse reactions (see Warnings). Do not administer IV unless a narcotic antagonist is immediately available.

*Continuous IV infusion:* 0.1 to 1 mg/mL in 5% Dextrose in Water by controlled-infusion device; higher concentrations have been used.

*Severe chronic pain associated with terminal cancer* – Prior to initiation of the morphine infusion (in concentrations between 0.2 to 1 mg/mL), a loading dose of ≥ 15 mg of morphine sulfate may be administered by IV push to alleviate pain.

The infusion dosage range is 0.8 to 80 mg/h, though doses up to 144 mg/h have been used. Thus, for the 1 mg/mL solution, the infusion may be run from 0.8 to 80 mg/h, and for a 0.5 mg/mL solution, the infusion may be run from 1.6 to 160 mL/h.

A constant infusion rate must be maintained with an infusion pump in order to assure proper dosage control. Take care to avoid overdosage (respiratory depression) or abrupt cessation of therapy, which may give rise to withdrawal symptoms.

*Open-heart surgery* – Administer large doses (0.5 to 3 mg/kg) of morphine IV as the sole anesthetic or with a suitable anesthetic agent. The patients are given oxygen and cardiovascular function is not depressed by morphine, as long as adequate ventilation is maintained.

*MI pain* – 8 to 15 mg administered parenterally. For very severe pain, additional smaller doses may be given every 3 to 4 hours as needed.

*Rectal* – 10 to 30 mg every 4 hours as needed or as directed by physician.

*Epidural (Duramorph, Astramorph PF)* –

*Adults:* Initial injection of 5 mg in the lumbar region may provide satisfactory pain relief for up to 24 hours. If adequate pain relief is not achieved within 1 hour, carefully administer incremental doses of 1 to 2 mg at intervals sufficient to assess effectiveness. Give no more than 10 mg/24 hours.

For continuous infusion, an initial dose of 2 to 4 mg/24 hours is recommended. Further doses of 1 to 2 mg may be given if pain relief is not achieved initially.

*Aged or debilitated patients:* Administer with extreme caution (see Warnings). Doses less than 5 mg may provide satisfactory pain relief for up to 24 hours.

*Infumorph, Duramorph, Astramorph PF:* Employ doses greater than 20 mg/day with caution because they may be associated with a higher likelihood of serious side effects. The starting dose must be individualized. The recommended initial epidural dose in patients who are not tolerant to opioids range from 3.5 to 7.5 mg/day. The usual starting dose for continuous epidural infusion, based upon limited data in patients who have some degree of opioid tolerance, is 4.5 to 10 mg/day. The dose requirements may increase significantly during treatment, frequently to 20 to 30 mg/day.

*Intrathecal* –

*Adult:* Intrathecal dosage is usually 1/10 that of epidural dosage. A single injection of 0.2 to 1 mg may provide satisfactory pain relief for up to 24 hours. (Caution: This is only 0.4 to 2 mL of the 0.5 mg/mL potency or 0.2 to 1 mL of the 1 mg/mL potency.) Do not inject intrathecally 2 mL of the 0.5 mg/mL potency or 1 mL of the 1 mg/mL potency. Use in lumbar area only. Repeated intrathecal injections are not recommended. A constant IV infusion of 0.6 mg/h naloxone for 24 hours after intrathecal injection may reduce incidence of potential side effects.

*Infumorph:* Familiarize with the continuous microinfusion device. To minimize risk from glass or other particles, the product must be filtered through a 5 micron or less microfilter before injecting into the microinfusion device. If dilution is required, 0.9% NaCl injection is recommended. Individualize the starting dose. The recommended initial lumbar intrathecal dose range in patients with no tolerance to opioids is 0.2 to 1 mg/day. The published range of doses for individuals who have some degree of opioid tolerance varies from 1 to 10 mg/day. Limited experience with continuous intrathecal infusion of morphine has shown that the daily doses have to be increased over time.

*Aged or debilitated:* Use extreme caution. Lower dose is usually satisfactory.

*Repeat dosage:* If pain recurs, consider alternative administration routes because experience with repeated doses by this route is limited.

*Intraventricular* – Currently available data indicate that this route of administration is effective in select patients with a short life expectancy and recalcitrant pain caused by head and neck malignancies and tumors (eg, superior sulcus tumors, breast carcinoma) that affect the brachial plexus. One to 2 doses/day are generally administered.

OPIUM:

Caution – Opium tincture contains 25 times more morphine than paregoric. Do not confuse opium tincture with paregoric; this may lead to an overdose of morphine.

Opium tincture –

Adults: 0.6 mL (equiv. to 6 mg morphine) 4 times/day; maximum 6 mL/day.

Paregoric –

Adults: 5 to 10 mL 1 to 4 times/day.

Children: 0.25 to 0.5 mL/kg 1 to 4 times/day.

OXYCODONE HCl:

Warning – Controlled-release oxycodone is an opioid agonist and a Schedule II controlled substance with an abuse liability similar to morphine.

Oxycodone can be abused in a manner similar to other opioid agonists, legal or illicit. This should be considered when prescribing or dispensing oxycodone controlled-release tablets in situations where the physician or pharmacist is concerned about an increased risk of misuse, abuse, or diversion.

Oxycodone controlled-release tablets are indicated for the management of moderate to severe pain when a continuous, around-the-clock analgesic is needed for an extended period of time.

Oxycodone controlled-release tablets are not intended for use as a prn (as needed) analgesic.

Oxycodone 80 and 160 mg controlled-release tablets are for use in opioid-tolerant patients only. These tablet strengths may cause fatal respiratory depression when administered to patients not previously exposed to opioids.

Immediate-release tablets –

Adults: 10 to 30 mg every 4 hours (5 mg every 6 hours for OxyIR, oxycodone immediate-release capsules, and OxyFast) as needed. Individualize dosage.

OxyFAST 20 mg/mL solution is a highly concentrated solution. Take care in prescribing and dispensing this solution strength.

Children: Not recommended for use in children.

5 to 15 mg every 4 to 6 hours as needed for pain. Titrate the dose based upon the individual patient's response. Patients with chronic pain should have their dosage given on an around-the-clock basis to prevent the reoccurrence of pain rather than treating the pain after it has occurred. This dose can then be adjusted to an acceptable level of analgesia, taking into account side effects experienced by the patient.

For control of severe chronic pain, administer on a regularly scheduled basis, every 4 to 6 hours, at the lowest dosage level that will achieve adequate analgesia.

As with any potent opioid, it is critical to adjust the dosing regimen for each patient individually, taking into account the patient's prior analgesic treatment experience.

Controlled-release tablets – Swallow tablets whole; do not break, chew, or crush. Taking broken, chewed, or crushed tablets could lead to the rapid release and absorption of a potentially fatal dose of oxycodone.

One 160 mg tablet is comparable to two 80 mg tablets when taken on an empty stomach. However, with a high-fat meal there is a 25% greater peak plasma concentration following one 160 mg tablet. Use dietary caution when patients are initially titrated to 160 mg tablets.

Take care to use low initial doses of controlled-release tablets in patients who are not already opioid tolerant, especially those who are receiving concurrent treatment with muscle relaxants, sedatives, or other CNS-active medications.

Patients not already taking opioids (opioid näive): A reasonable starting dose for most patients who are opioid näive is 10 mg every 12 hours. If a nonopioid analgesic (eg, aspirin, acetaminophen, NSAID) is being provided, it may be continued.

Patients currently on opioid therapy:

1.) Using standard conversion ratio estimates (see table below), multiply the mg/day of the previous opioids by the appropriate multiplication factors to obtain the equivalent total daily dose of oral oxycodone.

2.) Divide this 24-hour oxycodone dose in half to obtain the twice a day (every 12 hours) dose of controlled-release tablets.

3.) Round down to a dose that is appropriate for the tablet strengths available (10, 20, 40, 80, and 160 mg tablets).

4.) Discontinue all other around-the-clock opioid drugs when controlled-release tablet therapy is initiated.

No fixed conversion ratio is likely to be satisfactory in all patients, especially patients receiving large opioid doses. The recommended doses shown in the following table are only a starting point, and close observation and frequent titration are indicated until patients are stable in the new therapy.

| Multiplication Factors for Converting the Daily Dose of Prior Opioids to the Daily Dose of Oral Oxycodone[1] | | |
|---|---|---|
| Mg/day prior opioid × factor = mg/day oral oxycodone | | |
| | Oral prior opioid | Parenteral prior opioid |
| Oxycodone | 1 | — |
| Codeine | 0.15 | — |
| Fentanyl TTS | see below | see below |
| Hydrocodone | 0.9 | — |
| Hydromorphone | 4 | 20 |
| Levorphanol | 7.5 | 15 |
| Meperidine | 0.1 | 0.4 |
| Methadone | 1.5 | 3 |
| Morphine | 0.5 | 3 |

[1] To be used only for conversion to oral oxycodone. For patients receiving high-dose parenteral opioids, a more conservative conversion is warranted. For example, for high-dose parenteral morphine, use 1.5 instead of 3 as a multiplication factor.

*Special instructions for 80 and 160 mg controlled-release tablets:* For use in opioid-tolerant patients only.

Controlled-release tablets, 80 and 160 mg, are for use only in opioid-tolerant patients requiring daily oxycodone equivalent dosages of 160 mg or more for the 80 mg tablet and 320 mg or more for the 160 mg tablet. Take care in the prescribing of this tablet strength. Instruct patients against use by individuals other than the patient for whom it was prescribed, as such inappropriate use may have severe medical consequences.

*Therapy cessation:* When the patient no longer requires therapy with the controlled-release tablets, taper doses gradually over several days to prevent signs and symptoms of withdrawal in the physically dependent patient.

*Conversion from controlled-release tablets to parenteral opioids:* To avoid overdose, follow conservative dose conversion ratios. For patients receiving high-dose parenteral opioids, a more conservative conversion is warranted.

OXYMORPHONE HCl: Use smaller doses of oxymorphone than those recommended below for debilitated and elderly patients and those with severe liver disease.

*IV* – Initially, 0.5 mg.

*Subcutaneously or IM* – Initially, 1 to 1.5 mg every 4 to 6 hours, as needed. For analgesia during labor, give 0.5 to 1 mg IM.

*Rectal* – 5 mg every 4 to 6 hours.

Safety for use in children younger than 12 years of age has not been established.

PROPOXYPHENE:

Warning –

Fatalities:

• Do not prescribe propoxyphene for patients who are suicidal or addiction-prone.

• Prescribe propoxyphene with caution for patients taking tranquilizers or antidepressant drugs and patients who use alcohol in excess.

• Tell patients not to exceed the recommended dose and to limit alcohol intake.

Propoxyphene products in excessive doses, either alone or in combination with other CNS depressants (including alcohol), are a major cause of drug-related deaths. Fatalities within the first hour of overdosage are not uncommon. In a survey of deaths caused by overdosage conducted in 1975, in approximately 20% of fatal cases, death occurred within the first hour (5% within 15 minutes). Do not take propoxyphene in higher doses than those recommended by the physician. Judicious prescribing of propoxyphene is essential for safety. Consider nonnarcotic analgesics for depressed or suicidal patients. Do not prescribe propoxyphene for suicidal or addiction-prone patients. Caution patients about the concomitant use of propoxyphene products and alcohol because of potentially serious CNS-additive effects of these agents. Because of added CNS depressant effects, cautiously prescribe with concomitant sedatives, tranquilizers, muscle relaxants, antidepressants, or other CNS-depressant drugs. Advise patients of the additive depressant effects of these combinations.

Many propoxyphene-related deaths have occurred in patients with histories of emotional disturbances, suicidal ideation or attempts, or misuse of tranquilizers, alcohol, and other CNS-active drugs. Deaths have occurred as a consequence of the accidental ingestion of excessive quantities of propoxyphene alone or in combination with other drugs. Do not exceed the recommended dosage.

Because of differences in molecular weight, 100 mg of propoxyphene napsylate is required to supply propoxyphene equivalent to 65 mg of the HCl. In hepatic or renal impairment, reduce total daily dosage.

*Propoxyphene HCl –*
  *Usual dose:* 65 mg every 4 hours as needed. Do not exceed 390 mg/day.
*Propoxyphene napsylate –*
  *Usual dose:* 100 mg every 4 hours as needed. Do not exceed 600 mg/day.
*Elderly –* Propoxyphene metabolism rate may be reduced in some patients. Consider increased dosing interval.

REMIFENTANIL HCl: For IV use only. Individualize dosage.

Administer continuous infusions of remifentanil only by an infusion device. The injection site should be close to the venous cannula. Clear all IV tubing at the time of discontinuation of infusion.

*During general anesthesia –* Remifentanil is not recommended as the sole agent in general anesthesia because loss of consciousness cannot be assured and because of a high incidence of apnea, muscle rigidity, and tachycardia. Remifentanil is synergistic with other anesthetics and doses of thiopental, propofol, isoflurane, and midazolam have been reduced by up to 75% with the coadministration of remifentanil.

| Remifentanil Dosing Guidelines - General Anesthesia and Continuing as an Analgesic into the Postoperative Care Unit or Intensive Care Setting | | | |
|---|---|---|---|
| Phase | Continuous IV infusion (mcg/kg/min) | Infusion dose range (mcg/kg/min) | Supplemental IV bolus dose (mcg/kg) |
| Induction of anesthesia (through intubation) | 0.5 to 1[1] | NA[2] | NA[2] |
| Maintenance of anesthesia with: | | | |
| Nitrous oxide (66%) | 0.4 | 0.1 - 2 | 1 |
| Isoflurane (0.4 to 1.5 MAC) | 0.25 | 0.05 - 2 | 1 |
| Propofol (100 to 200 mcg/kg/min) | 0.25 | 0.05 - 2 | 1 |
| Continuation as an analgesic into the immediate postoperative period | 0.1 | 0.025 - 0.2 | not recommended |

[1] An initial dose of 1 mcg/kg may be administered over 30 to 60 seconds.
[2] No data available.

*During induction of anesthesia –* Administer at an infusion rate of 0.5 to 1 mcg/kg/min with a hypnotic or volatile agent for the induction of anesthesia. If endotracheal intubation is to occur less than 8 minutes after the start of infusion of remifentanil, then an initial dose of 1 mcg/kg may be administered over 30 to 60 seconds.

*During maintenance of anesthesia* – After endotracheal intubation, decrease the infusion rate of remifentanil in accordance with the dosing guidelines in the table above. Because of the rapid onset and short duration of action of remifentanil, the rate of administration during anesthesia can be titrated upward in 25% to 100% increments or downward in 25% to 50% decrements every 2 to 5 minutes to attain the desired level of μ-opioid effect. In response to light anesthesia or transient episodes of intense surgical stress, supplemental bolus doses of 1 mcg/kg may be administered every 2 to 5 minutes. At infusion rates more than 1 mcg/kg/min, consider increases in the concomitant anesthetic agents to increase the depth of anesthesia.

*Continuation as an analgesic into the immediate postoperative period under the direct supervision of an anesthesia practitioner* – Remifentanil infusions may be continued into the immediate postoperative period for select patients for whom later transition to longer-acting analgesics may be desired. The use of bolus injections of remifentanil to treat pain during the postoperative period is not recommended. When used as an IV analgesic in the immediate postoperative period, administer remifentanil initially by continuous infusion at a rate of 0.1 mcg/kg/min. The infusion rate may be adjusted every 5 minutes in 0.025 mcg/kg/min increments to balance the patient's level of analgesia and respiratory rate. Infusion rates more than 0.2 mcg/kg/min are associated with respiratory depression (respiratory rate less than 8 breaths/min).

*Individualization of dosage* –

*Elderly:* Decrease the starting doses of remifentanil by 50% in elderly patients (older than 65 years of age). Cautiously titrate to effect.

*Children:* The same doses (per kg) as adults are recommended for pediatric patients 2 years of age and older.

*Obesity:* Base the starting dose of remifentanil on ideal body weight (IBW) in obese patients (more than 30% over their IBW).

SUFENTANIL CITRATE: In obese patients (more than 20% above ideal total body weight), determine dosage on the basis of lean body weight. Reduce dosage in the elderly or debilitated. Monitor vital signs routinely.

For IV injection.

*Adult dosage range: Total dosage* –

*1 to 2 mcg/kg:* Administer with nitrous oxide/oxygen in patients undergoing general surgery for up to 8 hours in which endotracheal intubation and mechanical ventilation are required. Expected duration of anesthesia is 1 to 2 hours.

*Maintenance* – 10 to 25 mcg (0.2 to 0.5 mL) as needed for surgical stress/lightening of analgesia.

*2 to 8 mcg/kg:* Administer with nitrous oxide/oxygen in more complicated major surgical procedures. Expected duration of anesthesia is 2 to 8 hours.

*Maintenance* – 10 to 50 mcg (0.2 to 1 mL) for stress/lightening of analgesia.

*8 to 30 mcg/kg (anesthetic doses):* Administer with 100% oxygen and a muscle relaxant. Sufentanil produces sleep at dosages 8 mcg/kg or more and maintains a deep level of anesthesia without additional agents.

*Maintenance* – 0.5 to 10 mcg/kg for stress and lightening of anesthesia.

*Epidural use in labor and delivery* – 10 to 15 mcg administered with 10 mL bupivacaine 0.125% with or without epinephrine. Mix sufentanil and bupivacaine together before administration. Doses can be repeated twice (for a total of 3 doses) at 1-hour or more intervals until delivery.

Administer sufentanil by slow injection. Closely monitor respiration following each administration of an epidural injection of sufentanil.

*Children (younger than 12 years of age)* – For induction and maintenance of anesthesia in children undergoing cardiovascular surgery, a dose of 10 to 25 mcg/kg administered with 100% oxygen is recommended. Supplemental dosages of up to 25 to 50 mcg are recommended for maintenance.

**Actions**

Pharmacology:

| Narcotic Agonist Comparative Pharmacology[1] | | | | | | | |
|---|---|---|---|---|---|---|---|
| Drug | Analgesic | Antitussive | Constipation | Respiratory depression | Sedation | Emesis | Physical dependence |
| *Phenanthrenes* | | | | | | | |
| Codeine | + | +++ | + | + | + | + | ÷ |
| Hydrocodone | + | +++ | nd[2] | + | nd[2] | nd[2] | ÷ |
| Hydromorphone | ++ | +++ | + | ++ | + | + | ++ |
| Levorphanol | ++ | ++ | ++ | ++ | ++ | + | ++ |
| Morphine | ++ | +++ | ++ | ++ | ++ | ++ | ++ |
| Oxycodone | ++ | +++ | ++ | ++ | ++ | ++ | ++ |
| Oxymorphone | ++ | + | ++ | +++ | nd[2] | +++ | +++ |
| *Phenylpiperidines* | | | | | | | |
| Alfentanil | ++ | nd[2] | nd[2] | nd[2] | nd[2] | nd[2] | nd[2] |
| Fentanyl | ++ | nd[2] | nd[2] | + | nd[2] | + | nd[2] |
| Meperidine | ++ | + | + | ++ | + | nd[2] | ++ |
| Sufentanil | +++ | nd[2] | nd[2] | nd[2] | nd[2] | nd[2] | nd[2] |
| *Diphenylheptanes* | | | | | | | |
| Methadone | ++ | ++ | ++ | ++ | + | + | ÷ |
| Propoxyphene | + | nd[2] | nd[2] | + | + | + | ÷ |
| *Anilidopiperidines* | | | | | | | |
| Remifentanil | +++ | nd[2] | + | ++ | nd[2] | ++ | ÷ |

[1] Table adapted from Catalano RB. The medical approach to management of pain caused by cancer. *Semin Oncol* 1975;2:379-92 and Reuler JB, et al. The chronic pain syndrome: Misconceptions and management. *Ann Intern Med* 1980;93:588-96.
[2] nd = No data available.

Pharmacokinetics: Pharmacokinetic profiles are summarized in the table below using morphine as the standard. Data based on IM administration unless otherwise noted.

| Pharmacokinetics of Narcotic Agonist Analgesics[1] | | | | | | |
|---|---|---|---|---|---|---|
| Drug | Onset (minutes) | Peak (hours) | Duration[2] (hours) | t½ (hours) | Approximate equianalgesic doses[3] (mg) | |
| | | | | | Parenteral | Other |
| Alfentanil | immediate | nd[4] | nd[4] | 1 to 2[5] | IM 0.4 to 0.8 | nd[4] |
| Codeine | 10 to 30 | 0.5 to 1 | 4 to 6 | 3 | IM 120 to 130 SC 120 | Oral 180 - 200[6] |
| Fentanyl | 7 to 8 | nd[4] | 1 to 2 | 1.5 to 6 | IM 0.1 to 0.2 | Transdermal 25 mcg/h |
| Hydrocodone | nd[4] | nd[4] | 4 to 6 | 3.3 to 4.5 | nd[4] | Oral 30 |
| Hydromorphone | 15 to 30 | 0.5 to 1 | 4 to 5 | 2 to 3 | IM 1.3 to 1.5 SC 1 to 1.5 | Oral 7.5 |
| Levorphanol | 30 to 90 | 0.5 to 1 | 6 to 8 | 11 to 16 | IM 2 SC 2 | Oral 4 |
| Meperidine | 10 to 45 | 0.5 to 1 | 2 to 4 | 3 to 4 | IM 75 SC 75 to 100 | Oral 300[6] |
| Methadone | 30 to 60 | 0.5 to 1 | 4 to 6[7] | 15 to 30 | IM 10 SC 8 to 10 | Oral 10 to 20 |
| Morphine | 15 to 60[8] | 0.5 to 1 | 3 to 7 | 1.5 to 2 | IM 10 SC 10 | Oral 30 to 60 |
| Oxycodone | 15 to 30 | 1 | 4 to 6 | nd[4] | IM 10 to 15 SC 10 to 15 | Oral 30[6] |
| Oxymorphone | 5 to 10 | 0.5 to 1 | 3 to 6 | nd[4] | IM 1 SC 1 to 1.5 | Rectal 5, 10 |
| Propoxyphene (PO) | 30 to 60 | 2 to 2.5 | 4 to 6 | 6 to 12 | nd[4] | Oral 130[9] |

| Pharmacokinetics of Narcotic Agonist Analgesics[1] | | | | | | |
| | | | | | Approximate equianalgesic doses[3] (mg) | |
| Drug | Onset (minutes) | Peak (hours) | Duration[2] (hours) | t½ (hours) | Parenteral | Other |
|---|---|---|---|---|---|---|
| Remifentanil | 1 | 1 min | short[10] | ≈ 3 to 10 min | nd[4] | nd[4] |
| Sufentanil | 1.3 to 3[5] | nd[4] | nd[4] | 2.5 | IM 0.01 to 0.04 | nd[4] |

[1] Caution: Recommended doses do not apply for adult patients with body weight < 50 kg. Recommended doses do not apply to patients with renal or hepatic insufficiency or other conditions affecting drug metabolism and kinetics.
[2] After IV administration, peak effects may be more pronounced but duration is shorter. Duration of action may be longer with the oral route.
[3] Based on morphine 10 mg IM or subcutaneously. The initial dose of the new drug is given at ½ to ⅔ of the calculated dose because opioid-specific tolerance may occur, and the new drug may have more relative effectiveness (and more side effects) than the drug being discontinued.
[4] nd = No data available.
[5] Data based on IV administration.
[6] Starting doses lower (codeine, 30 mg; oxycodone, 5 mg; meperidine, 50 mg).
[7] Duration and half-life increase with repeated use because of cumulative effects.
[8] Data based on intrathecal or epidural administration.
[9] Starting doses lower (propoxyphene, 65 to 130 mg). In equimolar doses (100 mg of napsylate equals 65 mg of HCl).
[10] The duration of action does not increase with prolonged administration.

## Contraindications

Hypersensitivity to narcotics; diarrhea caused by poisoning until the toxic material has been eliminated; acute bronchial asthma; upper airway obstruction.

Morphine, epidural, or intrathecal: Presence of infection at injection site; anticoagulant therapy; bleeding diathesis; parenterally administered corticosteroids within a 2-week period or other concomitant drug therapy or medical condition that would contraindicate the technique of epidural or intrathecal analgesia.

Morphine, injection: Heart failure secondary to chronic lung disease; cardiac arrhythmias; brain tumor; acute alcoholism; delirium tremens; idiosyncrasy to the drug. Because of its stimulating effect on the spinal cord, do not use morphine in convulsive states (eg, status epilepticus, tetanus, strychnine poisoning).

Morphine, immediate release oral solution: Respiratory insufficiency; severe CNS depression; heart failure secondary to chronic lung disease; cardiac arrhythmias; increased intracranial or cerebrospinal pressure; head injuries; brain tumor; acute alcoholism; delirium tremens; convulsive disorders; after biliary tract surgery; suspected surgical abdomen; surgical anastomosis; idiosyncrasy to the drug; concomitantly with monoamine oxidase inhibitors (MAOIs) or within 14 days of such treatment.

Levorphanol: Acute alcoholism; bronchial asthma; increased intracranial pressure; respiratory depression; anoxia.

Meperidine: In patients taking MAOIs or in those who have received such agents within 14 days.

Hydromorphone injection: In patients not already receiving large amounts of parenteral narcotics; patients with respiratory depression in the absence of resuscitative equipment; status asthmaticus; use as obstetrical analgesia.

Fentanyl:
Transdermal – Hypersensitivity to fentanyl and adhesives; in the management of acute or postoperative pain, including use in outpatient surgeries; in the management of mild or intermittent pain responsive to PRN or nonopioid therapy; in doses exceeding 25 mcg/hour at the initiation of opioid therapy; in children younger than 12 years of age or patient younger than 18 years of age who weigh less than 50 kg, except in an authorized investigational research setting.
Transmucosal – In children who weigh less than 10 kg; treatment of acute or chronic pain (safety for use in these patients have not been established); doses greater than 15 mcg/kg in children and greater than 5 mcg/kg in adults because of the excessive frequency of significant hypoventilation at higher doses; for use at home or in any other setting outside a hospital setting.

*Opium:* Opium tincture in children; diarrhea caused by poisoning until the toxic material has been eliminated.

*Oxycodone:* Hypercarbia; paralytic ileus.

*Oxymorphone:* Paralytic ileus; treatment of pulmonary edema secondary to a chemical respiratory irritant.

*Remifentanil:* Epidural or intrathecal administration.

## Warnings

*Respiratory depression:* Narcotics may be expected to produce serious or potentially fatal respiratory depression if given in an excessive dose, too frequently, or in full dosage to compromised or vulnerable patients because the doses required to produce analgesia in the general clinical population may cause serious respiratory depression in vulnerable patients.

Reduce the initial dose by more than 50% when the drug is given to patients with any condition affecting respiratory reserve or in conjunction with other drugs affecting the respiratory center. Individually titrate subsequent doses according to the patient's response. Respiratory depression can be reversed by naloxone, a specific antagonist.

*Asthma and other respiratory conditions* – Use with extreme caution in patients with acute asthma, bronchial asthma, chronic obstructive pulmonary disease, or cor pulmonale, a substantially decreased respiratory reserve, and with preexisting respiratory depression, hypoxia, or hypercapnia.

*Excessive doses:* These products given in excessive doses, either alone or in combination with other CNS depressants (including alcohol), are a major cause of drug-related deaths.

*Suicide:* Do not prescribe propoxyphene for patients who are suicidal or addiction-prone.

*Head injury and increased intracranial pressure:* Narcotics may obscure the clinical course of patients with head injuries. The respiratory depressant effects and the capacity to elevate cerebrospinal fluid pressure may be markedly exaggerated in the presence of head injury, brain tumor, other intracranial lesions or a preexisting elevated intracranial pressure.

*Parenteral therapy:* Give by very slow IV injection, preferably as a diluted solution. The patient should be lying down. Rapid IV injection increases the incidence of adverse reactions. Use caution when injecting subcutaneously or IM in chilled areas or in patients with hypotension or shock because impaired perfusion may prevent complete absorption.

Limit epidural or intrathecal administration of **morphine** to the lumbar area.

*Hydrochlorides of opium alkaloids* – Do not administer IV.

*Hypotensive effect:* Narcotic analgesics may cause severe hypotension in individuals whose ability to maintain blood pressure has been compromised by a depleted blood volume, or coadministration of drugs such as phenothiazines or general anesthetics.

*Renal/Hepatic function impairment:* Renal and hepatic dysfunction may cause a prolonged duration and cumulative effect; smaller doses may be necessary.

*Meperidine* – In patients with renal dysfunction, normeperidine (an active metabolite of meperidine) may accumulate, resulting in increased CNS adverse reactions.

*Pregnancy: Category C.*

*Labor* – Narcotics cross the placental barrier and can produce depression of respiration and psycho-physiologic effects in the neonate.

*Lactation:* Most of these agents appear in breast milk, but effects on the infant may not be significant. Some recommend waiting 4 to 6 hours after use before nursing.

*Children:* Safety and efficacy of **sufentanil** in children younger than 2 years of age undergoing cardiovascular surgery have been documented in a limited number of cases. Safety and efficacy of **fentanyl** in children younger than 2 years of age are not established. Hypotension has occurred in neonates with respiratory distress syndrome on **alfentanil** 20 mcg/kg.

Do not use **oxycodone** in children; **propoxyphene** use is not recommended in children. **Methadone** is not recommended as an analgesic in children; documented clinical experience is insufficient to establish suitable dosage regimens. Safety of **oxymorphone** and **hydromorphone** is not established in children.

**Precautions**

*Acute abdominal conditions:* Narcotics may obscure diagnosis or clinical course.

*Special risk patients:* Exercise caution in elderly and debilitated patients and in those suffering from conditions accompanied by hypoxia or hypercapnia when even moderate therapeutic doses may dangerously decrease pulmonary ventilation. Also exercise caution in patients sensitive to CNS depressants, including those with cardiovascular disease; myxedema; convulsive disorders; increased ocular pressure; acute alcoholism; delirium tremens; cerebral arteriosclerosis; ulcerative colitis; fever; decreased respiratory reserve (eg, emphysema, severe obesity); hypothyroidism; kyphoscoliosis; Addison's disease; prostatic hypertrophy; urethral stricture; CNS depression; coma; gallbladder disease; recent GI or GU tract surgery; toxic psychosis.

*Skeletal muscle rigidity:* **Alfentanil**, **fentanyl**, and **sufentanil** may cause skeletal muscle rigidity, particularly of the truncal muscles. The incidence and severity of muscle rigidity is usually dose-related. Alfentanil, fentanyl, and sufentanil may produce muscular rigidity that involves all skeletal muscles, including those of the neck and extremities.

*Supraventricular tachycardias:* Use with caution in atrial flutter and other supraventricular tachycardias; vagolytic action may increase the ventricular response rate.

*Seizures:* Seizures may be aggravated or may occur in individuals without a history of convulsive disorders if dosage is substantially increased because of tolerance.

*Suppressed cough reflex:* Exercise caution when using narcotic analgesics postoperatively and in patients with pulmonary disease because cough reflex is suppressed.

*Tolerance:* Some patients develop tolerance to the narcotic analgesic. This may occur after days or months of continuous therapy. The dose generally needs to be increased to obtain adequate analgesia.

*Cross-tolerance* – Cross-tolerance is not complete. Switching to another narcotic agonist, starting with half the predicted equianalgesic dose, may circumvent the cross-tolerance.

*Drug abuse and dependence:* Narcotic analgesics have abuse potential. Psychological dependence and physical tolerance and dependence may develop upon repeated use. However, most patients who receive opiates for medical reasons do not develop dependence syndromes.

Infants born to mothers physically dependent on narcotics will also be physically dependent and may exhibit respiratory difficulties and withdrawal symptoms.

*Acute abstinence syndrome (withdrawal)* – Severity is related to the degree of dependence, the abruptness of withdrawal and the drug used. Generally, withdrawal symptoms develop at the time the next dose would ordinarily be given.

Do not use a narcotic antagonist to detect dependence. If a narcotic antagonist must be used for serious respiratory depression in a physically dependent patient, give with extreme care, using $\frac{1}{10}$ to $\frac{1}{5}$ the usual initial dose.

With morphine, cerebral and spinal receptors may develop tolerance/dependence independently, as a function of local dosage. Take care to avert withdrawal in those patients who have been maintained on parenteral/oral narcotics when epidural or intrathecal administration is considered. Withdrawal may occur following chronic epidural or intrathecal administration, as well as the development of tolerance to morphine by these routes.

*Hazardous tasks:* May produce drowsiness or dizziness; observe caution while driving or performing other tasks requiring alertness or physical dexterity.

## Drug Interactions

*Drug/Drug interactions:* Drugs that may affect narcotic analgesics include amitriptyline, barbiturate anesthetics, protease inhibitors, cimetidine, chlorpromazine, erythromycin, hydantoins, diazepam, droperidol, and rifampin. Charcoal and cigarette smoking may also affect narcotic analgesics. Drugs that may be affected by narcotic analgesics include carbamazepine, warfarin, MAOIs, furazolidone, nitrous oxide, beta blockers, and calcium channel blockers.

*Drug/Lab test interactions:* Determinations of plasma amylase or lipase levels may be unreliable for 24 hours after narcotic administration.

## Adverse Reactions

*Major hazards* – Respiratory depression; apnea; circulatory depression; respiratory arrest; coma; shock; cardiac arrest; hypoventilation. Most cases of serious or fatal adverse events involving **levorphanol** reported to the manufacturer or the FDA have involved either the administration of large initial doses or too frequent doses of the drug to non-opioid-tolerant patients, or the simultaneous administration of levorphanol with other drugs affecting respiration. Reduce the initial levorphanol dose by approximately more than 50% when it is given to patients along with another drug affecting respiration.

*Most frequent* – Respiratory depression; skeletal muscle rigidity; apnea; bradycardia; lightheadedness; dizziness; sedation; nausea; vomiting; sweating. Symptoms are more prominent in ambulatory patients and in those without severe pain. Use lower doses in these patients. Some reactions may be alleviated if the ambulatory patient lies down.

# NARCOTIC AGONIST-ANTAGONIST ANALGESICS

There are 2 types of narcotic agonist-antagonists: 1) Drugs which are antagonists at the μ receptor and are agonists at other receptors (ie, pentazocine), 2) partial agonists (ie, buprenorphine) that have limited agonist activity at the μ receptor. The narcotic agonist-antagonist analgesics are potent analgesic agents with a lower abuse potential than pure narcotic agonists. Because of their narcotic antagonist activity, these agents may precipitate withdrawal symptoms in those with opiate dependence.

| Narcotic Agonist-Antagonist Pharmacokinetics | | | | | | | |
|---|---|---|---|---|---|---|---|
| Agonist/Antagonist | | Onset (min) | Peak (min) | Duration (h) | $t^{1/2}$ (h) | Equivalent dose[1] (mg) | Relative antagonist activity |
| Buprenorphine | IM | 15 | 60 | 6 | 2.2-3.5 | 0.3 | equipotent with naloxone |
| | IV[2] | | | | | | |
| Butorphanol | IM | <10 | 30-60 | 3-4 | 2.5-4 | 2-3 | 30× pentazocine or $^1/_{40}$ naloxone |
| Dezocine | IM | ≤ 30 | 30-150 | 2-4[3] | nd | 10 | greater than pentazocine |
| | IV | ≤ 15 | | | 2.4[4] | | |
| Nalbuphine | IM | < 15[5] | 60 | 3-6 | 5 | 10 | 10× pentazocine |
| | IV | 12-30[2] | 30 | | | | |
| Pentazocine | IM | 15-20[2] | 15-60[1] | 3 | 2.2-3.5 | 30 | weak |
| | IV | 12-30[2] | nd | | | | |
| | oral | 15-30[2] | 60-180 | | | | |

[1] Parenteral dose equivalent to 10 mg morphine.
[2] Time to onset and peak effect shorter.
[3] Dose related.
[4] For 10 or 20 mg dose; 1.7 h for 5 mg dose.
[5] Also for subcutaneous administration.
* nd – no data

# PENTAZOCINE

**Injection**: 30 mg (as lactate) per mL (c-iv)          *Talwin* (Sanofi Winthrop)
**Tablets**: 50 mg (as HCl) and 0.5 mg naloxone HCl (c-iv)          *Talwin NX* (Sanofi Winthrop)

---

**Warning:**
    *Talwin Nx:* Talwin Nx is intended for oral use only. Severe, potentially lethal reactions (eg, pulmonary emboli, vascular occlusion, ulceration and abscesses, withdrawal symptoms in narcotic-dependent individuals) may result from misuse of this drug by injection or in combination with other substances.

---

**Indications**
    *Oral and parenteral:* Relief of moderate to severe pain.

    *Parenteral:* For preoperative or preanesthetic medication; supplement to surgical anesthesia.

**Administration and Dosage**
    *Oral:*
        *Adults* – Initially, 50 mg every 3 or 4 hours; increase to 100 mg if necessary. Do not exceed a total daily dosage of 600 mg. When anti-inflammatory or antipyretic effects are desired in addition to analgesia, aspirin can be administered concomitantly.
        *Children (younger than 12 years of age)* – Clinical experience is limited; use is not recommended.
        Pentazocine tablets are intended for oral use only. Severe, potentially lethal reactions may result from misuse by injection or when combined with other substances.

Oral pentazocine tablets contain 0.5 mg naloxone, a narcotic antagonist, to aid in elimination of the abuse potential.

*Parenteral:*

*Adults* – 30 mg IM, subcutaneously or IV; may repeat every 3 to 4 hours. Doses in excess of 30 mg IV or 60 mg IM or subcutaneously are not recommended. Do not exceed a total daily dosage of 360 mg.

Use subcutaneously only when necessary; severe tissue damage is possible at injection sites. When frequent injections are needed, administer IM, constantly rotating injection sites.

*Patients in labor* – A single 30 mg IM dose is most common. A 20 mg IV dose, given 2 or 3 times at 2- to 3-hour intervals, has resulted in adequate pain relief when contractions become regular.

*Children (younger than 12 years of age)* – Clinical experience is limited; use is not recommended.

*Admixture incompatibility* – Do not mix pentazocine in the same syringe with soluble barbiturates because precipitation will occur.

## Actions

*Pharmacology:* Pentazocine, a potent analgesic, weakly antagonizes the effects of morphine, meperidine, and other opiates at the μ-opioid receptor.

*Talwin NX* – Talwin NX tablets, which contain naloxone, produce analgesic effects when administered orally because naloxone has poor bioavailability.

*Pharmacokinetics:* Pentazocine is well absorbed from the GI tract and from subcutaneous and IM sites. Oral bioavailability is less than 20%; concentrations in plasma coincide closely with onset, intensity and duration of analgesia. It is excreted via the kidney, less than 5% unchanged.

## Contraindications

Hypersensitivity to pentazocine, naloxone (in *Talwin NX*) or any product component.

## Warnings

*Tissue damage:* Severe sclerosis of skin, subcutaneous tissues, and underlying muscle has occurred at injection sites following multiple doses of pentazocine lactate.

*Head injury and increased intracranial pressure:* Pentazocine can produce effects that may obscure the clinical course of head injury patients. Use with extreme caution and only if essential.

*MI:* Exercise caution in the IV use of pentazocine for patients with acute MI accompanied by hypertension or left ventricular failure. Use the oral form with caution in MI patients who have nausea or vomiting.

*Acute CNS manifestations:* Patients receiving therapeutic doses have experienced hallucinations (usually visual), disorientation, and confusion that have cleared spontaneously.

Seizures have occurred with the use of pentazocine.

*Renal/Hepatic function impairment:* The drug is metabolized in liver and excreted by the kidney; administer with caution to patients with such impairment. Extensive liver disease predisposes to greater side effects and may be the result of decreased drug metabolism.

*Pregnancy: Category C.*

*Labor* – Use with caution in women delivering premature infants.

*Lactation:* Safety for use in the nursing mother has not been established.

*Children:* Safety and efficacy in children younger than 12 years of age have not been established.

## Precautions

*Respiratory conditions:* Use caution and low dosage in patients with respiratory depression, severely limited respiratory reserve, severe bronchial asthma, obstructive respiratory conditions, and cyanosis.

*Biliary tract pressure elevation:* Biliary tract pressure elevation generally occurs for varying periods following narcotic use. However, some evidence suggests pentazocine causes little or no elevation in biliary tract pressures.

*Patients receiving narcotics:* Pentazocine is a mild narcotic antagonist. Some patients previously given narcotics, including methadone for the daily treatment of narcotic dependence, have experienced withdrawal symptoms after receiving pentazocine.

*Drug abuse and dependence:* Exercise special care in prescribing to emotionally unstable patients and to those with history of drug abuse; closely supervise when therapy exceeds 4 or 5 days.

"Ts and Blues" – Injection IV of oral preparations of **pentazocine** (*Talwin*, "Ts") and **tripelennamine** (PBZ, "Blues"), an $H_1$-blocking antihistamine has become a common form of drug abuse as a "substitute" for heroin.

*Hazardous tasks:* May produce sedation, dizziness, and occasional euphoria; observe caution while driving or performing other tasks requiring alertness, coordination, or physical dexterity.

**Drug Interactions**
Drugs that may interact with pentazocine include alcohol and barbiturate anesthetics.

**Adverse Reactions**
Significant adverse reactions include nausea; dizziness or lightheadedness; drowsiness; vomiting; euphoria; constipation; cramps; abdominal distress; anorexia; diarrhea; dry mouth; taste alteration; sedation; headache; weakness or faintness; depression; disturbed dreams; insomnia; syncope; hallucinations; tremor; irritability; excitement; tinnitus; disorientation; confusion; blurred vision; focusing difficulty; nystagmus; diplopia; miosis; edema of the face; sweating; anaphylactic reaction; rash; urticaria; soft tissue induration; nodules; cutaneous depression; ulceration (sloughing); severe sclerosis of the skin and subcutaneous tissues; diaphoresis; stinging on injection; flushed skin; dermatitis; pruritus; toxic epidermal necrolysis; decrease in blood pressure; tachycardia; circulatory depression; shock; hypertension; respiratory depression; dyspnea; transient apnea in newborns whose mothers received parenteral pentazocine during labor; depression of white blood cells (especially granulocytes); urinary retention; paresthesia; chills; neuromuscular and psychiatric muscle tremors; alterations in rate or strength of uterine contractions during labor (parenteral form).

## PENTAZOCINE COMBINATIONS

| | |
|---|---|
| **Tablets**: 12.5 mg (as HCl) and 325 mg aspirin (*c-iv*) | *Talwin Compound Caplets* (Sanofi Winthrop) |
| **Tablets**: 25 mg (as HCl) and 650 mg acetaminophen (*c-iv*) | *Talacen Caplets* (Sanofi Winthrop) |

**Administration and Dosage**
*Adults:*
Pentazocine and aspirin – 2 tablets 3 or 4 times/day.
Pentazocine and acetaminophen – 1 tablet every 4 hours, up to 6 tablets/day.
*Children:* Not recommended for children younger than 12 years of age.

## NALBUPHINE HCl

| | |
|---|---|
| **Injection**: 10 and 20 mg/mL (*Rx*) | Various, *Nubain* (Endo) |

**Indications**
Relief of moderate to severe pain.

For preoperative analgesia, as a supplement to balanced analgesia, to surgical and postsurgical anesthesia and for obstetrical analgesia during labor and delivery.

## Administration and Dosage

*Pain:*

*Adults* – Usual dose is 10 mg/70 kg administered subcutaneously, IM, or IV every 3 to 6 hours as necessary. Individualize dosage. In nontolerant individuals, the recommended single maximum dose is 20 mg, with a maximum total daily dose of 160 mg.

*Supplement to anesthesia:*

*Induction doses* – 0.3 to 3 mg/kg IV administered over a 10 to 15 minute period.

*Maintenance dose* – 0.25 to 0.5 mg/kg in a single IV administration.

*Patients dependent on narcotics:* Patients dependent on narcotics may experience withdrawal symptoms upon the administration of nalbuphine. If unduly troublesome, control by slow IV administration of small increments of morphine until relief occurs. If the previous analgesic was morphine, meperidine, codeine or another narcotic with similar duration of activity, administer 25% the anticipated nalbuphine dose initially. Observe for signs of withdrawal. If untoward symptoms do not occur, progressively increase doses at appropriate intervals until analgesia is obtained.

## Actions

*Pharmacology:* Nalbuphine is a potent analgesic with narcotic agonist and antagonist actions. Its analgesic potency is essentially equivalent to that of morphine on a milligram basis.

*Pharmacokinetics:* Onset of action occurs within 2 to 3 minutes after IV administration, and in less than 15 minutes following subcutaneous or IM injection. Nalbuphine is metabolized in the liver; plasma half-life is 5 hours. The duration of analgesic activity ranges from 3 to 6 hours. Approximately 7% is excreted unchanged in the urine.

## Contraindications

Hypersensitivity to nalbuphine.

## Warnings

*Administration:* Nalbuphine should be given as a supplement to general anesthesia only by persons specifically trained in the use of IV anesthetics and management of the respiratory effects of potent opioids.

*Head injury and increased intracranial pressure:* The possible respiratory depressant effects and the potential of potent analgesics to elevate cerebrospinal fluid pressure may be markedly exaggerated in the presence of head injury, intracranial lesions, or a preexisting increase in intracranial pressure.

*Renal/Hepatic function impairment:* Because nalbuphine is metabolized in the liver and excreted by the kidneys, use nalbuphine with caution in patients with renal or liver dysfunction and administer in reduced amounts.

*Pregnancy: Category* B. (*Category D* in prolonged use or in high doses at term). Safe use in pregnancy has not been established.

*Labor and delivery* – May produce fetal bradycardia, respiratory depression, apnea, cyanosis, and hypotonia in the neonate. Maternal administration of naloxone during labor has normalized these effects in some cases. Use with caution in women delivering premature infants.

*Lactation:* Exercise caution when nalbuphine is administered to a nursing woman.

*Children:* Not recommended in patients younger than 18 years of age.

## Precautions

*Respiratory depression:* At the usual adult dose of 10 mg/70 kg, nalbuphine causes respiratory depression approximately equal to that produced by equal doses of morphine. However, nalbuphine exhibits a ceiling effect; increases in dosage beyond 30 mg produce no further respiratory depression. Respiratory depression induced by nalbuphine can be reversed by naloxone. Administer nalbuphine with caution at low doses to patients with impaired respiration (eg, from other medication, uremia, bronchial asthma, severe infection, cyanosis, or respiratory obstructions).

*MI:* Use with caution in patients with MI who have nausea or vomiting.

*Biliary tract surgery:* Use with caution in patients about to undergo biliary tract surgery because it may cause spasm of the sphincter of Oddi.

*Cardiovascular effects:* During evaluation of nalbuphine in anesthesia, a higher incidence of bradycardia has been reported in patients who did not receive atropine preoperatively.

*Drug abuse and dependence:* Observe caution in prescribing nalbuphine to emotionally unstable patients or to individuals with a history of opioid abuse. Closely supervise such patients when long-term therapy is contemplated.

Abrupt discontinuation after prolonged use has been followed by symptoms of narcotic withdrawal.

*Hazardous tasks:* May produce drowsiness. Observe caution while driving or performing other tasks requiring alertness, coordination or physical dexterity.

**Drug Interactions**
Drugs that may interact with nalbuphine HCl include barbiturate anesthetics, cimetidine, CNS depressants.

**Adverse Reactions**
Adverse reactions occurring in 3% or more of patients include sedation; sweaty/clammy feeling; nausea; vomiting; dizziness; vertigo; dry mouth; headache.

## BUPRENORPHINE HCl

**BUPRENORPHINE HCl**

| | |
|---|---|
| **Tablets, sublingual:** 2 and 8 mg (as base) *(c-III)* | *Subutex* (Reckitt Benckiser) |
| **Injection:** 0.324 mg (equiv. to 0.3 mg buprenorphine) per mL *(c-III)* | Various, *Buprenex* (Reckitt Benckiser) |

**BUPRENORPHINE HCl COMBINATIONS**

| | |
|---|---|
| **Tablets, sublingual:** 2 mg buprenorphine base/0.5 mg naloxone, 8 mg buprenorphine base/2 mg naloxone *(c-III)* | *Suboxone* (Reckitt Benckiser) |

**Indications**
*Tablets, sublingual:* Treatment of opioid dependence.

*Injection:* Relief of moderate to severe pain.

*Buprenorphine/Naloxone combination:* Treatment of opioid dependence.

**Administration and Dosage**
*Tablets:* Administer sublingually as a single daily dose in the range of 12 to 16 mg/day. When taken sublingually, buprenorphine and buprenorphine/naloxone have similar clinical effects and are interchangeable. Buprenorphine tablets contain no naloxone and are preferred for use during induction.

*Administration* – Place tablets under the tongue until they are dissolved. The patient should continue to hold the tablets under the tongue until they dissolve; swallowing the tablets reduces the bioavailability of the drug.

*Induction* – To avoid precipitating withdrawal, undertake induction with buprenorphine when objective and clear signs of withdrawal are evident.

*Patients taking heroin or other short-acting opioids:* At treatment initiation, administer the dose of buprenorphine at least 4 hours after the patient last used opioids or, preferably, when early signs of withdrawal appear.

*Patients taking methadone or other long-acting opioids:* Withdrawal appears more likely in patients maintained on higher doses of methadone (more than 30 mg) and when the first buprenorphine dose is administered shortly after the last methadone dose.

*Maintenance* – Buprenorphine/Naloxone is the preferred medication for maintenance treatment because of the presence of naloxone in the formulation.

*Reducing dosage and stopping treatment* – Make the decision to discontinue therapy with buprenorphine or buprenorphine/naloxone after a period of maintenance or brief stabilization as part of a comprehensive treatment plan. Gradual and abrupt discontinuation have been used but there is not a best method of tapering the dose at the end of treatment.

*Injection:*
   *Patients 13 years of age and older* – 0.3 mg IM or slow IV, every 6 hours, as needed.
Repeat once (up to 0.3 mg) if required, 30 to 60 minutes after initial dosage, giving consideration to previous dose pharmacokinetics; use thereafter only as needed.
In high-risk patients (eg, elderly, debilitated, presence of respiratory disease) or in patients where other CNS depressants are present, such as in the immediate postoperative period, reduce dose by about 50%. Exercise extra caution with the IV route of administration, particularly with the initial dose.
   Occasionally, it may be necessary to give up to 0.6 mg. Data are insufficient to recommend single IM doses more than 0.6 mg for long-term use.
   *Children* – Buprenorphine has been used in children 2 to 12 years of age at doses between 2 and 6 mcg/kg of body weight given every 4 to 6 hours. There is insufficient experience to recommend a dose in infants below 2 years of age, single doses greater than 6 mcg/kg of body weight, or the use of a repeat or second dose at 30 to 60 minutes (such as is used in adults).

## Actions
*Pharmacology:* Buprenorphine is a semisynthetic centrally acting opioid analgesic derived from thebaine; a 0.3 mg dose is approximately equivalent to 10 mg morphine in analgesic effects. Buprenorphine exerts its analgesic effect via high affinity binding of CNS opiate receptors.
   Its narcotic antagonist activity is approximately equipotent to naloxone.
   *Cardiovascular* – Buprenorphine may cause a decrease or, rarely, an increase in pulse rate and blood pressure in some patients.
   *Respiratory effects* – A therapeutic dose of 0.3 mg buprenorphine can decrease respiratory rate similarly to an equianalgesic dose of morphine (10 mg).
*Pharmacokinetics:* Onset of analgesic effect occurs 15 minutes after IM injection, peaks in about 1 hour, and persists up to 6 hours. When given IV, the time to onset and peak is shortened.
   Buprenorphine is metabolized by the liver mediated by cytochrome P450 3A4, and its clearance is related to hepatic blood flow. Plasma protein binding is about 96%. The mean elimination half-life from plasma is 37 hours.

## Contraindications
Hypersensitivity to buprenorphine.

## Warnings
*Narcotic-dependent patients:* Because of the narcotic antagonist activity of buprenorphine, use in physically dependent individuals may result in withdrawal effects. Buprenorphine, a partial agonist, has opioid properties that may lead to psychic dependence because of a euphoric component of the drug. The drug may not be substituted in acutely dependent narcotic addicts because of its antagonist component.

*Respiratory effects:* There have been occasional reports of clinically significant respiratory depression associated with buprenorphine.

*Head injury/increased intracranial pressure:* Buprenorphine may elevate cerebrospinal fluid (CSF) pressure; use with caution in head injury, intracranial lesions, and other states where CSF pressure may be increased. Buprenorphine can produce miosis and changes in consciousness levels that may interfere with patient evaluation.

*Hepatitis:* Cases of cytolytic hepatitis and hepatitis with jaundice have been observed in the addict population receiving buprenorphine both in clinical trials and in postmarketing adverse event reports.

*Allergic reactions:* Cases of acute and chronic hypersensitivity to buprenorphine have been reported in clinical trials and in the postmarketing experience. The most common signs and symptoms include rash, hives, and pruritus. Cases of bronchospasm, angioneurotic edema, and anaphylactic shock have been reported.

*Hepatic function impairment:* Buprenorphine is metabolized by the liver; the activity may be altered in those individuals with impaired hepatic function.

*Pregnancy: Category* C.

*Labor and delivery* – Safety and efficacy have not been established.

*Lactation:* It is not known whether buprenorphine is excreted in breast milk.

*Children:* Safety and efficacy for use in children have not been established.

### Precautions

*Use with caution in the following:* Elderly or debilitated; severe impairment of hepatic, pulmonary or renal function; myxedema or hypothyroidism; adrenal cortical insufficiency; CNS depression or coma; toxic psychoses; prostatic hypertrophy or urethral stricture; acute alcoholism; delirium tremens; or kyphoscoliosis. Naloxone may not be effective in reversing respiratory depression.

*Biliary tract dysfunction:* Buprenorphine increases intracholedochal pressure to a similar degree as other opiates; administer with caution.

*Acute abdominal conditions:* As with other μ-opioid receptor agonists, the administration of buprenorphine or buprenorphine/naloxone may obscure the diagnosis or clinical course of patients with acute abdominal conditions.

*Hazardous tasks:* May cause dizziness or drowsiness; observe caution while driving or performing other tasks requiring alertness.

### Drug Interactions

Drugs that may interact with buprenorphine HCl include barbiturate anesthetics, benzodiazepines, CNS depressants, CYP3A4 inducers and inhibitors, and MAOIs.

### Adverse Reactions

Adverse reactions occurring in at least 3% of patients include sedation, dizziness/vertigo, headache, hypotension, nausea/vomiting, hypoventilation, miosis, sweating.

# TRAMADOL HCl

| Tablets: 50 mg (Rx) | Ultram (Ortho-McNeil) |
| --- | --- |

## Indications

*Pain:* Management of moderate to moderately severe pain.

## Administration and Dosage

For the treatment of painful conditions, 50 to 100 mg can be administered as needed for relief every 4 to 6 hours, not to exceed 400 mg/day. For moderate pain, 50 mg may be adequate as the initial dose, and for more severe pain, 100 mg is usually more effective as the initial dose.

*Elderly:* Available data do not suggest that a dosage adjustment is necessary in elderly patients 65 to 75 years of age unless they also have renal or hepatic impairment. For elderly patients older than 75 years of age, less than 300 mg/day in divided doses as above is recommended.

*Renal function impairment:* In all patients with Ccr less than 30 mL/min, it is recommended that the dosing interval be increased to 12 hours, with a maximum daily dose of 200 mg. Because only 7% of an administered dose is removed by hemodialysis, dialysis patients can receive their regular dose on the day of dialysis.

*Hepatic function impairment:* The recommended dose for patients with cirrhosis is 50 mg every 12 hours.

## Actions

*Pharmacology:* Tramadol is a centrally acting synthetic analgesic compound. Although its mode of action is not completely understood, from animal tests 2 complementary mechanisms appear applicable: Binding to μ-opioid receptors and inhibition of reuptake of norepinephrine and serotonin.

Onset of analgesia is evident within 1 hour after administration and reaches a peak in approximately 2 to 3 hours.

*Pharmacokinetics:*

*Absorption* – Tramadol is rapidly and almost completely absorbed after oral administration.

*Distribution* – Binding to human plasma proteins is approximately 20% and appears to be independent of concentration up to 10 mcg/mL.

*Metabolism* – Tramadol is extensively metabolized after oral administration. Approximately 30% of the dose is excreted in the urine as unchanged drug.

*Excretion* – The plasma elimination half-life of tramadol is approximately 6 to 7 hours.

## Contraindications

Hypersensitivity to tramadol; acute intoxication with alcohol, hypnotics, centrally acting analgesics, opioids, or psychotropic drugs.

## Warnings

*Seizure:* Administration of tramadol may enhance the seizure risk in patients taking MAO inhibitors, neuroleptics, other drugs that reduce the seizure threshold, patients with epilepsy or patients otherwise at increased risk for seizure.

*Anaphylactoid reactions:* Serious and rarely fatal anaphylactoid reactions have been reported in patients receiving tramadol therapy. Other reported reactions include pruritus, hives, bronchospasm, and angioedema. Patients with a history of anaphylactoid reactions to codeine and other opioids may be at increased risk and therefore should not receive tramadol.

*Concomitant CNS depressants:* Use with caution and in reduced dosages when administering to patients receiving CNS depressants such as alcohol, opioids, anesthetic agents, phenothiazines, tranquilizers, or sedative hypnotics.

*Concomitant MAO inhibitors:* Use with great caution in patients taking MAO inhibitors.

*Pregnancy: Category C.*

*Lactation:* Tramadol is not recommended for obstetrical preoperative medication or for postdelivery analgesia in nursing mothers.

*Children:* Not recommended in children younger than 16 years of age.

### Precautions

*Increased intracranial pressure or head trauma:* Use with caution in patients with increased intracranial pressure or head injury. Pupillary changes (miosis) from tramadol may obscure the existence, extent, or course of intracranial pathology.

*Acute abdominal conditions:* Tramadol may complicate the clinical assessment of patients with acute abdominal conditions.

*Opioid dependence:* Tramadol is not recommended for patients who are dependent on opioids.

*Drug abuse and dependence:* Do not use tramadol in opioid-dependent patients. Tramadol has been shown to reinitiate physical dependence in some patients that have been previously dependent on other opioids.

### Drug Interactions

Drugs that may interact with tramadol include carbamazepine, MAO inhibitors, and quinidine.

*Drug/Food interactions:* Food does not affect rate or extent of absorption; tramadol can be administered without regard to meals.

### Adverse Reactions

Adverse reactions occurring in 3% or more of patients include dizziness/vertigo; nausea; constipation; headache; somnolence; vomiting; pruritus; CNS stimulation; asthenia; sweating; dyspepsia; dry mouth; diarrhea; malaise; vasodilation; abdominal pain; anorexia; flatulence; rash; visual disturbance; urinary retention/frequency; menopausal symptoms; hypertonia.

# ACETAMINOPHEN (N-Acetyl-P-Aminophenol, APAP)

## ACETAMINOPHEN

**Suppositories:** 80, 120, 125, 300, 325, and 650 mg (*otc*) — Various, *Acetaminophen Uniserts* (Upsher-Smith), *Acephen* (G & W Labs), *Neopap* (PolyMedica)

**Tablets, chewable:** 80 mg (*otc*) — Various, *St. Joseph Aspirin-Free for Children* (Schering-Plough), *Tylenol, Children's, Tylenol, Junior Strength* (McNeil-CPC)

**Capsules:** 80, 160, and 500 mg (*otc*) — Various, *Feverall Sprinkle Caps* (Upsher-Smith), *Dapa Extra Strength* (Ferndale)

**Granules:** 80 mg (*otc*) — *Snaplets-FR Granules* (Baker Cummins)

**Caplets:** 160 mg (*otc*) — *Junior Strength Panadol* (Sterling Health)

**Caplets, extended release:** 650 mg (*otc*) — *Tylenol Extended Relief* (McNeil-CPC)

**Tablets:** 160, 325, 500, and 650 mg (*otc*) — Various, *Tylenol Regular Strength Tablets* (McNeil-CPC), *Aspirin Free Anacin Maximum Strength* (Whitehall)

**Elixir:** 80, 120, 130, 160, and 325 mg/5 mL (*otc*) — Various, *Ridenol* (RID), *Dolanex* (Lannett), *Ora-phen-PD* (Great Southern), *Tylenol Children's* (McNeil-CPC)

**Liquid:** 160 mg/5 mL and 500 mg/15 mL (*otc*) — Various, *St. Joseph Aspirin-Free Fever Reducer for Children* (Schering-Plough), *Tylenol Extra Strength* (McNeil-CPC)

**Solution:** 100 mg/mL and 120 mg/2.5 mL (*otc*) — Various, *Tempra Drops* (Mead Johnson Nutritional), *Liquiprin Infants' Drops* (Menley & James)

**Suspension:** 80 mg/0.8 mL and 160 mg/5 mL (*otc*) — *Tylenol Infants' Drops* (McNeil-CPC), *Tylenol, Children's* (McNeil-CPC)

## ACETAMINOPHEN, BUFFERED

**Effervescent granules:** 325 mg w/2.781 g sodium bicarbonate & 2.224 g citric acid/dose measure (*otc*) — *Bromo Seltzer* (Warner-Lambert)

## Indications

An analgesic-antipyretic in the presence of aspirin allergy, hemostatic disturbances (including anticoagulant therapy), bleeding diatheses (eg, hemophilia), upper GI disease (eg, ulcer, gastritis, hiatus hernia), and gouty arthritis; variety of arthritic and rheumatic conditions involving musculoskeletal pain, as well as in other painful disorders; diseases accompanied by discomfort and fever such as the common cold, "flu" and other bacterial or viral infections.

*Unlabeled uses:* Prophylactic APAP use in children receiving DTP vaccination appears to decrease incidence of fever and injection site pain. A dose immediately following vaccination and every 4 to 6 h thereafter for 48 to 72 h is suggested.

## Administration and Dosage

*Oral:*

    *Adults* – 325 to 650 mg every 4 to 6 hours, or 1 g 3 to 4 times/day. Do not exceed 4 g/day.

    *Children* – May repeat doses 4 or 5 times/day; do not exceed 5 doses in 24 hours.

| Acetaminophen Dosage for Children | | | |
| --- | --- | --- | --- |
| Age | Dosage (mg) | Age (years) | Dosage (mg) |
| 0-3 months | 40 | 4-5 | 240 |
| 4-11 months | 80 | 6-8 | 320 |
| 1-2 years | 120 | 9-10 | 400 |
| 2-3 years | 160 | 11 | 480 |

A 10 mg/kg/dose schedule has also been recommended.

*Suppositories:*

    *Adults* – 650 mg every 4 to 6 h. Give no more than 6 in 24 hours.

    *Children* –

        *(3 to 11 months of age):* 80 mg every 6 hours.

        *(1 to 3 years of age):* 80 mg every 4 hours.

        *(3 to 6 years of age):* 120 to 125 mg every 4 to 6 hours. Give no more than 720 mg/24 hours.

*(6 to 12 years of age)*: 325 mg every 4 to 6 hours. Give no more than 2.6 g/24 hours.

### Actions

*Pharmacology:* The site and mechanism of the analgesic effect is unclear. APAP reduces fever by a direct action on the hypothalamic heat-regulating centers, which increases dissipation of body heat (via vasodilatation and sweating). APAP is almost as potent as aspirin in inhibiting prostaglandin synthetase in the CNS, but its peripheral inhibition of prostaglandin synthesis is minimal.

APAP does not inhibit platelet aggregation, affect prothrombin response, or produce GI ulceration.

*Pharmacokinetics:*

*Absorption* – Absorption of acetaminophen is rapid and almost complete from the GI tract.

*Distribution* – Usual analgesic doses produce total serum concentrations of 5 to 20 mcg/mL.

*Metabolism/Excretion* – Average elimination half-life is 1 to 3 hours; half-life is slightly prolonged in neonates (2.2 to 5 hours) and in cirrhotics.

### Contraindications

Hypersensitivity to acetaminophen.

### Warnings

Do not exceed recommended dosage. Consult physician for use in children younger than 3 years of age, or for oral use longer than 5 days (children), 10 days (adults) or 3 days for fever. Chronic excessive use (more than 4 g/day) eventually may lead to transient hepatotoxicity. The kidneys may undergo tubular necrosis; the myocardium may be damaged.

*Hepatic function impairment:* Hepatotoxicity and severe hepatic failure occurred in chronic alcoholics following therapeutic doses. Caution chronic alcoholics to limit acetaminophen intake to 2 g/day or less.

*Pregnancy:* Acetaminophen crosses the placenta. It is routinely used during all stages of pregnancy; when used in therapeutic doses, it appears safe for short-term use.

*Lactation:* Acetaminophen is excreted in breast milk. No adverse effects in nursing infants were reported.

### Precautions

If a sensitivity reaction occurs, discontinue use.

Severe or recurrent pain or high or continued fever may indicate serious illness. If pain persists for more than 5 days, if redness is present or in arthritic and rheumatic conditions affecting children younger than 12 years of age, consult physician immediately.

### Drug Interactions

Drugs that may affect APAP include barbiturates, carbamazepine, hydantoins, isoniazid, rifampin, sulfinpyrazone, ethyl alcohol, and activated charcoal.

*Drug/Lab test interactions:* Acetaminophen may interfere with *Chemstrip bG, Dextrostix,* and *Visidex II* home blood glucose measurement systems; decreases of > 20% in mean glucose values may be noted. This effect appears to be drug-, concentration-, and system-dependent.

### Adverse Reactions

Used as directed, acetaminophen rarely causes severe toxicity or side effects.

# SALICYLATES

### ASPIRIN

**Tablets, chewable:** 81 mg (*otc*)
*Bayer Children's Aspirin* (Glenbrook), *St. Joseph Adult Chewable Aspirin* (Schering-Plough)

**Gum tablets:** 227.5 mg (*otc*)
*Aspergum* (Schering-Plough)

**Tablets:** 325 and 500 mg (*otc*)
Various, *Genuine Bayer Aspirin Tablets and Caplets* (Glenbrook), *Empirin* (Burroughs Wellcome), *Genprin* (Goldline), *Maximum Bayer Aspirin Tablets and Caplets* (Glenbrook), *Norwich Extra-Strength* (Procter & Gamble Pharm.)

**Tablets, enteric-coated:** 325 mg (*otc*)
Various, *Ecotrin Tablets and Caplets* (GlaxoSmith-Kline), *Regular Strength Bayer Enteric Coated Caplets* (Sterling Health)

**Tablets, enteric-coated:** 81, 165, 500, 650, and 975 mg (*otc*)
Various, *Bayer Low Adult Strength* (GlaxoSmith-Kline), ½ *Halfprin* (Kramer), *Ecotrin Maximum Strength Tablets and Caplets* (GlaxoSmithKline), *Extra Strength Bayer Enteric 500 Aspirin* (Sterling Health), *Easprin* (Parke-Davis)

**Tablets, timed-release:** 650 mg (*otc*)
*8-hour Bayer Timed-Release Caplets* (Glenbrook)

**Tablets, controlled-release:** 800 mg (*Rx*)
*ZORprin* (Boots)

**Suppositories:** 120 mg, 200 mg, 300 mg, and 600 mg (*otc*)
Various

### ASPIRIN (Acetylsalicylic Acid; ASA), BUFFERED

**Tablets:** 325 mg with buffers (*otc*)
Various, *Bayer Buffered Aspirin* (Sterling Health), *Magnaprin* (Rugby), *Regular Strength Ascriptin* (Aventis), *Bufferin* (Bristol-Myers), *Asprimox* (Invamed), *Adprin-B* (Pfeiffer), *Asprimox Extra Protection for Arthritis Pain* (Bristol-Myers), *Buffex* (Roberts Med.)

**Tablets, coated:** 500 mg with buffers (*otc*)
*Extra Strength Adprin-B* (Pfeiffer), *Extra Strength Bayer Plus Caplets* (Sterling Health), *Ascriptin Extra Strength* (Aventis), *Cama Arthritis Pain Reliever* (Sandoz), *Arthritis Pain Formula* (Whitehall)

**Tablets, effervescent:** 325 and 500 mg with buffers (*otc*)
*Alka-Seltzer with Aspirin, Alka-Seltzer Extra Strength with Aspirin* (Miles)

### CHOLINE SALICYLATE

**Liquid:** 870 mg/5 mL (*otc*)
*Arthropan* (Purdue Frederick)

### MAGNESIUM SALICYLATE

**Tablets:** 325, 467, 500, 545, 580, and 600 mg (*otc*)
*Original Doan's* (Ciba Consumer), *Backache Maximum Strength Relief* (B-M Squibb), *Extra Strength Doan's* (Ciba Consumer), *Magan* (Adria), *Bayer Select Maximum Strength Backache* (Sterling Health), *Mobidin* (Ascher)

### SALSALATE (Salicylsalicyclic Acid)

**Capsules:** 500 mg (*Rx*)
*Amigesic* (Amide), *Disalcid* (3M)

**Tablets:** 500 mg (*Rx*)
Various, *Disalcid* (3M), *Salflex* (Carnrick), *Salsitab* (Upsher-Smith)

**750 mg (*Rx*)**
Various, *Disalcid* (3M), *Salsitab* (Upsher-Smith), *Salflex* (Carnrick), *Marthritic* (Marnel)

### SODIUM SALICYLATE

**Tablets, enteric-coated:** 325 mg and 650 mg (*otc*)
Various

### SODIUM THIOSALICYLATE

**Injection:** 50 mg/mL (*Rx*)
Various, *Rexolate* (Hyrex)

### SALICYLATE COMBINATIONS

**Tablets:** 500 mg salicylate (as 293 mg choline salicylate and 362 mg Mg salicylate), 750 mg salicylate (as 440 mg choline salicylate and 544 mg Mg salicylate), 1000 mg salicylate (as 587 mg choline salicylate, 725 mg Mg salicylate) (*Rx*)
*Choline Magnesium Trisalicylate* (Sidmak), *Tricosal* (Invamed)

**Warning:**
Children and teenagers should not use salicylates for chickenpox or flu symptoms before a doctor is consulted about Reye's syndrome, a rare but serious illness.

### Indications
Mild to moderate pain; fever; various inflammatory conditions such as rheumatic fever, rheumatoid arthritis and osteoarthritis.

*Aspirin:* Aspirin, for reducing the risk of recurrent transient ischemic attacks (TIAs) or stroke in men who have had transient ischemia of the brain because of fibrin platelet emboli. It has not been effective in women and is of no benefit for completed strokes.

To reduce the risk of death or nonfatal myocardial infarction (MI) in patients with previous infarction or unstable angina pectoris.

### Administration and Dosage
ASPIRIN (*Acetylsalicylic Acid; ASA*):

*Minor aches and pains* – 325 to 650 mg every 4 hours as needed. Some extra strength (500 mg) products suggest 500 mg every 3 hours or 1000 mg every 6 hours.

*Arthritis, other rheumatic conditions (eg, osteoarthritis)* – 3.2 to 6 g/day in divided doses.

*Juvenile rheumatoid arthritis:* 60 to 110 mg/kg/day in divided doses (every 6 to 8 hours). When starting at lower doses (eg, 60 mg/kg/day), may increase by 20 mg/kg/day after 5 to 7 days, followed by 10 mg/kg/day after another 5 to 7 days.

Maintain a serum salicylate level of 150 to 300 mcg/mL.

*Acute rheumatic fever –*

*Adults:* 5 to 8 g/day, initially.

*Children:* 100 mg/kg/day for 2 weeks, then decreased to 75 mg/kg/day for 4 to 6 weeks.

*Therapeutic salicylate level:* Therapeutic salicylate levels 150 to 300 mcg/mL.

*Transient ischemic attacks in men* – 1300 mg/day in divided doses (650 mg 2 times/day, or 325 mg 4 times/day). One study indicated that a dose of 300 mg/day is as effective as the larger dose and may be associated with fewer side effects.

*MI prophylaxis* – 300 or 325 mg/day. This use applies to solid oral doseforms (buffered and plain) and to buffered aspirin in solution.

*Children –*

*Analgesic/antipyretic dosage:* 10 to 15 mg/kg/dose every 4 hours (see table), up to 60 to 80 mg/kg/day.

| Recommended Aspirin Dosage in Children | | | | | |
|---|---|---|---|---|---|
| Age (years) | Weight | | Dosage (mg every 4 hours) | No. of 81 mg tablets (every 4 hours) | No. of 325 mg tablets (every 4 hours) |
| | lbs | kg | | | |
| 2-3 | 24-35 | 10.6-15.9 | 162 | 2 | ½ |
| 4-5 | 36-47 | 16-21.4 | 243 | 3 | |
| 6-8 | 48-59 | 21.5-26.8 | 324 | 4 | 1 |
| 9-10 | 60-71 | 26.9-32.3 | 405 | 5 | |
| 11 | 72-95 | 32.4-43.2 | 486 | 6 | 1½ |
| 12-14 | ≥ 96 | ≥ 43.3 | 648 | 8 | 2 |

*Kawasaki disease (mucocutaneous lymph node syndrome):* For acute febrile period, 80 to 180 mg/kg/day; very high doses may be needed to achieve therapeutic levels. After the fever resolves, dosage may be adjusted to 10 mg/kg/day.

ASPIRIN, BUFFERED: The addition of small amounts of antacids may decrease GI irritation and increase the dissolution and absorption rates of these products. Dosing is the same as with unbuffered aspirin.

CHOLINE SALICYLATE: Has fever GI side effects than aspirin.

*Adults and children (older than 12 years of age)* – 870 mg every 3 to 4 hours; maximum 6 times/day. Rheumatoid arthritis patients may start with 5 to 10 mL, up to 4 times/day.

MAGNESIUM SALICYLATE: A sodium free salicylate derivative that may have a low incidence of GI upset. The product labeling and dosage are expressed as magnesium salicylate anhydrous. The possibility of magnesium toxicity exists in people with renal insufficiency.

Usual dose is 650 mg every 4 hours or 1090 mg, 3 times a day. May increase to 3.6 to 4.8 g/day in 3 or 4 divided doses.

Safety and efficacy for use in children have not been established.

SALSALATE *(Salicylsalicylic Acid)*: After absorption, the drug is partially hydrolyzed into two molecules of salicylic acid. Insoluble in gastric secretions, it is not absorbed until it reaches the small intestine.

Usual adult dose is 3000 mg/day given in divided doses.

SODIUM SALICYLATE: Less effective than an equal dose of aspirin in reducing pain or fever. Patients hypersensitive to aspirin may be able to tolerate sodium salicylate. Each gram contains 6.25 mEq sodium.

*Usual dose* – 325 to 650 mg every 4 hours.

SODIUM THIOSALICYLATE: Intramuscular administration is preferred.

*Acute gout* – 100 mg every 3 to 4 hours for 2 days, then 100 mg/day until asymptomatic.

*Muscular pain, musculoskeletal disturbances* – 50 to 100 mg/day or on alternate days.

*Rheumatic fever* – 100 to 150 mg every 4 to 8 hours for 3 days, then reduce to 100 mg twice/day. Continue until patient is aymptomatic.

## Actions

*Pharmacology:* Salicylates have analgesic, antipyretic, anti-inflammatory, and antirheumatic effects. Salicylates lower elevated body temperature through vasodilation of peripheral vessels, thus enhancing dissipation of excess heat. The anti-inflammatory and analgesic activity may be mediated through inhibition of the prostaglandin synthetase enzyme complex.

*Aspirin* – Aspirin differs from the other agents in this group in that it more potently inhibits prostaglandin synthesis, has greater anti-inflammatory effects and irreversibly inhibits platelet aggregation.

*Irreversible inhibition of platelet aggregation (aspirin)* – Single analgesic aspirin doses prolong bleeding time. Aspirin (no other salicylates) inhibits platelet aggregation for the life of the platelet (7 to 10 days).

Low doses of aspirin inhibit platelet aggregation and may be more effective than higher doses. Larger doses inhibit cyclooxygenase in arterial walls, interfering with prostacyclin production, a potent vasodilator and inhibitor of platelet aggregation.

*Pharmacokinetics:*

*Absorption/Distribution* – Salicylates are rapidly and completely absorbed after oral use. Bioavailability is dependent on the dosage form, presence of food, gastric emptying time, gastric pH, presence of antacids or buffering agents and particle size. Bioavailability of some enteric coated products may be erratic. Absorption from rectal suppositories is slower, resulting in lower salicylate levels. Protein binding of salicylates is concentration-dependent.

*Metabolism/Excretion* – Salicylic acid is eliminated by renal excretion.

## Contraindications

Hypersensitivity to salicylates or nonsteroidal anti-inflammatory drugs (NSAIDs). Use extreme caution in patients with history of adverse reactions to salicylates. Cross-sensitivity may exist between aspirin and other NSAIDs that inhibit prostaglandin synthesis, and aspirin, and tartrazine. Aspirin cross-sensitivity does not appear to occur with sodium salicylate, salicylamide, or choline salicylate. Aspirin hypersensitivity is more prevalent in those with asthma, nasal polyposis, chronic urticaria.

In hemophilia, bleeding ulcers and hemorrhagic states.

*Magnesium salicylate:* Magnesium salicylate in advanced chronic renal insufficiency because of $Mg^{++}$ retention.

### Warnings

*Otic effects:* Discontinue use if dizziness, ringing in ears (tinnitus), or impaired hearing occurs. Tinnitus probably represents blood salicylic acid levels reaching or exceeding the upper limit of the therapeutic range.

*Use in surgical patients:* Avoid aspirin, if possible, for 1 week prior to surgery because of the possibility of postoperative bleeding.

*Hypersensitivity reactions:* Aspirin intolerance, manifested by acute bronchospasm, generalized urticaria/angioedema, severe rhinitis, or shock occurs in 4% to 19% of asthmatics. Symptoms occur within 3 hours after ingestion. Have epinephrine 1:1000 immediately available.

    *Foods* – Foods may contribute to a reaction. Some foods with 6 mg/100 g salicylate include curry powder, paprika, licorice, Benedictine liqueur, prunes, raisins, tea, and gherkins. A typical American diet contains 10 to 200 mg/day salicylate.

*Hepatic function impairment:* Use caution in liver damage, preexisting hypoprothrombinemia, and vitamin K deficiency.

*Pregnancy:* Category D (aspirin); Category C (salsalate, magnesium salicylate). Avoid use during pregnancy, especially in third trimester.

*Lactation:* Salicylates are excreted in breast milk in low concentrations.

*Children:* Safety and efficacy of **magnesium salicylate** or **salsalate** have not been established. Administration of **aspirin** to children (including teenagers) with acute febrile illness has been associated with the development of Reye's syndrome. Dehydrated febrile children appear more prone to salicylate intoxication.

### Precautions

*Renal effects:* Use with caution in chronic renal insufficiency; aspirin may cause a transient decrease in renal function, and may aggravate chronic kidney diseases (rare).

    In patients with renal impairment, take precautions when administering **magnesium salicylate**.

*GI effects:* Use caution in those intolerant to salicylate because of GI irritation, and in gastric ulcers, peptic ulcer, mild diabetes, gout, erosive gastritis, or bleeding tendencies. **Salsalate** and **choline salicylate** may cause less GI irritation than aspirin.

    Although fecal blood loss is less with enteric coated aspirin than with uncoated, give enteric coated aspirin with caution to patients with GI distress, ulcer, or bleeding problems.

*Hematologic effects:* Aspirin interferes with hemostasis. Avoid use if patients have severe anemia, history of blood coagulation defects, or take anticoagulants.

*Long-term therapy:* To avoid potentially toxic concentrations, warn patients on long-term therapy not to take other salicylates (nonprescription analgesics, etc).

*Salicylism:* Salicylism may require dosage adjustment.

*Controlled-release aspirin:* Controlled-release aspirin, because of its relatively long onset of action, is not recommended for antipyresis or short-term analgesia. Not recommended in children older than 12 years of age; contraindicated in all children with fever accompanied by dehydration.

### Drug Interactions

Drugs that may affect aspirin include activated charcoal, ammonium chloride, ascorbic acid or methionine, antacids and urinary alkalinizers, carbonic anhydrase inhibitors, corticosteroids, and nizatidine. Drugs that may be affected by aspirin include alcohol, ACE inhibitors, anticoagulants (oral), beta-adrenergic blockers, heparin, loop diuretics, methotrexate, nitroglycerin, NSAIDs, probenecid and sulfinpyrazone, spironolactone, sulfonylureas and exogenous insulin, and valproic acid.

*Drug/Lab test interactions:* Salicylates compete with thyroid hormone for binding sites on thyroid binding pre-albumin and possibly thyroid binding globulin resulting in increases in **protein bound iodine**. Salicylates probably do not interfere with $T_3$ resin uptake.

*Serum uric acid* – Serum uric acid levels are elevated by salicylate levels less than 10 mg/dL and decreased by levels more than 10 mg/dL.

Salicylates in moderate to large (anti-inflammatory) doses cause false-negative readings for **urine glucose** by the glucose oxidase method and false-positive readings by the copper reduction method.

Salicylates in the urine interfere with **5-HIAA** determinations by fluorescent methods, but not by the nitrosonaphthol colorimetric method.

Salicylates in the urine interact with **urinary ketone** determinations by the ferric chloride (Gerhardt) method producing a reddish color.

Large doses may decrease urinary excretion of **phenolsulfonphthalein**.

Salicylates in the urine result in falsely elevated **vanillylmandelic acid (VMA)** with most tests, but falsely decrease VMA determinations by the Pisano method.

### Adverse Reactions

Adverse reactions include the following: Hives; rashes; angioedema; nausea, dyspepsia (5% to 25%); heartburn; epigastric discomfort; anorexia; massive GI bleeding; occult blood loss; potentiation of peptic ulcer; persistent iron deficiency anemia; prolongation of bleeding time; leukopenia; thrombocytopenia; purpura; decreased plasma iron concentration; shortened erythrocyte survival time; fever; thirst; dimness of vision.

*Miscellaneous:*

*Mild "salicylism"* – Mild "salicylism" may occur after repeated use of large doses and consists of dizziness, tinnitus, difficulty hearing, nausea, vomiting, diarrhea, mental confusion, CNS depression, headache, sweating, hyperventilation, and lassitude. Salicylate serum concentrations correlate with pharmacological actions and adverse effects observed.

# DIFLUNISAL

**Tablets:** 250 mg and 500 mg (*Rx*)        Various, *Dolobid* (Merck)

### Indications

Acute or long-term symptomatic treatment of mild to moderate pain, rheumatoid arthritis, and osteoarthritis.

### Administration and Dosage

*Mild to moderate pain:* Initially, 1 g, followed by 500 mg every 8 to 12 hours. A lower dosage may be appropriate; for example, 500 mg initially, followed by 250 mg every 8 to 12 hours.

*Osteoarthritis/rheumatoid arthritis:* 500 mg to 1 g/day in 2 divided doses. Individualize dosage. Do not exceed maintenance doses higher than 1.5 g/day.

### Actions

*Pharmacology:* Diflunisal, a salicylic acid derivative, is a nonsteroidal, peripherally acting, nonnarcotic analgesic with anti-inflammatory and antipyretic properties. Chemically, it differs from aspirin and is not metabolized to salicylic acid. Its mechanisms are unknown. Diflunisal is a prostaglandin synthetase inhibitor.

*Pharmacokinetics:* Diflunisal is rapidly and completely absorbed following oral administration; peak plasma concentrations occur between 2 to 3 hours, producing significant analgesia within 1 hour and maximum analgesia within 2 to 3 hours. The first dose tends to have a slower onset of pain relief than other drugs achieving comparable peak effects. Time required to achieve steady state increases with dosage, from 3 to 4 days with 125 mg twice/day to 7 to 9 days with 500 mg twice/day. An initial loading dose shortens the time to reach steady-state levels.

## Contraindications

Hypersensitivity to diflunisal.

Patients in whom acute asthmatic attacks, urticaria, or rhinitis are precipitated by aspirin or other nonsteroidal anti-inflammatory drugs.

## Warnings

*Peptic ulceration:* Peptic ulceration and GI bleeding have been reported. Fatalities occurred rarely.

*Renal function impairment:* Because diflunisal is eliminated primarily by the kidneys, monitor patients with significant renal impairment; use a lower daily dosage.

*Pregnancy: Category C.*

*Lactation:* Diflunisal is excreted in breast milk. Because of the potential for adverse reactions in nursing infants, discontinue either nursing or the drug.

*Children:* Use in children younger than 12 years of age is not recommended.

## Precautions

*Platelet function:* Platelet function and bleeding time are inhibited by diflunisal at higher doses.

*Ophthalmologic effects:* Ophthalmologic effects have been reported with these agents.

*Peripheral edema:* Peripheral edema has been observed. Use with caution in patients with compromised cardiac function, hypertension, or other conditions predisposing to fluid retention.

*Acetylsalicylic acid:* Acetylsalicylic acid has been associated with Reye's syndrome. Because diflunisal is a salicylic acid derivative, the possibility of its association with Reye's syndrome cannot be excluded.

## Drug Interactions

Drug interactions with diflusinol include acetaminophen; anticoagulants, oral; hydrochlorothiazide; indomethacin; sulindac.

## Adverse Reactions

Adverse reactions that occur in 3% or more include nausea, dyspepsia, GI pain, diarrhea, vomiting, headache, rash, fatigue/tiredness, tinnitus.

# DICLOFENAC SODIUM AND MISOPROSTOL

**Tablets**: 50 mg diclofenac sodium/200 mcg misoprostol and    *Arthrotec* (Searle)
75 mg diclofenac sodium/200 mcg misoprostol (*Rx*)

---

**Warning:**

The administration of this product by any route is contraindicated in pregnant women because its misoprostol component can cause abortion.

Reports, primarily from Brazil, of congenital anomalies and fetal death subsequent to use of misoprostol alone, as an abortifacient, have been received.

Patients must be advised of the abortifacient property and warned not to give the drug to others.

Uterine rupture has been reported when misoprostol was administered intravaginally in pregnant women to induce labor or to induce abortion beyond the first trimester of pregnancy.

Uterine perforation has been reported following administration of combined vaginal and oral misoprostol in pregnant women to induce abortion. In each of these reported cases, the gestational age of the pregnancies was unknown.

Do not use in women with childbearing potential unless the patient requires non-steroidal anti-inflammatory drug (NSAID) therapy and is at high risk of developing gastric or duodenal ulceration or of developing complications from gastric or duodenal ulcers associated with the use of the NSAID. In such patients, this drug may be prescribed if the patient:

- Had a negative serum pregnancy test within 2 weeks prior to beginning therapy;
- is capable of complying with effective contraceptive measures;
- has received both oral and written warnings of the hazards of misoprostol, the risk of possible contraception failure, and the danger to other women of childbearing potential should the drug be taken by mistake;
- will begin using this product only on the second or third day of the next normal menstrual period.

---

### Indications

*Arthritis patients at high risk of ulcers:* Treatment of the signs and symptoms of osteoarthritis or rheumatoid arthritis in patients at high risk of developing NSAID-induced gastric and duodenal ulcers and their complications.

### Administration and Dosage

Swallow tablets whole; do not chew, crush, or dissolve. Tablets may be taken with meals to minimize GI effects. Avoid coadministration with magnesium-containing antacids.

Do not exceed a total misoprostol dose of 800 mcg/day, and do not administer more than 200 mcg of misoprostol at any one time.

*Osteoarthritis:* The recommended dose is 50 mg diclofenac/200 mcg misoprostol 3 times/day. For patients who experience intolerance, 50 mg/200 mcg or 75 mg/200 mcg twice/day can be used, but are less effective in preventing ulcers. Do not exceed 150 mg of diclofenac per day.

*Rheumatoid arthritis:* Recommended dose is 50 mg diclofenac/200 mcg misoprostol 3 or 4 times/day. For patients who experience intolerance, 50 mg/200 mcg or 75 mg/200 mcg twice/day can be used, but are less effective in preventing ulcers. Do not exceed 225 mg of diclofenac per day.

*Special dosing considerations:* For gastric ulcer prevention, 200 mcg 3 and 4 times/day are therapeutically equivalent but more protective than the twice-daily regimen. For duodenal ulcer prevention, 4 times/day is more protective than the 2 or 3 times/day regimens. However, the 4 times/day regimen is less well tolerated.

Dosages may be individualized using the separate products (misoprostol and diclofenac), after which the patient may be changed to the appropriate diclofenac/misoprostol dose. If clinically indicated, misoprostol co-therapy with diclofenac/misoprostol or use of the individual components to optimize the misoprostol dose or frequency of administration may be appropriate.

### Actions
*Pharmacology:* This product is a combination containing diclofenac sodium, an NSAID with analgesic properties, and misoprostol, a GI mucosal protective prostaglandin $E_1$ analog.

*Pharmacokinetics:* The pharmacokinetics following oral administration of a single dose or multiple doses of diclofenac/misoprostol to healthy subjects under fasted conditions are similar to the pharmacokinetics of the 2 individual components. Food decreases the multiple-dose bioavailability profile of both formulations.

### Contraindications
Hypersensitivity to diclofenac or to misoprostol or other prostaglandins. Do not give to patients who have experienced asthma, urticaria, or other allergic-type reactions after taking aspirin or other NSAIDs.

### Warnings
*Pregnancy:* Category X.

*Lactation:* Diclofenac sodium is found in the milk of breastfeeding mothers. Because of the potential for serious adverse reactions in nursing infants, this product is not recommended for breastfeeding mothers.

*Children:* Safety and efficacy in patients younger than 18 years of age have not been established.

### Adverse Reactions
Adverse reactions reported in at least 3% of patients include the following: Abdominal pain, diarrhea, dyspepsia, nausea, flatulence.

# NAPROXEN AND LANSOPRAZOLE

**Tablets and Capsules, delayed release:** 375 naproxen/ 15 mg lansoprazole and 500 mg naproxen/15 mg lansoprazole (*Rx*)
*Prevacid NapraPAC 375* and *Prevacid NapraPAC 500** (TAP Pharmaceuticals)

* In weekly (7-day) blister cards containing 14 *Naprosyn* tablets and 7 *Prevacid* capsules and in 1-month administration packs containing 4 weekly blister cards.

### Indications
*Nonsteroidal anti-inflammatory drug (NSAID)-associated gastric ulcers:* For reducing the risk of NSAID-associated gastric ulcers in patients with a history of documented gastric ulcer who require the use of an NSAID for treatment of the signs and symptoms of rheumatoid arthritis, osteoarthritis, and ankylosing spondylitis.

### Administration and Dosage
Each daily dose consists of one 15 mg lansoprazole capsule and 2 of either 375 or 500 mg naproxen tablets. Take the lansoprazole capsule and 1 of the naproxen tablets before eating in the morning with a glass of water. Take the second naproxen tablet in the evening with a glass of water. The maximum daily naproxen dose of naproxen/lansoprazole is 1000 mg.

Swallow lansoprazole delayed-release capsules whole. Do not chew or crush.

*Dosage adjustment:* For naproxen/lansoprazole, no adjustment of the 15 mg lansoprazole component is necessary in patients with renal insufficiency or for the elderly. However, consider dose adjustment for the naproxen component for patients with renal insufficiency, liver disease, or the elderly.

# NONSTEROIDAL ANTI-INFLAMMATORY AGENTS

**CELECOXIB**
**Capsules**: 100 and 200 mg (*Rx*) — *Celebrex* (Searle)

**DICLOFENAC**
**Tablets**: 50 mg (as potassium) (*Rx*) — Various, *Cataflam* (Novartis)
**Tablets, delayed-release**: 25, 50, and 75 mg (as sodium) (*Rx*) — Various, *Voltaren* (Novartis)
**Tablets, extended-release**: 100 mg (as sodium) (*Rx*) — *Voltaren-XR* (Novartis)

**ETODOLAC**
**Capsules**: 200 and 300 mg (*Rx*) — Various, *Lodine* (Wyeth-Ayerst)
**Tablets**: 400 and 500 mg (*Rx*) — Various, *Lodine* (Wyeth-Ayerst)
**Tablets, extended-release**: 400, 500, and 600 mg — *Lodine XL* (Wyeth-Ayerst)

**FENOPROFEN CALCIUM**
**Capsules**: 200 and 300 mg (*Rx*) — Various, *Nalfon Pulvules* (Ranbaxy)
**Tablets**: 600 mg (*Rx*) — Various

**FLURBIPROFEN**
**Tablets**: 50 and 100 mg (*Rx*) — Various, *Ansaid* (Pharmacia)

**IBUPROFEN**
**Tablets**: 100 mg (*otc*) — *Junior Strength Motrin* (McNeil)
200 mg (*otc*) — Various, *Advil* (Whitehall-Robins), *Genpril* (Goldline), *Maximum Strength Midol* (Bayer), *Menadol* (Rugby), *Motrin IB* (McNeil), *Nuprin* (Bristol-Myers Squibb)
400, 600, and 800 mg (*Rx*) — Various, *Motrin* (Pharmacia)
**Tablets, chewable**: 50 and 100 mg (*otc*) — *Children's Advil* (Whitehall-Robins), *Children's Motrin* (McNeil), *Jr. Strength Motrin* (McNeil), *Jr. Strength Advil* (Whitehall-Robins)
**Capsules**: 200 mg (*otc*) — *Advil Liqui-Gels* (Whitehall-Robins)
**Suspension**: 100 mg/5 mL (*Rx*) — *Children's Advil* (Wyeth-Ayerst)
100 mg/5 mL (*otc*) — Various, *Children's Motrin* (McNeil-CPC), *PediaCare Fever* (Pharmacia)
100 mg/2.5 mL (*otc*) — *Pediatric Advil Drops* (Wyeth-Ayerst)
**Oral drops**: 40 mg/mL (*otc*) — *Infants' Motrin* (McNeil), *PediaCare Fever* (Pharmacia)

**INDOMETHACIN**
**Capsules**: 25 and 50 mg (*Rx*) — Various, *Indocin* (Merck)
**Capsules, sustained-release**: 75 mg (*Rx*) — Various, *Indocin SR* (Forte Pharma)
**Oral suspension**: 25 mg/5 mL (*Rx*) — *Indocin* (Merck)
**Suppositories**: 50 mg (*Rx*) — *Indocin* (Merck)

**KETOPROFEN**
**Tablets**: 12.5 mg (*otc*) — *Orudis KT* (Whitehall-Robins)
**Capsules**: 25, 50, and 75 mg (*Rx*) — Various, *Orudis* (Wyeth-Ayerst)
**Capsules, extended-release**: 100, 150, and 200 mg (*Rx*) — *Oruvail* (Wyeth-Ayerst)

**KETOROLAC TROMETHAMINE**
**Tablets**: 10 mg (*Rx*) — Various, *Toradol* (Roche)
**Injection**: 15 and 30 mg/mL (*Rx*) — *Toradol* (Roche)

**MECLOFENAMATE SODIUM**
**Capsules**: 50 and 100 mg (as sodium) (*Rx*) — Various

**MEFENAMIC ACID**
**Capsules**: 250 mg (*Rx*) — *Ponstel* (Parke-Davis)

**MELOXICAM**
**Tablets**: 7.5 mg (*Rx*) — *Mobic* (Boehringer Ingelheim/Abbott)

**NABUMETONE**
**Tablets**: 500 and 750 mg (*Rx*) — Various, *Relafen* (GlaxoSmithKline)

## NAPROXEN

| | |
|---|---|
| **Tablets**: 200 mg (as naproxen sodium) (*otc*) | Various, *Aleve* (Bayer) |
| 250 and 500 mg (as naproxen sodium) (*Rx*) | Various, *Anaprox* (Roche) |
| 250, 375, and 500 mg (*Rx*) | Various, *Naprosyn* (Roche) |
| **Tablets, delayed-release**: 375 and 500 mg (*Rx*) | Various, *EC-Naprosyn* (Roche) |
| **Tablets, controlled-release**: 375 (412.5 mg naproxen sodium) and 500 mg (550 mg naproxen sodium) (*Rx*) | *Naprelan* (Carnrick Laboratories) |
| **Suspension**: 125 mg/5 mL (*Rx*) | Various, *Naprosyn* (Roche) |

## OXAPROZIN

| | |
|---|---|
| **Tablets**: 600 mg (*Rx*) | *Daypro* (Searle) |

## PIROXICAM

| | |
|---|---|
| **Capsules**: 10 and 20 mg (*Rx*) | Various, *Feldene* (Pfizer) |

## SULINDAC

| | |
|---|---|
| **Tablets**: 150 and 200 mg (*Rx*) | Various, *Clinoril* (Merck) |

## TOLMETIN SODIUM

| | |
|---|---|
| **Tablets**: 200 and 600 mg (as sodium) (*Rx*) | Various, *Tolectin 200*, *Tolectin 600* (McNeil) |
| **Capsules**: 400 mg (as sodium) (*Rx*) | Various |

## VALDECOXIB

| | |
|---|---|
| **Tablets**: 10 and 20 mg (*Rx*) | *Bextra* (Searle) |

### Indications

**NSAIDs: Summary of Indications**

| Indications (✔ - Labeled) | Celecoxib | Diclofenac potassium | Diclofenac sodium/ Diclofenac sodium XR | Etodolac | Fenoprofen | Flurbiprofen | Ibuprofen | Indomethacin | Indomethacin SR | Ketoprofen | Ketoprofen SR | Ketorolac | Meclofenamate | Mefenamic acid | Meloxicam | Nabumetone | Naproxen | Oxaprozin | Piroxicam | Sulindac | Tolmetin | Valdecoxib |
|---|---|---|---|---|---|---|---|---|---|---|---|---|---|---|---|---|---|---|---|---|---|---|
| Rheumatoid arthritis (RA) | ✔ | ✔ | ✔ | ✔ | ✔ | ✔ | ✔ | ✔ | ✔ | ✔ | ✔ | | ✔ | | | ✔ | ✔ | ✔ | ✔ | ✔ | ✔ | ✔ |
| Osteoarthritis (OA) | ✔ | ✔ | ✔ | ✔ | ✔ | ✔ | ✔ | ✔ | ✔ | ✔ | ✔ | | ✔ | | ✔ | ✔ | ✔ | ✔ | ✔ | ✔ | ✔ | ✔ |
| Ankylosing spondylitis | | ✔ | ✔[1] | | | | | ✔ | ✔ | | | | | | | | ✔ | | | ✔ | | |
| Mild to moderate pain | | ✔ | | | ✔ | ✔ | | ✔ | | | | | ✔ | ✔[2] | | | ✔ | | | | | |
| Moderately severe acute pain | | | | | | | | | | | | ✔[3] | | | | | | | | | | |
| Primary dysmenorrhea | | ✔ | | | | | ✔ | | | ✔ | | | ✔ | ✔ | | | ✔ | | | | | ✔ |
| Juvenile RA | | | | | | | ✔ | | | | | | | | | | ✔ | | | | ✔ | |
| Tendinitis | | | | | | | | ✔ | ✔ | | | | | | | | ✔ | | | ✔ | | |
| Bursitis | | | | | | | | ✔ | ✔ | | | | | | | | ✔ | | | ✔ | | |
| Acute painful shoulder | | | | | | | | ✔ | ✔ | | | | | | | | | | | ✔ | | |
| Acute gout | | | | | | | | ✔ | | | | | | | | | ✔ | | | ✔ | | |
| Fever | | | | | | | ✔[4] | | | | | | | | | | | | | | | |
| Closure of persistent patent ductus arteriosus | | | | | | | | ✔[5] | | | | | | | | | | | | | | |

[1] Sodium only, not sodium XR.
[2] Therapy not to exceed 1 week.
[3] Therapy not to exceed 5 days.
[4] In children only.
[5] IV formulation only.

*Rheumatoid arthritis (RA) (except **ketorolac, mefenamic acid,** and **meloxicam**) and osteoarthritis (OA) (except ketorolac and mefenamic acid):* Relief of signs and symptoms; treatment of acute flares and exacerbation; long-term management.

*Concomitant therapy* – Concomitant therapy with other second-line drugs (eg, gold salts) demonstrates additional therapeutic benefit. Whether they can be used with partially effective doses of corticosteroids for a "steroid-sparing" effect and result in greater improvement is not established.

Use with salicylates is not recommended; greater benefit is not achieved, and the potential for adverse reactions is increased. The use of aspirin with nonsteroidal anti-inflammatory agents (NSAIDs) may cause a decrease in blood levels of the nonaspirin drug.

*Juvenile RA* – **Tolmetin, naproxen.**

*Mild to moderate pain (**diclofenac potassium, etodolac, fenoprofen, ibuprofen, ketoprofen, ketorolac, meclofenamate, mefenamic acid, naproxen, naproxen sodium**):* Postextraction dental pain, postsurgical episiotomy pain, and soft tissue athletic injuries.

*Primary dysmenorrhea:* **Diclofenac potassium, ibuprofen, ketoprofen, mefenamic acid, naproxen, naproxen sodium, valdecoxib.**

*Idiopathic heavy menstrual blood loss:* **Meclofenamate sodium.**

*Familial adenomatous polyposis (FAP) (**celecoxib**):* To reduce the number of adenomatous colorectal polyps in FAP as an adjunct to usual care (eg, endoscopic surveillance, surgery). It is not known whether there is a clinical benefit from a reduction in the number of colorectal polyps in FAP patients. It also is not known whether the effects of celecoxib treatment will persist after celecoxib is discontinued. The efficacy and safety of celecoxib treatment in patients with FAP longer than 6 months have not been studied.

## Administration and Dosage

CELECOXIB: Seek the lowest dose for each patient. Safety and efficacy in children younger than 18 years of age have not been evaluated.

*Osteoarthritis* – Recommended oral dosage is 200 mg/day administered as a single dose or as 100 mg twice a day.

*Rheumatoid arthritis* – Recommended oral dosage is 100 to 200 mg twice a day.

*FAP* – Continue usual medical care for FAP patients while on celecoxib. To reduce the number of adenomatous colorectal polyps in patients with FAP, the recommended oral dose is 400 mg/day. Take with food.

DICLOFENAC:

*Osteoarthritis* – 100 to 150 mg/day in divided doses (50 mg twice/day or 3 times/day [diclofenac sodium or potassium] or 75 mg twice/day [diclofenac sodium]). Dosages greater than 200 mg/day have not been studied.

*Rheumatoid arthritis* – 150 to 200 mg/day in divided doses (50 mg 3 or 4 times/day [diclofenac sodium or potassium] or 75 mg twice/day [diclofenac sodium]). Dosages greater than 225 mg/day of the delayed-release diclofenac sodium formulation and dosages greater than 200 mg/day of immediate-release diclofenac potassium formulation are not recommended.

*Ankylosing spondylitis* – 100 to 125 mg/day as 25 mg 4 times/day, with an extra 25 mg dose at bedtime, if necessary. Dosages greater than 125 mg/day have not been studied.

*Analgesia and primary dysmenorrhea (diclofenac potassium only)* – Recommended starting dose is 50 mg 3 times/day. In some patients, an initial dose of 100 mg followed by 50 mg doses will provide better relief. After the first day, when the maximum recommended dose may be 200 mg, the total daily dose generally should not exceed 150 mg.

ETODOLAC:

*Osteoarthritis* – Initially 600 to 1200 mg/day in divided doses, followed by adjustment in the range of 600 to 1200 mg/day in divided doses (400 mg 2 or 3 times/day; 300 mg 2, 3, or 4 times/day; 200 mg 3 or 4 times/day). Do not exceed 1200 mg/day.

*Patients weighing 60 kg or less:* Do not exceed 20 mg/kg.

*Analgesia* –

*Acute pain:* 200 to 400 mg every 6 to 8 hours. Do not exceed 1200 mg/day.

*Patients weighing 60 kg or less:* Do not exceed 20 mg/kg.

FENOPROFEN: Do not exceed 3.2 g/day. If GI upset occurs, take with meals or milk.

*Rheumatoid arthritis and osteoarthritis* – 300 to 600 mg 3 or 4 times/day.

*Mild to moderate pain* – 200 mg every 4 to 6 hours, as needed.

FLURBIPROFEN:
   *Rheumatoid arthritis and osteoarthritis* – Initial recommended total daily dose is 200 to 300 mg; administer in divided doses 2, 3, or 4 times/day. The largest recommended single dose in a multiple-dose daily regimen is 100 mg. Doses greater than 300 mg/day are not recommended.

IBUPROFEN:
   *Adults* – Do not exceed 3.2 g/day. If GI upset occurs, take with meals or milk.
      *Rheumatoid arthritis and osteoarthritis:* 1.2 to 3.2 g/day (300 mg 4 times/day or 400, 600, or 800 mg 3 or 4 times/day).
      *Mild to moderate pain:* 400 mg every 4 to 6 hours, as necessary.
      *Primary dysmenorrhea:* 400 mg every 4 hours, as necessary.
      *OTC use (minor aches and pains, dysmenorrhea, fever reduction):* 200 mg every 4 to 6 hours while symptoms persist. If pain or fever do not respond to 200 mg, 400 mg may be used. Do not exceed 1.2 g in 24 hours. Do not take for pain for longer than 10 days or for fever for longer than 3 days unless directed.
   *Children* –
      *Juvenile arthritis:* Usual dose is 30 to 40 mg/kg/day in 3 or 4 divided doses; 20 mg/kg/day may be adequate for milder disease. Doses greater than 50 mg/kg/day are not recommended.
      *Fever reduction/pain relief in children 6 months to 12 years of age:* Adjust dosage on the basis of the initial temperature level. If baseline temperature is 39.2°C (102.5°F) or lower, recommended dose is 5 mg/kg; if baseline temperature is higher than 39.2°C (102.5°F), recommended dose is 10 mg/kg. Duration of fever reduction is longer with the higher dose. Maximum daily dosage is 40 mg/kg.

INDOMETHACIN:
   *Moderate to severe rheumatoid arthritis (including acute flares of chronic disease), ankylosing spondylitis, and osteoarthritis* – 25 mg 2 or 3 times/day. If this is well tolerated, increase the daily dose by 25 or 50 mg (if required by continuing symptoms) at weekly intervals until a satisfactory response is obtained or until a daily dose of 150 to 200 mg is reached. Doses above this amount generally do not increase the effectiveness of the drug.
   In patients who have persistent night pain or morning stiffness, giving a large portion, up to a maximum of 100 mg of the total daily dose at bedtime, may help to relieve pain. The total daily dose should not exceed 200 mg.
   In acute flares of chronic rheumatoid arthritis, it may be necessary to increase the dosage by 25 or 50 mg/day.
   *Acute painful shoulder (bursitis or tendinitis)* – 75 to 150 mg/day in 3 or 4 divided doses. Discontinue the drug after inflammation has been controlled for several days. Usual course of therapy is 7 to 14 days.
   *Acute gouty arthritis* – 50 mg 3 times/day until pain is tolerable, then rapidly reduce the dose to complete cessation of the drug. Definite relief of pain usually occurs within 2 to 4 hours. Tenderness and heat usually subside in 24 to 36 hours, and swelling gradually disappears in 3 to 5 days. Do not use sustained-release form.
   *Sustained-release form* – Do not crush. The 75 mg sustained-release capsule can be taken once/day as an alternative to the 25 mg capsule 3 times/day. In addition, one 75 mg sustained-release capsule twice/day can be substituted for the 50 mg capsule 3 times/day. Do not use sustained-release form in acute gouty arthritis.
   *Children* – Efficacy in children 14 years of age and younger has not been established except in circumstances that warrant the risk. When using in children 2 years of age and older, closely monitor liver function. Suggested starting dose is 2 mg/kg/day in divided doses. Do not exceed 4 mg/kg/day or 150 to 200 mg/day, whichever is less.

KETOPROFEN: Take with antacids, food, or milk to minimize adverse GI effects.
   *Rheumatoid arthritis and osteoarthritis* – Do not exceed 300 mg/day for regular-release formulation or 200 mg/day for extended-release capsules.
      *Daily dose:* 150 to 300 mg divided into 3 or 4 doses.
      *Starting dose:* 75 mg 3 times/day or 50 mg 4 times/day. Reduce initial dose to ½ to ⅓ in elderly or debilitated patients or those with impaired renal function.

*Mild to moderate pain, primary dysmenorrhea* – 25 to 50 mg every 6 to 8 hours as needed. Give smaller dosages initially to smaller patients, the elderly, and those with renal or liver disease. Doses above 50 mg may be given, but doses above 75 mg do not display added therapeutic effects. Do not exceed 300 mg/day.

*OTC* –

*Adults:* 12.5 mg with a full glass of liquid every 4 to 6 hours. If pain or fever persists after 1 hour, follow with 12.5 mg. With experience, some patients may find an initial dose of 25 mg will give better relief. Do not exceed 25 mg in a 4- to 6-hour period or 75 mg in a 24-hour period.

*Children:* Do not give to those younger than 16 years of age unless directed by a physician.

KETOROLAC TROMETHAMINE: The combined duration of ketorolac IV/IM and oral is not to exceed 5 days. Oral use is only indicated as combination therapy to IV/IM.

*IV/IM* – When administering IV/IM, the IV bolus must be given over no less than 15 seconds. Give IM administration slowly and deeply into the muscle.

*Single-dose treatment:* Limit following regimen to single administration use only.

IM dosing –

*Younger than 65 years of age:* One 60 mg dose.

*65 years of age or older, renal impairment, or weight less than 50 kg (110 lbs):* One 30 mg dose.

IV dosing –

*Younger than 65 years of age:* One 30 mg dose.

*65 years of age or older, renal impairment, or weight less than 50 kg (110 lbs):* One 15 mg dose.

*Multiple-dose treatment:*

*Younger than 65 years of age* – The recommended dose is 30 mg every 6 hours. The maximum daily dose should not exceed 120 mg.

*65 years of age or older, renal impairment, or weight less than 50 kg (110 lbs)* – The recommended dose is 15 mg every 6 hours. The maximum daily dose for these populations should not exceed 60 mg.

*Oral* – Indicated only as continuation therapy to ketorolac IV/IM.

*Transition from IV/IM to oral:*

*Younger than 65 years of age* – 20 mg as a first oral dose for patients who received 60 mg IM single dose, 30 mg single IV dose, or 30 mg multiple dose IV/IM followed by 10 mg every 4 to 6 hours, not to exceed 40 mg in 24 hours.

*65 years of age or older, renal impairment, or weight less than 50 kg (110 lbs)* – 10 mg as a first oral dose for patients who received a 30 mg IM single dose, 15 mg IV single dose, or 15 mg multiple dose IV/IM followed by 10 mg every 4 to 6 hours, not to exceed 40 mg in 24 hours.

MECLOFENAMATE SODIUM:

*Mild to moderate pain* – 50 mg every 4 to 6 hours. Doses of 100 mg may be required for optimal pain relief. Do not exceed daily dosage of 400 mg.

*Excessive menstrual blood loss and primary dysmenorrhea* – 100 mg 3 times/day for up to 6 days, starting at the onset of menstrual flow.

*Rheumatoid arthritis and osteoarthritis* –

*Usual dosage:* 200 to 400 mg/day in 3 or 4 equal doses.

*Initial dosage:* Initiate at lower dosage; increase as needed to improve response. Do not exceed 400 mg/day.

*Children* – Safety and efficacy in children younger than 14 years of age are not established.

MEFENAMIC ACID:

*Acute pain* –

*Adults (14 years of age or older):* 500 mg, then 250 mg every 6 hours, as needed, usually not to exceed 1 week. Give with food.

*Primary dysmenorrhea* – 500 mg, then 250 mg every 6 hours. Start with the onset of bleeding and associated symptoms. Should not be necessary for longer than 2 to 3 days.

*Children* – Safety and efficacy in children younger than 14 years have not been established.

MELOXICAM:

*Osteoarthritis* – Use the lowest dosage for each patient. For treatment of osteoarthritis, the recommended starting and maintenance dose is 7.5 mg once/day. Some patients may receive additional benefit by increasing the dose to 15 mg once/day. The maximum recommended dose is 15 mg/day. Meloxicam may be taken without regard to meals.

NABUMETONE: Recommended starting dose is 1000 mg as a single dose with or without food. Some patients may obtain more symptomatic relief from 1500 to 2000 mg/day. Nabumetone can be given either once or twice/day. Dosages greater than 2000 mg/day have not been studied.

NAPROXEN:

*Rx* – Do not exceed 1.25 g/day naproxen (1.375 g/day naproxen sodium).

*Rheumatoid arthritis, osteoarthritis, ankylosing spondylitis, pain, dysmenorrhea, acute tendinitis, and bursitis:*

*Naproxen* – 250 to 500 mg twice/day. May increase to 1.5 g/day for limited periods.

*Delayed-release naproxen (EC-Naprosyn)* – 375 to 500 mg twice/day. Do not break, crush, or chew tablets.

*Controlled-release naproxen (Naprelan)* – 750 mg or 1500 mg once/day. Do not exceed 1000 mg/day.

*Naproxen sodium* – 275 to 550 mg twice/day. May increase to 1.65 g for limited periods.

*Juvenile arthritis:*

*Naproxen only (not naproxen sodium)* – Total daily dose is approximately 10 mg/kg in 2 divided doses.

*Suspension:* Use the following as a guide:

| Naproxen Suspension: Children's Dose | |
| --- | --- |
| Child's weight | Dose |
| 13 kg (29 lb) | 2.5 mL (0.5 tsp) bid |
| 25 kg (55 lb) | 5 mL (1 tsp) bid |
| 38 kg (84 lb) | 7.5 mL (1.5 tsp) bid |

*Acute gout:*

*Naproxen* – 750 mg, followed by 250 mg every 8 hours until attack subsides.

*Naproxen sodium* – 825 mg, then 275 mg every 8 hours until attack subsides.

*Controlled-release naproxen (Naprelan)* – 1000 to 1500 mg once/day on the first day, followed by 1000 mg once/day until the attack has subsided.

*Mild to moderate pain, primary dysmenorrhea, acute tendinitis, and bursitis:*

*Naproxen* – 500 mg, followed by 250 mg every 6 to 8 hours. Do not exceed a 1.25 g total daily dose. Thereafter, total daily dose should not exceed 1000 mg.

*Naproxen sodium* – 550 mg, followed by 275 mg every 6 to 8 hours. Do not exceed a 1.375 g total daily dose.

*Controlled-release naproxen (Naprelan)* – 1000 mg once daily. For patients requiring greater analgesic benefit, 1500 mg/day may be used for a limited period.

*Children:* Safety and efficacy in children younger than 2 years of age have not been established.

OTC –

*Adults:* 200 mg with a full glass of liquid every 8 to 12 hours while symptoms persist. With experience, some patients may find that an initial dose of 400 mg followed by 200 mg 12 hours later, if necessary, will give better relief. Do not exceed 600 mg in 24 hours unless otherwise directed.

*Elderly (older than 65 years of age):* Do not take greater than 200 mg every 12 hours.

*Children:* Do not give to children younger than 12 years of age except under the advice and supervision of a physician.

OXAPROZIN:
 *Rheumatoid arthritis* – 1200 mg once/day.

 *Osteoarthritis* – 1200 mg once/day. For patients of low body weight or with milder disease, an initial dosage of 600 mg once/day may be appropriate.

 *Maximum dose* – 1800 mg/day (or 26 mg/kg, whichever is lower) in divided doses.

PIROXICAM: Initiate and maintain at a single daily dose of 20 mg. May divide daily dose. Do not assess effect of therapy for 2 weeks.

 *Children* – Use in children has not been established.

SULINDAC: Administer twice/day with food. The usual maximum dosage is 400 mg/day. Dosages above 400 mg/day are not recommended.

 *Osteoarthritis, rheumatoid arthritis, and ankylosing spondylitis* – Initial dosage is 150 mg twice a day.

 *Acute painful shoulder (acute subacromial bursitis/supraspinatus tendinitis) and acute gouty arthritis* – 200 mg twice/day. After satisfactory response, reduce dosage accordingly.

 *Children* – Safety and efficacy have not been established.

TOLMETIN SODIUM:
 *Adults* –

  *Rheumatoid arthritis and osteoarthritis:* Initially, 400 mg 3 times/day; preferably include dose on arising and at bedtime. Control is usually achieved at doses of 600 to 1800 mg/day generally in 3 divided doses. Doses greater than 1800 mg/day are not recommended.

 *Children* –

  *(2 years of age or older):* Initially, 20 mg/kg/day in 3 or 4 divided doses. When control is achieved, usual dosage ranges from 15 to 30 mg/kg/day. Doses greater than 30 mg/kg/day are not recommended.

VALDECOXIB:
 *Osteoarthritis/Adult rheumatoid arthritis* – 10 mg once/day.

 *Primary dysmenorrhea* – 20 mg twice/day, as needed.

**Actions**

 *Pharmacology:* Nonsteroidal anti-inflammatory drugs have analgesic, antipyretic, and anti-inflammatory activities. Major mechanism is believed to be inhibition of cyclooxygenase activity and prostaglandin synthesis.

 Two COX isoenzymes have been identified: COX-1 and COX-2. Inhibition of COX-1 activity is considered a major contributor to NSAID GI toxicity. The function of the COX-2 isoenzyme is induced during pain and inflammatory stimuli.

 Many NSAIDs inhibit both COX-1 and COX-2. Most NSAIDs are mainly COX-1 selective (eg, **aspirin, ketoprofen, indomethacin, piroxicam, sulindac**). Others are considered slightly selective for COX-1 (eg, **ibuprofen, naproxen, diclofenac**) and others may be considered slightly selective for COX-2 (eg, **etodolac, nabumetone**). The mechanism of action of **celecoxib** and **valdecoxib** is primarily selective inhibition of COX-2.

*Pharmacokinetics:*

| Pharmacokinetic Parameters/Maximum Dosage Recommendations of NSAIDs | | | | | | | | |
|---|---|---|---|---|---|---|---|---|
| NSAID | Bioavailability (%) | Half-life (hours) | Volume of distribution | Clearance | Peak (hours) | Protein binding (%) | Renal elimination (%) | Fecal elimination (%) |
| *Acetic acids* | | | | | | | | |
| Diclofenac | 50 to 60 | 2 | 0.1 to 0.2 L/kg | 350 mL/min | 2 | > 99 | 65 | - |
| Indomethacin | 98 | 4.5 | 0.29 L/kg | 0.084 L/h/kg | 2 | 90 | 60 | 33 |
| Sulindac | 90 | 7.8 | NS[1] | ≈ 2.71 L/h | 2 to 4 | > 93 | 50 | 25 |
| Tolmetin | NS[1] | 2 to 7 | NS[1] | NS[1] | 0.5 to 1 | NS [1] | ≈ 100 | - |

| Pharmacokinetic Parameters/Maximum Dosage Recommendations of NSAIDs | | | | | | | | |
|---|---|---|---|---|---|---|---|---|
| NSAID | Bioavail-ability (%) | Half-life (hours) | Volume of distri-bution | Clearance | Peak (hours) | Protein binding (%) | Renal elimina-tion (%) | Fecal elimina-tion (%) |
| *COX-2 inhibitors* | | | | | | | | |
| Celecoxib | NS[1] | 11 | 400 L | 27.7 L/h | 3 | 97 | 27 | 57 |
| Valdecoxib | 83 | 8 to 11 | ≈ 86 L | ≈ 6 L/h | ≈ 3 | ≈ 98 | ≈ 90 | < 5 |
| *Fenamates* | | | | | | | | |
| Meclofena-mate | ≈ 100 | 1.3 | 23 L | 206 mL/min | 0.5 to 2 | > 99 | 70 | 30 |
| Mefenamic acid | NS[1] | 2 | 1.06 L/kg | 21.23 L/h | 2 to 4 | > 90 | 52 | 20 |
| *Naphthylalkanones* | | | | | | | | |
| Nambum-etone | > 80 | 22.5 | 0.1 to 0.2 L/kg | 26.1 mL/min | 9 to 12 | > 99 | 80 | 9 |
| *Oxicams* | | | | | | | | |
| Piroxicam | NS[1] | 50 | 0.15 L/kg | 0.002 to 0.003 L/kg/h | 3 to 5 | 98.5 | NS[1] | NS[1] |
| Meloxicam | 89 | 15 to 20 | 10 L | 7 to 9 mL/min | 4 to 5 | 99.4 | 50 | 50 |
| *Propionic acids* | | | | | | | | |
| Fenoprofen | NS[1] | 3 | NS[1] | NS[1] | 2 | 99 | 90 | - |
| Flurbiprofen | NS[1] | 5.7 | 0.1 to 0.2 L/kg | 1.13 L/h | ≈ 1.5 | > 99 | > 70 | - |
| Ibuprofen | > 80 | 1.8 to 2 | 0.15 L/kg | ≈ 3 to 3.5 L/h | 1 to 2 | 99 | 45 to 79 | - |
| Ketoprofen | 90 | 2.1 | 0.1 L/kg | 6.9 L/h | 0.5 to 2 | > 99 | 80 | - |
| Ketoprofen ER | 90 | 5.4 | 0.1 L/kg | 6.8 L/h | 6 to 7 | > 99 | 80 | - |
| Naproxen | 95 | 12 to 17 | 0.16 L/kg | 0.13 mL/min/kg | 2 to 4 | > 99 | 95 | - |
| Oxaprozin | 95 | 42 to 50 | 10 to 12.5 L | 0.25 to 0.34 L/h | 3 to 5 | > 99 | 65 | 35 |
| *Pyranocarboxylic acid* | | | | | | | | |
| Etodolac | ≥ 80 | 7.3 | 0.362 L/kg | 47 mL/h/kg | ≈ 1.5 | > 99 | 72 | 16 |
| *Pyrrolizine carboxylic acid* | | | | | | | | |
| Ketorolac | 100 | 5 to 6 | ≈ 0.2 L/kg | ≈ 0.025 L/h/kg | 2 to 3 | 99 | 91 | 6 |

[1] NS = Not studied.

**Contraindications**

*NSAID hypersensitivity:* Because of potential cross-sensitivity to other NSAIDs, do not give these agents to patients in whom aspirin or other NSAIDs have induced symptoms of asthma, rhinitis, urticaria, nasal polyps, angioedema, bronchospasm, and other symptoms of allergic or anaphylactoid reactions. Severe, rarely fatal, anaphylactic-like and asthmatic reactions have been reported in such patients receiving NSAIDs.

*Fenoprofen or mefenamic acid:* Pre-existing renal disease.

*Mefenamic acid:* Active ulceration or chronic inflammation of the upper or lower GI tract.

*Indomethacin suppositories:* History of proctitis or recent rectal bleeding.

*Valdecoxib and celecoxib:* Hypersensitivity to sulfonamides.

*Ketorolac:* Active peptic ulcer disease; recent GI bleeding or perforation; history of peptic ulcer disease or GI bleeding; advanced renal impairment or patients at risk for renal failure because of volume depletion; labor and delivery; nursing mothers; previously demonstrated hypersensitivity to ketorolac tromethamine; as prophylactic analgesic before any major surgery; intraoperatively when hemostasis is critical because of the increased risk of bleeding; suspected or confirmed cerebrovascular bleeding, hemorrhagic diathesis, incomplete hemostasis, and those at high risk of bleeding; patients currently receiving ASA or NSAIDs because of the cumulative risks of inducing serious NSAID-related adverse events; for neuraxial (epidural or intrathecal) administration; concomitant use with probenecid. Severe, rarely fatal anaphylactic-like and asthmatic reactions have been reported in such patients receiving NSAIDs.

**Warnings**

*Ketorolac tromethamine:* Ketorolac is indicated for the short-term (up to 5 days) management of moderately severe acute pain that requires analgesia at the opioid level. It is not indicated for minor or chronic painful conditions. Increasing the dose beyond the label recommendations will not provide better efficacy but will result in increasing risk of developing serious adverse events.

*GI effects* – Do not use ketorolac in active peptic ulcer disease, recent GI bleeding or perforation, a history of peptic ulcer disease, or GI bleeding.

*Renal effects* – Ketorolac is contraindicated in patients with advanced renal impairment and in patients at risk for renal failure because of volume depletion.

*Risk of bleeding* – Ketorolac inhibits platelet function and, therefore, is contraindicated in patients with suspected or confirmed cerebrovascular bleeding, hemorrhagic diathesis, and incomplete hemostasis, and in those at high risk of bleeding.

Ketorolac is contraindicated as prophylactic analgesia before any major surgery and is contraindicated intra-operatively when hemostasis is critical because of the increased risk of bleeding.

*Hypersensitivity* – Hypersensitivity reactions, ranging from bronchospasm to anaphylactic shock, have occurred.

*Intrathecal or epidural administration* – Ketorolac is contraindicated for intrathecal or epidural administration because of its alcohol content.

*Labor and delivery and lactation* – Use in labor and delivery and lactation is contraindicated.

*Concomitant use with NSAIDs* – Ketorolac is contraindicated in patients currently receiving aspirin or other NSAIDs because of the cumulative risk of inducing serious NSAID-related side effects; ketorolac also is contraindicated with the concomitant use of probenecid.

*Administration and dosage* – Ketorolac (oral) is indicated only as continuation therapy to ketorolac IV/IM; the combined duration of use of IV/IM and oral is not to exceed 5 days because of the increased risk of serious adverse events.

*Special populations* – Adjust dosage for patients 65 years of age and older, for patients weighing less than 50 kg (110 lbs), and for patients with moderately elevated serum creatinine. IV/IM doses are not to exceed 60 mg/day in these patients.

*GI effects:* Serious GI toxicity such as bleeding, ulceration, and perforation can occur at any time, with or without warning symptoms, in patients treated chronically with NSAID therapy. Higher doses of **meloxicam** (eg, 30 mg/day) were associated with increased risk of serious GI effects. Do not exceed daily doses of 15 mg.

If diarrhea occurs with **mefenamic acid** or diarrhea, GI irritation, and abdominal pain occur with **meclofenamate**, reduce dosage or temporarily discontinue use. Some patients may be unable to tolerate further therapy with these agents.

*CNS effects:* **Indomethacin** may aggravate depression or other psychiatric disturbances, epilepsy, and parkinsonism. Some of these agents also may cause headaches (highest incidence with **fenoprofen**, indomethacin, **ketorolac**, and **celecoxib**).

*Hypersensitivity reactions:* A potentially fatal apparent hypersensitivity syndrome has occurred with **sulindac**.

Anaphylactoid reactions have occurred in patients without known exposure to NSAIDs, but they typically occur in asthmatic patients who experience rhinitis with or without nasal polyps, or who exhibit severe, potentially fatal bronchospasm after taking aspirin or other NSAIDs.

*Serious skin reactions* – Serious skin reactions, including exfoliative dermatitis, Stevens-Johnson syndrome, and toxic epidermal necrolysis, have been reported through postmarketing surveillance in patients receiving valdecoxib. Fatalities due to Stevens-Johnson syndrome and toxic epidermal necrolysis have been reported. Discontinue valdecoxib at the first appearance of skin rash or any other sign of hypersensitivity.

*Renal function impairment:* NSAID metabolites are eliminated primarily by kidneys; use with caution in those with renal function impairment. In cases of advanced kidney disease, treatment with **piroxicam**, **meloxicam**, and **valdecoxib** is not recommended. Reduce dosage to avoid excessive accumulation.

Use **sulindac** with caution in patients with a history of renal lithiasis and keep patients well hydrated while receiving the drug.

*Hepatic function impairment:* Dose reduction may be needed with **naproxen**. Use caution in patients with impaired hepatic function or a history of liver disease.

**Valdecoxib** plasma concentrations are significantly increased (130%) in patients with moderate (Child-Pugh class B) hepatic impairment. In clinical trials, doses of valdecoxib above those recommended have been associated with fluid retention. The use of valdecoxib in patients with severe hepatic impairment (Child-Pugh class C) is not recommended.

*Elderly:* Age appears to increase the possibility of adverse reactions to NSAIDs. The risk of serious ulcer disease is increased; this risk appears to increase with dose. **Ketorolac** is cleared more slowly by the elderly; use caution and reduce dosage.

*Pregnancy:* Category B (ketoprofen, naproxen, naproxen sodium, flurbiprofen, diclofenac, fenoprofen, ibuprofen, indomethacin, meclofenamate, sulindac). Category C (etodolac, ketorolac, mefenamic acid, meloxicam, nabumetone, oxaprozin, tolmetin, piroxicam, celecoxib, valdecoxib). All NSAIDs are Category D if used in the third trimester or near delivery. Avoid during pregnancy, especially in the third trimester.

*Lactation:* Most NSAIDs are excreted in breast milk. In general, do not use in nursing mothers because of effects on infant's cardiovascular system.

*Children:* **Mefenamic acid** and **meclofenamate** are not recommended in children younger than 14 years of age. **Indomethacin** is not recommended in children 14 years of age and younger, except in circumstances that warrant the risk. Safety and efficacy of **meloxicam** and **valdecoxib** have not been established in children younger than 18 years of age. **Tolmetin** and **naproxen** are the only agents labeled for juvenile rheumatoid arthritis. Safety and efficacy of tolmetin in infants younger than 2 years of age are not established. Safety and efficacy of other NSAIDs in children are not established.

**Precautions**

*Monitoring:* Assess renal function before and during therapy. Monitor serum creatinine or creatinine clearance.

*Steroid dosage:* If reduced or eliminated during therapy, reduce slowly and observe patient closely for evidence of adverse effects, including adrenal insufficiency and exacerbation of symptoms.

*Porphyria:* Avoid the use of NSAIDs in patients with hepatic porphyria.

*Platelet aggregation:* NSAIDs can inhibit platelet aggregation; the effect is quantitatively less and of shorter duration than that seen with aspirin. These agents prolong bleeding time (within normal range) in healthy subjects.

*Preexisting asthma:* About 10% of patients with asthma may have aspirin-sensitive asthma. Because cross reactivity, including bronchospasm, between aspirin and other NSAIDs has been reported in such aspirin-sensitive patients, do not administer NSAIDs to patients with this form of aspirin sensitivity, and use the drug with caution in patients with preexisting asthma.

*Hematologic effects:* Decreased hemoglobin or hematocrit levels rarely have required discontinuation.

*Aseptic meningitis:* Aseptic meningitis with fever and coma has been observed on rare occasions in patients on NSAIDs therapy, although it is probably more likely to occur in patients with SLE.

*Cardiovascular effects:* May cause fluid retention and peripheral edema. Use caution in compromised cardiac function, hypertension, in patients on chronic diuretic therapy, or other conditions predisposing to fluid retention. Agents may be associated with significant deterioration of circulatory hemodynamics in severe heart failure and hyponatremia, presumably because of inhibition of prostaglandin-dependent compensatory mechanisms.

*Ophthalmologic effects:* Effects include blurred or diminished vision, scotomata, changes in color vision, corneal deposits, and retinal disturbances, including maculas.

*Infection:* NSAIDs may mask the usual signs of infection.

*Renal effects:* Acute renal insufficiency, interstitial nephritis with hematuria, nephrotic syndrome, proteinuria, hyperkalemia, hyponatremia, renal papillary necrosis, and other renal medullary changes may occur.

*Hepatic effects:* Borderline liver function test elevations may occur in about 15% of patients and may progress, remain essentially unchanged, or become transient with continued therapy.

*Pancreatitis:* Pancreatitis has occurred in patients receiving **sulindac**.

*Auditory effects:* Perform periodic auditory function tests during chronic **fenoprofen** therapy in patients with impaired hearing.

*Heavy menstrual blood loss evaluation:* Prior to prescribing **meclofenamate** for heavy blood flow and primary dysmenorrhea, make a thorough risk/benefit assessment.

*Dermatologic effects:* Promptly discontinue **mefenamic acid** if rash occurs. A combination of dermatologic and allergic signs and symptoms suggestive of serum sickness occasionally have occurred in conjunction with the use of **piroxicam**.

*Concomitant therapy:* Do not use **naproxen sodium** and **naproxen** concomitantly; both drugs circulate as naproxen anion.

Do not use **diclofenac** immediate-release, delayed-release, and extended-release tablets concomitantly with other diclofenac-containing products because they also circulate in plasma as diclofenac anion.

*Photosensitivity:* Photosensitivity may occur.

### Drug Interactions

Drugs that affect NSAIDs include the following: Bisphosphonates, cholestyramine, cimetidine, colestipol, cyclosporine, diflunisal, DMSO, fluconazole, ketoconazole, phenobarbital, phenylbutazone, probenecid, rifampin, ritonavir, salicylates, sucralfate.

Drugs that may be affected by NSAIDs include the following: Aminoglycosides, anticoagulants, ACE inhibitors, beta blockers, cyclosporine, dextromethorphan, digoxin, dipyridamole, hydantoins, lithium, loop diuretics, methotrexate, penicillamine, potassium-sparing diuretics, sympathomimetics, theophylline, thiazide diuretics.

*Drug/Lab test interactions:* Naproxen use may result in increased urinary values for 17-ketogenic steroids. Although 17-hydroxycorticosteroid measurements (Porter-Silber test) do not appear to be artificially altered, temporarily discontinue naproxen therapy 72 hours before adrenal function tests are performed.

*Naproxen* – Naproxen may interfere with some urinary assays of 5-hydroxy indole-acetic acid.

*Tolmetin* – Tolmetin metabolites in urine give positive tests for proteinuria using acid precipitation tests (eg, sulfosalicylic acid).

*Mefenamic acid* – A false-positive reaction for urinary bile, using the diazo tablet test, may result.

*Fenoprofen* – Amerlex-M kit assay values of total and free triiodothyronine in patients on fenoprofen have been reported as falsely elevated.

*Oxaprozin* – False-positive urine immunoassay screening tests for benzodiazepines have been reported in patients taking oxaprozin. This is because of the lack of specificity of the screening tests. False-positive test results may be expected for several days following discontinuation of oxaprozin therapy.

NSAIDs by decreasing platelet adhesion and aggregation, can prolong bleeding time by about 3 to 4 minutes.

*Drug/Food interactions:* Administration of **tolmetin** with milk decreased total tolmetin bio-availability by 16%. When tolmetin was taken immediately after a meal, peak plasma concentrations were reduced by 50%, while total bioavailability was again decreased by 16%. Peak concentration of **etodolac** is reduced by about 50% and the time to peak is increased by 1.4 to 3.8 hours following administration with food; however, the extent of absorption is not affected. Food may reduce the rate of absorption of **oxaprozin**, but the extent is unchanged.

## Adverse Reactions

*Cardiovascular:* CHF; hypotension; hypertension (**ketorolac**); palpitations; arrhythmias; tachycardia; vasodilation; peripheral edema; fluid retention.

*CNS:* Dizziness (**mefenamic acid, meloxicam, piroxicam, flurbiprofen, diclofenac, fenoprofen**); headache (**ketorolac, fenoprofen, indomethacin, diclofenac, flurbiprofen, meclofenamate, meloxicam, nabumetone, naproxen, tolmetin, ketoprofen, sulindac, celecoxib, valdecoxib, mefenamic acid, piroxicam, ibuprofen**); somnolence/drowsiness (**fenoprofen, naproxen**); asthenia (**tolmetin, etodolac**); malaise (**etodolac**); fatigue (**indomethacin**); insomnia (**meloxicam**).

*Dermatologic:* Rash/dermatitis, including maculopapular type (**ibuprofen, sulindac, meclofenamate, oxaprozin, nabumetone, mefenamic acid, meloxicam**); desquamation; angioneurotic edema; ecchymosis; petechiae; purpura; alopecia; pruritus (**nabumetone, naproxen**); eczema; skin discoloration; hyperpigmentation; skin irritation; peeling; skin eruptions (**naproxen**).

*GI:* Common GI adverse reactions include the following: Nausea; vomiting; diarrhea; constipation; abdominal distress/cramps/pain; dyspepsia; flatulence; anorexia; stomatitis.

    *Ulcer* – Gastric or duodenal ulcer with bleeding or perforation (**mefenamic acid**).

    *Bleeding* – Occult blood in the stool (**fenoprofen**).

    *Hepatic* – Elevated liver enzymes (**piroxicam, mefenamic acid**).

    *Other* – Gastritis (**etodolac**); pyrosis (**meclofenamate**); heartburn (**naproxen, meclofenamate, ibuprofen, mefenamic acid, piroxicam**); GI distress (**tolmetin**); epigastric pain (**ibuprofen** ); indigestion (**ibuprofen**); GI tract fullness (**ibuprofen**); GI pain (**sulindac**); gross bleeding (**mefenamic acid**).

*Hematologic:* Neutropenia; eosinophilia; leukopenia; pancytopenia; thrombocytopenia; agranulocytosis; granulocytopenia; aplastic anemia; hemolytic anemia; epistaxis; menorrhagia; hemorrhage; bruising; hemolysis, ecchymosis (**naproxen**).

*Metabolic:* Decreased or increased appetite; weight decrease or increase (**tolmetin**); glycosuria; hyperglycemia; hypoglycemia; hyperkalemia; hyponatremia; flushing or sweating.

*Renal:* Urinary tract infection (**flurbiprofen, meloxicam**); elevated BUN (**ketoprofen**); hematuria; cystitis; azotemia; nocturia; proteinuria; polyuria; dysuria; urinary frequency; pyuria; oliguria; anuria.

*Respiratory:* Dyspnea (**naproxen**); upper respiratory tract infection (**celecoxib, meloxicam, valdecoxib**); pharyngitis; bronchospasm; rhinitis; shortness of breath.

*Special senses:* Blurred vision; photophobia; amblyopia; swollen, dry, or irritated eyes; conjunctivitis; iritis; reversible loss of color vision; hearing disturbances or loss; ear pain; change in taste (metallic or bitter); diplopia; tinnitus.

*Miscellaneous:* Edema (**flurbiprofen, naproxen, meloxicam**); thirst; pyrexia (fever and chills); sweating; breast changes; gynecomastia; muscle cramps; facial edema; menstrual disorders; impotence; vaginal bleeding; influenza-like disease/symptoms (**meloxicam**).

# SULFASALAZINE

| | |
|---|---|
| **Tablets**: 500 mg (*Rx*) | Various, *Azulfidine* (Pharmacia) |
| **Tablets, delayed-release**: 500 mg (*Rx*) | *Azulfidine EN-tabs* (Pharmacia) |

For complete prescribing information, refer to the monograph in the GI chapter.

### Indications

*Rheumatoid arthritis (RA; enteric-coated tablets):* Treatment of patients with RA who have responded inadequately to salicylates or other nonsteroidal anti-inflammatory drugs (NSAIDs).

*Juvenile rheumatoid arthritis (JRA; enteric-coated tablets):* In the treatment of pediatric patients 6 years of age or older with polyarticular-course JRA who have responded inadequately to salicylates or other NSAIDs.

*Ulcerative colitis:* In the treatment of mild to moderate ulcerative colitis, and as adjunctive therapy in severe ulcerative colitis; for the prolongation of the remission period between acute attacks of ulcerative colitis (refer to the sulfasalazine monograph in the GI chapter).

*Unlabeled uses:* Psoriatic arthritis (2 g/day).

### Administration and Dosage

Give the drug in evenly divided doses over each 24-hour period; intervals between nighttime doses should not exceed 8 hours, with administration after meals recommended when feasible. Swallow tablets whole; do not crush or chew. Experience suggests that with daily dosages of 4 g or more, the incidence of adverse effects tends to increase.

Some patients may be sensitive to treatment with sulfasalazine. Various desensitization-like regimens have been reported to be effective. These regimens suggest starting with a total daily dose of 50 to 250 mg initially, and doubling it every 4 to 7 days until the desired therapeutic level is achieved. If the symptoms of sensitivity recur, discontinue sulfasalazine. Do not attempt desensitization in patients who have a history of agranulocytosis, or who have experienced an anaphylactoid reaction while previously receiving sulfasalazine.

*Rheumatoid arthritis:*

*Adults* – 2 g daily in 2 evenly divided doses. It is advisable to initiate therapy with a lower dosage (eg, 0.5 to 1 g/day) to reduce possible GI intolerance. A suggested dosing schedule is given below.

| Adult RA Sulfasalazine Dosing Schedule | | |
|---|---|---|
| | Number of delayed-release tablets | |
| Week of treatment | Morning | Evening |
| 1 | — | 1 |
| 2 | 1 | 1 |
| 3 | 1 | 2 |
| 4 | 2 | 2 |

A therapeutic response has been observed as early as 4 weeks after starting treatment, but treatment for 12 weeks may be required in some patients before clinical benefit is noted. Give consideration to increasing the daily dose to 3 g if the clinical response after 12 weeks is inadequate. Careful monitoring is recommended for doses more than 2 g/day.

*JRA-polyarticular course:*

*Children 6 years of age and older* – 30 to 50 mg/kg of body weight daily in 2 evenly divided doses. Typically, the maximum dose is 2 g/day. To reduce possible GI intolerance, begin with a quarter to a third of the planned maintenance dose and increase weekly until reaching the maintenance dose at 1 month.

### Adverse Reactions

Adverse reactions occurring in 3% or more of patients with RA include the following: Nausea, dyspepsia, rash, headache, abdominal pain, vomiting, fever, dizziness, stomatitis, pruritus, abnormal liver function tests, and leukopenia. One report showed a 10% rate of immunoglobulin suppression, which was slowly reversible and rarely accompanied by clinical findings.

# AGENTS FOR GOUT

In addition to the agents in this section, sulindac and indomethacin (see Nonsteroidal Anti-inflammatory Agents monograph) and phenylbutazone and oxyphenbutazone (see individual monographs) are indicated for the treatment of gout.

# PROBENECID

**Tablets:** 0.5 g *(Rx)*                    Various, *Benemid* (Merck), *Probalan* (Lannett)

### Indications
*Hyperuricemia:* Treatment of hyperuricemia associated with gout and gouty arthritis.

*Plasma levels:* Adjuvant to therapy with penicillins or cephalosporins, for elevation and prolongation of plasma levels of the antibiotic.

### Administration and Dosage
*Gout:* Do not start therapy until an acute gouty attack has subsided. However, if an acute attack is precipitated during therapy, probenecid may be continued. Give full therapeutic doses of colchicine or other appropriate therapy to control the acute attack.

*Adults* – 0.25 g twice/day for 1 week; 0.5 g twice/day thereafter. Gastric intolerance may indicate overdosage, and may be reduced by decreasing dosage.

*Renal impairment* – Some degree of renal impairment may be present in patients with gout. A daily dosage of 1 g may be adequate. However, if necessary, the daily dosage may be increased by 0.5 g increments every 4 weeks within tolerance (usually not more than 2 g/day) if symptoms of gouty arthritis are not controlled or the 24 hour urate excretion is not more than 700 mg. Probenecid may not be effective in chronic renal insufficiency, particularly when the glomerular filtration rate is 30 mL/minute or less.

*Urinary alkalinization* – Urates tend to crystallize out of an acid urine; therefore, a liberal fluid intake is recommended, as well as sufficient sodium bicarbonate (3 to 7.5 g/day) or potassium citrate (7.5 g/day) to maintain an alkaline urine; continue alkalization until the serum uric acid level returns to normal limits and tophaceous deposits disappear. Thereafter, urinary alkalization and the restriction of purine-producing foods may be relaxed.

*Maintenance therapy* – Continue the dosage that maintains normal serum uric acid levels. When there have been no acute attacks for 6 months or more and serum uric acid levels have remained within normal limits, decrease the daily dosage by 0.5 g every 6 months. Do not reduce the maintenance dosage to the point where serum uric acid levels increase.

*Penicillin or cephalosporin therapy:* The PSP excretion test may be used to determine the effectiveness of probenecid in retarding penicillin excretion and maintaining therapeutic levels. The renal clearance of PSP is reduced to about the normal rate when dosage of probenecid is adequate.

*Adults* – 2 g/day in divided doses. Reduce dosage in older patients in whom renal impairment may be present. Not recommended in conjunction with penicillin or a cephalosporin in the presence of known renal impairment.

*Children (2 to 14 years of age)* – Initial dose 25 mg/kg or 0.7 g/m². Maintenance dose 40 mg/kg/day or 1.2 g/m², divided into 4 doses. For children weighing more than 50 kg (110 lb), use the adult dosage. Do not use in children younger than 2 years of age.

*Gonorrhea (uncomplicated)* – Give probenecid as a single 1g dose immediately before or with 4.8 million units penicillin G procaine, aqueous, divided into at least 2 doses.

*Neurosyphilis* – Aqueous procaine penicillin G, 2 to 4 million units/day IM plus probenecid 500 mg 4 times/day, both for 10 to 14 days.†

*Pelvic inflammatory disease (PID)* – Cefoxitin 2 g IM plus probenecid, 1 g orally in a single dose concurrently.

† CDC 1993 Sexually Transmitted Diseases Treatment Guidelines. *MMWR.* 1993;42 (No. RR-14).

### Actions

*Pharmacology:* A uricosuric and renal tubular blocking agent, probenecid inhibits the tubular reabsorption of urate, thus increasing the urinary excretion of uric acid and decreasing serum uric acid levels.

Probenecid also inhibits the tubular secretion of most penicillins and cephalosporins and usually increases plasma levels by any route the antibiotic is given.

*Pharmacokinetics:* Probenecid is well absorbed after oral administration and produces peak plasma concentrations in 2 to 4 hours. It is highly protein bound (85% to 95%). Probenecid is excreted in the urine primarily as metabolites.

### Contraindications

Hypersensitivity to probenecid; children younger than 2 years of age; blood dyscrasias or uric acid kidney stones. Do not start therapy until an acute gouty attack has subsided.

### Warnings

*Exacerbation of gout:* Exacerbation of gout following therapy with probenecid may occur; in such cases, colchicine or other appropriate therapy is advisable.

*Salicylates:* Use of salicylates is contraindicated in patients on probenecid therapy. Salicylates antagonize probenecid's uricosuric action.

*Sulfa drug allergy:* Probenecid is a sulfonamide; patients with a history of allergy to sulfa drugs may react to probenecid.

*Hypersensitivity reactions:* Rarely, severe allergic reactions and anaphylaxis have occurred. Most of these occur within several hours after readministration following prior use of the drug.

*Renal function impairment:* Dosage requirements may be increased in renal impairment. Probenecid may not be effective in chronic renal insufficiency, particularly when the glomerular filtration rate is 30 mL/minute or less. Probenecid is not recommended in conjunction with a penicillin in the presence of known renal impairment.

*Pregnancy:* Category B.

*Children:* Do not use in children younger than 2 years of age.

### Precautions

*Alkalinization of urine:* Hematuria, renal colic, costovertebral pain, and formation of urate stones associated with use in gouty patients may be prevented by alkalization of urine and liberal fluid intake; monitor acid-base balance.

*Peptic ulcer history:* Use with caution.

### Drug Interactions

Drugs that may affect probenecid include salicylates.

Drugs that may be affected by probenecid include acyclovir; allopurinol; barbiturates; benzodiazepines; clofibrate; dapsone; dyphylline; methotrexate; NSAIDs; pantothenic acid; penicillamine; rifampin; sulfonamides; sulfonylureas; zidovudine; salicylates.

*Drug/Lab test interactions:* A reducing substance may appear in the urine during therapy. Although this disappears with discontinuation, a false diagnosis of glycosuria may be made. Confirm suspected glycosuria by using a test specific for glucose.

Falsely high determination of **theophylline** has occurred in vitro using the Schack and Waxler technique, when therapeutic concentrations of theophylline and probenecid were added to human plasma.

Probenecid may inhibit the renal excretion of: **Phenolsulfonphthalein (PSP), 17-ketosteroids,** and **sulfobromophthalein (BSP).**

### Adverse Reactions

Adverse reactions may include headache; anorexia; nausea; vomiting; urinary frequency; hypersensitivity reactions; sore gums; flushing; dizziness; anemia; hemolytic anemia (possibly related to G-6-PD deficiency); nephrotic syndrome; hepatic necrosis; aplastic anemia; exacerbation of gout; uric acid stones with or without hematuria; renal colic or costovertebral pain.

# ALLOPURINOL

**Tablets:** 100 and 300 mg (*Rx*)                    Various, *Zyloprim* (Prometheus)

### Indications

Gout: Management of signs and symptoms of primary or secondary gout.

Malignancies: Management of patients with leukemia, lymphoma, and malignancies receiving therapy which causes elevations of serum and urinary uric acid. Discontinue allopurinol when the potential for overproduction of uric acid is no longer present.

Calcium oxalate calculi: Management of patients with recurrent calcium oxalate calculi whose daily uric acid excretion exceeds 800 mg/day (males) or 750 mg/day (females). Carefully assess therapy initially and periodically to determine that treatment is beneficial and that the benefits outweigh the risks.

Unlabeled uses: In a limited number of patients, the use of an allopurinol mouthwash (20 mg in 3% methylcellulose; 1 mg/mL) after fluorouracil administration prevented stomatitis, a major dose-limiting toxicity of fluorouracil. However, another report indicated that allopurinol mouthwash is not effective. Further study is needed.

### Administration and Dosage

Control of gout and hyperuricemia: The average dose is 200 to 300 mg/day for mild gout and 400 to 600 mg/day for moderately severe tophaceous gout. Divide doses in excess of 300 mg. The minimum effective dose is 100 to 200 mg/day; the maximum recommended dose is 800 mg/day.

Children (6 to 10 years of age) – In secondary hyperuricemia associated with malignancy, give 300 mg/day; those younger than 6 years of age are generally given 150 mg/day. Evaluate response after approximately 48 hours of therapy and adjust dosage if necessary.

Another suggested dose is 1 mg/kg/day divided every 6 hours, to a maximum of 600 mg/day. After 48 hours of treatment, titrate dose according to serum uric acid levels.

Prevention of uric acid nephropathy during vigorous therapy of neoplastic disease: 600 to 800 mg/day for 2 to 3 days together with a high fluid intake. Similar considerations govern dosage regulation for maintenance purposes in secondary hyperuricemia.

To reduce the possibility of flare-up of acute gouty attacks: Start with 100 mg/day and increase at weekly intervals by 100 mg (without exceeding the maximum recommended dosage) until a serum uric acid level of 6 mg/dL or less is attained.

Serum uric acid levels: Normal serum urate levels are usually achieved in 1 to 3 weeks. The upper limit of normal is about 7 mg/dL for men and postmenopausal women and 6 mg/dL for premenopausal women. Do not rely on a single reading since estimation of uric acid may be difficult. By selecting the appropriate dose, and using uricosuric agents in certain patients, it is possible to reduce the serum uric acid level to normal and, if desired, to hold it as low as 2 to 3 mg/dL indefinitely.

Renal impairment: Accumulation of allopurinol and its metabolites can occur in renal failure; consequently, reduce the dose. With a Ccr of 10 to 20 mL/min, 200 mg/day is suitable. When the Ccr is less than 10 mL/min, do not exceed 100 mg/day. With extreme renal impairment (Ccr less than 3 mL/min) the interval between doses may also need to be increased. The correct dosage is best determined by using the serum uric acid level as an index.

Other suggested doses include: Ccr 60 mL/min, 200 mg/day; Ccr 40 mL/min, 15 mg/day; Ccr 20 mL/min, 100 mg/day; Ccr 10 mL/min, 100 mg on alternate days. Ccr less than 10 mL/min, 100 mg 3 times a week.

Concomitant therapy: In patients treated with colchicine or anti-inflammatory agents, continue therapy while adjusting the allopurinol dosage until a normal serum uric acid level and freedom from acute attacks have been maintained for several months.

*Replacement therapy:* In transferring a patient from a uricosuric agent to allopurinol, gradually reduce the dose of the uricosuric agent over several weeks and gradually increase the dose of allopurinol until a normal serum uric acid level is maintained.

*Recurrent calcium oxalate stones:* For hyperuricosuric patients, 200 to 300 mg/day in single or divided doses. Adjust dose up or down depending upon the resultant control of the hyperuricosuria based upon subsequent 24 hour urinary urate determinations. Patients may also benefit from dietary changes such as reduction of animal protein, sodium, refined sugars, oxalate-rich foods and excessive calcium intake as well as increase in oral fluids and dietary fiber.

### Actions

*Pharmacology:* Allopurinol inhibits xanthine oxidase, the enzyme responsible for the conversion of hypoxanthine to xanthine to uric acid. Allopurinol acts on purine catabolism, reducing the production of uric acid, without disrupting the biosynthesis of vital purines.

Administration generally results in a fall in both serum and urinary uric acid within 2 to 3 days. The magnitude of this decrease is dose-dependent. One week or more of treatment may be required before the full effects of the drug are manifested; likewise, uric acid may return to pretreatment levels slowly following cessation of therapy.

*Pharmacokinetics:* Allopurinol is approximately 90% absorbed from the GI tract.

Effective xanthine oxidase inhibition is maintained over 24 hours with single daily doses. Allopurinol is cleared essentially by glomerular filtration; oxipurinol is reabsorbed in the kidney tubules in a manner similar to the reabsorption of uric acid.

### Contraindications

Patients who have developed a severe reaction should not be restarted on the drug.

### Warnings

*Asymptomatic hyperuricemia:* Generally, do not use to treat asymptomatic hyperuricemia. Treatment should be considered with persitent hyperuricemia characterized by a serum urate concentration of greater than 13 mg/dL. High serum urate may be nephrotoxic.

*Hepatotoxicity:* A few cases of reversible clinical hepatotoxicity have occurred; in some patients, asymptomatic rises in serum alkaline phosphatase or serum transaminase levels have been observed. If anorexia, weight loss or pruritus develop in patients on allopurinol, evaluation of liver function should be part of their diagnostic workup. Perform periodic liver function tests during early stages of therapy.

*Hypersensitivity reactions:* Discontinue at first appearance of skin rash or other signs of allergic reactions. In some instances, rash may be followed by more severe hypersensitivity reactions such as exfoliative, urticarial or purpuric lesions, or Stevens-Johnson syndrome, generalized vasculitis, irreversible hepatotoxicity and rarely, death.

*Renal function impairment:* Some patients with preexisting renal disease or poor urate clearance have increased BUN during allopurinol administration. Patients with impaired renal function require less drug and careful observation during the early stages of treatment; reduce dosage or discontinue therapy if increased abnormalities in renal function appear and persist.

Renal failure in association with allopurinol has been observed among patients with hyperuricemia secondary to neoplastic diseases. Concurrent conditions such as multiple myeloma and congestive myocardial disease were present. Renal failure is also frequently associated with gouty nephropathy and rarely with allopurinol-associated hypersensitivity reactions. Albuminuria has occurred among patients who developed clinical gout following chronic glomerulonephritis and chronic pyelonephritis.

In patients with severely impaired renal function or decreased urate clearance, the plasma half-life of oxipurinol is greatly prolonged. A dose of 100 mg/day or

300 mg twice a week, or less, may be sufficient to maintain adequate xanthine oxidase inhibition to reduce serum urate levels.

*Pregnancy:* Category C.

*Lactation:* Allopurinol and oxipurinol have been found in breast milk. Exercise caution when administering to a nursing woman.

*Children:* Allopurinol is rarely indicated for use in children, with the exception of those with hyperuricemia secondary to malignancy or to certain rare inborn errors of purine metabolism.

### Precautions

*Monitoring:* Periodically determine liver and kidney function especially during the first few months of therapy. Perform BUN, serum creatinine, or Ccr and reassess the patient's dosage.

*Acute attacks of gout:* Acute attacks of gout have increased during the early stages of allopurinol administration when normal or subnormal serum uric acid levels have been attained; in general, give maintenance doses of colchicine prophylactically when allopurinol is begun. In addition, start patient at a low dose of allopurinol (100 mg/day) and increase at weekly intervals by 100 mg until a serum uric acid level of 6 mg/dL or less is attained without exceeding the maximum recommended dose. The attacks usually become shorter and less severe after several months of therapy.

*Fluid intake:* Fluid intake sufficient to yield a daily urinary output of at least 2 L and the maintenance of a neutral or slightly alkaline urine are desirable to avoid the theoretical possibility of formation of xanthine calculi under the influence of allopurinol therapy and to help prevent renal precipitation of urates in patients receiving concomitant uricosurics.

*Drowsiness:* Drowsiness has occurred occasionally. Patients should observe caution while driving or performing other tasks requiring alertness, coordination, or physical dexterity.

*Bone marrow depression:* Bone marrow depression has occurred in patients receiving allopurinol, most of whom received concomitant drugs with the potential for causing this reaction. This has occurred as early as 6 weeks to as long as 6 years after the initiation of therapy. Rarely, a patient may develop varying degrees of bone marrow depression, affecting one or more cell lines, while receiving allopurinol alone.

### Drug Interactions

Drugs that may affect allopurinol include ACE inhibitors; aluminum salts; thiazide diuretics; uricosuric agents.

Drugs that may be affected by allopurinol include ampicillin; anticoagulants; cyclophosphamide; theophyllines; thiopurines.

### Adverse Reactions

Adverse reactions may include skin rash; fever; chills; arthralgias; cholestatic jaundice; eosinophilia; mild leukocytosis; leukopenia; vesicular bullous dermatitis; eczematoid dermatitis; pruritus; urticaria; onycholysis; lichen planus; Stevens-Johnson syndrome; purpura; toxic epidermal necrolysis; nausea; vomiting; diarrhea; intermittent abdominal pain; gastritis; dyspepsia; increased alkaline phosphatase, AST and ALT; hepatomegaly; cholestatic jaundice; granulomatous hepatitis; hepatic necrosis; leukopenia; leukocytosis; eosinophilia; thrombocytopenia; headache; peripheral neuropathy; neuritis; paresthesia; somnolence; arthralgia; acute attacks of gout; ecchymosis; fever; myopathy; epistaxis; taste loss or perversion; renal failure; uremia; alopecia; hypersensitivity vasculitis; necrotizing angiitis.

# COLCHICINE

**Tablets:** 0.5 mg (1/120 g) and 0.6 mg (1/100 g) *(Rx)*   *Colchicine* (Abbott)

### Indications
*Gout:* Relieves pain of acute attacks, especially if adequate doses are given early in the attack. Many therapists use colchicine as interval therapy to prevent acute attacks. Recommended for regular prophylactic use between attacks and is often effective in aborting an attack when taken at the first sign of articular discomfort.

### Administration and Dosage
*Acute gouty arthritis:* Begin at the first warning of an acute attack. Usual initial dose is 1 to 1.2 mg; follow with 0.5 to 1.2 mg every 1 to 2 hours, until pain is relieved, or nausea, vomiting, or diarrhea occurs. (Opiates may be needed to control diarrhea.) After 1 or more attacks, patients can often judge their requirements accurately enough to stop before the "diarrheal dose."

The total amount of colchicine needed to control pain and inflammation during an acute attack is 4 to 8 mg. Articular pain and swelling typically abate within 12 hours and are usually gone in 24 to 48 hours. Wait 3 days before initiating a second course to minimize the possibility of cumulative toxicity.

If ACTH is used to treat a gouty arthritis attack, give colchicine 1 mg/day or more, and continue for a few days after ACTH is withdrawn.

*Prophylaxis during intercritical periods:* To reduce the frequency and severity of paroxysms, administer continuously. If patients have less than 1 attack/year, usual dose is 0.5 or 0.6 mg/day for 3 or 4 days a week; if more than 1 attack/year, usual dose is 0.5 or 0.6 mg/day. Severe cases may require 1 to 1.8 mg/day.

*Prophylaxis in patients undergoing surgery:* In patients with gout, an attack may be precipitated by even a minor surgical procedure. Administer 0.5 or 0.6 mg 3 times/day for 3 days before and 3 days after surgery.

*Prophylaxis or maintenance of recurrent or chronic gouty arthritis:* 0.5 to 1 mg once or twice/day.

### Actions
*Pharmacology:* The exact mechanism of action of colchicine in gout is not known. Colchicine apparently exerts its effect by reducing the inflammatory response to the deposited crystals and also by diminishing phagocytosis. Colchicine diminishes lactic acid production by leukocytes directly and by diminishing phagocytosis and thereby interrupts the cycle of urate crystal deposition and inflammatory response that sustains the acute attack.

*Pharmacokinetics:* Colchicine is rapidly absorbed after oral administration; peak plasma concentrations occur in 0.5 to 2 hours. High colchicine concentrations are found in the kidney, liver, and spleen. It is metabolized in the liver. Excretion occurs primarily by biliary and renal routes.

### Contraindications
Hypersensitivity to colchicine; serious GI, renal, hepatic, or cardiac disorders; blood dyscrasias.

### Warnings
*Hepatic function impairment:* Increased colchicine toxicity may occur.

*Fertility impairment:* Colchicine arrests cell division in animals and plants. It has adversely affected spermatogenesis in humans and in some animal species.

*Elderly:* Administer colchicine with great caution to elderly and debilitated patients.

*Pregnancy: Category C.*

*Lactation:* It is not known whether this drug is excreted in breast milk. Exercise caution when administering colchicine to a nursing woman.

*Children:* Safety and efficacy for use in children have not been established.

### Precautions
*Monitoring:* Perform periodic blood counts in patients receiving long-term therapy.

GI *effects:* Vomiting, diarrhea, abdominal pain, and nausea may occur, especially with maximum doses. These may be particularly troublesome in the presence of peptic ulcer or spastic colon. At toxic doses, colchicine may cause severe diarrhea, generalized vascular damage, and renal damage with hematuria and oliguria. To avoid more serious toxicity, discontinue use when these symptoms appear, regardless of whether joint pain has been relieved.

*Myopathy and neuropathy:* Colchicine myoneuropathy appears to be a common cause of weakness in patients on standard therapy who have elevated plasma levels caused by altered renal function. It is often unrecognized and misdiagnosed as polymyositis or uremic neuropathy. Proximal weakness and elevated serum creatine kinase are generally present, and resolve in 3 to 4 weeks following drug withdrawal.

*Malabsorption of vitamin $B_{12}$:* Colchicine induces reversible malabsorption of vitamin $B_{12}$, apparently by altering the function of ileal mucosa.

### Drug Interactions
*Drug/Lab test interactions:* Decreased **thrombocyte** values may be obtained. Colchicine may cause false-positive results when testing urine for **RBC** or **hemoglobin**.

### Adverse Reactions
Adverse reactions may include bone marrow depression with aplastic anemia; agranulocytosis or thrombocytopenia (long-term therapy); peripheral neuritis; purpura; myopathy; loss of hair; reversible azoospermia; dermatoses; hypersensitivity; vomiting; diarrhea; abdominal pain; nausea; elevated alkaline phosphatase and AST.

# PROBENECID AND COLCHICINE

**Tablets:** 500 mg probenecid/0.5 mg colchicine *(Rx)*  Probenecid and Colchicine (Ivax, Schein)

For complete prescribing information see the individual probenecid and colchicine monographs.

### Indications
For the treatment of chronic gouty arthritis when complicated by frequent, recurrent acute attacks of gout.

### Administration and Dosage
Do not start therapy with probenecid and colchicine until an acute gouty attack has subsided. However, if an acute attack is precipitated during therapy, probenecid and colchicine may be continued without changing the dosage and additional colchicine or other appropriate therapy given to control the acute attack.

The recommended adult dosage is 1 tablet/day for 1 week followed by 1 tablet twice daily.

# AGENTS FOR MIGRAINE

In addition to the agents on the following pages, **propanolol** and **timolol** are indicated for migraine prophylaxis.

# SEROTONIN 5-HT₁ RECEPTOR AGONISTS

| | |
|---|---|
| **ALMOTRIPTAN MALATE** | |
| **Tablets**: 6.25 and 12.5 mg (*Rx*) | *Axert* (Ortho-McNeil) |
| **ELETRIPTAN HBr** | |
| **Tablets**: 24.2 and 48.5 mg (*Rx*) | *Relpax* (Pfizer) |
| **FROVATRIPTAN SUCCINATE** | |
| **Tablets**: 2.5 mg (as base) (*Rx*) | *Frova* (Elan) |
| **NARATRIPTAN** | |
| **Tablets**: 1 and 2.5 mg (as HCl) (*Rx*) | *Amerge* (GlaxoSmithKline) |
| **RIZATRIPTAN BENZOATE** | |
| **Tablets**: 5 and 10 mg (*Rx*) | *Maxalt* (Merck) |
| **Tablets, orally disintegrating**: 5 and 10 mg (*Rx*) | *Maxalt-MLT* (Merck) |
| **SUMATRIPTAN** | |
| **Tablets**: 25, 50, and 100 mg (as succinate) (*Rx*) | *Imitrex* (GlaxoSmithKline) |
| **Injection**: 12 mg/mL (as succinate) (*Rx*) | |
| **Spray, nasal**: 5 and 20 mg (*Rx*) | |
| **ZOLMITRIPTAN** | |
| **Tablets**: 2.5 and 5 mg (*Rx*) | *Zomig* (MedPointe) |
| **Tablets, orally disintegrating**: 2.5 mg (*Rx*) | *Zomig ZMT* (MedPointe) |
| **Spray, nasal**: 5 mg (*Rx*) | *Zomig* (MedPointe) |

### Indications

*Migraine:* Acute treatment of migraine attacks with or without aura.

*Cluster headache (sumatriptan injection only):* Acute treatment of cluster headache episodes.

Not intended for the prophylactic therapy of migraine or for use in the management of hemiplegic or basilar migraine. Safety and efficacy have not been established for cluster headache, which is present in an older, predominantly male population (**almotriptan, eletriptan, frovatriptan, sumatriptan** tablets and spray, **zolmitriptan**).

### Administration and Dosage

ALMOTRIPTAN: Doses of 6.25 and 12.5 mg were effective for the acute treatment of migraines in adults, with the 12.5 mg dose tending to be a more effective dose. Individuals may vary in response to doses of almotriptan; therefore, individualize the dosage.

If the headache returns, the dose may be repeated after 2 hours, but do not give more than 2 doses within a 24-hour period. Controlled trials have not adequately established the efficacy of a second dose if the initial dose is ineffective.

The safety of treating an average of more than 4 headaches in a 30-day period has not been established.

*Hepatic function impairment* – The maximum decrease expected in the clearance of almotriptan caused by hepatic impairment is 60%. Therefore, do not exceed the maximum daily dose of 12.5 mg over a 24-hour period, and use a starting dose of 6.25 mg.

*Renal function impairment* – In patients with severe renal impairment, the clearance of almotriptan was decreased. Therefore, do not exceed the maximum daily dose of 12.5 mg over a 24-hour period, and use a starting dose of 6.25 mg.

ELETRIPTAN: Individualize dose. Single doses of 20 and 40 mg were effective for the acute treatment of migraine in adults, with a greater proportion of patients having a response following a 40 mg dose. Individuals may vary in response to doses of eletriptan tablets. An 80 mg dose, although also effective, was associated with an increased incidence of adverse events. Therefore, the maximum recommended single dose is 40 mg.

If, after the initial dose, the headache improves but then returns, a repeat dose may be beneficial. If a second dose is required, it should be taken at least 2 hours after the initial dose. If the initial dose is ineffective, controlled clinical trials have not shown the second dose to be beneficial in treating the same attack. The maximum daily dose should not exceed 80 mg.

The safety of treating an average of more than 3 headaches in a 30-day period has not been established.

*Hepatic function impairment* – Do not give eletriptan to patients with severe hepatic impairment because the effect of severe hepatic impairment on eletriptan metabolism was not evaluated. No dose adjustment is necessary in mild to moderate impairment.

FROVATRIPTAN: The recommended dosage is a single tablet (2.5 mg) taken orally with fluids.

If the headache recurs after initial relief, a second tablet may be taken, providing there is an interval of 2 or more hours between doses. The total daily dose of frovatriptan should not exceed 3 tablets (3 × 2.5 mg/day).

There is no evidence that a second dose of frovatriptan is effective in patients who do not respond to a first dose of the drug for the same headache.

The safety of treating an average of more than 4 migraine attacks in a 30-day period has not been established.

NARATRIPTAN: Single doses of 1 and 2.5 mg taken with fluid were effective for the acute treatment of migraine in adults. A greater proportion of patients had headache response following a 2.5 mg dose than following a 1 mg dose. Individualize dosage, weighing the possible benefit of the 2.5 mg dose with the potential for a greater risk of adverse events. If the headache returns or if the patient has only partial response, the dose may be repeated once after 4 hours, for a maximum dose of 5 mg in a 24-hour period. There is evidence that doses of 5 mg do not provide a greater effect than 2.5 mg.

*Renal/hepatic function impairment* – The use of naratriptan is contraindicated in patients with severe renal impairment (Ccr less than 15 mL/min) or severe hepatic impairment (Child-Pugh grade C) because of decreased clearance of the drug. In patients with mild to moderate renal or hepatic impairment, the maximum daily dose should not exceed 2.5 mg over a 24-hour period and a lower starting dose should be considered.

RIZATRIPTAN: Single doses of 5 and 10 mg were effective for the acute treatment of migraines in adults. There is little evidence that the 10 mg dose may provide a greater effect than the 5 mg dose. The choice of dose should be made on an individual basis, weighing the possible benefit of the 10 mg dose with the potential risk for increased adverse events.

*Redosing* – Doses should be separated by at least 2 hours; no more than 30 mg should be taken in any 24-hour period.

*Propranolol patients* – In patients receiving propranolol, use the 5 mg dose of rizatriptan benzoate tablets, up to a maximum of 3 doses in 24 hours.

*Orally disintegrating tablets* – Administration with liquid is not necessary. The orally disintegrating tablet is packaged in a blister within an outer aluminum pouch. Instruct patients not to remove the blister from the outer pouch until just prior to dosing. The blister pack should then be peeled open with dry hands and the orally disintegrating tablet placed on the tongue, where it will dissolve and be swallowed with saliva.

SUMATRIPTAN:

*Oral* – Single doses of 25, 50, or 100 mg tablets are effective for the acute treatment of migraine in adults. There is evidence that doses of 50 and 100 mg may provide a greater effect than 25 mg. Doses of 100 mg have not been proven to provide a greater effect than 50 mg. Individualize dosage, weighing the possible benefit of a higher dose with the potential for a greater risk of adverse events. If headache returns, or the patient has a partial response to the initial dose, additional doses may be taken at intervals of 2 hours or more up to a daily maximum of 200 mg. If headache returns following an initial treatment with the injection, additional doses of single tablets (up to 100 mg/day) may be given with an interval of 2 hours or more between tablet doses.

*Hepatic function impairment:* Maximum single dose up to 50 mg.

*MAO inhibitors:* Because of the potential of MAO-A inhibitors to cause unpredictable elevations in the bioavailability of oral sumatriptan, their combined use is contraindicated.

The safety of treating an average of more than 4 headaches in a 30-day period has not been established.

*Injection –* The maximum single adult dose is 6 mg injected subcutaneously.

Trials failed to show a clear benefit associated with the administration of a second 6 mg dose in patients who have failed to respond to a first injection. The maximum recommended dose that may be given in 24 hours is two 6 mg injections separated by 1 hour or more. If side effects are dose-limiting, lower doses may be used. In patients receiving doses less than 6 mg, use only the single-dose vial dosage form. An auto-injection device is available for use with 6 mg prefilled syringes to facilitate self-administration in patients in whom this dose is deemed necessary. With this device, the needle penetrates approximately ¼ inch (5 to 6 mm). Because the injection is intended to be given subcutaneously, intramuscular or intravascular delivery should be avoided. Patients should be directed to use injection sites with an adequate skin and subcutaneous thickness to accommodate the length of the needle.

*MAO inhibitors:* Consider decreased doses of sumatriptan in patients receiving MAO inhibitors.

*Intranasal –* A single dose of 5, 10, or 20 mg administered in 1 nostril is effective for the acute treatment of migraine in adults. A greater proportion of patients had headache response following a 20 mg dose than following a 5 to 10 mg dose. Weigh the possible benefit of the 20 mg dose with the potential for a greater risk of adverse events. A 10 mg dose may be achieved by administering a single 5 mg dose in each nostril. There is evidence that doses more than 20 mg do not provide a greater effect than 20 mg. If headache returns, the dose may be repeated once after 2 hours, not to exceed a total daily dose of 40 mg.

The safety of treating an average of more than 4 headaches in a 30-day period has not been established.

ZOLMITRIPTAN: Initial recommended dose is up to 2.5 mg (achieved by manually breaking a 2.5 mg tablet in half). If the headache returns, the dose may be repeated after 2 hours, not to exceed 10 mg within a 24-hour period. Response is greater following the 2.5 or 5 mg dose compared with 1.25 mg, with little added benefit and increased side effects associated with the 5 mg dose.

*Orally disintegrating tablets –* A single dose of 2.5 mg was effective for the acute treatment of migraines in adults. If the headache returns, the dose may be repeated after 2 hours, not to exceed 10 mg within a 24-hour period. Trials have not adequately established the efficacy of a second dose if the initial dose is ineffective.

Administration with a liquid is not necessary. The orally disintegrating tablet is packaged in a blister. Instruct patients not to remove the tablet from the blister until just prior to dosing. The blister pack should then be peeled open, and the orally disintegrating tablet placed on the tongue, where it will dissolve and be swallowed with the saliva. It is not recommended to break the orally disintegrating tablet.

On average, the safety of treating more than 3 headaches in a 30-day period has not been established.

*Nasal spray –* Administer 1 dose of 5 mg for the treatment of acute migraine. If the headache returns, the dose may be repeated after 2 hours. Do not exceed a maximum daily dose of 10 mg in any 24-hour period. Individuals may vary in response to zolmitriptan. The pharmacokinetics of a 5 mg nasal spray dose is similar to the 5 mg oral formulations. Doses lower than 5 mg can only be achieved through the use of an oral formulation. Therefore, choose the dose and route of administration on an individual basis. The efficacy of a second dose has not been established in placebo-controlled trials.

The safety of treating an average of more than 4 headaches in a 30-day period has not been established.

*Hepatic function impairment* – Administer zolmitriptan with caution in patients with liver disease, generally using doses less than 2.5 mg. Patients with moderate to severe hepatic impairment have decreased clearance of zolmitriptan; significant elevation in blood pressure was observed in some patients.

## Actions
*Pharmacology:* **Naratriptan, rizatriptan, sumatriptan, frovatriptan, almotriptan, eletriptan,** and **zolmitriptan** are selective agonists for a vascular 5-hydroxytryptamine₁ (serotonin) receptor subtype. Use of 5-HT₁ agonists results in cranial vessel constriction and inhibition of pro-inflammatory neuropeptide release, which correlates with the relief of migraine.

*Pharmacokinetics:*

| Pharmacokinetic Parameters of Triptans in Healthy Volunteers and in Patients with Migraine | | | | | | | |
|---|---|---|---|---|---|---|---|
| Drug | Dose and route of administration | $T_{max}$ (h) | $C_{max}$ (mcg/L) | Bioavail-ability (%) | $t_{1/2}$ (h) | AUC (mcg/L•h) | Plasma protein binding (%) |
| Almotriptan | 12.5 mg PO | 2.5 | 49.5 | 80 | 3.1 | 266 | ≈ 35 |
| | 25 mg PO | 2.7 | 64 | 69 | 3.6 | 443 | |
| Eletriptan | 20 mg PO | 2 | – | ≈ 50 | ≈ 4 | – | ≈ 85 |
| Frovatriptan | 2.5 mg PO | 3 | 4.2/7[a] | 29.6 | 25.7 | 94 | ≈ 15 |
| | 40 mg PO | 5 | 24.7/53.4[a] | 17.5 | 29.7 | 881 | |
| Naratriptan | 2.5 mg PO | 2 | 12.6 | 74 | 5.5 | 98 | ≈ 28 |
| Rizatriptan | 10 mg PO | 1, 1.6 to 2.5[b] | 19.8 | 40 | 2 | 50 | 14 |
| Sumatriptan | 6 mg SC | 0.17 | 72 | 96 | 2 | 90 | 14 to 21 |
| | 100 mg PO | 1.5 | 54 | 14 | 2 | 158 | |
| | 20 mg IN | 1.5 | 13 | 15.8 | 1.8 | 48 | |
| | 25 mg PR | 1.5 | 27 | 19.2 | 1.8 | 78 | |
| Zolmitriptan | 2.5 mg PO | 1.5, 3[b] | 3.3/3.8[a] | 39 | 2.3/2.6[a] | 18/21[a] | ≈ 25 |
| | 5 mg PO | 1.5, 3[b] | 10 | 46 | 3 | 42 | |
| | 5 mg IN | 3 | 3.93[c] | 102[d] | ≈ 3 | 22.4[c] | |

† Adapted from *Drugs.* 2000;60:1267.
[a] Value for men and women, respectively.
[b] Orally disintegrating tablets.
[c] Values based on 2.5 mg dose.
[d] Compared with oral tablet.

*Injection (Sumatriptan)* – Following a 6 mg subcutaneous injection, distribution half-life was 15 minutes, terminal half-life was 115 minutes, and Vd central compartment was 50 L. The $T_{max}$ or amount absorbed were not significantly altered by either the site or technique of injection (deltoid vs thigh).

## Contraindications
Injectable preparations used IV, because of the potential to cause coronary vasospasm; patients with ischemic heart disease (angina pectoris, history of MI, silent MI, strokes, transient ischemic attacks [TIAs], or documented silent ischemia); Prinzmetal's variant angina or other significant underlying cardiovascular disease (see Warnings); patients with signs or symptoms consistent with ischemic heart disease or coronary artery vasospasm; patients with uncontrolled hypertension; concurrent use of (or use within 24 hours of) ergotamine-containing preparations (or ergot-type medications such as dihydroergotamine or methysergide); concurrent MAO inhibitor therapy (or within 2 weeks of discontinuing an MAOI [except for **eletriptan**]; see Drug Interactions); within 24 hours of another 5-HT₁ agonist; hypersensitivity to the product or any of its ingredients; management of hemiplegic or basilar migraine; ischemic bowel disease.

*Naratriptan and sumatriptan:* Cerebrovascular or peripheral vascular syndromes, severe hepatic impairment (Child-Pugh grade C); severe renal impairment (Ccr less than 15 mL/min) (naratriptan only).

*Frovatriptan and eletriptan:* Peripheral vascular disease including but not limited to ischemic bowel disease.

*Eletriptan:* Severe hepatic impairment.

**Warnings**

Use 5-HT$_1$ agonists only where a clear diagnosis of migraine has been established.

*Risk of myocardial ischemia or infarction and other adverse cardiac events:* Because of the potential of this class of compounds to cause coronary vasospasm, do not give these agents to patients with documented ischemic or vasospastic coronary artery disease (CAD).

It is recommended that patients who are intermittent long-term users of 5-HT$_1$ agonists who have or acquire risk factors predictive of CAD undergo periodic interval cardiovascular evaluation as they continue use.

*Zolmitriptan –* Patients with symptomatic Wolff-Parkinson-White syndrome or arrhythmias associated with other cardiac accessory conduction pathway disorders should not receive zolmitriptan.

*Cardiac events and fatalities associated with 5-HT$_1$ agonists:* Serious adverse cardiac events, including acute MI, life-threatening disturbances of cardiac rhythm, and death have been reported within a few hours following the administration of other 5-HT$_1$ agonists.

*Cerebrovascular events and fatalities with 5-HT$_1$ agonists:* Cerebral hemorrhage, subarachnoid hemorrhage, stroke, and other cerebrovascular events have been reported in patients treated with 5-HT$_1$ agonists, and some have resulted in fatalities. In a number of cases, it appears possible that the cerebrovascular events were primary, the agonist having been administered in the incorrect belief that the symptoms experienced were a consequence of migraine, when they were not. It should be noted that patients with migraine may be at increased risk of certain cerebrovascular events (eg, stroke, hemorrhage, TIA).

*CYP3A4 inhibitors:* In vitro studies have shown that **eletriptan** is metabolized by the CYP3A4 enzyme. A clinical study has shown that coadministration of eletriptan with ketoconazole, erythromycin, verapamil, and fluconazole increased the C$_{max}$ and AUC of eletriptan 3- and 6-fold, 2- and 4-fold, 2- and 3-fold, and 1.4- and 2-fold, respectively. Do not use eletriptan within 72 hours of taking drugs that have demonstrated potent CYP3A4 inhibition.

*Other vasospasm-related events:* Peripheral vascular ischemia and colonic ischemia with abdominal pain and bloody diarrhea have been reported with 5-HT$_1$ agonists.

*Increases in blood pressure:* Significant elevations in systemic blood pressure, including hypertensive crisis, have been reported on rare occasions in patients with and without a history of hypertension treated with 5-HT$_1$ agonists.

*Local irritation:* Approximately 5% noted irritation in the nose and throat after using **sumatriptan** nasal spray. The symptoms were transient and, in approximately 60% of the cases, resolved in less than 2 hours.

*Hypersensitivity reactions:* Hypersensitivity reactions have occurred on rare occasions, and severe anaphylaxis/anaphylactoid reactions have occurred. Such reactions can be life-threatening or fatal. Refer to Management of Acute Hypersensitivity Reactions.

*Renal function impairment:* Use **rizatriptan** and **sumatriptan** with caution in dialysis patients because of a decrease in the clearance.

*Hepatic function impairment:* Administer with caution to patients with diseases that may alter the absorption, metabolism, or excretion of drugs. The bioavailability may be markedly increased in patients with liver disease. No dosage adjustment is necessary when **frovatriptan** or **eletriptan** is given to patients with mild to moderate hepatic impairment. Do not use eletriptan in severe hepatic impairment.

*Elderly:* Pharmacokinetics in the elderly are similar to those seen in younger adults.

*Pregnancy:* Category C.

*Lactation:* **Sumatriptan** and **eletriptan** are excreted in breast milk. **Zolmitriptan, naratriptan, almotriptan, frovatriptan,** and **rizatriptan** are excreted in rat milk.

*Children:* Safety and efficacy in children have not been established. 5-HT₁ receptor agonists are not recommended in patients younger than 18 years of age.

### Precautions

*Chest, jaw, or neck tightness:* Chest, jaw, or neck tightness is relatively common after 5-HT₁ agonist administration, and atypical sensations over the precordium (tightness, pressure, heaviness) have occurred, but have only rarely been associated with ischemic ECG changes.

*Seizures:* There have been rare reports of seizures following **sumatriptan** use.

*Binding to melanin-containing tissues:* Accumulation in melanin-rich tissues (such as the eye) could occur over time, raising the possibility that toxicity in these tissues could occur after extended use.

*Corneal opacities:* **Sumatriptan, eletriptan, naratriptan,** and **almotriptan** cause corneal opacities and defects in dogs, raising the possibility that these changes may occur in humans.

*Phenylketonurics:* **Rizatriptan** and **zolmitriptan** orally disintegrating tablets contain phenylalanine (a component of aspartame). Each 5 mg rizatriptan orally disintegrating tablet contains 1.05 mg phenylalanine, and each 10 mg orally disintegrating tablet contains 2.1 mg phenylalanine. Each 2.5 mg zolmitriptan orally disintegrating tablet contains 2.81 mg phenylalanine.

*Photosensitivity:* Photosensitization may occur. Caution patients to take protective measures against exposure to sunlight or ultraviolet light until tolerance is determined.

### Drug Interactions

Drugs that may affect 5-HT₁ receptor agonists include the following: Cimetidine, ergot-containing drugs, MAO inhibitors, oral contraceptives, potent CYP3A4 inhibitors (eg, ketoconazole), sibutramine, other 5-HT₁ receptor agonists, and propranolol. SSRIs may be affected by 5-HT₁ receptor agonists.

### Adverse Reactions

Adverse reactions occurring in 3% or more of patients include the following: asthenia, chest pain/pressure, dizziness, drowsiness, dry mouth, dyspepsia, fatigue, headache, heaviness, miscellaneous CNS effects, miscellaneous sensations, myasthenia, nausea, neck/throat/jaw pain/pressure, pain in specified/unspecified locations, paresthesia, skeletal pain/pressure, somnolence, vertigo, warm/cold sensation, warm/hot sensation.

*Zolmitriptan nasal spray:* Asthenia, discomfort of the nasal cavity, dizziness, hyperesthesia, nausea, pain, paresthesia, somnolence, throat pain, unusual taste.

# ERGOTAMINE DERIVATIVES

### DIHYDROERGOTAMINE

| | |
|---|---|
| **Spray, nasal:** 4 mg/mL (*Rx*) | *Migranal* (Xcel) |
| **Injection:** 1 mg/mL (*Rx*) | *D.H.E. 45* (Xcel) |

### ERGOTAMINE TARTRATE

| | |
|---|---|
| **Tablets, sublingual:** 2 mg (*Rx*) | *Ergomar* (Lotus Biochemical) |

### Indications

*Headache:* To abort or prevent vascular headaches such as migraine, migraine variant, and cluster headache (histaminic cephalalgia).

*Dihydroergotamine:* For the acute treatment of migraine headaches with or without aura and the acute treatment of cluster headache episodes (injection only). Dihydroergotamine nasal spray is not intended for the prophylactic therapy of migraine or for the management of hemiplegic or basilar migraine.

## Administration and Dosage

DIHYDROERGOTAMINE:

*Nasal spray* – Start with 1 spray (0.5 mg) in each nostril; repeat in 15 minutes for a total dosage of 4 sprays (2 mg). Studies have shown no additional benefit from acute doses greater than 2 mg for a single migraine administration. The safety of doses greater than 3 mg in a 24-hour period and 4 mg in a 7-day period has not been established. Do not use for chronic daily administration.

*Injection* – Administer in a dose of 1 mL IV, IM, or subcutaneously; may be repeated as needed at 1-hour intervals to a total dose of 3 mL for IM or subcutaneous delivery or 2 mL for IV delivery in a 24-hour period. Do not exceed a total weekly dosage of 6 mL. Do not use for chronic daily administration.

ERGOTAMINE: Initiate therapy as soon as possible after the first symptoms of an attack. Place 1 tablet under the tongue; take subsequent doses at 30 minute intervals if necessary. Do not exceed 3 tablets/24 hours. Do not exceed 10 mg/week.

## Actions

*Pharmacology:* Ergotamine has partial agonist or antagonist activity against tryptaminergic, dopaminergic and alpha-adrenergic receptors, depending upon their site; it is a highly active uterine stimulant. It constricts peripheral and cranial blood vessels and depresses central vasomotor centers.

Ergotamine reduces extracranial blood flow, causes a decline in the amplitude of pulsation in the cranial arteries and decreases hyperperfusion of the basilar artery territory. Ergotamine is a potent emetic that stimulates the chemoreceptor trigger zone.

Dihydroergotamine, a hydrogenated derivative of ergotamine, differs mainly in its degree of activity. It has less vasoconstrictive action than ergotamine, is 12 times less active as an emetic and has less oxytocic effect.

*Pharmacokinetics:*

*Absorption/Distribution* – GI and sublingual absorption of ergotamine is incomplete and erratic; following oral administration, peak blood levels are reached in about 2 hours. Following intranasal administration, however, the mean bioavailability of dihydroergotamine mesylate is 32% relative to the injectable administration.

Onset of action occurs in 15 to 30 minutes following IM administration of dihydroergotamine and persists for 3 to 4 hours.

*Metabolism/Excretion* – Ergotamine is metabolized by the liver; 90% of the metabolites are excreted in the bile. Although plasma half-life is about 2 hours, ergotamine has long-lasting effects which may be caused by tissue storage.

## Contraindications

Pregnancy (ergotamine's powerful uterine stimulant actions may cause fetal harm); hypersensitivity to ergot alkaloids; peripheral vascular disease (eg, thromboangiitis obliterans, leutic arteritis, severe arteriosclerosis, thrombophlebitis, Raynaud's disease); hepatic or renal impairment; severe pruritus; coronary artery disease; hypertension; sepsis. The use of potent CYP3A4 inhibitors (ritonavir, nelfinavir, indinavir, erythromycin, clarithromycin, troleandomycin, ketoconazole, itraconazole) with dihydroergotamine is contraindicated.

Do not give dihydroergotamine to patients with ischemic heart disease (angina pectoris, history of MI, documented silent ischemia) or to patients who have clinical symptoms or findings consistent with coronary artery vasospasm, including Prinzmetal variant angina.

Dihydroergotamine may increase blood pressure; do not give to patients with uncontrolled hypertension.

Do not use dihydroergotamine, 5-HT$_1$ agonists (eg, sumatriptan), ergotamine-containing or ergot-type medications, or methysergide within 24 hours of each other.

Do not administer dihydroergotamine to patients with hemiplegic or basilar migraine.

Dihydroergotamine should not be used by nursing mothers.

Do not use dihydroergotamine with peripheral and central vasoconstrictors because the combination may result in additive or synergistic elevation of blood pressure.

## Warnings

*CYP3A4 inhibitors (eg, macrolide antibiotics, protease inhibitors):* There have been rare reports of serious adverse events in connection with the coadministration.

*Fibrotic complications:* There have been reports of pleural and retroperitoneal fibrosis in patients following prolonged daily use of injectable dihydroergotamine.

*Risk of myocardial ischemia and/or MI and other adverse cardiac events:* Do not use dihydroergotamine in patients with documented ischemic or vasospastic coronary artery disease.

*Cardiac events and fatalities:* Serious adverse cardiac events, including acute MI, life-threatening disturbances of cardiac rhythm, and death have been reported following the administration of dihydroergotamine.

*Drug-associated cerebrovascular events and fatalities:* Cerebral hemorrhage, subarachnoid hemorrhage, stroke, and other cerebrovascular events have been reported in patients treated with dihydroergotamine; some have resulted in fatalities.

*Other vasospasm-related events:* Dihydroergotamine, like other ergot alkaloids, may cause vasospastic reactions other than coronary artery vasospasm. Myocardial and peripheral vascular ischemia have been reported with dihydroergotamine.

*Increase in blood pressure:* Significant elevation in blood pressure has been reported on rare occasions in patients with and without a history of hypertension.

*Local irritation:* Approximately 30% of patients using dihydroergotamine nasal spray (compared with 9% of placebo patients) have reported irritation in the nose or throat and/or disturbance in taste.

*Pregnancy:* Category X.

*Lactation:* Ergotamine is secreted into breast milk and has caused symptoms of ergotism (eg, vomiting, diarrhea) in the infant. Excessive dosing or prolonged administration may inhibit lactation.

*Children:* Safety and efficacy for use in children have not been established.

## Precautions

*Coronary artery vasospasm:* Dihydroergotamine may cause coronary artery vasospasm; patients who experience signs or symptoms suggestive of angina following its administration should, therefore, be evaluated for the presence of CAD or a predisposition to variant angina before receiving additional doses.

*Recommended dosage:* Exercise care to remain within the limits of recommended dosage.

*Drug abuse and dependence:* Patients who take ergotamine for extended periods of time may become dependent upon it and require progressively increasing doses for relief of vascular headaches and for prevention of dysphoric effects that follow withdrawal.

## Drug Interactions

Drugs that may affect ergot alkaloids include beta blockers, CYB3A4 inhibitors (see Contraindications), nicotine, and sibutramine.

Drugs that may be affected by ergot alkaloids include nitrates, $5HT_1$ receptor agonists, and vasoconstrictors.

## Adverse Reactions

*Dihydroergotamine nasal spray:* Adverse reactions occurring in at least 3% of patients include rhinitis, nausea, altered sense of taste, dizziness, vomiting, somnolence, pharyngitis, application site reaction.

*Ergotamine tartrate:* Nausea and vomiting occur in up to 10% of patients. Numbness and tingling of fingers and toes; muscle pain in the extremities; pulselessness; weakness in the legs; precordial pain; transient tachycardia or bradycardia; localized edema; itching.

*Miscellaneous:* Numbness and tingling of fingers and toes; muscle pain in the extremities; pulselessness; weakness in the legs; precordial distress and pain; transient tachycardia or bradycardia; localized edema; itching.

  *Large doses* – Large doses raise arterial pressure, produce coronary vasoconstriction, and slow the heart by both a direct action and a vagal effect.

# ISOMETHEPTENE MUCATE/DICHLORALPHENAZONE/ACETAMINOPHEN

**Capsules**: 65 mg isometheptene mucate, 100 mg dichloralphenazone, 325 mg APAP (*Rx*)

Various, *Duradrin* (Barr), *Midrin* (Women First HealthCare), *Migratine* (Major)

### Indications
For relief of tension and vascular headaches.

Based on a review of this drug (isometheptene mucate) by the National Academy of Sciences-National Research Council or other information, FDA has classified the other indication as "possibly" effective in the treatment of migraine headache. Final classification of the less-than-effective indication requires further investigation.

### Administration and Dosage
*Migraine headache:* Usual dosage is 2 capsules at once followed by 1 capsule every hour until relieved, up to 5 capsules within a 12 hour period.

*Tension headache:* Usual dosage is 1 or 2 capsules every 4 hours, up to 8 capsules/day.

### Actions
*Pharmacology:* Isometheptene mucate acts by constricting dilated cranial and cerebral arterioles, thus reducing the stimuli that lead to vascular headaches.

Dichloralphenazone, a mild sedative, reduces the patient's emotional reaction to the pain of both vascular and tension headaches.

Acetaminophen raises the threshold to painful stimuli, thus exerting an analgesic effect against all types of headaches.

### Contraindications
Glaucoma; severe cases of renal disease; hypertension; organic heart disease; hepatic disease; MAO inhibitor therapy.

### Warnings
*CNS effects:* Because of dichloralphenazone's structural similarity to chloral hydrate, there is a potential for CNS depressant effects.

*Drug abuse and dependence:* There have been no published reports of withdrawal signs or other signs of abuse. The risk of dependence is increased in patients with a history of alcoholism, drug abuse, or in patients with marked personality disorders.

### Precautions
*Observe caution:* Observe caution in hypertension, peripheral vascular disease, and after recent cardiovascular attacks.

### Drug Interactions
Drugs that may interact include MAO inhibitors.

### Adverse Reactions
Adverse reactions may include transient dizziness and skin rash.

# ANTIEMETIC/ANTIVERTIGO AGENTS

### CHLORPROMAZINE
| | |
|---|---|
| **Tablets:** 10, 25, 50, 100, and 200 mg (Rx) | Various, *Thorazine* (GlaxoSmithKline) |
| **Capsules, sustained release:** 30, 75, 150, 200, and 300 mg (Rx) | *Thorazine Spansules* (GlaxoSmithKline) |
| **Syrup:** 10 mg/5 mL (Rx) | *Chlorpromazine HCl* (Geneva) |
| **Concentrate:** 30 and 100 mg/mL (Rx) | Various, *Thorazine* (GlaxoSmithKline) |
| **Injection:** 25 mg/mL (Rx) | Various, *Ormazine* (Hauck), *Thorazine* (GlaxoSmithKline) |

### METOCLOPRAMIDE
| | |
|---|---|
| **Tablets:** 5 mg (Rx) | Various, *Reglan* (Robins) |
| **Tablets:** 10 mg (Rx) | Various, *Clopra* (Quantum), *Maxolon* (GlaxoSmithKline), *Octamide* (Adria), *Reclomide* (Major), *Reglan* (Robins) |
| **Syrup:** 5 mg/5 mL (Rx) | Various, *Reglan* (Robins), *Maxolon* (GlaxoSmithKline) |
| **Concentrated solution:** 10 mg/mL (Rx) | *Metoclopramide Intensol* (Roxane) |
| **Injection:** 5 mg/mL (Rx) | Various, *Octamide PFS* (Adria), *Reglan* (Robins) |

### PERPHENAZINE
| | |
|---|---|
| **Tablets:** 2, 4, 8, and 16 mg (Rx) | Various |

### PROCHLORPERAZINE
| | |
|---|---|
| **Tablets (as maleate):** 5, 10, and 25 mg (Rx) | Various, *Compazine* (GlaxoSmithKline) |
| **Capsules, sustained release:** 10, 15, and 30 mg (Rx) | *Compazine Spansules* (GlaxoSmithKline) |
| **Suppositories:** 2.5, 5, and 25 mg (Rx) | Various, *Compazine* (GlaxoSmithKline) |
| **Syrup:** 5 mg/5 mL (Rx) | *Compazine* (GlaxoSmithKline) |
| **Injection (as edisylate):** 5 mg/mL (Rx) | Various, *Prochlorperazine* (Wyeth-Ayerst), *Compazine* (GlaxoSmithKline) |

### THIETHYLPERAZINE
| | |
|---|---|
| **Supppositories:** 10 mg (Rx) | *Torecan* (Roxane) |

### TRIFLUPROMAZINE
| | |
|---|---|
| **Injection:** 10 and 20 mg/mL (Rx) | *Vesprin* (Princeton) |

### Administration and Dosage
*CHLORPROMAZINE HCl:*
>*Adults –*
>>*Nausea and vomiting:*
>>>*Oral* – 10 to 25 mg every 4 to 6 hours, as needed; increase if necessary.
>>>*Rectal* – 50 to 100 mg every 6 to 8 hours, as needed.
>>>*IM* – 25 mg. If no hypotension occurs, give 25 to 50 mg every 3 to 4 hours, as needed, until vomiting stops. Then switch to oral dosage.

>>*Intractable hiccoughs:* Orally, 25 to 50 mg 3 or 4 times/day. If symptoms persist 2 to 3 days, give 25 to 50 mg IM. If still persistent, use slow IV infusion with patient flat in bed. Give 25 to 50 mg in 500 to 1000 mL saline. Monitor blood pressure.
>*Children –*
>>*Nausea and vomiting:* Do not use in children younger than 6 months of age except where potentially lifesaving. Do not use in conditions for which specific children's dosages have not been established. The activity following IM use may last 12 hours.
>>>*Oral* – 0.25 mg/lb (0.55 mg/kg) every 4 to 6 hours.
>>>*Rectal* – 0.5 mg/lb (1.1 mg/kg) every 6 to 8 hours, as needed.
>>>*IM* – 0.25 mg/lb (0.55 mg/kg) every 6 to 8 hours, as needed.
>>*Maximum IM dosage –*
>>>*Children up to 5 years of age:* 40 mg/day.
>>>*Children 5 to 12 years of age:* 75 mg/day, except in severe cases.

*METOCLOPRAMIDE:*
>*Prevention of chemotherapy-induced emesis –* For doses in excess of 10 mg, dilute injection in 50 mL of a parenteral solution (Dextrose 5% in Water, Sodium Chloride Injection, Dextrose 5% in 0.45% Sodium Chloride, Ringer's or Lactated Ringer's Injection). Infuse slowly IV over not less than 15 minutes, 30 minutes before beginning cancer chemotherapy; repeat every 2 hours for 2 doses, then every 3 hours for 3 doses.

The initial 2 doses should be 2 mg/kg if highly emetogenic drugs such as cisplatin or dacarbazine are used alone or in combination. For less emetogenic regimens, 1 mg/kg/dose may be adequate.

Metoclopramide may have some potential value (10 mg orally or IV 30 minutes before each meal and at bedtime) in nausea and vomiting of a variety of etiologies (uncontrolled studies report 80% to 90% efficacy), including emesis during pregnancy and labor (5 to 10 mg orally or 5 to 20 mg IV or IM, 3 times a day).

PERPHENAZINE:
Oral – 8 to 16 mg/day in divided doses; occasionally, 24 mg may be necessary. Early dosage reduction is desirable.

IM – Give to seated or recumbent patient; observe patient for a short period afterward.

Adults: 5 mg repeated every 6 hours as necessary. Do not exceed 15 mg in ambulatory or 30 mg in hospitalized patients. For severe conditions, an initial dose of 10 mg may be given. Place patients on oral therapy as soon as possible, usually within 24 hours. In general, reserve higher dosages for hospitalized patients.

Children (older than 12 years of age): The lowest adult dose (5 mg). Pediatric dose not established.

IV – Use only when necessary to control severe vomiting, intractable hiccoughs or acute conditions such as violent retching during surgery. Limit use to recumbent hospitalized adults in doses not exceeding 5 mg. Give as a diluted solution by either fractional injection or slow drip infusion. In the surgical patient, slow infusion is preferred. When administered in divided doses, dilute to 0.5 mg/mL (1 mL mixed with 9 mL saline solution) and give not more than 1 mg per injection at not less than 1 to 2 minute intervals. Discontinue as soon as symptoms are controlled. Do not exceed 5 mg.

PROCHLORPERAZINE: Do not crush or chew sustained release preparations.
Adults: Control of severe nausea and vomiting –
Oral: Usually, 5 or 10 mg, 3 or 4 times/day; sustained release -15 mg on arising or 10 mg every 12 hours.

Rectal: 25 mg twice/day.

IM: Initially, 5 to 10 mg. If necessary, repeat every 3 or 4 hours. Do not exceed 40 mg/day.

Subcutaneous: Do not administer subcutaneously because of local irritation.

Adult surgery: Control of severe nausea and vomiting – Total parenteral dosage should not exceed 40 mg/day. Hypotension may occur if the drug is given IV or by infusion.

IM: 5 to 10 mg, 1 to 2 hours before induction of anesthesia (may repeat once in 30 minutes), or to control acute symptoms during and after surgery (may repeat once).

IV injection: 5 to 10 mg, 15 to 30 minutes before induction of anesthesia, or to control acute symptoms during or after surgery. Repeat once if necessary. Prochlorperazine may be administered either undiluted or diluted in isotonic solution, but do not exceed 10 mg in a single dose of the drug. Do not exceed 5 mg/mL/min. Do not use bolus injection.

IV infusion: 20 mg/L of isotonic solution. Do not dilute in less than 1 L of isotonic solution. Add to IV infusion 15 to 30 minutes before induction.

Children (over 20 pounds or 2 years of age): Control of severe nausea and vomiting –
Oral or rectal: More than one day of therapy is seldom necessary.
9.1 to 13.2 kg – 2.5 mg 1 or 2 times/day (not to exceed 7.5 mg/day).
13.6 to 17.7 kg – 2.5 mg 2 or 3 times/day (not to exceed 10 mg/day).
18.2 to 38.6 kg – 2.5 mg 3 times/day or 5 mg twice/day (not to exceed 15 mg/day).

IM: 0.06 mg/lb (0.132 mg/kg). Give by deep IM injection. Control is usually obtained with one dose. Duration of action may be 12 hours. Subsequent doses may be given if necessary.

PROMETHAZINE: For a complete listing of promethazine products, refer to the Antihistamines monograph in the Respiratory chapter.

*Oral and rectal –*

*Motion sickness:* The average adult dose is 25 mg twice/day. Take the initial dose 1 hour before travel, and repeat 8 to 12 hours later, if necessary. On succeeding days, administer 25 mg on arising and again before the evening meal. For children, administer 12.5 to 25 mg twice/day.

*Nausea and vomiting:* The average dose for active therapy in children or adults is 25 mg. Repeat as necessary in doses of 12.5 to 25 mg at 4 to 6 hour intervals.

*Children* – 0.25 to 0.5 mg/kg every 4 to 6 hours rectally, as needed. Do not use in children younger than 2 years of age. Adjust dose based on age, weight, and severity of condition.

*Parenteral –* Administer preferably by deep IM injection. Proper IV administration is well tolerated, but hazardous. When used IV, give in a concentration no greater than 25 mg/mL, and at a rate not to exceed 25 mg/min; it is preferable to inject through an appropriate site in tubing of an IV infusion set.

*Motion sickness:* 12.5 to 25 mg; may repeat as necessary 3 or 4 times a day.

*Nausea and vomiting:* 12.5 to 25 mg; do not repeat more frequently than every 4 hours. For postoperative nausea and vomiting, administer IM or IV.

In children younger than 12 years of age, do not exceed half the adult dose. As an adjunct to premedication, use 0.5 mg/lb (1.1 mg/kg) with an equal dose of narcotic or barbiturate and the appropriate dose of an atropine-like drug. Do not use in premature infants or neonates or in vomiting of unknown etiology in children.

*THIETHYLPERAZINE:* Do not use IV (may cause severe hypotension). Use of this drug has not been studied following intracardiac or intracranial surgery.

When used for nausea or vomiting associated with anesthesia and surgery, administer by deep IM injection at, or shortly before, termination of anesthesia.

*Adults –*

*Oral and Rectal:* 10 to 30 mg/day in divided doses.

*IM:* 2 mL, 1 to 3 times/day.

*Children –* Dosage not determined. Not recommended in children younger than 12 years of age.

*TRIFLUPROMAZINE HCl:*

*Adults –*

*IM (range):* 5 to 15 mg repeated every 4 hours, up to 60 mg maximum daily dose.

*Elderly or debilitated –* 2.5 mg; maximum daily dose, 15 mg.

*IV (range):* 1 mg, up to 3 mg total daily dose.

*Children (over 2½ years of age) –*

*IM:* 0.2 to 0.25 mg/kg; maximum 10 mg/day. The duration of activity following IM administration may last up to 12 hours. Do not administer IV.

## Actions

*Pharmacology:* Drug-induced vomiting (eg, drugs, radiation, metabolic disorders) is generally stimulated through the chemoreceptor trigger zone (CTZ), which in turn stimulates the vomiting center (VC) in the brain. Nausea of motion sickness is initiated by stimulation of labyrinthine mechanism of the ear, which sends impulses to CTZ. VC may also be stimulated directly by GI irritation, motion sickness, vestibular neuritis.

The following table indicates manufacturers' recommended uses for agents in this group. Several of these are indicated for uses other than as antiemetic/antivertigo agents.

| Recommended Uses for Antiemetic/Antivertigo Agents | | | |
|---|---|---|---|
| | Indications | | |
| Drug | Nausea and Vomiting | Motion Sickness | Vertigo |
| **ANTIDOPAMINERGICS** | | | |
| *Phenothiazines* — Chlorpromazine [1] | ✓ | | |
| Triflupromazine | ✓ | | |
| Perphenazine [1] | ✓ | | |
| Prochlorperazine | ✓ | | |
| Promethazine[2] | ✓ | ✓ | |
| Thiethylperazine | ✓ | | |
| *Other* — Metoclopramide | ✓ | | |
| **ANTICHOLINERGICS** | | | |
| *Antihistamines* — Cyclizine | ✓ | ✓ | |
| Meclizine | ✓ | ✓ | ✓[3] |
| Buclizine | ✓ | ✓ | |
| Diphenhydramine | | ✓ | |
| Dimenhydrinate | ✓ | ✓ | ✓ |
| *Other* — Trimethobenzamide | ✓ | | |
| Scopolamine | | ✓ | |
| **MISCELLANEOUS** | | | |
| *Miscellaneous* — Diphenidol | ✓ | | ✓ |
| Benzquinamide | ✓ | | |
| Phosphorated Carbohydrate Solution | ✓ | | |
| Hydroxyzine HCl | ✓[4] | | |
| Corticosteroids | ✓[4] | | |
| Cannabinoids | ✓ | | |

[1] Also indicated for relief of intractable hiccoughs.
[2] For complete listing of promethazine products refer to Antihistamine Product Pages.
[3] Classified "possibly effective" by the FDA.
[4] This is an *unlabeled* use.

**Warnings**

*Children:* Not recommended for uncomplicated vomiting in children; limit use to prolonged vomiting of known etiology.

Children with acute illnesses (eg, chickenpox, CNS infections, measles, gastroenteritis) or dehydration seem to be much more susceptible to neuromuscular reactions, particularly dystonias, than are adults. Do not use dimenhydrinate in children under 2 years of age unless directed by a doctor.

*Severe emesis* – Severe emesis should not be treated with an antiemetic drug alone; where possible, establish cause of vomiting. Direct primary emphasis toward restoration of body fluids and electrolyte balance, and relief of fever and causative disease process. Avoid overhydration which may result in cerebral edema.

# CYCLIZINE AND MECLIZINE

| **CYCLIZINE** | |
|---|---|
| **Tablets**: 50 mg (as HCl) (otc) | *Marezine* (Himmel) |
| **MECLIZINE** | |
| **Tablets**: 12.5, 25, and 50 mg (Rx) | Various, *Antivert* (Roerig), *Ru-Vert*-M (Solvay), *Dramamine II* (Pharmacia) |
| **Tablets, chewable**: 25 mg (Rx) | Various |
| **Tablets, chewable**: 25 mg (otc) | Various |
| **Capsules**: 25 mg (Rx) | Various, *Meni-D* (Seatrace) |
| **Capsules**: 30 mg (otc) | *Vergon* (Marnel) |

### Indications

*Motion sickness, vestibular system disease:* Prevention and treatment of nausea, vomiting, and dizziness of motion sickness.

Meclizine is "possibly effective" for the management of vertigo associated with diseases affecting the vestibular system.

### Administration and Dosage

CYCLIZINE:

Oral –

*Adults:* 50 mg taken ½ hour before departure; repeat every 4 to 6 hours. Do not exceed 200 mg/day.

*Children (6 to 12 years of age):* 25 mg, up to 3 times/day.

*Parenteral* – For IM use only. Not recommended for use in children.

*Adults:* 50 mg every 4 to 6 hours, as necessary.

MECLIZINE:

*Motion sickness* – Take an initial dose of 25 to 50 mg, 1 hour prior to travel. May repeat dose every 24 hours for the duration of the journey.

*Vertigo* – 25 to 100 mg/day in divided doses.

### Actions

*Pharmacology:* Cyclizine and meclizine have antiemetic, anticholinergic, and antihistaminic properties.

Cyclizine and meclizine have an onset of action of 30 to 60 minutes, depending on dosage; their duration of action is 4 to 6 hours and 12 to 24 hours, respectively.

### Contraindications

Hypersensitivity to cyclizine or meclizine.

### Warnings

*Pregnancy: Category* B. Meclizine presents the lowest risk of teratogenicity and is the drug of first choice in treating nausea and vomiting during pregnancy.

*Lactation:* Safety for use in the nursing mother has not been established.

*Children:* Safety and efficacy for use in children have not been established. Not recommended for use in children younger than 12 years of age.

### Precautions

*Hazardous tasks:* May produce drowsiness; patients should observe caution while driving or performing other tasks requiring alertness.

Because of the anticholinergic action of these agents, use with caution and with appropriate monitoring in patients with glaucoma, obstructive disease of the GI or GU tract, and in elderly males with possible prostatic hypertrophy. These drugs may have a hypotensive action, which may be confusing or dangerous in postoperative patients.

May have additive effects with alcohol and other CNS depressants (eg, hypnotics, sedatives, tranquilizers, antianxiety agents); use with caution.

### Adverse Reactions

Adverse reactions include the following: Hypotension; palpitations; tachycardia; drowsiness; restlessness; excitation; nervousness; insomnia; euphoria; blurred vision; diplopia; vertigo; tinnitus; auditory and visual hallucinations (particularly when dosage recommendations are exceeded); urticaria; rash; dry mouth; anorexia; nausea; vomiting; diarrhea; constipation; cholestatic jaundice (cyclizine); urinary frequency; difficult urination; urinary retention; dry nose and throat.

# BUCLIZINE HCl

**Tablets:** 50 mg *(Rx)*                    *Bucladin-S Softabs* (Stuart)

### Indications
For the control of nausea, vomiting, and dizziness of motion sickness.

### Administration and Dosage
Tablets can be taken without swallowing water. Place tablet in mouth and allow to dissolve, or chew or swallow whole.

*Adults:* A 50 mg dose usually alleviates nausea. In severe cases, 150 mg/day may be taken. Usual maintenance dose is 50 mg, 2 times/day. In prevention of motion sickness, take 50 mg at least hour before beginning travel. For extended travel, a second 50 mg dose may be taken after 4 to 6 hours.

### Actions
*Pharmacology:* Acts centrally to suppress nausea and vomiting.

### Contraindications
Hypersensitivity to buclizine HCl; pregnancy (see Warnings).

### Warnings
*Pregnancy:* Clinical data are not adequate to establish safety in early pregnancy.

*Children:* Safety and efficacy for use in children have not been established.

### Adverse Reactions
Drowsiness, dry mouth, headache, and jitteriness.

# DIPHENHYDRAMINE

For complete prescribing information and product availability, see Antihistamines group monograph.

### Indications
Treatment and prophylaxis (oral only) of motion sickness.

### Administration and Dosage
*Oral:* Adults – 25 to 50 mg 3 or 4 times/day.

*Children > 20 lbs (9.1 kg)* – 12.5 to 25 mg 3 or 4 times/day (5 mg/kg/24 h, or 150 mg/m$^2$/24 h. Do not exceed 300 mg.

Give first dose 30 minutes before exposure to motion and repeat before meals and upon retiring for the duration of journey.

*Parenteral:* For use only when the oral form is impractical.

*Adults* – 10 to 50 mg IV or deep IM; 100 mg if required. Maximum daily dosage is 400 mg.

*Children* – 5 mg/kg/24 h or 150 mg/m$^2$/24 h, in 4 divided doses, IV or deep IM. Maximum daily dosage is 300 mg.

# DIMENHYDRINATE

| | |
|---|---|
| **Tablets:** 50 mg (*Rx*) | *Dimetabs* (Jones Medical) |
| 50 mg (*otc*) | Various, *Calm-X* (Republic Drug), *Dramamine* (Pharmacia), *Triptone Caplets* (Commerce) |
| **Tablets, chewable:** 50 mg (*otc*) | *Dramamine* (Pharmacia) |
| **Capsules:** 50 mg (*otc*) | *Vertab* (UAD) |
| **Injection:** 50 mg/mL (*Rx*) | Various, *Dinate* (Seatrace), *Dramamine* (Pasadena), *Dymenate* (Keene), *Hydrate* (Hyrex) |
| **Liquid:** 12.5 mg/4 mL (*otc*) | Various, *Dramamine* (Pharmacia), |
| 12.5 mg/5 mL (*otc*) | *Children's Dramamine* (Pharmacia) |
| 15.62 mg/5 mL (*Rx*) | *Dramamine* (Pharmacia) |

## Indications

For the prevention and treatment of nausea, vomiting, dizziness, or vertigo of motion sickness.

## Administration and Dosage

*Adults:*

Oral – 50 to 100 mg every 4 to 6 hours. Do not exceed 400 mg in 24 hours.

IM – 50 mg, as needed.

IV – 50 mg in 10 mL Sodium Chloride Injection given over 2 minutes. Do not inject intra-arterially.

*Children:*

Oral (6 to 12 years of age) – 25 to 50 mg every 6 to 8 hours; do not exceed 150 mg in 24 hours.

Oral (2 to 6 years of age) – Up to 12.5 to 25 mg every 6 to 8 hours; do not exceed 75 mg in 24 hours.

IM – 1.25 mg/kg or 37.5 mg/m$^2$ 4 times/day; do not exceed 300 mg/day.

*Children (younger than 2 years of age):* Only on advice of a physician.

## Actions

*Pharmacology:* Dimenhydrinate consists of equimolar proportions of diphenhydramine and chlorotheophylline.

*Pharmacokinetics:* Dimenhydrinate has a depressant action on hyperstimulated labyrinthine function. The precise mode of action is not known. The antiemetic effects are believed to be caused by the diphenhydramine, an antihistamine also used as an antiemetic agent.

## Contraindications

Neonates; patients hypersensitive to dimenhydrinate or its components.

*Note:* Most IV products contain Benzyl Alcohol, which has been associated with a fatal "gasping syndrome" in premature infants and low birth weight infants.

## Warnings

*Pregnancy:* Category B.

*Lactation:* Small amounts of dimenhydrinate are excreted in breast milk.

*Children:* For infants and children especially, an overdose of antihistamines may cause hallucinations, convulsions, or death. Mental alertness may be diminished. In the young child, dimenhydrinate may produce excitation. Do not give to children under 2 years of age unless directed by a physician.

## Precautions

Use with caution in conditions which might be aggravated by anticholinergic therapy (eg, prostatic hypertrophy, stenosing peptic ulcer, pyloroduodenal obstruction, bladder neck obstruction, narrow angle glaucoma, bronchial asthma, cardiac arrhythmias).

## Drug Interactions

Drugs that may interact with dimenhydrinate may include CNS depressants and antibiotics.

**Adverse Reactions**

Adverse reactions may include drowsiness; confusion; nervousness; restlessness; headache; insomnia (especially in children); tingling, heaviness and weakness of hands; vertigo; dizziness; lassitude; excitation; nausea; vomiting; diarrhea; epigastric distress; constipation; anorexia; blurring of vision; diplopia; palpitations; hypotension; tachycardia; anaphylaxis; photosensitivity; urticaria; drug rash; hemolytic anemia; difficult or painful urination; nasal stuffiness; tightness of chest; wheezing; thickening of bronchial secretions; dryness of mouth, nose, and throat.

# TRIMETHOBENZAMIDE HCl

| | |
|---|---|
| **Capsules**: 100 mg (*Rx*) | *Tigan* (Roberts), *Trimazide* (Major) |
| 250 mg (*Rx*) | Various, *Tigan* (Roberts) |
| **Pediatric suppositories**: 100 mg (*Rx*) | Various, *Pediatric Triban* (Great Southern), *Tebamide* (G&W Labs), *T-Gen* (Goldline), *Tigan* (Roberts), *Trimazide* (Major) |
| **Suppositories**: 200 mg (*Rx*) | Various, *Tebamide* (G&W), *T-Gen* (Goldline), *Tigan* (Roberts), *Triban* (Great Southern), *Trimazide* (Major) |
| **Injection**: 100 mg/mL (*Rx*) | Various, *Pediatric Triban* (Great Southern), *Ticon* (Hauck), *Tigan* (Roberts) |

**Indications**

Control of nausea and vomiting.

**Administration and Dosage**

*Oral:*

*Adults* – 250 mg, 3 or 4 times/day.

*Children (30 to 90 lbs; 13.6 to 40.9 kg)* – 100 to 200 mg, 3 or 4 times/day.

*Rectal:*

*Adults* – 200 mg, 3 or 4 times/day.

*Children (30 to 90 lbs; 13.6 to 40.9 kg)* – 100 to 200 mg, 3 or 4 times/day.

*(less than 30 lbs)* – 100 mg, 3 or 4 times/day. Do not use in premature or newborn infants.

*Injection:* For IM use only.

*Adults* – 200 mg 3 or 4 times/day. Pain, stinging, burning, redness, and swelling may develop at injection site.

**Actions**

*Pharmacokinetics:* Mechanism is obscure, but may be mediated through the chemoreceptor trigger zone; direct impulses to vomiting center are not inhibited.

**Contraindications**

Hypersensitivity to trimethobenzamide, benzocaine or similar local anesthetics; parenteral use in children; suppositories in premature infants or neonates.

**Warnings**

*Pregnancy:* Safety for use has not been established.

*Lactation:* Safety for use in the nursing mother has not been established.

**Precautions**

Encephalitides, gastroenteritis, dehydration, electrolyte imbalance (especially in children and the elderly or debilitated), and CNS reactions have occurred when used during acute febrile illness.

Exercise caution when giving the drug with alcohol and other CNS-acting agents such as phenothiazines, barbiturates, and belladonna derivatives.

**Adverse Reactions**

Adverse reactions may include: Hypersensitivity reactions; parkinson-like symptoms; hypotension or pain following IM injection; blood dyscrasias; blurred vision; coma; convulsions; depression; diarrhea; disorientation; dizziness; drowsiness; headache; jaundice; muscle cramps; opisthotonos; allergic-type skin reactions.

# DRONABINOL

**Gelatin capsules:** 2.5, 5, and 10 mg (*c-iii*)                    *Marinol* (Roxane)

### Indications
*Antiemetic:* Treatment of nausea and vomiting associated with cancer chemotherapy in patients not responding adequately to conventional antiemetic treatment.

*Appetite stimulation:* Treating anorexia associated with weight loss in AIDS patients.

### Administration and Dosage
*Antiemetic:* Initially, give 5 mg/m$^2$ 1 to 3 hours prior to the administration of chemotherapy, then every 2 to 4 hours after chemotherapy is given, for a total of 4 to 6 doses/day. If the 5 mg/m$^2$ dose is ineffective, and there are no significant side effects, increase the dose by 2.5 mg/m$^2$ increments to a maximum of 15 mg/m$^2$ per dose. Use caution, however, as the incidence of disturbing psychiatric symptoms increases significantly at this maximum dose. Administration with phenothiazines may improve efficacy (vs either drug alone) without additional toxicity.

*Appetite stimulation:* Initially, give 2.5 mg twice/day before lunch and supper. For patients who cannot tolerate 5 mg/day, reduce dosage to 2.5 mg/day as a single evening or bedtime dose. When adverse reactions are absent or minimal and further therapeutic effect is desired, increase to 2.5 mg before lunch and 5 mg before supper (or 5 mg at lunch and 5 mg after supper). Although most patients respond to 2.5 mg twice/day, 10 mg twice/day has been tolerated in about 50% of patients. The dosage may be increased to a maximum of 20 mg/day in divided doses. Use caution in escalating the dosage because of the increased frequency of dose-related adverse reactions at higher dosages.

### Actions
*Pharmacology:* Dronabinol is the principal psychoactive substance present in *Cannabis sativa* L (marijuana). The mechanism of action is unknown.

Cannabinoids have complex CNS effects, including central sympathomimetic activity.

*Pharmacokinetics:*

*Absorption/Distribution* – Following oral administration, dronabinol is almost completely absorbed (90% to 95%). It has an onset of action of approximately 0.5 to 1 hour and peak effect at 2 to 4 hours. Duration for psychoactive effects is 4 to 6 hours, but the appetite stimulant effect may continue for 24 hours or more after administration.

*Metabolism/Excretion* – Dronabinol undergoes extensive first-pass hepatic metabolism.

Biliary excretion is the major route of elimination. Extended use at the recommended doses may cause accumulation of toxic amounts of dronabinol and its metabolites.

### Contraindications
Hypersensitivity to dronabinol, marijuana, or sesame oil.

### Warnings
*Tolerance:* Following 12 days of dronabinol, tolerance to the cardiovascular and subjective effects developed at doses ≥10 mg/day or less. An initial tachycardia induced by dronabinol was replaced successively by normal sinus rhythm and then bradycardia. A fall in supine blood pressure, made worse by standing, was also observed initially. Within days, these effects disappeared, indicating development of tolerance. Tachyphylaxis and tolerance did not, however, appear to develop to the appetite stimulant effect.

*Patient supervision:* Because of individual variation, determine clinically the period of patient supervision required.

*Elderly:* Use caution because the elderly are generally more sensitive to the psychoactive effects. In antiemetic studies, no difference in tolerance or efficacy was apparent in patients older than 55 years of age.

*Pregnancy: Category B.*

*Lactation:* Dronabinol is concentrated and excreted in breast milk; nursing mothers should not use dronabinol.

*Children:* Not recommended for AIDS-related anorexia in children because it has not been studied in this population. Dosage for chemotherapy-induced emesis is the same as in adults. Use caution in children because of the psychoactive effects.

**Precautions**
*Hypertension or heart disease:* Use with caution since dronabinol may cause a general increase in central sympathomimetic activity.

*Psychiatric patients:* In manic, depressive, or schizophrenic patients, symptoms of these disease states may be exacerbated by the use of cannabinoids.

*Drug abuse and dependence:* Dronabinol is highly abusable. Limit prescriptions to the amount necessary for a single cycle of chemotherapy.

A withdrawal syndrome consisting of irritability, insomnia, and restlessness was observed in some subjects within 12 hours following abrupt withdrawal of dronabinol. The syndrome reached its peak intensity at 24 hours when subjects exhibited hot flashes, sweating, rhinorrhea, loose stools, hiccoughs, and anorexia. The syndrome was essentially complete within 96 hours. EEG changes following discontinuation were consistent with a withdrawal syndrome. Several subjects reported impressions of disturbed sleep for several weeks after discontinuing high doses.

*Hazardous tasks:* Because of its profound effects on mental status, warn patients not to drive, operate complex machinery, or engage in any activity requiring sound judgment and unimpaired coordination while receiving treatment. Effects may persist for a variable and unpredictable period of time.

**Drug Interactions**
Drugs that may be affected by dronabinol include amphetamines, cocaine, sympathomimetics, anticholinergics, antihistamines, tricyclic antidepressants, alcohol, sedatives, hypnotics, psychomimetics, disulfiram, fluoxetine, and theophylline.

**Adverse Reactions**
Adverse reactions occurring in 3% or more of patients include euphoria, nausea, vomiting, dizziness, paranoid reaction, and somnolence.

# 5-HT₃ RECEPTOR ANTAGONISTS

**ALOSETRON HCl**
Tablets: 1 mg (1.124 mg alosetron HCl equiv. to 1 mg alosetron) (*Rx*)   *Lotronex* (GlaxoSmithKline)

**DOLASETRON**
Tablets: 50 and 100 mg (*Rx*)   *Anzemet* (Aventis)
Injection: 20 mg/mL (*Rx*)

**GRANISETRON**
Tablets: 1 mg (1.12 mg as HCl) (*Rx*)   *Kytril* (Roche)
Solution, oral: 1 mg/5 mL (1.12 mg/5 mL as HCl) (*Rx*)
Injection: 1 mg/mL (1.12 mg/mL as HCl) (*Rx*)

**ONDANSETRON**
Tablets: 4, 8, 24 mg (as HCl dihydrate) (*Rx*)   *Zofran* (GlaxoSmithKline)
Solution, oral: 4 mg/5 mL (5 mg as HCl) (*Rx*)
Injection: 2 mg/mL and 32 mg/50 mL (pre-mixed) (as HCl dihydrate) (*Rx*)
Tablets, orally disintegrating: 4 and 8 mg (as base) (*Rx*)   *Zofran ODT* (GlaxoSmithKline)

**PALONOSETRON HCl**
Injection: 0.25 mg/5 mL (as base)   *Aloxi* (MGI Pharma)

**Warning:**
Serious GI adverse events, some fatal, have been reported with the use of **alosetron**. These events, including ischemic colitis and serious complications of constipation, have resulted in hospitalization, blood transfusion, surgery, and death.

- Only physicians who have enrolled in GlaxoSmithKline's Prescribing Program for *Lotronex*, based on their attestation of qualifications and acceptance of responsibilities, should prescribe alosetron (see Administration and Dosage).
- Alosetron is indicated only for women with severe diarrhea-predominant irritable bowel syndrome (IBS) who have failed to respond to conventional therapy (see Indications). Less than 5% of IBS is considered severe. Before receiving the initial prescription for alosetron, the patient must read and sign the Patient-Physician Agreement.
- Alosetron should be discontinued immediately in patients who develop constipation or symptoms of ischemic colitis. Physicians should instruct patients to immediately report constipation or symptoms of ischemic colitis. Alosetron should not be resumed in patients who develop ischemic colitis. Physicians should instruct patients who report constipation to immediately contact them if the constipation does not resolve after discontinuation of alosetron. Patients with resolved constipation should resume alosetron only on the advice of their treating physician.

## Indications

*Antiemetic:* Prevention of nausea and vomiting associated with initial and repeat courses of emetogenic cancer therapy (including moderately and highly emetogenic cancer chemotherapy), including high-dose cisplatin; prevention of postoperative nausea or vomiting (**ondansetron** and **dolasetron**); for the prevention of acute or delayed nausea and vomiting associated with initial and repeat courses of moderately and highly emetogenic cancer chemotherapy (**palonosetron**); treatment of postoperative nausea or vomiting (**dolasetron** and **granisetron** injection); prevention of nausea and vomiting associated with radiotherapy in patients receiving total body irradiation, single high-dose fraction, or daily fractions to the abdomen (oral **ondansetron** and **granisetron**).

*IBS (alosetron):* Because of serious GI adverse events, some fatal, alosetron is indicated only for women with severe diarrhea-predominant IBS who have:
- chronic IBS symptoms (generally lasting 6 months or longer),
- had anatomic or biochemical abnormalities of the GI tract excluded, and
- failed to respond to conventional therapy.

Diarrhea-predominant IBS is severe if it includes diarrhea and 1 or more of the following:
- frequent and severe abdominal pain/discomfort,
- frequent bowel urgency or fecal incontinence,
- disability or restriction of daily activities because of IBS.

Less than 5% of IBS is considered severe.

*Unlabeled uses:*
    *Granisetron* – Acute nausea and vomiting following surgery (1 to 3 mg IV).
    *Dolasetron* – Radiotherapy-induced nausea and vomiting (40 mg IV or 0.3 mg/kg IV).

## Administration and Dosage

*ALOSETRON:* For safety reasons, alosetron is approved with marketing restrictions. Physicians must attest that they are able and willing to:
- diagnose and treat IBS,
- diagnose and manage ischemic colitis,
- diagnose and manage constipation and complications of constipation,

- understand the risks and benefits of treatment with alosetron for severe diarrhea-predominant IBS,
- educate patients on the risks and benefits of treatment with alosetron,
- report serious adverse events to GlaxoSmithKline at (888) 825-5249 or to the Food and Drug Administration's MedWatch Program at (800) FDA-1088.
- affix program stickers to all prescriptions for alosetron (ie, the original and all subsequent refill prescriptions). No telephone, facsimile, or computerized prescriptions are permitted with this program.

To enroll in the Prescribing Program for *Lotronex*, call (888) 825-5249 or visit www.LOTRONEX.com.

*Usual adult dose* – Start alosetron at a dosage of 1 mg orally once/day for 4 weeks. If, after 4 weeks, the 1 mg once daily dosage is well tolerated but does not adequately control IBS symptoms, then the dosage can be increased to 1 mg twice/day. Discontinue alosetron in patients who have not had adequate control of IBS symptoms after 4 weeks of treatment with 1 mg twice/day. Alosetron can be taken with or without food.

Discontinue alosetron immediately in patients who develop constipation or signs of ischemic colitis. Do not restart alosetron in patients who develop ischemic colitis.

*Children* – Safety and effectiveness have not been established in pediatric patients.

*Elderly* – Postmarketing experience suggests that elderly patients may be at greater risk for complications of constipation; therefore, exercise appropriate caution and follow-up if alosetron is prescribed for these patients.

DOLASETRON:

*Cardiac effects* – Administer dolasetron with caution in patients who have or may develop prolongation of cardiac conduction intervals, particularly $QT_c$.

*Infusion rate* – Dolasetron injection can be safely infused IV as rapidly as 100 mg/ 30 seconds or diluted in a compatible IV solution to 50 mL and infused over a period of up to 15 minutes.

*Chemotherapy-induced nausea and vomiting, prevention* –
IV:
*Adults* – 1.8 mg/kg as a single dose about 30 minutes before chemotherapy. Alternatively, a fixed dose of 100 mg can be administered over 30 seconds.

*Children (2 to 16 years of age)* – 1.8 mg/kg as a single dose about 30 minutes before chemotherapy, up to a maximum of 100 mg.

Oral:
*Adults* – 100 mg within 1 hour before chemotherapy.

*Children (2 to 16 years of age)* – 1.8 mg/kg within 1 hour before chemotherapy, up to a maximum of 100 mg.

*Postoperative nausea or vomiting, prevention/treatment* –
IV:
*Adults* – 12.5 mg as a single dose about 15 minutes before the cessation of anesthesia or as soon as nausea or vomiting presents.

*Children (2 to 16 years of age)* – 0.35 mg/kg as a single dose about 15 minutes before the cessation of anesthesia or as soon as nausea or vomiting presents, up to a maximum of 12.5 mg.

Oral (prevention only) –
*Adults:* 100 mg 2 hours before surgery.

*Children (2 to 16 years of age):* 1.2 mg/kg within 2 hours before surgery, up to a maximum of 100 mg.

GRANISETRON:

Oral –
*Emetogenic chemotherapy:* Adult dosage of 2 mg once daily or 1 mg twice daily. In the 2 mg once-daily regimen, two 1 mg tablets or 10 mL of oral solution are given up to 1 hour before chemotherapy. In the 1 mg twice-daily regimen, give the first 1 mg tablet or 1 teaspoonful (5 mL) of oral solution up to 1 hour before chemotherapy and the second tablet or second teaspoonful (5 mL) oral solution 12 hours

after the first. Either regimen is administered only on the day(s) chemotherapy is given. Continued treatment while not on chemotherapy has not been found to be useful.

*Radiation (total body irradiation or fractionated abdominal radiation):* Adult dose of 2 mg once daily. Two 1 mg tablets or 10 mL of oral solution are taken within 1 hour of radiation.

IV –

*Prevention of chemotherapy-induced nausea and vomiting:*

*Adults and children 2 years of age or older* – 10 mcg/kg administered IV within 30 minutes before initiation of chemotherapy, and only on the day(s) chemotherapy is given.

*Infusion preparation* – May be administered IV either undiluted over 30 seconds or diluted with 0.9% sodium chloride or 5% dextrose and infused over 5 minutes.

As a general precaution, do not mix solution with other drugs.

*Prevention and treatment of postoperative nausea and vomiting:*

*Adults* –

*Prevention:* 1 mg undiluted granisetron, administered IV over 30 seconds, before induction of anesthesia or immediately before reversal of anesthesia.

*Treatment:* After surgery, 1 mg undiluted granisetron administered IV over 30 seconds.

ONDANSETRON:

*Prevention of nausea/vomiting associated with cancer chemotherapy* –

*Parenteral:* The recommended IV dosage is three 0.15 mg/kg doses or a single 32 mg dose. With the 3 dose regimen, the first dose is infused over 15 minutes beginning 30 minutes before the start of emetogenic chemotherapy. Subsequent doses are administered 4 and 8 hours after the first dose. The single 32 mg dose is infused over 15 minutes beginning 30 minutes before the start of emetogenic chemotherapy.

*Children* – The dosage in children 4 to 18 years of age should be three 0.15 mg/kg doses (see above). Little information is available about dosage in children 3 years of age or younger.

*Oral (moderately emetogenic cancer chemotherapy):* In patients greater than 12 years of age, the recommended dose is 8 mg twice/day. Administer the first dose 30 minutes before the start of emetogenic chemotherapy, with a subsequent dose 8 hours after the first dose. Administer 8 mg twice a day (every 12 hours) for 1 to 2 days after completion of chemotherapy.

*Children* – Dosage is same as adults; for children 4 to 11 years, use 4 mg 3 times a day. Give the first dose 30 minutes before chemotherapy, with subsequent doses 4 and 8 hours after the first dose. Give 4 mg 3 times a day (every 8 hours) for 1 to 2 days after completion of chemotherapy.

*Prevention of nausea and vomiting associated with radiotherapy (oral)* – 8 mg 3 times/day.

*Total body irradiation:* 8 mg 1 to 2 hours before each fraction of radiotherapy administered each day.

*Single high-dose fraction radiotherapy to the abdomen:* 8 mg 1 to 2 hours before radiotherapy, with subsequent doses every 8 hours after the first dose for 1 to 2 days after completion of radiotherapy.

*Daily fractionated radiotherapy to the abdomen:* 8 mg 1 to 2 hours before radiotherapy, with subsequent doses every 8 hours after the first dose for each day radiotherapy is given.

*Prevention of postoperative nausea or vomiting* –

*Parenteral:* Immediately before induction of anesthesia, or postoperatively if the patient experiences nausea or vomiting shortly after surgery, administer 4 mg undiluted IV in not less than 30 seconds, preferably over 2 to 5 minutes. Alternatively, 4 mg undiluted may be administered IM as a single injection in adults. In patients who do not achieve adequate control, administration of a second IV dose of 4 mg ondansetron postoperatively does not provide additional control of nausea and vomiting.

*Children* – Patients 2 to 12 years of age weighing 40 kg or less may receive 0.1 mg/kg IV; give a single 4 mg dose for those weighing more than 40 kg. Administer over not less than 30 seconds, preferably over 2 to 5 minutes.

*Oral:* 16 mg given as a single dose 1 hour before induction of anesthesia.

*Children:* There is no experience in children.

*Prevention of nausea and vomiting associated with highly emetogenic cancer chemotherapy (oral)* – The recommended adult oral dosage is 24 mg administered 30 minutes before the start of single-day highly emetogenic chemotherapy, including cisplatin greater than 50 mg/m$^2$. Efficacy of the 32 mg single dose beyond 24 hours in these patients has not been established.

*Hepatic function impairment* – Do not exceed an 8 mg oral dose. For IV use, a single maximum daily dose of 8 mg infused over 15 minutes beginning 30 minutes before the start of emetogenic chemotherapy is recommended.

PALONOSETRON:

*Adults* – The recommended dosage of palonosetron is 0.25 mg administered as a single dose approximately 30 minutes before the start of chemotherapy. Repeated dosing of palonosetron within a 7-day interval is not recommended because the safety and efficacy of frequent (consecutive or alternate day) dosing in patients have not been evaluated.

*Administration:* Infuse IV over 30 seconds. Do not mix palonosetron with other drugs. Flush the infusion line with normal saline before and after administration of palonosetron.

## Actions

*Pharmacology:* Selective 5-hydroxytryptamine$_3$ (5-HT$_3$) receptor antagonists are antinauseant and antiemetic agents with little or no affinity for other serotonin receptors, alpha- or beta-adrenergic, dopamine-D$_2$, histamine-H$_1$, benzodiazepine, picrotoxin, or opioid receptors. 5-HT$_3$ receptor antagonists such as **alosetron** inhibit activation of nonselective cation channels, which results in the modulation of the enteric nervous system.

*Pharmacokinetics:* The elimination half-lives of these drugs range from 4 to 8 hours. Elimination is primarily via hepatic metabosim. Plasma concentrations of **alosetron** are 30% to 50% lower and less variable in men compared with women given the same dose. Plasma protein binding is 82% for alosetron, 65% for **granisetron** and 70% to 76% for **ondansetron**. The terminal elimination half-life of alosetron is approximately 1.5 hours.

## Contraindications

*Dolasetron:* Hypersensitivity to the drug or components of the product; markedly prolonged QTc or atrioventricular block II to III; patients receiving class I or III antiarrhythmic agents.

*Alosetron:* Do not initiate alosetron in patients with constipation. Alosetron is contraindicated in patients:

- with a history of chronic or severe constipation or with a history of sequelae from constipation,
- with a history of intestinal obstruction, stricture, toxic megacolon, GI perforation, or adhesions,
- with a history of ischemic colitis, impaired intestinal circulation, thrombophlebitis, or hypercoagulable state,
- with current or a history of Crohn's disease or ulcerative colitis,
- with active diverticulitis or a history of diverticulitis,
- who are unable to understand or comply with the Patient-Physician Agreement,
- with known hypersensitivity to any component of the product.

## Warnings

*Ischemic colitis:* Ischemic colitis has been reported in patients receiving **alosetron**. Immediately discontinue alosetron in patients with signs of ischemic colitis, such as rectal bleeding, bloody diarrhea, or new or worsening abdominal pain. Do not resume alosetron in patients who develop ischemic colitis.

*Constipation:* Serious complications of constipation, including obstruction, perforation, impaction, toxic megacolon, secondary colonic ischemia, and death have been reported with use of **alosetron**. Immediately discontinue alosetron treatment in patients who develop constipation.

*Postoperatively:* Routine prophylaxis is not recommended for patients in whom there is little expectation that nausea or vomiting will occur postoperatively. In patients where nausea or vomiting must be avoided postoperatively, IV **ondansetron** is recommended even where the incidence of postoperative nausea or vomiting is low. For patients who have postoperative nausea or vomiting, ondansetron may be given to prevent further episodes.

*Cardiac effects:* Acute, usually reversible, ECG changes (PR and QTc prolongation; QRS widening) caused by **dolasetron** have been observed. Dolasetron appears to prolong depolarization and, to a lesser extent, repolarization time. The magnitude and frequency of the ECG changes increased with dose. These ECG interval prolongations usually returned to baseline within 6 to 8 hours but in some patients were present at 24-hour follow up.

Administer dolasetron with caution in patients who have or may develop prolongation of cardiac conduction intervals, particularly QTc. These include patients with hypokalemia or hypomagnesemia, patients taking diuretics with potential for inducing electrolyte abnormalities, patients with congenital QT syndrome, patients taking antiarrhythmic drugs or other drugs that lead to QT prolongation and cumulative high dose anthracycline therapy.

*Peristalsis:* Ondansetron does not stimulate gastric or intestinal peristalsis. Do not use instead of nasogastric suction. Use in abdominal surgery may mask a progressive ileus or gastric distension.

*Hypersensitivity reactions:* Rare cases of hypersensitivity reactions, sometimes severe, have occurred.

*Hepatic function impairment:* Increased exposure to alosetron is likely to occur in patients with hepatic insufficiency.

*Pregnancy: Category B.*

*Lactation:* It is not known whether 5-HT₃ antagonists are excreted in breast milk.

*Children:*

    *Granisetron* – Safety and efficacy of the injection in children less than 2 years of age have not been established. Safety and efficacy of the oral doseform in children have not been established.

    *Ondansetron* – Little information is available about dosage in children 3 years of age or younger.

    *Dolasetron* – Safety and efficacy in children less than 2 years of age have not been established. See Administration and Dosage for use in children 2 years of age or older.

    *Alosetron* – Safety and efficacy in pediatric patients have not been established.

    *Palonosetron –*

      *Children:* A recommended IV dosage has not been established for pediatric patients.

### Precautions

*Benzyl alcohol:* Some of these products contain benzyl alcohol, which has been associated with a fatal "gasping syndrome" in premature infants.

### Drug Interactions

Inducers or inhibitors of P450 enzymes may change the clearance and, hence, the half-life of 5-HT₃ antagonists. No dosage adjustment is recommended for patients on these drugs. **Dolasetron** may be affected by atenolol, cimetidine, and rifampin. **Ondansetron** may be affected by rifampin.

## Adverse Reactions

Adverse reactions occurring in at least 3% of patients:

*Ondansetron:* Abdominal pain; anxiety/agitation; arrhythmias; increased AST and ALT; chills/shivering; constipation; diarrhea; dizziness; drowsiness/sedation; extrapyramidal syndrome; malaise/fatigue; fever/pyrexia; gynecological disorder; headache; hypotension; hypoxia; injection site reaction; musculoskeletal pain; pruritus; urinary retention; wound problem.

*Granisetron:* Abdominal pain; alopecia; anemia; decreased appetite; increased AST and ALT; asthenia; CNS stimulation; constipation; diarrhea; headache; leukopenia; nausea/vomiting; somnolence; shivers; thrombocytopenia.

*Dolasetron:* Abdominal pain; increased AST and ALT; bradycardia/tachycardia; dizziness; dyspepsia; fever/pyrexia; headache; hypotension; malaise/fatigue; pruritus.

*Alosetron:* Abdominal pain; constipation; GI discomfort/pain; nausea.

# APREPITANT

| **Capsules:** 80 and 125 mg *(Rx)* | *Emend* (Merck) |
| --- | --- |

## Indications

*Antiemetic:* Aprepitant, in combination with other antiemetic agents, is indicated for the prevention of acute and delayed nausea and vomiting associated with initial and repeat courses of highly emetogenic cancer chemotherapy, including high-dose cisplatin.

## Administration and Dosage

*Dosage regimen:* Aprepitant is given for 3 days as part of a regimen that includes a corticosteroid and a 5-HT$_3$ antagonist. The recommended dose of aprepitant is 125 mg orally 1 hour prior to chemotherapy treatment (day 1) and 80 mg once daily in the morning on days 2 and 3. Aprepitant has not been studied for the treatment of established nausea and vomiting.

Chronic continuous administration is not recommended. Aprepitant may be taken with or without food.

*Concomitant therapy:* The oral dexamethasone doses should be reduced by approximately 50% when coadministered with aprepitant.

The IV methylprednisolone dose should be reduced by approximately 25%, and the oral methylprednisolone dose should be reduced by approximately 50% when coadministered with aprepitant.

## Actions

*Pharmacology:* Aprepitant is a selective high-affinity antagonist of human substance P/neurokinin 1 (NK$_1$) receptors. Aprepitant has little or no affinity for serotonin (5-HT$_3$), dopamine, and corticosteroid receptors, the targets of existing therapies for chemotherapy-induced nausea and vomiting (CINV).

Studies show that aprepitant augments the antiemetic activity of the 5-HT$_3$-receptor antagonist ondansetron and the corticosteroid dexamethasone and inhibits both the acute and delayed phases of cisplatin-induced emesis.

*Pharmacokinetics:*

*Absorption* – The mean absolute oral bioavailability of aprepitant is approximately 60% to 65% and the mean peak plasma concentration (C$_{max}$) of aprepitant occurred at approximately 4 hours (T$_{max}$).

*Distribution* – Aprepitant is greater than 95% bound to plasma proteins. The mean apparent volume of distribution at steady state (Vd$_{ss}$) is approximately 70 L.

Aprepitant crosses the placenta in rats and rabbits and crosses the blood-brain barrier in humans.

*Metabolism* – Aprepitant undergoes extensive metabolism. In vitro studies using human liver microsomes indicate that aprepitant is metabolized primarily by CYP3A4 with minor metabolism by CYP1A2 and CYP2C19. No metabolism by CYP2D6, CYP2C9, or CYP2E1 was detected.

*Excretion* – Aprepitant is eliminated primarily by metabolism; aprepitant is not renally excreted. The apparent plasma clearance of aprepitant ranged from approximately 62 to 90 mL/min. The apparent terminal half-life ranged from approximately 9 to 13 hours.

## Contraindications

Aprepitant is a moderate CYP3A4 inhibitor. Aprepitant should not be used concurrently with pimozide or cisapride. Inhibition of cytochrome P450 isoenzyme 3A4 (CYP3A4) by aprepitant could result in elevated plasma concentrations of these drugs, potentially causing serious or life-threatening reactions. Aprepitant is contraindicated in patients who are hypersensitive to any component of the product.

## Warnings

*Pregnancy:* Category B.

*Lactation:* It is not known whether this drug is excreted in human milk. A decision should be made whether to discontinue nursing or to discontinue the drug, taking into account the importance of the drug to the mother.

*Children:* Safety and efficacy of aprepitant in children have not been established.

## Precautions

*Long-term therapy:* Chronic continuous use of aprepitant for prevention of nausea and vomiting is not recommended.

## Drug Interactions

Aprepitant is a substrate, a moderate inhibitor, and an inducer of CYP3A4. Aprepitant is also an inducer of CYP2C9. Use aprepitant with caution in patients receiving concomitant medicinal products, including chemotherapy agents that are primarily metabolized through CYP3A4 (docetaxel, paclitaxel, etoposide, irinotecan, ifosfamide, imatinib, vinorelbine, vinblastine, and vincristine).

Drugs that may affect aprepitant include CYP 3A4 inhibitors (eg, clarithromycin, diltiazem, itraconazole, ketoconazole, nefazodone, nelfinavir, ritonavir, troleandomycin), CYP3A4 inducers (eg, carbamazepine, phenytoin, rifampin), and paroxetine.

Aprepitant may be affected by paroxetine, CYP2C9 substrates (eg, phenytoin, tolbutamide, warfarin), CYP3A4 substrates (eg, alprazolam, cisapride, dexamethasone, docetaxel, etoposide, ifosfamide, imatinib, irinotecan, methylprednisolone, midazolam, paclitaxel, pimozide, triazolam, vinblastine, vincristine, vinorelbine), and oral contraceptives.

## Adverse Reactions

Adverse reactions occurring in at least 3% of aprepitant patients include the following: Abdominal pain, anorexia, ALT/AST/BUN/Serum creatinine increased, asthenia/fatigue, constipation, dehydration, diarrhea, dizziness, epigastric discomfort, gastritis, headache, heartburn, hiccoughs, nausea, neutropenia, proteinuria, tinnitus, vomiting.

# MEPROBAMATE

| **Tablets:** 200, 400, and 600 mg (c-IV) | Various, *Equanil* (Wyeth-Ayerst), *Miltown* (Wallace) |

## Indications
Management of anxiety disorders or short-term relief of the symptoms of anxiety.

## Administration and Dosage
*Adults:* 1.2 to 1.6 g/day in 3 to 4 divided doses; do not exceed 2.4 g/day.

*Children:* 100 to 200 mg 2 or 3 times/day.

## Actions
*Pharmacology:* Meprobamate has selective effects at multiple sites in the CNS, including the thalamus and limbic system. It also appears to inhibit multineuronal spinal reflexes. Meprobamate is mildly tranquilizing, and has some anticonvulsant and muscle relaxant properties.

*Pharmacokinetics:*

    *Absorption/Distribution* – Meprobamate is well absorbed from the GI tract; peak plasma concentrations are reached within 1 to 3 hours.

    *Metabolism/Excretion* – The liver metabolizes 80% to 92% of the drug; the remainder is excreted unchanged in the urine. Excretion is mainly renal (90%), with less than 10% appearing in feces.

## Contraindications
Acute intermittent porphyria; allergic or idiosyncratic reactions to meprobamate or related compounds.

## Warnings
*Hypersensitivity reactions:* Usually seen between the first to fourth dose in patients having no previous exposure to the drug.

*Renal function impairment:* Use with caution to avoid accumulation, since meprobamate is metabolized in the liver and excreted by the kidney.

*Elderly:* To avoid oversedation, use lowest effective dose.

*Pregnancy: Category D.*

*Lactation:* Meprobamate is excreted into breast milk at concentrations 2 to 4 times that of maternal plasma.

*Children:* Do not administer to children younger than 6 years of age. The 600 mg tablet is not intended for use in children.

## Precautions
*Epilepsy:* May precipitate seizures in epileptic patients.

*Drug abuse and dependence:* Physical and psychological dependence and abuse may occur. Abrupt discontinuation after prolonged and excessive use may precipitate a recurrence of pre-existing symptoms or withdrawal syndrome characterized by anxiety, anorexia, insomnia, vomiting, ataxia, tremors, muscle twitching, confusional states, and hallucinations. Generalized seizures occur in about 10% of cases and are more likely to occur in people with CNS damage or preexistent or latent convulsive disorders. Onset of withdrawal symptoms usually occurs within 12 to 48 hours after drug discontinuation; symptoms usually cease in the next 12 to 48 hours.

When excessive dosage has continued for weeks or months, reduce gradually over a period of 1 or 2 weeks rather than stopping abruptly.

*Hazardous tasks:* May produce drowsiness, dizziness, or blurred vision; patients should observe caution while driving or performing other tasks requiring alertness.

## Drug Interactions
*Alcohol:* Acute ingestion may result in a decreased clearance of meprobamate through inhibition of hepatic metabolic systems; enhanced CNS depressant effects may occur.

**Adverse Reactions**

Adverse reactions may include drowsiness; ataxia; dizziness; slurred speech; headache; vertigo; weakness; impairment of visual accommodation; euphoria; overstimulation; paradoxical excitement; nausea; vomiting; diarrhea; palpitations; tachycardia; various arrhythmias; syncope; hypotensive crises; allergic/idiosyncratic reactions; leukopenia; acute nonthrombocytopenic purpura; petechiae; ecchymoses; eosinophilia; peripheral edema; fever; hyperpyrexia; chills; angioneurotic edema; bronchospasm; oliguria; anuria; anaphylaxis; erythema multiforme; exfoliative dermatitis; stomatitis; proctitis; Stevens-Johnson syndrome; bullous dermatitis; paresthesias; agranulocytosis; aplastic anemia; thrombocytopenic purpura.

# BENZODIAZEPINES

**ALPRAZOLAM**

| | |
|---|---|
| **Tablets:** 0.25, 0.5, 1, and 2 mg (*c-IV*) | Various, *Xanax* (Pfizer) |
| **Tablets, extended-release:** 0.5, 1, 2, and 3 mg (*c-IV*) | *Xanax XR* (Pfizer) |
| **Oral solution:** 1 mg/mL (*c-IV*) | *Alprazolam Intensol* (Roxane) |

**CHLORDIAZEPOXIDE**

| | |
|---|---|
| **Capsules:** 5, 10, and 25 mg (*c-IV*) | Various, *Librium* (ICN Pharmaceuticals) |
| **Powder for injection:** 100 mg (*c-IV*) | *Librium* (ICN Pharmaceuticals) |

**CLONAZEPAM**

| | |
|---|---|
| **Tablets:** 0.5, 1, and 2 mg (*Rx*) | Various, *Klonopin* (Roche) |
| **Tablets, orally disintegrating:** 0.125, 0.25, 0.5, 1, and 2 mg (*Rx*) | Various, *Klonopin* (Roche) |

**CLORAZEPATE DIPOTASSIUM**

| | |
|---|---|
| **Tablets:** 3.75, 7.5, and 15 mg (*c-IV*) | Various, *Tranxene T-tab* (Ovation) |
| **Tablets, extended-release:** 11.25 and 22.5 mg (*c-IV*) | *Tranxene-SD Half Strength* , *Tranxene-SD* (Ovation) |

**DIAZEPAM**

| | |
|---|---|
| **Tablets:** 2, 5, and 10 mg (*c-IV*) | Various, *Valium* (Roche) |
| **Oral solution:** 5 mg/5 mL, 5 mg/mL (*c-IV*) | *Diazepam, Diazepam Intensol* (Roxane) |
| **Injection:** 5 mg/mL (*c-IV*) | Various |

**LORAZEPAM**

| | |
|---|---|
| **Tablets:** 0.5, 1, and 2 mg (*c-IV*) | Various |
| **Concentrated oral solution:** 2 mg/mL (*c-IV*) | *Lorazepam Intensol* (Roxane) |
| **Injection:** 2 and 4 mg/mL (*c-IV*) | Various, *Ativan* (Baxter) |

**OXAZEPAM**

| | |
|---|---|
| **Capsules:** 10, 15, and 30 mg (*c-IV*) | Various |

**Indications**

*Anxiety:* For the management of anxiety disorders or for the short-term relief of the symptoms of anxiety (anxiety associated with depression is also responsive) (alprazolam immediate-release and intensol, clorazepate, chlordiazepoxide, diazepam, lorazepam, oxazepam); for the management of anxiety, tension, agitation, and irritability in older patients (oxazepam).

*Panic disorder:* Treatment of panic disorder, with or without agoraphobia (alprazolam immediate-release and extended-release, clonazepam).

*Acute alcohol withdrawal:* For the symptomatic relief of acute alcohol withdrawal (clorazepate, chlordiazepoxide, oxazepam); may be useful in symptomatic relief of acute agitation, tremor, impending or acute delirium, tremens, and hallucinosis (diazepam).

*Anticonvulsant:* As adjunctive therapy in the management of partial seizures (clorazepate); adjunctively in status epilepticus and severe recurrent convulsive seizures (diazepam IV); adjunctively in convulsive disorders (diazepam oral).

*Preoperative:* For preoperative apprehension and anxiety (chlordiazepoxide, diazepam IV); prior to cardioversion for the relief of anxiety and tension and to diminish patient's recall (diazepam IV); adjunctively prior to endoscopic procedures for apprehension, anxiety, or acute stress reactions and to diminish patient's recall (diazepam); for preanesthetic medication to produce sedation, anxiety relief, and a decreased ability to recall surgery-related events (lorazepam).

*Muscle relaxant:* As an adjunct for the relief of skeletal muscle spasm because of reflex spasm caused by local pathology, spasticity caused by uppermotor neuron disorders, athetosis, stiff-man syndrome, used parenterally in the treatment of tetanus (diazepam).

*Seizure disorder:* Alone or as an adjunct in the treatment of the Lennox-Gastaut syndrome (petit mal variant), akinetic, and myoclonic seizures. May be useful in patients with absence seizures (petit mal) who have failed to respond to succinimides (see Anticonvulsant section).

*Status epilepticus:* For the treatment of status epilepticus (lorazepam).

### Administration and Dosage

ALPRAZOLAM: The necessary duration of treatment for responding patients is unknown. However, periodic reassessment is advised.

Reduce gradually when terminating or decreasing daily dose. Decrease by no more than 0.5 mg every 3 days.

*Anxiety disorders (immediate-release and intensol)* – Initial dose is 0.25 to 0.5 mg 3 times/day. Titrate to max total dose of 4 mg/day in divided doses at intervals of 3 to 4 days. If side effects occur with starting dose, decrease dose.

*Panic disorder (Xanax and Xanax XR)* –

*Immediate-release tablets:* Initial dose is 0.5 mg 3 times/day. Depending on response, increase dose at intervals of 3 to 4 days in increments of no more than 1 mg/day.

Successful treatment has required doses more than 4 mg/day; in controlled studies, doses in the range of 1 to 10 mg/day were used.

*Extended-release tablets:* Administer once daily, preferably in the morning. Take the tablets intact; do not chew, crush, or break.

Treatment may be initiated with 0.5 to 1 mg once daily. The suggested total daily dose ranges between 3 and 6 mg/day. The suggested total daily dosages will meet the needs of most patients; however, there will be some who require doses greater than 6 mg/day.

*Dose maintenance* – Most patients showed efficacy in the range of 3 to 6 mg/day. Occasionally as much as 10 mg/day was required to achieve successful response.

*Immediate/Extended-release tablets:*

*Dose titration* – Depending on response, the dose may be increased at intervals of 3 to 4 days in increments of no more than 1 mg/day. Slower titration to the dose levels may be advisable to allow full expression of the pharmacodynamic effect. Advance dose until an acceptable therapeutic response (ie, a substantial reduction in or total elimination of panic attacks) is achieved, intolerance occurs, or the maximum recommended dose is attained.

*Switching from immediate-release to extended-release tablets* – Patients currently treated with divided doses of immediate-release tablets (eg, 3 to 4 times/day) may be switched to extended-release tablets at the same total daily dose taken once daily. If the therapeutic response after switching is inadequate, dosage may be titrated as outlined above.

*Elderly or debilitated patients* –

*Immediate release and intensol:* 0.25 mg, given 2 or 3 times/day. Gradually increase if needed and tolerated.

*Extended-release:* The usual starting dose is 0.5 mg once/day. Gradually increase if needed and tolerated. The elderly may be especially sensitive to the effects of benzodiazepines.

*Administration of oral solution* – Alprazolam intensol is a concentrated oral solution. It is recommended that the oral solution be mixed with liquids or semi-solid food such as water, juices, soda or soda-like beverages, applesauce, and puddings. Use only the calibrated dropper provided with this product. Draw into the dropper the amount prescribed for a single dose. Then squeeze the dropper contents into a liquid or semi-solid food. Stir the liquid or food gently for a few seconds. The formulation blends quickly and completely. Consume the entire amount of the mixture of drug and liquid or drug and food immediately. Do not store for future use.

CLONAZEPAM:

*Panic disorder* – The initial dose for adults is 0.25 mg twice daily. An increase to the target dose for most patients of 1 mg/day may be made after 3 days. Higher doses of 2, 3, and 4 mg/day in a study were less effective than the 1 mg/day dose and were associated with more adverse effects. Nevertheless, it is possible that some individual patients may benefit from doses of up to a maximum dose of 4 mg/day and, in those instances, the dose may be increased in increments of 0.125 to 0.25 mg twice daily every 3 days until panic disorder is controlled or until side effects make further increases undesired. To reduce the inconvenience of somnolence, administration of one dose at bedtime may be desirable.

*Discontinuation* – Discontinue treatment gradually, with a decrease of 0.125 mg twice daily every 3 days until the drug is completely withdrawn. Periodically reevaluate the long-term usefulness of the drug for the individual patient.

*Administration* – Administer the tablets with water by swallowing the tablet whole. Administer the orally disintegrating tablet as follows: After opening the pouch, peel back the foil on the blister. Do not push the tablet through foil. Immediately upon opening the blister, using dry hands, remove the tablet and place it in the mouth. Tablet disintegration occurs rapidly in saliva so it can be easily swallowed with or without water.

CHLORDIAZEPOXIDE:

Oral –

*Mild to moderate anxiety:* 5 or 10 mg 3 or 4 times/day.

*Severe anxiety:* 20 or 25 mg 3 or 4 times/day.

*Geriatric patients or patients with debilitating disease:* 5 mg 2 to 4 times/day.

*Preoperative apprehension and anxiety:* On days preceding surgery, 5 to 10 mg 3 or 4 times/day.

*Acute alcohol withdrawal:* 50 to 100 mg; repeat as needed (up to 300 mg/day). Parenteral form usually used initially. Reduce to maintenance levels.

*Children:* Initially, 5 mg 2 to 4 times/day (may be increased in some children to 10 mg 2 or 3 times/day). Not recommended in children under 6 years of age.

A dosage of 0.5 mg/kg/day every 6 to 8 hours in children older than 6 years of age has also been recommended.

*Parenteral* – Use lower doses (25 or 50 mg) for elderly or debilitated patients and for older children. A dosage of 0.5 mg/kg/day every 6 to 8 hours IM in children older than 12 years of age has also been recommended. Acute symptoms may be rapidly controlled by parenteral administration; subsequent treatment, if necessary, may be given orally. While 300 mg may be given during a 6 hour period, do not exceed this dose in any 24 hour period. Not recommended in children younger than 12 years of age.

*Acute alcohol withdrawal:* 50 to 100 mg IM or IV initially; repeat in 2 to 4 hours if necessary.

*Acute or severe anxiety:* 50 to 100 mg IM or IV initially; then 25 to 50 mg 3 or 4 times/day if necessary.

*Preoperative apprehension/anxiety:* 50 to 100 mg IM 1 hour prior to surgery.

CLORAZEPATE DIPOTASSIUM:

*Anxiety* – 30 mg/day in divided doses. Adjust gradually within the range of 15 to 60 mg/day. May be administered as a single daily dose of 15 mg initially at bedtime.

*Symptomatic relief of acute alcohol withdrawal (immediate-release tablets)* –

*Day 1:* 30 mg initially, followed by 30 to 60 mg in divided doses.

*Day 2:* 45 to 90 mg in divided doses.

*Day 3:* 22.5 to 45 mg in divided doses.

*Day 4:* 15 to 30 mg in divided doses.

Thereafter, gradually reduce the dose to 7.5 to 15 mg once/day. Discontinue drug as soon as patient's condition is stable.

The maximum recommended total daily dose is 90 mg. Avoid excessive reductions in the total amount of drug administered on successive days.

*Elderly or debilitated patients* – Initiate treatment at a dose of 7.5 to 15 mg/day.

*Extended-release tablets* –

*Maintenance therapy:* Give the 22.5 mg tablet in a single daily dose as an alternate dosage form for patients stabilized on 7.5 mg 3 times/day. Do not use to initiate therapy. The 11.25 mg tablet may be administered as a single dose every 24 hours as an alternate dosage form for patients stabilized on a dose of 3.75 mg tablets 3 times/day. Not to be used to initiate therapy.

DIAZEPAM:

*Oral* –

*Management of anxiety disorders and relief of symptoms of anxiety (depending upon severity of symptoms):* 2 to 10 mg 2 to 4 times/day.

*Acute alcohol withdrawal:* 10 mg 3 or 4 times during the first 24 hours; reduce to 5 mg 3 or 4 times/day, as needed.

*Adjunct in skeletal muscle spasm:* 2 to 10 mg 3 or 4 times/day.

*Adjunct in convulsive disorders:* 2 to 10 mg 2 to 4 times/day.

*Elderly patients or in the presence of debilitating disease:* 2 to 2.5 mg 1 or 2 times/day initially; increase gradually as needed and tolerated.

*Children:* 1 to 2.5 mg 3 or 4 times/day initially; increase gradually as needed and tolerated. Not for use in children under 6 months. For sedation or muscle relaxation, a dosage of 0.12 to 0.8 mg/kg/24 hours divided 3 to 4 times a day has been recommended.

*Oral solution:* Dosage same as oral tablets.

*Intensol* – The **Intensol** is a concentrated oral solution as compared to standard oral liquid medications. It is recommended that the **Intensol** be mixed with liquid or semisolid food such as water, juices, soda or soda-like beverages, applesauce, and puddings. Use only the calibrated dropper provided with the product.

*Parenteral* –

*Children:* Administer slowly over 3 minutes. Do not exceed 0.25 mg/kg. After an interval of 15 to 30 minutes, the initial dose can be repeated.

*Moderate anxiety disorders and symptoms of anxiety:* 2 to 5 mg IM or IV. Repeat in 3 to 4 hours if necessary.

*Severe anxiety disorders and symptoms of anxiety:* 5 to 10 mg IM or IV. Repeat in 3 to 4 hours if necessary.

*Acute alcohol withdrawal:* 10 mg IM or IV initially; then 5 to 10 mg in 3 to 4 hours if necessary.

*Endoscopic procedures:*

*IV* – 10 mg or less is usually adequate; up to 20 mg may be used, especially when concomitant narcotics are omitted.

*IM* – 5 to 10 mg 30 minutes prior to procedure if IV route cannot be used.

*Muscle spasm:* 5 to 10 mg IM or IV initially; then 5 to 10 mg in 3 to 4 hours if necessary. Tetanus may require larger doses.

*Status epilepticus and severe recurrent convulsive seizures:* The IV route is preferred; administer slowly. Use the IM route if IV administration is impossible. Administer 5 to 10 mg initially; repeat if necessary at 10 to 15 minute intervals up to maximum dose of 30 mg. If necessary, repeat therapy in 2 to 4 hours. A dose of 0.2 to 0.5 mg/kg every 15 to 30 minutes for 2 to 3 doses (maximum dose, 30 mg).

*Infants (over 30 days of age) and children (under 5 years of age):* Inject 0.2 to 0.5 mg slowly every 2 to 5 minutes up to a maximum of 5 mg; 0.2 to 0.5 mg/kg/dose every 15 to 30 minutes for 2 to 3 doses (maximum dose, 5 mg) has been recommended.

*Neonates:* 0.3 to 0.75 mg/kg/dose every 15 to 30 minutes for 2 to 3 doses has been suggested.

*Preoperative medication:* 10 mg IM before surgery.

*Cardioversion:* 5 to 15 mg IV, 5 to 10 minutes prior to procedure.

*Tetanus:*

*Infants (over 30 days of age)* – 1 to 2 mg IM or IV slowly, repeated every 3 to 4 hours as necessary.

*Children (5 years of age and older)* – 5 to 10 mg repeated every 3 to 4 hours may be required.

*Sedation or muscle relaxation:*
*Children* – 0.04 to 0.2 mg/kg/dose every 2 to 4 hours, maximum of 0.6 mg/kg within an 8-hour period.

*Adults* – 2 to 10 mg/dose every 3 to 4 hours as needed.

LORAZEPAM:
*Oral* – 2 to 6 mg/day (varies from 1 to 10 mg/day) given in divided doses; take the largest dose before bedtime.

*Anxiety:* Initial dose, 2 to 3 mg/day given 2 or 3 times/day.

*Insomnia caused by anxiety or transient situational stress:* 2 to 4 mg at bedtime.

*Elderly or debilitated patients:* Initial dose, 1 to 2 mg/day in divided doses.

*Parenteral* –
*Status epilepticus:* The usual recommended dose is 4 mg given slowly (2 mg/min). If seizures continue or recur after a 10- to 15-minute observation period, an additional 4 mg IV dose may be slowly administered.

*Preanesthetic:* Reduce the doses of other CNS depressant drugs.

IM – 0.05 mg/kg up to a maximum of 4 mg. For optimum effect, administer at least 2 hours before operative procedure.

IV – Initial dose is 2 mg total or 0.044 mg/kg (0.02 mg/lb), whichever is smaller. This will sedate most adults; ordinarily, do not exceed in patients older than 50 years of age. If a greater lack of recall would be beneficial, doses as high as 0.05 mg/kg up to a total of 4 mg may be given. For optimum effect, give 15 to 20 minutes before the procedure.

*Children (younger than 18 years of age)* – Parenteral use is not recommended.

OXAZEPAM:
*Mild to moderate anxiety, with associated tension, irritability, agitation, or related symptoms of functional origin or secondary to organic disease* – 10 to 15 mg 3 or 4 times/day.

*Severe anxiety syndromes, agitation, or anxiety associated with depression* – 15 to 30 mg 3 or 4 times/day.

*Older patients with anxiety, tension, irritability and agitation* – Initial dosage is 10 mg 3 times/day. If necessary, increase cautiously to 15 mg 3 or 4 times/day.

*Alcoholics with acute inebriation, tremulousness, or anxiety on withdrawal* – 15 to 30 mg 3 or 4 times/day.

*Children (6 to 12 years of age)* – Dosage is not established.

## Actions

*Pharmacology:* Benzodiazepines appear to potentiate the effects of gamma-aminobutyrate (GABA) (ie, they facilitate inhibitory GABA neurotransmission) and other inhibitory transmitters by binding to specific benzodiazepine receptor sites.

*Pharmacokinetics:*

| | Benzodiazepine Pharmacokinetics | | | | | |
|---|---|---|---|---|---|---|
| Drug | Dosage range (mg/day)[1] | Peak plasma level (h)[1] | Elimination t½ (h) | Metabolites | Speed of onset[1] | Protein binding |
| Alprazolam | 0.75-4 | 1-2 | 6.3-26.9 | Alpha-hydroxy-alprazolam; Benzophenone | intermediate | 80% |
| Chlordiazepoxide | 15-100 | 0.5-4 | 5-30 | Desmethyl chlordiazepoxide;[2] Demoxepam; Desmethyldiazepam | intermediate | 96% |
| Clonazepam | 1.5-20 | 1-2 | 18-50 | Inactive 7-amino or 7-acetyl-amino derivatives[2] | intermediate | 97% |
| Clorazepate | 15-60 | 1-2 | 40-50 | Desmethyldiazepam | fast | 97%-98% |
| Diazepam | 4-40 | 0.5-2 | 20-80 | Desmethyldiazepam;[2] nordiazepam | very fast | 98% |

| Benzodiazepine Pharmacokinetics | | | | | | |
| --- | --- | --- | --- | --- | --- | --- |
| Drug | Dosage range (mg/day)[1] | Peak plasma level (h)[1] | Elimination t½ (h) | Metabolites | Speed of onset[1] | Protein binding |
| Lorazepam | 2-4 | 2-4 | 10-20 | Inactive glucuronide conjugate | intermediate | 85% |
| Oxazepam | 30-120 | 2-4 | 5-20 | Inactive glucuronide conjugate | slow | 87% |

[1] Oral administration.
[2] Major metabolite.
[3] Nordiazepam (active metabolite).

## Contraindications

Hypersensitivity to benzodiazepines; psychoses; acute narrow-angle glaucoma; patients with clinical or biochemical evidence of significant liver disease; intra-arterial use (lorazepam injection); children younger than 6 months of age, lactation (diazepam); coadministration with ketoconazole and itraconazole caused by inhibition of cytochrome P450 3A.

## Warnings

*Psychiatric disorders:* These agents are not intended for use in patients with a primary depressive disorder or psychosis, nor in those psychiatric disorders in which anxiety is not a prominent feature.

*Renal function impairment:* Observe usual precautions in the presence of impaired renal or hepatic function to avoid accumulation of these agents.

*Elderly:* The initial dose should be small and dosage increments made gradually, in accordance with the response of the patient, to preclude ataxia or excessive sedation.

*Pregnancy:* Category D.

*Lactation:* Benzodiazepines are excreted in breast milk (**lorazepam** not known). Chronic **diazepam** use in nursing mothers reportedly caused infants to become lethargic and to lose weight; do not give to nursing mothers.

*Children:*
    *Chlordiazepoxide* – Chlordiazepoxide is not recommended in children younger than 6 years of age (oral) or 12 years of age (injectable).
    *Alprazolam* – Safety and efficacy for use in patients younger than 18 years of age have not been established.
    *Lorazepam* – Do not use in patients younger than 18 years of age (injection); safety and efficacy for use in patients younger than 12 years of age are not established (oral).
    *Clorazepate* – Not recommended for use in patients younger than 9 years of age.
    *Diazepam* – Not for use in children younger than 6 months of age (oral); safety and efficacy have not been established in the neonate (30 days of age or younger; injectable).

## Precautions

*Monitoring:* Because of isolated reports of neutropenia and jaundice, perform periodic blood counts, and liver function tests during long-term therapy.

*Suicide:* In those patients in whom depression accompanies anxiety, suicidal tendencies may be present, and protective measures may be required.

*Paradoxical reactions:* Excitement, stimulation, and acute rage have occurred in psychiatric patients and hyperactive aggressive children. These reactions may be secondary to relief of anxiety and usually appear in the first 2 weeks of therapy.

*Drug abuse and dependence:* Prolonged use of therapeutic doses can lead to dependence. Withdrawal syndrome has occurred after as little as 4 to 6 weeks of treatment. It is more likely if the drug was short-acting (eg, alprazolam), if it was taken regularly for more than 3 months and if it was abruptly discontinued. Higher dosages may not be a factor affecting withdrawal.

*Parenteral administration* – Parenteral (IM or IV) therapy is indicated primarily in acute states. Keep patients under observation, preferably in bed, for up to 3 hours.

*Hazardous tasks:* May produce drowsiness or dizziness; observe caution while driving or performing other tasks requiring alertness.

**Drug Interactions**
Drugs that may affect benzodiazepines include alcohol, antacids, barbiturates, cimetidine, disulfiram, fluoxetine, isoniazid, ketoconazole, metoprolol, oral contraceptives, narcotics, probenecid, propoxyphene, propranolol, ranitidine, rifampin, scopolamine, theophylline, and valproic acid.

Drugs that may be affected by benzodiazepines include digoxin, levodopa, neuromuscular blocking agents, and phenytoin.

**Adverse Reactions**
*Cardiovascular:* Bradycardia; cardiovascular collapse; edema; hypertension; hypotension; palpitations; tachycardia.

*CNS:* Agitation; anterograde amnesia; apathy; ataxia; coma; confusion; crying; depression; delirium; difficulty in concentration; disorientation; dizziness; euphoria; fatigue; headache; hypoactivity; inability to perform complex mental functions; incoordination; irritability; lethargy; lightheadedness; memory impairment; nervousness; restlessness; rigidity; sedation and sleepiness; seizures; slurred speech; sobbing; stupor; syncope; tremor; unsteadiness; vertigo; vivid dreams; weakness.

*Dermatologic:* Ankle and facial edema; dermatitis; hair loss; hirsutism; pruritus; skin rash; urticaria.

*GI:* Anorexia; change in appetite; constipation; diarrhea; difficulty in swallowing; dry mouth; gastritis; increased salivation; nausea; sore gums; vomiting.

*GU:* Changes in libido; incontinence; menstrual irregularities; urinary retention.

*Ophthalmic:* Diplopia; nystagmus; visual disturbances.

*Psychiatric:* Behavior problems; hysteria; psychosis; suicidal tendencies.

*Respiratory:* Nasal congestion; respiratory disturbances.

*Miscellaneous:* Anemia; auditory disturbances; blood dyscrasias including agranulocytosis; dehydration; depressed hearing; diaphoresis; eosinophilia; fever; galactorrhea; gynecomastia; hiccoughs; increase or decrease in body weight; joint pain; leukopenia; muscular disturbance; paresthesias; thrombocytopenia.

# BUSPIRONE HCl

| **Tablets:** 5, 7.5, 10, 15, and 30 mg *(Rx)* | Various, *BuSpar* (Bristol-Myers Squibb) |
|---|---|

**Indications**
*Anxiety disorders:* Management of anxiety disorders or short-term relief of symptoms of anxiety.

**Administration and Dosage**
*Initial dose:* 15 mg/day (7.5 mg 2 times/day).

To achieve an optimal therapeutic response, increase the dosage 5 mg/day, at intervals of 2 to 3 days, as needed. Do not exceed 60 mg/day. Divided doses of 20 to 30 mg/day have been commonly used.

The bioavailability of buspirone is increased when given with food as compared with the fasted state. Consequently, patients should take buspirone in a consistent manner with regard to the timing of dosing; either always with or always without food.

*Concomitant therapy:* When buspirone is to be given with a potent inhibitor of CYP3A4, the dosage recommendations described in the Drug Interactions section should be followed.

**Actions**
*Pharmacology:* Mechanism of action is unknown. It differs from benzodiazepines in that it does not exert anticonvulsant or muscle relaxant effects. It also lacks prominent

sedative effects associated with more typical anxiolytics. Buspirone has effects on serotonin, dopamine, and norephinephrine.

*Pharmacokinetics:* Buspirone is rapidly absorbed and undergoes extensive first-pass metabolism. Approximately 95% of buspirone is plasma protein bound. In a single dose study, 29% to 63% of the dose was excreted in the urine within 24 hours.

## Contraindications
Hypersensitivity to buspirone HCl.

## Warnings
Buspirone has no established antipsychotic activity; do not employ in lieu of appropriate antipsychotic treatment.

*Physical and psychological dependence:* Buspirone has shown no potential for abuse or diversion and there is no evidence that it causes tolerance or physical or psychological dependence. However, carefully evaluate patients for a history of drug abuse and follow such patients closely, observing them for signs of misuse or abuse (eg, tolerance, drug-seeking behavior).

*Renal/Hepatic function impairment:* Because buspirone is metabolized by the liver and excreted by the kidneys, do not use in patients with severe hepatic or renal impairment.

*Pregnancy:* Category B.

*Lactation:* The extent of the excretion in breast milk of buspirone or its metabolites is not known.

*Children:* Safety and efficacy of buspirone were evaluated in 2 placebo-controlled 6-week trials involving a total of 559 pediatric patients (ranging from 6 to 17 years of age) with generalized anxiety disorder (GAD). Doses studied were 7.5 to 30 mg twice/day (15 to 60 mg/day). There were no significant differences between buspirone and placebo with regard to the symptoms of GAD.

## Precautions
*Monitoring:* Effectiveness for more than 3 to 4 weeks has not been demonstrated in controlled trials. However, patients have been treated for a year without ill effect. If used for extended periods, periodically reassess the usefulness of the drug.

*Interference with cognitive and motor performance:* Buspirone is less sedating than other anxiolytics and does not produce significant functional impairment. However, its CNS effect may not be predictable. Therefore, caution patients about driving or using complex machinery until they are certain that buspirone does not affect them adversely.

*Withdrawal reactions:* Withdraw patients from their prior treatment gradually before starting buspirone, especially patients who have been using a CNS depressant chronically.

*Dopamine receptor binding:* Buspirone can bind to central dopamine receptors.

*Monitoring:* Patients have been treated for several months without ill effect. If used for extended periods, periodically reassess the usefulness of the drug.

## Drug Interactions
*CYP450 system:* Substances that inhibit CYP3A4, such as ketoconazole or ritonavir, may inhibit buspirone metabolism and increase plasma concentrations of buspirone while substances that induce CYP3A4, such as dexamethasone or certain anticonvulsants (eg, phenytoin, phenobarbital, carbamazepine), may increase the rate of buspirone metabolism. If a patient has been titrated to a stable dosage on buspirone, a dose adjustment of buspirone may be necessary to avoid adverse events attributable to buspirone or diminished anxiolytic activity. Consequently, when administered with a potent inhibitor of CYP3A4, a low dose of buspirone used cautiously is recommended. When used in combination with a potent inducer of CYP3A4 the dosage of buspirone may need adjusting to maintain anxiolytic effect.

Drugs that may interact with buspirone include alcohol, cimetidine, CYP3A4 inhibitors and inducers, diazepam, fluoxetine, haloperidol, nefazodone, monoamine oxidase inhibitors, and trazodone.

*Drug/Food interactions:* The bioavailability of buspirone is increased when given with food as compared with the fasted state.

*Grapefruit juice* – Coadministration of buspirone (10 mg as a single-dose) with grapefruit juice (200 mL double-strength twice/day for 2 days) increased plasma buspirone concentrations (4.3-fold increase in $C_{max}$; 9.2-fold increase in AUC). Advise patients receiving buspirone to avoid drinking large amounts of grapefruit juice.

**Adverse Reactions**

Adverse reactions occurring in at least 3% of patients include dizziness, drowsiness, dry mouth, fatigue, headache, insomnia, lightheadedness, nausea, nervousness.

# HYDROXYZINE

| | |
|---|---|
| **Tablets:** 10, 25, and 50 mg (as HCl) (*Rx*) | Various |
| **Capsules:** 25, 50, and 100 mg (as pamoate equivalent to HCl) (*Rx*) | Various, *Vistaril* (Pfizer) |
| **Syrup:** 10 mg/5 mL (as HCl) (*Rx*) | Various |
| **Oral suspension:** 25 mg/5 mL (as pamoate equiv. to HCl) (*Rx*) | *Vistaril* (Pfizer) |
| **Injection:** 25 and 50 mg/mL (as HCl) (*Rx*) | Various, *Vistaril* (Pfizer) |

**Indications**

Symptomatic relief of anxiety and tension associated with psychoneurosis and as an adjunct in organic disease states in which anxiety is manifest.

Management of pruritus caused by allergic conditions such as chronic urticaria, atopic and contact dermatoses and in histamine-mediated pruritus.

As a sedative when used as premedication and following general anesthesia.

*IM only:* For the acutely disturbed or hysterical patient; the acute or chronic alcoholic with anxiety withdrawal symptoms or delirium tremens; allay anxiety; adjunctive therapy in asthma.

*Antiemetic (parenteral only)* – In controlling nausea and vomiting (excluding nausea and vomiting of pregnancy). As pre- and postoperative and pre- and postpartum adjunctive medication to control emesis.

*Analgesia, adjunctive therapy (parenteral only)* – As pre- and postoperative and pre- and postpartum adjunctive medication to permit reduction in narcotic dosage.

**Administration and Dosage**

*Parenteral:* Hydroxyzine is for deep IM administration only and may be given without further dilution. Avoid IV, subcutaneous, or intra-arterial administration (see Warnings). Inject well within the body of a relatively large muscle. In adults, the preferred site is the upper outer quadrant of the buttock or the midlateral thigh. In children, inject into the midlateral muscles of the thigh. In infants and small children, use the periphery of the upper outer quadrant of the gluteal region only when necessary, such as in burn patients, in order to minimize the possibility of sciatic nerve damage.

Use the deltoid area only if well developed, and then only with caution to avoid radial nerve injury. Do not inject into the lower and mid-third of the upper arm.

Start patients on IM therapy when indicated. Maintain on oral therapy whenever practicable. Adjust dosage according to patient's response.

*Anxiety* –
    *Adults:* 50 to 100 mg 4 times a day.

*Pruritus* –
    *Adults:* 25 mg 3 or 4 times a day.

*Sedative (as premedication and following general anesthesia)* –
   *Adults:* 50 to 100 mg.
   *Children:* 0.6 mg/kg.
*Antiemetic/Analgesia, adjunctive therapy (parenteral only)* –
   *Adults:* 25 to 100 mg IM as pre- and postoperative/pre- and postpartum adjunctive medication to permit reduction of narcotic dosage. Reduce dosage of concomitant CNS depressants by 50%.
   *Children:* 1.1 mg/kg (0.5 mg/lb) IM to control emesis or as pre- and postoperative adjunctive medication to permit reduction of narcotic dosage. Reduce dosage of concomitant CNS depressants by 50%.
*Oral:*
   *Anxiety* – The efficacy of hydroxyzine as an antianxiety agent for long-term use (longer than 4 months) has not been assessed; periodically reevaluate its usefulness.
      *Adults:* 50 to 100 mg 4 times a day.
      *Children (older than 6 years of age):* 50 to 100 mg/day in divided doses.
      *Children (younger than 6 years of age):* 50 mg/day in divided doses.
   *Pruritus* –
      *Adults:* 25 mg 3 or 4 times/day.
      *Children (older than 6 years of age):* 50 to 100 mg/day in divided doses.
      *Children (younger than 6 years of age):* 50 mg/day in divided doses.
   *Sedative (as premedication and following general anesthesia)* –
      *Adults:* 50 to 100 mg.
      *Children:* 0.6 mg/kg.

## Actions

*Pharmacology:* Hydroxyzine is not a cortical depressant; its action may be caused by suppressing activity in subcortical areas of CNS.

   Bronchodilator activity, antihistaminic, and analgesic effects have been confirmed. Hydroxyzine has antispasmodic properties, and an antiemetic effect has been demonstrated.

*Pharmacokinetics:* Oral hydroxyzine is rapidly absorbed from the GI tract; clinical effects are usually noted within 15 to 30 minutes after administration. Mean elimination half-life is 3 hours; half-life may be longer in elderly patients. Hydroxyzine is mainly metabolized by the liver.

## Contraindications

Hypersensitivity to hydroxyzine; early pregnancy, lactation.

Hydroxyzine injection is for IM use only. Do not inject subcutaneously, IV or intra-arterially.

## Warnings

*Administration:* For deep IM administration only; avoid subcutaneous, IV or intra-arterial injection. Tissue necrosis has been associated with subcutaneous or intra-arterial injection; hemolysis has occurred following IV administration.

*Hypersensitivity reactions:* Hypersensitivity reactions have occurred.

*Pregnancy:* Do not use in pregnancy.

*Lactation:* It is not known whether this drug is excreted in breast milk.

## Precautions

*ECG changes:* ECG abnormalities, particularly alterations in T-waves.

*Porphyria:* May exacerbate porphyria and is considered unsafe in porphyric patients.

*Hazardous tasks:* May produce drowsiness.

## Drug Interactions

Drugs that may interact with hydroxyzine include CNS depressants.

## Adverse Reactions

Adverse reactions may include dry mouth; drowsiness; involuntary motor activity, including rare instances of tremor and convulsions; hypersensitivity reactions, including wheezing, dyspnea, and chest tightness.

# DOXEPIN HCl

Doxepin is a tricyclic antidepressant which also has antianxiety effects. The following is an abbreviated monograph for doxepin. For complete information, refer to the Tricyclic Antidepressants monograph.

**Indications**

For the treatment of psychoneurotic patients with depression or anxiety; depression or anxiety associated with alcoholism or organic disease; psychotic depressive disorders with associated anxiety including involutional depression and manic-depressive disorders.

The target symptoms of psychoneurosis that respond to doxepin include anxiety, tension, depression, somatic symptoms and concerns, insomnia, guilt, lack of energy, fear, apprehension, and worry.

**Administration and Dosage**

The total daily dosage may be given on a divided or once-a-day dosage schedule. If the once-a-day schedule is employed, the maximum recommended dose is 150 mg/day, given at bedtime.

Not recommended in children younger than 12 years of age.

*Mild to moderate severity:* Start with 75 mg/day. The optimum dose range is 75 to 150 mg/day.

*More severely ill:* Gradual increase to 300 mg/day may be necessary. Additional therapeutic effect is rarely obtained by exceeding a dose of 300 mg/day.

*Very mild symptoms or emotional symptoms accompanying organic disease:* Some of these patients have been controlled on doses as low as 25 to 50 mg/day.

*Dilution the oral concentrate:* Dilute the oral concentrate with 120 mL of liquid (eg, water, milk and orange, grapefruit, tomato, prune, or pineapple juices) just prior to administration; not compatible with a number of carbonated beverages. For patients on methadone maintenance taking oral doxepin, mix the concentrate with methadone and lemonade, orange juice, water, and sugar water. *Do not mix with grape juice.* Preparation and storage of bulk dilutions are not recommended.

# ANTIDEPRESSANTS

| Antidepressant Pharmacologic and Pharmacokinetic Parameters | | | | | | | | | |
|---|---|---|---|---|---|---|---|---|---|
| | Major side effects | | | Amine uptake blocking activity | | | | | |
| 0 - none<br>+ - slight<br>++ - moderate<br>+++ - high<br>++++ - very high<br>+++++ - highest | Anticholinergic | Sedation | Orthostatic hypotension | Norepinephrine | Serotonin | Half-life (hours) | Therapeutic plasma level (ng/mL) | Time to reach steady state (days) | Dose range (mg/day) |
| **Tricyclics - Tertiary Amines** | | | | | | | | | |
| Amitriptyline | ++++ | ++++ | ++ | ++ | ++++ | 31-46 | 110-250[1] | 4-10 | 50-300 |
| Clomipramine | +++ | +++ | ++ | ++ | +++++ | 19-37 | 80-100 | 7-14 | 25-250 |
| Doxepin | ++ | +++ | ++ | + | ++ | 8-24 | 100-200[1] | 2-8 | 25-300 |
| Imipramine | ++ | ++ | +++ | ++[2] | ++++ | 11-25 | 200-350[1] | 2-5 | 30-300 |
| Trimipramine | ++ | +++ | ++ | + | + | 7-30 | 180[1] | 2-6 | 50-300 |
| **Tricyclics - Secondary Amines** | | | | | | | | | |
| Amoxapine[3] | +++ | ++ | + | +++ | ++ | 8[4] | 200-500 | 2-7 | 50-600 |
| Desipramine | + | + | + | ++++ | ++ | 12-24 | 125-300 | 2-11 | 25-300 |
| Nortriptyline | ++ | ++ | + | ++ | +++ | 18-44 | 50-150 | 4-19 | 30-100 |
| Protriptyline | +++ | + | + | ++++ | ++ | 67-89 | 100-200 | 14-19 | 15-60 |
| **Phenethylamine** | | | | | | | | | |
| Venlafaxine | 0 | 0 | 0 | +++ | +++ | 5-11 [1] | - | 3-4 | 75-375 |
| **Tetracyclic** | | | | | | | | | |
| Maprotiline | ++ | ++ | + | +++ | 0/+ | 21-25 | 200-300[1] | 6-10 | 50-225 |
| Mirtazapine | ++ | +++ | ++ | +++ | +++ | 20-40 | - | 5 | 15-45 |
| **Triazolopyridine** | | | | | | | | | |
| Trazodone | + | ++++ | ++ | 0 | +++ | 4-9 | 800-1600 | 3-7 | 150-600 |
| **Aminoketone** | | | | | | | | | |
| Bupropion[5] | ++ | ++ | + | 0/+ | 0/+ | 8-24 | - | 1.5-8 | 200-450 |
| **Selective Serotonin Reuptake Inhibitors** | | | | | | | | | |
| Citalopram | 0/+ | 0/+ | 0/+ | 0/+ | ++++ | 33 | - | 7 | 20-60 |
| Fluoxetine | 0/+ | 0/+ | 0/+ | 0/+ | +++++ | 1-16 days[1] | - | 2-4 weeks | 20-80 |
| Fluvoxamine | 0/+ | 0/+ | 0 | 0/+ | +++++ | 15.6 | - | ≈ 7 | 50-300 |
| Paroxetine | 0 | 0/+ | 0 | 0/+ | +++++ | 10-24 | - | 7-14 | 10-50 |
| Sertraline | 0 | 0/+ | 0 | 0/+ | +++++ | 1-4 days[1] | - | 7 | 50-200 |
| **Monoamine Oxidase Inhibitors** | | | | | | | | | |
| Tranylcypromine | + | + | 0 | - | - | 2.4-2.8 | - | - | 30-60 |
| Phenelzine | + | + | + | - | - | - | - | - | 45-90 |
| **Miscellaneous** | | | | | | | | | |
| Nefazodone | 0/+ | ++ | + | 0/+ | +++++ | 2-4 | - | 4-5 | 200-600 |

[1] Parent compound plus active metabolite.
[2] Via desipramine, the major metabolite.
[3] Also blocks dopamine receptors.
[4] 30 hours for major metabolite 8-hydroxyamoxapine.
[5] Inhibits dopamine uptake.

# TRICYCLIC COMPOUNDS

| | |
|---|---|
| **AMITRIPTYLINE** | |
| **Tablets:** 10, 25, 50, 75, 100, and 150 mg (*Rx*) | Various, *Elavil* (Zeneca) |
| **AMOXAPINE** | |
| **Tablets:** 25, 50, 100, and 150 mg (*Rx*) | Various, *Asendin* (Lederle) |
| **CLOMIPRAMINE HCl** | |
| **Capsules:** 25, 50, and 75 mg (*Rx*) | Various, *Anafranil* (Novartis) |
| **DESIPRAMINE HCl** | |
| **Tablets:** 10, 25, 50, 75, 100, and 150 mg (*Rx*) | Various, *Norpramin* (Aventis) |
| **DOXEPIN HCl** | |
| **Capsules:** 10, 25, 50, 75, 100, and 150 mg (*Rx*) | Various, *Sinequan* (Roerig) |
| **Oral concentrate:** 10 mg/mL (*Rx*) | Various |
| **IMIPRAMINE HCl** | |
| **Tablets:** 10, 25, and 50 mg (*Rx*) | Various, *Tofranil* (Novartis) |
| **IMIPRAMINE PAMOATE** | |
| **Capsules:** 75, 100, 125, and 150 mg (as imipramine HCl equivalent) (*Rx*) | *Tofranil-PM* (Novartis) |
| **NORTRIPTYLINE HCl** | |
| **Capsules:** 10, 25, 50, and 75 mg (*Rx*) | Various, *Aventyl HCl Pulvules* (Eli Lilly), *Pamelor* (Novartis) |
| **Solution:** 10 mg (as base)/5 mL (*Rx*) | *Pamelor* (Novartis) |
| **PROTRIPTYLINE HCl** | |
| **Tablets:** 5 and 10 mg (*Rx*) | Various, *Vivactil* (Merck) |
| **TRIMIPRAMINE MALEATE** | |
| **Capsules:** 25, 50, and 100 mg (*Rx*) | *Surmontil* (Wyeth) |

## Indications

Relief of symptoms of depression (except clomipramine). The activating properties of **protriptyline** make it particularly suitable for withdrawn and anergic patients.

Agents with significant sedative action may be useful in depression associated with anxiety and sleep disturbances. The activating properties of **protriptyline** make it particularly suitable for withdrawn and anergic patients.

*Amoxapine:* Relief of depressive symptoms in patients with neurotic or reactive depressive disorders and endogenous and psychotic depression; depression accompanied by anxiety or agitation.

*Doxepin:* Treatment of psychoneurotic patients with depression or anxiety; depression or anxiety associated with alcoholism (not to be taken concomitantly with alcohol); depression or anxiety associated with organic disease (the possibility of drug interaction should be considered if the patient is receiving other drugs concomitantly); psychotic depressive disorders with associated anxiety including involutional depression and manic-depressive disorders. The target symptoms of psychoneurosis that respond particularly well to doxepin include anxiety, tension, depression, somatic symptoms and concerns, sleep disturbances, guilt, lack of energy, fear, apprehension, and worry.

*Imipramine:* Treatment of enuresis in children 6 years of age or older as temporary adjunctive therapy.

*Clomipramine:* Only for treatment of Obsessive-Compulsive Disorder (OCD).

## Administration and Dosage

*Plasma levels:* Determination of plasma levels may be useful in identifying patients who appear to have toxic effects and may have excessively high levels, or those in whom lack of absorption or noncompliance is suspected. Make adjustments in dosage according to patient's clinical response and not based on plasma levels.

*Adolescent, elderly, and outpatients:* Initiate therapy at a low dosage and increase gradually. Most antidepressant drugs have a lag period of 10 days to 4 weeks before a therapeutic response is noted. Increasing the dose will not shorten this period but rather increase the incidence of adverse reactions. Following remission, maintenance medication may be required for a longer time at the lowest dose that will maintain remission. Continue maintenance therapy ≥ 3 months to decrease the possibility of relapse.

AMITRIPTYLINE HCl:

*Outpatients* – 75 mg/day in divided doses. May increase to 150 mg/day. Alternatively, initiate therapy with 50 to 100 mg at bedtime. Increase by 25 to 50 mg as necessary, to a total of 150 mg/day.

*Hospitalized patients:* Hospitalized patients may require 100 mg/day initially. Gradually increase to 200 to 300 mg, if necessary.

*Adolescent and elderly patients* – 10 mg 3 times a day with 20 mg at bedtime may be satisfactory in adolescent and elderly patients who cannot tolerate higher doses.

*Maintenance* – 40 to 100 mg/day. Total daily dosage may be given in a single dose, preferably at bedtime.

*IM* – Do not administer IV. Initially, 20 to 30 mg IM, 4 times a day. The effects may be more rapid with IM than with oral administration.

*Children* – Not recommended for children younger than 12 years of age.

AMOXAPINE: Amoxapine is not recommended for patients younger than 16 years of age.

Usual effective dose range is 200 to 300 mg/day. If no response is seen at 300 mg, increase dosage, depending upon tolerance, to 400 mg/day. Hospitalized patients refractory to antidepressant therapy and who have no history of convulsive seizures may have dosage cautiously increased up to 600 mg/day in divided doses.

*Adults* – Initially, 50 mg 2 or 3 times/day. Depending upon tolerance, increase dosage to 100 mg 2 or 3 times/day by the end of the first week. Increase above 300 mg/day only if 300 mg/day has been ineffective for at least 2 weeks. Once an effective dosage is established, the drug may be given in a single bedtime dose (not to exceed 300 mg). If the total daily dosage exceeds 300 mg, give in divided doses.

*Elderly patients* – Initially, 25 mg 2 or 3 times a day. If tolerated, dosage may be increased by the end of the first week to 50 mg 2 or 3 times a day. Although 100 to 150 mg/day may be adequate for many elderly patients, some may require higher dosage; carefully increase up to 300 mg/day. Once an effective dosage is established, give amoxapine in a single bedtime dose, not to exceed 300 mg.

CLOMIPRAMINE HCl: Administer in divided doses with meals to reduce GI side effects. After titration, the total daily dose may be given once/day at bedtime to minimize daytime sedation.

*Adults* – Initiate at 25 mg/day and gradually increase, as tolerated, to approximately 100 mg during the first 2 weeks. Thereafter, the dosage may be increased gradually over the next several weeks to a maximum of 250 mg/day.

*Children and adolescents* – Initiate at 25 mg/day and gradually increase during the first 2 weeks, as tolerated, to a daily maximum of 3 mg/kg or 100 mg, whichever is smaller. Thereafter, the dosage may be increased to a daily maximum of 3 mg/kg or 200 mg, whichever is smaller.

DESIPRAMINE HCl: Not recommended for use in children younger than 12 years of age.

*Adults* – 100 to 200 mg/day. Initial therapy may be given in divided doses or as a single daily dose. In more severely ill patients, gradually increase to 300 mg/day, if necessary. Do not exceed 300 mg/day.

*Elderly and adolescents* – 25 to 100 mg/day. Dosages greater than 150 mg not recommended.

DOXEPIN HCl: Not recommended for use in children younger than 12 years of age.

*Mild to moderate anxiety or depression* – Initially, 75 mg/day. Usual optimum dosage is 75 to 150 mg/day. Alternatively, the total daily dosage, up to 150 mg, may be given at bedtime.

*Mild symptomatology or emotional symptoms accompanying organic disease* – 25 to 50 mg/day as often as effective.

*More severe anxiety or depression* – Higher doses (eg, 50 mg 3 times/day) may be required; if necessary, gradually increase to 300 mg/day.

*Oral concentrate* – Dilute oral concentrate with approximately 120 mL of water, milk or fruit juice prior to administration. Do not mix with carbonated beverages.

*IMIPRAMINE HCl:*
    *Depression –*
        *Hospitalized patients:* Initially, 100 orally in divided doses; gradually increase to 200 mg/day, as required. If no response occurs after 2 weeks, increase to 250 to 300 mg/day. Administer the total daily dosage once/day at bedtime.
        *Outpatients:* Initially, 75 mg/day, increased to 150 mg/day. Do not exceed 200 mg/day. Give once/day, preferably at bedtime.
        *Maintenance –* 50 to 150 mg/day or lowest dose that will maintain remission.
        *Adolescent and elderly patients:* Initially, 30 to 40 mg/day orally; it is generally not necessary to exceed 100 mg/day.
        *Childhood enuresis (6 years of age or older) –* Initially, 25 mg/day 1 hour before bedtime. If no satisfactory response in 1 week, increase up to 50 mg/night if younger than 12 years of age; up to 75 mg/night if older than 12 years of age. A dose more than 75 mg/day does not enhance efficacy and increases side effects. Do not exceed 2.5 mg/kg/day. In early night bedwetters, it may be more effective given earlier and in divided amounts (25 mg midafternoon and bedtime).

*IMIPRAMINE PAMOATE:*
    *Hospitalized patients –* Initiate therapy at 100 to 150 mg/day; may be increased to 200 mg/day. If there is no response after 2 weeks, increase dosage to 250 to 300 mg/day.
    *Outpatients –* Initiate therapy at 75 mg/day. If necessary, dosage may be increased to 200 mg/day.
    *Adult maintenance dosage –* The usual maintenance dose is 75 to 150 mg/day.
    *Adolescent and geriatric patients –* Initiate therapy in these age groups with imipramine HCl at a total daily dosage of 25 to 50 mg because imipramine pamoate does not come in these strengths. Dosage may be increased according to response and tolerance, but it is generally unnecessary to exceed 100 mg/day in these patients. Imipramine pamoate capsules may be used when total daily dosage is established at 75 mg or more.

*NORTRIPTYLINE:*
    *Adults –* 25 mg 3 or 4 times/day; begin at a low level and increase as required. Total daily dose can be given at bedtime. Doses above 150 mg/day are not recommended.
    *Elderly and adolescent patients –* 30 to 50 mg/day in divided doses or once/day. Not recommended for use in children.

*PROTRIPTYLINE HCl:* Not recommended for use in children.
    *Adults –* 15 to 40 mg/day divided into 3 or 4 doses. May increase to 60 mg/day. Dosages above 60 mg/day are not recommended. Make any increases in the morning dose.
    *Adolescent and elderly patients –* Initially, 5 mg 3 times/day; increase gradually, if necessary. In elderly patients, monitor the cardiovascular system closely if dose exceeds 20 mg/day.

*TRIMIPRAMINE MALEATE:* Not recommended for use in children.
    *Adult outpatients –* Initially, 75 mg/day in divided doses; increase to 150 mg/day. Do not exceed 200 mg/day. The total dosage requirement may be given at bedtime.
    *Adult hospitalized patients –* Initially, 100 mg/day in divided doses, increased gradually in a few days to 200 mg/day depending upon individual response and tolerance. If improvement does not occur in 2 to 3 weeks, increase to a maximum dose of 250 to 300 mg/day.
    *Adolescent and elderly patients –* Initially, 50 mg/day, with gradual increments up to 100 mg/day.
    *Maintenance –* Maintenance medication may be required at the lowest dose that will maintain remission (range 50 to 150 mg/day). Administer as a single bedtime dose.

**Actions**
    *Pharmacology:* The tricyclic antidepressants (TCAs), structurally related to the phenothiazine antipsychotic agents, possess 3 major pharmacologic actions in varying degrees: Blocking of the amine pump, sedation, and peripheral and central anticholinergic action. In contrast to phenothiazines, which act on dopamine receptors, TCAs inhibit reuptake of norepinephrine or serotonin (5-hydroxytryptamine,

5-HT) at the presynaptic neuron. Amoxapine, a metabolite of loxapine, retains some of the postsynaptic dopamine receptor-blocking action of neuroleptics.

*Other pharmacological effects* – Clinical effects, in addition to antidepressant effects, include sedation, anticholinergic effects, mild peripheral vasodilator effects and possible "quinidine-like" actions.

*Pharmacokinetics:*

*Absorption/Distribution* – The TCAs are well absorbed from the GI tract with peak plasma concentrations occurring in 2 to 4 hours; they undergo a significant first-pass effect. They are highly bound (more than 90%) to plasma proteins, are lipid soluble and are widely distributed in tissues, including the CNS.

*Metabolism/Excretion* – Metabolism of TCAs occurs in the liver by demethylation, hydroxylation and glucuronidation, and it varies for each patient. Some intermediate active metabolites include:

Amitriptyline ➡ nortriptyline
Amoxapine ➡ 7 hydroxy and 8 hydroxyamoxapine
Clomipramine ➡ desmethylclomipramine
Doxepin ➡ desmethyldoxepin
Imipramine ➡ desipramine

Because of the long half-life, a single daily dose may be given. Up to 2 to 4 weeks may be required to achieve maximal clinical response.

## Contraindications

Prior sensitivity to any tricyclic drug. Not recommended for use during the acute recovery phase following myocardial infarction. Concomitant use of monoamine oxidase inhibitors (MAOIs) is generally contraindicated.

*Doxepin:* Patients with glaucoma or a tendency for urinary retention.

Cross-sensitivity may occur among the dibenzazepines (**clomipramine, desipramine, imipramine, nortriptyline, and trimipramine**). In addition, dibenzoxepines (**doxepin, amoxapine**) may produce cross-sensitivity.

## Warnings

*Tardive dyskinesia:* Tardive dyskinesia, a syndrome consisting of potentially irreversible, involuntary, dyskinetic movements may develop in patients treated with neuroleptics (eg, antipsychotics). Amoxapine is not an antipsychotic, but it has substantive neuroleptic activity.

*Neuroleptic malignant syndrome (NMS):* NMS is a potentially fatal condition reported in association with antipsychotic drugs and with **amoxapine**.

Hyperthermia has occurred with **clomipramine**; most cases occurred when it was used with other drugs (eg, neuroleptics) and may be examples of an NMS.

*Seizure disorders:* Because TCAs lower the seizure threshold, use with caution in patients with a history of seizures or other predisposing factors (eg, brain damage of varying etiology, alcoholism, concomitant drugs known to lower the seizure threshold). However, seizures have occurred both in patients with and without a history of seizure disorders. Seizure was identified as the most significant risk of **clomipramine** use.

*Anticholinergic effects:* Use with caution in patients with a history of urinary retention, urethral or ureteral spasm; narrow-angle glaucoma, angle-closure glaucoma, or increased intraocular pressure.

*Cardiovascular disorders:* Use with extreme caution in patients with cardiovascular disorders because of the possibility of conduction defects, arrhythmias, CHF, sinus tachycardia, MI, strokes, and tachycardia. These patients require cardiac surveillance at all dose levels of the drug. In high doses, TCAs may produce arrhythmias, sinus tachycardia, conduction defects, and prolonged conduction time. Tachycardia and postural hypotension may occur more frequently with **protriptyline**.

*Hyperthyroid patients:* Hyperthyroid patients or those receiving thyroid medication require close supervision because of the possibility of cardiovascular toxicity, including arrhythmias.

*Psychiatric patients:* Schizophrenic or paranoid patients may exhibit a worsening of psychosis with TCA therapy, and manic-depressive patients may experience a shift to a hypomanic or manic phase; this may also occur when switching antidepressants and withdrawing them. In overactive or agitated patients, increased anxiety or agitation may occur. Paranoid delusions, with or without associated hostility, may be exaggerated. Reduction of TCA dosage and concomitant antipsychotic therapy may be necessary.

The possibility of suicide in depressed patients remains during treatment and until significant remission occurs. Patients should not have easy access to large quantities of the drug; prescribe small quantities of TCAs.

*Mania/Hypomania:* Hypomanic or manic episodes may occur, particularly in patients with cyclic disorders. Such reactions may necessitate discontinuation of the drug.

*MAOIs:* Do not give MAOIs with or immediately following TCAs. Allow at least 14 days to elapse between MAOI discontinuation and TCA institution. Some TCAs have been used safely and successfully with MAOIs. Initiate TCA cautiously with gradual dosage increase until achieving optimum response.

*Rash:* Antidepressant drugs can cause skin rashes or "drug fever" in susceptible individuals. They are more likely to occur during the first few days of treatment but may also occur later. Discontinue if rash or fever develop.

*Renal/Hepatic function impairment:* Use with caution and in reduced doses in patients with hepatic impairment; metabolism may be impaired, leading to drug accumulation. Use with caution in patients with significantly impaired renal function.

*Elderly:* Be cautious in dose selection for an elderly patient, usually starting at the low end of the dosing range. Elderly patients may be sensitive to the anticholinergic side effects of TCAs.

Elderly patients taking **amitriptyline** may be at increased risk for falls; start on low doses of amitriptyline and observe closely.

*Pregnancy:* (*Category D* - amitriptyline, imipramine, nortriptyline; *Category C* - amoxapine, clomipramine, desipramine, doxepin, protriptyline, trimipramine).

*Lactation:* These agents are excreted into breast milk in low concentrations.

*Children:* Not recommended for patients younger than 12 years of age. Safety and efficacy are not established for **amoxapine** in children younger than 16 years of age or **trazodone** or **clomipramine** in children younger than 10 years of age. The safety and efficacy of **imipramine** as temporary adjunctive therapy for nocturnal enuresis in pediatric patients younger than 6 years of age have not been established. The safety of the drug for long-term, chronic use as adjunctive therapy for nocturnal enuresis in pediatric patients 6 years of age and older has not been established. Safety and efficacy are not established in the pediatric age group for **trimipramine, nortriptyline, protriptyline,** and **desipramine**.

Do not exceed 2.5 mg/kg/day of **imipramine**.

### Precautions

*Monitoring:* Perform baseline and periodic leukocyte and differential counts and liver function studies. Fever or sore throat may signal serious neutrophil depression; discontinue therapy if there is evidence of pathological neutropenia.

*Monitor ECG* – Monitor ECG prior to initiation of large doses of TCAs and at appropriate intervals thereafter.

*Electroconvulsive therapy:* Electroconvulsive therapy with coadministration of TCAs may increase the hazards of therapy.

*Elective surgery:* Discontinue therapy for as long as possible before elective surgery.

*Blood sugar levels:* Elevated and lowered blood sugar levels have occurred.

*Sexual dysfunction:* Sexual dysfunction was markedly increased in male patients with OCD taking clomipramine (42% ejaculatory failure, 20% impotence) compared to placebo. Sexual dysfunction also occurs with other TCAs.

*Weight changes:* Weight gain occurred in 18% of patients receiving **clomipramine**. Some patients had weight gain in excess of 25% of their initial body weight. Weight gain also occurs with other TCAs.

*Serotonin syndrome:* Some TCAs inhibit neuronal reuptake of serotonin and can increase synaptic serotonin levels (eg, **clomipramine**, **amitriptyline**). Either therapeutic or excessive doses of these drugs, in combination with other drugs that also increase synaptic serotonin levels (such as MAOIs), can cause a serotonin syndrome consisting of tremor, agitation, delirium, rigidity, myoclonus, hyperthermia, and obtundation.

*Hazardous tasks:* May impair mental or physical abilities required for the performance of potentially hazardous tasks.

*Photosensitivity:* Photosensitization (photoallergy or phototoxicity) may occur.

**Drug Interactions**

*P450 system:* Concomitant use of TCAs with other drugs metabolized by cytochrome P450 2D6 may require lower doses than those usually prescribed for either the TCA or the other drug.

Drugs that may affect tricyclic compounds include barbiturates, carbamazepine, charcoal, cimetidine, haloperidol, histamine $H_2$-antagonists, MAO inhibitors, rifamycins, SSRIs, smoking, and valproic acid.

Drugs that may be affected by tricyclic compounds include anticholinergics, carbamazepine, clonidine, dicumarol, grepafloxacin, guanethidine, levodopa, quinolones, sparfloxacin, and sympathomimetics.

**Adverse Reactions**

Sedation and anticholinergic effects are reported most frequently.

*Withdrawal symptoms* – Although not indicative of addiction, abrupt cessation after prolonged therapy may produce nausea, headache, vertigo, nightmares, and malaise. Gradual dosage reduction may produce, within 2 weeks, transient symptoms including irritability, restlessness, dreams, and sleep disturbance.

*Enuretic children* – Consider adverse reactions reported with adult use. Most common are nervousness, sleep disorders, tiredness, and mild GI disturbances. These usually disappear with continued therapy or dosage reduction.

*Cardiovascular:*

*General* – Arrhythmias; changes in AV conduction; ECG changes (most frequently with toxic doses); flushing; heart block; hot flushes; hypertension; hypotension; orthostatic hypotension; palpitations; precipitation of CHF; premature ventricular contractions; stroke; sudden death; syncope; tachycardia.

*Desipramine* – Hypertensive episodes during surgery. There have been reports of sudden death in children.

*CNS:*

*General* – Agitation; akathisia; alterations in EEG patterns; anxiety; ataxia; coma; confusion (especially in the elderly); disorientation; disturbed concentration; dizziness; drowsiness; dysarthria; exacerbation of psychosis; excitement; excessive appetite; extrapyramidal symptoms including abnormal involuntary movements and tardive dyskinesia; fatigue; hallucinations; delusions; headache; hyperthermia; hypomania; incoordination; insomnia; mania; nervousness; neuroleptic malignant syndrome; nightmares; numbness; panic; paresthesias of extremities; peripheral neuropathy; restlessness; tremors; seizures; tingling; weakness.

*GU:* Gynecomastia and testicular swelling in the male; breast enlargement, menstrual irregularity and galactorrhea in the female; increased or decreased libido; painful ejaculation; impotence; nocturia; urinary frequency.

*GI:* Nausea and vomiting; anorexia; epigastric distress; diarrhea; flatulence; dysphagia; increased salivation; stomatitis; glossitis; parotid swelling; abdominal cramps; pancreatitis; black tongue.

*Hematologic:* Bone marrow depression including agranulocytosis; eosinophilia; purpura; thrombocytopenia; leukopenia.

*Clomipramine* – Anemia; leukemoid reaction; lymphadenopathy; lymphoma-like disorder.

*Hypersensitivity:*
    General – Cross-sensitivity with other TCAs; drug fever; edema (general or of face and tongue); itching; petechiae; photosensitization; pruritus; rash; urticaria; vasculitis.

*Respiratory:*
    General – Exacerbation of asthma.

*Special senses:* Tinnitus; abnormal lacrimation.

*Miscellaneous:*
    General – Alopecia; fever; hyperthermia; hyperpyrexia; local edema; nasal stuffiness; increased perspiration; proneness to falling; weight gain or loss.

    *Clomipramine* – Abnormal skin odor; arthralgia; back pain; chest pain; chills; dependent edema; general edema; fever; halitosis; increased susceptibility to infection; malaise; muscle weakness; myalgia; pain; thirst; withdrawal syndrome.

# TETRACYCLIC COMPOUNDS

| **MAPROTILINE** | |
|---|---|
| **Tablets**: 25, 50, and 75 mg (*Rx*) | Various |
| **MIRTAZAPINE** | |
| **Tablets**: 15, 30, and 45 mg (*Rx*) | *Remeron* (Organon) |
| **Tablets, orally disintegrating**: 15, 30, and 45 mg (*Rx*) | *Remeron SolTab* (Organon) |

## Indications
*Depression:* Treatment of depression.

## Administration and Dosage
MAPROTILINE HCl: May be given as a single daily dose or in divided doses. Therapeutic effects are sometimes seen within 3 to 7 days, although as long as 2 to 3 weeks are usually necessary before improvement is observed.

*Initial adult dosage –*

    *Mild to moderate depression:* An initial dose of 75 mg/day is suggested for outpatients. In some patients, especially the elderly, an initial dose of 25 mg/day may be used. Because of the long half-life of maprotiline, maintain initial dosage for 2 weeks. The dosage may then be increased gradually in 25 mg increments, as required and tolerated. Most patients respond to a dose of 150 mg/day, but doses as high as 225 mg/day may be required.

    *Severe depression:* Give hospitalized patients an initial daily dose of 100 to 150 mg, which may be gradually increased, as required and tolerated. Most hospitalized patients with moderate to severe depression respond to a daily dosage of 150 mg, although doses as high as 225 mg may be required. Do not exceed 225 mg/day.

    *Maintenance* – Dosage may be reduced to 75 to 150 mg/day with adjustment depending on therapeutic response.

    *Elderly* – In general, lower doses are recommended for patients older than 60 years of age. Doses of 50 to 75 mg/day are satisfactory as maintenance therapy for elderly patients who do not tolerate higher amounts.

    Maprotiline is not recommended for patients younger than 18 years of age.

MIRTAZAPINE:

    *Initial treatment* – The recommended starting dose for mirtazapine is 15 mg/day administered in a single dose, preferably in the evening prior to sleep. Patients not responding to the initial 15 mg dose may benefit from dosage increases up to a maximum of 45 mg/day. Do not change dose at intervals of less than 1 or 2 weeks.

    *Maintenance/Extended treatment* – Treatment for acute episodes of depression should continue for 6 months or more.

    *Switching to or from a monoamine oxidase inhibitor (MAOI)* – At least 14 days should elapse between discontinuation of an MAOI and initiation of therapy with mirtazapine. In addition, allow at least 14 days after stopping mirtazapine before starting an MAOI.

*Elderly and renal/hepatic function impairment* – The clearance of mirtazapine is reduced in elderly patients and in patients with moderate to severe renal or hepatic impairment.

*Administration of orally disintegrating tablets* – Open tablet blister pack with dry hands and place tablet on tongue. The tablet will disintegrate rapidly on the tongue and can be swallowed with saliva. Use the tablet immediately after removal from the blister; it cannot be scored. No water is needed. Do not attempt to split the tablet. Use orally disintegrating tablets immediately upon opening individual tablet blisters.

### Actions

*Pharmacology:* Tetracyclics enhance central noradrenergic and serotonergic activity. They do not inhibit monoamine oxidase. Although maprotiline and mirtazapine are in the same chemical class, they each affect different neurotransmitters and thus have different side effect profiles. Maprotiline primarily acts by blocking reuptake of norepinephrine at nerve endings.

Mirtazapine is a potent antagonist of $5\text{-}HT_2$ and $5\text{-}HT_3$ receptors. It is a potent antagonist of histamine ($H_1$) receptors and a moderate antagonist at muscarinic receptors.

*Pharmacokinetics:*

*Maprotiline* – The mean time to peak is 12 hours. The elimination half-life averages 43 hours. Binding to serum proteins is approximately 88%. Maprotiline is metabolized in the liver and excreted via the bile.

*Mirtazapine* – Mirtazapine is rapidly and completely absorbed following oral administration and has a half-life of approximately 20 to 40 hours, with females of all ages exhibiting significantly longer elimination half-lives than males (37 vs 26 hours). Steady-state plasma levels of mirtazapine are attained within 5 days. Mirtazapine is approximately 85% bound to plasma protein.

*Metabolism/Excretion:* Mirtazapine has an absolute bioavailability of approximately 50%. It is eliminated predominantly via urine (75%) with 15% in feces.

### Contraindications

Hypersensitivity to maprotiline or mirtazapine; coadministration with monamine oxidase inhibitors (MAOIs).

*Maprotiline:* Known or suspected seizure disorders; during acute phase of MI.

### Warnings

*Anticholinergic properties:* Maprotiline should be administered with caution in patients with increased intraocular pressure, history of urinary retention, or history of narrow-angle glaucoma because of the drug's anticholinergic properties.

*Monoamine oxidase inhibitors (MAOIs):* Do not give tetracyclics with MAOIs. Allow a minimum of 14 days to elapse after discontinuation of MAOIs before starting a tetracyclic.

*Seizures:* Seizures are rare. The risk of seizures may be increased when tetracyclics are taken concomitantly with phenothiazines, when the dosage of benzodiazepines is rapidly tapered in patients receiving tetracyclics or when the recommended dosage of the tetracyclic is exceeded.

*Cardiovascular:* Use with caution in patients with a history of MI and angina because of the possibility of conduction defects, arrhythmia, MI, strokes, and tachycardia. Use with caution in patients predisposed to hypotension.

*Electroshock therapy:* Avoid concurrent administration of maprotiline with electroshock therapy because of the lack of experience in this area.

*Agranulocytosis:* In clinical trials, two patients treated with mirtazapine developed agranulocytosis and a third patient developed severe neutropenia. All 3 patients recovered after mirtazapine was stopped.

*Renal/Hepatic function impairment:* Use mirtazapine with caution in patients with impaired renal and hepatic function.

*Elderly:* Oral clearance was reduced in the elderly compared with the younger subjects. Caution is indicated in administering mirtazapine to elderly patients.

*Pregnancy: Category* B (maprotiline); *Category* C (mirtazapine).

*Lactation:*

> *Maprotiline* – Maprotiline is excreted in breast milk. At steady state, the concentration in milk corresponds closely to the concentrations in whole blood.
>
> *Mirtazapine* – It is not known if mirtazapine is excreted in breast milk.

*Children:* Safety and efficacy in children (younger than 18 years of age for **maprotiline**) have not been established.

### Precautions

*Monitoring:* Discontinue **maprotiline** if there is evidence of pathological neutrophil depression. Perform leukocyte and differential counts in patients who develop fever and sore throat during therapy.

*Somnolence:* Somnolence was reported in 54% of patients treated with mirtazapine.

*Dizziness:* Dizziness was reported in 7% of patients treated with mirtazapine.

*Increased appetite/Weight gain:* Appetite increase was reported in 17% of patients treated with mirtazapine. In some trials, weight gain of 7% or more of body weight occurred in 7.5% of patients treated.

*Cholesterol/Triglycerides:* Nonfasting cholesterol increases to 20% or more above the upper limits of normal and nonfasting triglyceride increases to 500 mg/dL or more were observed.

*Mania/Hypomania:* Use carefully in patients with a history of mania/hypomania.

*Suicidal ideation:* Closely supervise high-risk patients during initial drug therapy.

*Elective surgery:* Prior to elective surgery, discontinue **maprotiline** for as long as possible, because little is known about the interaction between maprotiline and general anesthetics.

*Orthostatic hypotension:* Orthostatic hypotension was infrequently observed in clinical trials with depressed patients.

*Lab test abnormalities:* Clinically significant ALT elevations (3 times or more the upper limit of the normal range) were observed in 2% of patients exposed to mirtazapine.

*Hazardous tasks:* Caution patients about engaging in hazardous activities until they are reasonably certain that tetracyclics do not adversely affect their ability to engage in such activities.

### Drug Interactions

Drugs that may affect maprotiline include thyroid hormones, benzodiazepines, and phenothiazines. Drugs that may be affected by maprotiline include anticholinergics, guanethidine, and sympathomimetics. Drugs that may be affected by mirtazapine include alcohol and diazepam.

### Adverse Reactions

Adverse reactions include asthenia; flu syndrome; dry mouth; constipation; increased appetite; weight gain; abnormal dreams; anxiety; dizziness; drowsiness; headache; nervousness; somnolence; abnormal thinking; tremor; weakness and fatigue; blurred vision.

# TRAZODONE HCl

| | |
|---|---|
| **Tablets**: 50 and 100 mg (*Rx*) | Various, *Desyrel* (Mead Johnson) |
| 150 and 300 mg (*Rx*) | Various, *Desyrel Dividose* (Mead Johnson) |

### Indications
Treatment of depression.

### Administration and Dosage
Initiate dosage at a low level and increase gradually. Drowsiness may require the administration of a major portion of the daily dose at bedtime or a reduced dosage. Take shortly after a meal or light snack.

*Adults:* An initial dose is 150 mg/day in divided doses. This may be increased by 50 mg/day every 3 to 4 days. The maximum dose for outpatients usually should not exceed 400 mg/day in divided doses. Inpatients or more severely depressed subjects may be given up to, but not in excess of, 600 mg/day in divided doses.

*Maintenance:* Keep dosage at the lowest effective level. Once an adequate response has been achieved, dosage may be gradually reduced with subsequent adjustment depending on response.

### Actions
*Pharmacology:* Trazodone is not a monoamine oxidase inhibitor and does not stimulate the CNS. In animals, it selectively inhibits serotonin uptake by brain synaptosomes and potentiates the behavioral changes induced by the serotonin precursor, 5–hydroxytryptophan.

*Pharmacokinetics:*

*Absorption/Distribution* – Trazodone is well absorbed after oral administration. Peak plasma levels occur in approximately 1 hour when taken on an empty stomach or in 2 hours when taken with food.

*Metabolism/Excretion* – Trazodone is extensively metabolized in the liver and is a CYP3A4 substrate. Elimination is biphasic, with a half-life of 3 to 6 hours and 5 to 9 hours, respectively, and is unaffected by food.

### Contraindications
Hypersensitivity to trazodone; initial recovery phase of MI.

### Warnings
*Preexisting cardiac disease:* Not recommended for use during the initial recovery phase of MI. Trazodone may be arrhythmogenic in some patients. Arrhythmias identified include isolated PVCs, ventricular couplets, and short episodes (3 to 4 beats) of ventricular tachycardia. Closely monitor patients with preexisting cardiac disease, particularly for cardiac arrhythmias.

*Priapism:* Patients with prolonged or inappropriate penile erection should discontinue use immediately and consult a physician or go to an emergency room. Priapism of the clitoris has also occurred.

*Pregnancy: Category* C.

*Lactation:* The drug may be excreted in breast milk.

*Children:* Safety and efficacy for use in children younger than 18 years of age are not established.

### Precautions
*Suicide:* The possibility of suicide in seriously depressed patients is inherent in the illness and may persist until significant remission occurs.

*Hypotension:* Hypotension, including orthostatic hypotension and syncope, has occurred.

*Elective surgery:* There is little known about the interaction between trazodone and general anesthetics; therefore, prior to elective surgery, discontinue trazodone for as long as clinically feasible.

*Electroconvulsive therapy:* Avoid concurrent administration with electroconvulsive therapy because of the absence of experience in this area.

*Lab test abnormalities:* Discontinue the drug in any patient whose white blood cell count or absolute neutrophil count falls below normal levels. White blood cell and differential counts are recommended for patients who develop fever and sore throat (or other signs of infection) during therapy.

*Hazardous tasks:* May produce drowsiness, dizziness, or blurred vision.

**Drug Interactions**
Trazodone may affect CNS depressants (alcohol, barbiturates), digoxin, monoamine oxidase inhibitors, phenytoin, and warfarin. Trazodone may be affected by carbamazepine, phenothiazines, and SSRIs.

**Adverse Reactions**
Adverse reactions occurring in 3% or more of patients include: Hypotension, syncope, tachycardia/palpitations, anger/hostility, confusion, dizziness/lightheadedness, drowsiness, excitement, fatigue, headache, incoordination, insomnia, nervousness, nightmares/vivid dreams, tremors, abdominal/gastric disorder, constipation, diarrhea, dry mouth, nausea/vomiting, blurred vision, allergic skin condition/edema, aches/pains, decreased appetite, nasal/sinus congestion, weight gain/loss.

# BUPROPION HCl

| | |
|---|---|
| **Tablets**: 75 and 100 mg (*Rx*) | Various, *Wellbutrin* (GlaxoSmithKline) |
| **Tablets, sustained-release**: 100, 150, and 200 mg | *Wellbutrin SR* (GlaxoSmithKline) |
| **Tablets, extended-release**: 100, 150 and 300 mg | *Wellbutrin XL* (GlaxoSmithKline) |

**Indications**
*Depression:* Treatment of depression. Effectiveness of bupropion in long-term use (more than 6 weeks) has not been evaluated.

**Administration and Dosage**
*General:* It is particularly important to administer bupropion in a manner most likely to minimize the risk of seizure (see Warnings). Do not exceed dose increases of 100 mg/day of the immediate-release formulation in a 3-day period. Gradual escalation of dosage also is important to minimize agitation, motor restlessness, and insomnia often seen during the initial days of treatment. If necessary, these effects may be managed by temporary reduction of dose or the short-term administration of an intermediate- to long-acting sedative-hypnotic. A sedative-hypnotic usually is not required beyond the first week of treatment. Insomnia also may be minimized by avoiding bedtime doses. If distressing, untoward effects supervene, stop dose escalation.

*Bupropion immediate-release (IR):* Do not exceed dose increases of 100 mg/day in a 3-day period. No single dose of bupropion should exceed 150 mg. Administer 3 times/day, preferably with at least 6 hours between successive doses.

*Adults* – 300 mg/day, given 3 times/day. Begin dosing at 200 mg/day, given as 100 mg twice/day. Based on clinical response, this dose may be increased to 300 mg/day, given as 100 mg 3 times/day no sooner than 3 days after beginning therapy.

| **Bupropion Dosage Regimen** | | | | | |
|---|---|---|---|---|---|
| | | | Number of tablets | | |
| Treatment day | Total daily dose | Tablet strength | Morning | Midday | Evening |
| 1 | 200 mg | 100 mg | 1 | 0 | 1 |
| 4 | 300 mg | 100 mg | 1 | 1 | 1 |

*Increasing the dosage above 300 mg/day* – An increase in dosage up to a maximum of 450 mg/day given in divided doses of not more than 150 mg each may be considered for patients in whom no clinical improvement is noted after several weeks of treatment at 300 mg/day. Dosing above 300 mg/day may be accomplished using the 75 or 100 mg tablets. The 100 mg tablets must be administered 4 times/day with at least 4 hours between successive doses in order not to exceed the limit of

150 mg in a single dose. Discontinue in patients who do not demonstrate an adequate response after an appropriate period of 450 mg/day.

*Bupropion sustained-release (SR):* The usual adult target dosage is 300 mg/day given as 150 mg twice/day. Begin dosing with 150 mg/day given as a single daily dose in the morning. If the 150 mg initial dose is adequately tolerated, increase to 300 mg/day given as 150 mg twice/day as early as day 4 of dosing. Allow at least 8 hours between successive doses. Swallow whole; do not crush, divide, or chew.

    *Increasing the dosage above 300 mg/day* – As with other antidepressants, the full antidepressant effect of the SR formula may not be evident until 4 weeks of treatment or longer. Consider an increase in dosage to the maximum of 400 mg/day given as 200 mg twice/day for patients in whom no clinical improvement is noted after several weeks of 300 mg/day treatment.

*Bupropion XL:* The usual adult target dose is 300 mg/day, given once daily in the morning. Dosing should begin at 150 mg/day, given as a single daily dose in the morning. If the 150 mg initial dose is adequately tolerated, an increase to the 300 mg/day target dose, given once daily, may be made as early as day 4 of dosing. There should be an interval of at least 24 hours between successive doses. Swallow whole; do not crush, divide, or chew.

    *Increasing the dosage above 300 mg/day* – As with other antidepressants, the full antidepressant effect of the XL formula may not be evident until 4 weeks of treatment or longer. An increase in dosage to the maximum of 450 mg/day, given as a single dose, may be considered for patients in whom no clinical improvement is noted after several weeks of treatment at 300 mg/day.

    *Switching to Bupropion XL* – When switching patients from bupropion tablets to XL tablets or from SR tablets to XL tablets, give the same total daily dose when possible. Patients who are currently being treated with bupropion tablets at 300 mg/day (eg, 100 mg 3 times/day) may be switched to XL tablets 300 mg once daily. Patients who are currently being treated with SR tablets at 300 mg/day (eg, 150 mg twice daily) may be switched to XL tablets 300 mg once daily.

*Maintenance:* Use the lowest dose that maintains remission. Although it is not known how long the patient should remain on bupropion, acute episodes of depression generally require several months or longer of treatment.

*Hepatic impairment:* Use bupropion with extreme caution in patients with severe hepatic cirrhosis. The dose should not exceed 75 mg once/day (100 mg every day or 150 mg every other day for bupropion SR; 150 mg every other day for XL) in these patients. Use bupropion with caution in patients with hepatic impairment (including mild to moderate hepatic cirrhosis); consider a reduced frequency or dose in patients with mild to moderate hepatic cirrhosis.

*Renal impairment:* Use bupropion with caution in patients with renal impairment and consider a reduced frequency or dose.

## Actions

*Pharmacology:* The mechanism of the antidepressant effect of bupropion is not known. Bupropion does not inhibit monoamine oxidase. It is a weak blocker of the neuronal uptake of serotonin and norepinephrine; it also inhibits the neuronal reuptake of dopamine to some extent.

*Pharmacokinetics:*

    *Absorption/Distribution* – Following oral administration, peak plasma concentrations usually are achieved within 2 hours for bupropion, 3 hours for bupropion SR, and 5 hours for bupropion XL, followed by a biphasic decline. The half-life of the second (postdistributional) phase of bupropion ranges 8 to 24 hours; mean elimination half-life for bupropion SR is 21 hours.

## Contraindications

Hypersensitivity to the drug; seizure disorder; current or prior diagnosis of bulimia or anorexia nervosa (because of a higher incidence of seizures noted in such patients treated with bupropion); concurrent administration of a monoamine oxidase inhibitor (MAOI) (at least 14 days should elapse between discontinuation of an

MAOI and initiation of treatment with bupropion); in patients being treated with other bupropion products (eg, for smoking cessation) because of the incidence of dose-dependent seizures; in patients undergoing abrupt discontinuation of alcohol or sedatives (including benzodiazepines).

### Warnings

*Other bupropion medications:* Bupropion, bupropion SR, and bupropion XL contain the same active ingredient found in Zyban, used as an aid to smoking cessation treatment. Do not use bupropion in combination with Zyban or any other medications that contain bupropion.

*Anorexia nervosa/bulimia:* Do not give with current or prior diagnosis of bulimia or anorexia nervosa because of a higher incidence of seizures noted in patients treated for bulimia with the IR formulation of bupropion.

*Seizures:* Bupropion immediate-release is associated with seizures in approximately 0.4% of patients treated at doses up to 450 mg/day. This incidence of seizures may exceed that of other marketed antidepressants by as much as 4-fold. The estimated seizure incidence increases almost 10-fold between 450 and 600 mg/day. Given the wide variability among individuals and their capacity to metabolize and eliminate drugs, this disproportionate increase in seizure incidence with dose incrementation calls for caution in dosing.

Data for bupropion SR tablets revealed a seizure incidence of approximately 0.1% in patients treated at doses up to 300 mg/day and increases to approximately 0.4% at the maximum recommended dose of 400 mg/day. The risk of seizure appears to be strongly associated with dose. Bupropion XL, while not formally evaluated in clinical trials, may be similar to that presented for the IR and SR formulations of bupropion.

*Recommendations for reducing seizure risk* – (1) The total daily dose does not exceed 450 mg (400 mg SR; 450 mg XL); (2) the daily dose is administered 3 times/day, with each single dose not to exceed 150 mg to avoid high peak concentrations of bupropion or its metabolites (twice/day for SR tablets with each single dose not to exceed 200 mg to avoid high peak concentrations of bupropion and its metabolites); and (3) the rate of incrementation of dose is very gradual.

Use extreme caution when administering to patients with a history of seizure, cranial trauma, or other predisposition toward seizure, or prescribed with other agents (eg, antipsychotics, other antidepressants, theophylline, systemic steroids) that lower seizure threshold.

*Hepatotoxicity:* In animals receiving large doses of bupropion chronically, there was an increased incidence of hepatic hyperplastic nodules, hepatocellular hypertrophy, and histologic changes with laboratory tests that suggested mild hepatocellular injury.

*Hypersensitivity reactions:* Anaphylactoid reactions characterized by symptoms such as pruritus, urticaria, angioedema, and dyspnea requiring medical treatment have been reported. In addition, there have been rare spontaneous postmarketing reports of erythema multiforme, Stevens-Johnson syndrome, and anaphylactic shock associated with bupropion.

*Renal function impairment:* Use bupropion with caution in patients with renal impairment and consider a reduced frequency or dose as bupropion and its metabolites could accumulate in such patients to a greater extent than usual. Closely monitor the patient for adverse effects that could indicate possible high drug or metabolite levels.

*Hepatic function impairment:* Use bupropion with extreme caution in patients with severe hepatic cirrhosis. In these patients, a reduced dose or frequency is required, as peak bupropion levels are substantially increased and accumulation is likely to occur in such patients to a greater extent than usual. Do not exceed 75 mg once a day (100 mg every day or 150 mg every other day for bupropion SR; 150 mg every other day for bupropion XL) in these patients.

*Elderly:* Because elderly patients are more likely to have decreased renal function, take care in dose selection; it may be useful to monitor renal function (see Precautions, Administration and Dosage).

*Pregnancy: Category B.*

*Lactation:* Bupropion and its metabolites are secreted in breast milk.

*Children:* Safety and efficacy in children under 18 years of age have not been established.

### Precautions

*CNS symptoms:* A substantial proportion of patients experience some degree of increased restlessness, agitation, anxiety, and insomnia, especially shortly after initiation of treatment.

*Neuropsychiatric phenomena:* Patients have shown a variety of neuropsychiatric signs and symptoms including delusions, hallucinations, psychotic episodes, confusion, and paranoia.

*Activation of psychosis or mania:* Antidepressants can precipitate manic episodes in bipolar manic depressive patients during the depressed phase of their illness and may activate latent psychosis in other susceptible patients.

*Altered appetite and weight:* A weight loss of more than 5 pounds occurred in 28% of patients treated with immediate-release formulation of bupropion and in at least 14% of patients treated with bupropion SR.

*Suicide:* The possibility of a suicide attempt is inherent in depression and may persist until significant remission occurs. Accordingly, write prescriptions for the smallest number of tablets consistent with good patient management.

*Cardiac effects:* Hypertension, in some cases severe, requiring acute treatment, has been reported in patients receiving bupropion alone and in combination with nicotine replacement therapy. Monitoring of blood pressure is recommended in patients who receive the combination of bupropion and nicotine replacement. Exercise care if bupropion is used in in patients with a recent history of MI or unstable heart disease.

*Drug abuse and dependence:* Studies in healthy volunteers, subjects with a history of multiple drug abuse, and depressed patients showed some increase in motor activity and agitation/excitement. In individuals experienced with drugs of abuse, a single dose of 400 mg bupropion produced mild amphetamine-like activity as compared with placebo.

*Photosensitivity:* Photosensitization may occur; therefore, caution patients to take protective measures (ie, sunscreens, protective clothing) against exposure to ultraviolet light or sunlight until tolerance is determined.

### Drug Interactions

Drugs that may interact with bupropion include alcohol, amantadine, carbamazepine, MAOIs and levodopa, nicotine replacement products, ritonavir, tricyclic antidepressants, and warfarin.

*CYP450:* Exercise care when administering drugs known to affect hepatic drug metabolizing enzyme systems (eg, carbamazepine, cimetidine, phenobarbital, phenytoin).

In vitro studies indicate that bupropion is primarily metabolized to hydroxybupropion by the cytochrome P450 2B6 isoenzyme. Therefore, the potential exists for a drug interaction between bupropion and drugs that affect the cytochrome P450 2B6 metabolism (eg, orphenadrine, cyclophosphamide).

Approach with caution coadministration of bupropion with drugs that are metabolized by the cytochrome P450 2D6 (CYP2D6) isoenzyme, including certain antidepressants, antipsychotics, beta blockers, and Type 1C antiarrhythmics, and initiate coadministration at the lower end of the dose range of the concomitant medication. If bupropion is added to the treatment regimen of a patient already receiving a drug metabolized by CYP2D6, consider the need to decrease the dose of the original medication, particularly for those concomitant medications with a narrow therapeutic index.

Use caution during coadministration of bupropion and agents (eg, antipsychotics, other antidepressants, theophylline, systemic steroids) or treatment regimens (eg, abrupt discontinuation of benzodiazepines) that lower seizure threshold. Use low initial dosing and small gradual dose increases.

**Adverse Reactions**

Adverse reactions occurring in at least 3% of patients include abdominal pain; agitation; akinesia/bradykinesia; amblyopia; anorexia; anxiety; appetite increase; arthralgia; arthritis; asthenia; auditory disturbance; blurred vision; cardiac arrythmias; chest pain; confusion; constipation; decreased libido; diarrhea; disturbed concentration; dizziness; dry mouth; dyspepsia; excessive sweating; fatigue; flushing; gustatory disturbance; hostility; headache/migraine; hot flashes; hypertension; hypotension; impaired sleep quality; impotence; increased salivary flow; infection; insomnia; irritability; memory decreased; menstrual complaints; muscle spasms; myalgia; nausea/vomiting; nervousness; pain; palpitations; pharyngitis; pruritus; rash; sedation; sensory disturbance; sinusitis; somnolence; tachycardia; taste perversion; tinnitus; tremor; upper respiratory complaints; urinary frequency; weight loss/gain.

# VENLAFAXINE

**Tablets:** 25, 37.5, 50, 75, and 100 mg (Rx)          *Effexor* (Wyeth-Ayerst)
**Capsules, extended-release:** 37.5, 75, and 150 mg (Rx)          *Effexor* XR (Wyeth-Ayerst)

**Indications**

*Depression:* Treatment of depression.

*Anxiety:* Treatment of generalized anxiety disorder (GAD) and social anxiety disorder (SAD) (extended-release [ER] only).

**Administration and Dosage**

*Venlafaxine immediate-release:*

*Depression* – Administer venlafaxine ER in a single dose with food either in the morning or in the evening at approximately the same time each day. Swallow each capsule whole with fluid and not divided, crushed, chewed, or placed in water, or it may be administered by carefully opening the capsule and sprinkling the entire contents on a spoonful of applesauce. Swallow this drug/food mixture immediately without chewing, and follow with a glass of water to ensure complete swallowing of the pellets.

*Initial treatment:* The recommended starting dose is 75 mg/day, administered in 2 or 3 divided doses, taken with food. Depending on tolerability and the need for further clinical effect, the dose may be increased to 150 mg/day. If needed, further increase the dose up to 225 mg/day. When increasing the dose, make increments of up to 75 mg/day at intervals of at least 4 days. Certain patients, including more severely depressed patients, may respond more to higher doses, up to a maximum of 375 mg/day, generally in 3 divided doses.

*Discontinuing venlafaxine* – When discontinuing venlafaxine after more than 1 week of therapy, it is generally recommended that the dose be tapered to minimize the risk of discontinuation symptoms. Patients should have their dose tapered gradually over a 2-week period.

*Venlafaxine extended-release:*

*Depression* –

*Initial treatment:* The recommended starting dosage for venlafaxine extended-release is 75 mg/day administered in a single dose. For some new patients, it may be desirable to start at 37.5 mg/day for 4 to 7 days. Patients not responding to the initial 75 mg/day dosage may benefit from dose increases to a maximum of approximately 225 mg/day. Dose increases should be in increments of up to 75 mg/day as needed and should be made at intervals of at least 4 days.

*GAD* – For most patients, the recommended starting dose is 75 mg/day, administered in a single dose. For some patients, it may be desirable to start at 37.5 mg/day for 4 to 7 days before increasing to 75 mg/day. Certain patients not responding to the initial 75 mg/day dose may benefit from dose increases to a maximum of approximately 225 mg/day. Dose increases should be increments of up to 75 mg/day, as needed, and should be made at intervals of not less than 4 days.

*Discontinuing venlafaxine ER* – When discontinuing treatment after more than 1 week of therapy, taper the dose to minimize the risk of discontinuation symptoms. In clinical trials, tapering was achieved by reducing the daily dose by 75 mg at 1-week intervals.

*Renal/Hepatic function impairment:* It is recommended that the total daily dose be reduced by 50% in patients with moderate hepatic impairment and by 25% to 50% in patients with mild to moderate renal impairment. It is recommended that the total daily dose be reduced by 50% and the dose be withheld until the dialysis treatment is completed (4 hours) in patients undergoing hemodialysis.

*Switching patients from immediate- to extended-release venlafaxine:* Patients currently treated at a therapeutic dose with venlafaxine may be switched to the extended-release form at the nearest equivalent dose (mg/day; eg, 37.5 mg venlafaxine 2 times/day to 75 mg venlafaxine ER once daily).

*Switching patients to or from a monoamine oxidase inhibitor (MAOI):* At least 14 days should elapse between discontinuation of an MAOI and initiation of therapy with venlafaxine. In addition, allow at least 7 days after stopping venlafaxine before starting an MAOI.

## Actions

*Pharmacology:* Venlafaxine and its active metabolite, O-desmethylvenlafaxine (ODV), are potent inhibitors of neuronal serotonin and norepinephrine reuptake and weak inhibitors of dopamine reuptake.

*Pharmacokinetics:* Venlafaxine is well absorbed (at least 92%) and extensively metabolized in the liver. ODV is the only major active metabolite. Renal elimination of venlafaxine and its metabolites is the primary route of excretion. Venlafaxine ER provides a slower rate of absorption but the same extent of absorption compared with the immediate-release tablet.

## Contraindications

Hypersensitivity to venlafaxine or any ingredients of the product; concomitant use in patients taking monoamine oxidase inhibitors (MAOIs).

## Warnings

*MAO inhibitors:* Because venlafaxine is an inhibitor of norepinephrine and serotonin reuptake, it is recommended that venlafaxine not be used in combination with an MAOI or within 14 days of discontinuing treatment with an MAOI. Allow at least 7 days after stopping venlafaxine before starting an MAOI.

*Sustained hypertension:* There is a dose-dependent increase in the incidence of sustained hypertension for venlafaxine from 3% for doses less than 100 mg/day up to 13% for doses greater than 300 mg/day. It is recommended that patients receiving venlafaxine have regular monitoring of blood pressure. For patients who experience a sustained increase in food pressure, consider dose reduction or discontinuation.

*Renal/Hepatic function impairment:* In patients with renal impairment (GFR, 10 to 70 mL/min) or cirrhosis of the liver, a lower dose may be necessary.

*Pregnancy:* Category C.

*Lactation:* Venlafaxine and ODV are excreted in breast milk.

*Children:* Safety and efficacy in patients younger than 18 years of age for immediate-release or ER venlafaxine have not been established.

## Precautions

*Discontinuation:* Abrupt discontinuation or dose reduction of venlafaxine has been found to be associated with the appearance of new symptoms, the frequency of which increased with increased dose level and with longer duration of treatment. Reported symptoms include agitation, anorexia, anxiety, confusion, coordination impairment, diarrhea, dizziness, dry mouth, dysphoric mood, fasciculation, fatigue, headache, hypomania, insomnia, nausea, nervousness, nightmares, seizure, sensory disturbance (including shock-like electrical sensations), somnolence, sweating, tremor, vertigo, and vomiting. It is recommended that the dosage of venlafaxine ER be tapered gradually and the patient monitored.

*Anxiety and insomnia:* Anxiety, nervousness, and insomnia were reported for venlafaxine-treated patients, and led to drug discontinuation.

*Appetite/Weight changes:* Anorexia was reported for venlafaxine-treated patients. A dose-dependent weight loss often was noted in patients treated for several weeks.

*Mania/Hypomania:* Hypomania or mania has occurred in patients treated with venlafaxine.

*Seizures:* Seizures have been reported in venlafaxine-treated patients.

*Suicide:* The possibility of a suicide attempt is inherent in depression and may persist until significant remission occurs.

*Hyponatremia:* Hyponatremia and the syndrome of inappropriate antidiuretic hormone secretion (SIADH) may occur with venlafaxine.

*Mydriasis:* Mydriasis has been reported; monitor patients with raised intraocular pressure or those at risk of acute narrow angle glaucoma.

*Abnormal bleeding:* There have been reports of abnormal bleeding (most commonly ecchymosis) associated with venlafaxine treatment.

*Concomitant illness:* Exercise caution in patients whose underlying medical conditions might be compromised by increases in heart rate (eg, patients with hyperthyroidism, heart failure, or recent MI), particularly when using doses of venlafaxine more than 200 mg/day.

*Cardiac patients:* Venlafaxine has not been evaluated in patients with a recent history of MI or unstable heart disease.

*Drug abuse and dependence:* Carefully evaluate patients for history of drug abuse and follow such patients closely, observing them for signs of misuse or abuse of venlafaxine.

*Hazardous tasks:* Caution patients about operating hazardous machinery, including automobiles, until they are reasonably certain that venlafaxine therapy does not adversely affect their ability to engage in such activities.

### Drug Interactions
Drugs that may affect venlafaxine include cimetidine and MAOIs. Drugs that may be affected by venlafaxine include clozapine, desipramine, haloperidol, indinavir, St. John's wort, trazodone, sibutramine, sumatriptan, and warfarin.

Venlafaxine is metabolized to its active metabolite, ODV, by cytochrome P4502D$_6$. Therefore, the potential exists for a drug interaction between venlafaxine and drugs that inhibit this isoenzyme.

### Adverse Reactions
Adverse reactions occurring in at least 3% of patients include abdominal pain; abnormal dreams; abnormal ejaculation/orgasm; accidental injury; agitation; anorexia; anxiety; asthenia; blurred vision; chills; constipation; decreased libido; depression; diarrhea; dizziness; dry mouth; dyspepsia; flatulence; flu syndrome; headache; hypertonia; impotence; increased blood pressure/hypertension; insomnia; infection; nausea; nervousness; paresthesia; pharyngitis; rash; somnolence; sweating; tremor; urinary frequency; vasodilation; vomiting; weight loss; yawning.

# NEFAZODONE HCl

**Tablets**: 50, 100, 150, 200, and 250 mg (*Rx*)　　　　Various

> **Warning:**
> Cases of life-threatening hepatic failure have been reported in patients treated with nefazodone. The reported rate in the US is about 1 case of liver failure resulting in death or transplant per 250,000 to 300,000 patient-years of nefazodone treatment.
>
> Ordinarily, do not initiate treatment with nefazodone in individuals with active liver disease or with elevated baseline serum transaminases. There is no evidence that pre-existing liver disease increases the likelihood of developing liver failure; however, baseline abnormalities can complicate patient monitoring.
>
> Advise patients to be alert for signs and symptoms of liver dysfunction (eg, jaundice, anorexia, GI complaints, malaise) and to report them to their doctor immediately if they occur.
>
> Discontinue nefazodone if clinical signs or symptoms suggest liver failure. Patients who develop evidence of hepatocellular injury such as increased serum AST or serum ALT levels at least 3 times the upper limit of normal while on nefazodone should be withdrawn from the drug. These patients should be presumed to be at increased risk for liver injury if nefazodone is reintroduced. Accordingly, do not consider such patients for retreatment.

## Indications
*Depression:* Treatment of depression.

## Administration and Dosage
*Initial treatment:* Recommended starting dose is 200 mg/day, administered in 2 divided doses. In clinical trials, the effective dose range was generally 300 to 600 mg/day. Increase doses in increments of 100 to 200 mg/day, again on a twice/day schedule, at intervals of no less than 1 week.

*Elderly/Debilitated patients:* The recommended initial dose is 100 mg/day on a twice/day schedule.

*Maintenance/Continuation/Extended treatment:* There is no evidence to indicate how long the depressed patient should be treated with nefazodone. However, it is generally agreed that pharmacologic treatment for acute episodes of depression should continue for at least 6 months. Whether the dose of antidepressant needed to induce remission is identical to the dose needed to maintain euthymia is unknown. In clinical trials, more than 250 patients were treated for at least 1 year.

## Actions
*Pharmacology:* Nefazodone is an antidepressant with a chemical structure unrelated to available antidepressant agents. The mechanism of action is unknown. Nefazodone inhibits neuronal uptake of serotonin and norepinephrine.

*Pharmacokinetics:*
　*Absorption/Distribution* – Nefazodone is rapidly and completely absorbed. Its absolute bioavailability is low (about 20%) and variable. Food delays absorption of nefazodone and decreases the bioavailability about 20%. Peak plasma concentrations occur at about 1 hour.

　*Metabolism/Excretion* – Nefazodone is extensively metabolized after oral administration by less than 1% is excreted unchanged in urine. The mean half-life of nefazodone ranged between 11 and 24 hours. Nefazodone is extensively (more than 99%) bound to human plasma proteins in vitro.

## Contraindications
Coadministration with cisapride, pimozide, or carbamazepine (see Warnings and Drug Interactions); patients who were withdrawn from nefazodone because of evidence

of liver injury (see Warning box, Warnings); hypersensitivity to nefazodone or other phenylpiperazine antidepressants.

Coadministration of triazolam and nefazodone causes a significant increase in the plasma level of triazolam; a 75% reduction in the initial triazolam dosage is recommended. Avoid the coadministration of triazolam and nefazodone for most patients, including the elderly.

## Warnings

*Hepatotoxicity:* See Warning box. Cases of life-threatening hepatic failure have been reported in patients treated with nefazodone. The time to liver injury resulting in death or transplant generally ranged from 2 weeks to 6 months on nefazodone therapy. Advise patients to be alert for signs and symptoms of liver dysfunction (eg, jaundice, anorexia, GI complaints, malaise) and to report them to their doctor immediately if they occur. Discontinue nefazodone if clinical signs or symptoms suggest liver failure. Patients who develop evidence of hepatocellular injury such as increased serum AST or serum ALT levels 3 times or more the upper limit of normal, while on nefazodone should be withdrawn from the drug. Such patients should not be considered for retreatment.

*Long-term use:* The effectiveness of nefazodone in long-term use (ie, for more than 6 to 8 weeks) has not been systematically evaluated.

*Serious interactions:*

*MAO inhibitors* – Because nefazodone is an inhibitor of both serotonin and norepinephrine reuptake, it is recommended that nefazodone not be used in combination with an MAOI, or within 14 days of discontinuing treatment with an MAOI. Allow at least 1 week after stopping nefazodone before starting an MAOI.

*Triazolobenzodiazepines* – Triazolam and alprazolam, metabolized by cytochrome P450 3A4, have increased plasma concentrations when administered concomitantly with nefazodone. If triazolam is coadministered with nefazodone, a 75% reduction in the initial triazolam dosage is recommended. It is recommended that triazolam not be used in combination with nefazodone. No dosage adjustment is required for nefazodone.

*Antihistamines, nonsedating/cisapride/pimozide* – Cisapride and pimozide are metabolized by the cytochrome P450 3A4 isozyme; inhibitors of 3A4 can block the metabolism of these drugs, resulting in increased plasma concentrations of parent drug, which is associated with QT prolongation and with rare cases of serious cardiovascular adverse events, including death, because of ventricular tachycardia of the torsades de pointes type. In vitro, nefazodone inhibits 3A4. It is recommended that nefazodone not be used in combination with cisapride or pimozide.

*Hepatic function impairment:* Rare cases of severe idiosyncratic hepatocellular injury have occurred. It is suggested that routine liver chemistries be obtained prior to initiating therapy and monitored routinely throughout the course of treatment. Obtain liver function tests for patients at the first symptoms suggestive of hepatic dysfunction (eg, nausea, vomiting, abdominal pain, fatigue, anorexia, dark urine).

*Pregnancy: Category C.*

*Lactation:* It is not known whether nefazodone or its metabolites are excreted in breast milk.

*Children:* Safety and efficacy in individuals less than 18 years of age have not been established.

## Precautions

*Use in patients with concomitant illness:* Nefazodone has not been evaluated or used to any appreciable extent in patients with a recent history of MI or unstable heart disease. Sinus bradycardia, defined as heart rate up to 50 bpm and a decrease of at least 15 bpm from baseline, was observed in 1.5% of nefazodone-treated patients compared with 0.4% of placebo-treated patients ($P \leq 0.05$). Treat patients with a recent history of MI or unstable heart disease with caution.

*Postural hypotension:* Use nefazodone with caution in patients with known cardiovascular or cerebrovascular disease that could be exacerbated by hypotension and conditions that would predispose patients to hypotension.

*Mania/Hypomania:* As with all antidepressants, use nefazodone cautiously in patients with a history of mania.

*Suicide:* The possibility of a suicide attempt is inherent in depression and may persist until significant remission occurs.

*Seizures:* Rare occurrences of convulsions (including grand mal seizures) following nefazodone administration have been reported since market introduction. A causal relationship to nefazodone has not been established.

*Priapism:* If patients present with prolonged or inappropriate erections, they should discontinue therapy immediately and consult their physicians.

*Hepatic cirrhosis:* In patients with cirrhosis of the liver, the AUC values of nefazodone and its metabolite HO-NEF were increased by about 25%.

*Visual disturbances:* There have been reports of visual disturbances associated with the use of nefazodone, including blurred vision, scotoma, and visual trails.

*Drug abuse and dependence:* Carefully evaluate patients for a history of drug abuse and follow such patients closely, observing them for signs of misuse or abuse of nefazodone.

*Hazardous tasks:* Caution patients about operating hazardous machinery, including automobiles, until they are reasonably certain that nefazodone therapy does not adversely affect their ability to engage in such activities.

*Photosensitivity:* Photosensitization (photoallergy or phototoxicity) may occur; therefore, caution patients to take protective measures (ie, sunscreens, protective clothing) against exposure to sunlight or ultraviolet light (eg, tanning beds) until tolerance is determined.

## Drug Interactions

Drugs that affect nefazadone include general anesthetics, sibutramine, sumatriptan, buspirone, carbamazepine, and propranolol. Drugs that may be affected by nefazodone include alcohol, benzodiazepines, buspirone, carbamazepine, cisapride, pimozide, digoxin, haloperidol, HMG-CoA reductase inhibitors, MAOIs, pimozide, propranolol, St. John's wort, cyclosporine, and tacrolimus.

*Potential interaction with drugs that inhibit or are metabolized by cytochrome P450 (3A4 and 2D6) isozymes:* Caution is indicated in the combined use of nefazodone with any drugs known to be metabolized by the 3A4 isozyme (in particular, cisapride or pimozide).

*Drugs highly bound to plasma protein:* Administration to a patient taking another drug that is highly protein bound may cause increased free concentrations of the other drug, potentially resulting in adverse events. Conversely, adverse effects could result from displacement of nefazodone by other highly bound drugs.

*Drug/Food interactions:* Food delays absorption of nefazodone and decreases the bioavailability by about 20%.

## Adverse Reactions

Adverse reactions occurring in at least 3% of patients include nausea; headache; asthenia; flu syndrome; dry mouth; constipation; dyspepsia; diarrhea; increased appetite; peripheral edema; pharyngitis; cough; blurred vision; abnormal vision; somnolence; dizziness; insomnia; lightheadedness; confusion; memory impairment; paresthesia; vasodilation; concentration decreased; postural hypotension; infection; abnormal dreams.

# DULOXETINE HYDROCHLORIDE

| **Capsules:** 20, 30, and 60 mg (*Rx*) | *Cymbalta* (Eli Lilly) |
| --- | --- |

### Indications

*Diabetic peripheral neuropathic (DPN) pain:* For the management of neuropathic pain associated with diabetic peripheral neuropathy.

*Major depressive disorder (MDD):* For the treatment of MDD as defined in the DSM-IV.

### Administration and Dosage

Duloxetine should be swallowed whole and should not be chewed or crushed, nor should the contents be sprinkled on food or mixed with liquids.

*Diabetic peripheral neuropathic pain:*

*Initial treatment* – Administer as a total dose of 60 mg/day given once daily without regard to meals.

*Maintenance/Continuation/Extended treatment* – Because the progression of diabetic peripheral neuropathy is highly variable and management of pain is empirical, assess the effectiveness of duloxetine individually. Efficacy beyond 12 weeks has not been studied.

*MDD:*

*Initial treatment* – Administer as a total dose of 40 mg/day (given as 20 mg twice daily) to 60 mg/day (given either once a day or as 30 mg twice daily) without regard to meals.

*Maintenance/Continuation/Extended treatment* – Acute episodes of major depression require several months or longer of sustained pharmacologic therapy. Periodically reassess patients to determine the need for maintenance treatment and the appropriate dose for such treatment.

*Switching patients to or from a monoamine oxidase inhibitor (MAOI)* – At least 14 days should elapse between discontinuation of an MAOI and initiation of therapy with duloxetine. In addition, at least 5 days should be allowed after stopping duloxetine before starting an MAOI.

### Actions

*Pharmacology:* Although the mechanism of the antidepressant and central pain inhibitory action of duloxetine in humans is unknown, it is believed to be related to its potentiation of serotonergic and noradrenergic activity in the CNS. Preclinical studies have shown that duloxetine is a potent inhibitor of neuronal serotonin and norepinephrine reuptake and a less potent inhibitor of dopamine reuptake. Duloxetine has no significant affinity for dopaminergic, adrenergic, cholinergic, histaminergic, opioid, glutamate, and gamma-aminobutyric acid (GABA) receptors in vitro and does not inhibit MAO.

*Pharmacokinetics:*

*Absorption/Distribution* – Orally administered duloxetine is well absorbed. There is a median 2-hour lag until absorption begins, with $C_{max}$ occurring 6 hours postdose. Food does not affect the $C_{max}$ of duloxetine but delays the time to reach peak concentration from 6 to 10 hours. The apparent volume of distribution averages approximately 1,640 L. Duloxetine is highly bound (more than 90%) to proteins in human plasma, binding primarily to albumin and $\alpha_1$-acid glycoprotein. Steady-state plasma concentrations are typically achieved after 3 days of dosing.

*Metabolism/Excretion* – Duloxetine undergoes extensive metabolism and has an elimination half-life of approximately 12 hours (range, 8 to 17 hours). Elimination of duloxetine is mainly through hepatic metabolism involving two P450 isozymes, CYP2D6 and CYP1A2.

### Contraindications

Known hypersensitivity to duloxetine or any ingredient of the product; concomitant use in patients taking MAOIs; use in patients with uncontrolled narrow-angle glaucoma.

**Warnings**

*Suicide risk:* Patients with MDD, both adult and pediatric, may experience worsening of their depression and/or the emergence of suicidal ideation and behavior (suicidality), whether or not they are taking antidepressant medications, and this risk may persist until significant remission occurs. Closely observe patients being treated with antidepressants for clinical worsening and suicidality, especially at the beginning of a course of drug therapy or at the time of dose changes. Consider changing the therapeutic regimen, including possibly discontinuing the medication, in patients whose depression is persistently worse or whose emergent suicidality is severe, abrupt in onset, or was not part of the patient's presenting symptoms.

*MAOIs:* In patients receiving a serotonin reuptake inhibitor in combination with an MAOI, there have been reports of serious, sometimes fatal, reactions including hyperthermia, rigidity, myoclonus, autonomic instability with possible rapid fluctuations of vital signs, and mental status changes that include extreme agitation progressing to delirium and coma. These reactions also have been reported in patients who have recently discontinued serotonin reuptake inhibitors and are then started on an MAOI. Some cases presented with features resembling neuroleptic malignant syndrome. It is recommended that duloxetine not be used in combination with an MAOI, or within at least 14 days of discontinuing treatment with an MAOI. Based on the half-life of duloxetine, at least 5 days should be allowed after stopping duloxetine before starting an MAOI.

*Renal function impairment:* Increased plasma concentrations of duloxetine, and especially of its metabolites, occur in patients with end-stage renal disease (ESRD) and severe renal impairment (Ccr less than 30 mL/min). Duloxetine is not recommended for patients with ESRD.

*Hepatic function impairment:*

    *Hepatotoxicity* – Duloxetine increases the risk of elevation of serum transaminase levels. The combination of transaminase elevations and elevated bilirubin, without evidence of obstruction, is generally recognized as an important predictor of severe liver injury. Because it is possible that duloxetine and alcohol may interact to cause liver injury, duloxetine should ordinarily not be prescribed to patients with substantial alcohol use.

    Do not administer duloxetine to patients with hepatic insufficiency; markedly increased exposure occurs.

*Elderly:* Caution should be exercised in treating elderly patients. When individualizing the dosage, take extra care when increasing the dose.

*Pregnancy:* Category C.

*Lactation:* It is unknown whether or not duloxetine and/or its metabolites are excreted into human milk; nursing while taking duloxetine is not recommended.

*Children:* Safety and efficacy have not been established.

**Precautions**

*Monitoring:* Monitor patients for the emergence of agitation, irritability, and other symptoms, as well as the emergence of suicidality; monitor blood pressure (BP) prior to initiation and periodically during treatment.

*BP effects:* In clinical trials, duloxetine treatment was associated with mean increases in BP, averaging 2 mm Hg systolic and 0.5 mm Hg diastolic and an increase in the incidence of at least 1 measurement of systolic BP over 140 mm Hg compared with placebo. Measure BP prior to initiating treatment and periodically throughout treatment.

*Discontinuation of treatment:* Symptoms associated with discontinuation of duloxetine and other SSRIs and SNRIs have been reported. Monitor patients for symptoms including dizziness, nausea, headache, paresthesia, vomiting, irritability, and nightmares when discontinuing treatment.

    A gradual reduction in the dose rather than abrupt cessation is recommended whenever possible. If intolerable symptoms occur following a decrease in the dose or discontinuation of treatment, resuming the previously prescribed dose may be considered. Subsequently, the physician may continue decreasing the dose, but at a more gradual rate.

*Special risk:*

*Mania/Hypomania activation* – In placebo-controlled trials in patients with MDD, activation of mania or hypomania was reported in 0.1% of duloxetine-treated patients and 0.1% of placebo-treated patients. Use cautiously in patients with a history of mania.

*Seizures* – In placebo-controlled clinical trials in patients with MDD, seizures occurred in 0.1% of patients treated with duloxetine and 0% of patients treated with placebo. Prescribe duloxetine with care in patients with a history of a seizure disorder.

*Controlled narrow-angle glaucoma* – In clinical trials, duloxetine was associated with an increased risk of mydriasis; therefore, use cautiously in patients with controlled narrow-angle glaucoma.

*Concomitant illness* – Duloxetine is rapidly hydrolyzed in acidic media to naphthol; use caution in patients with conditions that may slow gastric emptying.

*Diabetes* – In clinical trials, small increases in fasting blood glucose were observed in duloxetine-treated patients; however, overall diabetic control did not worsen as evidenced by stable $HbA_{1c}$ values.

*Drug abuse and dependence:* Duloxetine has not been systematically studied in humans for its potential for abuse. Physicians should carefully evaluate patients for a history of drug abuse and follow such patients closely, observing them for signs of misuse or abuse (eg, development of tolerance, incrementation of dose, drug-seeking behavior).

*Hazardous tasks:* Caution patients about operating hazardous machinery, including automobiles, until they are reasonably certain that duloxetine therapy does not adversely affect their ability to engage in such activities.

## Drug Interactions

Drugs that may affect duloxetine include inhibitors of CYP1A2 (eg, fluvoxamine, quinolone antibiotics), inhibitors of CYP2D6 (eg, fluoxetine, quinidine, paroxetine), and alcohol.

Drugs that may be affected by duloxetine include drugs extensively metabolized by CYP2D6 (eg, flecainide, phenothiazines, propafenone, tricyclic antidepressants, thioridazine), alcohol, CNS-acting drugs, MAOIs, and drugs highly bound to plasma proteins (eg, warfarin).

## Adverse Reactions

Small mean increases from baseline to endpoint in ALT, AST, CPK, and alkaline phosphatase have occurred.

Duloxetine is in a class of drugs known to affect urethral resistance.

*MDD:* Adverse reactions occurring in at least 3% of patients include the following: abnormal orgasm, anxiety, blurred vision, constipation, decreased appetite/anorexia, decreased libido, delayed ejaculation, diarrhea, dizziness, dry mouth, ejaculatory dysfunction, erectile dysfunction, fatigue, increased sweating, insomnia, nausea, somnolence, tremor, vomiting.

*Diabetic peripheral neuropathic pain:* Adverse reactions occurring in at least 3% of patients include the following: anorexia, asthenia, constipation, cough, decrease appetite, diarrhea, dizziness, dry mouth, dyspepsia, erectile dysfunction, fatigue, headache, hyperhydrosis, insomnia, loose stools, muscle cramp, myalgia, nasopharyngitis, nausea, pharyngolaryngeal pain, pollakiuria, pyrexia, somnolence, tremor, vomiting.

# SELECTIVE SEROTONIN REUPTAKE INHIBITORS

| | |
|---|---|
| **CITALOPRAM HBr** | |
| **Tablets:** 10, 20, 40 mg as base (*Rx*) | *Celexa* (Forest) |
| **Solution, oral:** 10 mg/5 mL (*Rx*) | |
| **ESCITALOPRAM OXALATE** | |
| **Tablets:** 5, 10, 20 mg (as base) (*Rx*) | *Lexapro* (Forest) |
| **Solution, oral:** 5 mg (as base)/5 mL (*Rx*) | |
| **FLUOXETINE HCl** | |
| **Tablets:** 10 and 20 mg as base (*Rx*) | Various, *Prozac* (Dista) |
| **Capsules:** 10, 20, and 40 mg as base (*Rx*) | Various, *Prozac Pulvules* (Eli Lilly/Dista), *Sarafem Pulvules* (Eli Lilly) |
| **Capsules, delayed-release:** 90 mg (*Rx*) | *Prozac Weekly* (Eli Lilly) |
| **Solution, oral:** 20 mg/5 mL (*Rx*) | Various, *Prozac* (Dista) |
| **FLUVOXAMINE MALEATE** | |
| **Tablets:** 25, 50, and 100 mg (*Rx*) | Various, *Luvox* (Solvay) |
| **PAROXETINE HCl** | |
| **Tablets:** 10, 20, 30, and 40 mg (*Rx*) | Various, *Paxil* (GlaxoSmithKline) |
| **Tablets, controlled-release:** 12.5, 25, and 37.5 mg (*Rx*) | *Paxil CR* (GlaxoSmithKline) |
| **Suspension:** 10 mg/5 mL (*Rx*) | *Paxil* (GlaxoSmithKline) |
| **PAROXETINE MESYLATE** | |
| **Tablets:** 10, 20, 30, and 40 mg (*Rx*) | *Pexeva* (Synthon) |
| **SERTRALINE HCl** | |
| **Tablets:** 25, 50, and 100 mg (*Rx*) | *Zoloft* (Roerig) |
| **Oral concentrate:** 20 mg/mL (*Rx*) | |

## Indications

*Bulimia nervosa:* Fluoxetine.

*Depression:* Citalopram, escitalopram, fluoxetine, paroxetine (immediate- and controlled-release), sertraline.

*Obsessive-compulsive disorder (OCD):* Fluoxetine; fluvoxamine; paroxetine (immediate-release), sertraline.

*Panic disorder:* Paroxetine (immediate- and controlled-release), sertraline, fluoxetine.

*Posttraumatic stress disorder (PTSD):* Paroxetine (immediate-release), sertraline.

*Premenstrual dysphoric disorder (PMDD):* Fluoxetine, paroxetine (controlled-release), sertraline.

*Social anxiety disorder/generalized anxiety disorder (GAD):* Paroxetine (immediate- and controlled-release), sertraline, escitalopram

*Unlabeled uses:*

*Fluoxetine* – Alcoholism (20 to 80 mg/day); anorexia nervosa; bipolar depression (10 mg every other day to 20 mg/day); personality disorder (20 mg/day); cataplexy (20 to 60 mg/day); chronic daily headache, tension-type and migraine headache prophylaxis (10 to 80 mg/day); posttraumatic stress disorder (10 to 80 mg/day); levodopa-induced dyskinesia; fibromyalgia (10 to 80 mg/day); Raynaud phenomenon (20 to 60 mg/day); diabetic neuropathy (20 to 60 mg/day); generalized anxiety disorder (20 mg/day).

*Citalopram* – Panic disorder (20 to 30 mg/day); impulsive aggression in children (20 to 40 mg/day)

## Administration and Dosage

CITALOPRAM HBr:

*Initial therapy* – 20 mg once/day in the morning or evening with or without food. Dose increases usually should occur in increments of 20 mg at intervals of no less than 1 week. Doses greater than 40 mg/day are not recommended.

*Maintenance therapy* – Antidepressant efficacy is maintained for periods of up to 24 weeks following 6 or 8 weeks of initial treatment (32 weeks total). Periodically re-evaluate the long-term usefulness of the drug for the individual patient if citalopram is used for extended periods.

*Elderly/Hepatic function impairment* – 20 mg/day is the recommended dose for most elderly patients and patients with hepatic impairment, with titration to 40 mg/day only for nonresponding patients.

*Renal impairment* – Use with caution in patients with severe renal impairment.

*Switching to or from a monoamine oxidase inhibitor (MAOI)* – Allow at least 14 days to elapse between discontinuation of an MAOI and initiation of citalopram. Similarly, allow at least 14 days after stopping citalopram before starting an MAOI.

ESCITALOPRAM OXALATE:

GAD –

*Initial therapy:* 10 mg once daily. If the dose is increased to 20 mg, this should occur after a minimum of 1 week.

*Maintenance therapy:* GAD is recognized as a chronic condition. The efficacy of escitalopram in the treatment of GAD beyond 8 weeks has not been systematically studied. The physician who elects to use escitalopram for extended periods should periodically reevaluate the long-term usefulness of the drug for the individual patient.

*Major depressive disorder* –

*Initial therapy:* 10 mg once daily. There is no greater benefit of 20 over 10 mg. If the dose is increased to 20 mg, this should occur after a minimum of 1 week.

Administer once daily in the morning or evening, with or without food.

*Maintenance therapy:* Antidepressant efficacy was maintained on 10 or 20 mg/day in clinical trials for periods of up to 36 weeks following 8 weeks of initial treatment. Periodically reassess to determine the need for maintenance treatment.

*Elderly/Hepatic function impairment* – 10 mg/day is the recommended dose for most elderly patients and patients with hepatic impairment.

*Renal impairment* – Use with caution in patients with severe renal impairment; no dosage adjustment is necessary for patients with mild or moderate renal impairment.

*Switching to or from a monoamine oxidase inhibitor (MAOI)* – Allow at least 14 days to elapse between discontinuation of an MAOI and initiation of escitalopram therapy. Similarly, allow at least 14 days after stopping escitalopram before starting an MAOI.

FLUOXETINE HCl:

*Depression* –

*Initial:*

*Adults* – 20 mg/day in the morning. Consider a dose increase after several weeks if no clinical improvement is observed. Administer doses greater than 20 mg/day on a once (morning) or twice (eg, morning and noon) daily schedule. Do not exceed a maximum dose of 80 mg/day.

*Children (8 up to 18 years of age)* – Initiate treatment with a dose of 10 or 20 mg/day. After 1 week at 10 mg/day, increase the dose to 20 mg/day. However, because of higher plasma levels in lower weight children, the starting and target dose in this group may be 10 mg/day. A dose increase to 20 mg/day may be considered after several weeks if insufficient clinical improvement is observed.

*Weekly dosing:* Initiate Prozac Weekly 7 days after the last 20 mg/day dose. If satisfactory response is not maintained, consider re-establishing a daily dosing regimen.

*Maintenance:* Optimal duration of fluoxetine therapy remains speculative. Acute episodes of depression generally require several months or longer of sustained pharmacological therapy.

*Obsessive-compulsive disorder* –

*Initial:*

*Adults* – 20 mg/day in the morning. Consider a dose increase after several weeks if insufficient clinical improvement is observed. Administer doses greater than 20 mg/day on a once (morning) or twice (morning and noon) daily schedule. A dose range of 20 to 60 mg/day is recommended; however, doses of up to 80 mg/day have been well tolerated. Do not exceed 80 mg/day.

*Children (8 to 18 years of age)* – In adolescents and higher weight children, initiate treatment with a dose of 10 mg/day. After 2 weeks, increase the dose to 20 mg/day. A dose range of 20 to 60 mg/day is recommended.

In lower weight children, initiate treatment with a dose of 10 mg/day. Additional dose increases may be considered after several more weeks if insufficient clinical improvement is observed. A dose range of 20 to 30 mg/day is recommended. Experience with daily doses greater than 20 mg is very minimal; there is no experience with doses greater than 60 mg.

*Maintenance:* Patients have been continued on therapy for an additional 6 months without loss of benefit.

*Bulimia nervosa* –

*Initial:* The recommended dose is 60 mg/day, administered in the morning. For some patients it may be advisable to titrate up to this target dose over several days. Fluoxetine doses greater than 60 mg/day have not been studied systematically in patients with bulimia.

*Maintenance:* Patients have been continued on therapy for an additional 52 weeks without loss of benefit. Make dosage adjustments to maintain the patient on the lowest effective dosage and periodically reassess the patient to determine the need for treatment.

*Panic disorder* –

*Initial:* Initiate treatment with a dose of 10 mg/day. After 1 week, increase the dose to 20 mg/day. The most frequently administered dose in the 2 flexible-dose clinical trials was 20 mg/day. Fluoxetine doses above 60 mg/day have not been systematically evaluated in patients with panic disorder.

*Maintenance:* Panic disorder is a chronic condition and it is reasonable to consider continuation for a responding patient. Nevertheless, periodically reassess patients to determine the need for continued treatment.

*PMDD (Sarafem)* –

*Initial:* 20 mg/day given continuously (every day of the menstrual cycle) or intermittently (defined as starting a daily dose 14 days prior to the anticipated onset of menstruation through the first full day of menses and repeating with each new cycle). Do not exceed a maximum dose of 80 mg/day.

*Maintenance/Continuation:* Systemic evaluation has shown that its efficacy is maintained for periods of up to 6 months at a dose of 20 mg/day. Reassess patients periodically to determine the need for continued treatment.

*Hepatic function impairment* – Use a lower or less frequent dosage.

*Special risk patients* – Consider a lower or less frequent dosage for patients, such as the elderly, with concurrent disease or on multiple medications.

*Switching patients to a TCA* – Dosage of TCA may need to be reduced, and plasma TCA concentrations may need to be monitored temporarily when fluoxetine is coadministered or has been recently discontinued.

*Switching patients to or from a monoamine oxidase inhibitor (MAOI)* – At least 14 days should elapse between discontinuation of an MAOI and initiation of therapy with fluoxetine. In addition, allow at least 5 weeks, perhaps longer after stopping fluoxetine before starting an MAOI.

*Thioridazine* – Do not administer thioridazine with fluoxetine or within a minimum of 5 weeks after fluoxetine has been discontinued.

FLUVOXAMINE MALEATE:

*Initial therapy* – Recommended starting dose is 50 mg as a single bedtime dose. Increase dose in 50 mg increments every 4 to 7 days, as tolerated, until maximum therapeutic benefit is achieved, not to exceed 300 mg/day. It is advisable to give total daily doses greater than 100 mg in 2 divided doses; if doses are unequal, give larger dose at bedtime.

*Pediatric therapy* – In patients 8 to 17 years of age, the starting dose is 25 mg as a single daily dose at bedtime. Increase the dose in 25 mg increments every 4 to 7 days as tolerated until maximum therapeutic benefit is achieved (not to exceed 200 mg/day). Divide total daily doses greater than 50 mg into 2 doses. If the 2 divided doses are not equal, give the larger dose at bedtime.

*Maintenance therapy* – Although efficacy has not been documented for more than 10 weeks in controlled trials, OCD is a chronic condition and it is reasonable to consider continuation for a responding patient.

*Elderly/Hepatic function impairment* – These patients have been observed to have decreased fluvoxamine clearance. It may be appropriate to modify initial dose and subsequent titration.

PAROXETINE HCl:
   *Depression* –
    *Initial dose:*
      *Immediate-release* – 20 mg/day. Administer as a single daily dose, usually in the morning. Usual range is 20 to 50 mg/day. Some patients not responding to a 20 mg dose may benefit from dose increases in 10 mg/day increments up to a maximum of 50 mg/day. Dose changes should occur at intervals of at least 1 week.

      *Controlled-release* – 25 mg/day. Administer as a single daily dose with or without food, usually in the morning. Usual range is 25 to 62.5 mg/day. As with all drugs, the full effect may be delayed. Some patients not responding to a 25 mg dose may benefit from dose increases in 12.5 mg/day increments up to a maximum of 62.5 mg/day. Change doses at intervals of at least 1 week. Swallow controlled-release tablet whole; do not chew or crush.

    *Maintenance therapy:* It is generally agreed that acute episodes of depression require several months or longer of sustained pharmacologic therapy. Efficacy has been maintained for period up to 1 year with doses that averaged about 30 mg.

   *OCD (immediate-release)* –
    *Initial:* 20 mg/day. Administer as a single daily dose, usually in the morning. Start with 20 mg/day and may be increased in 10 mg/day increments. Dose changes should occur at intervals of at least 1 week. Usual range is 20 to 60 mg/day. The maximum dosage should not exceed 60 mg/day.

    *Maintenance therapy:* Patients have been continued on therapy for 6 months without loss of benefit. However, make dosage adjustments to maintain the patient on the lowest effective dosage and periodically reassess the patient to determine the need for treatment.

   *Panic disorder* –
    *Initial:*
      *Immediate-release* – 10 mg/day; the recommended target dose is 40 mg/day. Administer as a single daily dose, usually in the morning. Start with 10 mg/day and may be increased in 10 mg/day increments. Dose changes should occur at intervals of at least 1 week. Usual range is 10 to 60 mg/day. The maximum dosage should not exceed 60 mg/day.

      *Controlled-release* – 12.5 mg/day. Administer as a single daily dose, usually in the morning. Dose changes occur in 12.5 mg/day increments. Usual range is 12.5 to 75 mg/day. Do not exceed the maximum dosage of 75 mg/day. Change doses at intervals of at least 1 week. Swallow controlled-release tablet whole; do not chew or crush.

    *Maintenance therapy:* Long-term maintenance of efficacy has been demonstrated for 3 months. Make dosage adjustments to maintain the patient on the lowest effective dosage and reassess the patients periodically to determine the need for continued treatment.

   *Social anxiety disorder* –
    *Immediate-release:* 20 mg/day administered as a single daily dose with or without food, usually in the morning. Usual range is 20 to 60 mg/day.

    *Controlled-release:* 12.5 mg/day. Administer as a single daily dose with or without food, usually in the morning. Usual range is 12.5 to 37.5 mg/day. If necessary, increase dose at intervals of at least 1 week, in increments of 12.5 mg/day up to a maximum of 37.5 mg/day. Swallow controlled-release tablets whole; do not chew or crush.

    *Maintenance:* Although the efficacy beyond 12 weeks of dosing has not been demonstrated in controlled clinical trials, social anxiety disorder is recognized as a chronic condition, and it is reasonable to consider continuation of treatment for a responding patient. Make dosage adjustments to maintain the patient on the lowest effective dosage, and periodically reassess patients to determine the need for continued treatment.

*Generalized anxiety disorder (immediate-release)* –

*Initial:* 20 mg/day administered as a single daily dose with or without food, usually in the morning. Usual range is 20 to 50 mg/day. Change doses in 10 mg/day increments and at intervals of at least 1 week. There is not sufficient evidence to suggest a greater benefit to doses higher than 20 mg/day.

*Maintenance:* Continued therapy for up to 24 weeks has demonstrated a benefit of such maintenance. Generalized anxiety disorder is recognized as a chronic condition, and it is reasonable to consider continuation of treatment for a responding patient.

*PTSD (immediate-release)* –

*Initial:* 20 mg/day. Administer as a single daily dose with or without food, usually in the morning. Usual range is 20 to 50 mg/day. Change doses, if indicated, in 10 mg/day increments and at intervals of at least 1 week. There is not sufficient evidence to suggest a greater benefit for a dose of 40 mg/day compared with 20 mg/day.

*Maintenance:* Although the efficacy beyond 12 weeks of dosing has not been demonstrated, PTSD is recognized as a chronic condition, and it is reasonable to consider continuation of treatment for a responding patient. Maintain the patient on the lowest effective dosage and periodically reassess patients to determine the need for continued treatment.

*PMDD (controlled-release)* –

*Initial:* 12.5 mg/day. Administer as a single daily dose with or without food, usually in the morning. Usual range is 12.5 mg/day and 25 mg/day. Change doses at intervals of at least 1 week. Swallow controlled-release tablet whole; do not chew or crush.

*Maintenance:* The effectiveness for a period exceeding 3 menstrual cycles has not been systematically evaluated in controlled trials. It is reasonable to consider continuation of treatment for a responding patient, and periodically reassess patients to determine the need for continued treatment.

*Elderly or debilitated or patients with severe renal or hepatic impairment* – The recommended initial dose is 10 mg/day (immediate-release) or 12.5 mg/day (controlled-release). Increases may be made if indicated. Do not exceed 40 mg/day (immediate-release) or 50 mg/day (controlled-release).

*Switching patients to or from a monoamine oxidase inhibitor (MAOI)* – Allow at least 14 days between discontinuation of an MAOI and initiation of paroxetine therapy. Similarly, allow at least 14 days after stopping paroxetine before starting an MAOI.

*Discontinuation of treatment* – When discontinuing treatment, monitor for symptoms such as dizziness, sensory disturbances (eg, paresthesias such as electric shock sensations), agitation, anxiety, nausea, and sweating. A gradual reduction in the dose rather than abrupt cessation is recommended whenever possible.

SERTRALINE HCl:

*Adults* –

*Initial treatment:*

*Depression and OCD* – 50 mg once/day.

*Panic disorder, social anxiety disorder, and PTSD* – 25 mg once/day. After 1 week, increase the dose to 50 mg once/day.

Patients were dosed in a range of 50 to 200 mg/day in the clinical trials. Patients not responding to a 50 mg dose may benefit from dose increases up to a maximum of 200 mg/day. Given the 24-hour elimination half-life of sertraline, dose changes should not occur at intervals of less than 1 week.

*PMDD* – 50 mg/day, either daily throughout the menstrual cycle or limited to the luteal phase of the menstrual cycle, depending on physician assessment.

Patients not responding to a 50 mg/day dose may benefit from dose increases (at 50 mg increments/menstrual cycle) up to 150 mg/day when dosing daily throughout the menstrual cycle, or 100 mg/day when dosing during the luteal phase of the menstrual cycle. If a 100 mg/day dose has been established with luteal phase dosing, utilize a 50 mg/day titration step for 3 days at the beginning of each luteal phase dosing period.

*Maintenance/Continuation/Extended treatment* –

*Major depressive disorder:* It is generally agreed that acute episodes of depression require several months or longer of sustained pharmacologic therapy. Systematic evaluation of sertraline has shown that the antidepressant efficacy is maintained for a period of up to 44 weeks following 8 weeks of open-label acute treatment (52 weeks total) at doses of 50 to 200 mg/day.

*Social anxiety disorder:* Social anxiety disorder is a chronic condition that may require several months or longer of sustained pharmacological therapy beyond response to initial treatment. Systematic evaluation of sertraline has demonstrated that its efficacy in social anxiety disorder is maintained for periods of up to 24 weeks following 20 weeks of treatment at a dose of 50 to 200 mg/day. Make dosage adjustments to maintain patients on the lowest effective dose and periodically reassess patients to determine the need for long-term treatment.

*OCD, panic disorder:* Although the efficacy of sertraline beyond 10 to 12 weeks of dosing for OCD and panic disorder has not been documented in controlled trials, all are chronic conditions and it is reasonable to consider continuation of a responding patient. Dosage adjustments may be needed to maintain the patient on the lowest effective dosage, and patients should be periodically reassessed to determine the need for continued treatment.

*PTSD:* It generally is agreed that PTSD requires several months or longer of sustained pharmacological therapy beyond response to initial treatment.

*Long-term use* – Systematic evaluation of sertraline has demonstrated that its efficacy in PTSD is maintained for periods of up to 28 weeks following 24 weeks of treatment at a dose of 50 to 200 mg/day. Physicians periodically should re-evaluate the long-term usefulness of the drug for the individual patient.

*PMDD:* The effectiveness of sertraline in long-term use (that is, for more than 3 menstrual cycles) has not been systematically evaluated in controlled trials. However, as women commonly report that symptoms worsen with age until relieved by the onset of menopause, it is reasonable to consider continuation of a responding patient. Dosage adjustments, which may include changes between dosage regimens (eg, daily throughout the menstrual cycle vs during the luteal phase of the menstrual cycle), may be needed to maintain the patient on the lowest effective dosage. Periodically reassess patients to determine the need for continued treatment.

*Children* –

*OCD:* Initiate dosage with 25 mg once/day for children (6 to 12 years of age) and 50 mg once/day in adolescents (13 to 17 years of age) in the morning or evening. Patients were dosed in a range of 25 to 200 mg/day in trials for pediatric patients 6 to 17 years of age with OCD. Patients not responding to an initial dose of 25 or 50 mg/day may benefit from dose increases up to a maximum of 200 mg/day. For children with OCD, take into account the generally lower body weights compared with adults when increasing the dose to avoid excess dosing. Given the 24-hour elimination half-life, dose changes should not occur at intervals of less than 1 week.

*Hepatic function impairment* – Give a lower or less-frequent dosage in patients with hepatic impairment. Use with caution in these patients.

*Oral concentrate* – Dilute prior to use with 4 oz. (½ cup) of water, ginger ale, lemon/lime soda, lemonade, or orange juice only. Administer the dose immediately after mixing; do not mix in advance.

## Actions

*Pharmacology:* These agents are potent and selective inhibitors of neuronal serotonin reuptake and they also have a weak effect on norepinephrine and dopamine neuronal reuptake.

*Pharmacokinetics:*

| SSRI Pharmacokinetics | | | | | | | |
|---|---|---|---|---|---|---|---|
| SSRIs | Time to peak plasma concentration (h) | Peak plasma concentration (ng/mL) | Half-life (h) | Protein binding (%) | Time to reach steady state (days) | Primary route of elimination | Bioavailability (%) |
| Citalopram | ≈ 4 | nd[1] | ≈ 35 | ≈ 80 | ≈ 7 | 20% renal, fecal | ≈ 80 |
| Escitalopram | 5 | nd | 27 - 32 | ≈ 56 | ≈ 7 | 7% renal | 80[2] |
| Fluoxetine | 6 - 8 | 15 - 55 | 24 - 384[3] | ≈ 94.5 | ≈ 28 | hepatic | nd |
| Fluvoxamine | 3 - 8 | 88 - 546 | 13.6 - 15.6 | ≈ 80 | ≈ 7 | ≈ 94% renal | 53 |
| Paroxetine | 5.2 | 61.7 | 21 | ≈ 93-95 | ≈10 | 64% renal, 36% fecal | 100 |
| Paroxetine CR | 6 - 10 | 30 | 15 - 20 | | 14 | | |
| Sertraline | 4.5 - 8.4 | nd | 26 - 104[3] | 98 | ≈ 7 | 40% - 45% renal, 40% - 45% fecal | nd |

[1] nd = No data.
[2] Based on citalopram data.
[3] t½ includes the active metabolite.

### Contraindications

Hypersensitivity to SSRIs; in combination with a monoamine oxidase inhibitor (MAOI), or within 14 days of discontinuing an MAOI; administration of thioridazine with **fluoxetine** or within a minimum of 5 weeks after fluoxetine has been discontinued; coadministration of **fluvoxamine** with cisapride, thioridazine or pimozide; concomitant use of thioridazine with **paroxetine**; concomitant use of pimozide with **sertraline**; coadministration of sertraline oral concentrate and disulfiram.

### Warnings

*Long-term use:* The effectiveness of long-term use of SSRIs for OCD, panic disorder, and bulimia has not been systematically evaluated. However, the long-term use of SSRIs for depression has been evaluated and demonstrated to maintain antidepressant response for up to 1 year.

*MAOIs:* It is recommended that SSRIs not be used in combination with an MAOI or within 14 days of discontinuing treatment with an MAOI. Allow at least 2 weeks after stopping the SSRIs before starting an MAOI.

*Platelet function:* Altered platelet function or abnormal results from laboratory studies have occurred in patients taking **fluoxetine**, **paroxetine**, or **sertraline**.

*Suicide risk:* Patients with major depressive disorder, both adult and pediatric, may experience worsening of their depression and/or the emergence of suicidal ideation and behavior (suicidality), whether or not they are taking antidepressant medications, and this risk may persist until significant remission occurs. Consider changing the therapeutic regimen, including possibly discontinuing the medication, in patients whose depression is persistently worse or whose emergent suicidality is severe, abrupt in onset, or was not part of the patient's presenting symptoms.

*Rash and accompanying events:* Seven percent of patients taking **fluoxetine** have developed a rash or urticaria; about 33% were withdrawn from treatment. Most patients improved promptly with discontinuation of fluoxetine or adjunctive treatment with antihistamines or steroids; all patients recovered completely. Several other patients have had systemic syndromes suggestive of serum sickness.

Systemic events, possibly related to vasculitis, have developed in patients with rash. Although rare, these events may be serious, involving lung, kidney, or liver. Death has been associated with the events.

*Renal function impairment:* No dose adjustment of **citalopram**, **fluoxetine**, or **fluvoxamine** in renally impaired patients is routinely necessary.

Reduce the initial dosage of **paroxetine** in patients with severe renal impairment.

Use **sertraline** and **escitalopram** with caution in patients with severe renal impairment.

*Hepatic function impairment:* SSRIs are metabolized extensively by the liver. Use with caution in patients with severe liver impairment.

In subjects with hepatic impairment, clearance of racemic citalopram was decreased and plasma concentrations were increased. The recommended dose of **escitalopram** in hepatically impaired patients is 10 mg/day.

*Elderly:* Clearance of **fluvoxamine** is decreased by about 50% in elderly patients. A lower starting dose of **paroxetine** is recommended. Sertraline plasma clearance may be lower. In 2 pharmacokinetic studies, **citalopram** AUC was increased by 23% and 30%, respectively, in elderly subjects as compared with younger subjects, and its half-life was increased by 30% and 50%, respectively. In 2 pharmacokinetic studies, **escitalopram** half-life was increased by approximately 50% in elderly subjects as compared with young subjects and $C_{max}$ was unchanged.

*Pregnancy: Category* C.

*Lactation:* **Escitalopram, fluoxetine, fluvoxamine, citalopram,** and **paroxetine** are excreted in breast milk. It is not known whether **sertraline** or its metabolites are excreted in breast milk.

*Children:* Safety and efficacy in children (younger than 18 years of age) have not been established.

The efficacy of **sertraline** for the treatment of OCD was demonstrated in a 12-week, multicenter, placebo-controlled study with 187 outpatients 6 to 17 years of age. The efficacy of sertraline in pediatric patients with depression, panic disorder, PTSD, PMDD, or social anxiety disorder has not been established.

The efficacy of **fluvoxamine** for the treatment of OCD was demonstrated in a 10-week, multicenter, placebo-controlled study with 120 outpatients 8 to 17 years of age. The adverse event profile was similar to that observed in adult studies. The risks, if any, that may be associated with fluvoxamine's extended use in children and adolescents with OCD have not been systematically assessed. Have the prescriber be mindful that the evidence supporting fluvoxamine use in children and adolescents derives from relatively short-term clinical studies and from extrapolation of experience gained with adult patients.

## Precautions

*Anxiety, nervousness, and insomnia:* Anxiety, nervousness, and insomnia occurred in 2% to 22% of patients treated with an SSRI.

*Altered appetite and weight:* Significant weight loss, especially in underweight depressed patients, has occurred. Approximately 3% to 17% of patients treated with an SSRI experienced anorexia during initial therapy.

*Abnormal bleeding:* Altered platelet function and/or abnormal results from laboratory studies in patients taking **fluoxetine, paroxetine,** or **sertraline** have occurred. There have been reports of abnormal bleeding or purpura in several patients; it is unclear whether the SSRIs had a causative role.

*Mania/Hypomania:* Activation of mania/hypomania occurred infrequently in about 0.1% to 2.2% of patients taking SSRIs. Use cautiously in patients with a history of mania.

*Seizures:* Seizures have occurred with **fluoxetine** (0.1%), **fluvoxamine** (0.2%), **paroxetine** (0.1%), **sertraline** (0.2%), and **citalopram** (0.3%). These percentages appear similar to the rate associated with other antidepressants. Use with care in patients with history of seizures. Discontinue therapy if seizures occur.

*Suicide:* The possibility of a suicide attempt is inherent in depression and may persist until significant remission occurs.

*Concomitant illness:* Use caution in patients with diseases or conditions that could affect metabolism or hemodynamic responses.

*Cardiac effects:* SSRIs have not been systematically evaluated in patients with a recent history of MI or unstable heart disease. Patients with these diagnoses were generally excluded from clinical studies during the product's premarketing testing. However, the ECGs of patients who received SSRIs in clinical trials were evaluated and the data indicate that they are not associated with the development of clinically significant ECG abnormalities.

*Fluoxetine dose changes:* The long elimination half-life of **fluoxetine** and norfluoxetine means that changes in dose will not be fully reflected in plasma for several weeks, affecting titration to final dose and withdrawal from treatment.

*Glaucoma:* Mydriasis has been reported infrequently in premarketing studies with SSRIs. A few cases of acute angle-closure glaucoma associated with **paroxetine** therapy have been reported in the literature. As mydriasis can cause acute angle closure in patients with narrow-angle glaucoma, use caution when SSRIs are prescribed for patients with narrow-angle glaucoma.

*Effects of smoking:* Smokers had a 25% increase in the metabolism of **fluvoxamine** compared with nonsmokers.

*Electroconvulsive therapy (ECT):* There are no clinical studies establishing the benefit of the combined use of ECT and SSRIs. Rare prolonged seizure in patients on **fluoxetine** has occurred.

*Hyponatremia:* Several cases of SSRI-induced hyponatremia (some with serum sodium less than 110 mmol/L) have occurred. The hyponatremia appeared to be reversible when the drug was discontinued. The majority of these occurrences have been in older patients and in patients taking diuretics or who were otherwise volume-depleted.

*Diabetes:* **Fluoxetine** may alter glycemic control. Hypoglycemia has occurred during therapy, and hyperglycemia has developed following discontinuation of the drug. The dosage of insulin or the sulfonylurea may need to be adjusted when fluoxetine is started or discontinued.

*Uricosuric effect:* **Sertraline** is associated with a mean decrease in serum uric acid of about 7%. The clinical significance of this weak uricosuric effect is unknown. There have been no reports of acute renal failure with sertraline.

*Discontinuation of SSRIs:* During marketing of SSRIs and SNRIs, there have been spontaneous reports of adverse events occurring upon discontinuation of these drugs, particularly when abrupt, including the following: agitation, anxiety, confusion, dizziness, dysphoric mood, emotional lability, headache, hypomania, insomnia, irritability, lethargy, and sensory disturbances (eg, paresthesias such as electric shock sensations). While these events are generally self-limiting, there have been reports of serious discontinuation symptoms.

*Drug abuse and dependence:* Before staring an SSRI, carefully evaluate patients for history of drug abuse and follow such patients closely, observing them for signs of misuse or abuse.

*Hazardous tasks:* SSRIs may cause dizziness or drowsiness. Instruct patients to observe caution while driving or performing tasks requiring alertness, coordination, or physical dexterity.

*Photosensitivity:* Photosensitization may occur.

### Drug Interactions

*Drugs highly bound to plasma protein:* Because SSRIs are highly bound to plasma protein, administration to a patient taking another drug that is highly protein-bound may cause increased free concentrations of the other drug, potentially resulting in adverse events. Conversely, adverse effects could result from displacement of SSRIs by other highly bound drugs.

*P450 system:* Concomitant use of SSRIs with drugs metabolized by cytochrome P4502D6 may require lower doses than usually prescribed for either **paroxetine** or the other drug because paroxetine may significantly inhibit the activity of this isozyme.

Hepatic metabolism of **citalopram** and **escitalopram** occurs primarily through cytochrome P450 3A4 and 2C19 isoenzymes. Inhibitors of 3A4 (eg, azole antifungals, macrolide antibiotics) and 2C19 (eg, omeprazole) would be expected to increase plasma citalopram levels. Inducers of 3A4 (eg, carbamazepine) would be expected to decrease citalopram and escitalopram levels.

*Serotonin syndrome:* The serotonin syndrome is a rare complication of therapy with serotonergic drugs. When this problem occurs with SSRIs, it is most commonly in the setting of other concurrent medications that increase serotonin by different mechanisms.

*Drugs that may affect SSRIs:* Drugs that may affect SSRIs include azole antifungals, barbiturates, carbamazepine, cimetidine, cyproheptadine, , lithium, macrolides, MAOIs, metoclopramide, phenytoin, sibutramine, smoking, St. John's wort, tramadol, linezolid, L-tryptophan.

*Drugs that may be affected by SSRIs:* Drugs that may be affected by SSRIs include alcohol, benzodiazepines, beta blockers, buspirone, carbamazepine, cisapride, clozapine, cyclosporine, diltiazem, digoxin, haloperidol, hydantoins, lithium, methadone, mexiletine, nonsedating antihistamines, NSAIDs, olanzapine, phenothiazines, phenytoin, pimozide, procyclidine, ritonavir, ropivacaine, sumatriptan, sulfonylureas, sympathomimetics, tacrine, theophylline, tolbutamide, tricyclic antidepressants, and warfarin.

*Drug/Food interactions:* In one study following a single dose of **sertraline** with and without food, sertraline AUC was slightly increased and $C_{max}$ was 25% greater. Time to reach peak plasma level decreased from 8 hours post-dosing to 5.5 hours.

Food does not appear to affect systemic bioavailability of **fluoxetine** although it may delay absorption. **Fluvoxamine** and **citalopram** bioavailability is not affected by food. Thus, fluoxetine, fluvoxamine, and citalopram may be given with or without food.

## Adverse Reactions

| SSRIs Adverse Reactions (%)[a] | | | | | | |
|---|---|---|---|---|---|---|
| Adverse reaction | Citalopram | Escitalopram | Fluoxetine | Fluvoxamine | Paroxetine IR/CR | Sertraline |
| *Cardiovascular* | | | | | | |
| Chest pain | — | ≥ 1 | ≥ 1 | — | 3 | 1 | ≥ 1 |
| Hot flushes | 0.1 - 1 | ≥ 1 | — | — | — | — | 0.1 - 1 |
| Hypertension | 0.1 - 1 | ≥ 1 | ≥ 1 | ≥ 1 | ≥ 1 | 2 | 0.1 - 1 |
| Hypotension (postural) | ≥ 1 | — | 0.1 - 1 | ≥ 1 | — | 0.1 - 1 | 0.1 - 1 |
| Palpitations | — | ≥ 1 | 1 - 3 | 3 | 2 - 3 | 0.1 - 1 | ≥ 1 |
| Syncope | 0.1 - 1 | 0.1 - 1 | 0.1 - 1 | ≥ 1 | ≥ 1 | — | 0.1 - 1 |
| Tachycardia | ≥ 1 | 0.1 - 1 | 0.1 - 1 | ≥ 1 | ≥ 1 | 1 - 2 | 0.1 - 1 |
| Vasodilation | — | — | 2 - 3 | 3 | 2 - 4 | 2 - 3 | < 0.1 |
| *CNS* | | | | | | |
| Abnormal dreams | — | 3 | 3 | — | 3 - 4 | 1 | 0.1 - 1 |
| Abnormal thinking | — | — | 2 - 6 | — | 0.1 - 1 | 0.1 - 1 | — |
| Agitation | 3 | 0.1 - 1 | ≥ 1 | 2 | 3 - 6 | 2 - 3 | 1 - 6 |
| Amnesia | ≥ 1 | 0.1 - 1 | ≥ 1 | ≥ 1 | 2 | 0.1 - 1 | 0.1 - 1 |
| Anxiety | 4 | — | 12 - 13 | 1 - 5 | 2 - 6 | 2 - 5 | 4 |
| Apathy | ≥ 1 | 0.1 - 1 | — | ≥ 1 | — | — | 0.1 - 1 |
| CNS stimulation | — | — | 0.1 - 1 | 2 | — | — | — |
| Concentration, decreased/impaired | ≥ 1 | ≥ 1 | — | — | 3 - 4 | 1 - 3 | — |
| Confusion | ≥ 1 | 0.1 - 1 | ≥ 1 | — | 1 | 1 | 0.1 - 1 |
| Depersonalization | 0.1 - 1 | 0.1 - 1 | 0.1 - 1 | 0.1 - 1 | 3 | 0.1 - 1 | — |
| Depression | ≥ 1 | 0.1 - 1 | — | 2 | — | 2 | 0.1 - 1 |
| Dizziness | — | 4 - 7 | 2 - 11 | 2 - 11 | 6 - 14 | 6 - 14 | 6 - 17 |
| Drugged feeling | — | — | — | — | 2 | — | — |
| Emotional lability | 0.1 - 1 | 0.1 - 1 | ≥ 1 | 0.1 - 1 | ≥ 1 | 0.1 - 1 | 0.1 - 1 |
| Fatigue | 5 | 2-8 | — | — | — | — | 10 - 16 |
| Headache | — | 24 | 13 - 24 | 3 - 22 | 17 - 18 | 15 - 27 | 25 |
| Hypertonia | 0.1 - 1 | — | 0.1 - 1 | 2 | 0.1 - 1 | 2 - 3 | ≥ 1 |
| Hypoesthesia | 0.1 - 1 | — | 0.1 - 1 | — | 0.1 - 1 | 0.1 - 1 | ≥ 1 |
| Hypo-/Hyperkinesia | 0.1 - 1 | — | — | ≥ 1 | 0.1 - 1 | 0.1 - 1 | 0.1 - 1 |
| Insomnia | 15 | 7 - 14 | 9 - 24 | 4 - 21 | 11 - 24 | 7 - 20 | 12 - 23 |

| SSRIs Adverse Reactions (%)[a] | | | | | | |
|---|---|---|---|---|---|---|
| Adverse reaction | Citalopram | Escitalopram | Fluoxetine | Fluvoxamine | Paroxetine IR/CR | | Sertraline |
| Libido decreased | 1 - 4 | 3 - 7 | 3 - 9 | 2 | 3 - 12 | 7 - 12 | 1 - 11 |
| Manic reaction | — | — | — | ≥ 1 | — | — | — |
| Myoclonus/twitching | — | 0.1 - 1 | 0.1 - 1 | ≥ 1 | 2 - 3 | 1 - 2 | 0.1 - 1 |
| Nervousness | — | 0.1 - 1 | 3 - 14 | 2 - 12 | 3 - 9 | 2 - 8 | 5 |
| Paresthesia | ≥ 1 | 2 | — | — | 4 | 1 - 3 | 2 |
| Psychotic reaction | — | — | — | ≥ 1 | — | — | — |
| Sleep disorder | — | — | ≥ 1 | 0.1-1 | — | — | — |
| Somnolence | 18 | 4 - 13 | 12 - 13 | 4 - 22 | 13 - 24 | 3 - 22 | 2 - 15 |
| Tremor | 8 | 0.1 - 1 | 9 - 12 | 5 | 4 - 15 | 4 - 8 | < 1 - 11 |
| Vertigo | 0.1 - 1 | 0.1 - 1 | — | 0.1 - 1 | ≥ 1 | 2 | 0.1 - 1 |
| *Dermatologic* | | | | | | | |
| Acne | 0.1 - 1 | 0.1 - 1 | 0.1 - 1 | 0.1 - 1 | 0.1 - 1 | 0.1 - 1 | 0.1 - 1 |
| Pruritus | ≥ 1 | 0.1 - 1 | 3 | — | ≥ 1 | 0.1 - 1 | 0.1 - 1 |
| Rash | ≥ 1 | ≥ 1 | 4 - 5 | — | 2 - 3 | ≥ 1 | 3 |
| Sweating, excessive/ increased | 11 | 3 - 8 | 7 - 8 | 7 | 1 - 14 | 6 - 14 | 3 - 11 |
| *GI* | | | | | | | |
| Abdominal pain | 3 | 2 | 6 | 1 | 4 | 3-7 | 2-7 |
| Anorexia | 4 | — | 10 - 11 | 1 - 6 | — | — | 3-11 |
| Constipation | — | 3 - 6 | 5 | 10 | 5 - 16 | 2 - 13 | 1 - 8 |
| Decreased appetite | — | 3 | — | — | 2 - 9 | 1 - 12 | — |
| Diarrhea/loose stools | 8 | 6 - 14 | 2 - 11 | 1 - 11 | 9 - 19 | 6 - 18 | 13 - 24 |
| Dry mouth | 20 | 4 - 9 | 9 - 11 | 1 - 14 | 9 - 21 | 2 - 18 | 6 - 16 |
| Dyspepsia | 5 | 2 - 6 | 7 - 8 | 1 - 10 | 2 - 5 | 2 - 13 | 6 - 13 |
| Dysphagia | 0.1 - 1 | — | 0.1 - 1 | 2 | 0.1 - 1 | — | 0.1 - 1 |
| Flatulence | ≥ 1 | 2 | 3 | 4 | 4 | 6 - 8 | — |
| Gastroenteritis | 0.1 - 1 | ≥ 1 | 0.1 - 1 | 0.1 - 1 | 0.1 - 1 | 0.1 - 1 | 0.1 - 1 |
| Increased appetite | ≥ 1 | ≥ 1 | ≥ 1 | — | 2 - 4 | — | ≥ 1 |
| Melena | — | — | 0.1 - 1 | — | — | — | < 0.1 |
| Nausea | 21 | 15 - 18 | 9 - 27 | 9 - 40 | 15 - 36 | 17 - 23 | 13 - 30 |
| Oropharynx disorder | — | — | — | — | 2 | — | — |
| Tooth disorder/caries | — | 2 | — | 3 | < 0.1 | 0.1 - 1 | 0.1 - 1 |
| Vomiting | 4 | 3 | 1 - 3 | 2 - 5 | 2 - 3 | 2 | 4 |
| *GU* | | | | | | | |
| Abnormal ejaculation | 6 | 9 - 14 | — | 8 | 6 - 28 | 15 - 27 | 7 - 19 |
| Female genital disorders | — | — | — | — | 2 - 9 | 2 - 10 | — |
| Male genital disorders, others | — | — | — | — | 4 - 10 | — | — |
| Menstrual disorder | — | 2 | — | — | — | 1 - 2 | 0.1 - 1 |
| Sexual dysfunction/ impotence/ anorgasmia | 1 - 3 | 2 - 6 | 0.1 - 1 | 2 | 2 - 13 | 5 - 10 | ≥ 1 |
| Urinary frequency | — | ≥ 1 | 2 | 3 | 2 - 3 | 2 | 0.1 - 1 |
| Urinary tract infection | — | ≥ 1 | — | 0.1 - 1 | 2 | 3 | — |
| Urination disorder/ retention | 0.1 - 1 | — | 0.1- 1 | 1 | 3 | 2 | 0.1 - 1 |
| *Musculoskeletal* | | | | | | | |
| Arthralgia | 2 | ≥ 1 | — | 0.1 - 1 | ≥ 1 | 2 | 0.1 - 1 |
| Myalgia | 2 | ≥ 1 | — | — | 2 - 4 | 5 | ≥ 1 |
| Myasthenia | — | — | < 0.1 | 0.1 - 1 | 1 | < 0.1 | — |
| Myopathy | — | — | < 0.1 | < 0.1 | 2 | < 0.1 | — |
| *Respiratory* | | | | | | | |
| Bronchitis | 0.1 - 1 | ≥ 1 | — | 0.1 - 1 | 0.1 - 1 | 1 - 2 | < 0.1 |
| Cough (increased) | ≥ 1 | ≥ 1 | — | ≥ 1 | ≥ 1 | 1 - 2 | 0.1 - 1 |
| Dyspnea | 0.1 - 1 | — | — | 2 | 0.1 - 1 | — | 0.1 - 1 |
| Pharyngitis | — | — | 6 - 10 | — | 4 | 8 | — |
| Respiratory disorder | — | — | — | — | 7 | — | — |
| Rhinitis | 5 | 5 | 16 - 23 | — | 3 | 4 | ≥ 1 |
| Sinusitis | 3 | 3 | — | ≥ 1 | 4 | 4 - 8 | 0.1 - 1 |

| SSRIs Adverse Reactions (%)[a] | | | | | | |
|---|---|---|---|---|---|---|
| Adverse reaction | Citalopram | Escitalopram | Fluoxetine | Fluvoxamine | Paroxetine IR/CR | | Sertraline |
| Upper respiratory tract infection | 5 | — | — | 9 | — | — | 0.1 - 1 |
| Yawn | 2 | 2 | 3 - 5 | 2 | 2 - 5 | 2 - 5 | ≥ 1 |
| *Special senses* | | | | | | | |
| Amblyopia | — | — | — | 3 | — | — | — |
| Taste perversion/ change | ≥ 1 | 0.1 - 1 | ≥ 1 | 3 | 2 | 2 | — |
| Tinnitus | 0.1 - 1 | ≥ 1 | ≥ 1 | — | ≥ 1 | 0.1 - 1 | ≥ 1 |
| Vision disturbances/ blurred vision/ abnormal vision | ≥ 1 | ≥ 1 | 2 - 3 | — | 2 - 8 | 1 - 5 | 3 |
| *Miscellaneous* | | | | | | | |
| Accidental injury/ trauma | — | — | 1 - 8 | ≥ 1 | 3 - 6 | 3 - 8 | — |
| Allergy/allergic reac- tion | — | ≥ 1 | — | 0.1 - 1 | 0.1 - 1 | 2 | < 0.1 |
| Asthenia | — | 0.1 - 1 | 8 - 14 | 2 - 14 | 3 - 22 | 14 - 18 | ≥ 1 |
| Back pain | — | — | — | — | 3 | 4 - 5 | ≥ 1 |
| Chills | — | 0.1 - 1 | ≥ 1 | 2 | 2 | 0.1 - 1 | — |
| Edema | 0.1 - 1 | — | — | ≥ 1 | 0.1 - 1 | 0.1 - 1 | 0.1 - 1 |
| Fever | 2 | ≥ 1 | 2 - 5 | — | — | 0.1 - 1 | 0.1 - 1 |
| Flu syndrome | 0.1 - 1 | 5 | 3 - 12 | 3 | 5 - 6 | 6 - 8 | — |
| Malaise | — | 0.1 - 1 | 0.1 - 1 | ≥ 1 | 0.1 - 1 | 0.1 - 1 | < 1 - 10 |
| Pain | — | — | 3 - 9 | — | — | 3 | 1 - 6 |
| Weight gain | ≥ 1 | ≥ 1 | ≥ 1 | ≥ 1 | ≥ 1 | 1 - 3 | ≥ 1 |
| Weight loss | ≥ 1 | 0.1 - 1 | 2 - 3 | ≥ 1 | 0.1 - 1 | 1 | 0.1 - 1 |

[a] Data are pooled from different studies and are not necessarily comparable.

# MONOAMINE OXIDASE INHIBITORS

## ISOCARBOXAZID
**Tablets:** 10 mg (*Rx*)      *Marplan* (Hoffman-La Roche)

## PHENELZINE
**Tablets:** 15 mg (as sulfate) (*Rx*)      *Nardil* (Parke-Davis)

## TRANYLCYPROMINE
**Tablets:** 10 mg (as sulfate) (*Rx*)      *Parnate* (GlaxoSmithKline)

### Indications
*Depression:* In general, the MAOIs appear to be indicated in patients with atypical (exogenous) depression, and in some patients unresponsive to other antidepressive therapy. They are rarely a drug of first choice.

### Administration and Dosage
ISOCARBOXAZID:
    *Initial dosage* – 10 mg twice daily. Increase dosage by 10 mg every 2 to 4 days to achieve a dosage of 40 mg by the end of the first week. Increase by increments of up to 20 mg/week, to a maximum recommended dosage of 60 mg/day. Daily dosage should be divided into 2 to 4 doses.
    *Maintenance dosage* – After maximum clinical response is achieved, attempt to reduce the dosage slowly over a period of several weeks without jeopardizing therapeutic response. Beneficial effect may not be seen in some patients for 3 to 6 weeks. If no response is obtained by then, discontinue therapy.
    Because of the limited experience with systematically monitored patients receiving isocarboxazid at the higher end of the currently recommended dose range of up to 60 mg/day, caution is indicated in patients for whom a dose of 40 mg/day is exceeded.
PHENELZINE:
    *Initial dose* – 15 mg 3 times/day.

*Early phase treatment* – Increase dosage to 60 mg/day or more at a fairly rapid pace consistent with patient tolerance. It may be necessary to increase dosage up to 90 mg/day to obtain sufficient MAO inhibition. Many patients do not show a clinical response until treatment at 60 mg has been continued for at least 4 weeks.

*Maintenance dose* – After maximum benefit is achieved, reduce dosage slowly over several weeks. Maintenance dose may be as slow as 15 mg/day or every other day; continue for as long as required.

TRANYLCYPROMINE: The usual effective dosage is 30 mg/day in divided doses. If there is no improvement after 2 weeks, increase dosage in 10 mg/day increments of 1 to 3 weeks. Dosage range may be extended to a maximum of 60 mg/day from the usual 30 mg/day. Withdrawal from tranylcypromine should be gradual.

## Actions

*Pharmacology:* These drugs are non-selective MAOIs and cause an increase in the concentration of endogenous epinephrine, norepinephrine, and serotonin (5HT) in storage sites throughout the nervous system.

*Pharmacokinetics:* Phenelzine and tranylcypromine are well absorbed orally. The clinical effects of phenelzine may continue for up to 2 weeks after discontinuation of therapy. When tranylcypromine is withdrawn, MAO activity is recovered in 3 to 5 days (possibly up to 10 days), although the drug is excreted in 24 hours.

## Contraindications

Hypersensitivity to these agents; pheochromocytoma; CHF; a history of liver disease or abnormal liver function tests; severe impairment of renal function; confirmed or suspected cerebrovascular defect; cardiovascular disease; hypertension; history of headache; in patients over 60 because of the possibility of existing cerebral sclerosis with damaged vessels; coadministration with other MAOIs; dibenzazepine-related agents including tricyclic antidepressants, carbamazepine, and cyclobenzaprine; buproprion; SSRIs; buspirone; sympathomimetics; meperidine; dextromethorphan; anesthetic agents; CNS depressants; antihypertensives; caffeine; cheese or other foods with high tyramine content (see Warnings and Drug Interactions).

## Warnings

*Hypertensive crises:* The most serious reactions involve changes in blood pressure; it is inadvisable to use these drugs in elderly or debilitated patients or in the presence of hypertension, cardiovascular, or cerebrovascular disease. Not recommended in patients with frequent or severe headaches because headache during therapy may be the first symptom of a hypertensive reaction.

*Warning to the patient* – Warn all patients against eating foods with high tyramine or tryptophan content and for 2 weeks after discontinuing MAOIs. Also warn patients against drinking alcoholic beverages and against self-medication with certain proprietary agents such as cold, hay fever, or weight reduction preparations containing sympathomimetic amines while undergoing therapy. Instruct patients not to consume excessive amounts of caffeine in any form and to report promptly the occurrence of headache or other unusual symptoms.

*Concomitant antidepressants:* In patients receiving a selective serotonin reuptake inhibitor (SSRIs) in combination with an MAOI, there have been reports of serious, sometimes fatal, reactions including hyperthermia, rigidity, myoclonus, autonomic instability with possible rapid fluctuations of vital signs, and mental status changes that include extreme agitation progressing to delirium and coma. It is recommended that SSRIs not be used in combination with an MAOI, or within 14 days of an MAOI. Allow 2 weeks or longer after stopping the SSRIs before starting an MAOI. Allow 5 weeks or longer after stopping fluoxetine before starting an MAOI.

MAOIs should not be administered together with or immediately following tricyclic antidepressants (TCAs). At least 14 days should elapse between the discontinuation of the MAOIs and the institution of a TCA. Some TCAs have been used safely and successfully in combination with MAOIs.

*Withdrawal:* Withdrawal may be associated with nausea, vomiting, and malaise.

*Coexisting symptoms:* **Tranylcypromine** and **isocarboxazid** may aggravate coexisting symptoms in depression, such as anxiety and agitation.

*Renal function impairment:* Observe caution in patients with impaired renal function because there is a possibility of cumulative effects in such patients.

*Elderly:* Older patients may suffer more morbidity than younger patients during and following an episode of hypertension or malignant hyperthermia with MAOI use. Use with caution in the elderly.

*Pregnancy:* Category C.

*Lactation:* Safety for use during lactation has not been established. **Tranylcypromine** is excreted in breast milk.

*Children:* Not recommended for patients younger than 16 years of age.

## Precautions

*Hypotension:* Follow all patients for symptoms of postural hypotension. Blood pressure usually returns to pretreatment levels rapidly when the drug is discontinued or the dosage is reduced.

*Hypomania:* Hypomania has been the most common severe psychiatric side effect reported. This has been largely limited to patients in whom disorders characterized by hyperkinetic symptoms coexist with, but are obscured by, depressive affect.

*Diabetes:* There is conflicting evidence as to whether MAOIs affect glucose metabolism or potentiate hypoglycemic agents. Consider this if used in diabetics.

*Epilepsy:* The effect of MAOIs on the convulsive threshold may vary. Do not use with metrizamide; discontinue MAOI 48 hours or more prior to myelography and resume ≥ 24 hours postprocedure.

*Hepatic complications:* Perform periodic liver function tests, such as bilirubins, alkaline phosphatase, or transaminases during therapy; discontinue at the first sign of hepatic dysfunction or jaundice.

*Myocardial ischemia:* MAOIs may suppress anginal pain that would otherwise serve as a warning of myocardial ischemia.

*Hyperthyroid patients:* Use **tranylcypromine** and **isocarboxazid** cautiously because of increased sensitivity to pressor amines.

*Switching MAOIs:* In several case reports, hypertensive crisis, cerebral hemorrhage and death have possibly resulted from switching from one MAOI to another without a waiting period. However, in other patients no adverse reactions occurred. Nevertheless, a waiting period of 10 to 14 days is recommended when switching from one MAOI to another.

*Drug abuse and dependence:* There have been reports of drug dependency in patients using doses of **tranylcypromine** and **isocarboxazid** significantly in excess of the therapeutic range.

## Drug Interactions

Drugs that may affect MAOIs include dibenzazepine-related entities, disulfiram, methylphenidate, metrizamide, and sulfonamide.

Drugs that may be affected by MAOIs include anesthetics, antidepressants, antidiabetic agents, barbiturates, beta blockers, bupropion, buspirone, carbamazepine, cyclobenzapine, dextromethorphan, guanethidine, levodopa, meperidine, methyldopa, rauwolfia alkaloids, sulfonamide, sumatriptan, sympathomimetics, thiazide diuretics, and L-tryptophan.

*Drug/Food interactions:* Warn all patients against eating foods with a high **tyramine** content. Hypertensive crisis may result (see Warnings).

## Adverse Reactions

*Cardiovascular:* Orthostatic hypotension, associated in some patients with falling; disturbances in cardiac rate and rhythm.

*CNS:* Dizziness; vertigo; headache; overactivity; hyperreflexia; tremors; muscle twitching; mania; hypomania; jitteriness; confusion; memory impairment; sleep disturbances including hypersomnia and insomnia; weakness; myoclonic movements; fatigue; drowsiness; restlessness; overstimulation including increased anxiety, agitation and manic symptoms.

*GI:* Constipation; nausea; diarrhea; abdominal pain.

*Miscellaneous:* Edema; dry mouth; blurred vision; hyperhidrosis; elevated serum transaminases; minor skin reactions such as skin rashes; anorexia; weight changes.

# ANTIPSYCHOTIC AGENTS

> **Warning:**
> *Clozapine:*
>   *Agranulocytosis* – Because of a significant risk of agranulocytosis, a potentially life-threatening adverse event, reserve **clozapine** use in 1) the treatment of severely ill patients with schizophrenia who fail to show an acceptable response to adequate courses of standard antipsychotic drug treatment, or 2) for reducing the risk of recurrent suicidal behavior in patients with schizophrenia or schizoaffective disorder who are judged to be at risk of re-experiencing suicidal behavior.
>
>   Patients being treated with clozapine must have a baseline white blood cell (WBC) and differential count before initiation of treatment, as well as regular WBC counts during treatment and for 4 weeks after discontinuation of treatment.
>
>   Clozapine is available only through a distribution system that ensures monitoring of WBC counts according to the schedule described below, prior to delivery of the next supply of medication.
>
>   *Seizures* – Seizures have been associated with the use of **clozapine**. Dose appears to be an important seizure predictor, with a greater likelihood at higher clozapine doses. Use caution when administering clozapine to patients with a history of seizures or other predisposing factors. Advise patients not to engage in any activity where sudden loss of consciousness could cause serious risk to themselves or others.
>
>   *Myocarditis* – Analyses of postmarketing safety databases suggest **clozapine** is associated with an increased risk of fatal myocarditis, especially during, but not limited to, the first month of therapy. In patients in whom myocarditis is suspected, discontinue clozapine treatment promptly.
>
>   *Other adverse cardiovascular and respiratory effects* – Orthostatic hypotension, with or without syncope, can occur with **clozapine** treatment. Rarely, collapse can be profound and accompanied by respiratory and/or cardiac arrest. Orthostatic hypotension is more likely to occur during initial titration in association with rapid dose escalation. In patients who have had even a brief interval off clozapine (2 or more days since the last dose), start treatment with 12.5 mg once or twice daily (see Warnings).
>
>   Because collapse, respiratory arrest, and cardiac arrest during initial treatment have occurred in patients receiving benzodiazepines or other psychotropic drugs, caution is advised when clozapine is initiated in patients taking a benzodiazepine or any other psychotropic drug.

## Indications

| | | | | | | | | | | | | | | | | | |
|---|---|---|---|---|---|---|---|---|---|---|---|---|---|---|---|---|---|
| | | | | | | | | **Antipsychotics — Summary of Indications**[a] | | | | | | | | | |
| Indications<br><br>✔ = labeled<br>X = unlabeled | Aripiprazole | Chlorpromazine | Clozapine | Fluphenazine | Haloperidol | Loxapine | Mesoridazine | Molindone | Olanzapine | Perphenazine | Pimozide | Prochlorperazine | Quetiapine | Risperidone | Thioridazine | Thiothixene | Trifluoperazine | Ziprasidone |
| Acute agitation associated with bipolar I mania | | | | | | | | | ✔ (IM)[b] | | | | | | | | | |
| Acute agitation in schizophrenia | | | | | | | | | ✔ (IM)[b] | | | | | | | | | ✔ (IM)[b] |
| Acute intermittent porphyria | | ✔ | | | | | | | | | | | | | | | | |

## Antipsychotics — Summary of Indications[a]

| Indications  ✓ = labeled  X = unlabeled | Aripiprazole | Chlorpromazine | Clozapine | Fluphenazine | Haloperidol | Loxapine | Mesoridazine | Molindone | Olanzapine | Perphenazine | Pimozide | Prochlorperazine | Quetiapine | Risperidone | Thioridazine | Thiothixene | Trifluoperazine | Ziprasidone |
|---|---|---|---|---|---|---|---|---|---|---|---|---|---|---|---|---|---|---|
| Acute manic and/or mixed episodes associated with bipolar disorder | ✓ | ✓ | X | | | | | | ✓ | | | | ✓ | ✓ | | | | ✓ |
| Hyperactivity (pediatric patients) | | ✓ | | ✓ | | | | | | | | | | | | | | |
| Intractable hiccoughs | | ✓ | | | X | | | | | | | | | | | | | |
| Nausea/Vomiting | | ✓ | | X | X | | | | | ✓ | | ✓ | | | | | | |
| Nonpsychotic anxiety | | | | | | | | | | | | ✓ | | | | | ✓ | |
| Presurgical apprehension/restlessness | | ✓ | | | | | | | | | | | | | | | | |
| Psychotic disorders | | | | ✓ | ✓ | | | | | ✓ | | | | | | | | |
| Recurrent suicidal behavior | | | ✓ | | | | | | | | | | | | | | | |
| Schizophrenia | ✓ | ✓ | ✓ | ✓ | | ✓ | ✓ | ✓ | ✓ | ✓ | X | ✓ | ✓ | ✓ | ✓ | ✓ | ✓ | ✓ |
| Severe behavioral problems (pediatric patients) | | ✓ | | | ✓ | | | | | | | | | X | | | | |
| Tetanus | | ✓ | | | | | | | | | | | | | | | | |
| Tourette disorder | | | | | ✓ | | | | | | ✓ | | | | | | | |
| *Unlabeled uses* | | | | | | | | | | | | | | | | | | |
| Behavioral problems associated with autism | | | | | | | | | | | | | | X | | | | |
| Migraines (acute treatment) | | X | | | | | | | | | | X | | | | | | |
| Obsessive-compulsive disorder (refractory to SSRIs) | | | | | | | | | X | | | | | X | | | | |
| PCP-induced psychosis | | | | | X | | | | | | | | | | | | | |
| Psychosis/Agitation in dementia or Alzheimer disease | | | X | | X | | | | X | | | | X | X | X | | | X |
| Psychosis in Parkinson disease | | | X | | | | | | | | | | X | X | | | | |

[a] For more detailed information, see the information below and individual drug monographs.
[b] IM = intramuscular

### Actions
*Pharmacology:*

| Antipsychotic Receptor Affinity | |
|---|---|
| Antipsychotic agent | Receptor affinity |
| *Conventional agents* | |
| Chlorpromazine | **High** — adrenergic  **Weak** — peripheral anticholinergic, histaminergic, serotonergic |
| Fluphenazine | Dopamine $D_2$, histamine $H_1$, alpha-adrenergic, serotonin 5-$HT_2$ |
| Haloperidol | Dopamine $D_2$, alpha-adrenergic, serotonin 5-$HT_2$ |
| Loxapine | Dopamine $D_2$, histamine $H_1$, alpha-adrenergic, muscarinic $M_1$ |
| Mesoridazine | Dopamine $D_2$, histamine $H_1$, alpha-adrenergic, muscarinic $M_1$ |
| Molindone | **Low** — dopamine $D_2$, alpha-adrenergic, serotonin 5-$HT_2$ |

| Antipsychotic Receptor Affinity | |
|---|---|
| Antipsychotic agent | Receptor affinity |
| Perphenazine | Dopamine $D_2$, histamine $H_1$, alpha-adrenergic |
| Pimozide | Dopamine $D_2$, alpha-adrenergic, serotonin 5-$HT_2$ |
| Prochlorperazine | Dopamine $D_2$, histamine $H_1$, alpha- $D_2$adrenergic, serotonin 5-$HT_2$ |
| Promethazine[1] | Histamine $H_1$, muscarinic, some serotonin |
| Thioridazine | Dopamine $D_2$, histamine $H_1$, alpha-adrenergic, muscarinic $M_1$, serotonin 5-$HT_2$ |
| Thiothixene | High — dopamine $D_2$<br>Low — histamine $H_1$, alpha-adrenergic |
| Trifluoperazine | Dopamine $D_2$, histamine $H_1$, alpha-adrenergic, muscarinic $M_1$, serotonin 5-$HT_2$ |
| Atypical agents | |
| Aripiprazole | High — dopamine $D_2$[2], $D_3$, serotonin 5-$HT_{1A}$[2], 5-$HT_{2A}$<br>Moderate — dopamine $D_4$, 5-$HT_{2C}$, 5-$HT_7$, alpha$_1$-adrenergic, histamine $H_1$ |
| Clozapine | High — dopamine $D_4$<br>Other receptors — dopamine $D_1$, $D_2$, $D_3$, $D_5$, adrenergic, cholinergic, histaminergic, serotonergic |
| Olanzapine | High — serotonin 5-$HT_{2A}$, 5-$HT_{2C}$, dopamine $D_1$, $D_2$, $D_3$, $D_4$, muscarinic $M_1$, $M_2$, $M_3$, $M_4$, $M_5$, histamine $H_1$, alpha$_1$adrenergic<br>Weak — $GABA_A$, benzodiazepine receptor, beta-adrenergic |
| Quetiapine | Serotonin 5-$HT_{1A}$, 5-$HT_2$, dopamine $D_1$, $D_2$, alpha$_1$ and $_2$-adrenergic, histamine $H_1$ |
| Risperidone | High — dopamine $D_2$, serotonin 5-$HT_2$<br>Low to moderate — 5-$HT_{1C}$, 5-$HT_{1D}$, 5-$HT_{1A}$, histamine $H_1$, alpha-adrenergic<br>Weak — $D_1$, haloperidol-sensitive sigma site |
| Ziprasidone | High — dopamine $D_2$, $D_3$, 5-$HT_{2A}$, 5-$HT_{2C}$, 5-$HT_{1A}$[1], 5-$HT_{1D}$, alpha$_1$adrenergic<br>Moderate — histamine $H_1$ |

[1] Promethazine is classified as a phenothiazine but not indicated as an antipsychotic.
[2] Partial agonist activity.

| Pharmacological Parameters of Antipsychotics | | | | | | | |
|---|---|---|---|---|---|---|---|
| Antipsychotic agent | Approx. equiv. dose (mg) | Usual oral adult daily dose range (mg) | Sedation | EPS | Anticholinergic effects | Orthostatic hypotension | Weight gain |
| **Phenothiazines** | | | | | | | |
| *Aliphatic* | | | | | | | |
| Chlorpromazine | 100 | 30-800 | +++ | ++ | ++ | +++ | |
| *Piperazine* | | | | | | | |
| Fluphenazine | 2 | 1-40 | + | ++++ | + | + | |
| Perphenazine | 10 | 12-64 | ++ | ++ | + | + | |
| Prochlorperazine | | 15-150 | | | | | |
| Trifluoperazine | 5 | 2-15 | + | +++ | + | + | |
| *Piperidines* | | | | | | | |
| Mesoridazine | 50 | 100-400 | +++ | + | +++ | ++ | |
| Thioridazine | 100 | 150-800 | +++ | + | +++ | +++ | |
| **Thioxanthenes** | | | | | | | |
| Thiothixene | 4 | 6-60 | + | +++ | + | + | |
| **Phenylbutylpiperadines** | | | | | | | |
| *Butyrophenone* | | | | | | | |
| Haloperidol | 2 | 1-100 | + | ++++ | + | + | |
| *Diphenylbutylpiperadine* | | | | | | | |
| Pimozide | | 1-10 | + | +++ | ++ | + | |

| Pharmacological Parameters of Antipsychotics | | | | | | | |
|---|---|---|---|---|---|---|---|
| Antipsychotic agent | Approx. equiv. dose (mg) | Usual oral adult daily dose range (mg) | Sedation | EPS | Anticholinergic effects | Orthostatic hypotension | Weight gain |
| **Dihydroindolones** | | | | | | | |
| Molindone | 10 | 15-225 | + | ++ | + | + | |
| Ziprasidone | | 40-200 | ++ | ++ | + | ++ | + |
| **Dibenzepines** | | | | | | | |
| *Dibenzoxazepines* | | | | | | | |
| Loxapine | 10 | 20-250 | + | ++ | + | + | |
| *Dibenzodiazepine* | | | | | | | |
| Clozapine | 50 | 300-900 | +++ | 0 | +++ | +++ | ++++ |
| *Thienbenzodiazepine* | | | | | | | |
| Olanzapine | | 5-20 | ++ | + | ++ | ++ | ++++ |
| *Dibenzothiazepine* | | | | | | | |
| Quetiapine | | 50-800 | ++ | 0 | 0-+ | ++ | +++ |
| **Benzisoxazole** | | | | | | | |
| Risperidone | | 4-16 | + | ++ | 0-+ | ++ | +++ |
| **Quinolinone** | | | | | | | |
| Aripiprazole | | 10-30 | ++ | 0 | 0-+ | + | +++ |

++++ = Very high incidence of side effects, +++ = High incidence of side effects, ++ = Moderate incidence of side effects, + = Low incidence of side effects

The exact mechanism of action of the antipsychotic agents is unknown; however, it is thought to be due to their antagonistic actions on the receptors of several neurotransmitters.

*Pharmacokinetics:*
*Absorption* – Oral absorption tends to be erratic and variable. Peak plasma levels are seen 2 to 6 hours after oral use.

*Distribution* – These agents are widely distributed in tissues; CNS concentrations exceed those in plasma. They are highly bound to plasma proteins (91% to 99%).

*Metabolism* – CYP2D6 is the enzyme responsible for metabolism of many antipsychotics. Extensive biotransformation occurs in the liver.

*Excretion* – One-half of the excretion of these agents occurs via the kidneys and the other half occurs through enterohepatic circulation. Elimination half-lives range from 10 to 20 hours or more.

### Contraindications

Hypersensitivity to drug or any other component of the product (cross-sensitivity between phenothiazines may occur); comatose or greatly depressed states because of CNS depressants or from any other cause (phenothiazines, **clozapine, loxapine, molindone, pimozide, haloperidol**); coadministration with other drugs that prolong the QT interval and in patients with congenital long QT syndrome or history of cardiac arrhythmias (**mesoridazine, thioridazine, pimozide, ziprasidone**; see Drug Interactions).

*Phenothiazines:* Suspected or established subcortical brain damage (**fluphenazine**); blood dyscrasias (**perphenazine, trifluoperazine, fluphenazine**); bone marrow depression (**perphenazine, trifluoperazine, fluphenazine**); preexisting liver damage (**perphenazine, trifluoperazine, fluphenazine**); pediatric surgery (**prochlorperazine**); hypertensive or hypotensive heart disease of extreme degree (**thioridazine**).

*Thiothixene:* Circulatory collapse; blood dyscrasias.

*Haloperidol:* Parkinson disease.

*Pimozide:* Treatment of simple tics or tics other than those associated with Tourette disorder; in combination with drugs (eg, pemoline, methylphenidate, amphetamines) that may themselves cause motor or phonic tics until it is determined whether or not the drugs, rather than Tourette disorder, are responsible for the tics.

*Clozapine:* Myeloproliferative disorders; uncontrolled epilepsy; history of **clozapine**-induced agranulocytosis or severe granulocytopenia; should not be used with other agents having a well-known potential to cause agranulocytosis or suppress bone marrow function.

*Ziprasidone:* Recent acute MI; uncompensated heart failure.

## Warnings

*Tardive dyskinesia (TD):* TD, a syndrome consisting of potentially irreversible, involuntary dyskinetic movements, may develop in patients treated with antipsychotic drugs. Both the risk of developing TD and the likelihood that it will become irreversible are increased as duration of treatment and total cumulative dose administered increase.

*Extrapyramidal symptoms (EPS):* Dystonic reactions develop primarily with the use of traditional antipsychotics. EPS has occurred during the administration of **haloperidol** and **pimozide** frequently, often during the first few days of treatment.

*Neuroleptic malignant syndrome (NMS):* A potentially fatal symptom complex sometimes referred to as NMS has been reported in association with administration of antipsychotic drugs. Clinical manifestations of NMS are hyperpyrexia, muscle rigidity, altered mental status, and evidence of autonomic instability (irregular pulse or BP, tachycardia, diaphoresis, cardiac dysrhythmia). Additional signs may include elevated creatine phosphokinase, myoglobinuria (rhabdomyolysis), and acute renal failure.

*CNS effects:* These agents may impair mental or physical abilities, especially during the first few days. Drowsiness may occur during the first or second week, after which it generally disappears. If troublesome, lower the dosage. Caution patients against activities requiring alertness (ie, operating vehicles or machinery).

*Encephalopathic syndrome* – An encephalopathic syndrome (characterized by weakness, lethargy, fever, tremulousness and confusion, extrapyramidal symptoms, leukocytosis, elevated serum enzymes, BUN, fasting blood sugar) has occurred in a few patients treated with lithium plus an antipsychotic (**haloperidol**).

*Cardiovascular:* Use with caution in patients with cardiovascular disease, cerebrovascular disease, conditions that would predispose patients to hypotension, or mitral insufficiency. Increased pulse rates occur in most patients.

*ECG changes* – A minority of **clozapine** patients experience ECG repolarization changes similar to those seen with other antipsychotic drugs, including S-T segment depression and flattening or inversion of T waves, which all normalize after discontinuation of clozapine.

**Ziprasidone, pimozide, mesoridazine,** and **thioridazine** have been shown to prolong the QT interval, and drugs with this potential have been associated with torsade de pointes-type arrhythmias and sudden death. Certain circumstances may increase the risk of torsade de pointes and/or sudden death in association with the used of drugs that prolong the QT interval, including the following: 1) Bradycardia; 2) hypokalemia or hypomagnesemia; 3) concomitant use of other drugs that prolong the QT interval; and 4) presence of congenital prolongation of the QT interval. Perform a baseline ECG and measure serum potassium and magnesium before initiation of treatment and periodically during treatment, especially during a period of dose adjustment. Patients with QT interval over 450 msec should not receive mesoridazine or thioridazine. Ziprasidone should be avoided in patients with histories of significant cardiovascular illness (eg, QT prolongation, recent acute MI, uncompensated heart failure, cardiac arrhythmia). Replete patients with low potassium and/or magnesium with those electrolytes before proceeding with treatment. Discontinue treatment if the QT interval is over 500 msec. Patients who experience symptoms that may be associated with the occurrence of torsade de pointes (eg, dizziness, palpitations, syncope) may warrant further cardiac evaluation; in particular, consider Holter monitoring.

Nonspecific ECG changes, usually reversible Q- and T-wave distortions, have been observed in some patients receiving phenothiazines. Nonspecific ECG changes have been observed in some patients receiving **thiothixene**.

**Haloperidol** has been associated with ECG changes, including QT interval prolongation and ECG pattern changes compatible with the polymorphous configuration of torsade de pointes.

Rare, transient, nonspecific T-wave changes have been reported on ECG in patients taking **molindone**.

Prolongation of the QT interval and torsade de pointes have been reported with risperidone overdoses.

*Myocarditis* – Postmarketing **clozapine** surveillance data from 4 countries revealed cases of myocarditis, some fatal.

*Cardiomyopathy* – Cases of cardiomyopathy have been reported in patients treated with **clozapine**.

*Pulmonary embolism* – Consider the possibility of pulmonary embolism in patients receiving **clozapine** who present with deep vein thrombosis, acute dyspnea, chest pain, or with other respiratory signs and symptoms.

*Hypotension* – Orthostatic hypotension with or without syncope can occur, especially during initial titration in association with rapid dose escalation, and may represent a continuing risk in some patients. In 1 report, initial **clozapine** doses as low as 12.5 mg were associated with collapse and respiratory arrest. Carefully watch patients who are undergoing surgery, and who are on large doses of phenothiazines, for hypotensive phenomena. The hypotensive effects may occur after the first injection of the antipsychotic, occasionally after subsequent injections, and rarely after the first oral dose. Recovery is usually spontaneous and symptoms disappear within 0.5 to 2 hours.

*Tachycardia* – Tachycardia, which may be sustained, also has been observed in approximately 25% of patients taking clozapine.

*Cerebrovascular effects:* Cerebrovascular adverse events (eg, stroke, transient ischemic attack), including fatalities, were reported in patients (mean, 85 years of age; range, 73 to 97 years of age) in trials of **risperidone** in elderly patients with dementia-related psychosis. In placebo-controlled trials, there was a significantly higher incidence of cerebrovascular adverse events in patients treated with risperidone compared with patients treated with placebo. **Risperidone** is not approved for the treatment of patients with dementia-related psychosis.

*Sudden death:* Previous brain damage or seizures may be predisposing factors; avoid high doses in known seizure patients.

*Priapism:* Rare cases of priapism have been associated with **risperidone, ziprasidone, quetiapine, aripiprazole,** and **olanzapine**.

*Hyperprolactinemia:* Antipsychotic drugs elevate prolactin levels; the elevation persists during chronic administration.

*Hyperglycemia and diabetes mellitus:* Hyperglycemia, in some cases extreme and associated with ketoacidosis or hyperosmolar coma or death, has been reported in patients treated with atypical antipsychotics.

Regularly monitor patients with an established diagnosis of diabetes mellitus who are started on atypical antipsychotics for worsening of glucose control. Patients with risk factors for diabetes mellitus (eg, obesity, family history of diabetes) who are starting treatment with atypical antipsychotics should undergo fasting blood glucose testing at baseline and periodically during treatment. Monitor any patient treated with atypical antipsychotics for symptoms of hyperglycemia, including polydipsia, polyuria, polyphagia, and weakness. Patients who develop symptoms of hyperglycemia during treatment with atypical antipsychotics should undergo fasting blood glucose testing. In some cases, hyperglycemia resolved when the atypical antipsychotic was discontinued; however, some patients required continuation of antidiabetic treatment despite discontinuation of the suspect drug.

*Antiemetic effects:* Drugs with antiemetic effect can obscure signs of toxicity of other drugs, or mask symptoms of disease (eg, brain tumor, intestinal obstruction, Reye's syndrome). They can suppress the cough reflex; aspiration of vomitus is possible.

*Pulmonary:* Cases of bronchopneumonia (some fatal) have followed the use of antipsychotic agents. Lethargy and decreased sensation of thirst caused by central inhibition may lead to dehydration, hemoconcentration, and reduced pulmonary ventilation.

*Agranulocytosis:* Agranulocytosis, defined as an ANC of less than 500/mm³, occurs in association with **clozapine** use at a cumulative incidence at 1 year of about 1.3%. This reaction could prove fatal if not detected early and therapy interrupted.

*Ophthalmic:* Use with caution in patients with a history of glaucoma. During prolonged therapy, ocular changes may occur; these include particle deposition in the cornea and lens, progressing in more severe cases to star-shaped lenticular opacities. Pigmentary retinopathy occurs most frequently in patients receiving **thioridazine** dosages more than 1 g/day.

*Pigmentary retinopathy* – Careful observation should be made for pigmentary retinopathy and lenticular pigmentation (fine lenticular pigmentation has been noted in a small number of patients treated for prolonged periods. Pigmentary retinopathy, which has been observed primarily in patients taking larger than recommended thioridazine doses, is characterized by diminution of visual acuity, brownish coloring of vision, and impairment of night vision; examination of the fundus discloses deposits of pigment.

*Cataracts* – Lens changes also have been observed in patients taking **quetiapine** during long-term treatment. Examination of the lens by methods adequate to detect cataract formation, such as slit-lamp exam, is recommended at initiation of treatment or shortly thereafter, and at 6-month intervals.

*Seizure disorders:* These drugs can lower the convulsive threshold and may precipitate seizures. Use cautiously in patients with a history of epilepsy and only when absolutely necessary.

*GI dysmotility:* Esophageal dysmotility and aspiration have been associated with antipsychotic drug use. Aspiration pneumonia is a common cause of morbidity and mortality in elderly patients, in particular those with advanced Alzheimer dementia. Use **quetiapine**, **ziprasidone**, **risperidone**, **olanzapine**, **aripiprazole**, and others cautiously in patients at risk for aspiration pneumonia.

*Hypersensitivity reactions:* Patients who have demonstrated a hypersensitivity reaction (eg, blood dyscrasias, jaundice) with a phenothiazine should not be re-exposed to any phenothiazine unless the potential benefits of treatment outweigh the possible hazards.

*Renal function impairment:* Administer cautiously to those with diminished renal function.

*Hepatic function impairment:* Use with caution in patients with impaired hepatic function. Patients with a history of hepatic encephalopathy caused by cirrhosis have increased sensitivity to the CNS effects of antipsychotic drugs (ie, impaired cerebration and abnormal slowing of the EEG). Dosage adjustments may be necessary in patients receiving **quetiapine** who are hepatically impaired.

*Carcinogenesis:* Neuroleptic drugs (except **promazine**) elevate prolactin levels which persist during chronic use. Tissue culture experiments indicate approximately one third of human breast cancers are prolactin-dependent in vitro, a factor of potential importance if use of these drugs is contemplated in a patient with previously detected breast cancer.

*Elderly:* Dosages in the lower range are sufficient for most elderly patients. Monitor response and adjust dosage accordingly. Increase dosage gradually in elderly patients.

*Pregnancy:* Category C. (Category B, clozapine).

*Lactation:* Decide whether to discontinue nursing or discontinue the drug, taking into account the importance of the drug to the mother.

*Children:* In general, these products are not recommended for children younger than 12 years of age. Children seem more prone to develop extrapyramidal reactions, even at moderate doses. Therefore, use the lowest effective dosage.

**Precautions**

*Anticholinergic effects:* Most antipsychotic agents are associated with constipation, dry mouth, and tachycardia, all adverse events possibly related to cholinergic antagonism. Anticholinergic effects of **clozapine** are very potent. Use caution in patients with clinically significant prostatic hypertrophy, narrow-angle glaucoma or a history of paralytic ileus.

*Cholesterol:* Decreased serum cholesterol has occurred with some agents; however, **quetiapine** may raise plasma cholesterol and triglycerides.

*Concomitant conditions:* Use with caution in patients: Exposed to extreme heat or phosphorus insecticides; atropine or related drugs because of additive anticholinergic effects; in a state of alcohol withdrawal; with dermatoses or other allergic reactions to phenothiazine derivatives because of the possibility of cross-sensitivity; who have exhibited idiosyncrasy to other centrally acting drugs.

*Hematologic:* Various blood dyscrasias have occurred.

*Myelography:* Discontinue phenothiazines at least 48 hours before myelography because of the possibility of seizures; do not resume therapy for at least 24 hours postprocedure.

*Thrombotic thrombocytopenic purpura (TTP):* A single case of TTP was reported with **risperidone**. The relationship to therapy is unknown.

*Thyroid:* Severe neurotoxicity (rigidity, inability to walk or talk) may occur in patients with thyrotoxicosis who are also receiving antipsychotics.

 *Hypothyroidism* – **Quetiapine** demonstrated a dose-related decrease in total and free thyroxine ($T_4$) of approximately 20% at the higher end of the therapeutic dose range that was maximal in the first 2 to 4 weeks of treatment and maintained without adaptation or progression during more chronic therapy.

*Hyperpyrexia:* A significant, not otherwise explained rise in body temperature may indicate intolerance to antipsychotics.

*Abrupt withdrawal:* These drugs are not known to cause psychic dependence and do not produce tolerance or addiction. However, following abrupt withdrawal of high dose therapy, symptoms such as gastritis, nausea, vomiting, dizziness, headache, tachycardia, insomnia, and tremulousness have occurred. These symptoms can be reduced by gradual reduction of the dosage or by continuing antiparkinson agents for several weeks after the antipsychotic is withdrawn.

*Suicide:* Suicide possibility in depressed patients remains during treatment and until significant remission occurs. This type of patient should not have access to large quantities of the drug.

*Cutaneous pigmentation changes:* Rare instances of skin pigmentation have occurred, primarily in females on long-term, high dose therapy. These changes, restricted to exposed areas of the skin, range from almost imperceptible darkening to a slate gray color, sometimes with a violet hue. Pigmentation may fade following drug discontinuation.

*Phenylketonurics:* Inform phenylketonuric patients that some of these products contain phenylalanine.

*Benzyl alcohol:* Some of these products contain benzyl alcohol, which has been associated with a fatal "gasping syndrome" in premature infants.

*Drug abuse and dependence:* Evaluate patients for history of drug abuse, and observe such patients closely for signs of misuse or abuse (eg, development of tolerance, increases in dose, drug-seeking behavior).

*Photosensitivity:* Because photosensitivity has been reported (rarely with thioridazine), undue exposure to the sun should be avoided during phenothiazine treatment.

*Sulfite sensitivity:* Some of these products contain sulfites that may cause allergic-type reactions, including anaphylactic symptoms and life-threatening or less severe asthmatic episodes in certain susceptible persons. The overall prevalence of sulfite sensitivity in the general population is unknown and probably low. It is seen more frequently in asthmatic or atopic nonasthmatic persons.

### Drug Interactions

| Antipsychotics and Enzymes Involved with Metabolism ||
|---|---|
| Antipsychotic agent | Enzyme(s) |
| Aripiprazole | CYP3A4, 2D6 |
| Clozapine | CYP1A2, 2D6, 3A4 |
| Olanzapine | CYP1A2, 2D6 |
| Perphenazine | CYP2D6 |
| Pimozide | CYP3A, 1A2 |
| Quetiapine | CYP3A4 |
| Risperidone | CYP2D6 |
| Thioridazine | CYP2D6 |
| Ziprasidone | Aldehyde oxidase, CYP3A4, 1A2 |

*CYP450:* Several antipsychotics are metabolized by the cytochrome P450 (CYP450) enzyme system. Therefore, several drug interactions may be possible involving drugs that are potent inhibitors or inducers of this enzyme system. Monitor and adjust therapy as needed when these antipsychotics are coadministered with potent inhibitors or inducers of the following isoenzymes.

Drugs that may affect phenothiazines include anticholinergics, beta blockers, meperidine, paroxetine, ritonavir, and thiazide diuretics.

Drugs that may be affected by phenothiazines include anticholinergics, beta blockers, guanethidine, meperidine, oral anticoagulants, phenytoin, thiazide diuretics, and dofetilide.

Drugs that may affect the antipsychotics include carbamazepine, charcoal, cimetidine, clozapine, fluoxetine, methyldopa, phenobarbital, and phenytoin.

Drugs that may be affected by antipsychotics include antiarrhythmics, anticholinergics, antihypertensive agents, CNS depressants, dopamine, epinephrine, levodopa, lorazepam, phenothiazines, and thioridazine.

Drugs that may interact with the atypical antipsychotics include the following: carbamazepine, cimetidine, CYP1A2 inducers/inhibitors, CYP3A4 inhibitors, dopamine agonists, famotidine, levodopa, lorazepam, phenytoin, quinidine, ritonavir, SSRIs, thioridazine, and valproate.

Drugs that may interact with clozapine include caffeine, SSRIs, benzodiazepines, risperidone, CYP1A2 induces/inhibitors, CYP3A4 inhibitors, phenobarbital, ritonavir, and risperidone.

Drugs that may interact with haloperidol include anticholinergic agents, azole antifungal agents, carbamazepine, lithium, rifamycins, and fluoxetine.

*Drug/Lab test interactions:* Phenothiazines may produce false-positive phenylketonuria (PKU) test results. Phenothiazines may cause false-positive pregnancy test results.

### Adverse Reactions

Adverse reactions occurring in at least 3% of patients include the following:

*Typical antipsychotic agents:*
  CNS – Akathesia; akinesia; asthenia; bizarre dreams; depression; drowsiness; headache; insomnia; hyperkinesia; sedation; somnolence.
  *Miscellaneous* – Impotence; rash.

*Atypical antipsychotic agents:*
  *Cardiovascular* – Chest pain; hypertension; hypotension; tachycardia.
  CNS – Agitation; akathisia; akinesia; anxiety; asthenia; confusion; dizziness; drowsiness; dystonia; extrapyramidal symptoms; gait abnormal; headache; hyperkinesia; hypokinesia; insomnia; libido decreased; restlessness; syncope; tremor; vertigo.
  *Dermatologic* – Ecchymosis; eczema; rash.

GI – Abdominal pain/discomfort; altered taste; appetite increased; constipation; diarrhea; dry mouth; dyspepsia; gastroesophageal reflux; nausea; salivation; vomiting; weight gain.

GU – Ejaculation disorders; impotence; menorrhagia.

*Respiratory* – Coughing; pharyngitis; rhinitis.

*Special senses* – Abnormal vision; blurred vision; visual disturbances.

*Miscellaneous* – Accidental injury; arthralgia; back pain; diaphoresis; edema (peripheral); fever; hypertonia; joint pain; leukopenia; muscle pain; rigidity.

## PHENOTHIAZINE AND THIOXANTHENE DERIVATIVES

### PHENOTHIAZINE DERIVATIVES
**CHLORPROMAZINE HCl**

| | |
|---|---|
| **Tablets**: 10, 25, 50, 100, and 200 mg (*Rx*) | Various, *Thorazine* (GlaxoSmithKline) |
| **Oral concentrate**: 100 mg/mL (*Rx*) | Various |
| **Suppositories (as base)**: 100 mg (*Rx*) | *Thorazine* (GlaxoSmithKline) |
| **Injection**: 25 mg/mL (*Rx*) | Various, *Thorazine* (GlaxoSmithKline) |

**FLUPHENAZINE**

| | |
|---|---|
| **Tablets**: 1, 2.5, 5, and 10 mg (*Rx*) | Various |
| **Elixir**: 2.5 mg/5 mL (*Rx*) | Various |
| **Injection**: 2.5 mg/mL, 25 mg/mL (*Rx*) | Various, *Prolixin Decanoate* (Apothecon) |

**PERPHENAZINE**

| | |
|---|---|
| **Tablets**: 2, 4, 8, and 16 mg (*Rx*) | Various |
| **Oral concentrate**: 16 mg per 5 mL (*Rx*) | (Pharmaceutical Associates) |

**PROCHLORPERAZINE**

| | |
|---|---|
| **Tablets**: 5 and 10 mg (as maleate) (*Rx*) | Various, *Compazine* (GlaxoSmithKline) |
| **Capsules, sustained release**: 10 and 15 mg (as maleate) (*Rx*) | *Compazine* (GlaxoSmithKline) |
| **Syrup**: 5 mg/5 mL (as edisylate) (*Rx*) | *Compazine* (GlaxoSmithKline) |
| **Suppositories**: 2.5, 5, and 25 mg (*Rx*) | Various, *Compazine* (GlaxoSmithKline), *Compro* (Paddock) |
| **Injection**: 5 mg/mL (as edisylate) | Various, *Compazine* (GlaxoSmithKline) |

**THIORIDAZINE HCl**

| | |
|---|---|
| **Tablets**: 10, 15, 25, 50, 100, 150, and 200 mg (*Rx*) | Various |

**TRIFLUOPERAZINE**

| | |
|---|---|
| **Tablets**: 1, 2, 5, and 10 mg (*Rx*) | Various |

### THIOXANTHENE DERIVATIVES
**THIOTHIXENE**

| | |
|---|---|
| **Capsules**: 1, 2, 5, 10, and 20 mg (*Rx*) | Various, *Navane* (Roerig) |

**Indications**

*Chlorpromazine HCl:*

*Behavioral problems* – For the treatment of severe behavioral problems in children 1 to 12 years of age marked by combativeness and/or explosive hyperexcitable behavior (out of proportion to immediate provocations).

*Emesis/Hiccoughs* – For the control of nausea and vomiting and relief of intractable hiccoughs.

*Hyperactivity* – For the short-term treatment of hyperactive children who show excessive motor activity with accompanying conduct disorders consisting of some or all of the following symptoms: Impulsivity, difficulty sustaining attention, aggressivity, mood lability, and poor frustration tolerance.

*Manic-depressive illness* – For the control of manifestations of the manic type of manic-depressive illness.

*Porphyria, acute intermittent* – For the treatment of acute intermittent porphyria.

*Schizophrenia* – For the treatment of schizophrenia.

*Surgery* – Relief of restlessness and apprehension prior to surgery.

*Tetanus* – An adjunct in treatment of tetanus.

*Fluphenazine:*

> *Psychotic disorders* – For the management of manifestations of psychotic disorders; esterified formulations (decanoate) are indicated for patients requiring prolonged and parenteral neuroleptic therapy (eg, chronic schizophrenic patients).

*Perphenazine:*

> *Emesis* – To control severe nausea and vomiting and intractable hiccoughs.
>
> *Psychotic disorders* – For the treatment of schizophrenia (tablets); management of manifestations of psychotic disorders (oral concentrate).

*Prochlorperazine:*

> *Emesis* – To control severe nausea and vomiting. (*Compro* is only indicated for severe nausea and vomiting in adults.)
>
> *Nonpsychotic anxiety* – Short-term treatment of generalized nonpsychotic anxiety; however, prochlorperazine is not the first drug of choice for this indication.
>
> *Schizophrenia* – For the treatment of schizophrenia.

*Trifluoperazine HCl:*

> *Nonpsychotic anxiety* – Short-term treatment of nonpsychotic anxiety (not the drug of choice in most patients).
>
> *Schizophrenia* – For the management of schizophrenia.

*Thioridazine HCl:*

> *Schizophrenia* – For the management of schizophrenic patients who fail to respond adequately to treatment with other antipsychotic drugs. Before initiating treatment with thioridazine, it is strongly recommended that a patient be given at least 2 trials, each with a different antipsychotic drug product, at an adequate dose and for an adequate duration.

*Thiothixene:*

> *Schizophrenia* – For the management of schizophrenia.

## Administration and Dosage

CHLORPROMAZINE: Individualize dosage based on condition severity. Increase dosage until symptoms are controlled, then gradually reduce dosage to the lowest effective maintenance level. Increase parenteral dosage only if hypotension has not occurred.

> *Oral concentrate* – Add desired dosage to 60 mL or more of diluent just prior to administration. Suggested vehicles are tomato or fruit juice, milk, simple syrup, orange syrup, carbonated beverages, coffee, tea, or water. Semisolid foods (eg, soups, puddings) may also be used.
>
> *Injection* – Subcutaneous administration is not advised. Inject IM slowly, deep into upper outer quadrant of buttock. Because of possible hypotensive effects, reserve for bedfast patients or for acute ambulatory cases and keep patient recumbent for at least ½ hour after injection. If irritation is a problem, dilute injection with saline or 2% procaine; do not mix with other agents in the syringe. Avoid injecting undiluted into vein. Use the IV route only for severe hiccoughs, surgery, and tetanus. Slight yellowing will not alter potency. Discard if markedly discolored.
>
> Because of the possibility of contact dermatitis, avoid getting solution on hands or clothing.
>
> *Psychotic disorders* – Maximum improvement may not be seen for weeks or even months. Continue optimum dosage for 2 weeks, then gradually reduce to lowest effective maintenance level; 200 mg/day is not unusual. Some patients require higher dosages (eg, 800 mg/day is not uncommon in discharged mental patients).
>
> > *Hospitalized patients:*
> >
> > Acute schizophrenic or manic states –
> >
> > > IM: 25 mg initially. If necessary, give an additional 25 to 50 mg injection in 1 hour. Increase gradually over several days (up to 400 mg every 4 to 6 hours in exceptionally severe cases) until patient is controlled. Patient usually becomes quiet and cooperative within 24 to 48 hours. Substitute oral dosage and increase until the patient is calm; 500 mg/day is usually sufficient. While gradual increases to 2000 mg or more/day may be necessary, little therapeutic gain is achieved by exceeding 1000 mg/day for extended periods.

*Less acutely disturbed* –
Oral: 25 mg 3 times/day. Increase gradually until effective dose is reached, usually 400 mg/day.

*Outpatients:*
Oral – Initial oral dose is 10 mg 3 or 4 times/day or 25 mg 2 or 3 times/day.

*More severe cases:*
Oral – Give 25 mg 3 times/day. After 1 or 2 days, daily dosage may be increased by 20 to 50 mg at semiweekly intervals until patient becomes calm and cooperative.

*Prompt control of severe symptoms:*
IM – 25 mg; if necessary, repeat in 1 hour. Give subsequent doses orally, 25 to 50 mg 3 times/day.

*Behavioral disorders/Hyperactivity* – Generally, do not use chlorpromazine in children younger than 6 months of age except where potentially lifesaving. It should not be used in conditions for which specific children's dosages have not been established.

*Outpatients:*
Oral – 0.5 mg/kg (0.25 mg/lb) every 4 to 6 hours, as needed.
Rectal – 1 mg/kg (0.5 mg/lb) every 6 to 8 hours, as needed.
IM – 0.5 mg/kg (0.25 mg/lb) every 6 to 8 hours, as needed.

*Hospitalized patients:*
Oral – Start with low doses and increase gradually. In severe behavior disorders, 50 to 100 mg/day, or in older children, 200 mg/day or more may be necessary. There is little evidence that improvement in severely disturbed mentally retarded patients is enhanced by doses beyond 500 mg/day.

IM –
*5 years of age or younger or 50 lbs:* Do not exceed 40 mg/day.
*5 to 12 years of age or 50 to 100 lbs:* Do not exceed 75 mg/day, except in unmanageable cases.

*Surgery* –
*Adults:*
*Preoperative apprehension* – 25 to 50 mg orally 2 to 3 hours before surgery or 12.5 to 25 mg IM 1 to 2 hours before surgery.

*Intraoperative (to control acute nausea/vomiting)* –
IM: 12.5 mg. Repeat in ½ hour if necessary and if no hypotension occurs.
IV: 2 mg per fractional injection at 2-minute intervals. Do not exceed 25 mg (dilute 1 mg/mL with saline).

*Children:*
*Preoperative apprehension* – 0.5 mg/kg (0.25 mg/lb) orally 2 to 3 hours before operation or 0.5 mg/kg (0.25 mg/lb) IM 1 to 2 hours before operation.

*Intraoperative (to control acute nausea/vomiting)* –
IM: 0.25 mg/kg (0.125 mg/lb); repeat in ½ hour if needed and if no hypotension occurs.
IV: 1 mg per fractional injection at 2-minute intervals; do not exceed IM dosage. Always dilute to 1 mg/mL with saline.

*Tetanus* –
*Adults:* 25 to 50 mg IM 3 or 4 times/day, usually with barbiturates. For IV use, 25 to 50 mg diluted to at least 1 mg/mL and administered at a rate of 1 mg/min.

*Children:* 0.5 mg/kg (0.25 mg/lb) IM or IV every 6 to 8 hours. When given IV, dilute to at least 1 mg/mL and administer at a rate of 1 mg per 2 minutes. In children up to 23 kg (50 lbs), do not exceed 40 mg/day; 23 to 45 kg (50 to 100 lbs), do not exceed 75 mg/day, except in severe cases.

*Acute intermittent porphyria (adults)* – 25 to 50 mg orally 3 or 4 times/day or 25 mg IM 3 or 4 times/day until patient can take oral therapy.

*Elderly/Debilitated/Emaciated* – Lower initial doses and more gradual adjustments are recommended.

FLUPHENAZINE HCl: Individualize dosage. The oral dose is approximately 2 to 3 times the parenteral dose. Institute treatment with a low initial dosage; increase as necessary. Therapeutic effect is often achieved with doses under 20 mg/day. However, daily doses up to 40 mg may be needed.

*Oral –*

*Adults:* Initially administer 2.5 to 10 mg/day in divided doses at 6 to 8 hour intervals. When symptoms are controlled, reduce dosage gradually to daily maintenance doses of 1 or 5 mg, often given as a single daily dose. Continued treatment is needed to achieve maximum therapeutic benefits; further adjustments in dosage may be necessary during the course of therapy to meet the patient's requirements.

*Elderly –* Initially, 1 to 2.5 mg/day, adjusted according to response.

For psychotic patients stabilized on a fixed daily dosage of orally administered fluphenazine, conversion from oral therapy to the long-acting injectable fluphenazine decanoate may be indicated.

*Injection –*

*Hydrochloride formulation:* Administer IM. Average starting dose for adult patients is 1.25 mg (0.5 mL) IM. Initial total daily dose may range from 2.5 to 10 mg and should be divided and given at 6- to 8-hour intervals. Use dosages exceeding 10 mg per day with caution. When symptoms are controlled, oral maintenance therapy can generally be instituted often with single daily doses.

*Decanoate formulation:* Administer IM or subcutaneously. Use a dry syringe and needle of at least 21 gauge. A wet needle or syringe may cause the solution to become cloudy. Initiate with 12.5 to 25 mg (0.5 to 1 mL). The onset of action generally appears between 24 and 72 hours after injection, and the effects of the drug on psychotic symptoms become significant within 48 to 96 hours. Determine subsequent injections and dosage interval in accordance with patient response. When administered as maintenance therapy, a single injection may be effective in controlling schizophrenic symptoms up to 4 weeks or longer. The response to a single dose has been found to last as long as 6 weeks in a few patients on maintenance therapy.

Initially, treat patients who have never taken phenothiazines with a shorter-acting form of the drug before administering the decanoate. This helps to determine the response to fluphenazine and to establish appropriate dosage.

No precise formula can be given to convert to fluphenazine decanoate use. However, in a controlled multicenter study, oral 20 mg/day fluphenazine HCl was equivalent to 25 mg fluphenazine decanoate every 3 weeks. This is an approximate conversion ratio of 0.5 mL (12.5 mg) decanoate every 3 weeks for every 10 mg fluphenazine HCl daily. Do not exceed 100 mg. If doses greater than 50 mg are needed, increase succeeding doses cautiously in 12.5 mg increments.

Once conversion to fluphenazine decanoate is made, careful clinical monitoring of the patient and appropriate dosage adjustment should be made at the time of each injection.

*Severely agitated patients –* Initially treat with a rapid-acting phenothiazine. When acute symptoms subside, administer 25 mg of the fluphenazine decanoate; adjust subsequent dosage as necessary.

*"Poor risk" patients –* In "poor risk" patients (known phenothiazine hypersensitivity or with disorders predisposing to undue reactions), cautiously initiate oral or parenteral fluphenazine. When appropriate dosage is established, give equivalent dose of fluphenazine decanoate.

PERPHENAZINE:

*Moderately disturbed nonhospitalized patients with schizophrenia –* 4 to 8 mg 3 times/day; reduce as soon as possible to minimum effective dosage.

*Hospitalized patients –* 8 to 16 mg 2 to 4 times/day; avoid dosages more than 64 mg/day.

Reserve prolonged administration of doses exceeding 24 mg/day for hospitalized patients or patients under continued observation for early detection and management of adverse reactions. An antiparkinsonian agent, such as trihexyphenidyl HCl or benztropine mesylate, is valuable in controlling drug-induced extrapyramidal symptoms.

*Oral concentrate* – Dilute perphenazine oral solution (concentrate) only with water, saline, 7-Up, homogenized milk, carbonated orange drink, and pineapple, apricot, prune, orange, V-8, tomato, and grapefruit juices. Do not mix perphenazine oral solution (concentrate) with beverages containing caffeine (eg, coffee, cola), tannics (eg, tea), or pectinates (eg, apple juice) because physical incompatibility may result. Suggested dilution is approximately 2 fluid ounces of diluent for each 5 mL (16 mg) or teaspoonful of perphenazine oral solution (concentrate). A graduated dropper marked to measure 8 mg or 4 mg is supplied with each bottle.

*Children* – Not recommended for children younger than 12 years of age.

*Elderly* – Geriatric patients are particularly sensitive to the side effects of antipsychotics. Start on lower doses and observe closely.

PROCHLORPERAZINE:

*Adults* – Increase dosage more gradually in debilitated or emaciated patients.

*Schizophrenia:* Adjust dosage in adult psychiatric disorders to the response of the individual and according to the severity of the condition. Begin with the lowest recommended dose. Although response is ordinarily seen within a day or 2, longer treatment is usually required before maximal improvement is seen.

*Oral –*

*Mild conditions:* 5 or 10 mg 3 or 4 times/day.

*Moderate to severe conditions:* 10 mg 3 or 4 times/day. Gradually Increase dosage until symptoms are controlled or side effects become bothersome. When dosage is increased by small increments over 2 or 3 days, side effects either do not occur or are easily controlled. Some patients respond satisfactorily on 50 to 75 mg/day.

*Severe conditions:* 100 to 150 mg/day.

*IM* – Subcutaneous administration is not advisable because of local irritation.

Inject an initial dose of 10 to 20 mg (2 to 4 mL) deeply into the upper outer quadrant of the buttock. Many patients respond shortly after the first injection. Repeat the initial dose every 2 to 4 hours (or, in resistant cases, every hour) to gain control of the patient, if necessary. More than 3 or 4 doses are seldom necessary. After control is achieved, switch patient to an oral form of the drug at the same dosage levels or higher. If, in rare cases, parenteral therapy is needed for a prolonged period, give 10 to 20 mg (2 to 4 mL) every 4 to 6 hours.

*Nonpsychotic anxiety in adults:*

*Oral* – 5 mg 3 to 4 times/day; by spansule capsule, usually one 15 mg capsule on arising or one 10 mg capsule every 12 hours. Do not administer in doses of more than 20 mg/day or for longer than 12 weeks.

*Children* – Do not use in pediatric patients under 20 lb or younger than 2 years of age. Do not use in conditions for which children's dosages have not been established.

Children seem more prone to develop extrapyramidal reactions, even on moderate doses. Use the lowest effective dose. Occasionally the patients may react to the drug with signs of restlessness and excitement. Do not administer additional doses if this occurs. Take particular precaution in administering the drug to children with acute illnesses or dehydration.

Adjust dosage and frequency of administration according to the severity of the symptoms and the response of the patient. The duration of activity following IM administration may last up to 12 hours. Subsequent doses may be given by the same route if necessary.

*Schizophrenia in children:*

*Oral or rectal* – For children 2 to 12 years of age, starting dosage is 2½ mg 2 or 3 times/day. Do not give more than 10 mg on the first day. Then increase dosage according to the patient's response. When writing a prescription for the 2½ mg size suppository, write "2½", not "2.5". This will help avoid confusion with the 25 mg adult size.

*Children (2 to 5 years of age):* Usual total daily dose does not exceed 20 mg.

*Children (6 to 12 years of age):* Usual total daily dose does not exceed 25 mg.

IM – For ages under 12, calculate the dose on the basis of 0.06 mg/lb of body weight; give by deep IM injection. Control is usually obtained with 1 dose. After control is achieved, switch the patient to an oral form of the drug at the same dosage level or higher.

*Elderly* – Dosages in the lower range are sufficient for most elderly patients. Because they appear to be more susceptible to hypotension and neuromuscular reactions, observe such patients closely. Tailor dosage to the individual, carefully monitor response, and adjust dose accordingly. Increase dosage more gradually in elderly patients.

*Compatibility* – Do not mix prochlorperazine injection with other agents in the syringe.

THIORIDAZINE: Dosage must be individualized and the smallest effective dosage should be determined for each patient.

*Adults* – Starting dose is 50 to 100 mg 3 times/day with a gradual increment to a maximum of 800 mg/day, if necessary. Once effective control of symptoms has been achieved, the dosage may be reduced gradually to determine the minimum maintenance dose. The total daily dosage ranges from 200 to 800 mg, divided into 2 to 4 doses.

*Children* – For patients unresponsive to other agents, the recommended initial dose is 0.5 mg/kg/day given in divided doses. Dosage may be increased gradually until optimum therapeutic effect is obtained or the maximum dose of 3 mg/kg/day has been reached.

*Oral concentrate* – Concentrate may be diluted with distilled or acidified tap water or suitable juices. Dilute each dose just prior to administration; preparation and storage of bulk dilutions is not recommended.

TRIFLUOPERAZINE: Individualize dosage. Increase dosage more gradually in debilitated or emaciated patients. When maximum response is achieved, reduce dosage gradually to a maintenance level. Use the lowest effective dosage. Patients may be controlled with once- or twice-daily administration.

*Schizophrenia* –
Oral:
*Adults* – 2 to 5 mg orally twice daily. Start small or emaciated patients on the lower dosage. Most patients will show optimum response with 15 or 20 mg/day, although a few may require 40 mg/day or more. Optimum therapeutic dosage levels should be reached within 2 or 3 weeks.

*Children (6 to 12 years of age)* – Adjust dosage to the weight of the child and severity of the symptoms. These dosages are for children 6 to 12 years of age who are hospitalized or under close supervision. Initial dose is 1 mg once or twice daily. Dosage may be increased gradually until symptoms are controlled or until side effects become troublesome. While it is usually not necessary to exceed 15 mg/day, older children with severe symptoms may require higher doses.

*Nonpsychotic anxiety* – 1 or 2 mg twice daily. Do not administer more than 6 mg/day or for longer than 12 weeks because trifluoperazine use at higher doses or for longer intervals may cause persistent tardive dyskinesia that may prove irreversible.

*Elderly patients* – Usually, lower dosages are sufficient. The elderly appear more susceptible to hypotension and neuromuscular reactions; observe closely and increase dosage gradually.

THIOTHIXENE: Not recommended in children younger than 12 years of age.

*Mild conditions* – Initially, 2 mg 3 times/day. If indicated, an increase to 15 mg/day is often effective.

*Severe conditions* – Initially, 5 mg twice/day. Optimal is 20 to 30 mg/day. If indicated, 60 mg/day is often effective. Exceeding 60 mg/day rarely increases response.

# PHENYLBUTYLPIPERADINE DERIVATIVES

**HALOPERIDOL**

| | |
|---|---|
| **Tablets:** 0.5, 1, 2, 5, 10, and 20 mg (*Rx*) | Various |
| **Oral concentrate:** 2 mg/mL (as lactate) (*Rx*) | Various |
| **Injection:** 5 mg/mL (as lactate) (*Rx*) | Various, *Haldol* (McNeil) |
| 50 mg (equiv. to 70.5 mg decanoate)/mL (*Rx*) | Various, *Haldol Decanoate 50* (McNeil, Bedford) |
| 100 mg (equiv. to 141.04 mg decanoate)/mL (*Rx*) | Various, *Haldol Decanoate 100* (McNeil) |

**PIMOZIDE**

| | |
|---|---|
| **Tablets:** 1 and 2 mg (*Rx*) | *Orap* (Teva) |

### Indications

*Haloperidol:*

*Psychotic disorder* – For the treatment of psychotic disorders (eg, schizophrenia). Haloperidol decanoate is for patients who require prolonged parenteral antipsychotic therapy.

*Behavioral problems* – For the treatment of behavioral problems in children with combative, explosive hyperexcitability that cannot be accounted for by immediate provocation. Reserve for use in these children only after failure to respond to psychotherapy or medications other than antipsychotics.

*Hyperactivity* – For short-term treatment of hyperactive children who show excessive motor activity with accompanying conduct disorders consisting of impulsivity, difficulty sustaining attention, aggression, mood lability, or poor frustration tolerance. Reserve for use in these children only after failure to respond to psychotherapy or medications other than antipsychotics.

*Tourette disorder* – For the control of tics and vocal utterances in Tourette disorder.

*Pimozide:*

*Tourette disorder* – For suppression of motor and phonic tics in patients with Tourette disorder who have failed to respond satisfactorily to standard treatment. Pimozide is not intended as a treatment of first choice, nor is it intended for the treatment of tics that are merely annoying or cosmetically troublesome. Pimozide should be reserved for use in Tourette disorder patients whose development or daily life function is severely compromised by the presence of motor and phonic tics.

### Administration and Dosage

HALOPERIDOL: Individualize dosage. Children, debilitated, or geriatric patients and those with a history of adverse reactions to neuroleptic drugs may require less haloperidol.

*Psychotic disorders –*

*Adults: Initial dosage:* Moderate symptoms or geriatric or debilitated patients: 0.5 to 2 mg given 2 or 3 times/day; severe symptoms or chronic or resistant patients: 3 to 5 mg 2 or 3 times/day. To achieve prompt control, higher doses may be required.

Patients who remain severely disturbed or inadequately controlled may require dosage adjustment. Daily dosages up to 100 mg may be necessary. Infrequently, doses more than 100 mg have been used for severely resistant patients; however, safety of prolonged administration of such doses has not been demonstrated.

*Children (3 to 12 years of age):* Do not use in children younger than 3 years of age. Initial dose is 0.5 mg/day (25 to 50 mcg/kg/day). If required, increase in 0.5 mg increments each 5 to 7 days up to 0.15 mcg/kg/day or until therapeutic effect is obtained. Total dose may be divided and given 2 or 3 times/day. The dose in this age group has not been well established.

*IM administration:* 2 to 5 mg haloperidol lactate for prompt control of the acutely agitated patient with moderately severe to very severe symptoms. Depending on response, administer subsequent doses as often as every 60 minutes, although 4- to 8-hour intervals may be satisfactory.

The safety and efficacy of IM administration in children have not been established.

The oral form should replace the injectable as soon as it is feasible. For an approximation of the total daily dose required, use the parenteral dose administered in the preceding 24 hours; carefully monitor the patient for the first several days. Give the first oral dose within 12 to 24 hours following the last parenteral dose.

*Tourette disorder* –

*Adults:* A starting dose of 0.5 to 1.5 mg 3 times/day by mouth has been suggested; up to about 10 mg/day may be needed. Requirements vary considerably and the dose must be very carefully adjusted to obtain the optimum response.

*Children (3 to 12 years of age; 15 to 40 kg):* 0.05 to 0.075 mg/kg/day. Severely disturbed psychotic children may require higher doses.

*Behavioral disorders/hyperactivity* –

*Children (3 to 12 years of age; 15 to 40 kg):* 0.05 to 0.075 mg/kg/day. Severely disturbed psychotic children may require higher doses.

In severely disturbed, nonpsychotic children or in hyperactive children with conduct disorders, short-term administration may suffice. There is little evidence that behavior improvement is further enhanced by dosages more than 6 mg/day.

*Haloperidol decanoate injection* – Individualize dosage and provide close clinical supervision during initiation and stabilization of therapy. The recommended interval between doses is monthly or every 4 weeks. However, variation in patient response may dictate a need for adjustment of the dosing interval as well as the dose. To determine the minimum effective dose, begin with lower initial doses and adjust the dose upward as needed.

Intended for use in chronic psychotic patients who require prolonged parenteral antipsychotic therapy. These patients should be previously stabilized on antipsychotic medication, and should have been treated with, and well tolerated on short-acting haloperidol in order to exclude the possibility of an unexpected adverse sensitivity to haloperidol. Close clinical supervision is required during the initial period of dose adjustment in order to minimize the risk of overdosage or reappearance of psychotic symptoms before the next injection. During dose adjustment or episodes of exacerbation of psychotic symptoms, haloperidol decanoate therapy can be supplemented with short-acting forms of haloperidol.

| Haloperidol Decanoate Dosing Recommendations[1] | | |
|---|---|---|
| Patients | 1st Month[2] | Monthly maintenance |
| Stabilized on low daily oral doses (≤ 10 mg/day) | 10 to 15 × daily oral dose | 10 to 15 × previous daily oral dose |
| Elderly or debilitated | | |
| Stabilized on higher doses; risk of relapse | 20 × daily oral dose | 10 to 15 × previous daily oral dose |
| Tolerant to oral haloperidol | | |

[1] Clinical experience with doses greater than 450 mg/month has been limited.
[2] Initial dose should not exceed 100 mg. See below.

*Initial dosage:* The initial dose should not exceed 100 mg regardless of previous antipsychotic dose requirements. If the conversion requires more than 100 mg of haloperidol decanoate as an initial dose, administer that dose in 2 injections (maximum of 100 mg initially followed by the balance in 3 to 7 days).

*Maintenance dosage:* Individualize with titration upward or downward based on therapeutic response.

*Administration:* Administer by deep IM injection. A 21-gauge needle is recommended. The maximum volume per injection site should not exceed 3 mL. Do not administer IV.

*Elderly/Debilitated* – Lower initial doses and more gradual adjustments are recommended.

PIMOZIDE: Introduce the drug slowly and gradually. Perform ECG at baseline and periodically thereafter, especially during dosage adjustment.

*Tourette disorder* –

*Adults:*

*Initial dose* – 1 to 2 mg/day in divided doses. Thereafter, increase dose every other day.

*Maintenance dose* – Less than 0.2 mg/kg/day or 10 mg/day, whichever is less. Do not exceed 0.2 mg/kg/day or 10 mg/day.

*Children:* Although Tourette's disorder most often has its onset between the ages of 2 and 15 years, information on the use and efficacy of pimozide in patients less than 12 years of age is limited.

Initiate at a dose of 0.05 mg/kg, preferably taken once at bedtime; the dose may be increased every third day to a maximum of 0.2 mg/kg, not to exceed 10 mg/day.

*Gradual withdrawal* – Periodically attempt to reduce dosage to see if tics persist. Increases of tic intensity and frequency may represent a transient, withdrawal-related phenomenon rather than a return of symptoms. Allow 1 or 2 weeks to elapse before concluding that an increase in tic manifestations is caused by the underlying disease rather than drug withdrawal. A gradual withdrawal is recommended in any case.

# MOLINDONE HCl

| **Tablets:** 5, 10, 25, and 50 mg (*Rx*) | *Moban* (Endo) |
|---|---|

### Indications
*Schizophrenia:* Management of schizophrenia.

### Administration and Dosage
*Initial dosage:* 50 to 75 mg/day, increased to 100 mg/day in 3 or 4 days. Individualize dosage; patients with severe symptoms may require up to 225 mg/day.

Start elderly and debilitated patients on lower dosage.

*Maintenance therapy:*
Mild – 5 to 15 mg 3 or 4 times/day;
Moderate – 10 to 25 mg 3 or 4 times/day;
Severe – 225 mg/day may be required.

# ATYPICAL ANTIPSYCHOTICS

| *BENZISOXAZOLE DERIVATIVES* | |
|---|---|
| **RISPERIDONE** | |
| **Tablets:** 0.25, 0.5, 1, 2, 3, and 4 mg (*Rx*) | *Risperdal* (Janssen) |
| **Tablets, orally disintegrating:** 0.5, 1, and 2 mg | *Risperdal* M-TAB (Janssen) |
| **Oral solution:** 1 mg/mL (*Rx*) | *Risperdal* (Janssen) |
| **Powder for injection:** 25, 37.5, and 50 mg (*Rx*) | *Risperdal* Consta (Janssen) |
| **ZIPRASIDONE** | |
| **Capsules:** 20, 40, 60, and 80 mg (as HCl) (*Rx*) | *Geodon* (Pfizer) |
| **Powder for injection:** 20 mg (as mesylate) (*Rx*) | |
| *DIBENZAPINE DERIVATIVES* | |
| **CLOZAPINE** | |
| **Tablets:** 12.5, 25, and 100 mg (*Rx*) | Various, *Clozaril* (Novartis) |
| **Tablets, orally disintegrating:** 25 and 100 mg | *FazaClo* (Alamo) |
| **LOXAPINE** | |
| **Capsules:** 5, 10, 25, and 50 mg (*Rx*) | Various, *Loxitane* (Watson) |
| **OLANZAPINE** | |
| **Tablets:** 2.5, 5, 7.5, 10, 15, and 20 mg (*Rx*) | *Zyprexa* (Eli Lilly) |
| **Tablets, orally disintegrating:** 5, 10, 15, and 20 mg (*Rx*) | *Zyprexa* Zydis (Eli Lilly) |
| **Powder for injection:** 10 mg (*Rx*) | *Zyprexa* IntraMuscular (Eli Lilly) |
| **QUETIAPINE FUMARATE** | |
| **Tablets:** 25, 100, 200, and 300 mg (*Rx*) | *Seroquel* (AstraZeneca) |
| *QUINOLINONE DERIVATIVES* | |
| **ARIPIPRAZOLE** | |
| **Tablets:** 5, 10, 15, 20, and 30 mg (*Rx*) | *Abilify* (Bristol-Myers Squibb/Otsuka America) |

**Warning:**
*Clozapine:*

*Agranulocytosis* – Because of a significant risk of agranulocytosis, a potentially life-threatening adverse event, reserve clozapine for use in the treatment of severely ill schizophrenic patients who fail to show an acceptable response to adequate courses of standard antipsychotic drug treatment because of insufficient effectiveness or the inability to achieve an effective dose because of intolerable adverse effects from those drugs. Consequently, before initiating treatment with clozapine, it is strongly recommended that a patient be given at least 2 trials, each with a different standard antipsychotic drug product, at an adequate dose and for an adequate duration.

Patients who are being treated with clozapine must have a baseline white blood cell (WBC) and differential count before initiation of treatment and regular WBC counts during treatment and for 4 weeks after the discontinuation of clozapine.

Clozapine is available only through a distribution system that ensures monitoring of WBC counts according to the schedule described below prior to delivery of the next supply of medication.

*Seizures* – Seizures have been associated with the use of clozapine. Dose appears to be an important predictor of seizure, with a greater likelihood at higher clozapine doses. Use caution when administering clozapine to patients having a history of seizures or other predisposing factors. Advise patients not to engage in any activity where sudden loss of consciousness could cause serious risk to themselves or others.

*Myocarditis* – Clozapine may be associated with an increased risk of fatal myocarditis, especially during, but not limited to, the first month of therapy. If myocarditis is suspected, promptly discontinue clozapine treatment.

*Other adverse cardiovascular and respiratory effects* – Orthostatic hypotension, with or without syncope, can occur with clozapine treatment. Rarely, collapse can be profound and be accompanied by respiratory or cardiac arrest. Orthostatic hypotension is more likely to occur during initial titration in association with rapid dose escalation. In patients who have had even a brief interval off clozapine (ie, 2 or more days since the last dose), start treatment with 12.5 mg once or twice/day (see Administration and Dosage).

Because collapse, respiratory arrest, and cardiac arrest during initial treatment have occurred in patients who were being administered benzodiazepines or other psychotropic drugs, caution is advised when clozapine is initiated in patients taking a benzodiazepine or any other psychotropic drug (see Warnings in Antipsychotic Agents group monograph).

**Indications**
*Aripiprazole:*

*Bipolar mania* – For the treatment of acute manic and mixed episodes associated with bipolar disorder.

*Schizophrenia* – For the treatment of schizophrenia.

*Clozapine:*

*Schizophrenia* – For the management of severely ill schizophrenic patients who fail to respond adequately to standard antipsychotic drug treatment.

*Recurrent suicidal behavior (except orally disintegrating tablets)* – For reducing the risk of recurrent suicidal behavior in patients with schizophrenia or schizoaffective disorder who are judged to be at chronic risk for re-experiencing suicidal behavior, based on history and recent clinical state. Continue clozapine treatment to reduce the risk of suicidal behavior for at least 2 years.

*Loxapine:*

*Schizophrenia* – For the treatment of schizophrenia.

*Olanzapine:*
> *Bipolar disorder (oral) –*
>> *Monotherapy:* For the treatment of acute mixed or manic episodes associated with bipolar I disorder and for the maintenance monotherapy of bipolar disorder.
>> *Combination therapy:* In combination with lithium or valproate for the short-term treatment of acute manic episodes associated with bipolar I disorder.
> *Schizophrenia (oral) –* For the treatment of schizophrenia.
> *Agitation associated with schizophrenia and bipolar I mania (injection) –* For the treatment of agitation associated with schizophrenia and bipolar I mania.

*Quetiapine fumarate:*
> *Schizophrenia –* For the treatment of schizophrenia.
> *Bipolar mania –* For short-term treatment of acute manic episodes associated with bipolar I disorder, as monotherapy or adjunct therapy to lithium or divalproex.

*Risperidone:*
> *Schizophrenia –* For the treatment of schizophrenia.
> *Bipolar mania (oral only) –*
>> *Monotherapy:* For the short-term treatment of acute manic or mixed episodes associated with bipolar I disorder, as defined in the *DSM-IV.*
>> *Combination therapy:* The combination of risperidone with lithium or valproate is indicated for the short-term treatment of acute manic or mixed episodes associated with bipolar I disorder, as defined in the *DSM-IV.*

*Ziprasidone:*
> *Acute agitation (injection only) –* For the treatment of acute agitation in schizophrenic patients for whom treatment with ziprasidone is appropriate and who need IM antipsychotic medication for rapid control of the agitation.
> *Bipolar mania (oral only) –* For the treatment of acute manic or mixed episodes associated with bipolar disorder, with or without psychotic features.
> *Schizophrenia –* For the treatment of schizophrenia.

## Administration and Dosage
ARIPIPRAZOLE:
> *Bipolar mania –*
>> *Usual dose:* In clinical trials, the starting dose was 30 mg given once a day. A dose of 30 mg/day was found to be effective. Approximately 15% of patients had their dose decreased to 15 mg based on assessment of tolerability. The safety of doses above 30 mg/day has not been evaluated in clinical trials.
>> *Maintenance:* There is no body of evidence available from controlled trials to guide a clinician in the longer-term management of a patient who improves during treatment of an acute manic episode with aripiprazole. While it is generally agreed that pharmacological treatment beyond an acute response in mania is desirable, for maintenance of the initial response and prevention of new manic episodes, there are no systematically obtained data to support the use of aripiprazole in such longer-term treatment (ie, beyond 3 weeks).
> *Schizophrenia –*
>> *Usual dose:* The recommended starting and target dose is 10 or 15 mg/day administered on a once-daily schedule without regard to meals. Aripiprazole has been systematically evaluated and shown to be effective in a dose range of 10 to 30 mg/day; however, doses higher than 10 or 15 mg/day (the lowest doses in these trials) were not more effective than 10 or 15 mg/day. Dosage increases should not be made before 2 weeks, the time needed to achieve steady state.
>> *Maintenance therapy:* Systematic evaluation of patients with schizophrenia who had been symptomatically stable on other antipsychotic medications for periods of 3 months or longer, were discontinued from those medications, and were then administered 15 mg/day aripiprazole and observed for relapse during a period of up to 26 weeks. These patients demonstrated a benefit of such maintenance treatment. Periodically reassess patients to determine the need for maintenance treatment.

*Concomitant use with potential CYP3A4 inhibitors* – When coadministration of ketoconazole with aripiprazole occurs, reduce the aripiprazole dose to one-half of the usual dose. When the CYP3A4 inhibitor is withdrawn from combination therapy, increase aripiprazole dose.

*Concomitant use with potential CYP2D6 inhibitors* – When coadministration of potential CYP2D6 inhibitors such as quinidine, fluoxetine, or paroxetine with aripiprazole occurs, reduce the aripiprazole dose to at least one-half of its normal dose. When the CYP2D6 inhibitor is withdrawn from combination therapy, increase the aripiprazole dose.

*Concomitant use with potential CYP3A4 inducers* – When a potential CYP3A4 inducer such as carbamazepine is added to aripiprazole therapy, double the aripiprazole dose to 20 to 30 mg. Base additional dose increases on clinical evaluation. When carbamazepine is withdrawn from combination therapy, reduce the aripiprazole dose to 10 to 15 mg.

*Switching from other antipsychotics* – There are no systemically collected data to specifically address switching patients with schizophrenia from other antipsychotics to aripiprazole or concerning coadministration with other antipsychotics. While immediate discontinuation of the previous antipsychotic treatment may be acceptable for some patients with schizophrenia, gradual discontinuation may be more appropriate for others. In all cases, minimize the period of overlapping antipsychotic administration.

CLOZAPINE: Clozapine is available only through a distribution system that ensures monitoring of WBC counts according to the schedule described below prior to delivery of the next supply of medication. For more information, call (800) 448-5938. Upon initiation of clozapine therapy, up to a 1 week supply of additional tablets may be provided to the patient to be held for emergencies (eg, weather, holidays).

Drug dispensing ordinarily should not exceed a weekly supply. If a patient is eligible for WBC testing every other week, then a 2-week supply can be dispensed. Dispensing should be contingent on the results of a WBC count.

*Monitoring* – Patients must have a blood sample drawn for a WBC count before initiation of treatment with clozapine and must have subsequent WBC counts done at least weekly for the first 6 months of continuous treatment. If WBC counts remain acceptable (WBC at least 3000/mm$^3$, ANC at least 1500/mm$^3$) during this period, WBC counts may be monitored every other week thereafter. After the discontinuation of clozapine, continue weekly WBC counts for an additional 4 weeks.

*Initial* – 12.5 mg once or twice/day, then continued with daily dosage increments of 25 to 50 mg/day, if well tolerated, to achieve a target dose of 300 to 450 mg/day by the end of 2 weeks. Make subsequent dosage increments no more than once or twice weekly, in increments not to exceed 100 mg. Cautious titration and a divided dosage schedule are necessary to minimize the risks of hypotension, seizure, and sedation.

In a multicenter study, patients were titrated during the first 2 weeks up to a maximum dose of 500 mg/day on a 3 times/day basis and were then dosed in a total daily dose range of 100 to 900 mg/day on a 3 times/day basis thereafter, with clinical response and adverse effects as guides to correct dosing.

| Clozapine Therapy Guidelines Based on WBC and ANC[1] | | |
|---|---|---|
| WBC count (mm$^3$) | ANC (mm$^3$) | Guidelines |
| < 3500, or history of myeloproliferative disorder, or previous clozapine-induced agranulocytosis or granulocytopenia | | Do not initiate treatment. |
| < 3500, or > 3500 with a substantial drop[2] from baseline, following initiation of treatment | | Repeat WBC and differential counts. Symptoms of infection include the following: Lethargy, weakness, fever, sore throat. |

| Clozapine Therapy Guidelines Based on WBC and ANC[1] | | |
|---|---|---|
| WBC count (mm³) | ANC (mm³) | Guidelines |
| 3000 to 3500 on subsequent counts | > 1500 | Perform twice weekly WBC and differential counts. |
| < 3000 | or < 1500 | Interrupt therapy, monitor for flu-like symptoms or other symptoms of infection. May resume therapy if no signs of infection develop, WBC count > 3000, and granulocyte count > 1500. However, continue twice/wk WBC and differential counts until WBC returns to 3500. |
| < 2000 | < 1000 | Monitor WBC count and differential daily. Consider bone marrow aspiration to ascertain granulopoietic status. If granulopoiesis is deficient, consider protective isolation. If infection develops, perform cultures and institute antibiotics. Do not rechallenge with clozapine because agranulocytosis may develop with a shorter latency. |

[1] See manufacturer's product labeling for more specific recommendations.
[2] A substantial drop is defined as a single drop of 3000 or more in the WBC count or a cumulative drop of 3000 or more within 3 weeks.

*Dose adjustment* – Continue daily dosing on a divided basis to an effective and tolerable dose level. While many patients may respond adequately at doses between 300 to 600 mg/day, it may be necessary to raise the dose to the 600 to 900 mg/day range. Do not exceed 900 mg/day. The mean and median clozapine doses are approximately 600 mg/day for schizophrenia and 300 mg/day for reducing recurrent suicidal behavior.

Because of the possibility of increased adverse reactions at higher doses, particularly seizures, give patients adequate time to respond to a given dose level before escalation to a higher dose.

Because of the significant risk of agranulocytosis and seizure, events that present a continuing risk over time, avoid the extended treatment of patients failing to show an acceptable level of clinical response.

*Maintenance* – Continue clozapine at the lowest level needed to maintain remission. Periodically reassess patients to determine the need for maintenance treatment.

*Discontinuation* – In the event of planned termination of clozapine therapy, gradual reduction in dose is recommended over a 1- to 2-week period. However, should a patient's medical condition require abrupt discontinuation (eg, leukopenia), carefully observe the patient for the recurrence of psychotic symptoms and symptoms related to cholinergic rebound (eg, headache, nausea, vomiting, diarrhea). After the discontinuation of clozapine, continue weekly WBC counts for an additional 4 weeks.

*Reinitiation of treatment* – When restarting patients who have had even a brief interval off clozapine (ie, 2 days or more since the last dose) it is recommended that treatment be reinitiated with one-half of a 25 mg tablet (12.5 mg) once or twice/day. If that dose is well tolerated, it may be feasible to titrate patients back to a therapeutic dose more quickly than is recommended for initial treatment. However, any patient who has previously experienced respiratory or cardiac arrest with initial dosing but was then able to be successfully titrated to a therapeutic dose should be retitrated with extreme caution after even 24 hours of discontinuation.

| | No abnormal blood event and break in therapy is ≤ 1 month | No abnormal blood event and break in therapy is > 1 month | Abnormal blood event and patient is rechallengeable | No abnormal blood event and break in therapy is ≤ 1 year | No abnormal blood event and break in therapy is > 1 year |
|---|---|---|---|---|---|
| **Monitoring Guidelines for Patients Reinitiated on Clozapine** | | | | | |
| Therapy duration | | | | | |
| < 6 months | Continue weekly monitoring left off to complete 6 months | Restart weekly monitoring for 6 months | Restart weekly monitoring for 6 months after recovery from event | — | — |
| ≥ 6 months | — | — | | Continue monitoring at every other week intervals | Restart weekly monitoring for 6 months |

Certain additional precautions seem prudent. Re-exposure of a patient might enhance the risk of an untoward event's occurrence and increase its severity. Patients discontinued for WBC counts below 2000/mm$^3$ or an ANC below 1000/mm$^3$ must not be restarted on clozapine (see Warnings in Antipsychotic Agents group monograph).

*Orally disintegrating tablets* – Do not push the orally disintegrating tablet through the foil. Just prior to use, peel the foil from the blister and gently remove the orally disintegrating tablet. Immediately place the tablet in the mouth, allow it to disintegrate, and swallow with saliva. No water is needed to take clozapine. Destroy half tablets.

LOXAPINE: Individualize dosage. Administer 2 to 4 times/day in divided doses.

*Initial dosage* – 10 mg twice/day. In severely disturbed patients, up to 50 mg/day may be desirable. Increase dosage fairly rapidly over the first 7 to 10 days until symptoms are controlled.

*Maintenance therapy* – Reduce dosage to the lowest level compatible with control of symptoms.

The usual therapeutic and maintenance range is 60 to 100 mg/day. Many patients have been maintained satisfactorily at dosages in the range of 20 to 60 mg/day. Dosage higher than 250 mg/day is not recommended.

OLANZAPINE:

*Bipolar mania* –

*Monotherapy:* Initial dose is 10 to 15 mg/day without regard to meals. Adjust dosage at 5 mg increments in intervals of not less than 24 hours if indicated.

Short-term (3 to 4 weeks) antimanic efficacy was demonstrated in a dose range of 5 to 20 mg/day. The safety of doses above 20 mg/day has not been evaluated.

*Maintenance monotherapy:* The benefit of maintaining bipolar patients on monotherapy with olanzapine at a dose of 5 to 20 mg/day, after achieving a responder status for an average duration of 2 weeks, was demonstrated in a controlled trial. Periodically reevaluate olanzapine use in patients taking the drug for extended periods.

*Combination therapy:* When coadministered with lithium or valproate, generally begin olanzapine dosing with 10 mg once daily without regard to meals.

Short-term (6 weeks) antimanic efficacy was demonstrated in a dose range of 5 to 20 mg/day in clinical trials. The safety of doses above 20 mg/day has not been evaluated in clinical trials.

*Schizophrenia (oral)* – Initial dose is 5 to 10 mg once daily without regard to meals, with a target dose of 10 mg/day within several days of initiation. Adjust dosage, if indicated, at 5 mg/day increments or decrements in intervals not less than 1 week.

Efficacy was demonstrated in a dose range of 10 to 15 mg/day in clinical trials. However, increases in efficacy were not demonstrated in doses above 10 mg/day. Doses above 10 mg/day are recommended only after clinical assessment. The safety of doses above 20 mg/day has not been evaluated in clinical trials.

*Maintenance treatment:* Periodically reassess patients to determine the need for maintenance treatment.

*Agitation associated with schizophrenia and bipolar I mania (IM)* –

*Usual dose:* The efficacy of IM olanzapine injection in controlling agitation in these disorders was demonstrated in a dose range of 2.5 to 10 mg. The recommended dose is 10 mg. A lower dose of 5 or 7.5 mg may be considered when clinical factors warrant. If agitation warranting additional IM doses persists following the initial dose, subsequent doses up to 10 mg may be given. The efficacy of repeated doses in agitated patients has not be systematically evaluated in controlled clinical trials. Maximal dosing of IM olanzapine (eg, three doses of 10 mg given 2 to 4 hours apart) may be associated with a substantial occurrence of significant orthostatic hypotension. Patients requiring subsequent IM injections should be assessed for orthostatic hypotension. The administration of an additional dose to a patient with a clinically significant postural change in systolic blood pressure is not recommended.

If ongoing olanzapine therapy is clinical indicated, oral olanzapine may be initiated in a range of 5 to 20 mg/day as soon as clinically appropriate.

*Administration of IM injection* – For IM use only. Do not administer IV or subcutaneously. Inject slowly, deep into the muscle mass.

*Preparation for administration* – Dissolve the contents of the vial using 2.1 mL sterile water for injection to provide a solution containing approximately 5 mg/mL olanzapine. The resulting solution should appear clear and yellow. Use immediately (within 1 hour) after reconstitution. Discard any unused portion. The following table provides injection volumes for delivering various doses of IM olanzapine for injection.

| IM Olanzapine Injection Volume | |
| --- | --- |
| Olanzapine dose (mg) | Volume of injection (mL) |
| 10 | Withdraw total contents of vial |
| 7.5 | 1.5 |
| 5 | 1 |
| 2.5 | 0.5 |

*Dosing in special populations* –

*Oral:* The recommended starting dose is 5 mg in patients who are debilitated, who have a predisposition to hypotensive reactions, who otherwise exhibit a combination of factors that may result in slower metabolism of olanzapine (eg, nonsmoking female patients at least 65 years of age), or who may be more pharmacodynamically sensitive to olanzapine.

*Injection:* Consider a dose of 5 mg per injection for geriatric patients or when other clinical factors warrant. Consider a lower dose of 2.5 mg per injection for patients who otherwise might be debilitated, be predisposed to hypotensive reactions, or be more pharmacodynamically sensitive to olanzapine.

*Administration of orally disintegrating tablets* – Peel back foil on blister; do not push tablet through foil. Using dry hands, remove from the foil and place the entire tablet in the mouth. The tablet will disintegrate with or without liquid.

QUETIAPINE FUMARATE:

*Schizophrenia* –

*Usual dose:* Initial dose of 25 mg twice/day, with increases in increments of 25 to 50 mg 2 or 3 times/day on the second and third day, as tolerated, to a target dose range of 300 to 400 mg/day by the fourth day, given 2 or 3 times/day. Further dosage adjustments should occur at intervals of at least 2 days. Dose increments/

decrements of 25 to 50 mg twice/day are recommended. Efficacy was demonstrated in a dose range of 150 to 750 mg/day. The safety of doses above 800 mg/day has not been evaluated.

*Bipolar mania –*

*Usual dose:* When used as monotherapy or adjunct therapy (with lithium or divalproex), initiate quetiapine in twice-daily doses totaling 100 mg/day on day 1, increased to 400 mg/day on day 4 in increments of up to 100 mg/day in twice daily divided doses. Further dosage adjustments up to 800 mg/day by day 6 should be in increments of no more than 200 mg/day. Data indicate that the majority of patients responded between 400 and 800 mg/day. The safety of doses above 800 mg/day has not been evaluated in clinical trials.

*Maintenance –* Continue quetiapine in responding patients, but at the lowest dose needed to maintain remission. Periodically reassess patients.

*Special populations –* Consider a slower rate of dose titration and a lower target dose in the elderly, patients with hepatic impairment, debilitated patients, or those who have a predisposition to hypotensive reactions. Perform dose escalation with caution.

*Hepatic function impairment –* Start patients with hepatic impairment on 25 mg/day. Increase the dose daily in increments of 25 to 50 mg/day to an effective dose, depending on the clinical response and tolerability of the patient.

*Reinitiation of treatment in patients previously discontinued –* When restarting patients who have had an interval of less than 1 week off quetiapine, titration of quetiapine is not required and the maintenance dose may be reinitiated. For patients who have been off quetiapine for more than 1 week, follow the initial titration schedule.

*Switching from other antipsychotics –* The period of overlapping antipsychotic administration should be minimized. When switching patients with schizophrenia from depot antipsychotics, if medically appropriate, initiate quetiapine therapy in place of the next scheduled injection. Periodically reevaluate the need for continuing existing EPS medication.

RISPERIDONE:

*Schizophrenia –*

*Initial dose:* Risperidone can be administered on a twice-daily or once-daily schedule. Initial dose is 1 mg twice daily (day 1), increasing by 1 mg twice daily as tolerated (on days 2 and 3), up to a target dose of 3 mg twice daily (by day 3). Regardless of which regimen is employed, a slower titration may be medically appropriate in some patients. Further dosage adjustments at 1 to 2 mg increments or decrements may be made at intervals of not less than 1 week.

Maximal effect was generally seen in a range of 4 to 8 mg/day. Doses above 6 mg/day for twice-daily dosing were associated with more extrapyramidal symptoms and other adverse effects and generally are not recommended. The safety of doses above 16 mg/day has not been evaluated in clinical trials.

*Maintenance therapy:* The effectiveness of risperidone 2 to 8 mg/day at delaying relapse was demonstrated in controlled trials in patients who had been clinically stable for at least 4 weeks and then were followed for a period of 1 to 2 years. Periodically, reassess patients to determine the need for maintenance treatment with appropriate dose.

*Bipolar mania (oral only) –*

*Usual dose:* Administer on a once-daily schedule, starting with 2 to 3 mg/day. If indicated, adjust dosage at intervals of not less than 24 hours and in dosage increments/decrements of 1 mg/day as studied in the short-term, placebo-controlled trials. In these trials, short-term (3 week) antimanic efficacy was demonstrated in a flexible dosage range of 1 to 6 mg/day. Risperidone doses higher than 6 mg/day were not studied.

*Maintenance therapy:* There is no evidence available from controlled trials to guide a clinician in the longer-term management of a patient who improves during treatment of an acute manic episode with risperidone. While it is generally agreed that pharmacological treatment beyond an acute response in mania is desirable, both for maintenance of the initial response and for prevention of new manic episodes, there are no systematically obtained data to support the use of risperidone in such longer-term treatment (ie, beyond 3 weeks).

*Reinitiation of treatment* – When restarting patients who have had an interval off risperidone, follow the initial titration schedule.

*Special populations (oral)* – The recommended initial dose is 0.5 mg twice daily in patients who are elderly, debilitated, have severe renal or hepatic impairment, are predisposed to hypotension, or in whom hypotension would pose a risk. Adjust dose at increments of no more than 0.5 mg twice daily. Give increases to dosages above 1.5 mg twice daily at intervals of at least 1 week. In some patients, slower titration may be medically appropriate.

Once-daily dosing in the elderly or debilitated may occur after the patient has been titrated on a twice-daily regimen for 2 to 3 days at the target dose.

*Switching from other antipsychotic agents* – When switching from other antipsychotic agents to risperidone, immediate discontinuation of the previous antipsychotic treatment may be acceptable for some patients; gradual discontinuation may be more appropriate for other patients. In all cases, minimize the period of overlapping antipsychotic administration. When switching patients from a depot antipsychotic, initiate risperidone therapy in place of the next scheduled injection. Reevaluate the need for continuing existing medications that treat extrapyramidal symptoms.

*Oral solution administration* – The oral solution can be mixed with water, coffee, orange juice, or low-fat milk; it is not compatible with cola or tea.

*Orally disintegrating tablet administration* – Do not open the blister until ready to administer. For single tablet removal, separate 1 of the 4 blister units by tearing apart at the perforation. Bend the corner where indicated. Peel back foil to expose the tablet. Do not push the tablet through the foil because this could damage the tablet. Using dry hands, remove the tablet from the blister unit, and immediately place the entire tablet on the tongue. Consume the tablet immediately, as the tablet cannot be stored once removed from the blister unit. Tablets disintegrate in the mouth within seconds and can be swallowed subsequently with or without liquid. Advise patients not to split or chew the tablet.

*Injection* – For patients who have never taken oral risperidone, establish tolerability with oral risperidone prior to initiating treatment with injectable risperidone.

The recommended dose is 25 mg IM every 2 weeks. Although dose response for effectiveness has not been established for risperidone injection, some patients not responding to 25 mg may benefit from a higher dose of 37.5 or 50 mg. The maximum dose should not exceed 50 mg risperidone injection every 2 weeks.

Give oral risperidone or another antipsychotic medication with the first risperidone injection and continue for 3 weeks (then discontinue) to ensure that adequate therapeutic plasma concentrations are maintained prior to the main release phase of risperidone from the injection site.

*Dose adjustments* – Do not make upward dosage adjustments more frequently than every 4 weeks. The clinical effects of this dose adjustment should not be anticipated earlier than 3 weeks after the first injection with the higher dose.

*Renal/Hepatic impairment* – Treat with titrated doses of oral risperidone prior to initiating treatment with risperidone injection. The recommended starting dose is 0.5 mg oral risperidone twice daily during the first week, which can be increased to 1 mg twice daily or 2 mg once daily during the second week. If a dose of at least 2 mg oral risperidone is well tolerated, an injection of 25 mg risperidone can be administered every 2 weeks. Continue oral supplementation for 3 weeks after the first injection until the main release of risperidone from the injection site has begun. In some patients, slower titration may be medically appropriate.

*Reinitiation of treatment* – When restarting patients who have had an interval off treatment with risperidone injection, supplement with oral risperidone or another antipsychotic medication.

*Switching from other antipsychotic agents* – Continue previous antipsychotic agents for 3 weeks after the first risperidone injection to ensure that therapeutic concentrations are maintained until the main release phase of risperidone from the injection site has begun. For schizophrenic patients who have never taken oral risperidone, establish tolerability with oral risperidone prior to initiating treatment with risperidone injection. As recommended with other antipsychotic medications, periodically reevaluate the need for continuing existing extrapyramidal symptom medication.

*Administration of* IM – Administer risperidone injection every 2 weeks by deep IM gluteal injection. A health care professional should administer each injection using the enclosed safety needle. Alternate injections between the 2 buttocks. Do not administer IV.

Do not combine 2 different dosage strengths of risperidone injection in a single administration.

ZIPRASIDONE:

*Schizophrenia* – When deciding among the alternative treatments available for schizophrenia, consider ziprasidone's greater capacity to prolong the $QT/QT_c$ interval compared with other antipsychotic drugs.

*Initial treatment:* Administer ziprasidone capsules at an initial daily dose of 20 mg twice/day with food. In some patients, daily dosage subsequently may be adjusted on the basis of individual clinical status up to 80 mg twice/day. Dosage adjustments, if indicated, generally should occur at intervals of not less than 2 days, as steady state is achieved within 1 to 3 days. In order to ensure use of the lowest effective dose, observe patients for improvement for several weeks before upward dosage adjustment.

*Maintenance treatment:* While there is no body of evidence available to answer the question of how long a patient should be treated with ziprasidone, systematic evaluation of ziprasidone has shown that its efficacy in schizophrenia is maintained for periods of up to 52 weeks at a dose of 20 to 80 mg twice/day. No additional benefit was demonstrated for doses greater than 20 mg twice/day.

*Acute agitation* – The recommended dose is 10 to 20 mg administered as required up to a maximum dose of 40 mg/day. Doses of 10 mg may be administered every 2 hours; doses of 20 mg may be administered every 4 hours up to a maximum of 40 mg/day. IM administration of ziprasidone for more than 3 consecutive days has not been studied.

If long-term therapy is indicated, oral ziprasidone capsules should replace IM administration as soon as possible.

Because there is no experience regarding the safety of administering ziprasidone IM to schizophrenic patients already taking oral ziprasidone, coadministration is not recommended.

*Bipolar mania* –

*Initial treatment:* Administer oral ziprasidone at an initial daily dose of 40 mg twice/day with food. Then, increase the dose to 60 or 80 mg twice/day on the second day of treatment and subsequently adjust on the basis of toleration and efficacy within the range of 40 to 80 mg twice/day. In the flexible-dose clinical trials, the mean daily dose administered was approximately 120 mg.

*Maintenance treatment:* There is no body of evidence available from controlled trials to guide a clinician in the longer-term management of a patient who improves during treatment of mania with ziprasidone. While it is generally agreed that pharmacological treatment beyond an acute response in mania is desirable, for maintenance of the initial response and prevention of new manic episodes, there are no systematically obtained data to support the use of ziprasidone in such longer-term treatment (ie, beyond 3 weeks).

## Contraindications

*Clozapine:* Hypersensitivity to clozapine or any other component of the drug; uncontrolled epilepsy; myeloproliferative disorders; history of clozapine-induced agranulocytosis or severe granulocytopenia; simultaneous administration with other agents having a well-known potential to cause agranulocytosis or otherwise suppress bone marrow function; severe CNS depression or comatose states from any cause.

Causative factors of agranulocytosis may interact synergistically to increase the risk or severity of bone marrow suppression.

# LITHIUM

| | |
|---|---|
| **Capsules:** 150 mg lithium carbonate (4.06 mEq lithium) (*Rx*) | *Lithium Carbonate* (Roxane) |
| 300 mg lithium carbonate (8.12 mEq lithium) (*Rx*) | Various, *Eskalith* (SKB), *Lithonate* (Solvay Pharm.) |
| 600 mg lithium carbonate (16.24 mEq lithium) (*Rx*) | *Lithium Carbonate* (Roxane) |
| **Tablets:** 300 mg lithium carbonate (8.12 mEq lithium) (*Rx*) | Various, *Eskalith* (GlaxoSmithKline), *Lithane* (Miles Pharm.), *Lithotabs* (Solvay Pharm.) |
| **Tablets, slow release:** 300 mg lithium carbonate (8.12 mEq lithium) (*Rx*) | *Lithobid* (Ciba) |
| **Tablets, controlled release:** 450 mg lithium carbonate (12.18 mEq lithium) (*Rx*) | *Eskalith CR* (GlaxoSmithKline) |
| **Syrup:** 8 mEq lithium (as citrate equivalent to 300 mg lithium carbonate) per 5 mL (*Rx*) | Various |

**Warning:**
Toxicity is closely related to serum lithium levels and can occur at therapeutic doses. Facilities for serum lithium determinations are required to monitor therapy.

## Indications
*Mania:* For the treatment of manic episodes of manic-depressive illness. Maintenance therapy prevents or diminishes the frequency and intensity of subsequent manic episodes in those manic-depressive patients with a history of mania.

*Unlabeled uses:* Lithium carbonate (300 to 1000 mg/day) has improved the neutrophil count in patients with cancer chemotherapy-induced neutropenia, in children with chronic neutropenia, and in AIDS patients receiving zidovudine.

## Administration and Dosage
Individualize dosage according to both serum levels and clinical response.

*Serum lithium levels:* Draw blood samples immediately prior to the next dose (8 to 12 hours after the previous dose) when lithium concentrations are relatively stable. Do not rely on serum levels alone.

*Acute mania:* Optimal patient response is usually established and maintained with 600 mg 3 times/day or 900 mg twice/day for the slow release form. Such doses normally produce an effective serum lithium level ranging between 1 and 1.5 mEq/L.

Determine serum levels twice weekly during the acute phase, and until the serum level and clinical condition of the patient have been stabilized.

*Long-term use:* The desirable serum levels are 0.6 to 1.2 mEq/L. Dosage will vary, but 300 mg 3 to 4 times/day will usually maintain this level. Monitor serum levels in uncomplicated cases on maintenance therapy during remission every 2 to 3 months.

## Actions
*Pharmacology:* Lithium alters sodium transport in nerve and muscle cells, and effects a shift toward intraneuronal catecholamine metabolism. The specific mechanism in mania is unknown, but it affects neurotransmitters associated with affective disorders. Its antimanic effects may be the result of increases in norepinephrine reuptake and increased serotonin receptor sensitivity.

*Pharmacokinetics:*
*Absorption/Distribution* – Lithium is readily absorbed from the GI tract. Peak serum levels occur in 0.5 to 3 hours and absorption is complete within 8 hours. Onset of action is slow (5 to 14 days). Until the desired therapeutic effect is attained, maintain a steady-state serum level of 0.8 to 1.4 mEq/L, then slowly decrease the lithium dose to a maintenance level. The therapeutic serum level range is from 0.4 to 1 mEq/L.

*Excretion* – About 95% of the lithium dose is eliminated by the kidney.

## Warnings

*High-risk patients:* The risk of lithium toxicity is very high in patients with significant renal or cardiovascular disease, severe debilitation, dehydration, or sodium depletion, or in patients receiving diuretics. Undertake treatment with extreme caution.

*Encephalopathic syndrome:* Encephalopathic syndrome has occurred in a few patients given lithium plus a neuroleptic. In some instances, irreversible brain damage occurred. Monitor closely for evidence of neurologic toxicity.

*Renal function impairment:* Morphologic changes with glomerular and interstitial fibrosis and nephron atrophy have occurred in patients on chronic lithium therapy. The relationship between such changes and renal function has not been established.

Acquired nephrogenic diabetes insipidus – Acquired nephrogenic diabetes insipidus unresponsive to vasopressin has been associated with chronic lithium administration. Polydipsia and polyuria occur frequently. The mechanism is thought to be the decreased response of the renal tubules to the antidiuretic hormone causing decreased reabsorption of water. Impairment of the concentrating ability of the kidneys is reversed when lithium therapy is discontinued. Management may involve decreasing the dose, discontinuing lithium, or the cautious use of a thiazide diuretic or amiloride. Monitor the patient's renal status.

*Elderly:* The decreased rate of excretion in the elderly contributes to a high incidence of toxic effects. Use lower doses and more frequent monitoring.

*Pregnancy:* Category D.

*Lactation:* Lithium is excreted in breast milk. Do not nurse during lithium therapy.

*Children:* Safety and efficacy for use in children younger than 12 years of age have not been established.

## Precautions

*Infection:* Concomitant infection with elevated temperature may necessitate a temporary reduction or cessation of medication.

*Hazardous tasks:* Observe caution while driving or performing other tasks requiring alertness.

*Tolerance of lithium:* Tolerance of lithium is greater during the acute manic phase and decreases when manic symptoms subside.

*Hypothyroidism:* Hypothyroidism may occur with long-term lithium administration. Patients may develop enlargement of thyroid gland and increased thyroid-stimulating hormone levels.

*Sodium depletion:* Lithium decreases renal sodium reabsorption, which could lead to sodium depletion. Therefore, the patient must maintain a normal diet (including salt) and an adequate fluid intake (2500 to 3000 mL).

*Parameters to monitor:* Perform the following laboratory tests prior to and periodically during lithium therapy: Serum creatinine; complete blood count; urinalysis; sodium and potassium; fasting glucose; electrocardiogram; and thyroid function tests. Check lithium serum levels weekly until dosage is stabilized. Once steady state has been reached, monitor the level weekly. Once the patient is on maintenance therapy, the level may be checked every 2 to 3 months.

## Drug Interactions

Drugs that may affect lithium include acetazolamide, carbamazepine, fluoxetine, haloperidol, loop diuretics, methyldopa, NSAIDs, osmotic diuretics, theophyllines, thiazide diuretics, urinary alkalinizers, and verapamil.

Drugs that may be affected by lithium include phenothiazines, sympathomimetics, iodide salts, neuromuscular blocking agents, and tricyclic antidepressants.

## Adverse Reactions

Adverse reactions may include arrhythmia; hypotension; peripheral circulatory collapse; bradycardia; sinus node dysfunction with severe bradycardia; ECG changes; tremor; muscle hyperirritability; ataxia; choreoathetotic movements; hyperactive deep tendon reflexes; pseudotumor cerebri; euthyroid goiter; hypothyroidism; EEG changes; blackout spells; epileptiform seizures; slurred speech; dizziness; vertigo; incontinence of urine or feces; somnolence; psychomotor retardation; restlessness; confusion; stupor; coma; acute dystonia; downbeat nystagmus; blurred vision; startled response; hypertonicity; slowed intellectual functioning; hallucinations; poor memory; tongue movements; tics; tinnitus; cog wheel rigidity; anorexia; nausea; vomiting; diarrhea; dry mouth; gastritis; salivary gland swelling; abdominal pain; excessive salivation; flatulence; indigestion; albuminuria; oliguria; glycosuria; decreased Ccr; symptoms of nephrogenic diabetes; drying and thinning of hair; anesthesia of skin; chronic folliculitis; xerosis cutis; alopecia; exacerbation of psoriasis; acne; angioedema; fatigue; lethargy; sleepiness; dehydration; weight loss; transient scotomata; impotence; sexual dysfunction; dysgeusia; taste distortion; tightness in chest; hypercalcemia; hyperparathyroidism; salty taste; swollen lips; swollen, painful joints; fever; polyarthralgia; dental caries; leukocytosis; headache; transient hyperglycemia; generalized pruritus with or without rash; cutaneous ulcers; worsening of organic brain syndromes; excessive weight gain; edematous swelling of ankles or wrists; thirst or polyuria, sometimes resembling diabetes insipidus; metallic taste; painful discoloration of fingers and toes and coldness of the extremities.

# MEMANTINE

| **Tablets:** 5 and 10 mg (*Rx*) | *Namenda* (Forest Laboratories) |

### Indications
*Alzheimer disease:* For the treatment of moderate to severe dementia of the Alzheimer type.

### Administration and Dosage
Memantine can be taken with or without food.

*Dosage:* The recommended starting dose of memantine is 5 mg once daily. The recommended target dose is 20 mg/day. Increase the dose in 5 mg increments to 10 mg/day (5 mg twice daily), 15 mg/day (5 mg and 10 mg as separate doses), and 20 mg/day (10 mg twice daily). The minimum recommended interval between dose increases is 1 week.

### Actions
*Pharmacology:* Persistent activation of CNS N-methyl-D-aspartate (NMDA) receptors by the excitatory amino acid glutamate has been hypothesized to contribute to the symptomatology of Alzheimer disease. Memantine is an NMDA receptor antagonist.

*Pharmacokinetics:*

*Absorption/Distribution* – Memantine is highly absorbed with peak concentrations reached in approximately 3 to 7 hours. The mean volume of distribution is 9 to 11 L/kg and the plasma protein binding is low (45%).

*Metabolism/Excretion* – Memantine undergoes little metabolism, with the majority (57% to 82%) of an administered dose excreted unchanged in urine. Memantine has a terminal elimination half-life of about 60 to 80 hours. Renal clearance involves active tubular secretion.

### Contraindications
Known hypersensitivity to memantine or to any excipients used in the formulation.

### Warnings
*GU conditions:* Conditions that raise urine pH may decrease the urinary elimination of memantine, resulting in increased plasma levels of memantine.

*Renal function impairment:* Consider dose adjustment in patients with mild, moderate, and severe renal impairment. The use of memantine in patients with severe renal impairment is not recommended.

*Pregnancy:* Category B.

*Lactation:* It is not known whether memantine is excreted in human breast milk.

*Children:* There are no adequate and well-controlled trials documenting the safety and efficacy of memantine in any illness occurring in children.

### Drug Interactions
*NMDA antagonists:* The combined use of memantine with other NMDA antagonists (amantadine, ketamine, and dextromethorphan) has not been systematically evaluated. Approach such use with caution.

*Drugs eliminated via renal mechanisms:* Coadministration of drugs that use the same renal cationic system, including hydrochlorothiazide (HCTZ), triamterene, cimetidine, ranitidine, quinidine, and nicotine, potentially could result in altered plasma levels of both agents.

*Drugs that make the urine alkaline:* Alterations of urine pH toward the alkaline condition may lead to an accumulation of the drug with a possible increase in adverse effects.

### Adverse Reactions
Adverse reactions occurring in at least 3% of patients include the following: back pain, confusion, constipation, coughing, dizziness, hallucination, headache, hypertension, pain, somnolence, vomiting.

# DEXMETHYLPHENIDATE HCl

| **Tablets**: 2.5, 5, and 10 mg (*c-II*) | *Focalin* (Novartis) |
| --- | --- |

**Warning:**
> *Drug dependence:* Give dexmethylphenidate cautiously to patients with a history of drug dependence or alcoholism. Chronic, abusive use can lead to marked tolerance and psychological dependence with varying degrees of abnormal behavior. Frank psychotic episodes can occur, especially with parenteral abuse. Careful supervision is required during drug withdrawal from abusive use because severe depression may occur. Withdrawal following chronic therapeutic use may unmask symptoms of the underlying disorder that may require follow-up.

## Indications

*Attention deficit hyperactivity disorder (ADHD):* For the treatment of ADHD. Dexmethylphenidate is indicated as an integral part of a total treatment program for ADHD that may include other measures (eg, psychological, educational, social) for patients with this syndrome. Drug treatment may not be indicated for all patients. Stimulants are not intended for use in the patient who exhibits symptoms secondary to environmental factors or other primary psychiatric disorders, including psychosis.

## Administration and Dosage

Administer twice/day, at least 4 hours apart, with or without food.

Individualize dosage according to the needs and responses of the patient.

*Patients new to methylphenidate:* The recommended starting dose of dexmethylphenidate for patients who are not currently taking racemic methylphenidate or for patients who are on stimulants other than methylphenidate is 5 mg/day (2.5 mg twice/day).

Dosage may be adjusted in 2.5 to 5 mg increments to a maximum of 20 mg/day (10 mg twice/day). In general, dosage adjustments may proceed at approximately weekly intervals.

*Patients currently using methylphenidate:* For patients currently using methylphenidate, the recommended starting dose of dexmethylphenidate is half the dose of racemic methylphenidate. The maximum recommended dose is 20 mg/day (10 mg twice/day).

*Dose reduction and discontinuation:* If paradoxical aggravation of symptoms or other adverse events occur, reduce the dosage, or, if necessary, discontinue the drug.

If improvement is not observed after appropriate dosage adjustment over a 1-month period, discontinue the drug.

## Actions

*Pharmacology:* Dexmethylphenidate HCl is a CNS stimulant. It is the more pharmacologically active enantiomer of the *d-* and *l-*enantiomers and is thought to block the reuptake of norepinephrine and dopamine into the presynaptic neuron and increase the release of these monoamines into the extraneuronal space.

*Pharmacokinetics:*

*Absorption* – Dexmethylphenidate HCl is readily absorbed following oral administration. In patients with ADHD, plasma dexmethylphenidate concentrations increase rapidly, reaching a maximum in the fasted state at approximately 1 to 1.5 hours postdose.

*Distribution* – Plasma dexmethylphenidate concentrations in children decline exponentially following oral administration.

*Metabolism* – Dexmethylphenidate is metabolized primarily to *d-α*-phenyl-piperidine acetic acid (also known as *d*-ritalinic acid) by de-esterification. This metabolite has little or no pharmacological activity.

In vitro studies showed that dexmethylphenidate did not inhibit cytochrome P450 isoenzymes.

*Excretion* – The mean plasma elimination half-life of dexmethylphenidate is approximately 2.2 hours.

## Contraindications

Patients with marked anxiety, tension, and agitation, because the drug may aggravate these symptoms; hypersensitivity to methylphenidate or other components of the product; patients with glaucoma, motor tics, or a family history or diagnosis of Tourette's syndrome; during treatment with monoamine oxidase inhibitors (MAOIs), and also within a minimum of 14 days following discontinuation of an MAOI (hypertensive crises may result).

## Warnings

*Depression:* Do not use dexmethylphenidate to treat severe depression.

*Fatigue:* Do not use dexmethylphenidate for the prevention or treatment of normal fatigue states.

*Long-term suppression of growth:* Although a causal relationship has not been established, suppression of growth (eg, weight gain, height) has been reported with long-term stimulant use in children.

*Psychosis:* In psychotic children, administration of methylphenidate may exacerbate symptoms of behavior disturbance and thought disorder.

*Seizures:* Methylphenidate may lower the convulsive threshold in patients with history of seizures, in patients with prior EEG abnormalities in the absence of a history of seizures, and, very rarely, in the absence of a history of seizures and no prior EEG evidence of seizures. In the presence of seizures, discontinue the drug.

*Hypertension and other cardiovascular conditions:* Use cautiously in patients with hypertension. Monitor blood pressure at appropriate intervals in all patients taking dexmethylphenidate, especially those with hypertension. Caution is indicated in treating patients whose underlying medical conditions might be compromised by increases in blood pressure or heart rate (eg, pre-existing hypertension, heart failure, recent MI, hyperthyroidism).

*Visual disturbance:* Difficulties with accommodation and blurring of vision have been reported.

*Carcinogenesis:* In a lifetime carcinogenicity study carried out in B6C3F1 mice, racemic methylphenidate caused an increase in hepatocellular adenomas and, in males only, an increase in hepatoblastomas at a daily dose of approximately 60 mg/kg/day. The significance to these results to humans is unknown.

*Pregnancy: Category C.*

*Lactation:* It is not known whether dexmethylphenidate is excreted in human milk.

*Children:* The safety and efficacy of dexmethylphenidate in children younger than 6 years of age have not been established.

## Precautions

*Monitoring:* Periodic CBC, differential, and platelet counts are advised during prolonged therapy.

## Drug Interactions

Drugs that may be affected by dexmethylphenidate or racemic methylphenidate include antihypertensive agents, pressor agents, coumarin anticoagulants, anticonvulsants, tricyclic antidepressants, selective serotonin reuptake inhibitors, and clonidine.

## Adverse Reactions

Adverse reactions occurring in 5% or more of patients include abdominal pain, anorexia, fever, and nausea.

*Adverse reactions with other methylphenidate HCl products* – Nervousness and insomnia are the most common adverse reactions reported with other methylphenidate products. In children, loss of appetite, abdominal pain, weight loss during prolonged therapy, insomnia, and tachycardia may occur more frequently; however, any of the other adverse reactions listed below also may occur.

# METHYLPHENIDATE HCl

| | |
|---|---|
| **Tablets**: 5, 10, and 20 mg (c-ii) | Various, Ritalin (Novartis), Methylin (Alliant) |
| **Tablets, chewable**: 2.5, 5, and 10 mg (c-ii) | Methylin (Alliant) |
| **Tablets, extended-release**: 10 mg (c-ii) | Metadate ER (Celltech), Methylin ER (Alliant) |
| 18 mg (c-ii) | Concerta (McNeil) |
| 20 mg (c-ii) | Various, Metadate ER (Celltech), Methylin ER (Alliant) |
| 27, 36, and 54 mg (c-ii) | Concerta (McNeil) |
| **Tablets, sustained-release**: 20 mg (c-ii) | Ritalin-SR (Novartis) |
| **Capsules, extended-release**: 20 mg (c-ii) | Metadate CD (Celltech) |
| 10, 20, 30, and 40 mg (c-ii) | Ritalin LA (Novartis) |

---

**Warning:**

> *Drug dependence:* Give methylphenidate cautiously to emotionally unstable patients, such as those with a history of drug dependence or alcoholism, because such patients may increase dosage on their own initiative.
>
> Chronic abuse can lead to marked tolerance and psychic dependence with varying degrees of abnormal behavior. Frank psychotic episodes can occur, especially with parenteral abuse. Careful supervision is required during drug withdrawal because severe depression, as well as the effects of chronic overactivity, can be unmasked. Long-term follow-up may be required because of the patient's basic personality disturbances.

---

## Indications

*Attention deficit disorders (ADD)/attention deficit hyperactivity disorders (ADHD):* As part of a total treatment program in children with a behavioral syndrome characterized by moderate to severe distractibility, short attention span, hyperactivity, emotional lability, and impulsivity.

*Narcolepsy (Ritalin, Ritalin SR, Metadate ER):* Treatment of narcolepsy.

## Administration and Dosage

*Adults:* Individualize dosage. Administer in divided doses 2 or 3 times/day, preferably 30 to 45 minutes before meals. Average dose is 20 to 30 mg/day. Dosage ranges from 10 to 15 mg/day to 40 to 60 mg/day. Patients who are unable to sleep if medication is taken late in the day should take the last dose before 6 pm.

*Children (6 years of age and older):* Start with small doses (eg, 5 mg before breakfast and lunch) with gradual increments of 5 to 10 mg/wk. Daily dosage above 60 mg is not recommended. If improvement is not observed after dosage adjustment over 1 month, discontinue use. If paradoxical aggravation of symptoms or other adverse effects occurs, reduce dosage or discontinue the drug.

Discontinue periodically to assess condition. Improvement may be sustained when the drug is temporarily or permanently discontinued. Drug treatment should not be indefinite and usually may be discontinued after puberty.

*All patients:* Sustained-release (SR) and Methylin ER tablets have a duration of approximately 8 hours and may be used in place of regular tablets when the 8-hour dosage of the SR tablets and Methylin ER corresponds to the titrated 8-hour dosage of the regular tablets. SR and Methylin ER tablets must be swallowed whole, never crushed or chewed. Take the chewable tablets (child or adult dose) with at least 8 oz (a full glass; 240 mL) of water or other fluid. Taking this product without enough liquid may cause choking.

*Maintenance/Extended treatment:* Discontinue periodically to assess condition. Improvement may be sustained when the drug is either temporarily or permanently discontinued. Drug treatment should not and need not be indefinite and usually may be discontinued after puberty.

*Dose reduction and discontinuation:* If paradoxical aggravation of symptoms or other adverse events occur, reduce dosage or discontinue the drug.

If improvement is not observed after appropriate dosage adjustment over a 1-month period, discontinue the drug.

*Concerta:* Administer orally once/day in the morning with or without food. Advise patients to swallow the capsules whole with the aid of liquids and not to chew, divide, or crush them. The tablet shell, along with insoluble core components, is eliminated from the body.

*Patients new to methylphenidate* – The recommended starting dose for patients who are not currently taking methylphenidate or for patients who are on stimulants other than methylphenidate is 18 mg once/day. Dosage may be adjusted in 18 mg increments at weekly intervals to a maximum of 54 mg/day taken once/day in the morning.

*Patients currently using methylphenidate* – The recommended dose for patients currently taking methylphenidate twice/day, 3 times/day, or SR doses of 10 to 60 mg/day is provided in the following table.

Dosage may be adjusted at weekly intervals to a maximum of 54 mg/day taken once/day in the morning.

| Recommended Dose Conversion from Methylphenidate Regimens to *Concerta* | |
| --- | --- |
| Previous methylphenidate daily dose | Recommended *Concerta* dose |
| 5 mg methylphenidate twice/day or 5 mg methylphenidate 3 times/day or 20 mg methylphenidate SR | 18 mg every morning |
| 10 mg methylphenidate twice/day or 10 mg methylphenidate 3 times/day or 40 mg methylphenidate SR | 36 mg every morning |
| 15 mg methylphenidate twice/day or 15 mg methylphenidate 3 times/day or 60 mg methylphenidate SR | 54 mg every morning |

A 27 mg dosage strength is available for physicians who wish to prescribe between the 18 and 36 mg dosages.

In other methylphenidate regimens, use clinical judgment when selecting the starting dose. Daily dosage above 54 mg is not recommended.

*Metadate CD:* Administer once daily in the morning before breakfast. The capsules may be swallowed whole with the aid of liquids or may be opened and the capsule contents sprinkled onto a small amount (tablespoon) of applesauce and given immediately; do not store for future use. The capsules and the capsule contents must not be crushed or chewed.

*Sprinkle administration* – Sprinkle onto a small amount of soft food (eg, applesauce). The entire capsule contents must be used as a single 20 mg dose. The dose cannot be split because the immediate-release and extended (continuous)-release beads cannot be physically distinguished from one another. Administer the dose immediately after sprinkling. Do not store for future use. The beads contained within the capsules must not be crushed or chewed.

*Initial treatment* – 20 mg once/day. Adjust dosage in weekly 20 mg increments to a maximum of 60 mg/day taken once/day in the morning, depending upon tolerability and degree of efficacy. Daily dosage above 60 mg is not recommended.

*Ritalin LA:* Individualize dosage.

*Initial treatment* – The recommended starting dose is 20 mg once/day. Dosage may be adjusted in weekly 10 mg increments to a maximum of 60 mg/day taken once/day in the morning, depending on tolerability and degree of efficacy observed. Daily dosage above 60 mg is not recommended. When a lower initial dose is appropriate, patients may begin treatment with an immediate-release methylphenidate product at a lower dose. After titration to 10 mg twice/day, these patients may be switched to *Ritalin LA* according to the guidelines in the table below.

*Patients currently using methylphenidate* – The recommended dose for patients currently taking methylphenidate twice/day or SR is provided below. Dosing recommendations are based on current dose regimen and clinical judgment.

| *Ritalin LA* Dosing Regimens in Current Methylphenidate Users | |
| --- | --- |
| Previous methylphenidate dose | Recommended *Ritalin LA* dose |
| 10 mg bid or 20 mg methylphenidate SR | 20 mg qd |
| 15 mg methylphenidate bid | 30 mg qd |
| 20 mg bid or 40 mg methylphenidate SR | 40 mg qd |
| 30 mg bid or 60 mg methylphenidate SR | 60 mg qd |

## Actions

*Pharmacology:* Methylphenidate is a mild CNS stimulant with actions similar to the amphetamines. The exact mechanism of action is not fully understood.

*Pharmacokinetics:* Rapidly and well absorbed from the GI tract, methylphenidate achieves peak blood levels in 1 to 3 hours. Peak plasma levels occur in children in 4.7 hours for the SR tablets and 1.9 hours for the regular tablets. The mean plasma half-life for methylphenidate HCl and *Concerta* tablets is approximately 3 to 3.5 hours. Plasma half-life for *Metadate CD* is reportedly 6.8 hours. SR and ER tablets are more slowly but as extensively absorbed as regular tablets.

## Contraindications

Marked anxiety, tension, and agitation (the drug may aggravate these symptoms); hypersensitivity to methylphenidate or other components of the product; glaucoma; motor tics or a family history or diagnosis of Tourette syndrome.

*Ritalin, Ritalin SR, Concerta, Metadate CD, Ritalin LA:* Concurrent treatment with monoamine oxidase inhibitors (MAOIs) and within a minimum of 14 days following discontinuation of an MAOI (hypertensive crisis may result).

## Warnings

*Seizure disorders:* Methylphenidate may lower the seizure threshold in patients with a history of seizures, with prior EEG abnormalities in absence of seizures, and, very rarely, in the absence of history of seizures and no prior EEG evidence of seizures. Safe concomitant use with anticonvulsants has not been established. If seizures occur, discontinue the drug.

*GI obstruction:* Because the *Concerta* tablet is nondeformable and does not appreciably change shape in the GI tract, do not administer to patients with pre-existing severe GI narrowing (eg, small bowel inflammatory disease, "short gut" syndrome because of adhesions or decreased transit time, history of peritonitis, cystic fibrosis, chronic intestinal pseudo-obstruction, Meckel's diverticulum). Because of the controlled-release design of the tablet, only use *Concerta* in patients who are able to swallow the tablet whole.

*Hypertension:* Use cautiously; monitor blood pressure in all patients, especially those with hypertension.

*Severe depression:* Do not use methylphenidate for severe depression of either exogenous or endogenous origin.

*Fatigue:* Do not use methylphenidate for the prevention or treatment of normal fatigue states.

*Long-term suppression of growth:* Suppression of growth has been reported with long-term use in children. Interrupt treatment for patients who are not growing or gaining weight as expected.

*Psychosis:* Methylphenidate may exacerbate symptoms of behavior disturbances and thought disorder.

*Visual disturbances:* Visual disturbances have been encountered rarely. Difficulties with accommodation and blurring of vision have been reported.

*Pregnancy: Category C.*

*Lactation:* The amount of methylphenidate excreted in breast milk is unknown.

*Children:* Do not use in children under 6 years of age because safety and efficacy have not been established. In psychotic children, the drug may exacerbate symptoms of behavior disturbance and thought disorder.

Safety and efficacy of long-term use in children are not established. Although a causal relationship has not been established, suppression of growth (eg, weight gain or height) has been reported with long-term use of stimulants in children. Carefully monitor patients on long-term therapy.

### Precautions

*Monitoring:* Perform periodic CBC, differential, and platelet counts during prolonged therapy.

*Phenylketonurics:* Each 2.5 mg chewable tablet contains 0.42 mg phenylalanine; each 5 mg chewable tablet contains 0.84 mg phenylalanine; and each 10 mg chewable tablet contains 1.68 mg phenylalanine.

*Agitation:* Patients with an element of agitation may react adversely; discontinue therapy if necessary.

*Prescribing:* Drug treatment is not indicated in all cases of this behavioral syndrome. The decision to prescribe methylphenidate should depend on chronicity and severity of symptoms and appropriateness for age.

*Acute stress:* When symptoms are associated with acute stress reactions, treatment with methylphenidate usually is not indicated.

*Drug abuse and dependence:* Give cautiously to emotionally unstable patients, such as those with a history of drug dependence or alcoholism, because they may increase dosage on their own initiative (see Warning Box).

### Drug Interactions

Drugs that may affect methylphenidate include MAOIs. Drugs that may be affected by methylphenidate HCl include guanethidine, anticonvulsants (eg, phenytoin, phenobarbital, primidone), selective serotonin reuptake inhibitors, coumarin anticoagulants, and tricyclic antidepressants.

### Adverse Reactions

Adverse reactions may include the following: Skin rash; urticaria; fever; arthralgia; exfoliative dermatitis; erythema multiforme with necrotizing vasculitis; thrombocytopenic purpura; dizziness; headache; dyskinesia; drowsiness; Tourette syndrome; toxic psychosis; blood pressure and pulse changes; tachycardia; angina; cardiac arrhythmias; palpitations; anorexia; nausea; abdominal pain; weight loss; nervousness; insomnia; leukopenia; anemia; hair loss; loss of appetite; abdominal pain; vomiting, upper respiratory tract infection; cough increased; pharyngitis; sinusitis.

# PEMOLINE

| | |
|---|---|
| **Tablets**: 18.75, 37.5, and 75 mg (c-iv) | *Pemoline* (Apothecon), *Cylert* (Abbott), *PemADD* (Mallinckrodt) |
| **Tablets, chewable**: 37.5 mg (c-iv) | *Cylert* (Abbott), *PemADD CT* (Mallinckrodt) |

**Warning:**
> Because of its association with life-threatening hepatic failure, pemoline should not ordinarily be considered as first-line drug therapy for attention deficit hyperactivity disorder (ADHD). Because pemoline provides an observable symptomatic benefit, patients who fail to show substantial clinical benefit within 3 weeks of completing dose titration should be withdrawn from therapy.
>
> Since pemoline's marketing in 1975, 15 cases of acute hepatic failure have been reported to the FDA. While the absolute number of reported cases is not large, the rate of reporting ranges from 4 to 17 times the rate expected in the general population. This estimate may be conservative because of underreporting and because the long latency between initiation of pemoline treatment and the occurrence of hepatic failure may limit recognition of the association. If only a portion of actual cases were recognized and reported, the risk could be substantially higher.
>
> Of the 15 cases reported as of December 1998, 12 resulted in death or liver transplantation, usually within 4 weeks of the onset of signs and symptoms of liver failure. The earliest onset of heptic abnormalities occurred 6 months after initiation of pemoline. Although some reports described dark urine and nonspecific prodromal symptoms (eg, anorexia, malaise, GI symptoms), in other reports it was not clear if any prodromol symptoms preceded the onset of jaundice.
>
> Initiate treatment with pemoline only in individuals without liver disease and with normal baseline liver function tests. It is not clear if baseline and periodic liver function testing are predictive of these instances of acute liver failure; however, it is generally believed that early detection of drug-induced hepatic injury along with immediate withdrawal of the suspect drug enhances the likelihood for recovery. Accordingly, the following liver monitoring program is recommended: Determine serum ALT levels at baseline and every 2 weeks thereafter. If pemoline therapy is discontinued and then restarted, perform liver function test monitoring at baseline and reinitiate at the frequency above.
>
> Discontinue pemoline if serum ALT is increased to a clinically significant level or any increase 2 times or more the upper limit of normal, or if clinical signs and symptoms suggest liver failure.
>
> The physician who elects to use pemoline should obtain written informed consent from the patient prior to initiation of pemoline therapy.

## Indications

*ADHD:* As part of a total treatment program in children with a behavioral syndrome characterized by moderate to severe distractibility, short attention span, hyperactivity, emotional lability, and impulsivity.

## Administration and Dosage

Administer as a single dose each morning. Recommended starting dose is 37.5 mg/day. Gradually increase at 1-week intervals using increments of 18.75 mg until desired response is obtained. Mean effective doses range from 56.25 to 75 mg/day. Maximum recommended dose is 112.5 mg/day.

Clinical improvement is gradual; significant benefit may not be evident until week 3 or 4 of administration.

Interrupt drug administration occasionally to determine if there is a recurrence of behavioral symptoms sufficient to require continued therapy.

## Actions

*Pharmacology:* Pemoline is a CNS stimulant. Although structurally dissimilar to the amphetamines and methylphenidate, it has pharmacologic activity similar to that of other stimulants but with minimal sympathomimetic effects. Although the exact mechanism of action is unknown, pemoline may act through dopaminergic mechanisms.

*Pharmacokinetics:* Pemoline is rapidly absorbed from the GI tract. Approximately 50% is protein bound. Peak serum levels occur within 2 to 4 hours after ingestion of a single dose. The serum half-life is approximately 12 hours. Steady state is reached in approximately 2 to 3 days. The drug is widely distributed throughout body tissues, including the brain. Pemoline is metabolized by the liver and primarily excreted by the kidneys. Approximately 50% is excreted unchanged and only minor fractions are present as metabolites.

## Contraindications

Known hypersensitivity or idiosyncrasy to pemoline; hepatic insufficiency.

## Warnings

*Renal function impairment:* Administer with caution to patients with significantly impaired renal function.

*Pregnancy: Category B.*

*Lactation:* It is not known whether pemoline is excreted in breast milk. Exercise caution when administering pemoline to a nursing woman.

*Children:* Safety and efficacy in children younger than 6 years of age have not been established.

In psychotic children, administration may exacerbate symptoms of behavior disturbance and thought disorder. CNS stimulants, including pemoline, can precipitate motor and phonic tics and Tourette's syndrome. Therefore, clinical evaluation for tics and Tourette's syndrome in children and their families should precede use of stimulants.

Chronic administration may be associated with growth inhibition; therefore, monitor growth during treatment. Long-term effects in children have not been well established.

Treatment is not indicated in all cases of ADHD; consider therapy only in light of complete history and evaluation of the child. The decision to prescribe pemoline should depend on the assessment of the chronicity and severity of the child's symptoms and their appropriateness for his or her age, and not depend solely on the presence of 1 or more of the behavioral characteristics.

## Precautions

*Hepatic effects:* See Black Box Warning.

*Drug abuse and dependence:* The pharmacologic similarity of pemoline to other psychostimulants with known dependence liability suggests that psychological or physical dependence might occur. There have been isolated reports of transient psychotic symptoms occurring in adults following the long-term misuse of excessive oral doses. Give with caution to emotionally unstable patients who may increase the dosage on their own initiative.

## Drug Interactions

Carefully monitor patients receiving pemoline with other drugs, especially drugs with CNS activity.

Decreased seizure threshold has been reported in patients receiving pemoline concomitantly with antiepileptic medications.

## Adverse Reactions

*Most frequent* – Insomnia usually occurs early in therapy prior to optimum therapeutic response; it is often transient or responds to dosage reduction.

*CNS:* Convulsive seizures; Tourette's syndrome; hallucinations; dyskinetic movements of tongue, lips, face, and extremities; abnormal oculomotor function (eg, nystagmus, oculogyric crisis); mild depression; dizziness; increased irritability; headache; drowsiness.

*GI:* Stomachache; nausea. Anorexia with weight loss may occur during the first weeks. In most cases it is transient; weight gain usually resumes within 3 to 6 months.

*Hepatic:* Hepatic dysfunction including elevated liver enzymes, hepatitis, jaundice, and fatal hepatic failure has occurred. Elevated liver enzymes are not rare and appear reversible upon drug discontinuance. Most patients with elevated liver enzymes were asymptomatic.

*Miscellaneous:* Growth suppression with long-term use of stimulants in children; skin rashes; aplastic anemia (rare).

# TACRINE HCl (Tetrahydroaminoacridine; THA)

**Capsules:** 10, 20, 30, and 40 mg (*Rx*)          *Cognex* (Parke-Davis)

## Indications
*Alzheimer disease:* Treatment of mild to moderate dementia of the Alzheimer type.

## Administration and Dosage
The rate of dose escalation may be slowed if a patient is intolerant to the recommended titration schedule. However, it is not advisable to accelerate the dose incrementation plan. Following initiation of therapy, or any dosage increase, observe patients carefully for adverse effects. Take between meals whenever possible; however, if minor GI upset occurs, take with meals to improve tolerability. Taking tacrine with meals can be expected to reduce plasma levels approximately 30% to 40%.

*Initiation of treatment:* The initial dose of tacrine is 40 mg/day (10 mg 4 times/day). Maintain this dose for 4 weeks or more with every other week monitoring of transaminase levels beginning at week 4 of therapy. It is important that the dose not be increased during this period because of the potential for delayed onset of transaminase elevations.

*Dose titration:* Following 4 weeks of treatment at 40 mg/day (10 mg 4 times/day), increase the dose to 80 mg/day (20 mg 4 times/day), providing there are no significant transaminase elevations and the patient is tolerating treatment. Titrate patients to higher doses (120 and 160 mg/day in divided doses on a 4 times/day schedule) at 4-week intervals on the basis of tolerance.

*Dose adjustment:* Monitor serum transaminase levels (specifically ALT) every other week from at least week 4 to week 16 following initiation of treatment, after which monitoring may be decreased to every 3 months. For patients who develop ALT elevations more than 2 times the upper limit of normal (ULN), the dose and monitoring regimen should be modified as described in the table below.

A full monitoring and dose titration sequence must be repeated in the event that a patient suspends treatment with tacrine for more than 4 weeks.

| Recommended Tacrine Dose and Monitoring Regimen Modification in Response to Transaminase Elevations | |
| --- | --- |
| Transaminase levels | Treatment and monitoring regimen |
| ≤ 2 × ULN | Continue treatment according to recommended titration and monitoring schedule. |
| > 2 to ≤ 3 × ULN | Continue treatment according to recommended titration. Monitor transaminase levels weekly until levels return to normal limits. |
| > 3 to ≤ 5 × ULN | Reduce the daily dose by 40 mg/day. Monitor ALT levels weekly. Resume dose titration and every other week monitoring when transaminase levels return to within normal limits. |

| Recommended Tacrine Dose and Monitoring Regimen Modification in Response to Transaminase Elevations ||
| Transaminase levels | Treatment and monitoring regimen |
| --- | --- |
| > 5 × ULN | Stop treatment. Monitor the patient closely for signs and symptoms associated with hepatitis and follow transaminase levels until within normal limits (see Rechallenge). |

Experience is limited in patients with ALT > 10 × ULN. The risk of rechallenge must be considered against demonstrated clinical benefit. Patients with clinical jaundice confirmed by a significant elevation in total bilirubin (more than 3 mg/dL) or those exhibiting clinical signs or symptoms of hypersensitivity (eg, rash or fever) in association with ALT elevations should immediately and permanently discontinue tacrine and not be rechallenged.

*Rechallenge:* Patients who are required to discontinue treatment because of transaminase elevations may be rechallenged once transaminase levels return to within normal limits. Rechallenge of patients exposed to transaminase elevations less than 10 × ULN has not resulted in serious liver injury. However, because experience in the rechallenge of patients who had elevations greater than 10 × ULN is limited, the risks associated with the rechallenge of these patients are not well characterized. Carefully and frequently (weekly) monitor serum ALT when rechallenging such patients. If rechallenged, give patients an initial dose of 40 mg/day (10 mg 4 times/day) and monitor transaminase levels weekly. If, after 6 weeks on 40 mg/day, the patient is tolerating the dosage with no unacceptable elevations in transaminases, recommended dose titration and transaminase monitoring may be resumed.

Continue weekly monitoring of ALT levels for a total of 16 weeks, after which monitoring may be decreased to monthly for 2 months and every 3 months thereafter.

**Actions**

*Pharmacology:* Tacrine is a centrally acting reversible cholinesterase inhibitor, commonly referred to as THA.

*Pharmacokinetics:*

  *Absorption* – Maximal plasma concentrations occur within 1 to 2 hours.

  *Distribution* – Mean volume of distribution of tacrine is approximately 349 L. Tacrine is approximately 55% bound to plasma proteins.

  *Metabolism* – Tacrine is extensively metabolized by the cytochrome P450 system.

  *Excretion* – The elimination half-life is approximately 2 to 4 hours.

**Contraindications**

Hypersensitivity to tacrine or acridine derivatives; patients previously treated with tacrine who developed treatment-associated jaundice; a serum bilirubin greater than 3 mg/dL; signs or symptoms of hypersensitivity (eg, rash or fever) in association with ALT elevations.

**Warnings**

*Anesthesia:* Tacrine is likely to exaggerate succinylcholine-type muscle relaxation during anesthesia.

*Cardiovascular conditions:* Tacrine may have vagotonic effects on the heart rate.

*GI disease/dysfunction:* Tacrine is an inhibitor of cholinesterase and may be expected to increase gastric acid secretion caused by increased cholinergic activity. Therefore, closely monitor patients at increased risk for developing ulcers for symptoms of active or occult GI bleeding.

*Hepatic effects:* Prescribe with care in patients with current evidence or history of abnormal liver function indicated by significant abnormalities in serum transaminase, bilirubin, and gamma-glutamyl transpeptidase levels.

The incidence of transaminase elevations is higher among females. There are no other known predictors of the risk of hepatocellular injury.

*GU effects:* Cholinomimetics may cause bladder outflow obstruction.

*Neurological conditions:*
   *Seizures* – Cholinomimetics are believed to have some potential to cause generalized convulsions; however, seizure activity may also be a manifestation of Alzheimer disease.
   *Cognitive function* – Worsening of cognitive function has been reported following abrupt discontinuation of tacrine or after a large reduction in total daily dose ( 80 mg/day or more).

*Pulmonary conditions:* Because of its cholinomimetic action, use tacrine with care in patients with a history of asthma.

*Hepatic disease:* Although studies in patients with liver disease have not been done, it is likely that functional hepatic impairment will reduce the clearance of tacrine and its metabolites.

*Pregnancy:* Category C.

*Lactation:* It is not known whether this drug is excreted in breast milk.

*Children:* There are no adequate and well controlled trials to document the safety and efficacy of tacrine in any dementing illness occurring in children.

### Precautions
*Monitoring:* Monitor serum transaminase levels (specifically ALT) every other week from at least week 4 to week 16 following initiation of treatment, after which monitoring may be decreased to every 3 months. Repeat a full monitoring sequence in the event that a patient suspends treatment with tacrine for more than 4 weeks. If transaminase elevations occur, modify the dose (see Administration and Dosage).
   Continue to monitor ALT levels weekly for a total of 16 weeks, then decrease to monthly for 2 months and to every 3 months thereafter.

*Hematology:* Decreased absolute neutrophil counts (ANC) less than 500 to 1500/mcL have been reported rarely. The total clinical experience in more than 12,000 patients does not indicate a clear association between tacrine treatment and serious white blood cell abnormalities.

### Drug Interactions
Drugs that may be affected by tacrine include anticholinergics, cholinomimetics, cholinesterase inhibitors, and theophylline.

Drugs that may affect tacrine include cimetidine.

Tacrine is primarily eliminated by hepatic metabolism via cytochrome P450 drug metabolizing enzymes. Drug interactions may occur when it is given concurrently with agents such as theophylline that undergo extensive metabolism via cytochrome P450 IA2.

### Adverse Reactions
Adverse reactions occurring in 3% or more of patients include elevated transaminases; nausea; vomiting; diarrhea; dyspepsia; myalgia; headache; fatigue; chest pain; weight decrease; agitation; depression; abnormal thinking; anxiety; anorexia; abdominal pain; flatulence; constipation; dizziness; confusion; ataxia; insomnia; somnolence; urinary incontinence; urinary tract infection; urination frequency; rash; facial flushing; coughing; upper respiratory tract infection; rhinitis.

## RIVASTIGMINE

**Capsules**: 1.5, 3, 4.5, 6 mg (as tartrate) (*Rx*)      *Exelon* (Novartis)
**Solution**: 2 mg/mL (as tartrate) (*Rx*)      *Exelon* (Novartis)

### Indications
*Alzheimer dementia:* For the treatment of mild to moderate dementia of the Alzheimer type.

### Administration and Dosage
The recommended starting dose of rivastigmine is 1.5 mg twice a day. If dose is well tolerated, after a minimum of 2 weeks of treatment, the dose may be increased to

3 mg twice a day. Subsequent increases to 4.5 and 6 mg twice/day should be attempted after a minimum of 2 weeks at the previous dose. If adverse effects (eg, nausea, vomiting, abdominal pain, loss of appetite) cause intolerance during treatment, instruct the patient to discontinue treatment for several doses and then restart at the same or next lower dose level. If treatment is interrupted for longer than several days, reinitiate treatment with the lowest daily dose and titrate as described above. The maximum dose is 6 mg twice/day (12 mg/day).

Take with food in divided doses in the morning and evening.

*Oral solution:* Each dose of rivastigmine may be swallowed directly from the syringe or first mixed with a small glass of water, cold fruit juice, or soda. Instruct patients to stir and drink the mixture.

Rivastigmine oral solution and capsules may be interchanged at equal doses.

*Storage/Stability:* When rivastigmine oral solution is combined with cold fruit juice or soda, the mixture is stable at room temperature for ≤ 4 hours.

## Actions

*Pharmacology:* While the precise mechanism of rivastigmine's action is unknown, it is postulated to exert its therapeutic effect by enhancing cholinergic function. This is accomplished by increasing the concentration of acetylcholine through reversible inhibition of its hydrolysis by cholinesterase. If this proposed mechanism is correct, rivastigmine's effect may lessen as the disease process advances and fewer cholinergic neurons remain functionally intact.

*Pharmacokinetics:*

*Absorption* – Rivastigmine is rapidly and completely absorbed with an absolute bioavailability of approximately 36% (3 mg dose). Peak plasma concentrations are reached in approximately 1 hour.

*Distribution* – Rivastigmine is widely distributed throughout the body with a volume of distribution in the range of 1.8 to 2.7 L/kg.

Rivastigmine is approximately 40% bound to plasma proteins.

*Metabolism* – Rivastigmine is rapidly and extensively metabolized, primarily via cholinesterase-mediated hydrolysis to the decarbamylated metabolite.

*Excretion* – The elimination half-life is approximately 1.5 hours, with most elimination as metabolites via the urine.

## Contraindications

Hypersensitivity to rivastigmine, other carbamate derivatives, or other components of the formulation.

## Warnings

*GI effects:* Rivastigmine is associated with significant GI adverse reactions, including nausea and vomiting, anorexia, and weight loss.

*Weight loss:* In the controlled trials, approximately 26% of women on high doses of rivastigmine (more than 9 mg/day) had weight loss of 7% or more of their baseline weight compared with 6% in the placebo-treated patients. Approximately 18% of the males in the high dose group experienced a similar degree of weight loss compared with 4% in placebo-treated patients. It is not clear how much of the weight loss was associated with anorexia, nausea, vomiting, and diarrhea associated with drug administration.

*Anorexia:* In the controlled clinical trials, of the patients treated with a rivastigmine dose of 6 to 12 mg/day, 17% developed anorexia compared with 3% of the placebo patients. Neither the time course nor the severity of the anorexia is known.

*Peptic ulcers/GI bleeding:* Because of their pharmacological action, cholinesterase inhibitors may be expected to increase gastric acid secretion caused by increased cholinergic activity. Therefore, monitor patients closely for symptoms of active or occult GI bleeding, especially those at increased risk for developing ulcers (eg, those with a history of ulcer disease or those receiving concurrent nonsteroidal anti-inflammatory drugs [NSAID]). Clinical studies of rivastigmine have shown no significant increase, relative to placebo, in the incidence of either peptic ulcer disease or GI bleeding.

*Anesthesia:* Rivastigmine, as a cholinesterase inhibitor, is likely to exaggerate succinylcholine-type muscle relaxation during anesthesia.

*Cardiovascular effects:* Drugs that increase cholinergic activity may have vagotonic effects on heart rates (eg, bradycardia). The potential for this action may be particularly important in patients with "sick sinus syndrome" or other supraventricular cardiac conduction conditions.

*Urinary obstruction:* Drugs that increase cholinergic activity may cause urinary obstruction.

*Seizures:* Drugs that increase cholinergic activity are believed to have some potential for causing seizures. However, seizure activity also may be a manifestation of Alzheimer disease.

*Pulmonary effects:* Like other drugs that increase cholinergic activity, use with care in patients with a history of asthma or obstructive pulmonary disease.

*Pregnancy: Category B.*

*Lactation:* It is not known whether rivastigmine is excreted in breast milk.

### Drug Interactions
Drugs that may interfere with rivastigmine include anticholinergics and cholinomimetics and other cholinesterase inhibitors.

### Adverse Reactions
Adverse reactions occurring in 3% or more of patients include the following: Dizziness; headache; insomnia; confusion; depression; anxiety; somnolence; hallucination; tremor; aggressive reaction; nausea; vomiting; diarrhea; anorexia; abdominal pain; dyspepsia; constipation; flatulence; accidental trauma; fatigue; urinary tract infection; asthenia; malaise; rhinitis; increased sweating; hypertension; influenza-like symptoms; syncope; weight decrease.

## GALANTAMINE HBr

**Tablets**: 4, 8, and 12 mg *(Rx)*    *Reminyl* (Janssen)
**Oral solution**: 4 mg/mL *(Rx)*

### Indications
*Alzheimer disease:* Treatment of mild to moderate dementia of the Alzheimer type.

### Administration and Dosage
*Dosage:* 16 to 32 mg/day given twice/day with morning and evening meals. The recommended dose range is 16 to 24 mg/day given twice/day.

Starting dose is 4 mg twice/day (8 mg/day). After a minimum of 4 weeks of treatment, if well tolerated, increase the dose to 8 mg twice/day (16 mg/day). Attempt a further increase to 12 mg twice/day (24 mg/day) only after a minimum of 4 weeks at the previous dose.

If therapy has been interrupted for several days or longer, the patient should be restarted at the lowest dose and the dose escalated to the current dose.

### Actions
*Pharmacology:* Galantamine is a competitive and reversible inhibitor of acetylcholinesterase. While the precise mechanism of galantamine's action is unknown, it may exert its therapeutic effect by enhancing cholinergic function.

*Pharmacokinetics:*

*Absorption/Distribution* – Galantamine is rapidly and completely absorbed with time-to-peak concentration in about 1 hour. Galantamine has an absolute oral bioavailability of about 90%. The plasma protein binding of galantamine is 18%.

*Metabolism/Excretion* – Galantamine is metabolized by hepatic cytochrome P450 CYP 2D6 and CYP 3A4 enzymes, glucuronidated, and excreted unchanged in the urine.

*Special populations –*

*Elderly:* Data from clinical trials in patients with Alzheimer disease indicated that galantamine concentrations are 30% to 40% higher than in healthy young subjects.

*Gender:* Galantamine clearance is about 20% lower in females than in males (explained by lower body weight in females).

## Contraindications

Known hypersensitivity to galantamine or to any excipients used in the formulation.

## Warnings

*Renal function impairment:* For patients with moderate renal impairment, the dose generally should not exceed 16 mg/day. In patients with severe renal impairment (Ccr less than 9 mL/min), the use of galantamine is not recommended.

*Hepatic function impairment:* In patients with moderately impaired hepatic function, the dose generally should not exceed 16 mg/day. The use of galantamine in patients with severe hepatic impairment is not recommended.

*Pregnancy:* Category B.

*Lactation:* It is not known whether galantamine is excreted in breast milk. Galantamine has no indication for use in nursing mothers.

*Children:* Safety and efficacy of galantamine in children have not been established.

## Precautions

*Special risk:*

*Anesthesia –* Galantamine is likely to exaggerate the neuromuscular blockade effects of succinylcholine-type and similar neuromuscular blocking agents during anesthesia.

*Cardiovascular conditions –* Cholinesterase inhibitors have vagotonic effects on the sinoatrial and atrioventricular nodes, leading to bradycardia and AV block. These actions may be particularly important to patients with supraventricular cardiac conduction disorders or to patients taking other drugs concomitantly that significantly slow heart rate. Consider all patients to be at risk for adverse effects on cardiac conduction.

*GI conditions –* Cholinomimetics may increase gastric acid secretion because of increased cholinergic activity. Therefore, monitor patients closely for symptoms of active or occult GI bleeding, especially those with an increased risk for developing ulcers.

Galantamine has been shown to produce nausea, vomiting, diarrhea, anorexia, and weight loss. In patients who experienced nausea, the median duration was 5 to 7 days.

*GU –* Although this was not observed in clinical trials with galantamine, cholinomimetics may cause bladder outflow obstruction.

*Neurological conditions –*

*Seizures:* Cholinesterase inhibitors are believed to have some potential to cause generalized convulsions.

*Pulmonary conditions:* Prescribe galantamine with care to patients with a history of severe asthma or obstructive pulmonary disease.

## Drug Interactions

Drugs that may affect galantamine include succinylcholine and bethanechol. Drugs that may be affected by galantamine include succinylcholine, bethanechol, cimetidine, ketoconazole, paroxetine, and erythromycin.

## Adverse Reactions

The most frequent adverse reactions leading to discontinuation of galantamine therapy included nausea, dizziness, vomiting, anorexia, and syncope.

Adverse events occurring in at least 5% of galantamine patients and at least 2 times placebo include nausea, diarrhea, anorexia, vomiting, and weight decrease. Other adverse events occurring in at least 3% of patients receiving galantamine include dizziness, headache, depression, insomnia, somnolence, tremor, abdominal pain, dyspepsia, urinary tract infection, hematuria, fatigue, rhinitis, and anemia.

# DONEPEZIL HCl

| Tablets: 5 and 10 mg (Rx) | Aricept (Eisai/Pfizer) |
|---|---|

### Indications

*Alzheimer disease:* The treatment of mild to moderate dementia of the Alzheimer type.

### Administration and Dosage

The dosages of donepezil are 5 and 10 mg once per day in the evening, just prior to retiring.

The higher dose of 10 mg did not provide a statistically significant clinical benefit greater than that of 5 mg. Do not increase to 10 mg until patients have been on a daily dose of 5 mg for 4 to 6 weeks.

Donepezil may be taken with or without food.

### Actions

*Pharmacology:* Donepezil enhances cholinergic function. This increase in cholinergic function is accomplished by increasing the concentration of acetylcholine through reversible inhibition of its hydrolysis by acetylcholinesterase (AChE). If this proposed mechanism of action is correct, donepezil's effect may lessen as the disease process advances and fewer cholinergic neurons remain functionally intact.

*Pharmacokinetics:*

    *Absorption* – Donepezil is well absorbed with a relative oral bioavailability of 100% and reaches peak plasma concentrations in 3 to 4 hours.

    *Distribution* – Following multiple dose administration, steady state is reached within 15 days. Donepezil is approximately 96% bound to human plasma proteins.

    *Metabolism* – Donepezil is excreted in urine. It is metabolized by CYP 450 isoenzyme 2D6 and 3A4 and undergoes glucuronidation.

    *Excretion* – The elimination half-life of donepezil is approximately 70 hours and the mean apparent plasma clearance is 0.13 L/h/kg.

### Contraindications

Hypersensitivity to donepezil or to piperidine derivatives.

### Warnings

*Anesthesia:* Donepezil, as a cholinesterase inhibitor, is likely to exaggerate succinylcholine-type muscle relaxation during anesthesia.

*Cardiovascular:* Cholinesterase inhibitors may have vagotonic effects on heart rate (eg, bradycardia). The potential for this action may be particularly important to patients with "sick sinus syndrome" or other supraventricular cardiac conduction conditions. Syncopal episodes have occurred in association with the use of donepezil.

*GI:* Through their primary action, cholinesterase inhibitors may be expected to increase gastric acid secretion because of increased cholinergic activity. Therefore, monitor patients closely for symptoms of active or occult GI bleeding, especially those at increased risk for developing ulcers.

*GU:* Cholinomimetics may cause bladder outflow obstruction.

*Seizures:* Cholinomimetics may have some potential to cause generalized convulsions. However, seizure activity also may be a manifestation of Alzheimer disease.

*Pulmonary:* Prescribe cholinesterase inhibitors with care for patients with a history of asthma or obstructive pulmonary disease.

*Pregnancy: Category* C.

*Lactation:* It is not known whether donepezil is excreted in breast milk.

*Children:* There are no adequate and well controlled tirals to document the safety and efficacy of donepezil in any illness occurring in children.

### Drug Interactions

Drugs that may affect donepezil are ketoconazole and quinidine. Drugs that may be affected by donepezil include anticholinergics, cholinometics/cholinesterase inhibitors, NSAIDs, furosemide, digoxin, warfarin, theophylline, and cimetidine.

**Adverse Reactions**
 Adverse reactions that may occur in 3% or more of patients include headache, whole body pain, fatigue, nausea, diarrhea, vomiting, anorexia, muscle cramps, insomnia, dizziness, depression, abnormal dreams, ecchymosis, and weight decrease.

# AMPHETAMINES

Amphetamine, dextroamphetamine, and methamphetamine also are indicated for attention deficit disorders in children, as part of a total treatment program. For complete prescribing information on the amphetamines for this and other uses, consult the general amphetamine monograph.

# ERGOLOID MESYLATES (Dihydrogenated Ergot Alkaloids, Dihydroergotoxine)

| | |
|---|---|
| **Tablets, oral:** 0.5 and 1 mg (*Rx*) | Various, *Gerimal* (Rugby), *Hydergine* (Sandoz) |
| **Tablets, sublingual:** 0.5 and 1 mg (*Rx*) | Various, *Gerimal* (Rugby), *Hydergine* (Sandoz) |
| **Liquid:** 1 mg/mL (*Rx*) | *Hydergine* (Sandoz) |

**Indications**
 *Age-related mental capacity decline:* Individuals older than 60 years of age who manifest signs and symptoms of an idiopathic decline in mental capacity. Patients who respond suffer from some process related to aging or have some underlying dementing condition.

**Administration and Dosage**
 The usual starting dose is 1 mg 3 times/day. Alleviation of symptoms usually is gradual; results may not be observed for 3 to 4 weeks. Doses up to 4.5 to 12 mg/day have been used. Up to 6 months of treatment may be necessary to determine efficacy, using doses of 6 mg/day or more. Do not chew or crush sublingual tablets.

**Actions**
 *Pharmacology:* Ergoloid mesylates contain equal proportions of dihydroergocornine mesylate, dihydroergocristine mesylate, and dihydroergocryptine mesylate.
 The mechanism by which ergoloid mesylates produce mental effects is unknown.

 *Pharmacokinetics:* Ergoloid mesylates are rapidly absorbed from the GI tract; peak plasma concentrations are achieved within 0.6 to 3 hours. The liquid capsule has a 12% greater bioavailability than the oral tablet. The mean half-life of unchanged ergoloid in plasma is about 2.6 to 5.1 hours.

**Contraindications**
 Hypersensitivity to ergoloid mesylates.

 Acute or chronic psychosis, regardless of etiology.

**Precautions**
 *Before prescribing:* Before prescribing ergoloid mesylates, exclude the possibility that the patient's signs and symptoms arise from a potentially reversible and treatable condition. Exclude delirium and dementiform illness secondary to systemic disease, primary neurological disease, or primary disturbance of mood.

 *Reassessment:* Periodically reassess the diagnosis and the benefit of current therapy to the patient.

**Adverse Reactions**
 Adverse reactions may include sublingual irritation; transient nausea and GI disturbances.

# ATOMOXETINE HCl

**Capsules:** 10, 18, 25, 40, and 60 mg (as base) *(Rx)*          *Strattera* (Eli Lilly)

## Indications
*Attention-deficit/hyperactivity disorder (ADHD):* For the treatment of ADHD.

## Administration and Dosage
The safety of single doses over 120 mg and total daily doses above 150 mg have not been systematically evaluated.

*Initial treatment:*
   *Children up to 70 kg* – Initiate at a total daily dose of approximately 0.5 mg/kg and increase after a minimum of 3 days to a target total daily dose of approximately 1.2 mg/kg administered as a single daily dose in the morning or as evenly divided doses in the morning and late afternoon/early evening. No additional benefit has been demonstrated for doses higher than 1.2 mg/kg/day. The total daily dose in children and adolescents should not exceed 1.4 mg/kg or 100 mg, whichever is less.

   *Adults and children over 70 kg* – Initiate at a total daily dose of 40 mg and increase after a minimum of 3 days to a target total daily dose of approximately 80 mg administered as a single daily dose in the morning or as evenly divided doses in the morning and late afternoon/early evening. After 2 to 4 additional weeks, the dose may be increased to a maximum of 100 mg in patients who have not achieved an optimal response. There are no data that support increased effectiveness at higher doses. The maximum recommended total daily dose in children over 70 kg and adults is 100 mg.

*Maintenance treatment:* There is no evidence available from controlled trials to indicate how long the patient with ADHD should be treated with atomoxetine. However, pharmacological treatment of ADHD may be needed for extended periods. Periodically re-evaluate the long-term usefulness of the drug for the individual patient.

*Hepatic function impairment:* For patients with moderate hepatic function impairment (Child-Pugh Class B), reduce initial and target doses to 50% of the normal dose. For patients with severe hepatic function impairment (Child-Pugh Class C), reduce initial and target doses to 25% of normal.

*Concomitant use:* In children up to 70 kg body weight administered strong CYP2D6 inhibitors, initiate atomoxetine at 0.5 mg/kg/day and only increase to the usual target dose of 1.2 mg/kg/day if symptoms fail to improve after 4 weeks and the initial dose is well-tolerated.

   In children over 70 kg body weight and adults administered strong CYP2D6 inhibitors, initiate atomoxetine at 40 mg/day and only increase to the usual target dose of 80 mg/day if symptoms fail to improve after 4 weeks and the initial dose is well-tolerated.

*Discontinuation:* Atomoxetine can be discontinued without being tapered.

## Actions
*Pharmacology:* Atomoxetine is a selective norepinephrine reuptake inhibitor. The precise mechanism by which it produces its therapeutic effects in ADHD is unknown, but it is thought to be related to selective inhibition of the presynaptic norepinephrine transporter, as determined in ex vivo uptake and neurotransmitter depletion studies.

*Pharmacokinetics:*
   *Absorption/Distribution* – Atomoxetine is well absorbed after oral administration and is minimally affected by food. It is rapidly absorbed after oral administration, with absolute bioavailability of about 63% in extensive metabolizers (EMs) and 94% in poor metabolizers (PMs). Maximal plasma concentrations ($C_{max}$) are reached approximately 1 to 2 hours after dosing. At therapeutic concentrations, 98% of atomoxetine in plasma is bound to protein, primarily albumin.

   *Metabolism/Excretion* – Atomoxetine is metabolized primarily through the CYP2D6 enzymatic pathway. In adult EMs, mean half-life is 5.2 hours. In PMs, mean half-life is 21.6 hours.

Atomoxetine is excreted primarily as 4-hydroxyatomoxetine-O-glucuronide, mainly in the urine (greater than 80%) and to a lesser extent in the feces (less than 17%).

*Special populations –*

*Hepatic function impairment:* Atomoxetine exposure (AUC) is increased, compared with normal subjects, in EM subjects with moderate (Child-Pugh Class B) (2-fold increase) and severe (Child-Pugh Class C) (4-fold increase) hepatic insufficiency. Dosage adjustment is recommended for patients with moderate or severe hepatic insufficiency (see Administration and Dosage).

## Contraindications

Patients known to be hypersensitive to atomoxetine or other constituents of the product; with a monoamine oxidase inhibitor (MAOI) or within 2 weeks after discontinuing an MAOI; narrow angle glaucoma (see Warnings).

## Warnings

*Long-term use:* The effectiveness of atomoxetine for long-term use (ie, for more than 9 weeks in child and adolescent patients and 10 weeks in adult patients) has not been systematically evaluated in controlled trials. Therefore, periodically re-evaluate the long-term usefulness of the drug for the individual patient.

*MAOIs:* Do not take atomoxetine with an MAOI or within 2 weeks after discontinuing an MAOI. Do not initiate treatment with an MAOI within 2 weeks after discontinuing atomoxetine. With other drugs that affect brain monoamine concentrations, there have been reports of serious, sometimes fatal, reactions (eg, hyperthermia, rigidity, myoclonus, autonomic instability with possible rapid fluctuations of vital signs, mental status changes that include extreme agitation progressing to delirium and coma) when taken in combination with an MAOI. Some cases presented with features resembling neuroleptic malignant syndrome. Such reactions may occur when these drugs are given concomitantly or in close proximity.

*Narrow angle glaucoma:* In clinical trials, atomoxetine use was associated with an increased risk of mydriasis; therefore, its use is not recommended in patients with narrow angle glaucoma.

*Growth:* Monitor growth during treatment with atomoxetine. During acute treatment studies (up to 9 weeks), atomoxetine-treated patients lost an average of 0.4 kg, while placebo patients gained an average of 1.5 kg. Weight and height were assessed during open-label studies of 12 and 18 months; mean rates of growth were compared with normal growth curves. Patients treated with atomoxetine for at least 18 months gained an average of 6.5 kg while mean weight percentile decreased slightly from 68 to 60. For this same group of patients, the average gain in height was 9.3 cm with a slight decrease in mean height percentile from 54 to 50. Whether final adult height or weight is affected by treatment with atomoxetine is unknown. Monitor patients requiring long-term therapy and consider interrupting therapy in patients who are not growing or gaining weight satisfactorily.

*Hypersensitivity reactions:* Although uncommon, allergic reactions (eg, angioneurotic edema, urticaria, rash) have been reported in patients taking atomoxetine.

*Pregnancy:* Category C.

*Lactation:* Atomoxetine and/or its metabolites were excreted in the milk of rats. It is not known if atomoxetine is excreted in human milk. Exercise caution if atomoxetine is administered to a nursing woman.

*Children:* The safety and efficacy of atomoxetine in pediatric patients less than 6 years of age have not been established. The efficacy of atomoxetine beyond 9 weeks and safety of atomoxetine beyond 1 year of treatment have not been systematically evaluated.

## Precautions

*Cardiac effects:* Use atomoxetine with caution in patients with hypertension, tachycardia, or cardiovascular or cerebrovascular disease because it can increase blood pressure and heart rate. Measure pulse and blood pressure at baseline, following dose increases, and periodically while on therapy.

*Urinary retention/hesitancy:* In adult ADHD controlled trials, the rates of urinary retention and urinary hesitation (3%, 7/269) were increased among atomoxetine subjects compared with placebo subjects (0%, 0/263). Consider a complaint of urinary retention or urinary hesitancy to be potentially related to atomoxetine.

*CYP2D6 metabolism:* PMs of CYP2D6 have a 10-fold higher AUC and a 5-fold higher peak concentration to a given dose of atomoxetine compared with EMs. Approximately 7% of the Caucasian population are PMs. The higher blood levels in PMs lead to a higher rate of some adverse events of atomoxetine.

*Sexual dysfunction:* Atomoxetine appears to impair sexual function in some patients. Changes in sexual desire, performance, and satisfaction are not well assessed in most clinical trials because they need special attention and because patients and physicians may be reluctant to discuss them. Accordingly, estimates of the incidence of untoward sexual experience and performance cited in product labeling are likely to underestimate the actual incidence.

### Drug Interactions
Drugs that may interact with atomoxetine include albuterol, CYP2D6 inhibitors, MAOIs, and pressor agents.

### Adverse Reactions
*Children and adolescents:*

*Commonly observed adverse events:* The most commonly observed adverse events in patients treated with atomoxetine were the following: Dyspepsia, nausea, vomiting, fatigue, decreased appetite, dizziness, mood swings.

Adverse events observed in at least 3% of patients in child and adolescent trials included the following: Headache, irritability, somonolence, dizziness (excluding vertigo), abdominal pain upper, appetite decreased, vomiting, dyspepsia, constipation, diarrhea, cough, rhinorrhea, dermatitis, fatigue, ear infection, influenza.

*Poor CYP2D6 metabolizers:* The following adverse events occurred in at least 2% of PM patients and were twice as frequent or statistically significantly more frequent in PM patients compared with EM patients: Decreased appetite, insomnia, sedation, depression, tremor, early morning awakening, pruritus, mydriasis.

*Adults:* Adverse events observed in at least 3% of patients in adult trials included the following: Palpitations, hot flushes, headache, insomnia and/or middle insomnia, dizziness, libido decreased, abnormal dreams, paresthesia, sleep disorder, sinus headache, sweating increased, dry mouth, nausea, appetite decreased, constipation, dyspepsia, urinary hesitation and/or urinary retention and/or difficulty in micturition, dysmenorrhea, erectile disturbance, ejaculation failure and/or ejaculation disorder, impotence, menstrual disorder, prostatitis, fatigue and/or lethargy, sinusitis, myalgia, pyrexia, rigors.

# OLANZAPINE AND FLUOXETINE HCl

**Capsules**: 6 mg olanzipine/25 mg fluoxetine, 6 mg olanzap-    *Symbyax* (Eli Lilly)
ine/50 mg fluoxetine, 12 mg olanzapine/25 fluoxetine, 12 mg
olanzapine/50 mg fluoxetine (*Rx*)

## Indications

*Bipolar disorder:* For the treatment of depressive episodes associated with bipolar disorder.

## Administration and Dosage

Administer once daily in the evening, generally beginning with the 6 mg/25 mg capsule. While food has no appreciable effect on the absorption of olanzapine and
fluoxetine given individually, the effect of food on the absorption of olanzapine/
fluoxetine has not been studied. Dosage adjustments, if indicated, can be made
according to efficacy and tolerability. Antidepressant efficacy was demonstrated with
olanzapine/fluoxetine in a dose range of olanzapine 6 to 12 mg and fluoxetine 25
to 50 mg. The safety of doses above 18 mg/75 mg has not been evaluated in clinical studies.

*Special populations:* Use a starting dose of 6 mg/25 mg for patients with a predisposition
to hypotensive reactions, patients with hepatic impairment, or patients who exhibit
a combination of factors that may slow the metabolism of olanzapine/fluoxetine
(eg, female gender, elderly, nonsmoking status). When indicated, perform dose escalation with caution in these patients. Olanzapine/fluoxetine has not been systemically studied in patients older than 65 years of age or in patients younger than
18 years of age.

# SEDATIVES/HYPNOTICS, NONBARBITURATE

To facilitate comparison, the products are divided into the following 2 groups: Miscellaneous nonbarbiturates and benzodiazepines. Although sedative doses can be given, these agents primarily are intended to be hypnotics.

In the table below, some pharmacokinetic properties of the nonbarbiturate sedative/hypnotics are compared. Do not use this table to predict exact duration of effect, but use as a guide in drug selection.

| Nonbarbiturate Sedative/Hypnotics Pharmacokinetic Parameters | | | | | | | |
|---|---|---|---|---|---|---|---|
| | Adult oral dose | | Onset (min) | Duration of action (h) | Half-life (h) | Protein binding (%) | Urinary excretion, unchanged (%) |
| Drug | Hypnotic | Sedative | | | | | |
| Miscellaneous nonbarbiturates | | | | | | | |
| Chloral hydrate | 0.5 to 1 g | 250 mg tid pc | 30 | nd | 7 to 10[1] | 35-41 | nd |
| Ethchlorvynol | 500 mg | 100 to 200 mg bid or tid | 15 to 60 | 5 | 10 to 20[2] | nd | 40[3] |
| Paraldehyde | 10 to 30 mL | 5 to 10 mL | 10 to 15 | 8 to 12 | 3.4 to 9.8 | nd | small |
| Propiomazine | nd | 10 to 20 mg | nd | nd | nd | nd | nd |
| Benzodiazepines | | | | | | | |
| Estazolam | 1 to 2 mg | na | nd | nd | 10 to 24 | 93 | < 5 |
| Flurazepam | 15 to 30 mg | na | 17 | 7 to 8 | 150 to 100[4] | 97 | < 1[4] |
| Quazepam | 15 mg | na | nd | nd | 25 to 41 | > 95 | trace |
| Temazepam | 15 to 30 mg | na | nd | nd | 10 to 17 | 98 | 1.5 |
| Triazolam | 0.125 to 0.5 mg | na | nd | nd | 1.5 to 5.5 | 90 | 2 |

[1] Trichloroethanol, the principal metabolite.
[2] In acute use, half-life of the distribution phase (1 to 3 hours) is more appropriate.
[3] Free and conjugated forms of the major metabolite, secondary alcohol of ethchlorvynol.
[4] Active metabolite, desalkylflurazepam.
ˉ na = Not applicable.
ˉ nd = No data.

# ZOLPIDEM TARTRATE

**Tablets:** 5 and 10 mg (c-IV)        *Ambien* (Searle)

### Indications
*Insomnia:* For the short-term treatment of insomnia.

### Administration and Dosage
*Adults:* Individualize dosage. Usual dose is 10 mg immediately before bedtime.
Downward dosage adjustment may be necessary when given with agents having known CNS-depressant effects because of the potentially additive effects.

*Elderly or debilitated patients:* Elderly or debilitated patients may be especially sensitive to the effects of zolpidem. Patients with hepatic insufficiency do not clear the drug as rapidly as healthy individuals. An initial 5 mg dose is recommended in these patients.

*Maximum dose:* The total dose should not exceed 10 mg.

### Actions
*Pharmacology:* Zolpidem is a nonbenzodiazepine hypnotic. While zolpidem is a hypnotic agent with a chemical structure unrelated to benzodiazepines, barbiturates, or other drugs with known hypnotic properties, it interacts with a GABA-BZ receptor complex and shares some of the pharmacological properties of the benzodiazepines.

*Pharmacokinetics:* The pharmacokinetic profile is characterized by rapid absorption from the GI tract and a short elimination half-life. Zolpidem is converted to inactive metabolites that are eliminated primarily by renal excretion.

## Warnings

*Duration of therapy:* Generally limit hypnotics to 7 to 10 days of use; re-evaluate the patient if they are to be taken for more than 2 to 3 weeks. Do not prescribe in quantities exceeding a 1 month supply.

*Psychiatric/Physical disorder:* Because sleep disturbances may be the presenting manifestation of a physical or psychiatric disorder, initiate symptomatic treatment of insomnia only after a careful evaluation of the patient.

*Abrupt discontinuation:* Following the rapid dose decrease or abrupt discontinuation of sedative/hypnotics, signs and symptoms similar to those associated with withdrawal from other CNS-depressant drugs have occurred.

*CNS-depressant effects:* Zolpidem, like other sedative/hypnotic drugs, has CNS-depressant effects. Because of the rapid onset of action, only ingest immediately prior to going to bed. Zolpidem had additive effects when combined with alcohol; therefore, do not take with alcohol.

*Renal function impairment:* Data in end-stage renal failure patients repeatedly treated with zolpidem did not demonstrate drug accumulation or alterations in pharmacokinetic parameters. No dosage adjustment in renally impaired patients is required; however, closely monitor these patients.

*Hepatic function impairment:* Modify dosing accordingly in patients with hepatic insufficiency.

*Elderly:* Closely monitor these patients. Impaired motor or cognitive performance after repeated exposure or unusual sensitivity to sedative/hypnotic drugs is a concern in the treatment of elderly or debilitated patients.

*Pregnancy:* Category B.

*Lactation:* The use of zolpidem in nursing mothers is not recommended.

*Children:* Safety and efficacy in children younger than 18 years of age have not been established.

## Precautions

*Respiratory depression:* Although preliminary studies did not reveal respiratory depressant effects at hypnotic doses in healthy individuals, observe caution if zolpidem is prescribed to patients with compromised respiratory function, since sedative/hypnotics have the capacity to depress respiratory drive.

*Depression:* As with other sedative/hypnotic drugs, administer zolpidem with caution to patients exhibiting signs or symptoms of depression. Suicidal tendencies may be present in such patients and protective measures may be required. Intentional overdosage is more common in this group of patients; therefore, prescribe the least amount of drug that is feasible for the patient at any one time.

*Drug abuse and dependence:* Sedative/hypnotics have produced withdrawal signs and symptoms following abrupt discontinuation. These reported symptoms range from mild dysphoria and insomnia to a withdrawal syndrome that may include abdominal and muscle cramps, vomiting, sweating, tremors, and convulsions. Zolpidem does not reveal any clear evidence for withdrawal syndrome.

Because individuals with a history of addiction to, or abuse of, drugs or alcohol are at risk of habituation and dependence, they should be under careful surveillance when receiving zolpidem or any other hypnotic.

## Drug Interactions

*Drug/Food interactions:* For faster sleep onset, do not administer with or immediately after a meal.

## Adverse Reactions

Adverse reactions occurring in 3% or more of patients include dizziness; drugged feelings; headache; allergy; back pain; headache; drowsiness; dizziness; lethargy; nausea; dyspepsia; diarrhea; myalgia; arthralgia; upper respiratory tract infection; sinusitis; pharyngitis; dry mouth.

# ZALEPLON

**Capsules:** 5 and 10 mg (c-iv)                    *Sonata* (Wyeth-Ayerst)

## Indications

*Insomnia:* For the short-term treatment of insomnia.

## Administration and Dosage

The recommended dose of zaleplon for most nonelderly adults is 10 mg. For certain low-weight individuals, 5 mg may be a sufficient dose. Although the risk of certain adverse events associated with zaleplon appears to be dose dependent, the 20 mg dose has been shown to be adequately tolerated and may be considered for the occasional patient who does not benefit from a trial of a lower dose. Doses greater than 20 mg have not been adequately evaluated and are not recommended. Hypnotics should generally be limited to 7 to 10 days of use, and re-evaluation of the patient is recommended if they are to be taken for longer than 2 to 3 weeks.

Take zaleplon immediately before bedtime or after going to bed and experiencing difficulty falling asleep. Taking it with or immediately after a heavy, high-fat meal results in slower absorption and would be expected to reduce the effect of zaleplon on sleep latency.

*Elderly/Debilitated:* Elderly and debilitated patients appear to be more sensitive to the effects of hypnotics; therefore, the recommended dose for these patients is 5 mg. Doses larger than 10 mg are not recommended.

*Hepatic function impairment:* Treat patients with mild to moderate hepatic impairment with zaleplon 5 mg because of reduced clearance. Do not use in patients with severe hepatic impairment.

*Renal function impairment:* No dose adjustment is necessary in patients with mild to moderate renal impairment.

*Concomitant cimetidine* – Give an initial dose of 5 mg to patients concomitantly taking cimetidine (see Drug Interactions).

## Actions

*Pharmacology:* Zaleplon is a nonbenzodiazepine hypnotic. Zaleplon has a chemical structure unrelated to benzodiazepines, barbiturates, or other drugs with known hypnotic properties.

Zaleplon binds selectively to the brain omega$_1$ receptor situated on the alpha subunit of the GABA$_A$ receptor complex and potentiates t-butyl-bicyclophosphorothionate (TBPS) binding.

*Pharmacokinetics:*

*Absorption* – Zaleplon is rapidly and almost completely absorbed following oral administration. Peak plasma concentrations are attained within approximately 1 hour after oral administration.

*Distribution* – Zaleplon is a lipophilic compound with a volume of distribution of approximately 1.4 L/kg following IV administration, indicating substantial distribution into extravascular tissues.

*Metabolism* – After oral administration, zaleplon is extensively metabolized with less than 1% of the dose excreted unchanged in urine.

*Excretion* – Following oral or IV administration, zaleplon is rapidly eliminated with a mean half-life of approximately 1 hour.

## Contraindications

None known.

## Warnings

*Duration of therapy:* Because sleep disturbances may be the presenting manifestation of a physical or psychiatric disorder, initiate symptomatic treatment of insomnia only after careful evaluation of the patient. The failure of insomnia to remit after 7 to 10 days of treatment may indicate the need for evaluation of a primary psychiatric or medical illness. Do not prescribe zaleplon in quantities exceeding a 1-month supply.

*Abnormal thinking/behavior changes:* A variety of abnormal thinking and behavior changes have been reported to occur in association with the use of sedatives/hypnotics.

*Rapid dose decrease/discontinuation:* Following rapid dose decrease or abrupt discontinuation of sedatives/hypnotics, there have been reports of signs and symptoms similar to those associated with withdrawal from other CNS-depressant drugs.

*CNS effects:* Zaleplon, like other hypnotics, has CNS-depressant effects. Caution patients receiving zaleplon against engaging in hazardous occupations requiring complete mental alertness or motor coordination (eg, operating machinery or driving a motor vehicle) after ingesting the drug, including potential impairment of the performance of such activities that may occur the day following zaleplon ingestion. Zaleplon, as well as other hypnotics, may produce additive CNS-depressant effects when coadministered with other psychotropic medications, anticonvulsants, antihistamines, ethanol, and other drugs that produce CNS depression. Do not take zaleplon with alcohol.

*Hepatic function impairment:* Zaleplon is metabolized primarily by the liver and undergoes significant presystemic metabolism. Consequently, the oral clearance of zaleplon was reduced by 70% and 87% in compensated and decompensated cirrhotic patients, respectively.

*Elderly:* Impaired motor or cognitive performance after repeated exposure or unusual sensitivity to sedative/hypnotic drugs is a concern in the treatment of elderly or debilitated patients.

*Pregnancy:* Category C.

*Lactation:* Because the effects of zaleplon on a nursing infant are not known, it is recommended that nursing mothers not take zaleplon.

*Children:* The safety and efficacy have not been established.

**Precautions**

*Timing of drug administration:* Take zaleplon immediately before bedtime or after going to bed and experiencing difficulty falling asleep. As with all sedatives/hypnotics, taking zaleplon while ambulatory may result in short-term memory impairment, hallucinations, impaired coordination, dizziness, and lightheadedness.

*Respiratory effects:* Although preliminary studies did not reveal respiratory depressant effects at hypnotic doses of zaleplon in healthy subjects, observe caution if zaleplon is prescribed to patients with compromised respiratory function because sedatives/hypnotics have the capacity to depress respiratory drive.

*Depression:* As with other sedative/hypnotic drugs, administer zaleplon with caution to patients exhibiting signs or symptoms of depression. Suicidal tendencies may be present in such patients and protective measures may be required. Intentional overdosage is more common in this group of patients; therefore, prescribe the least amount of the drug that is feasible for the patient at any one time.

*Drug abuse and dependence:*
   *Abuse* – Two studies assessed the abuse liability of zaleplon at doses of 25, 50, and 75 mg in subjects with known histories of sedative drug abuse. The results of these studies indicate that zaleplon has an abuse potential similar to benzodiazepine and benzodiazepine-like hypnotics.

**Drug Interactions**

*Drugs that induce CYP3A4:* CYP3A4 is a minor metabolizing enzyme of zaleplon. The CYP3A4-inducer rifampin reduced zaleplon $C_{max}$ and AUC by approximately 80%.

*Cimetidine:* Cimetidine inhibits aldehyde oxidase and CYP3A4, the primary and secondary enzymes, respectively, responsible for zaleplon metabolism. Use an initial dose of 5 mg for patients concomitantly treated with cimetidine.

*Drug/Food interactions:* The effects of zaleplon on sleep onset may be reduced if it is taken with or immediately after a high-fat/heavy meal.

**Adverse Reactions**

Adverse effects occurring in 3% or more of patients include the following: Amnesia; anxiety; dizziness; paresthesia; somnolence; dyspepsia; nausea; eye pain; abdominal pain; asthenia; headache; myalgia; dysmenorrhea.

# BENZODIAZEPINES

| | |
|---|---|
| **ESTAZOLAM** | |
| **Tablets:** 1 and 2 mg (c-IV) | *ProSom* (Abbott) |
| **FLURAZEPAM HCl** | |
| **Capsules:** 15 and 30 mg (c-IV) | Various, *Dalmane* (Valeant) |
| **QUAZEPAM** | |
| **Tablets:** 7.5 and 15 mg (c-IV) | *Doral* (Wallace) |
| **TEMAZEPAM** | |
| **Capsules:** 7.5, 15, and 30 mg (c-IV) | Various, *Restoril* (Sandoz) |
| **TRIAZOLAM** | |
| **Tablets:** 0.125 and 0.25 mg (c-IV) | Various, *Halcion* (Pharmacia) |

**Indications**

*Insomnia:* Insomnia characterized by difficulty in falling asleep, frequent nocturnal awakenings, or early morning awakening. Can be used for recurring insomnia or poor sleeping habits and in acute or chronic medical situations requiring restful sleep.

**Administration and Dosage**

ESTAZOLAM:

*Adults* – 1 mg at bedtime; however, some patients may need a 2 mg dose.

*Elderly* – If healthy, 1 mg at bedtime; initiate increases with particular care.

*Debilitated or small elderly patients* – Consider a starting dose of 0.5 mg, although this is only marginally effective in the overall elderly population.

FLURAZEPAM:

*Adults* – 30 mg before bedtime. In some patients, 15 mg may suffice.

*Elderly or debilitated* – Initiate with 15 mg until individual response is determined.

QUAZEPAM:

*Adults* – Initiate at 15 mg until individual responses are determined; may reduce to 7.5 mg in some patients.

*Elderly or debilitated* – Attempt to reduce nightly dosage after the first 1 or 2 nights.

TEMAZEPAM:

*Adults* – Give 15 to 30 mg before bedtime.

*Elderly or debilitated* – Initiate with 15 mg until individual response is determined.

TRIAZOLAM:

*Adults* – 0.125 to 0.5 mg before bedtime.

*Elderly or debilitated* – 0.125 to 0.25 mg. Initiate with 0.125 mg until individual response is determined.

**Actions**

*Pharmacology:* **Estazolam, flurazepam, quazepam, temazepam,** and **triazolam** are benzodiazepine derivatives useful as hypnotics. Benzodiazepines are believed to potentiate gamma aminobutyric acid (GABA) neuronal inhibition.

*Pharmacokinetics:*

| Select Benzodiazepine (Hypnotic) Pharmacokinetic Parameters | | | | |
|---|---|---|---|---|
| Drug | Usual adult oral dose (mg) | Time to peak plasma levels (h) | Half-life (h) | Protein binding (%) | Urinary excretion, unchanged (%) |
| Estazolam | 1 to 2 | 2 | 8 to 28 | 93 | < 5 |
| Flurazepam | 15 to 30 | 0.5 to 1 (7.6 to 13.6)[1] | 2 to 3 (47 to 100)[1] | 97 | < 1 |
| Quazepam | 7.5 to 15 | 2 (1 to 2) | 41 (47 to 100)[1] | > 95 | trace |

| Select Benzodiazepine (Hypnotic) Pharmacokinetic Parameters | | | | | |
|---|---|---|---|---|---|
| Drug | Usual adult oral dose (mg) | Time to peak plasma levels (h) | Half-life (h) | Protein binding (%) | Urinary excretion, unchanged (%) |
| Temaze-pam | 15 to 30 | 1.2 to 1.6 | 3.5 to 18.4 (9 to 15) | 96 | 0.2 |
| Triazolam | 0.125 to 0.5 | 1 to 2 | 1.5 to 5.5 | 78 to 89 | 2 |

[1] N-desalkylflurazepam, active metabolite.

## Contraindications

Hypersensitivity to other benzodiazepines; pregnancy (see Warnings); established or suspected sleep apnea (**quazepam**).

Concurrent use with ketoconazole, itraconazole, and nefazodone, medications that significantly impair the oxidative metabolism of **triazolam** mediated by cytochrome P450 3A (CYP3A).

## Warnings

*Anterograde amnesia:* Anterograde amnesia of varying severity and paradoxical reactions has occurred following therapeutic doses of **triazolam**. Although this effect generally occurred with a dose of 0.5 mg, it has also been reported with 0.125 and 0.25 mg doses. This effect may occur with some other benzodiazepines, but data suggest that it may occur at a higher rate with triazolam. Cases of "traveler's amnesia" have been reported by individuals who have taken triazolam to induce sleep while traveling.

*Renal/Hepatic function impairment:* Observe usual precautions under these conditions. Abnormal liver function tests as well as blood dyscrasias have been reported with benzodiazepines.

*Elderly:* The risk of developing oversedation, dizziness, confusion, or ataxia increases substantially with larger doses of benzodiazepines in elderly and debilitated patients. Initiate with lowest effective dose.

*Pregnancy: Category* X (estazolam, quazepam, temazepam, triazolam, flurazepam).

*Lactation:* Safety for use in the nursing mother has not been established.

*Children:*
> *Flurazepam* – Not for use in children younger than 15 years of age.
> *Estazolam, quazepam, temazepam, triazolam* – Not for use in children younger than 18 years of age.

## Precautions

*Monitoring:* When **triazolam** or **estazolam** treatment is protracted, obtain periodic blood counts, urinalysis, and blood chemistry analyses.

*Depression:* Administer with caution in severely depressed patients or in those in whom there is evidence of latent depression or suicidal tendencies. Signs or symptoms of depression may be intensified by hypnotic drugs.

*Sleep disorder:* Rebound sleep disorder, which is characterized by recurrence of insomnia to levels worse than before treatment began, may occur following abrupt withdrawal of triazolam, usually during the first 1 to 3 nights. Gradual rather than abrupt discontinuation of the drug may help avoid this syndrome.

*Nocturnal sleep:* Disturbed nocturnal sleep may occur for the first or second night after discontinuing use.

*Morning insomnia:* Early morning insomnia, or early morning awakenings, appears to be more common with the use of short half-life agents (**temazepam, triazolam**) than agents with intermediate or long half-lives (**estazolam, flurazepam, quazepam**). However, daytime sleepiness appears to be more prevalent with the long half-life agents.

*Respiratory depression and sleep apnea:* Observe caution. In patients with compromised respiratory function, respiratory depression and sleep apnea have occurred.

*Drug abuse and dependence:* Withdrawal symptoms following abrupt discontinuation of benzodiazepines have occurred in patients receiving excessive doses over extended periods of time. Gradual withdrawal is preferred.

*Hazardous tasks:* Observe caution while driving or performing tasks requiring alertness.

## Drug Interactions

Drugs that may affect benzodiazepines include alcohol/CNS depressants, cimetidine, oral contraceptives, disulfiram, isoniazid, probenecid, rifampin, smoking, theophyllines, and macrolides.

Drugs that may be affected by benzodiazepines include digoxin, neuromuscular blocking agents (nondepolarizing), and phenytoin.

## Adverse Reactions

Adverse reactions include the following: Palpitations; chest pains; tachycardia; headache; nervousness; apprehension; irritability; confusion; euphoria; relaxed feeling; weakness; tremor; lack of concentration; coordination disorders; confusional states/ memory impairment; depression; dreaming/nightmares; insomnia; paresthesia; restlessness; tiredness; dysesthesia; heartburn; nausea; vomiting; diarrhea; constipation; GI pain; anorexia; taste alterations; dry mouth; body/joint pain; tinnitus; GU complaints; cramps/pain; congestion.

*Estazolam:* Other adverse reactions reported only for estazolam include the following: Somnolence (42%); asthenia (11%); hypokinesia (8%); hangover (3%); cold symptoms, lower extremity/back/abdominal pain (1% to 3%).

# SEDATIVES AND HYPNOTICS, BARBITURATE

| | |
|---|---|
| **AMOBARBITAL SODIUM** | |
| **Powder for injection:** (c-ɪɪ) | *Amytal Sodium* (Lilly) |
| **APROBARBITAL** | |
| **Elixir:** 40 mg/5 mL (c-ɪɪɪ) | *Alurate* (Roche) |
| **BUTABARBITAL SODIUM** | |
| **Tablets:** 15, 30, 50, and 100 mg (c-ɪɪɪ) | Various, *Butisol Sodium* (Wallace) |
| **Elixir:** 30 mg/5 mL (c-ɪɪɪ) | Various, *Butisol Sodium* (Wallace) |
| **MEPHOBARBITAL** | |
| **Tablets:** 32, 50, and 100 mg (c-ɪv) | *Mebaral* (Sanofi Winthrop) |
| **PENTOBARBITAL SODIUM** | |
| **Capsules:** 50 and 100 mg (c-ɪɪ) | Various, *Nembutal Sodium* (Abbott) |
| **Suppositories:** 30, 60, 120, and 200 mg (c-ɪɪɪ) | *Nembutal Sodium* (Abbott) |
| **Injection:** 50 mg/mL (c-ɪɪ) | *Pentobarbital Sodium* (Wyeth-Ayerst), *Nembutal Sodium* (Abbott) |
| **PHENOBARBITAL** | |
| **Tablets:** 15, 16, 30, 60, and 100 mg (c-ɪv) | Various, *Solfoton* (ECR Pharm.) |
| **Capsules:** 16 mg (c-ɪv) | *Solfoton* (ECR Pharm.) |
| **Elixir:** 15 mg/5 mL and 20 mg/5 mL (c-ɪv) | Various |
| **Injection:** 30, 60, 65, and 130 mg/mL (c-ɪv) | Various, *Luminal Sodium* (Sanofi Winthrop) |
| **SECOBARBITAL SODIUM** | |
| **Capsules:** 100 mg (c-ɪɪ) | Various, *Seconal Sodium Pulvules* (Lilly) |
| **Injection:** 50 mg/mL (c-ɪɪ) | *Secobarbital Sodium* (Wyeth-Ayerst) |
| **ORAL COMBINATIONS** | |
| **Capsules:** 50 mg amobarbital sodium and 50 mg secobarbital sodium; 100 mg amobarbital sodium and 100 mg secobarbital sodium (c-ɪɪ) | *Tuinal 100 mg Pulvules, Tuinal 200 mg Pulvules* (Lilly) |

The following general discussion of the barbiturates refers to their use as sedative-hyp-notic agents and as anticonvulsants.

### Indications

*Acute convulsive episodes:* Emergency control of certain acute convulsive episodes (eg, those associated with status epilepticus, cholera, eclampsia, meningitis, tetanus, and toxic reactions to strychnine or local anesthetics).

*Anticonvulsant (mephobarbital, phenobarbital):* Treatment of partial and generalized tonic-clonic and cortical focal seizures.

*Hypnotic:* Short-term treatment of insomnia, because barbiturates appear to lose their effectiveness in sleep induction and maintenance after 2 weeks. If insomnia persists, seek alternative therapy (including nondrug) for chronic insomnia.

*Preanesthetic:* Used as preanesthetic sedatives.

*Sedation:* Although traditionally used as nonspecific CNS depressants for daytime sedation, the barbiturates have generally been replaced by the benzodiazepines.

### Administration and Dosage

*IM injection:* IM injection of the sodium salts should be made deeply into a large muscle. Do not exceed 5 mL at any one site because of possible tissue irritation. Monitor patient's vital signs.

*IV:* Restrict to conditions in which other routes are not feasible, either because the patient is unconscious or resists, or because prompt action is imperative. Slow IV injection is essential; observe patients carefully during administration.

*Rectal administration:* Rectally administered barbiturates are absorbed from the colon and are used occasionally in infants for prolonged convulsive states, or when oral or parenteral administration may be undesirable.

*Elderly/Debilitated:* Reduce dosage because these patients may be more sensitive to barbiturates.

*Hepatic/Renal function impairment:* Reduce dosage.

AMOBARBITAL SODIUM: The maximum single dose for an adult is 1 g.

*Sedative* – The usual adult dosage is 30 to 50 mg 2 or 3 times/day.

*Hypnotic* – The usual adult dose is 65 to 200 mg.

*IM* – The average IM dose ranges from 65 to 500 mg.

*IV* – Do not exceed the rate of 50 mg/min. Ordinarily, 65 to 500 mg may be given to a child 6 to 12 years of age.

*APROBARBITAL:*
    *Sedative* – 40 mg 3 times/day.
    *Mild insomnia* – 40 to 80 mg before retiring.
    *Pronounced insomnia* – 80 to 160 mg before retiring.

*BUTABARBITAL SODIUM:*
    *Adults* –
        *Daytime sedation:* 15 to 30 mg 3 or 4 times/day.
        *Bedtime hypnotic:* 50 to 100 mg
        *Preoperative sedation:* 50 to 100 mg, 60 to 90 minutes before surgery.
    *Children* –
        *Preoperative sedation:* 2 to 6 mg/kg/day (maximum 100 mg).

*MEPHOBARBITAL:*
    *Sedative* –
        *Adults:* 32 to 100 mg 3 or 4 times/day. Optimum dose is 50 mg 3 or 4 times/day.
        *Children:* 16 to 32 mg 3 or 4 times/day.
    *Epilepsy* –
        *Adults:* Average dose is 400 to 600 mg/day.
        *Children (younger than 5 years of age):* 16 to 32 mg 3 or 4 times/day.
        *Children (older than 5 years of age):* 32 to 64 mg 3 or 4 times/day.

Take at bedtime if seizures generally occur at night, and during the day if attacks are diurnal. Start treatment with a small dose and gradually increase over 4 or 5 days until optimum dosage is determined.

    *Combination drug therapy* – May be used in combination with phenobarbital, in alternating courses or concurrently. When the two are used at the same time, the dose should be approximately ½ the amount of each used alone. The average daily dose for an adult is 50 to 100 mg phenobarbital and 200 to 300 mg mephobarbital. May also be used with phenytoin. When used concurrently, a reduced dose of phenytoin is advisable, but the full dose of mephobarbital may be given. Satisfactory results have been obtained with an average daily dose of 230 mg phenytoin plus about 600 mg mephobarbital.

*PENTOBARBITAL SODIUM:*
    *Oral* –
        *Adults:*
            *Sedation* – 20 mg 3 or 4 times/day.
            *Hypnotic* – 100 mg at bedtime.
        *Children:*
            *Sedation/Preanesthetic* – 2 to 6 mg/kg/day (maximum 100 mg), depending on age, weight, and degree of sedation desired.
            *Hypnotic* – Base dosage on age and weight.
    *Rectal* – Do not divide suppositories.
        *Adults:* 120 to 200 mg.
        *Children:*
            *12 to 14 years of age (36.4 to 50 kg; 80 to 110 lbs)* – 60 or 120 mg.
            *5 to 12 years of age (18.2 to 36.4 kg; 40 to 80 lbs)* – 60 mg.
            *1 to 4 years of age (9 to 18.2 kg; 20 to 40 lbs)* – 30 or 60 mg.
            *2 months to 1 year of age (4.5 to 9 kg; 10 to 20 lbs)* – 30 mg.
    *Parenteral* –
        *IV:* Initially administer 100 mg in the 70 kg adult. Reduce dosage proportionally for pediatric or debilitated patients. At least 1 minute is necessary to determine the full effect. If needed, additional small increments of the drug may be given to a total of 200 to 500 mg for healthy adults.

IM: The usual adult dosage is 150 to 200 mg; children's dosage frequently ranges from 2 to 6 mg/kg as a single IM injection, not to exceed 100 mg.

PHENOBARBITAL:

*Anticonvulsant* – In infants and children, a loading dose of 15 to 20 mg/kg produces blood levels of approximately 20 mcg/mL shortly after administration.

Oral –

Adults:

*Sedation* – 30 to 120 mg/day in 2 to 3 divided doses. A single dose of 30 to 120 mg may be given at intervals; frequency is determined by response. It is generally considered that no more than 400 mg should be given during a 24-hour period.

*Hypnotic* – 100 to 200 mg.

*Anticonvulsant* – 60 to 100 mg/day.

Children:

*Anticonvulsant* – 3 to 6 mg/kg/day.

*Sedation* – 8 to 32 mg.

*Hypnotic* – Determined by age and weight.

Parenteral –

Adults:

*Sedation* – 30 to 120 mg/day IM or IV in 2 to 3 divided doses.

*Preoperative sedation* – 100 to 200 mg, IM only, 60 to 90 minutes before surgery.

*Hypnotic* – 100 to 320 mg IM or IV.

*Acute convulsions* – 200 to 320 mg IM or IV, repeat 6 hours as necessary.

Children:

*Preoperative sedation* – 1 to 3 mg/kg IM or IV.

*Anticonvulsant* – 4 to 6 mg/kg/day for 7 to 10 days to blood level of 10 to 15 mcg/mL, or 10 to 15 mg/kg/day, IV or IM.

*Status epilepticus* – 15 to 20 mg/kg IV over 10 to 15 minutes. It is imperative to achieve therapeutic levels as rapidly as possible. When given IV, it may require 15 minutes or longer to attain peak levels in the brain.

SECOBARBITAL SODIUM:

Oral –

Adults:

*Preoperative sedation* – 200 to 300 mg 1 to 2 hours before surgery.

*Bedtime hypnotic* – 100 mg.

Children: For preoperative sedation, 2 to 6 mg/kg (maximum 100 mg).

Parenteral –

Adults:

*Hypnotic* – Usual dose is 100 to 200 mg IM or 50 to 250 mg IV.

*Preoperative sedation* – For light sedation, 1 mg/kg (0.5 to 0.75 mg/lb) IM, 10 to 15 minutes before procedure.

*Dentistry* – In patients who are to receive nerve blocks, 100 to 150 mg IV.

Children:

*Preoperative sedation* – 4 to 5 mg/kg IM.

*Status epilepticus* – 15 to 20 mg/kg IV over 15 minutes.

## Actions

*Pharmacology:* These agents depress the sensory cortex, decrease motor activity, alter cerebellar function, and produce drowsiness, sedation, and hypnosis.

Barbiturates have little analgesic action at subanesthetic doses and may increase the reaction to painful stimuli. All barbiturates exhibit anticonvulsant activity in anesthetic doses. However, only phenobarbital and mephobarbital are effective as oral anticonvulsants in subhypnotic doses.

*Pharmacokinetics:*

| | Barbiturate | Half-Life (h) | | Oral dosage range (mg) | | Onset (minutes) | Duration (hours) |
|---|---|---|---|---|---|---|---|
| | | Range | Mean | Sedative[1] | Hypnotic | | |
| Long-acting | Mephobarbital | 11 to 67 | 34 | 32 to 200 | — | 30 to ≥ 60 | 10 to 16 |
| | Phenobarbital | 53 to 118 | 79 | 30 to 120 | 100 to 320 | | |
| Intermediate | Amobarbital[2] | 16 to 40 | 25 | — | — | 45 to 60 | 6 to 8 |
| | Aprobarbital | 14 to 34 | 24 | 120 | 40 to 160 | | |
| | Butabarbital | 66 to 140 | 100 | 45 to 120 | 50 to 100 | | |
| Short-acting | Pentobarbital | 15 to 50 | †[3] | 40 to 120 | 100 | 10 to 15 | 3 to 4 |
| | Secobarbital | 15 to 40 | 28 | — | 100 | | |

**Pharmacokinetics of Sedatives and Hypnotic Barbiturates**

[1] Total daily dose; administered in 2 to 4 divided doses.
[2] Available as injection only.
[3] May follow dose-dependent kinetics. Mean t½ is 50 hours for 50 mg and 22 hours for 100 mg.

## Contraindications

Barbiturate sensitivity; manifest or latent porphyria; marked impairment of liver function; severe respiratory disease when dyspnea or obstruction is evident; nephritic patients; patients with respiratory disease where dyspnea or obstruction is present; intra-arterial administration; subcutaneous administration; previous addiction to the sedative/hypnotic group.

## Warnings

*Habit forming:* Tolerance or psychological and physical dependence may occur with continued use. Administer with caution, if at all, to patients who are mentally depressed, have suicidal tendencies or a history of drug abuse. Limit prescribing and dispensing to the amount required for the interval until the next appointment.

*Withdrawal symptoms –* Withdrawal symptoms can be severe and may cause death.

*Treatment of dependence –* Treatment of dependence consists of cautious and gradual withdrawal of the drug that takes an extended period of time.

*IV administration:* Too rapid administration may cause respiratory depression, apnea, laryngospasm, or vasodilation with fall in blood pressure. Parenteral solutions of barbiturates are highly alkaline. Therefore, use extreme care to avoid perivascular extravasation or intra-arterial injection.

*Phenobarbital sodium –* Phenobarbital sodium may be administered IM or IV as an anticonvulsant for emergency use. When administered IV, it may require 15 minutes or more before reaching peak concentrations in the brain.

*Pain:* Exercise caution when administering to patients with acute or chronic pain, because paradoxical excitement could be induced or important symptoms could be masked.

*Seizure disorders:* Status epilepticus may result from abrupt discontinuation, even when administered in small daily doses in the treatment of epilepsy.

*Effects on vitamin D:* Barbiturates may increase vitamin D requirements, possibly by increasing the metabolism of vitamin D via enzyme induction.

*Renal function impairment:* Barbiturates are excreted either partially or completely unchanged in the urine and are contraindicated in impaired renal function.

*Hepatic function impairment:* Barbiturates are metabolized primarily by hepatic microsomal enzymes. Administer with caution and initially in reduced doses.

*Elderly:* May produce marked excitement, depression, and confusion.

*Pregnancy: Category D.*

*Lactation:* Exercise caution when administering to the nursing mother because small amounts are excreted in breast milk.

*Children:* In some people, especially children, barbiturates repeatedly produce excitement rather than depression. Barbiturates may produce irritability, excitability, inappropriate tearfulness, and aggression in children. Safety and efficacy of amobarbital (children younger than 5 years of age) and aprobarbital have not been established.

## Precautions

*Monitoring:* During prolonged therapy, perform periodic laboratory evaluation of organ systems, including hematopoietic, renal, and hepatic systems.

*Special risk patients:* Untoward reactions may occur in the presence of fever, hyperthyroidism, diabetes mellitus, and severe anemia. Use with caution.

Use **mephobarbital** with caution in myasthenia gravis and myxedema.

## Drug Interactions

Drugs that may affect barbiturates include alcohol, charcoal, chloramphenicol, MAO inhibitors, rifampin, and valproic acid. Drugs that may be affected by barbiturates include acetaminophen, anticoagulants, beta blockers, carbamazepine, chloramphenicol, clonazepam, oral contraceptives, corticosteroids, digitoxin, doxorubicin, doxycycline, felodipine, fenoprofen, griseofulvin, hydantoins, methoxyflurane, metronidazole, narcotics, phenmetrazine, phenylbutazone, quinidine, theophylline, and verapamil.

## Adverse Reactions

Adverse reactions may include somnolence; agitation; confusion; hyperkinesia; ataxia; CNS depression; nightmares; nervousness; psychiatric disturbance; hallucinations; insomnia; anxiety; dizziness; abnormal thinking; headache; fever (especially with chronic phenobarbital use); hypoventilation; apnea; bradycardia; hypotension; syncope; nausea; vomiting; constipation; liver damage, particularly with chronic phenobarbital use; skin rashes; angioedema (particularly following chronic phenobarbital use).

# ANTICONVULSANTS

| | Anticonvulsants: Indications and Pharmacokinetics | | | | | |
|---|---|---|---|---|---|---|
| | Drug | Labeled indications | Protein binding (%) | Metabolism/ Excretion | t½ (h) | Therapeutic serum levels (mcg/mL) |
| *Barbiturates* | Phenobarbital[1] (PB) | Status epilepticus Epilepsy, all forms Tonic-clonic | 40 to 60 | Liver; 25% eliminated unchanged in urine | 53 to 140 | 15 to 40 |
| *Hydantoins* | Phenytoin | Tonic-clonic Psychomotor | ≈90 | Liver; renal excretion. < 5% excreted unchanged | Dose-dependent[2] | 5 to 20 |
| *Hydantoins* | Mephenytoin | Tonic-clonic Psychomotor Focal Jacksonian | nd | Liver | 95 (active metabolite) | nd |
| *Hydantoins* | Ethotoin | Tonic-clonic Psychomotor | nd | Liver; renal excretion of metabolites | 3 to 9[3] | 15 to 50 |
| *Succinimides* | Ethosuximide | Absence | 0 | Liver; 25% excreted unchanged in urine | 30 (children 7 to 9 yrs) 40 to 60 (adults) | 40 to 100 |
| *Succinimides* | Methsuximide | Absence | nd | Liver; < 1% excreted unchanged in urine | < 2 (40, active metabolite) | nd |
| *Succinimides* | Phensuximide | Absence | nd | Urine, bile | 8 (active metabolite) | nd |
| *Sulfonamides* | Zonisamide | Partial[4] | 40 | Accetylation and reduction; excreted in urine | 63 | nd |
| *Oxazolidinediones* | Trimethadione | Absence | 0 | Demethylated to dimethadione; 3% excreted unchanged | 6 to 13 days (dimethadione) | ≥ 700 (dimethdione) |
| *Benzodiazepines* | Clonazepam | Absence Myoclonic Akinetic | 50 to 85 | 5 metabolites identified; urine is major excretion route | 18 to 60 | 20 to 80 ng/mL |
| *Benzodiazepines* | Clorazepate | Partial[4] | 97 | Hydrolyzed in stomach to desmethyldiazepam (active); metabolized in liver, renally excreted | 30 to 100 | nd |
| *Benzodiazepines* | Diazepam | Status epilepticus[4] Epilepsy, all forms[4] | 97 to 99 | Liver, active metabolites | 20 to 50 | nd |

**Anticonvulsants: Indications and Pharmacokinetics**

| Drug | | Labeled indications | Protein binding (%) | Metabolism/ Excretion | t½ (h) | Therapeutic serum levels (mcg/mL) |
|---|---|---|---|---|---|---|
| Miscellaneous | Primidone | Tonic-clonic Psychomotor Focal | 20 to 25 | Metabolized to PB and PEMA, both active | 5 to 15 (primidone) 10 to 18 (PEMA) 53 to 140 (PB) | 5 to 12 (primidone) 15 to 40 (PB) |
| | Valproic acid | Absence | 80 to 94 | Liver; excreted in urine | 5 to 20 | 50 to 150 |
| | Carbamazepine | Tonic-clonic Mixed Psychomotor | ≈ 75 | Liver to active 10, 11-epoxide. 72% excreted in urine, 28% in feces | 18 to 54 (initial) 10 to 20[5] ≈ 6 (10, 11-epoxide) | 4 to 12 |
| | Phenacemide | Severe mixed psychomotor | nd | Liver | nd | nd |
| | Felbamate[6] | Partial (adults) Partial/generalized assoc. with Lennox-Gastaut syndrome (children) | 22 to 25 | 40% to 50% unchanged in urine, 40% as unidentified metabolites and conjugates | 20 to 23 | nd[7] |
| | Oxcarbazepine | Partial | 40 | Reduced to 10-monohydroxy metabolite (active); excreted in urine (80%) | 2; 9 (MHD) | nd[7] |
| | Lamotrigine | Partial (adults) | ≈ 55 | Glucuronic acid conjugation to inactive metabolites; 94% excreted in urine, 2% in feces | ≈ 33[5] | nd |

[1] Other barbiturates are also used as anticonvulsants. See Sedatives/Hypnotics section.
[2] Exhibits dose-dependent, nonlinear pharmacokinetics.
[3] Below 8 mcg/mL; > 8 mcg/mL, t½ not defined because of dose-dependent, nonlinear pharmacokinetics.
[4] Recommended for adjunctive use.
[5] Undergoes autoinduction. Half-life after repeated doses.
[6] Because of cases of aplastic anemia, it has been recommended that the use of this drug be discontinued unless, in the judgment of the physician, continued therapy is warranted.
[7] Value of monitoring blood levels not established.

# HYDANTOINS

**ETHOTOIN**
**Tablets**: 250 and 500 mg (Rx) — *Peganone* (Abbott)
**FOSPHENYTOIN SODIUM**
**Injection**: 150 mg (100 mg phenytoin) and 750 mg (500 mg phenytoin) (Rx) — *Cerebyx* (Parke-Davis)
**PHENYTOIN, ORAL**
**Tablets, chewable**: 50 mg (Rx) — *Dilantin Infatab* (Parke-Davis)
**Oral suspension**: 30 and 125 mg/5 mL (Rx) — *Dilantin-30 or -125* (Parke-Davis)
**PHENYTOIN SODIUM, ORAL, PROMPT**
**Capsules**: 30 and 100 mg (Rx) — Various, *Diphenylan Sodium* (Lannett)
**PHENYTOIN SODIUM, EXTENDED**
**Capsules**: 30 and 100 mg (Rx) — *Dilantin Kapseals* (Parke-Davis)
**PHENYTOIN SODIUM, PARENTERAL**
**Injection**: 50 mg/mL (Rx) — Various, *Dilantin* (Parke-Davis)
**PHENYTOIN SODIUM WITH PHENOBARBITAL**
**Capsules**: 100 mg/16 and 32 mg (Rx) — *Dilantin with Phenobarbital Kapseals* (Parke-Davis)

**Indications**
Control of grand mal and psychomotor seizures.

*Phenytoin:* To prevent and treat seizures occurring during or following neurosurgery.
*Parenteral* – For the control of status epilepticus of the grand mal type.

## Administration and Dosage

ETHOTOIN: Administer in 4 to 6 divided doses/day. Take after food; space doses as evenly as practical.

Adults – The initial daily dose should be 1 g or less, with subsequent gradual dosage increases over several days. The usual adult maintenance dose is 2 to 3 g/day; less than 2 g/day is ineffective in most adults.

Pediatric – Initial dose should not exceed 750 mg/day. The usual maintenance dose in children ranges from 500 mg to 1 g/day, although occasionally 2 g or rarely 3 g/day may be necessary.

FOSPHENYTOIN: The dose, concentration in dosing solutions and infusion rate of IV fosphenytoin is expressed as phenytoin sodium equivalents (PE) to avoid the need to perform molecular weight-based adjustments when coverting between fosphenytoin and phenytoin sodium doses. Prescribe and dipense fosphenytoin in PEs. Fosphenytoin has important differences in administration from those for parenteral phenytoin sodium.

Dilute fosphenytoin in 5% Dextrose or 0.9% Saline Solution for Injection to a concentration ranging from 1.5 to 25 mg PE/mL.

Status epilepticus – The loading dose 15 to 20 mg PE/kg administered at 100 to 150 mg PE/min.

Because the full antiepileptic effect of phenytoin, whether given as fosphenytoin or parenteral phenytoin, is not immediate, other measures, including concomitant administration of an IV benzodiazepine, will usually be necessary for control of status epilepticus.

Nonemergent and maintenance dosing –

Loading dose: 10 to 20 mg PE/kg given IV or IM.

Maintenance dose: 4 to 6 mg PE/kg/day.

Because if the risk of hypotension, administer at a rate of 150 mg PE/min or less.

Continuously monitor the electrocardiogram, blood pressure, and respiratory function and observe the patient throughout the period of maximal serum phenytoin concentrations, approximately 10 to 20 minutes after the end of the infusion.

Renal/Hepatic function impairment – Because of an increased fraction of unbound phenytoin in patients with renal or hepatic disease, or in those with hypoalbuminemia, interpret total phenytoin plasma concentrations with caution. Unbound phenytoin concentrations may be more useful in these patients. After IV administration, fosphenytoin clearance to phenytoin may be increased without a similar increase in phenytoin clearance. This has the potential to increase the frequency and severity of adverse events.

Elderly – Age does not have a significant impact on the pharmacokinetics of fosphenytoin following administration. Phenytoin clearance is decreased slightly in elderly patients and lower or less frequent dosing may be required.

PHENYTOIN AND PHENYTOIN SODIUM, ORAL: Phenytoin sodium contains 92% phenytoin. Phenytoin and phenytoin sodium prompt are not for once/day dosing. Phenytoin sodium extended may be used for once/day dosing.

Loading dose – An oral loading dose of phenytoin may be used in adults who require rapid steady-state serum levels and where IV administration is not possible.

Initially, 1 g of phenytoin capsules is divided into 3 doses (400 mg, 300 mg, 300 mg) and administered at intervals of 2 hours. Normal maintenance dosage is then instituted 24 hours after the loading dose, with frequent serum level determinations.

Adults – Adults who have received no previous treatment may be started on 100 mg (125 mg suspension) 3 times/day. Satisfactory maintenance dosage is 300 to 400 mg/day. An increase to 600 mg/day (625 mg/day suspension) may be necessary.

Pediatric – Initially, 5 mg/kg/day in 2 or 3 equally divided doses with subsequent dosage individualized to a maximum of 300 mg/day. Daily maintenance dosage is 4 to 8 mg/kg. Children over 6 years may require the minimum adult dose (300 mg/day). If the daily dosage cannot be divided equally, give the larger dose before retiring.

*Single daily dosage* – In adults, if seizure control is established with divided doses of three 100 mg extended phenytoin sodium capsules daily, once/day dosage with 300 mg may be considered; patient compliance is essential on a once/day regimen. Only extended phenytoin sodium capsules are recommended once/day.

*Bioavailability* – Because of the potential bioavailability differences between products, brand interchange is not recommended. Dosage adjustments may be required when switching from the extended to the prompt products.

PHENYTOIN SODIUM, PARENTERAL:

*Status epilepticus* – In adults, administer loading dose of 10 to 15 mg/kg slowly. Follow by maintenance doses of 100 mg orally or IV every 6 to 8 hours. For neonates and children, oral absorption of phenytoin is unreliable; IV loading dose is 15 to 20 mg/kg in divided doses of 5 to 10 mg/kg.

*Neurosurgery (prophylactic dosage)* – 100 to 200 mg IM at approximately 4 hour intervals during surgery and the postoperative period.

## Actions

*Pharmacology:* The primary site of action of hydantoins appears to be the motor cortex, where spread of seizure activity is inhibited. Possibly by promoting sodium efflux from neurons, hydantoins tend to stabilize the threshold against hyperexcitability.

*Pharmacokinetics:*

*Absorption/Distribution* – Phenytoin is slowly absorbed from the small intestine. Rate and extent of absorption varies and is dependent on the product formulation. Bioavailability may differ among products of different manufacturers. Administration IM results in precipitation of phenytoin at the injection site, resulting in slow and erratic absorption, which may continue for up to 5 days or more. Plasma protein binding is 87% to 93% and is lower in uremic patients and neonates. Volume of distribution averages 0.6 L/kg.

Phenytoin's therapeutic plasma concentration is 10 to 20 mcg/mL, although many patients achieve complete seizure control at lower serum concentrations.

*Metabolism/Excretion* – Phenytoin is metabolized in the liver and excreted in the urine. The metabolism of phenytoin is capacity-limited and shows saturability. Elimination is exponential (first-order) at plasma concentrations less than 10 mcg/mL, and plasma half-life ranges from 6 to 24 hours.

## Contraindications

Hypersensitivity to hydantoins.

*Ethotoin:* Hepatic abnormalities or hematologic disorders.

*Phenytoin:* Because of its effect on ventricular automaticity, do not use phenytoin in sinus bradycardia, sino-atrial block, second- and third-degree AV block, or in patients with Adams-Stokes syndrome.

## Warnings

*Withdrawal:* Abrupt withdrawal in epileptic patients may precipitate status epilepticus.

*Other seizures:* Hydantoins are not indicated in seizures caused by hypoglycemia or other metabolic causes.

*Phenytoin:* Use with caution in hypotension and severe myocardial insufficiency.

*Hypersensitivity reactions:* Phenytoin hypersensitivity reactions are not typical; they may present as one of many different syndromes (eg, lymphoma, hepatitis, Stevens-Johnson syndrome) and may include such symptoms as fever, rash, arthralgias, or lymphadenopathy.

*Hepatic function impairment:* Biotransformation of hydantoins occurs in the liver; elderly patients or those with impaired liver function or severe illness may show early signs of toxicity.

*Induced abnormalities* – Phenytoin-induced hepatitis is one of the more commonly reported hypersensitivity syndromes.

*Pregnancy:* There is an association between use of anticonvulsant drugs by women with epilepsy and an elevated incidence of birth defects in children born to these women. The great majority of mothers receiving anticonvulsant medication deliver normal infants.

*Lactation:* These drugs are excreted in breast milk.

### Precautions

*Hematologic effects:* Perform blood counts and urinalyses when therapy is begun and at monthly intervals for several months thereafter. Blood dyscrasias have occurred.

*Dermatologic effects:* Discontinue these drugs if a skin rash appears. If the rash is exfoliative, purpuric, or bullous, do not resume use.

*Lymph node hyperplasia:* Lymph node hyperplasia has been associated with hydantoins, and may represent a hypersensitivity reaction.

*Hyperglycemia:* Hyperglycemia, resulting from the drug's inhibitory effect on insulin release, has occurred. Hydantoins also may raise blood sugar levels in hyperglycemic people.

*Cardiovascular:* Death from cardiac arrest has occurred after too-rapid IV administration, sometimes preceded by marked QRS widening. Administer cautiously in the presence of advanced AV block. Do not exceed an IV infusion rate of 50 mg/min.

*Osteomalacia:* Osteomalacia has been associated with phenytoin therapy.

*Acute intermittent porphyria:* Administer hydantoins cautiously to patients with acute intermittent porphyria.

### Drug Interactions

*Increased hydantoin effects:*

| Hydantoin Drug Interactions: Increased Hydantoin Effects | | | |
|---|---|---|---|
| Inhibit metabolism | | Displace anticonvulsant | Unknown |
| Amiodarone<br>Benzodiazepines<br>Chloramphenicol<br>Cimetidine<br>Disulfiram<br>Ethanol<br>(acute ingestion)<br>Fluconazole<br>Isoniazid | Metronidazole<br>Miconazole<br>Omeprazole<br>Phenacemide<br>Phenylbutazone<br>Succinimides<br>Sulfonamides<br>Trimethoprim<br>Valproic acid | Salicylates<br>Tricyclic antidepressants<br>Valproic acid | Chlorpheniramine<br>Ibuprofen<br>Phenothiazines |

*Decreased hydantoin effects:*

| Hydantoin Drug Interactions: Decreased Hydantoin Effects | | |
|---|---|---|
| Increase metabolism | Decrease absorption | Unknown |
| Barbiturates<br>Carbamazepine<br>Diazoxide<br>Ethanol<br>(chronic ingestion)<br>Rifampin<br>Theophylline | Antacids<br>Charcoal<br>Sucralfate | Antineoplastics<br>Folic acid<br>Influenza virus vaccine<br>Loxapine<br>Nitrofurantoin<br>Pyridoxine |

| Hydantoin Drug Interactions: Decreased Effects of Other Drugs | | |
|---|---|---|
| Increased metabolism by phenytoin | | Other |
| Acetaminophen<br>Amiodarone<br>Carbamazepine<br>Cardiac glycosides<br>Corticosteroids<br>Dicumarol<br>Disopyramide<br>Doxycycline<br>Estrogens | Haloperidol<br>Methadone<br>Metyrapone<br>Mexiletine<br>Oral contraceptives<br>Quinidine<br>Theophylline<br>Valproic acid | Cyclosporine<br>Dopamine<br>Furosemide<br>Levodopa<br>Levonorgestrel<br>Mebendazole<br>Nondepolarizing muscle relaxants<br>Phenothiazines<br>Sulfonylureas |

Drugs that may be affected by hydantoins include lithium, meperidine, primidone, and warfarin.

*Drug/Lab test interactions:* Phenytoin may interfere with the **metyrapone** and the 1 mg **dexamethasone** tests.

*Drug/Food interactions:* Several case reports and single-dose studies suggest that enteral nutritional therapy may decrease phenytoin concentrations; however, this has not been substantiated.

### Adverse Reactions
*Cardiovascular:*
> *Phenytoin IV* – Cardiovascular collapse; CNS depression; hypotension (when the drug is administered rapidly IV).

*CNS:* Nystagmus; ataxia; dysarthria; slurred speech; mental confusion; dizziness; insomnia; transient nervousness; motor twitchings; diplopia; fatigue; irritability; drowsiness; depression; numbness; tremor; headache.

*Dermatologic:* Manifestations sometimes accompanied by fever have included scarlatiniform, morbilliform, maculopapular, urticarial, and nonspecific rashes; a morbilliform rash is the most common.

*Endocrine:* Diabetes insipidus; hyperglycemia.

*GI:* Nausea; vomiting; diarrhea; constipation.

*GU:* Urinary retention; oliguria; dysuria; vaginitis; albuminuria; genital edema; kidney failure; polyuria; urethral pain; urinary incontinence; vaginal moniliasis.

*Hematologic:* Hematopoietic complications, some fatal, include thrombocytopenia, leukopenia, granulocytopenia, agranulocytosis, and pancytopenia. Macrocytosis and megaloblastic anemia usually respond to folic acid therapy. Eosinophilia; monocytosis; leukocytosis; simple anemia; hemolytic anemia; aplastic anemia; ecchymosis.

*Respiratory:* Pneumonia; pharyngitis; sinusitis; hyperventilation; rhinitis; apnea; aspiration pneumonia; asthma; dyspnea; atelectasis; increased cough/sputum; epistaxis; hypoxia; pneumothorax; hemoptysis; bronchitis; chest pain; pulmonary fibrosis.

*Special senses:* Tinnitus; diplopia; taste perversion; amblyopia; deafness; visual field defect; eye pain; conjunctivitis; photophobia; hyperacusis; mydriasis; parosmia; ear pain; taste loss.

*Lab test abnormalities:* Phenytoin may decrease serum thyroxine and free thyroxine concentrations.

*Miscellaneous:* Polyarthropathy; hyperglycemia; weight gain; chest pain; edema; fever; photophobia; conjunctivitis; gynecomastia.
> *Gingival hyperplasia* – Gingival hyperplasia occurs frequently with phenytoin.

# ZONISAMIDE

| **Capsules:** 25, 50, and 100 mg *(Rx)* | *Zonegran* (Eisai) |
| --- | --- |

### Indications
*Epilepsy:* Adjunctive therapy in the treatment of partial seizures in adults with epilepsy.

### Administration and Dosage
*Adults:* Individualize dose starting with 100 mg/day. The dose may be increased after at least 2 weeks to 200 mg/day. Additional dose increases to 300 and 400 mg/day may be made at 2-week intervals to achieve steady state. Administer zonisamide once or twice/day, except during the 100 mg dosage initiation. The prescriber may wish to prolong the duration of treatment at lower doses to fully assess the effects of zonisamide at steady state, noting that many of the side effects of zonisamide are more frequent at doses of 300 mg/day and above. Although there is some evidence of greater response at doses above 100 to 200 mg/day, the increase appears small, and formal dose-response studies have not been conducted. Evidence from con-

trolled trials suggests that zonisamide doses of 100 to 600 mg/day are effective, but there is no suggestion of increasing response above 400 mg/day. There is little experience with doses greater than 600 mg/day.

Zonisamide may be taken with or without food. Swallow the capsules whole. Use caution in patients with renal or hepatic disease.

*Discontinuation of therapy:* Abrupt withdrawal of zonisamide in patients with epilepsy may precipitate increased seizure frequency or status epilepticus. Gradually reduce dose.

## Actions

*Pharmacology:* The precise mechanism(s) of action is unknown. In vitro pharmacological studies suggest that zonisamide blocks sodium channels and reduces voltage-dependent, transient inward currents, stabilizing neuronal membranes and suppressing neuronal hypersynchronization. Zonisamide does not appear to potentiate the synaptic activity of GABA. In vivo studies demonstrated that zonisamide facilitates dopaminergic and serotonergic neurotransmission.

*Pharmacokinetics:* Peak plasma concentrations (range, 2 to 5 mcg/mL) in healthy volunteers occur within 2 to 6 hours. The apparent volume of distribution is approximately 1.45 L/kg. At concentrations of 1 to 7 mcg/mL, it is approximately 40% bound to human plasma proteins. The elimination half-life in plasma is approximately 63 hours. The elimination half-life in red blood cells is approximately 105 hours. Zonisamide is excreted primarily in urine.

## Contraindications

Hypersensitivity to sulfonamides or zonisamide.

## Warnings

*Oligohydrosis and hyperthermia in children:* Oligohydrosis, sometimes resulting in heat stroke and hospitalization, is associated with zonisamide in children.

Decreased sweating and elevated body temperature characterized these cases. Many cases were reported after exposure to elevated environmental temperatures. Heat stroke, requiring hospitalization, was diagnosed in some cases. There have been no reported deaths.

Children appear to be at an increased risk for zonisamide-associated oligohydrosis and hyperthermia. Closely monitor patients, especially children, treated with zonisamide for evidence of decreased sweating and increased body temperature, particularly in warm or hot weather. Use caution when zonisamide is prescribed with other drugs that predispose patients to heat-related disorders (eg, carbonic anhydrase inhibitors, drugs with anticholinergic activity).

*Cognitive/Neuropsychiatric adverse events:* Use of zonisamide was frequently associated with the following CNS-related adverse events: 1) Psychiatric symptoms, including depression and psychosis; 2) psychomotor slowing, difficulty with concentration, and speech or language problems, in particular, word-finding difficulties; and 3) somnolence or fatigue.

*Potentially fatal reactions to sulfonamides:* Fatalities have occurred, although rarely, as a result of severe reactions to sulfonamides (eg, zonisamide), including Stevens-Johnson syndrome, toxic epidermal necrolysis, fulminant hepatic necrosis, agranulocytosis, aplastic anemia, and other blood dyscrasias.

*Serious skin reactions:* Discontinue zonisamide in patients who develop an otherwise unexplained rash or observe them frequently.

*Serious hematological events:* Two confirmed cases of aplastic anemia and 1 confirmed case of agranulocytosis were reported in the first 11 years of marketing in Japan.

*Renal function impairment:* Zonisamide was associated with a statistically significant 8% mean increase from the baseline serum creatinine and blood urea nitrogen (BUN). The increase appeared to persist but was not progressive; this has been interpreted as an effect on glomerular filtration rate (GFR). The decrease in GFR appeared within the first 4 weeks of treatment. There is no information about reversibility of the effects of GFR after long-term use after drug discontinuation. Discontinue zonisamide in patients who develop acute renal failure or a clinically significant sustained increase in the creatinine/BUN concentration. Do not use zonisamide in patients with renal failure (estimated GFR less than 50 mL/min), as there has been insufficient experience concerning drug dosing and toxicity.

*Elderly:* Use caution in selecting a dose for an elderly patient, usually starting at the low end of the dosing range.

*Pregnancy: Category* C. Advise women of childbearing potential who are given zonisamide to use effective contraception.

*Lactation:* It is not known whether zonisamide is excreted in breast milk.

*Children:* Safety and efficacy of zonisamide in patients younger than 16 years of age have not been established. Zonisamide is not approved for pediatric use.

### Precautions
*Lab test abnormalities:* Monitor renal function periodically.

Zonisamide was associated with an increase in serum alkaline phosphatase, with a mean increase of approximately 8% over the baseline.

*Hazardous tasks:* Zonisamide may produce drowsiness, especially at higher doses. Advise patients not to drive a car or operate other complex machinery until the effect of zonisamide is known.

### Drug Interactions
*CYP 450:* Drugs that induce liver enzymes (eg, phenytoin, carbamazepine, phenobarbital) increase the metabolism and clearance of zonisamide and decrease its half-life. Concurrent medication with drugs that induce or inhibit CYP3A4 would be expected to alter serum concentrations of zonisamide. Zonisamide is not expected to interfere with the metabolism of other drugs that are metabolized by cytochrome P450 isozymes.

*Drug/Food interactions:* The time to maximum concentration of zonisamide is delayed in the presence of food, but no effect on bioavailability occurs.

### Adverse Reactions
The most commonly observed adverse events associated with the use of zonisamide were agitation/irritability, anorexia, dizziness, headache, nausea, and somnolence.

The adverse events most commonly associated with discontinuation were somnolence, fatigue, or ataxia (6%); anorexia (3%); difficulty concentrating (2%); difficulty with memory, mental slowing, nausea/vomiting (2%); and weight loss (1%). Many of these adverse events were dose-related.

Adverse reactions occurring in at least 3% of patients include the following: Abdominal pain, agitation/irritability, anorexia, anxiety, ataxia, confusion, depression, diarrhea, difficulty concentrating, difficulty with memory, diplopia, dizziness, dyspepsia, fatigue, flu syndrome, headache, insomnia, mental slowing, nausea, nystagmus, paresthesia, rash, somnolence, speech abnormalities, tiredness, weight loss.

## CLONAZEPAM

**Tablets:** 0.5, 1, and 2 mg (c-iv)  
**Tablets, orally disintegrating:** 0.125, 0.25, 0.5, 1, and 2 mg (c-iv)

Various, *Klonopin* (Roche)  
*Klonopin Wafers* (Roche)

For complete prescribing information, refer to the Benzodiazepines monograph in the Antianxiety Agents section.

### Indications
*Seizure disorders:* Used alone or as adjunctive treatment of Lennox-Gastaut syndrome (petit mal variant), akinetic, and myoclonic seizures. It may be useful in patients with absence (petit mal) seizures who have failed to respond to succinimides.

*Panic disorders:* For the treatment of panic disorder, with or without agoraphobia, as defined in DSM-IV (see Antianxiety Agents section).

**Administration and Dosage**

*Adults:* Initial dose should not exceed 1.5 mg/day in 3 divided doses. Increase in increments of 0.5 to 1 mg every 3 days until seizures are adequately controlled or until side effects preclude any further increase. Individualize maintenance dosage. Maximum recommended dosage is 20 mg/day.

*Infants and children (10 years of age or younger or 30 kg):* To minimize drowsiness, the initial dose should be between 0.01 to 0.03 mg/kg/day, not to exceed 0.05 mg/kg/day, given in 2 or 3 divided doses. Increase dosage by no more than 0.25 to 0.5 mg every third day until a daily maintenance dose of 0.1 to 0.2 mg/kg has been reached, unless seizures are controlled or side effects preclude further increase. When possible, divide the daily dose into 3 equal doses. If doses are not equally divided, give the largest dose at bedtime.

*Administration:* Swallow tablet whole with water. Administer the orally disintegrating tablet as follows: After opening the pouch, peel back the foil on the blister. Do not push the tablet through foil. Immediately upon opening the blister, using dry hands, remove the tablet and place it in the mouth. Tablet disintegration occurs rapidly in saliva so it can be easily swallowed with or without water.

## CLORAZEPATE DIPOTASSIUM

| | |
|---|---|
| **Tablets:** 3.75, 7.5, and 15 mg (c-iv) | Various, *Tranxene T-Tab* (Ovation) |
| **Tablets, extended release:** 11.25 mg (c-iv) | *Tranxene-SD Half Strength* (Abbott) |
| 22.5 mg (c-iv) | *Tranxene-SD* (Abbott) |

For complete prescribing information, refer to the Benzodiazepines monograph in the Antianxiety Agents section.

**Indications**

*Partial seizures:* As adjunctive therapy in the management of partial seizures.

*Alcohol withdrawal:* For the symptomatic relief of acute alcohol withdrawal (see monograph in the Antianxiety Agents section).

*Anxiety:* For the management of anxiety disorders or for the short-term relief of the symptoms of anxiety (see monograph in the Antianxiety Agents section).

**Administration and Dosage**

*Adults and children (older than 12 years of age):* The maximum initial dose is 7.5 mg 3 times/day. Increase dosage by 7.5 mg or less every week; do not exceed 90 mg/day.

*Children:* Maximum initial dose is 7.5 mg 2 times/day. Increase dosage by 7.5 mg or less every week; do not exceed 60 mg/day. Not recommended in patients younger than 9 years of age.

*Extended-release (ER) tablets:* A 22.5 mg ER tablet may be administered as a single dose once daily as an alternate dosage form for patients stabilized on a dose of 7.5 mg 3 times/day; do not use to initiate therapy.

The 11.25 mg ER tablet may be administered as a single dose once daily as an alternate dosage form for patients stabilized on a dose of 3.75 mg 3 times/day; do not use to initiate therapy.

## DIAZEPAM

| | |
|---|---|
| **Tablets:** 2, 5, and 10 mg (c-iv) | Various, *Valium* (Roche) |
| **Solution (Intensol):** 5 mg/mL (c-iv) | *Diazepam Intensol* (Roxane) |
| **Solution:** 1 mg/mL (c-iv) | *Diazepam* (Roxane) |
| **Injection:** 5 mg/mL (c-iv) | Various |
| **Gel, rectal:** 2.5 mg (pediatric), 5 mg (pediatric), 10 mg (pediatric and adult), 15 mg (adult), and 20 mg (adult) (c-iv) | *Diastat* (Xcel) |

For complete prescribing information, refer to the Benzodiazepines monograph in the Antianxiety Agents section.

## Indications

*Oral:* May be used adjunctively in convulsive disorders; it is not proven useful as sole therapy.

*Parenteral:* Adjunct in status epilepticus and severe recurrent convulsive seizures.

*Rectal:* For selected, refractory patients on stable regimens of anti-epileptic agents who require intermittent use of diazepam to control bouts of increased seizure activity.

## Administration and Dosage

*Oral (tablets, oral solution, and Intensol):* Adults – 2 to 10 mg 2 to 4 times/day.

    *Elderly or debilitated patients* – 2 to 2.5 mg once or twice/day initially.

    *Children* – Not for use in children younger than 6 months of age. Give 1 to 2.5 mg 3 or 4 times/day initially; increase gradually as needed and tolerated.

*Intensol preparation:* Mix with liquid or semisolid food such as water, juices, soda, applesauce, and puddings. Consume the entire amount immediately. Do not store.

*Parenteral:*

    *Administration* – The IV route is preferred in the convulsing patient. However, if IV administration is impossible, the IM route may be used. Inject deeply into the muscle. Inject IV slowly (at least 1 minute for each 5 mg). Do not use small veins (eg, dorsum of hand or wrist); avoid intra-arterial use and extravasation.

    *Adults* – Do not administer diazepam emulsified injection IM. Initially 5 to 10 mg. May be repeated at 10- to 15-minute intervals up to a maximum dose of 30 mg if necessary. Therapy may be repeated in 2 to 4 hours; however, residual active metabolites may persist.

    *Children 5 years of age or older* – 1 mg every 2 to 5 minutes up to a maximum of 10 mg. Repeat in 2 to 4 hours if necessary.

    *Infants older than 30 days of age and children younger than 5 years of age* – 0.2 to 0.5 mg slowly every 2 to 5 minutes up to a maximum of 5 mg. Safety and efficacy of parenteral diazepam have not been established in the neonate (30 days of age or younger).

    *Admixture incompatibility* – Do not mix or dilute with other solutions or drugs in syringe or infusion flask. Diazepam interacts with plastic containers and administration sets, significantly decreasing availability of drug delivered.

*Rectal:* 0.2 to 0.5 mg/kg depending on age.

    *2 to 5 years of age* – 0.5 mg/kg.

    *6 to 11 years of age* – 0.3 mg/kg.

    *12 years of age or older* – 0.2 mg/kg.

    Calculate the recommended dose by rounding upward to the next available unit dose. A second dose, when required, may be given 4 to 12 hours after the first dose. Do not treat more than 5 episodes per month or more than 1 episode every 5 days.

    *Elderly and debilitated* – Adjust dosage downward to reduce ataxia or oversedation.

| Diazepam Rectal Dosing Based on Age and Weight | | | |
|---|---|---|---|
| 2 to 5 years of age weight (kg) | 6 to 11 years of age weight (kg) | ≥ 12 years of age weight (kg) | Dose (mg) |
| 6 to 11 | 10 to 18 | 14 to 27 | 5 |
| 12 to 22 | 19 to 37 | 28 to 50 | 10 |
| 23 to 33 | 38 to 55 | 51 to 75 | 15 |
| 34 to 44 | 56 to 74 | 76 to 111 | 20 |

A 2.5 mg supplemental dose may be given for patients requiring more precise dose titration or as a partial replacement dose for patients who may expel a portion of the first dose.

# LAMOTRIGINE

**Tablets**: 25, 100, 150, and 200 mg (Rx)
**Tablets, chewable**: 2, 5, and 25 mg (Rx)

*Lamictal* (GlaxoSmithKline)
*Lamictal Chewable Dispersible Tablets* (GlaxoSmithKline)

---

**Warning:**

Serious rashes requiring hospitalization and discontinuation of treatment have been reported in association with lamotrigine use. The incidence of these rashes, which include Stevens-Johnson syndrome, is approximately 1% in pediatric patients (younger than 16 years of age) and 0.3% in adults.

In clinical trials of bipolar and other mood disorders, the rate of serious rash was 0.08% (0.8 per 1000) in adult patients receiving lamotrigine as initial monotherapy and 0.13% (1.3 per 1000) in adult patients receiving lamotrigine as adjunctive therapy.

Rare cases of toxic epidermal necrolysis or rash-related death have occurred, but their numbers are too few to permit a precise estimate of the rate.

Because the rate of serious rash is greater in pediatric patients than in adults, it bears emphasis that lamotrigine is approved only for use in pediatric patients younger than 16 years of age who have seizures associated with the Lennox-Gastaut syndrome (see Indications).

Other than age, no factors have been identified that are known to predict the risk of occurrence or the severity of rash associated with lamotrigine. It is suggested, yet to be proven, that the risk of rash may also be increased by 1) coadministration of lamotrigine with valproic acid (VPA), 2) exceeding the recommended initial dose of lamotrigine, or 3) exceeding the recommended dose escalation for lamotrigine. However, cases have been reported in the absence of these factors.

Nearly all cases of life-threatening rashes associated with lamotrigine have occurred within 2 to 8 weeks of treatment initiation. However, isolated cases have been reported after prolonged treatment (eg, 6 months). Accordingly, duration of therapy cannot be relied upon as a means to predict the potential risk heralded by the first appearance of a rash.

Although benign rashes also occur with lamotrigine, it is not possible to predict reliably which rashes will prove to be life-threatening. Accordingly, discontinue lamotrigine at the first sign of rash, unless the rash is clearly not drug-related. Discontinuation of treatment may not prevent a rash from becoming life-threatening or permanently disabling or disfiguring.

---

### Indications

*Epilepsy, adjunctive therapy:* Adjunctive therapy in the treatment of partial seizures in adults with epilepsy and as adjunctive therapy in the generalized seizures of Lennox-Gastaut syndrome in pediatric (at least 2 years of age) and adult patients.

*Epilepsy, monotherapy:* Indicated for conversion to monotherapy in adults with partial seizures who are receiving treatment with a single enzyme-inducing AED.

Safety and efficacy have not been established as initial monotherapy, for conversion to monotherapy from non-enzyme-inducing AEDs (eg, valproate), or for simultaneous conversion to monotherapy from 2 or more concomitant AEDs.

Safety and efficacy in patients younger than 16 years of age, other than those with partial seizures and the generalized seizures of Lennox-Gastaut syndrome, have not been established.

*Bipolar disorder:* For the maintenance treatment of Bipolar I Disorder to delay the time to occurrence of mood episodes (eg, depression, mania, hypomania, mixed episodes) in patients treated for acute mood episodes with standard therapy.

### Administration and Dosage

*General dosing considerations:* The risk of nonserious rash is increased when exceeding the recommended initial dose and/or the rate of dose escalation of lamotrigine. Therefore, closely follow the dosing recommendations.

It is recommended that lamotrigine not be restarted in patients who discontinued because of rash associated with prior treatment with lamotrigine, unless the potential benefits clearly outweigh the risks. If the decision is made to restart a patient who has discontinued lamotrigine, then assess the need to restart with the initial dosing recommendations. It is recommended that, the greater the interval of time since the previous dose, the greater consideration be given to restarting with the initial dosing recommendations. If a patient has discontinued lamotrigine for a period of more than 5 half-lives, it is recommended that initial dosing recommendations and guidelines be followed.

*Adjunctive therapy:* For dosing guidelines below, enzyme-inducing antiepileptic drugs (EIAEDs) include phenytoin, carbamazepine, phenobarbital, and primidone.

*Lamotrigine added to AEDs other than EIAEDs and VPA* – The effect of AEDs other than EIAEDs and VPA on the metabolism of lamotrigine cannot be predicted. Therefore, no specific dosing guidelines can be provided in that situation. Exercise conservative starting doses and dose escalations (as with concomitant VPA). Maintenance dosing would be expected to fall between the maintenance dose with VPA and the maintenance dose when added to EIAEDs without VPA.

*Patients 2 to 12 years of age:*

| Lamotrigine Added to an AED Regimen Containing VPA in Patients 2 to 12 Years of Age | | |
|---|---|---|
| Weeks 1 and 2 | 0.15 mg/kg/day in 1 or 2 divided doses, rounded down to the nearest whole tablet. | |
| Weeks 3 and 4 | 0.3 mg/kg/day in 1 or 2 divided doses, rounded down to the nearest whole tablet. | |
| Weight-based dosing can be achieved by using the following guide: | | |
| If the patient's weight is: | Give this daily dose using the most appropriate combination of lamotrigine 2 and 5 mg tablets | |
| Greater than | And less than | Weeks 1 and 2 | Weeks 3 and 4 |
| 6.7 kg | 14 kg | 2 mg every other day | 2 mg every day |
| 14.1 kg | 27 kg | 2 mg every day | 4 mg every day |
| 27.1 kg | 34 kg | 4 mg every day | 8 mg every day |
| 34.1 kg | 40 kg | 5 mg every day | 10 mg every day |
| Usual maintenance dose: 1 to 5 mg/kg/day (maximum 200 mg/day in 1 or 2 divided doses). To achieve the usual maintenance dose, increase subsequent doses every 1 to 2 weeks as follows: Calculate 0.3 mg/kg/day, round this amount down to the nearest whole tablet, and add this amount to the previously administered daily dose. | | | |

The smallest available strength of lamotrigine chewable dispersible tablets is 2 mg. Administer only whole tablets. If the calculated dose cannot be achieved using whole tablets, round down to the nearest whole tablet.

| Lamotrigine Added to EIAEDs (Without Valproic Acid) in Patients 2 to 12 Years of Age | |
|---|---|
| Weeks 1 and 2 | 0.6 mg/kg/day in 2 divided doses, rounded down to the nearest 5 mg. |
| Weeks 3 and 4 | 1.2 mg/kg/day in 2 divided doses, rounded down to the nearest 5 mg. |
| Usual maintenance dose: 5 to 15 mg/kg/day (maximum 400 mg/day in 2 divided doses). To achieve the usual maintenance dose, increase subsequent doses every 1 to 2 weeks as follows: Calculate 1.2 mg/kg/day, round this amount down to the nearest 5 mg, and add this amount to the previously administered daily dose. | |

*Patients older than 12 years of age:* Recommended dosing guidelines for lamotrigine added to valproic acid and guidelines for lamotrigine added to EIAEDs are summarized in the tables below.

| Lamotrigine Added to AED Regimen Containing Valproic Acid in Patients > 12 Years of Age | |
|---|---|
| Weeks 1 and 2 | 25 mg every other day |
| Weeks 3 and 4 | 25 mg every day |
| Usual maintenance dose: 100 to 400 mg/day (1 or 2 divided doses). To achieve maintenance, doses may be increased by 25 to 50 mg/day every 1 to 2 weeks. The usual maintenance dose in patients adding lamotrigine to valproic acid alone ranges from 100 to 200 mg/day. | |

| Lamotrigine Added to EIAEDs (Without Valproic Acid) in Patients > 12 Years of Age | |
|---|---|
| Weeks 1 and 2 | 50 mg/day |
| Weeks 3 and 4 | 100 mg/day in 2 divided doses |
| Usual maintenance dose: 300 to 500 mg/day (in 2 divided doses). To achieve maintenance, increase doses by 100 mg/day every 1 to 2 weeks. | |

*Conversion from a single EIAED to monotherapy with lamotrigine in patients 16 years of age or older:* The goal of the transition regimen is to effect the conversion to monotherapy with lamotrigine under conditions that ensure adequate seizure control while mitigating the risk of serious rash associated with the rapid titration of lamotrigine.

The recommended maintenance dose of lamotrigine as monotherapy is 500 mg/day given in 2 divided doses.

The conversion regimen involves first titrating lamotrigine to the target dose (500 mg/day in 2 divided doses) while maintaining the dose of the EIAED at a fixed level.

Withdraw concomitant EIAED by 20% decrements each week over a 4-week period.

Because of an increased risk of rash, do not exceed the recommended initial dose and subsequent dose escalations (see Warning Box).

*Usual maintenance dose:* In patients receiving multi-drug regimens employing EIAEDs without valproic acid, maintenance doses of adjunctive lamotrigine as high as 700 mg/day have been used. In patients receiving valproic acid alone, maintenance doses of adjunctive lamotrigine as high as 200 mg/day have been used.

*Renal function impairment:* Base initial doses on the patient's AED regimen (see above); reduced maintenance doses may be effective for patients with significant renal function impairment. Use with caution in these patients.

*Hepatic function impairment:* Generally, reduce initial, escalation, and maintenance doses by approximately 50% in patients with moderate (Child-Pugh Grade B) and 75% in patients with severe (Child-Pugh Grade C) hepatic impairment. Adjust escalation and maintenance doses according to clinical response.

*Dosage regimen for bipolar disorder:* The target dose of lamotrigine is 200 mg/day (100 mg/day in combination with valproate and 400 mg/day in combination with carbamazepine or other enzyme-inducing drugs). Doses above 200 mg/day are not recommended. Treatment with lamotrigine is introduced, based on concurrent medications, according to the regimen outlined in the following table.

| Escalation Regimen for Lamotrigine for Patients with Bipolar Disorder | | | |
|---|---|---|---|
| | For patients not taking carbamazepine (or other enzyme-inducing drugs) or valproic acid | For patients taking valproic acid | For patients taking carbamazepine (or other enzyme-inducing drugs) and not taking valproic acid |
| Weeks 1 and 2 | 25 mg daily | 25 mg every other day | 50 mg daily |
| Weeks 3 and 4 | 50 mg daily | 25 mg daily | 100 mg daily, in divided doses |
| Week 5 | 100 mg daily | 50 mg daily | 200 mg daily, in divided doses |

| Escalation Regimen for Lamotrigine for Patients with Bipolar Disorder | | | |
|---|---|---|---|
| | For patients not taking carbamazepine (or other enzyme-inducing drugs) or valproic acid | For patients taking valproic acid | For patients taking carbamazepine (or other enzyme-inducing drugs) and not taking valproic acid |
| Week 6 | 200 mg daily | 100 mg daily | 300 mg daily, in divided doses |
| Week 7 | 200 mg daily | 100 mg daily | up to 400 mg daily, in divided doses |

*Dosage adjustment for bipolar disorder:* If other psychotropic medications are withdrawn following stabilization, the dose of lamotrigine should be adjusted. For patients discontinuing valproate, the dose of lamotrigine should be doubled over a 2-week period in equal weekly increments (see following table). For patients discontinuing carbamazepine or other enzyme inducing agents, the dose of lamotrigine should remain constant for the first week and then should be decreased by half over a 2-week period in equal weekly decrements. The dose of lamotrigine may then be further adjusted to the target dose (200 mg) as clinically indicated.

If other drugs are subsequently introduced, the dose of lamotrigine may need to be adjusted. In particular, the introduction of valproate requires reduction in the dose of lamotrigine.

| Adjustments to Lamotrigine Dosing for Patients with Bipolar Disorder Following Discontinuation of Psychotropic Medications | | | |
|---|---|---|---|
| | Discontinuation of psychotropic drugs excluding valproic acid, carbamazepine, or other enzyme-inducing drugs | After discontinuation of valproic acid | After discontinuation of carbamazepine or other enzyme-inducing drugs |
| | | Current lamotrigine dose (mg/day) 100 | Current lamotrigine dose (mg/day) 400 |
| Week 1 | Maintain current lamotrigine dose | 150 | 400 |
| Week 2 | Maintain current lamotrigine dose | 200 | 300 |
| Week 3 onward | Maintain current lamotrigine dose | 200 | 200 |

*Discontinuation strategy:* For patients receiving lamotrigine in combination with other AEDs, consider a re-evaluation for all AEDs in the regimen if a change in seizure control or an appearance or worsening of adverse experiences is observed.

If a decision is made to discontinue therapy with lamotrigine, a stepwise reduction of dose over 2 weeks or more (approximately 50% per week) is recommended unless safety concerns require a more rapid withdrawal (see Precautions).

Discontinuing an EIAED prolongs the half-life of lamotrigine; discontinuing valproic acid shortens the half-life of lamotrigine.

*Target plasma levels:* A therapeutic plasma concentration range has not been established for lamotrigine. Base dosing of lamotrigine on therapeutic response.

*Administration of chewable dispersible tablets:* Swallow lamotrigine chewable dispersible tablets whole, chewed, or dispersed in water or diluted fruit juice. If chewed, consume a small amount of water or diluted fruit juice to aid in swallowing.

To disperse chewable dispersible tablets, add the tablets to a small amount of liquid (1 teaspoon or enough to cover the medication). Approximately 1 minute later, when the tablets are completely dispersed, swirl the solution and consume the entire quantity immediately. Do not attempt to administer partial quantities of the dispersed tablets.

### Actions

*Pharmacology:* Lamotrigine is chemically unrelated to existing AEDs. The precise mechanism(s) by which lamotrigine exerts its anticonvulsant action are unknown.

*Pharmacokinetics:*

*Absorption/Distribution* – Lamotrigine is rapidly and completely absorbed after oral administration.

*Metabolism/Excretion* – Lamotrigine is eliminated more rapidly in patients who have been taking hepatic EIAEDs.

Following multiple administrations (150 mg twice a day) to healthy volunteers taking no other medications, lamotrigine induced its own metabolism resulting in a 25% decrease (25.4 hours) in half-life and a 37% increase (0.58 mL/min/kg) in plasma clearance at steady state compared with values obtained in the same volunteers following a single dose.

### Contraindications

Hypersensitivity to the drug or its components.

### Warnings

*Withdrawal seizures:* Do not abruptly discontinue AEDs because of the possibility of increasing seizure frequency. Unless safety concerns require a more rapid withdrawal, taper the dose of lamotrigine over a period of at least 2 weeks.

*Organ failure:* Fatalities associated with multi-organ failure and various degrees of hepatic failure have been reported during premarketing development. These cases occurred in association with other serious events (eg, status epilepticus, overwhelming sepsis), making it impossible to identify the initiating cause.

*Addition of lamotrigine to a multidrug regimen that includes valproic acid:* Because valproic acid reduces the clearance of lamotrigine, the dosage of lamotrigine in the presence of valproic acid is less than half of that required in its absence.

*Dermatologic:* Use caution, especially in pediatric patients (see Warning Box).

There is evidence that the inclusion of valproate in a multidrug regimen increases the risk of serious, potentially life-threatening rash.

Serious rashes associated with hospitalization and discontinuation of lamotrigine have been reported. It is recommended that lamotrigine not be restarted in patients who discontinued use due to rash associated with prior treatment with lamotrigine unless the potential benefits clearly outweigh the risks. If the decision is made to restart a patient who has discontinued lamotrigine, assess the need to restart with the initial dosing recommendations (See Administration and Dosage).

*Hypersensitivity reactions:* Hypersensitivity reactions, some fatal or life-threatening, also have occurred. Some reactions have included clinical features of multiorgan dysfunction such as hepatic abnormalities and evidence of disseminated intravascular coagulation. It is important to note that early manifestations of hypersensitivity (eg, fever, lymphadenopathy) may be present even though a rash is not evident.

*Renal/Hepatic function impairment:* Use with caution.

*Elderly:* Exercise caution in dose selection for elderly patients.

*Pregnancy: Category* C.

*Lactation:* Preliminary data indicate that lamotrigine passes into breast milk.

*Children:* Lamotrigine is indicated as adjunctive therapy for partial seizures in patients above 2 years of age and for the generalized seizures of Lennox-Gastaut syndrome. Safety and efficacy for other uses in patients younger than 16 years of age have not been established. Safety and efficacy in patients below the age of 18 years with bipolar disorder have not been established.

### Precautions

*Monitoring:* The value of monitoring plasma concentrations of lamotrigine has not been established. Because of the possible pharmacokinetic interactions between lamotrigine and other AEDs being taken concomitantly, monitoring of the plasma levels of lamotrigine and concomitant AEDs may be indicated, particularly during dosage adjustments.

*Sudden unexplained death in epilepsy (SUDEP):* During premarketing development, 20 sudden and unexplained deaths were recorded among 4700 patients with epilepsy (5747 patient-years of exposure). Some of these could represent seizure-related deaths in which the seizure was not observed (eg, at night).

*Status epilepticus:* Valid estimates of the incidence of treatment-emergent status epilepticus among lamotrigine-treated patients are difficult to obtain. At a minimum, 7 of 2343 adult patients had episodes that could unequivocally be described as status epilepticus. In addition, variably defined episodes of seizure exacerbation (eg, seizure clusters, seizure flurries) were reported.

*Suicide:* The possibility of a suicide attempt is inherent in Bipolar Disorder, and close supervision of high-risk patients should accompany drug therapy. Write prescriptions for lamotrigine for the smallest quantity of tablets consistent with good patient management, in order to reduce the risk of overdose. Overdoses have been reported for lamotrigine, some of which have been fatal.

*Melanin-containing tissues:* Lamotrigine binds to melanin and may cause toxicity in these tissues after extended use. Be aware of the possibility of long-term ophthalmologic effects.

*Special risk:* Caution is advised when using lamotrigine in patients with diseases or conditions that could affect metabolism or elimination of the drug, such as renal or hepatic function impairment (see Warnings) or cardiac function impairment.

### Drug Interactions
Drugs that may affect lamotrigine include acetaminophen, carbamazepine, folate inhibitors, oral contraceptives, oxcarbazepine, phenobarbital, phenytoin, primidone, rifamycins, succinimides, and valproic acid.

Drugs that may be affected by lamotrigine include carbamazepine and valproic acid.

### Adverse Reactions
Approximately 11% of the 3378 adult patients who received lamotrigine in premarketing clinical trials discontinued treatment because of an adverse experience.

Adverse reactions occurring in 3% or more of patients include abdominal pain; accidental injury; anorexia; anxiety; asthenia; ataxia; blurred vision; constipation; convulsion; cough increased; depression; diarrhea; diplopia; dizziness; dysmenorrhea; dyspepsia; eczema; fever; flu syndrome; headache; hemorrhage; incoordination; infection; insomnia; irritability; nausea; pharyngitis; pneumonia; pruritus; rash; rhinitis; somnolence; speech disorder; tooth disorder; tremor; urinary tract infection; vaginitis; vision abnormality; vomiting.

With Lennox-Gastaut syndrome, 3.8% of patients on lamotrigine discontinued because of adverse experiences. The most common adverse experience that led to discontinuation was rash.

Approximately 10% of the 1136 pediatric patients with Lennox-Gastaut syndrome discontinued treatment because of an adverse experience. The adverse events most commonly associated with discontinuation were rash (3.9%), aggravated reaction (1.7%), and ataxia (0.9%).

# LEVETIRACETAM

**Tablets**: 250, 500, and 750 mg (*Rx*)
**Oral solution**: 100 mg/mL (*Rx*)

*Keppra* (UCB Pharma)

## Indications
*Epilepsy:* Adjunctive therapy in the treatment of partial onset seizures in adults with epilepsy.

## Administration and Dosage
Initiate treatment with 1,000 mg/day, given as twice/day dosing (500 mg twice per day). Additional dosing increments may be given (1,000 mg/day additional every 2 weeks) to a maximum recommended daily dose of 3,000 mg. Long-term experience at doses greater than 3,000 mg/day is relatively minimal, and there is no evidence that doses greater than 3,000 mg/day confer additional benefit.

Give orally with or without food.

*Renal function impairment:* Individualize dosing according to the patient's renal function status. Recommended doses and adjustment for dose are shown in the following table.

| Levetiracetam Dosing Adjustment Regimen for Patients with Impaired Renal Function | | | |
|---|---|---|---|
| Group | Ccr (mL/min) | Dosage (mg) | Frequency |
| Normal | > 80 | 500 to 1,500 | q 12 h |
| Mild | 50 to 80 | 500 to 1,000 | q 12 h |
| Moderate | 30 to 50 | 250 to 750 | q 12 h |
| Severe | < 30 | 250 to 500 | q 12 h |
| ESRD patients using dialysis | — | 500 to 1,000[a] | q 24 h |

[a] Following dialysis, a 250 to 500 mg supplemental dose is recommended.

*Hepatic function impairment:* No dose adjustment is needed for patients with hepatic impairment.

## Actions
*Pharmacology:* Levetiracetam is chemically unrelated to other antiepileptic drugs. The precise mechanism by which levetiracetam exerts its antiepileptic effect is unknown.

*Pharmacokinetics:* Absorption is rapid, with peak plasma concentrations occurring in approximately 1 hour following oral administration in fasted subjects. Steady state is achieved after 2 days of multiple twice/day dosing. Levetiracetam is not extensively metabolized. The plasma half-life in adults is approximately 7 hours. Levetiracetam is eliminated from the systemic circulation by renal excretion.

## Contraindications
Hypersensitivity to the drug or any of its ingredients.

## Warnings
*CNS effects:*

*Somnolence* – In controlled trials of patients with epilepsy, 14.8% of levetiracetam-treated patients reported somnolence compared with 8.4% of placebo patients.

*Asthenia* – In controlled trials of patients with epilepsy, 14.7% of levetiracetam-treated patients reported asthenia vs 9.1% with placebo.

*Coordination difficulties* – A total of 3.4% of levetiracetam-treated patients experienced coordination difficulties (reported as either ataxia, abnormal gait, or incoordination) vs 1.6% with placebo.

Somnolence, asthenia, and coordination difficulties occurred most frequently within the first 4 weeks of treatment.

*Psychotic symptoms* – In controlled trials of patients with epilepsy, 5 (0.7%) of levetiracetam-treated patients experienced psychotic symptoms compared with 1 (0.2%) placebo patient. A total of 13.3% of levetiracetam patients experienced other behavioral symptoms (eg, agitation, hostility, anxiety, apathy, emotional lability, depersonalization, depression) compared with 6.2% of placebo patients.

In addition, 4 (0.5%) levetiracetam-treated patients attempted suicide vs 0% with placebo.

*Withdrawal seizure:* Withdraw levetiracetam gradually to minimize the potential of increased seizure frequency.

*Renal function impairment:* Take caution in dosing patients with moderate and severe renal impairment and patients undergoing hemodialysis. Reduce dosage in patients with impaired renal function receiving levetiracetam, and give supplemental doses to patients after dialysis (see Actions and Administration and Dosage).

*Elderly:* No overall differences in safety were observed between subjects 65 years of age or older and younger subjects. There were insufficient numbers of elderly subjects in controlled trials of epilepsy to adequately assess the efficacy of levetiracetam in these patients. Because elderly patients are more likely to have decreased renal function, take care in dose selection; it may be useful to monitor renal function.

*Pregnancy:* Category C.

*Lactation:* Levetiracetam is excreted in breast milk. Because of the potential for serious adverse reactions in nursing infants, decide whether to discontinue nursing or discontinue the drug, taking into account the importance of the drug to the mother.

*Children:* Safety and efficacy in patients younger than 16 years of age have not been established.

## Precautions

*Hematologic effects:* Minor but statistically significant decreases compared with placebo in total mean RBC count ($0.03 \times 10^6/mm^2$), mean hemoglobin (0.09 g/dL), and mean hematocrit (0.38%), were seen in levetiracetam-treated patients in controlled trials.

A total of 3.2% of treated and 1.8% of placebo patients had at least 1 possibly significant ($2.8 \times 10^9/L$ or less) decreased WBC, and 2.4% of treated and 1.4% of placebo patients had at least 1 possibly significant ($1 \times 10^9/L$ or less) decreased neutrophil count. Of the treated patients with a low neutrophil count, all but 1 rose toward or to baseline with continued treatment. No patient was discontinued secondary to low neutrophil counts.

*Hazardous tasks:* Patients should use caution while driving or performing other tasks requiring alertness, coordination or physical dexterity.

## Drug Interactions

*Drug/Food interactions:* Food does not affect the extent of absorption of levetiracetam, but it decreases $C_{max}$ by 20% and delays $T_{max}$ by 1.5 hours.

## Adverse Reactions

The most frequently reported adverse events associated with the use of levetiracetam in combination with other AEDs were asthenia, dizziness, infection, and somnolence.

Adverse reactions occurring in at least 3% of patients include the following: Anorexia, asthenia, ataxia, depression, dizziness, headache, infection, nervousness, pain, pharyngitis, rhinitis, somnolence, vertigo.

Adverse reactions most commonly associated with discontinuation or dose reduction of levetiracetam in patients with epilepsy include convulsion and somnolence.

# PRIMIDONE

| | |
|---|---|
| **Tablets**: 50 mg *(Rx)* | *Mysoline* (Wyeth-Ayerst) |
| 250 mg *(Rx)* | Various, *Mysoline* (Wyeth-Ayerst) |
| **Oral Suspension**: 250 mg/5 mL *(Rx)* | *Mysoline* (Wyeth-Ayerst) |

### Indications
*Epilepsy:* For control of grand mal, psychomotor, or focal epileptic seizures, either alone or with other anticonvulsants. It may control grand mal seizures refractory to other anticonvulsants.

*Unlabeled uses:* Benign familial tremor (essential tremor, 750 mg/day).

### Administration and Dosage
Individualize dosage.

*Adults and children (older than 8 years of age):* Patients who have received no previous treatment may be started on primidone according to the following regimen:

Days 1 to 3 – 100 to 125 mg at bedtime.

Days 4 to 6 – 100 to 125 mg twice/day.

Days 7 to 9 – 100 to 125 mg 3 times/day.

Day 10 – maintenance – 250 mg 3 to 4 times/day. If required, increase dose to 250 mg 5 to 6 times/day, but do not exceed doses of 500 mg 4 times/day (2 g/day).

*Children (younger than 8 years of age):* The following regimen may be used to initiate therapy:

Days 1 to 3 – 50 mg at bedtime.

Days 4 to 6 – 50 mg twice/day.

Days 7 to 9 – 100 mg twice/day.

Day 10 – maintenance – 125 to 250 mg 3 times/day, or 10 to 25 mg/kg/day in divided doses.

*Patients already receiving other anticonvulsants:* Start primidone at 100 to 125 mg at bedtime; gradually increase to maintenance level as the other drug is gradually decreased. When therapy with primidone alone is the objective, the transition should not be completed in less than 2 weeks.

*Bioequivalence:* Bioequivalence problems have been documented for primidone products marketed by different manufacturers. Brand interchange is not recommended unless comparative bioavailability data are available.

### Actions
*Pharmacology:* Primidone's mechanism of antiepileptic action is not known.

Primidone and its 2 metabolites, phenobarbital and phenylethylmalonamide (PEMA) have anticonvulsant activity.

*Pharmacokinetics:* Primidone is readily absorbed from the GI tract. Phenobarbital appears in plasma after several days of continuous therapy. Therapeutic plasma concentrations are 5 to 12 mcg/mL for primidone and 15 to 40 mcg/mL for phenobarbital. PEMA and phenobarbital have longer half-lives (10 to 18 hours and 53 to 140 hours, respectively) and accumulate with chronic use. About 40% of primidone is excreted unchanged in the urine.

### Contraindications
Porphyria; hypersensitivity to phenobarbital.

### Warnings
*Status epilepticus:* Abrupt withdrawal of antiepileptic medication may precipitate status epilepticus.

*Therapeutic efficacy:* Therapeutic efficacy of a dosage regimen takes several weeks to assess.

*Pregnancy:* The effects of primidone in pregnancy are unknown.

*Lactation:* Primidone appears in breast milk in substantial quantities.

**Precautions**

*Monitoring:* Because therapy generally extends over prolonged periods, perform complete blood counts and a sequential multiple analysis test every 6 months.

*Hazardous tasks:* Patients should use caution while driving or performing other tasks requiring alertness, coordination, or physical dexterity.

**Drug Interactions**

Drugs that may affect primidone include acetazolamide, carbamazepine, hydantoins, isoniazid, nicotinamide, and succinimides.

Drugs that may be affected by primidone include carbamazepine.

**Adverse Reactions**

Adverse reactions may include ataxia, vertigo, fatigue, hyperirritability, emotional disturbances, diplopia, nystagmus, drowsiness, personality deterioration with mood changes, paranoia, nausea, anorexia, vomiting, megaloblastic anemia, thrombocytopenia, impotence, morbilliform or maculopapular skin eruptions, crystalluria.

# VALPROIC ACID and DERIVATIVES

| | |
|---|---|
| **Tablets, delayed-release**: 125, 250, and 500 mg (as divalproex sodium) (*Rx*) | *Depakote* (Abbott) |
| **Tablets, extended-release**: 250 and 500 mg (as divalproex sodium) | *Depakote* ER (Abbott) |
| **Capsules**: 250 mg (valproic acid) (*Rx*) | Various, *Depakene* (Abbott) |
| **Capsules, sprinkle**: 125 mg (as divalproex sodium) (*Rx*) | *Depakote* (Abbott) |
| **Syrup**: 250 mg (as sodium valproate)/5 mL (*Rx*) | Various, *Depakene* (Abbott) |
| **Injection**: 100 mg/mL (as valproate acid) (*Rx*) | *Depacon* (Abbott) |

**Warning:**

*Hepatotoxicity:* Hepatic failure resulting in fatalities has occurred in patients receiving valproic acid and its derivatives. Children under 2 years of age are at a considerably increased risk of developing fatal hepatotoxicity, especially those on multiple anticonvulsants and those with congenital metabolic disorders, severe seizure disorders accompanied by mental retardation, and organic brain disease. In this patient group, use with extreme caution and as a sole agent. Weigh benefits of seizure control against risks. Above this age group, the incidence of fatal hepatotoxicity decreases considerably in progressively older patient groups. These incidents usually have occurred during the first 6 months of treatment. Serious or fatal hepatotoxicity may be preceded by nonspecific symptoms such as loss of seizure control, malaise, weakness, lethargy, facial edema, anorexia, jaundice, and vomiting. Monitor patients closely for appearance of these symptoms. Perform liver function tests prior to therapy and at frequent intervals thereafter, especially during the first 6 months.

*Teratogenicity:* Valproate can produce teratogenic effects such as neural tube defects (eg, spina bifida). The use of divalproex sodium in women of childbearing potential requires that the benefits of its use be weighed against the risk of injury to the fetus. This is especially important when the treatment of a spontaneously reversible condition ordinarily not associated with permanent injury or risk of death (eg, migraine) is contemplated (see Warnings and Patient Information). An information sheet describing the teratogenic potential of valproate is available for patients.

---

**Warning: (cont.)**

*Pancreatitis:* Cases of life-threatening pancreatitis have been reported in children and adults receiving valproate. Some of the cases have been described as hemorrhagic with a rapid progression from initial symptoms to death. Cases have been reported shortly after initial use as well as after several years of use. Warn patients and guardians that abdominal pain, nausea, vomiting, or anorexia can be symptoms of pancreatitis that require prompt medical evaluation. If pancreatitis is diagnosed, discontinue valproate. Initiate alternative treatment for the underlying medical condition as clinically indicated.

---

## Indications

*Epilepsy:* For use as sole and adjunctive therapy in the treatment of simple and complex absence seizures and adjunctively in patients with multiple seizure types that include absence seizures; as monotherapy and adjunctive therapy in the treatment of patients with complex partial seizures that occur in isolation or in association with other types of seizures.

Valproate sodium injection is indicated as an IV alternative in patients for whom oral administration of valproate products is temporarily not feasible.

*Mania (divalproex sodium delayed-release tablets):* Treatment of manic episodes associated with bipolar disorder.

*Migraine (divalproex sodium delayed-release and ER tablets):* As prophylaxis of migraine headaches.

## Administration and Dosage

*Oral products:* Bedtime administration may minimize effects of CNS depression. GI irritation may be minimized by taking with food or by slowly increasing the dose. Delayed-release divalproex sodium may reduce the incidence of irritative GI effects. Swallow the extended-release tablets whole; do not crush or chew. Swallow the valproic acid capsules without chewing to avoid local irritation of the mouth and throat.

*Sprinkle capsules:* Capsules may be swallowed whole or opened and the entire contents sprinkled on a small amount (teaspoonful) of soft food such as applesauce or pudding. Swallow drug/food mixture immediately; do not chew. Do not store for future use.

*Valproic acid syrup or capsule dosing:* The following table is a guide for the initial daily dose of valproic acid (15 mg/kg/day) syrup and capsules.

| Valproic Acid Syrup and Capsule Initial Dosing Guide | | | | | |
|---|---|---|---|---|---|
| Weight | | Total daily dose (mg) | Number of capsules or teaspoonfuls of syrup | | |
| kg | lb | | Dose 1 | Dose 2 | Dose 3 |
| 10 to 24.9 | 22 to 54.9 | 250 | 0 | 0 | 1 |
| 25 to 39.9 | 55 to 87.9 | 500 | 1 | 0 | 1 |
| 40 to 59.9 | 88 to 131.9 | 750 | 1 | 1 | 1 |
| 60 to 74.9 | 132 to 164.9 | 1000 | 1 | 1 | 2 |
| 75 to 89.9 | 165 to 197.9 | 1250 | 2 | 1 | 2 |

*Injection:* For IV use only. Administer as a 60-minute infusion (but not more than 20 mg/min) with the same frequency as the oral products. Use of valproate sodium injection for periods of more than 14 days has not been studied. Switch patients to oral valproate products as soon as it is clinically feasible.

Rapid infusion of IV valproate sodium has been associated with an increase in adverse events.

*Conversion from oral products to injection:* When switching from oral products, the total daily dose of valproate sodium injection should be equivalent to the total daily dose of the oral product. Closely monitor patients receiving doses near the maximum recommended daily dose of 60 mg/kg/day, particularly those not receiving enzyme-inducing drugs. If the total daily dose exceeds 250 mg, give in a divided regimen.

*Younger children:* Younger children, especially those receiving enzyme-inducing drugs, will require larger maintenance doses to attain targeted valproic acid concentrations.

*Elderly:* Reduce the starting dose because of a decrease in unbound clearance of valproate; base therapeutic dose on clinical response.

*Dose-related adverse reactions:* Because the frequency of adverse effects (particularly elevated liver enzymes and thrombocytopenia) may be dose-related, weigh the benefit of improved therapeutic effect with higher doses against the possibility of a greater incidence of adverse reactions. The probability of thrombocytopenia appears to increase significantly at total valproate concentrations of 110 mcg/mL or more (females) or 135 mcg/mL or more (males).

*Complex partial seizures:*
   Monotherapy – Adults and children 10 years of age or older.
   Initiate therapy at 10 to 15 mg/kg/day; increase by 5 to 10 mg/kg/wk to achieve optimal clinical response. Ordinarily, optimal clinical response is achieved at daily doses below 60 mg/kg/day. If satisfactory clinical response has not been achieved, measure plasma levels to determine whether they are in the usually accepted therapeutic range (50 to 100 mcg/mL).
   *Conversion to monotherapy:* Initiate therapy at 10 to 15 mg/kg/day. Increase the dosage by 5 to 10 mg/kg/wk to achieve optimal clinical response. Ordinarily, optimal clinical response is achieved at daily doses less than 60 mg/kg/day. If satisfactory clinical response has not been achieved, measure plasma levels to determine whether they are in the usually accepted therapeutic range (50 to 100 mcg/mL). Concomitant antiepilepsy drug (AED) dosage ordinarily can be reduced by about 25% every 2 weeks. This reduction may be started at initiation of therapy or delayed by 1 to 2 weeks if there is a concern that seizures are likely to occur. Monitor patients closely during this period for increased seizure frequency.
   *Adjunctive therapy* – Divalproex sodium or valproic acid may be added to the patient's regimen at a dosage of 10 to 15 mg/kg/day. The dosage may be increased by 5 to 10 mg/kg/wk to achieve optimal clinical response. Ordinarily, optimal clinical response is achieved at daily doses less than 60 mg/kg/day. If satisfactory clinical response has not been achieved, measure plasma levels to determine whether they are in the usually accepted therapeutic range (50 to 100 mcg/mL). If the total daily dose exceeds 250 mg, administer in divided doses.

*Simple and complex absence seizures:* The recommended initial dose is 15 mg/kg/day; increase at 1-week intervals by 5 to 10 mg/kg/day until seizures are controlled or side effects preclude further increase. The maximum recommended dosage is 60 mg/kg/day. If the total daily dose is more than 250 mg, give in divided doses.
   In epileptic patients previously receiving valproic acid therapy, initiate divalproex sodium at the same daily dose and dosing schedule. After the patient is stabilized on divalproex tablets, a dosing schedule of 2 or 3 times/day may be elected in selected patients.

*Conversion from Depakote to Depakote ER:* In adult and pediatric patients 10 years of age and older, patients with epilepsy previously receiving *Depakote*, *Depakote ER* should be administered once daily using a dose 8% to 20% higher than the total daily dose of *Depakote*. For patients whose *Depakote* total daily dose cannot be directly converted to *Depakote ER*, consideration may be given at the clinician's discretion to increase the patient's *Depakote* total daily dose to the next higher dosage before converting to the appropriate total daily dose of *Depakote ER*.

| Dose Conversion from Depakote to Depakote ER | |
| --- | --- |
| Depakote total daily dose (mg) | Depakote ER (mg) |
| 500[1] to 625 | 750 |
| 750[1] to 875 | 1000 |
| 1000[1] to 1125 | 1250 |
| 1250 to 1375 | 1500 |
| 1500 to 1625 | 1750 |
| 1750 | 2000 |
| 1875 to 2000 | 2250 |
| 2125 to 2250 | 2500 |
| 2375 | 2750 |
| 2500 to 2750 | 3000 |
| 2875 | 3250 |
| 3000 to 3125 | 3500 |

[1] These total daily doses of Depakote cannot be directly converted to an 8% to 20% higher total daily dose of Depakote ER because the required dosing strengths of Depakote ER are not available. Consideration may be given at the clinician's discretion to increase the patient's Depakote total daily dose to the next higher dosage before converting to the appropriate total daily dose of Depakote ER.

Mania (divalproex sodium delayed-release tablets): 750 mg/day in divided doses; increase as rapidly as possible to achieve the lowest therapeutic dose that produces the desired clinical effect or the desired range of plasma concentrations (trough plasma concentrations 50 to 125 mcg/mL). Maximum concentrations generally were achieved within 14 days. Maximum recommended dosage is 60 mg/kg/day.

Migraine:

Divalproex sodium delayed-release tablets – The starting dose is 250 mg orally twice/day. Some patients may benefit from doses up to 1000 mg/day. There is no evidence that higher doses lead to greater efficacy.

Divalproex sodium ER tablets – The recommended starting dose is 500 mg once daily for 1 week, thereafter increasing to 1000 mg once daily. Although doses other than 1000 mg once daily have not been evaluated in patients with migraines, the effective dose range of delayed-released tablets in these patients is 500 to 1000 mg/day. As with other valproate products, individualize doses of the ER tablets and adjust the dose as necessary. When ER tablets are given in doses 8% to 20% higher than the total daily dose of the delayed-release tablets, the two formulations are bioequivalent. If a patient requires smaller dose adjustments than that available with the ER tablets, use the delayed-release tablets instead.

Therapeutic serum levels: Therapeutic serum levels for most patients with seizures will range from 50 to 100 mcg/mL; however, a good correlation has not been established between daily dose, serum level, and therapeutic effect.

### Actions

Pharmacology: This group includes valproic acid, sodium valproate (the sodium salt), and divalproex sodium (a compound containing equal proportions of valproic acid and sodium valproate). Regardless of form, dosage is expressed as valproic acid equivalents.

Valproic acid is chemically unrelated to other drugs used to treat seizure disorders. Although the mechanism of action is not established, its activity may be related to increased brain levels of gamma-aminobutyric acid (GABA).

Pharmacokinetics:

Absorption – Valproic acid is rapidly and almost completely absorbed from the GI tract. Absorption of the drug is delayed but not decreased by administration with meals; administration of the drug with milk products does not affect the rate or degree of absorption. The bioavailability of valproate from divalproex sodium delayed-release tablets and capsules containing coated particles has been shown to be equivalent to that of valproic acid capsules.

The absolute bioavailability of divalproex ER tablets administered as a single dose after a meal was approximately 90% relative to IV infusion. The ER tablet produced an average bioavailability of 89% relative to divalproex delayed-release tablets given 2, 3, or 4 times daily. Maximum valproate plasma concentrations in these studies were achieved on average 4 to 17 hours after the ER dose intake. The ER tablets are not bioequivalent to the delayed-release tablets.

*Distribution* – Valproic acid is rapidly distributed. Volume of distribution of total or free valproic acid is 11 or 92 L/1.73 m$^2$, respectively. Valproic acid has been detected in CSF (approximately 10% of total concentrations) and milk (about 1% to 10% of serum concentrations). Therapeutic range is commonly considered to be 50 to 100 mcg/mL of total valproate. The plasma protein binding of valproate is concentration-dependent. Protein binding of valproate is reduced in the elderly, in patients with chronic hepatic diseases, in patients with renal impairment, and in the presence of other drugs (eg, aspirin). Conversely, valproate may displace certain protein-bound drugs (eg, phenytoin, carbamazepine, warfarin, tolbutamide).

*Metabolism/Excretion* – Primarily metabolized in liver. Mean terminal half-life for valproate monotherapy ranges from 9 to 16 hours. Half-lives in the lower part of the range usually are found in patients taking other enzyme-inducing antiepileptic drugs.

## Contraindications

Hepatic disease or significant hepatic dysfunction; hypersensitivity to valproic acid; known urea cycle disorders (see Warnings).

## Warnings

*Pancreatitis:* Cases of life-threatening pancreatitis have been reported in children and adults receiving valproate. Some of the cases have been described as hemorrhagic with rapid progression from initial symptoms to death. Some cases have occurred shortly after initial use as well as after several years of use. Warn patients and guardians that abdominal pain, nausea, vomiting, or anorexia can be symptoms of pancreatitis that require prompt medical evaluation.

*Urea cycle disorders (UCDs):* Hyperammonemic encephalopathy, sometimes fatal, has been reported following initiation of valproate therapy in patients with UCDs, a group of uncommon genetic abnormalities, particularly ornithine transcarbamylase deficiency. Patients who develop symptoms of unexplained hyperammonemic encephalopathy while receiving valproate therapy should receive prompt treatment (including discontinuation of valproate therapy) and be evaluated for underlying urea cycle disorders (see Precautions).

*Thrombocytopenia:* The frequency of thrombocytopenia may be dose-related. The probability of thrombocytopenia increases significantly at total trough valproate plasma concentrations greater than or equal to 110 mcg/mL in females and 135 mcg/mL in males.

*Acute head injuries:* A study evaluating the effect of IV valproate in the prevention of posttraumatic seizures in patients with acute head injuries found a higher incidence of death in valproate treatment groups compared with the IV phenytoin treatment group. Until further information is available, it seems prudent not to use valproate sodium injection in patients with acute head trauma for the prophylaxis of posttraumatic seizures.

*Hepatotoxicity:* See Warning Box.

*Long-term use:* Safety and effectiveness for long-term use in mania (more than 3 weeks) have not been systematically evaluated in clinical trials.

*Discontinuation:* Do not abruptly discontinue in patients with major seizures because of the strong possibility of precipitating status epilepticus with hypoxia and threat to life.

*Elderly:* In elderly patients, increase dosage more slowly and with regular monitoring for fluid and nutritional intake, dehydration, somnolence, and other adverse events. Consider dose reductions or discontinuation of valproate in patients with decreased food or fluid intake and in patients with excessive somnolence. A reduced starting dose is recommended (see Administration and Dosage).

*Pregnancy:* Category D.

*Lactation:* Concentrations of valproic acid in breast milk are 1% to 10% of serum concentrations. Consider discontinuing nursing when valproate products are administered to a nursing woman.

*Children:* See Warning Box. The safety and efficacy of divalproex sodium for the treatment of acute mania has not been studied in individuals younger than 18 years of age. Divalproex sodium extended-release tablets are not recommended in children. Use of valproate sodium injection has not been studied in children below 2 years of age.

    *Migraine* – The safety and efficacy of divalproex sodium for the prophylaxis of migraines has not been studied in individuals under 16 years of age.

## Precautions

*Hematologic effects:* Thrombocytopenia, inhibition of the secondary phase of platelet aggregation, and abnormal coagulation parameters have occurred; determine platelet counts and bleeding time before initiating therapy, at periodic intervals, and prior to surgery.

*Hyperammonemia:* Hyperammonemia has been reported and may be present despite normal liver function tests. In patients who develop unexplained lethargy and vomiting or changes in mental status, measure an ammonia level.

*Suicidal ideation:* Suicidal ideation may be a manifestation of certain psychiatric disorders and may persist until significant remission of symptoms occurs.

*Hazardous tasks:* Patients should use caution while driving or performing other tasks requiring alertness, coordination, or physical dexterity.

## Drug Interactions

Drugs that may affect valproic acid include carbamazepine, charcoal, chlorpromazine, cholestyramine, cimetidine, erythromycin, ethosuximide, felbamate, lamotrigine, phenytoin, rifampin, and salicylates. Drugs that may be affected by valproic acid include carbamazepine, clonazepam, diazepam, ethosuximide, lamotrigine, phenobarbital, phenytoin, tolbutamide, tricyclic antidepressants, warfarin, and zidovudine.

*Drug/Lab test interactions:* Valproic acid is partially eliminated in the urine as a keto-metabolite, which may lead to a false interpretation of the urine ketone test. There have been reports of altered thyroid function tests associated with valproic acid.

## Adverse Reactions

Adverse reactions in at least 3% of patients include the following: Asthenia, somnolence, dizziness, tremor, ataxia, emotional lability, abnormal thinking, amnesia, euphoria, hypesthesia, nervousness, paresthesia, insomnia, depression, nausea, dyspepsia, diarrhea, vomiting, abdominal pain, increased appetite, constipation, anorexia, thrombocytopenia, ecchymosis, flu syndrome, infection, bronchitis, rhinitis, pharyngitis, dyspnea, nystagmus, diplopia, amblyopia/blurred vision, taste perversion, tinnitus, weight gain, back pain, alopecia, fever, weight loss, headache, peripheral edema, infection, rash.

# CARBAMAZEPINE

| | |
|---|---|
| **Tablets:** 200 mg (*Rx*) | Various, *Epitol* (Teva), *Tegretol* (Novartis) |
| **Tablets, chewable:** 100 mg (*Rx*) | Various, *Tegretol* (Novartis) |
| **Tablets, extended release:** 100, 200, and 400 mg (*Rx*) | *Tegretol-XR* (Novartis) |
| **Capsules, extended release:** 100, 200, and 300 mg (*Rx*) | *Carbatrol* (Shire) |
| **Suspension:** 100 mg/5 mL (*Rx*) | Various, *Tegretol* (Novartis) |
| 200 mg/10 mL (*Rx*) | *Carbamazepine* (Alpharma) |

**Warning:**
Aplastic anemia and agranulocytosis have been reported in association with carbamazepine therapy. The risk of developing these reactions is 5 to 8 times greater than in the general population. Consider discontinuation of the drug if any evidence of significant bone marrow depression develops.

### Indications

*Epilepsy:* Partial seizures with complex symptoms. Patients with these seizures appear to show greatest improvement. Generalized tonic-clonic seizures; mixed seizure patterns or other partial or generalized seizures.

*Trigeminal neuralgia:* Treatment of pain associated with true trigeminal neuralgia and glossopharyngeal neuralgia.

### Administration and Dosage

*Conversion from conventional tablets to extended-release tablets:* Extended-release carbamazepine is for twice/day administration. Administer the same total daily mg dose of extended-release carbamazepine. Swallow extended-release tablets whole; never crush or chew. Inspect extended-release tablets for chips or cracks; do not consume damaged tablets. Extended-release tablet coating is not absorbed and is excreted in the feces; these coatings may be noticeable in the stool.

*Epilepsy:*
Initial –
Adults and children (older than 12 years of age): 200 mg twice/day (100 mg 4 times/day of suspension). Increase at weekly intervals by 200 mg/day or less using a 3 or 4 times/day regimen (2 times/day with extended release) until the best response is obtained. Do not exceed 1,000 mg/day in children 12 to 15 years of age or 1,200 mg/day in patients older than 15 years of age. Doses 1,600 mg/day or less have been used in adults.

Children (6 to 12 years of age): 100 mg twice/day (50 mg 4 times/day of suspension). Increase at weekly intervals gradually by adding 100 mg/day or less using a 3 or 4 times/day regimen (2 times/day with extended release) until the best response is obtained. Do not exceed 1,000 mg/day.

Children (younger than 6 years of age): 10 to 20 mg/kg/day 2 or 3 times/day (4 times/day with suspension). Increase weekly to achieve optimal clinical response administered 3 or 4 times/day.

Maintenance –
Adults and children (older than 12 years of age): Adjust to minimum effective level, usually 800 to 1,200 mg/day.

Children (6 to 12 years of age): Adjust to minimum effective level, usually 400 to 800 mg/day. May also be calculated on basis of 20 to 30 mg/kg/day, in divided doses 3 or 4 times/day.

Children (younger than 6 years of age): Ordinarily, optimal clinical response is achieved at daily doses less than 35 mg/kg. If satisfactory clinical response has not been achieved, measure plasma levels to determine whether or not they are in the therapeutic range. No recommendation regarding the safety of carbamazepine for use at doses greater than 35 mg/kg/24 hours can be made.

Combination therapy – When adding to existing anticonvulsant therapy, do so gradually while other anticonvulsants are maintained or gradually decreased, except phenytoin, which may have to be increased.

*Trigeminal neuralgia:*
Initial – 100 mg twice/day on the first day (50 mg 4 times/day of suspension). May increase by up to 200 mg/day using 100 mg increments every 12 hours (50 mg 4 times/day of suspension) as needed. Do not exceed 1,200 mg/day.

Maintenance – Control of pain can usually be maintained with 400 to 800 mg/day (range, 200 to 1,200 mg/day). Attempt to reduce the dose to the minimum effective level or to discontinue the drug at least once every 3 months.

## Actions

*Pharmacology:* Carbamazepine's mechanism of action is unknown. It appears to act by reducing polysynaptic responses and blocking the posttetanic potentiation.

*Pharmacokinetics:*

*Absorption/Distribution* – Both the suspension and tablet deliver equivalent amounts of drug to the systemic circulation; however, the suspension is absorbed somewhat faster than the tablet. Carbamazepine is 76% bound to plasma proteins.

*Metabolism/Excretion* – Carbamazepine is metabolized in the liver to the 10,11-epoxide, which also has anticonvulsant activity. It may induce its own metabolism. Initial half-life ranges from 25 to 65 hours and decreases to 12 to 17 hours with repeated doses.

## Contraindications

History of bone marrow depression; hypersensitivity to carbamazepine and tricyclic antidepressants; concomitant use of monoamine oxidase (MAO) inhibitors. Discontinue MAO inhibitors for a minimum of 14 days before carbamazepine administration.

## Warnings

*Minor pain:* This drug is not a simple analgesic. Do not use for the relief of minor aches or pains.

*Dermatologic:* Severe dermatologic reactions, including toxic epidermal necrolysis (Lyell syndrome) and Stevens-Johnson syndrome, have been reported with carbamazepine. These reactions have been extremely rare; however, a few fatalities have been reported.

*Hematologic:* Patients with a history of adverse hematologic reaction to any drug may be particularly at risk.

*Anticholinergic effects:* Carbamazepine has shown mild anticholinergic activity; therefore, use with caution in patients with increased intraocular pressure.

*CNS effects:* Because of the drug's relationship to other tricyclic compounds, the possibility of activating latent psychosis, confusion, or agitation in elderly patients may occur.

*Hypersensitivity reactions:* Hypersensitivity reactions to carbamazepine have been reported in patients who previously experienced this reaction to anticonvulsants, including phenytoin and phenobarbital. Consider discontinuation of carbamazepine if any evidence of hypersensitivity develops.

*Carcinogenesis:* Carbamazepine administered to rats for 2 years at doses of 25 to 250 mg/kg/day resulted in a dose-related increase in the incidence of hepatocellular tumors in females and benign interstitial cell adenomas in the testes of males.

*Pregnancy:* Category D.

*Lactation:* Carbamazepine and its epoxide metabolite are transferred into breast milk. Because of the potential for serious adverse reactions, decide whether to discontinue nursing or to discontinue the drug, taking into account the importance of the drug to the mother.

*Children:* In children younger than 15 years of age, there is an inverse relationship between carbamazepine-10,11-epoxide/carbamazepine ratio and increasing age. The safety of carbamazepine in children has been studied up to 6 months of age.

## Precautions

*Hepatic effects:* Hepatic effects, ranging from slight elevations in liver enzymes to rare cases of hepatic failure have been reported. In some cases, hepatic effects may progress despite discontinuation of the drug.

*Hyponatremia:* Hyponatremia has been reported in association with carbamazepine use, either alone or in combination with other drugs.

*Absence seizures:* Absence seizures (petit mal) do not appear to be controlled by carbamazepine.

*Special risk:* Prescribe carbamazepine only after benefit-to-risk appraisal in patients with a history of the following: Cardiac, hepatic, or renal damage; adverse hematologic reaction to other drugs; interrupted courses of therapy with the drug.

*Lab test abnormalities:* Perform baseline liver function tests and periodic evaluations. Obtain baseline and periodic eye examinations (slit lamp, funduscopy, and tonometry), urinalysis, and BUN determinations.

Obtain complete pretreatment hematological testing as a baseline. Repeat these tests at monthly intervals during the first 2 months and, thereafter, obtain yearly or every-other-year CBC, white cell differential, and platelet count.

*Hazardous tasks:* May produce drowsiness, dizziness, or blurred vision; patients should observe caution while driving or performing other tasks requiring alertness.

## Drug Interactions

Drugs that can increase carbamazepine serum levels include cimetidine, danazol, diltiazem, erythromycin, felbamate, clarithromycin, fluoxetine, isoniazid, niacinamide, propoxyphene, ketaconazole, itraconazole, verapamil, valproate, troleandomycin, loratadine, nicotinamide, tricyclic antidepressants, SSRIs, nefazodone, protease inhibitors.

Drugs that can decrease carbamazepine serum levels include charcoal, cisplatin, doxorubicin, felbamate, hydantoins, rifampin, phenobarbital, primidone, theophylline.

The serum levels of oral contraceptives, haloperidol, bupropion, anticoagulants, felbamate, valproic acid, felodipine, tricyclic antidepressants, acetaminophen, ziprasidone, voriconazole, topiramate, tiagabine, olanzapine, and lamotrigine can be lowered by carbamazepine.

*Drug/Lab test interactions:*
   *Thyroid function –* Thyroid function tests show decreased values with carbamazepine.
   *Pregnancy tests –* Interference with some pregnancy tests has been reported.

*Drug/Food interactions:* Avoid coadministration of carbamazepine with grapefruit products. Serum carbamazepine levels may be elevated.

## Adverse Reactions

Adverse reactions may include abdominal pain, abnormal involuntary movements, abnormal liver function tests, aching joints or muscles, acute urinary retention, adenopathy or lymphadenopathy aggravation of coronary artery disease, aggravation of disseminated lupus erythematosus, agranulocytosis, albuminuria, alopecia, alterations in pigmentation, anorexia, aplastic anemia, arrhythmias, asthma, AV block, azotemia, behavioral changes in children, blurred vision, bone marrow depression, cardiovascular complications that have resulted in fatalities, cerebral arterial insufficiency, CHF, cholestatic/hepatocellular jaundice, confusion, conjunctivitis, constipation, depression with agitation, diaphoresis, diarrhea, disturbances of coordination, dizziness, drowsiness, dryness of mouth or pharynx, dyspnea, edema, elevated BUN, eosinophilia, erythema multiforme and nodosum, exfoliative dermatitis, fatigue, fever and chills, gastric distress, glossitis and stomatitis, glycosuria, headache, hepatitis, hyperacusis, hypotension, impotence, inappropriate antidiuretic hormone secretion syndrome (SIADH), leg cramps, leukocytosis, leukopenia, microscopic deposits in urine, nausea, nystagmus, oculomotor disturbances, oliguria with hypertension, pancytopenia, paralysis, peripheral neuritis and paresthesias, photosensitivity reactions, pneumonia, pneumonitis, primary thrombophlebitis, pruritic and erythematous rashes, pulmonary eosinophilia, purpura, recurrence of thrombophlebitis, renal failure, scattered, punctate cortical lens opacities, speech disturbances, Stevens-Johnson syndrome, syncope and collapse, talkativeness, thrombocytopenia, tinnitus, toxic epidermal necrolysis, transient diplopia, unsteadiness, urinary frequency, urticaria, visual hallucinations, vomiting.

# GABAPENTIN

| | |
|---|---|
| **Capsules**: 100, 300, and 400 mg (*Rx*) | *Neurontin* (Parke-Davis) |
| **Tablets**: 100, 300, and 400 mg (*Rx*) | *Gabarone* (Ivax) |
| **Tablets**: 600 and 800 mg (*Rx*) | *Neurontin* (Parke-Davis) |
| **Solution, oral**: 250 mg/5 mL (*Rx*) | *Neurontin* (Parke-Davis) |

## Indications

*Epilepsy:* Adjunctive therapy in the treatment of partial seizures with and without secondary generalization in patients more than 12 years of age with epilepsy. Also indicated as adjunctive therapy for partial seizures in children 3 to 12 years of age.

*Postherpetic neuralgia:* For management of postherpetic neuralgia in adults.

## Administration and Dosage

Take with or without food.

*Postherpetic neuralgia:* In adults with postherpetic neuralgia, gabapentin therapy may be initiated as a single 300 mg dose on day 1, 600 mg/day on day 2 (divided twice daily), and 900 mg/day on day 3 (divided 3 times daily). The dose can subsequently be titrated up as needed for pain relief to a daily dose of 1800 mg (divided 3 times daily).

*Epilepsy:* Recommended for add-on therapy in patients 3 years of age or older.

    *Patients more than 12 years of age* – The effective dose is 900 to 1800 mg/day in divided doses (3 times/day) using 300 or 400 mg capsules or 600 or 800 mg tablets. The starting dose is 300 mg 3 times/day. If necessary, the dose may be increased using 300 or 400 mg capsules or 600 or 800 mg tablets 3 times/day up to 1800 mg/day. Dosages up to 2400 mg/day have been well tolerated in long-term clinical studies. Doses of 3600 mg/day also have been administered to a small number of patients for a relatively short duration, and have been well tolerated. The maximum time between doses in the 3 times/day schedule should not exceed 12 hours.

    *Pediatric patients 3 to 12 years of age* – The starting dose should range from 10 to 15 mg/kg/day in 3 divided doses, and the effective dose reached by upward titration over a period of about 3 days. The effective dose of gabapentin in patients 5 years of age or older is 25 to 35 mg/kg/day and given in divided doses (3 times/day). The effective dose in pediatric patients 3 and 4 years of age is 40 mg/kg/day and given in divided doses (3 times/day). Gabapentin may be administered as the oral solution, capsule, tablet, or using combinations of these formulations. Dosages up to 50 mg/kg/day have been well tolerated in a long-term clinical study. The maximum time interval between doses should not exceed 12 hours.

It is not necessary to monitor gabapentin plasma concentrations to optimize therapy. Further, because there are no significant pharmacokinetic interactions with other commonly used anti-epileptic drugs, the addition of gabapentin does not alter the plasma levels of these drugs appreciably.

If gabapentin is discontinued or an alternate anticonvulsant medication is added to the therapy, this should be done gradually over a minimum of 1 week.

*Renal function impairment:*

| Gabapentin Dosage Based on Renal Function in Patients ≥ 12 Years of Age | | | | | | |
|---|---|---|---|---|---|---|
| Creatinine clearance (mL/min) | Total daily dose range (mg/day) | Dose regimen (mg) | | | | |
| ≥ 60 | 900 to 3600 | 300 tid | 400 tid | 600 tid | 800 tid | 1200 tid |
| > 30 to 59 | 400 to 1400 | 200 bid | 300 bid | 400 bid | 500 bid | 700 bid |
| > 15 to 29 | 200 to 700 | 200 qd | 300 qd | 400 qd | 500 qd | 700 qd |
| 15[1] | 100 to 300 | 100 qd | 125 qd | 150 qd | 200 qd | 300 qd |

| Gabapentin Dosage Based on Renal Function in Patients ≥ 12 Years of Age | | | | | | |
|---|---|---|---|---|---|---|
| Creatinine clearance (mL/min) | Total daily dose range (mg/day) | Dose regimen (mg) | | | | |
| Posthemodialysis supplemental dose (mg)[2] | | | | | | |
| Hemodialysis | | $125^2$ | $150^2$ | $200^2$ | $250^2$ | $350^2$ |

[1] For patients with creatinine clearance (Ccr) < 15 mL/min, reduce daily dose in proportion to Ccr (eg, patients with a Ccr of 7.5 mL/min should receive one-half the daily dose that patients with a Ccr of 15 mL/min receive.
[2] Patients on hemodialysis should receive maintenance doses based on estimates of Ccr as indicated in the upper portion of the table and a supplemental posthemodialysis dose administered after each 4 hours of hemodialysis as indicated in the lower portion of the table.

Use of gabapentin in patients under 12 years of age with compromised renal function has not been studied.

### Actions

*Pharmacology:* Gabapentin is an oral antiepileptic agent. The mechanism by which it exerts its anticonvulsant and analgesic actions is unknown.

*Pharmacokinetics:* Gabapentin bioavailability is not dose-proportional. It circulates largely unbound (less than 3%) to plasma protein and is eliminated from the systemic circulation by renal excretion as unchanged drug; it is not appreciably metabolized.

### Contraindications

Hypersensitivity to the drug or its ingredients.

### Warnings

*Neuropsychiatric adverse events (3 to 12 years of age):* Gabapentin use in pediatric patients with epilepsy 3 to 12 years of age is associated with the occurrence of CNS-related adverse events.

   Among the gabapentin-treated patients, most of the events were mild to moderate in intensity.

*Withdrawal-precipitated seizure:* Antiepileptic drugs should not be abruptly discontinued because of the possibility of increasing seizure frequency.

*Status epilepticus:* In the placebo controlled studies, the incidence of status epilepticus in patients receiving gabapentin was 0.6% vs 0.5% with placebo.

*Sudden and unexplained deaths:* During the course of premarketing development of gabapentin, 8 sudden and unexplained deaths were recorded among 2203 patients.

*Elderly:* No systematic studies in geriatric patients have been conducted. Adverse clinical events reported among 59 gabapentin-exposed patients more than 65 years of age did not differ in kind from those reported for younger individuals.

*Pregnancy: Category C.*

*Lactation:* Gabapentin is secreted into breast milk.

*Children:* Safety and efficacy in children less than 3 years of age has not been established.

### Drug Interactions

Drugs that may affect gabapentin include antacids, cimetidine, hydrocodone, and morphine. Drugs that may be affected by gabapentin include oral contraceptives and hydrocodone.

*Drug/Lab test interactions:* Because false-positive readings were reported with the *Ames N-Multistix SG* dipstick test for urinary protein when gabapentin was added to other antiepileptic drugs, the more specific sulfosalicylic acid precipitation procedure is recommended to determine the presence of urine protein.

### Adverse Reactions

Adverse reactions occurring in at least 3% of patients include somnolence, weight gain, hostility, emotional lability, nausea/vomiting, bronchitis, viral infections, fever, dizziness, ataxia, fatigue, nystagmus, rhinitis, diplopia, amblyopia, tremor, asthenia, headache, peripheral edema, diarrhea, constipation, dry mouth.

# TIAGABINE HCI

**Tablets**: 4, 12, 16, and 20 mg (*Rx*)                    *Gabitril Filmtabs* (Abbott)

## Indications
*Partial seizures:* Adjunctive therapy for treatment of partial seizures.

## Administration and Dosage
Tiagabine is given orally and should be taken with food.

*Children (12 to 18 years of age ):* Initiate tiagabine at 4 mg once/day. Modification of con-comitant antiepilepsy drugs is not necessary, unless clinically indicated. The total daily dose of tiagabine may be increased by 4 mg at the beginning of week 2. Thereafter, the total daily dose of may be increased by 4 to 8 mg at weekly inter-vals until clinical response is achieved or up to 32 mg/day. Give the total daily dose in 2 to 4 divided doses. Doses greater than 32 mg/day have been tolerated in a small number of adolescent patients for a relatively short duration.

*Adults and children older than 18 years of age:* Initiate tiagabine at 4 mg once/day. Modifica-tion of concomitant antiepilepsy drugs is not necessary, unless clinically indicated. The total daily dose of tiagabine may be increased by 4 to 8 mg at weekly inter-vals until clinical response is achieved or up to 56 mg/day. Give the total daily dose in 2 to 4 divided doses. Doses greater than 56 mg/day have not been systemati-cally evaluated in adequate well controlled trials.

Experience is limited in patients taking total daily doses greater than 32 mg/day using twice/day dosing. A typical dosing titration regimen for patients taking enzyme-inducing antiepilepsy drugs (EIAEDs) is provided.

| Typical Dosing Titration Regimen of Tiagabine for Patients Taking EIAEDs | | |
|---|---|---|
| Week | Initiation and titration schedule | Total daily dose |
| Week 1 | Initiate at 4 mg once/day | 4 mg/day |
| Week 2 | Increase total daily dose by 4 mg | 8 mg/day (in 2 divided doses) |
| Week 3 | Increase total daily dose by 4 mg | 12 mg/day (in 3 divided doses) |
| Week 4 | Increase total daily dose by 4 mg | 16 mg/day (in 2 to 4 divided doses) |
| Week 5 | Increase total daily dose by 4 to 8 mg | 20 to 24 mg/day (in 2 to 4 divided doses) |
| Week 6 | Increase total daily dose by 4 to 8 mg | 24 to 32 mg/day (in 2 to 4 divided doses) |
| Usual adult maintenance dose | 32 to 56 mg/day in 2 to 4 divided doses | |

## Actions
*Pharmacology:* The precise mechanism by which tiagabine exerts its antiseizure effect is unknown, although it is believed that it blocks GABA uptake into presynaptic neu-rons, permitting more GABA to be available for receptor binding on the sur-faces of postsynaptic cells.

*Pharmacokinetics:*

*Absorption/Distribution* – Absorption of tiagabine is rapid and nearly complete (more than 95%), with an absolute oral bioavailability of approximately 90%. Following multiple dosing, steady state is achieved within 2 days. Tiagabine is 96% bound to plasma proteins.

*Metabolism/Excretion* – Tiagabine is likely to be metabolized primarily by the P450 3A (CYP3A) isoform, although contributions to the metabolism of tiagabine from CYP 1A2, CYP 2D6, or CYP 2C19 have not been excluded. Approximately 2% of an oral dose of tiagabine is excreted unchanged, with 25% and 63% of the remaining dose excreted into the urine and feces, respectively, primarily as metabo-lites.

#### Contraindications

Hypersensitivity to the drug or its ingredients.

#### Warnings

*Withdrawal seizures:* Do not abruptly discontinue antiepilepsy drugs (AEDs) because of the possibility of increasing seizure frequency. Withdraw tiagabine gradually to minimize the potential for increased seizure frequency, unless safety concerns require a more rapid withdrawal.

*EEG abnormalities:* Patients with a history of spike and wave discharges on EEG have been reported to have exacerbations of their EEG abnormalities associated with these cognitive/neuropsychiatric events. This raises the possibility that these clinical events may, in some cases, be a manifestation of underlying seizure activity.

*Status epilepticus:* Among the patients treated with tiagabine across all epilepsy studies (controlled and uncontrolled), 5% had some form of status epilepticus. Of the 5%, 57% of patients experienced complex partial status epilepticus. A critical risk factor for status epilepticus was the presence of the condition history; 33% of patients with a history of status epilepticus had recurrence during tiagabine treatment.

*Sudden unexpected death in epilepsy (SUDEP):* There have been as many as 10 cases of SUDEP during the clinical development of tiagabine among 2531 patients with epilepsy (3831 patient-years of exposure).

The rate is within the range of estimates for the incidence of SUDEP not receiving tiagabine. The estimated SUDEP rates in patients receiving tiagabine are similar to those observed in patients receiving other AEDs, chemically unrelated to tiagabine, who underwent clinical testing in similar populations at about the same time. This evidence suggests that the SUDEP rates reflect population rates, not a drug effect.

*Hepatic function impairment:* Because the clearance of tiagabine is reduced in patients with liver disease (approximately 60%), dosage reduction or longer dosing intervals may be necessary in these patients.

*Pregnancy: Category C.*

*Lactation:* Tiagabine or its metabolites are excreted in the milk of rats. Use in women who are nursing only if the benefits clearly outweigh the risks.

*Children:* Safety and efficacy in children younger than 12 years of age have not been established.

#### Precautions

*Concomitant EIAED:* Virtually all experience with tiagabine has been obtained in patients receiving 1 or more concomitant EIAED. Use in noninduced patients (eg, patients receiving valproate monotherapy) may require lower doses or a slower dose titration of tiagabine for clinical response. Patients taking a combination of inducing and noninducing drugs (eg, carbamazepine and valproate) should be considered to be induced.

*Generalized weakness:* Moderately severe to incapacitating generalized weakness has been reported following administration of tiagabine in approximately 1% of patients with epilepsy. The weakness resolved in all cases after a reduction in dose or discontinuation of tiagabine.

*Ophthalmic effects:* Although no specific recommendations for periodic ophthalmologic monitoring exists, be aware of the possibility of long-term ophthalmologic effects.

*Therapeutic drug monitoring:* Because of the potential for pharmacokinetic interactions between tiagabine and drugs that induce or inhibit hepatic metabolizing enzymes, it may be useful to obtain plasma levels of tiagabine before and after changes are made in the therapeutic regimen.

#### Drug Interactions

Drugs that may affect tiagabine include valproate, carbamazepine, phenytoin, and phenobarbital. Valproate may be affected by tiagabine.

*Drug/Food interactions:* A high-fat meal decreases the rate, but not the extent (AUC), of tiagabine absorption.

### Adverse Reactions

Adverse reactions that occurred in 3% or more of patients include abdominal pain; pain (unspecified); dizziness; asthenia; somnolence; nervousness; tremor; insomnia; difficulty with concentration/attention; ataxia; confusion; speech disorder; difficulty with memory; parasthesia; depression; emotional lability; abnormal gait; nausea; diarrhea; vomiting; pharyngitis; cough increased; rash.

# TOPIRAMATE

**Tablets:** 25, 50, 100, and 200 mg (*Rx*)
**Capsules, sprinkle:** 15 and 25 mg (*Rx*)                    *Topamax* (Ortho-McNeil)

### Indications

*Epilepsy:*
   *Partial onset seizures* – Adjunctive therapy for partial onset seizure treatment in adults and children 2 to 16 years of age.
   *Tonic-clonic seizures* – Adjunctive therapy for primary generalized tonic-clonic seizures in adults and children 2 to 16 years of age.
   *Seizures associated with Lennox-Gastaut syndrome* – Adjunctive therapy in patients at least 2 years of age with seizures associated with Lennox-Gastaut syndrome.

*Migraine:* As prophylaxis of migraine headache in adults. The usefulness of topiramate in the acute treatment of migraine headache has not been studied.

### Administration and Dosage

It is not necessary to monitor topiramate plasma concentrations to optimize therapy.

Because of the bitter taste, do not break tablets.

Topiramate can be taken without regard to meals.

*Epilepsy:*
   *Adults (17 years of age and older): partial seizures, primary generalized tonic-clonic seizures, or Lennox-Gastaut syndrome* – The recommended total daily dose as adjunctive therapy is 200 to 400 mg/day in 2 divided doses in adults with partial seizures, and 400 mg/day in 2 divided doses in adults with tonic-clonic seizures. It is recommended that therapy be initiated at 25 to 50 mg/day followed by titration to an effective dose in increments of 25 to 50 mg/week. Titrating in increments of 25 mg/week may delay the time to reach an effective dose.
   Doses more than 400 mg/day (600, 800, and 1,000 mg/day) have not been shown to improve responses. Doses more than 1,600 mg/day have not been studied.
   *Pediatric patients (2 to 16 years of age): partial seizures, primary generalized tonic-clonic seizures, or Lennox-Gastaut syndrome* – The recommended total daily dose as adjunctive therapy is approximately 5 to 9 mg/kg/day in 2 divided doses. Begin titration at or below 25 mg (based on a range of 1 to 3 mg/kg/day) nightly for the first week. Then increase the dosage at 1- or 2-week intervals by increments of 1 to 3 mg/kg/day (administered in 2 divided doses) to achieve optimal clinical response. Guide dose titration by clinical outcome.

*Migraine:* The recommended total daily dose is 100 mg/day administered in 2 divided doses. The recommended titration rate 100 mg/day is:

|        | Morning dose | Evening dose |
|--------|--------------|--------------|
| Week 1 | None         | 25 mg        |
| Week 2 | 25 mg        | 25 mg        |
| Week 3 | 25 mg        | 50 mg        |
| Week 4 | 50 mg        | 50 mg        |

Guide dose titration rate by clinical outcome. If required, longer intervals between dose adjustments can be used.

*Concomitant therapy:* On occasion, the addition of topiramate to phenytoin may require an adjustment of the dose of phenytoin to achieve optimal clinical outcome. The addition or withdrawal of phenytoin and/or carbamazepine during adjunctive therapy with topiramate may require adjustment of the dose of topiramate.

*Sprinkle capsules:* Swallow whole or administer by carefully opening the capsule and sprinkling the entire contents on a small amount (teaspoon) of soft food. Swallow this drug/food mixture immediately; do not chew. Do not store for future use.

*Hepatic function impairment:* In hepatically impaired patients, topiramate plasma concentrations may be increased. Administer with caution.

*Renal function impairment:* In renally impaired subjects (Ccr less than 70 mL/min/1.73 m²), 50% of the usual adult dose is recommended. Such patients will require a longer time to reach steady state at each dose.

*Hemodialysis:* Topiramate is cleared by hemodialysis 4 to 6 times greater than in a healthy individual; a prolonged period of dialysis may cause topiramate levels to fall below that required to maintain an antiseizure effect. To avoid rapid drops in topiramate plasma concentration during hemodialysis, a supplemental dose of topiramate may be required. The actual adjustment should take into account 1) the duration of the dialysis period, 2) the clearance rate of the dialysis system being used, and 3) the effective renal clearance of topiramate in the patient being dialyzed.

## Actions

*Pharmacology:* The precise mechanism by which topiramate exerts its anticonvulsant and migraine prophylaxis effects are unknown. Topiramate, at pharmacologically relevant concentrations, blocks voltage-dependent sodium channels, augments the activity of the neurotransmitter gamma-aminobutyrate at some subtypes of the GABA-A receptor, antagonizes the AMPA/kainate subtype of the glutamate receptor, and inhibits the carbonic anhydrase enzyme, particularly isozymes II and IV.

*Pharmacokinetics:*

*Absorption/Distribution* – Absorption of topiramate is rapid, with peak plasma concentrations occurring at approximately 2 hours following a 400 mg oral dose. The relative bioavailability of topiramate from the tablet formulation is approximately 80% compared with a solution. The bioavailability of topiramate is not affected by food.

Steady state is reached in approximately 4 days in patients with normal renal function. Topiramate is 15% to 41% bound to human plasma proteins over the concentration range of 0.5 to 250 mcg/mL.

*Metabolism/Excretion* – Topiramate is not extensively metabolized and is primarily eliminated unchanged in the urine (approximately 70% of an administered dose). The mean plasma elimination half-life is 21 hours after single or multiple doses. Overall, plasma clearance is approximately 20 to 30 mL/min following oral administration.

*Bioequivalency* – The sprinkle formulation is bioequivalent to the immediate-release tablet formulation and, therefore, may be substituted as therapeutically equivalent.

## Contraindications

A history of hypersensitivity to any component of this product.

## Warnings

*Acute myopia and secondary-angle closure glaucoma:* A syndrome consisting of acute myopia associated with secondary-angle closure glaucoma has been reported in pediatric and adult patients receiving topiramate. Symptoms include acute onset of decreased visual acuity or ocular pain. Ophthalmologic findings can include myopia, anterior chamber shallowing, ocular hyperemia (redness), and increased intraocular pressure. Mydriasis may or may not be present. Symptoms typically occur within 1 month of initiating topiramate therapy. The primary treatment to reverse symptoms is discontinuation of topiramate as rapidly as possible, according to the judgment of the treating physician.

*Metabolic acidosis:* Hyperchloremic, nonanion gap, metabolic acidosis is associated with topiramate treatment. This metabolic acidosis is caused by renal bicarbonate loss because of the inhibitory effect of topiramate on carbonic anhydrase. Generally, topiramate-induced metabolic acidosis occurs early in treatment, although cases can occur at any time during treatment. Bicarbonate decrements usually are mild to moderate; rarely, patients can experience severe decrements to values below 10 mEq/L. Conditions or therapies that predispose to acidosis may be additive to the bicarbonate lowering effects of topiramate. If metabolic acidosis develops and persists, consider reducing the dose or discontinuing topiramate.

*Oligohydrosis and hyperthermia:* Oligohydrosis (decreased sweating), infrequently resulting in hospitalization, has been reported in association with topiramate use. Decreased sweating and an elevation in body temperature above normal characterized these cases. The majority of the reports have been in children.

Closely monitor patients, especially pediatric patients, treated with topiramate for evidence of decreased sweating and increased body temperature, especially in hot weather. Use caution when topiramate is prescribed with other drugs that predispose patients to heat-related disorders; these drugs include, but are not limited to, other carbonic anhydrase inhibitors and drugs with anticholinergic activity.

*Withdrawal:* Withdraw antiepileptic drugs, including topiramate, gradually to minimize the potential of increased seizure frequency.

*CNS-related adverse events:*

*Adults* – Adverse reactions most often associated with the use of topiramate were related to the CNS and were observed in both the epilepsy and migraine populations. In adults, the most frequent of these can be classified into 3 general categories:

1.) Cognitive-related dysfunction (eg, confusion; psychomotor slowing; difficulty with concentration/attention; difficulty with memory; speech or language problems, particularly word-finding difficulties).

2.) Psychiatric/behavioral disturbances (eg, depression, mood problems).

3.) Somnolence or fatigue.

*Children* – The incidences of cognitive/neuropsychiatric adverse events in pediatric patients generally were lower than previously observed in adults. These events included psychomotor slowing, difficulty with concentration/attention, speech disorders/related speech problems, and language problems. The most frequently reported neuropsychiatric events in this population were somnolence and fatigue.

*Sudden unexplained death in epilepsy:* Sudden and unexplained deaths were recorded among a cohort of treated patients (2,796 subject years of exposure). This represents an incidence of 0.0035 deaths per patient year.

*Renal function impairment:* The major route of elimination of unchanged topiramate and its metabolites is via the kidney. Dosage adjustment may be required.

*Hepatic function impairment:* In hepatically impaired patients, administer topiramate with caution because clearance may be decreased.

*Carcinogenesis:* An increase in urinary bladder tumors was observed in mice given topiramate (20, 75, and 300 mg/kg) for 21 months. The relevance of this finding to human carcinogenic risk is uncertain.

*Pregnancy: Category C.*

*Lactation:* Topiramate is excreted in the milk of lactating rats. Limited observations in patients suggest an extensive secretion of topiramate into breast milk. Weigh the potential benefit to the mother against the potential risk to the infant.

*Children:* Safety and efficacy in children younger than 2 years of age have not been established.

**Precautions**

*Monitoring:* Measurement of baseline and periodic serum bicarbonate during topiramate treatment is recommended.

*Hyperammonemia and encephalopathy associated with concomitant valproic acid use:* Administration of topiramate and valproic acid has been associated with hyperammonemia with or without encephalopathy in patients who have tolerated either drug alone. In most cases, symptoms and signs abated with discontinuation of either drug.

In patients who develop unexplained lethargy, vomiting, or changes in mental status, consider hyperammonemic encephalopathy and measure an ammonia level.

*Kidney stones:* A total of 1.5% patients exposed to topiramate during its development reported the occurrence of kidney stones; an incidence approximately 2 to 4 times that expected in a similar, untreated population. Kidney stones also have been reported in pediatric patients.

An explanation for the association of topiramate and kidney stones may lie in the fact that topiramate is a weak carbonic anhydrase inhibitor. Carbonic anhydrase inhibitors (eg, acetazolamide, dichlorphenamide) promote stone formation by reducing urinary citrate excretion and by increasing urinary pH. The concomitant use of topiramate with other carbonic anhydrase inhibitors or potentially in patients on a ketogenic diet may create a physiological environment that increases the risk of kidney stone formation and should be avoided.

Increased fluid intake increases urinary output, lowering substance concentration involved in stone formation. Hydration is recommended to reduce new stone formation.

*Paresthesia:* Paresthesia, an effect associated with the use of other carbonic anhydrase inhibitors, appears to be a common effect of topiramate.

*Photosensitivity:* Photosensitization may occur; therefore, caution patients to take protective measures against exposure to sunlight or ultraviolet light until tolerance is determined.

## Drug Interactions

Topiramate may affect alcohol, amitriptyline, CNS depressants, lithium, oral contraceptives, digoxin, estrogens, hydantoins, metformin, risperidone, and valproic acid.

Topiramate may be affected by carbamazepine, hydantoins, metformin, and valproic acid.

## Adverse Reactions

*Epilepsy* – Adverse reactions occurring in at least 3% of adult patients include abdominal pain, abnormal coordination, abnormal gait, abnormal vision, aggressive reaction, agitation, allergy, anorexia, apathy, asthenia, ataxia, back pain, breast pain, chest pain, cognitive problems, confusion, constipation, depression, difficulty with concentration/attention, difficulty with memory, diplopia, dizziness, dry mouth, dyspepsia, emotional lability, fatigue, influenza-like symptoms, language problems, leg pain, mood problems, nausea, nervousness, nystagmus, paresthesia, pharyngitis, psychomotor slowing, rhinitis, sinusitis, somnolence, speech disorders/related speech problems, taste perversion, tremor, urinary tract infection, weight decrease.

Adverse reactions occurring in at least 3% of pediatric patients include abnormal gait, aggressive reaction, anorexia, ataxia, confusion, constipation, difficulty with concentration/attention, difficulty with memory, dizziness, epistaxis, fatigue, gastroenteritis, hyperkinesia, increased saliva, injury, insomnia, nausea, nervousness, personality disorder (behavior problems), pneumonia, psychomotor slowing, purpura, skin disorder, somnolence, speech disorders/related speech problems, urinary incontinence, viral infection, weight decrease.

*Migraine* – Adverse reactions occurring in at least 3% of patients include the following: abdominal pain, anorexia, anxiety, arthralgia, blurred vision, bronchitis, confusion, coughing, depression, diarrhea, difficulty with memory, difficulty concentrating, dizziness, dyspepsia, dyspnea, dry mouth, ejaculation premature, fatigue, gastroenteritis, hypoesthesia, injury, insomnia, involuntary muscle contractions, language problems, menstrual disorder, mood problems, nausea, nervousness, paresthesia, pharyngitis, psychomotor slowing, pruritus, sinusitis, somnolence, taste perversion, upper respiratory infection, urinary tract infection, viral infection, vomiting, weight decrease.

# MAGNESIUM SULFATE

| | |
|---|---|
| **Injection**: 4% (0.325 mEq/mL) and 8% (0.65 mEq/mL) (*Rx*)<br>12.5% (1 mEq/mL) and 50% (4 mEq/mL) (*Rx*) | *Magnesium Sulfate* (Abbott)<br>Various |

### Indications

*Seizure:* Seizure prevention and control in severe pre-eclampsia or eclampsia without producing deleterious CNS depression in the mother or infant, and in convulsions associated with abnormally low levels of plasma magnesium as a contributing factor.

*Acute nephritis in children:* Acute nephritis in children to control hypertension, encephalopathy, and convulsions.

*Hypomagnesemia:* Magnesium deficiency, prevention and correction in total parenteral nutrition.

*Unlabeled uses:* Magnesium sulfate (2 g IV over 1 to 2 minutes for adults) has been shown to prevent recurrences of torsade de pointes by suppressing early-after depolarizations.

### Administration and Dosage

Individualize dosage. Monitor the patient's clinical status to avoid toxicity. Discontinue as soon as the desired effect is obtained. Repeat doses are dependent on continuing presence of the patellar reflex and adequate respiratory function.

*IM:* 4 to 5 g of a 50% solution every 4 hours as necessary.

*IV:* 4 g of a 10% to 20% solution, not exceeding 1.5 mL/min of a 10% solution.

*IV infusion:* 4 to 5 g in 250 mL of 5% dextrose or sodium chloride, not exceeding 3 mL/min.

*Children:* IM - 20 to 40 mg/kg in a 20% solution; repeat as necessary.

### Actions

*Pharmacology:* Magnesium prevents or controls convulsions by blocking neuromuscular transmission and decreasing the amount of acetylcholine liberated at the end plate by the motor nerve impulse.

One gram of magnesium sulfate provides 8.12 mEq of magnesium.

*Pharmacokinetics:* Approximately 1% to 2% of total body magnesium is located in the extracellular fluid space. Magnesium is 30% bound to albumin. With IV use, the onset of anticonvulsant action is immediate and lasts approximately 30 minutes. With IM use, onset occurs in 1 hour and persists for 3 to 4 hours. Effective anticonvulsant serum levels range from 2.5 or 3 to 7.5 mEq/L. Magnesium is excreted by the kidney.

### Contraindications

Heart block or myocardial damage; do not give in toxemia of pregnancy during the 2 hours preceding delivery.

### Warnings

*Aluminum toxicity:* Some products may contain aluminum. See individual product labeling for ingredients.

*IV use:* IV use in eclampsia is reserved for immediate control of life-threatening convulsions.

*Renal function impairment:* Because magnesium is excreted by the kidneys, parenteral use in the presence of renal insufficiency may lead to magnesium intoxication. Use with caution.

*Elderly:* Elderly patients often require reduced dosage because of impaired renal function.

*Pregnancy: Category A.*

*Lactation:* Because magnesium is distributed into milk, exercise caution when administering to a nursing mother. The American Academy of Pediatrics considers magnesium sulfate compatible with breastfeeding.

*Children:* Hypermagnesemia in the newborn may require resuscitation and assisted ventilation via endotracheal intubation or intermittent positive pressure ventilation as well as IV calcium. Elevated magnesium levels in the newborn may persist for up to 7 days; elimination half-life is approximately 43.2 hours.

### Precautions

*Monitoring:* Monitor serum magnesium levels and clinical status to avoid overdosage.

*Urine output:* Maintain at a level of 100 mL every 4 hours.

### Drug Interactions

*CNS depressants:* When barbiturates, narcotics, other hypnotics (or systemic anesthetics), or other CNS depressants are to be given in conjunction with magnesium, adjust their dosage with caution because of additive CNS depressant effects of magnesium.

*Neuromuscular blockers:* Magnesium sulfate potentiates the neuromuscular blockade produced by neuromuscular blocking agents.

### Adverse Reactions

Adverse reactions may include cardiac depression, circulatory collapse, CNS depression, depressed reflexes, flaccid paralysis, flushing, hypocalcemia, hypotension, hypothermia, magnesium intoxication, respiratory paralysis, sweating, tetany.

# OXCARBAZEPINE

**OXCARBAZEPINE**
**Tablets:** 150, 300, and 600 mg (*Rx*)                *Trileptal* (Novartis)
**Suspension:** 300 mg/5 mL (*Rx*)

### Indications

*Epilepsy:* For use as monotherapy or adjunctive therapy in the treatment of partial seizures in adults and children 4 to 16 years of age with epilepsy.

### Administration and Dosage

Oxcarbazepine may be taken with or without food.

*Withdrawal of antiepileptic drugs (AEDs)* · Withdraw gradually to minimize the potential of increased seizure frequency.

*Adults:*
  *Adjunctive therapy (600 mg/day twice/day)* – If clinically indicated, the dose may be increased by a maximum of 600 mg/day at approximately weekly intervals; the recommended daily dose is 1200 mg/day. Daily doses more than 1200 mg/day show somewhat greater effectiveness in controlled trials, but most patients were not able to tolerate the 2400 mg/day dose, primarily because of CNS effects. Observe and monitor closely the plasma levels of the concomitant AEDs during the period of oxcarbazepine titration, especially at oxcarbazepine doses more than 1200 mg/day.
  *Conversion to monotherapy (600 mg/day twice/day)* – Patients receiving concomitant AEDs may be converted to monotherapy by initiating treatment with oxcarbazepine at 300 mg twice daily while simultaneously initiating the reduction of the concomitant AED dose. Withdraw the concomitant AEDs over 3 to 6 weeks, while reaching the maximum dose of oxcarbazepine in approximately 2 to 4 weeks. Oxcarbazepine may be increased as clinically indicated by a maximum increment of 600 mg/day at approximate weekly intervals to achieve the recommended daily dose of 2400 mg/day. A daily dose of 1200 mg/day has been shown in 1 study to be effective in patients in whom monotherapy has been initiated with oxcarbazepine.
  *Initiation of monotherapy (600 mg/day twice/day)* – Increase by 300 mg/day every third day to a dose of 1200 mg/day. Controlled trials in these patients examined the effectiveness of a 1200 mg/day dose; a dose of 2400 mg/day has been shown to be effective in patients converted from other AEDs to oxcarbazepine monotherapy.

*Pediatric patients 4 to 16 years of age:*
  *Adjunctive therapy* – 8 to 10 mg/kg not to exceed 600 mg/day twice/day. Achieve the target maintenance dose of oxcarbazepine over 2 weeks, according to patient weight, using the following table.

| Oxcarbazepine Target Maintenance Doses for Pediatric Patients | |
| --- | --- |
| Patient weight (kg) | Target maintenance dose (mg/day) |
| 20 to 29 | 900 |
| 29.1 to 39 | 1200 |
| > 39 | 1800 |

In the clinical trial, in which the intention was to reach these target doses, the median daily dose was 31 mg/kg with a range of 6 to 51 mg/kg.

*Conversion to monotherapy:* Patients receiving concomitant AEDs may be converted to monotherapy by initiating treatment at approximately 8 to 10 mg/kg/day given in a twice-daily regimen, while simultaneously initiating the reduction of the dose of the concomitant AEDs. The concomitant AEDs can be completely withdrawn over 3 to 6 weeks, while oxcarbazepine may be increased as clinically indicated by a maximum increment of 10 mg/kg/day at approximately weekly intervals to achieve the recommended daily dose.

*Initiation of monotherapy:* Patients not currently being treated with antiepileptic drugs may have monotherapy initiated with oxcarbazepine. Initiate at a dose of 8 to 10 mg/kg/day given in a twice-daily regimen. Increase the dose by 5 mg/kg/day every third day to the recommended daily dose shown in the table below.

| Maintenance Doses of Oxcarbazepine for Children During Monotherapy | |
| --- | --- |
| Weight (kg) | Dose (mg/day) |
| 20 | 600 to 900 |
| 25 | 900 to 1200 |
| 30 | 900 to 1200 |
| 35 | 900 to 1500 |
| 40 | 900 to 1500 |
| 45 | 1200 to 1500 |
| 50 | 1200 to 1800 |
| 55 | 1200 to 1800 |
| 60 | 1200 to 2100 |
| 65 | 1200 to 2100 |
| 70 | 1500 to 2100 |

*Renal function impairment (Ccr less than 30 mL/min):* Initiate therapy at ½ the usual starting dose (300 mg/day) and increase slowly to achieve the desired clinical response.

**Actions**

*Pharmacology:* Oxcarbazepine activity is primarily exerted through the 10-monohydroxy metabolite (MHD) of oxcarbazepine. The precise mechanism by which oxcarbazepine and MHD exert their antiseizure effect is unknown.

*Pharmacokinetics:*

*Absorption* – Following oral administration of oxcarbazepine, it is completely absorbed and extensively metabolized to its pharmacologically active MHD metabolite.

*Distribution* – Approximately 40% of MHD is bound to serum proteins, predominantly to albumin.

*Metabolism* – Oxcarbazepine is rapidly reduced by cytosolic enzymes in the liver to its MHD, which is primarily responsible for the pharmacological effect of oxcarbazepine. MHD is metabolized further by conjugation with glucuronic acid.

*Excretion* – The half-life of the parent drug is approximately 2 hours, while the half-life of MHD is approximately 9 hours.

**Contraindications**

Known hypersensitivity to oxcarbazepine or any of its components.

**Warnings**

*Hyponatremia:* Clinically significant hyponatremia generally occurred during the first 3 months of treatment with oxcarbazepine, although there were patients who first developed a serum sodium less than 125 mmol/L greater than 1 year after initiation of therapy. Most patients who developed hyponatremia were asymptomatic, but patients in the clinical trials were frequently monitored and some had their oxcarbazepine dose reduced or discontinued or had their fluid intake restricted for hyponatremia. When oxcarbazepine was discontinued, normalization of serum sodium generally occurred within a few days without additional treatment.

Measure serum sodium levels for patients during maintenance treatment with oxcarbazepine.

*History of hypersensitivity reaction to carbamazepine:* Approximately 25% to 30% of patients who have had hypersensitivity reactions to carbamazepine will experience a hypersensitivity reaction with oxcarbazepine.

*Hepatic function impairment:* The pharmacokinetics of oxcarbazepine and MHD have not been evaluated in severe hepatic impairment. Adjust dose in renally impaired patients.

*Carcinogenesis:* In mice, a dose-related increase in the incidence of hepatocellular adenomas was observed with oxcarbazepine.

There was an increase in the incidence of benign testicular interstitial cell tumors and granular cell tumors in the cervix and vagina in rats.

*Mutagenesis:* Oxcarbazepine increased mutation frequencies in the Ames test in vitro in the absence of metabolic activation in 1 of 5 bacterial strains. Oxcarbazepine and MHD produced increases in chromosomal aberrations and polyploidy in the Chinese hamster ovary assay in vitro in the absence of metabolic activation.

*Fertility impairment:* In a fertility study in rats, estrous cyclicity was disrupted and numbers of corpora lutea, implantations, and live embryos were reduced in females receiving the highest dose (approximately 2 times the maximum recommended human dose on a mg/m$^2$ basis).

*Elderly:* Following administration of single (300 mg) and multiple (600 mg/day) doses of oxcarbazepine to elderly volunteers (60 to 82 years of age), the maximum plasma concentrations and AUC values of MHD were 30% to 60% higher than in younger volunteers (18 to 32 years of age).

*Pregnancy: Category* C.

*Lactation:* Oxcarbazepine and its active metabolite MHD are excreted in human breast milk.

*Children:* After a single-dose administration of 5 to 15 mg/kg of oxcarbazepine, the dose-adjusted AUC values of MHD were 30% to 40% lower in children younger than 8 years of age than in children older than 8 years of age. The clearance in children older than 8 years of age approaches that of adults.

Oxcarbazepine has been shown to be effective as adjunctive therapy or monotherapy for partial seizures in patients 4 to 16 years of age.

**Precautions**

*CNS effects:* Psychomotor slowing, difficulty with concentration, and speech or language problems; somnolence or fatigue; and coordination abnormalities, including ataxia and gait disturbances.

*Withdrawal of AEDs:* Withdraw gradually to minimize the potential of increased seizure frequency.

*Lab test abnormalities:* Serum sodium levels less than 125 mmol/L have been observed in patients treated with oxcarbazepine. Experience from clinical trials indicates that serum sodium levels return toward normal when the oxcarbazepine dosage is reduced or discontinued or when the patient was treated conservatively (eg, fluid restriction).

Laboratory data from clinical trials suggest that oxcarbazepine use was associated with decreases in $T_4$, without changes in $T_3$ or TSH.

**Drug Interactions**

*Cytochrome P450:* Oxcarbazepine inhibits CYP2C19 and induces CYP3A4/5 with potentially important effects on plasma concentrations of other drugs.

Strong inducers of cytochrome P450 enzymes (ie, carbamazepine, phenytoin, phenobarbital) have been shown to decrease the plasma levels of MHD (29% to 40%).

Cimetidine, erythromycin, and dextropropoxyphene had no effect on the pharmacokinetics of MHD. Results with warfarin show no evidence of interaction with either single or repeated doses of oxcarbazepine.

Drugs that may be affected by oxcarbazepine include felodipine, lamotrigine, oral contraceptives, phenobarbital, and phenytoin. Drugs that may affect oxcarbazepine include carbamazepine, phenobarbital, phenytoin, valproic acid, and verapamil.

**Adverse Reactions**

Adverse reactions that occurred in 3% or more of patients were as follows: Headache; dizziness; somnolence; anxiety; ataxia; nystagmus; abnormal gait; insomnia; tremor; amnesia; convulsions aggravated; emotional lability; hypoesthesia; nervousness; abnormal coordination; speech disorder; confusion; dysmetria; abnormal thinking; rash; nausea; vomiting; abdominal pain; anorexia; dry mouth; diarrhea; dyspepsia; constipation; urinary tract infection; hyponatremia; back pain; rhinitis; upper respiratory tract infection; coughing; bronchitis; pharyngitis; epistaxis; chest infection; sinusitis; diplopia; vertigo; taste perversion; abnormal vision; fatigue; fever; asthenia; falling down (nos); infection viral.

*Adjunctive therapy/monotherapy in adults previously treated with other AEDs* – The most commonly observed (5% or more) adverse experiences seen in association with oxcarbazepine and substantially more frequent than in placebo-treated patients were the following: Dizziness, somnolence, diplopia, fatigue, nausea, vomiting, ataxia, abnormal vision, abdominal pain, tremor, dyspepsia, abnormal gait.

Approximately 23% of these 1537 adult patients discontinued treatment because of an adverse experience. The adverse experiences most commonly associated with discontinuation were the following: Dizziness (6.4%), diplopia (5.9%), ataxia (5.2%), vomiting (5.1%), nausea (4.9%), somnolence (3.8%), headache (2.9%), fatigue (2.1%), abnormal vision (2.1%), tremor (1.8%), abnormal gait (1.7%), rash (1.4%), hyponatremia (1%).

*Adjunctive therapy/monotherapy in pediatric patients previously treated with other AEDs* – The most commonly observed (5% or more) adverse experiences seen in association with oxcarbazepine in pediatric patients were similar to those seen in adults.

Approximately 11% of the 456 pediatric patients discontinued treatment because of an adverse experience. The adverse experiences most commonly associated with discontinuation were the following: Somnolence (2.4%); vomiting (2%); ataxia (1.8%); diplopia, dizziness (1.3%); fatigue, nystagmus (1.1%).

*Monotherapy in adults not previously treated with other AEDs* – Approximately 9% of 295 adult patients discontinued treatment because of an adverse experience. The adverse experiences most commonly associated with discontinuation were the following: Dizziness, nausea, rash (1.7%); headache (1.4%).

*Monotherapy in pediatric patients not previously treated with other AEDs* – Approximately 9.2% of 152 pediatric patients discontinued treatment because of an adverse experience. The adverse experiences most commonly associated (at least 1%) with discontinuation were rash (5.3%) and maculopapular rash (1.3%).

# CYCLOBENZAPRINE HCl

**Tablets:** 10 mg (*Rx*)           Various, *Flexeril* (Merck)

### Indications
*Musculoskeletal conditions:* Adjunct to rest and physical therapy for relief of muscle spasm associated with acute painful musculoskeletal conditions.

*Unlabeled uses:* Cyclobenzaprine (10 to 40 mg/day) appears to be a useful adjunct in the management of the fibrositis syndrome.

### Administration and Dosage
Give 10 mg 3 times/day (range, 20 to 40 mg/day in divided doses). Do not exceed 60 mg/day. Do not use longer than 2 or 3 weeks.

### Actions
*Pharmacology:* Cyclobenzaprine, structurally related to the tricyclic antidepressants (TCAs), relieves skeletal muscle spasm of local origin without interfering with muscle function. It is ineffective in muscle spasm caused by CNS disease. The net effect is a reduction of tonic somatic motor activity, influencing both gamma and alpha motor systems.

*Pharmacokinetics:* Cyclobenzaprine is well absorbed after oral administration, but there is a large intersubject variation in plasma levels. The onset of action occurs in 1 hour with a duration of 12 to 24 hours. It is highly bound to plasma proteins, extensively metabolized and excreted primarily via the kidneys. Elimination half-life is 1 to 3 days.

### Contraindications
Hypersensitivity to cyclobenzaprine; concomitant use of monoamine oxidase (MAO) inhibitors or within 14 days after their discontinuation; acute recovery phase of MI and in patients with arrhythmias, heart block, or conduction disturbances or CHF; hyperthyroidism.

### Warnings
*Spasticity:* Cyclobenzaprine is not effective in the treatment of spasticity associated with cerebral or spinal cord disease, or in children with cerebral palsy.

*Duration:* Use only for short periods (up to 2 or 3 weeks); effectiveness for more prolonged use is not proven.

*Similarity to TCAs:* Cyclobenzaprine is closely related to the TCAs. In short-term studies for indications other than muscle spasm associated with acute musculoskeletal conditions, and usually at doses greater than those recommended, some of the more serious CNS reactions noted with the TCAs have occurred.

*Pregnancy:* Category B.

*Lactation:* It is not known whether cyclobenzaprine is excreted in breast milk.

*Children:* Safety and efficacy in children younger than 15 years of age have not been established.

### Precautions
*Anticholinergic effects:* Because of its anticholinergic action, use with caution in patients with a history of urinary retention, angle-closure glaucoma, and increased intraocular pressure.

*Hazardous tasks:* May impair mental or physical abilities required for performance of hazardous tasks; patients should observe caution while driving or performing other tasks requiring alertness, coordination, and physical dexterity.

### Drug Interactions
Drugs that may interact with cyclobenzaprine HCl include MAO inhibitors and TCAs.

### Adverse Reactions
Adverse reactions occurring in 3% or more of patients include drowsiness, dizziness, fatigue, tiredness, asthenia, blurred vision, headache, nervousness, confusion, dry mouth, nausea, constipation, dyspepsia, unpleasant taste, purpura, bone marrow depression, leukopenia, eosinophilia, thrombocytopenia, elevation and lowering of blood sugar levels, and weight gain or loss.

# DIAZEPAM

| | |
|---|---|
| **Tablets**: 2, 5, and 10 mg (c-iv) | Various, *Valium* (Roche) |
| **Oral solution**: 5 mg/5 mL (c-iv) | *Diazepam* (Roxane) |
| **Concentrated oral solution**: 5 mg/mL (c-iv) | *Diazepam Intensol* (Roxane) |
| **Injection**: 5 mg/mL (c-iv) | Various, *Valium* (Roche), *Zetran* (Hauck), *Dizac* (Ohmeda) |

The following is an abbreviated monograph. For complete prescribing information, refer to the Benzodiazepines monograph in the Antianxiety Agents section.

### Indications

An adjunct for the relief of skeletal muscle spasm caused by reflex spasm to local pathology (such as inflammation of the muscles or joints, or secondary to trauma); spasticity caused by upper motor neuron disorders; athetosis; stiff-man syndrome. Injectable diazepam may also be used as an adjunct in tetanus.

Also used as an antianxiety agent and an anticonvulsant.

### Administration and Dosage

*Oral:* Individualize dosage for maximum beneficial effect.

*Adults* – 2 to 10 mg 3 or 4 times/day.

*Geriatric or debilitated patients* – 2 to 2.5 mg 1 or 2 times/day initially, increasing as needed and tolerated.

*Children* – 1 to 2.5 mg 3 or 4 times/day initially, increasing as needed and tolerated (not for use in children older than 6 months of age).

*Intensol* – Dosages are same as those listed above. Mix with liquid or semi-solid food such as water, juices, soda or soda-like beverages, applesauce, and puddings. Stir in gently. Consume the entire mixture immediately. Do not store for future use.

*Sustained release* – 15 to 30 mg once/day.

*Parenteral:* Use lower doses (2 to 5 mg) and slow dosage increases for elderly or debilitated patients and when other sedatives are given. When acute symptoms are controlled with the injectable form, administer oral therapy if further treatment is required.

*Neonates (up to 30 days of age)* – Safety and efficacy have not been established. Prolonged CNS depression has been observed in neonates, apparently because of inability to biotransform diazepam into inactive metabolites.

*Children* – Give slowly over 3 minutes in a dosage not to exceed 0.25 mg/kg. After a 15 to 30 minute interval, the initial dosage can be safely repeated. If relief is not obtained after a third administration, begin adjunctive therapy appropriate to the condition being treated.

*IM:* Inject deeply into the muscle.

*IV:* Inject slowly, taking at least 1 minute for each 5 mg (1 mL). Do not use small veins (ie, dorsum of hand or wrist). Avoid intra-arterial administration or extravasation. Do not mix or dilute with other solutions or drugs.

*Adults* – 5 to 10 mg, IM or IV initially, then 5 to 10 mg in 3 to 4 hours, if necessary. For tetanus, larger doses may be required.

*Children* – For tetanus in infants older than 30 days of age, 1 to 2 mg IM or IV slowly; repeat every 3 to 4 hours as necessary. In children 5 years of age or older, 5 to 10 mg. Repeat every 3 to 4 hours if necessary to control tetanus spasms. Have respiratory assistance available.

### Actions

*Pharmacology:* Major muscle relaxant actions occur in the following 2 proposed sites: At the spinal level resulting in enhancement of GABA-mediated presynaptic inhibition, and at supraspinal sites, probably in the brain stem reticular formation.

# BACLOFEN

**Tablets:** 10 and 20 mg (*Rx*)                                    Various, *Lioresal* (Geigy)
**Intrathecal:** 10 mg/20 mL (500 mcg/mL) and 10 mg/5 mL    *Lioresal* (Medtronic)
(2000 mcg/mL) (*Rx*)

---

**Warning:**

Abrupt discontinuation of intrathecal baclofen, regardless of the cause, has resulted in sequelae that include high fever, altered mental status, exaggerated rebound spasticity, and muscle rigidity, which in rare cases has advanced to rhabdomyolysis, multiple organ-system failure, and death.

Prevention of abrupt discontinuation of intrathecal baclofen requires careful attention to programming and monitoring of the infusion system, refill scheduling and procedures, and pump alarms. Advise patients and caregivers of the importance of keeping scheduled refill visits and educate them on the early symptoms of baclofen withdrawal. Give special attention to patients at apparent risk (eg, spinal cord injuries at T-6 or above, communication difficulties, history of withdrawal symptoms from oral or intrathecal baclofen). Consult the technical manual of the implantable infusion system for additional postimplant clinician and patient information (see Warnings).

---

### Indications

*Oral:* Alleviation of signs and symptoms of spasticity resulting from multiple sclerosis, particularly for the relief of flexor spasms and concomitant pain, clonus, and muscular rigidity. Patients should have reversible spasticity so that treatment will aid in restoring residual function.

Oral baclofen may be of some value in patients with spinal cord injuries and other spinal cord diseases.

*Intrathecal:* Management of severe spasticity of spinal cord origin in patients who are unresponsive to oral baclofen therapy or experience intolerable CNS side effects at effective doses. Intended for use by the intrathecal route in single bolus test doses (via spinal catheter or lumbar puncture) and, for chronic use, only in implantable pumps approved by the FDA specifically for the administration of baclofen into the intrathecal space.

Intrathecal therapy may be considered an alternative to destructive neurosurgical procedures. Prior to implantation of a device for chronic intrathecal infusion, patients must show a response in a screening trial.

The efficacy as a treatment for spasticity of cerebral origin is not established.

*Unlabeled uses:*

*Oral –* Treatment of trigeminal neuralgia (50 to 60 mg/day).

*Intrathecal –* 25, 50, or 100 mcg appears to be beneficial in children for reducing spasticity in cerebral palsy.

### Administration and Dosage

*Oral:* Individualize dosage. Start at a low dosage and increase gradually until the optimum effect is achieved (usually 40 to 80 mg/day).

The following dosage schedule is suggested: 5 mg 3 times/day for 3 days; 10 mg 3 times/day for 3 days; 15 mg 3 times/day for 3 days; 20 mg 3 times/day for 3 days. Thereafter, additional increases may be necessary, but the total daily dose should not exceed 80 mg/day (20 mg 4 times/day).

The lowest effective dose is recommended. If benefits are not evident after a reasonable trial period, withdraw the drug slowly.

*Intrathecal:* Refer to the manufacturer's manual for the implantable intrathecal infusion pump for specific instructions and precautions for programming the pump or refilling the reservoir.

Consult complete *Drug Facts and Comparisons* monograph and/or manufacturer product information for full intrathecal dosing information.

*Dilution instructions* –

*Screening:* Both strengths (10 mg/5 mL and 10 mg/20 mL) must be diluted with sterile preservative-free Sodium Chloride for Injection, USP to a 50 mcg/mL concentration for bolus injection into the subarachnoid space.

*Maintenance:* For patients who require concentrations other than 500 or 2000 mcg/mL, baclofen intrathecal must be diluted with sterile, preservative free Sodium Chloride for Injection, USP.

*Delivery regimen* – Baclofen intrathecal is most often administered in a continuous infusion mode immediately following implant. For those patients implanted with programmable pumps who have achieved relatively satisfactory control on continuous infusion, further benefit may be attained using more complex schedules of delivery.

## Actions

*Pharmacology:* The precise mechanism of action is not known. Baclofen can inhibit mono- and polysynaptic reflexes at the spinal level, possibly by hyperpolarization of afferent terminals, although actions at supraspinal sites also may contribute to its clinical effect. Baclofen has CNS-depressant properties.

*Pharmacokinetics:*

*Oral* – Baclofen is rapidly and extensively absorbed. Absorption may be dose-dependent, reduced with increasing doses. Peak serum levels are reached in about 2 hours; half-life is 3 to 4 hours. It is excreted primarily by the kidney in unchanged form with intersubject variation in absorption or elimination.

*Intrathecal* –

*Bolus:* The onset of action is generally 0.5 to 1 hour after an intrathecal bolus dose. Peak spasmolytic effect is seen at about 4 hours after dosing and effects may last 4 to 8 hours. Onset, peak response, and duration of action may vary with individual patients depending on the dose and severity of symptoms.

*Continuous infusion:* The antispastic action is first seen at 6 to 8 hours after initiation of continuous infusion. Maximum activity is observed in 24 to 48 hours. The mean CSF clearance was about 30 mL/h in 10 patients on continuous intrathecal infusion.

## Contraindications

Hypersensitivity to baclofen.

*Oral:* Treatment of skeletal muscle spasm resulting from rheumatic disorders; stroke, cerebral palsy, and Parkinson's disease.

*Intrathecal:* IV, IM, subcutaneous, or epidural administration.

## Warnings

*Intrathecal administration:* Because of the possibility of potentially life-threatening CNS depression, cardiovascular collapse, or respiratory failure, physicians must be adequately trained and educated in chronic intrathecal infusion therapy.

*Infection:* Patients should be infection-free prior to the screening trial with baclofen injection because the presence of a systemic infection may interfere with an assessment of the patient's response.

Patients should be infection-free prior to pump implantation because the presence of infection may increase the risk of surgical complications. Moreover, a systemic infection may complicate attempts to adjust the pump's dosing rate.

*Abrupt drug withdrawal:*

*Oral* – Hallucinations and seizures have occurred on abrupt withdrawal. An isolated case of manic psychosis has been reported. Except in cases of serious adverse reactions, reduce dose slowly when drug is discontinued.

*Intrathecal* – Early symptoms of baclofen withdrawal may include return of baseline spasticity, pruritus, hypotension, and paresthesias. Some clinical characteristics of the advanced intrathecal baclofen withdrawal syndrome may resemble autonomic dysreflexia, infection (sepsis), malignant hyperthermia, neuroleptic-malignant syndrome, or other conditions associated with a hypermetabolic state or widespread rhabdomyolysis.

The suggested treatment for intrathecal baclofen withdrawal is the restoration of intrathecal baclofen at or near the same dosage as before therapy was interrupted.

*Stroke:* Baclofen has not significantly benefited patients with stroke; they also have poor drug tolerance.

*Renal function impairment:* Because baclofen is primarily excreted unchanged through the kidneys, administer with caution to patients with impaired renal function. Dosage reduction may be necessary.

*Pregnancy: Category C.*

*Lactation:* In mothers treated with oral baclofen in therapeutic doses, the active substance passes into the breast milk. It is not known whether detectable levels of drug are present in breast milk of nursing mothers receiving intrathecal baclofen.

*Children:*

Oral – Safety for use in children younger than 12 years of age has not been established. Oral baclofen is not recommended for use in children.

Intrathecal – Safety in children younger than 4 years of age has not been established.

## Precautions

*Epilepsy:* Monitor the clinical state and EEG at regular intervals because deterioration in seizure control and EEG changes have occurred in patients taking this drug.

*Need for spasticity:* Use with caution where spasticity is used to sustain upright posture and balance in locomotion or whenever spasticity is utilized to obtain increased function.

*Ovarian cysts:* Ovarian cysts have been found by palpation in about 4% of multiple sclerosis patients treated with baclofen for up to 1 year. In most cases, these cysts disappeared spontaneously while patients continued to receive the drug. Ovarian cysts are estimated to occur spontaneously in about 1% to 5% of the normal female population.

*Psychotic disorders:* Cautiously treat patients suffering from psychotic disorders, schizophrenia, or confusional states and keep under careful surveillance because exacerbations of these conditions have been observed with oral administration.

*Autonomic dysreflexia:* Use with caution in patients with a history of autonomic dysreflexia. The presence of nociceptive stimuli or abrupt withdrawal may cause an autonomic dysreflexic episode.

*Hazardous tasks:* Because of the possibility of sedation, patients should observe caution while driving or performing other tasks requiring alertness, coordination, or physical dexterity.

## Adverse Reactions

Adverse reactions occurring in at least 3% of patients include the following: Drowsiness, weakness of extremities, dizziness/lightheadedness, seizures, headache, nausea/vomiting, numbness/itching/tingling, hypotension, blurred vision, constipation, hypotonia, slurred speech, coma, lethargy/fatigue, confusion, insomnia, urinary frequency.

# DANTROLENE SODIUM

**Capsules**: 25, 50, and 100 mg (*Rx*)
**Powder for injection**: 20 mg/vial. Concentration following reconstitution is ≈ 0.32 mg/mL. In 70 mL vials. (*Rx*)

*Dantrium* (Procter & Gamble)
*Dantrium Intravenous* (Procter & Gamble)

---

**Warning:**
   Dantrolene has a potential for hepatotoxicity. Do not use in conditions other than those recommended. The incidence of symptomatic hepatitis (fatal and nonfatal) reported in patients taking up to 400 mg/day is much lower than in those taking 800 mg/day or more. Even sporadic short courses of these higher dose levels within a treatment regimen markedly increased the risk of serious hepatic injury. Liver dysfunction, as evidenced by liver enzyme elevations, has been observed in patients exposed to the drug for varying periods of time. Overt hepatitis has been most frequently observed between the third and twelfth months of therapy. Risk of hepatic injury appears to be greater in females, in patients older than 35 years of age, and in patients taking other medications in addition to dantrolene.

Monitor hepatic function, including frequent determinations of AST or ALT. If no observable benefit is derived from therapy after 45 days, discontinue use.

Use the lowest possible effective dose for each patient.

---

### Indications
*Spasticity:*
   *Oral* – For the control of clinical spasticity resulting from upper motor neuron disorders such as spinal cord injury, stroke, cerebral palsy, or multiple sclerosis. It is of particular benefit to the patient whose functional rehabilitation has been retarded by the sequelae of spasticity. Such patients must have presumably reversible spasticity where relief of spasticity will aid in restoring residual function.

*Malignant hyperthermia (MH):*
   *IV* – Management of the fulminant hypermetabolism of skeletal muscle characteristic of MH crisis, along with appropriate supportive measures.

   Preoperatively, and sometimes postoperatively, to prevent or attenuate the development of clinical and laboratory signs of MH in individuals judged to be susceptible to MH.

   *Oral* – Preoperatively to prevent or attenuate the development of signs of MH in susceptible patients who require anesthesia or surgery. Currently accepted clinical practices in the management of such patients must still be adhered to (careful monitoring for early signs of MH, minimizing exposure to triggering mechanisms, and prompt use of IV dantrolene and indicated supportive measures if signs of MH appear).

   Following a MH crisis to prevent recurrence of MH.

### Administration and Dosage
   Exercise caution at meals on the day of administration because difficulty swallowing and choking has been reported.

*Chronic spasticity:* Titrate and individualize dosage. In view of the potential for liver damage in long-term use, discontinue therapy if benefits are not evident within 45 days.

   *Adults* – Begin with 25 mg once/day, increase to 25 mg 2 to 4 times/day, then increase by increments of 25 mg up to as high as 100 mg 2 to 4 times/day if necessary. As most patients will respond to 400 mg/day or less, higher doses rarely are needed. Maintain each dosage level for 4 to 7 days to determine response. Adjust dosage to achieve maximal benefit without adverse effects.

   *Children* – Use a similar approach. Start with 0.5 mg/kg twice/day; increase to 0.5 mg/kg, 3 or 4 times/day; then by increments of 0.5 mg/kg, up to 3 mg/kg, 2 to 4 times/day if necessary. Do not exceed doses higher than 100 mg 4 times/day.

MH:

*Preoperative prophylaxis* – Dantrolene may be given orally or IV to patients judged susceptible to MH as part of the overall patient management to prevent or attenuate development of clinical and laboratory signs of MH.

*Oral* – Give 4 to 8 mg/kg/day orally in 3 or 4 divided doses for 1 or 2 days prior to surgery, with last dose given approximately 3 to 4 hours before scheduled surgery with a minimum of water. This dosage usually will be associated with skeletal muscle weakness and sedation (sleepiness or drowsiness) or excessive GI irritation (nausea or vomiting); adjust within the recommended dosage range to avoid incapacitation or excessive GI irritation.

*IV* – Dantrolene IV may decrease the grip strength and increase weakness of leg muscles, especially walking down stairs.

*Treatment* – As soon as the MH reaction is recognized, discontinue all anesthetic agents. Use of 100% oxygen is recommended. Administer dantrolene by continuous rapid IV push beginning at a minimum dose of 1 mg/kg, and continuing until symptoms subside or a maximum cumulative dose of 10 mg/kg has been reached. If the physiologic and metabolic abnormalities reappear, repeat the regimen. Administration should be continuous until symptoms subside.

*Children* – Dose is the same as for adults.

*Postcrisis follow-up* – Following a MH crisis, give 4 to 8 mg/kg/day orally, in 4 divided doses for 1 to 3 days to prevent recurrence. IV dantrolene may be used when oral administration is not practical. The IV dose must be individualized, starting with 1 mg/kg or more as the clinical situation dictates.

## Actions

*Pharmacology:* In isolated nerve-muscle preparation, dantrolene produced relaxation by affecting contractile response of the skeletal muscle at a site beyond the myoneural junction and directly on the muscle itself. In skeletal muscle, the drug dissociates the excitation-contraction coupling, probably by interfering with the release of calcium from the sarcoplasmic reticulum.

*MH* – Dantrolene may prevent changes within the muscle cell that result in MH syndrome by interfering with calcium release from the sarcoplasmic reticulum to the myoplasm.

*Pharmacokinetics:*

*Absorption/Distribution* – Absorption after oral administration is incomplete (approximately 70%) and slow but consistent, and dose-related blood levels are obtained.

*Metabolism* – Dantrolene is found in measurable amounts in blood and urine. Mean half-life in adults is 9 hours after a 100 mg oral dose and 4 to 8 hours after IV administration. Because it is probably metabolized by hepatic microsomal enzymes, metabolism enhancement by other drugs is possible.

## Contraindications

*Oral:* Active hepatic disease, such as hepatitis and cirrhosis; where spasticity is used to sustain upright posture and balance in locomotion or to obtain or maintain increased function; treatment of skeletal muscle spasm resulting from rheumatic disorders.

## Warnings

*Hepatic effects:* Fatal and nonfatal liver disorders of an idiosyncratic or hypersensitivity type may occur. At the start of therapy, perform baseline liver function studies. If abnormalities exist, the potential for hepatotoxicity could be enhanced.

Perform liver function studies at appropriate intervals during therapy. If such studies reveal abnormal values, generally discontinue therapy. Some laboratory values may return to normal with continued therapy; others may not.

If symptoms of hepatitis accompanied by liver function test abnormalities or jaundice appear, discontinue therapy. If caused by dantrolene and detected early, abnormalities may revert to normal when the drug is discontinued. See Warning Box.

*Long-term use:* Safety and efficacy have not been established.

Continued long-term administration is justified if use of the drug: Significantly reduces painful or disabling spasticity such as clonus; significantly reduces the intensity or degree of nursing care required; rids the patient of any annoying manifestation of spasticity considered important by the patient.

Brief withdrawal for 2 to 4 days will frequently demonstrate exacerbation of the manifestations of spasticity and may serve to confirm a clinical impression.

In view of the potential for liver damage in long-term use, discontinue therapy if benefits are not evident within 45 days.

*MH:* IV use is not a substitute for previously known supportive measures. These measures include discontinuing the suspect triggering agents, attending to increased oxygen requirements, managing the metabolic acidosis, instituting cooling when necessary, attending to urinary output, and monitoring electrolyte imbalance.

*Pregnancy: Category* C (parenteral).

*Lactation:* Do not use in nursing women.

*Children:* Safety for use in children younger than 5 years of age has not been established.

### Precautions

*Extravasation:* Because of the high pH of the IV formulation, prevent extravasation into the surrounding tissues.

*Special risk:* Use with caution in patients with impaired pulmonary function, particularly those with obstructive pulmonary disease; severely impaired cardiac function caused by myocardial disease; history of previous liver disease or dysfunction.

*Hazardous tasks:* Patients should use caution while driving or performing other tasks requiring alertness, coordination or physical dexterity.

*Photosensitivity:* Photosensitization may occur; therefore, caution patients to take protective measures against exposure to ultraviolet light or sunlight until tolerance is determined.

### Drug Interactions

Drugs that may interact with dantrolene include clofibrate, estrogens, warfarin, and verapamil.

Avoid alcohol and other CNS depressants.

### Adverse Reactions

Adverse reactions may include drowsiness; dizziness; weakness; general malaise; fatigue; diarrhea; constipation; GI bleeding; anorexia; dysphagia; gastric irritation; abdominal cramps; hepatitis; speech disturbance; seizure; headache; lightheadedness; visual disturbance; diplopia; taste alteration; insomnia; mental depression; confusion; increased nervousness; tachycardia; erratic blood pressure; phlebitis; increased urinary frequency; hematuria; crystalluria; difficult erection; urinary incontinence; nocturia; dysuria; urinary retention; abnormal hair growth; acne-like rash; pruritus; urticaria; eczematoid eruption; sweating; myalgia; backache; chills; fever; feeling of suffocation; excessive tearing; pleural effusion with pericarditis; severity: pulmonary edema developing during treatment of MH crisis; thrombophlebitis following IV dantrolene; urticaria; erythema; hepatitis; seizures; pleural effusion with pericarditis.

# PARKINSON DISEASE

Parkinsonism is a neurological disease with a variety of origins characterized by tremor, rigidity, akinesia, and disorders of posture and equilibrium. The onset is slow and progressive, with symptoms advancing over months to years.

| | | | | | | |
|---|---|---|---|---|---|---|
| **Drug Therapy for Parkinsonism** | | | | | | |
| | Indications | | | | | |
| Drugs | Post-encephalitic | Arterio-sclerotic | Idiopathic | Drug/chemical induced | Adjunct to Levodopa/carbidopa | Usual daily dose range (mg) |
| **Anticholinergics** | | | | | | |
| Procyclidine | ✔ | ✔ | ✔ | ✔ | | 7.5 to 20 |
| Trihexyphenidyl | ✔ | ✔ | ✔ | ✔ | ✔ | 1 to 15 |
| Benztropine | ✔ | ✔ | ✔ | ✔ | | 0.5 to 6.5 |
| Biperiden | ✔ | ✔ | ✔ | ✔ | | 2 to 8 |
| Ethopropazine | ✔ | ✔ | ✔ | ✔ | | 50 to 600 |
| Diphenhydramine | ✔ | ✔ | ✔ | ✔ | | 10 to 400 |
| **Dopaminergic Agents** | | | | | | |
| Levodopa | ✔ | ✔ | ✔ | ✔[1] | | 500 to 8000 |
| Carbidopa/Levodopa | ✔ | | ✔ | ✔[1] | | 10/100 to 200/2000 |
| Amantadine | ✔ | ✔ | ✔ | ✔ | | 200 to 400 |
| Bromocriptine | ✔ | | ✔ | | | 12.5 to 100 |
| Pergolide | | | | | ✔ | 1 to 5 |
| Selegiline | | | | | ✔ | 10 |
| Pramipexole | | | ✔ | | | 0.375 to 4.5 |
| Ropinirole | | | ✔ | | | 0.75 to 3 |

[1] Not effective in drug-induced extrapyramidal symptoms.

# ANTICHOLINERGICS

**BENZTROPINE MESYLATE**
**Tablets**: 0.5, 1, and 2 mg (*Rx*)　　　　Various, *Cogentin* (Merck)
**Injection**: 1 mg/mL (*Rx*)　　　　　　　*Cogentin* (Merck)
**BIPERIDEN**
**Tablets**: 2 mg (*Rx*)　　　　　　　　　　*Akineton* (Knoll)
**Injection**: 5 mg/mL (*Rx*)　　　　　　　*Akineton* (Knoll)
**ETHOPROPAZINE HCl**
**Tablets**: 10 and 50 mg (*Rx*)　　　　　*Parsidol* (Parke-Davis)
**PROCYCLIDINE**
**Tablets**: 5 mg (*Rx*)　　　　　　　　　　*Kemadrin* (GlaxoSmithKline)
**TRIHEXYPHENIDYL HCl**
**Tablets**: 2 and 5 mg (*Rx*)　　　　　　　Various, *Artane* (Lederle)
**Capsules, sustained release**: 5 mg (*Rx*)　*Artane Sequels* (Lederle)
**Elixir**: 2 mg/5 mL (*Rx*)　　　　　　　　*Artane* (Lederle)

### Indications
Adjunctive therapy in all forms of parkinsonism (postencephalitic, arteriosclerotic and idiopathic) and in the control of drug-induced extrapyramidal disorders.

### Administration and Dosage
Give before or after meals, as determined by patient's reaction. Postencephalitic patients (more prone to excessive salivation) may prefer to take it after meals and may, in addition, require small amounts of atropine. If the mouth dries excessively, take before meals, unless it causes nausea. If taken after meals, thirst can be allayed by mint candies, chewing gum, or water.

*BENZTROPINE MESYLATE:* Because there is not significant difference in onset of action after IV or IM injection, there is usually no need to use the IV route. In emergency situations, when the condition of the patients is alarming, 1 to 2 mL will normally provide quick relief.

*Dosage titration* – Because of cumulative action, initiate therapy with a low dose, increase in increments of 0.5 mg gradually at 5 or 6 day intervals to the smallest amount necessary for optimal relief. Maximum daily dose is 6 mg.

*Dose intervals* – Some patients experience greatest relief by taking the entire dose at bedtime; others react more favorably to divided doses, 2 to 4 times/day.

*Parkinsonism* – 1 to 2 mg/day, with a range of 0.5 to 6 mg/day, orally or parenterally.

*Idiopathic parkinsonism:* Start with 0.5 to 1 mg at bedtime; 4 to 6 mg/day may be required.

*Postencephalitic parkinsonism:* 2 mg/day in 1 dose or more. In highly sensitive patients, begin therapy with 0.5 mg at bedtime; increase as necessary.

*Drug-induced extrapyramidal disorders* – Administer 1 to 4 mg once or twice/day.

*Acute dystonic reactions:* 1 to 2 mL IM or IV usually relieves the condition quickly. After that, 1 to 2 mL orally 2 times/day usually prevents recurrence.

Extrapyramidal disorders which develop soon after initiating treatment with neuroleptic drugs are likely to be transient. A dosage of 1 to 2 mg orally 2 or 3 times a day usually provides relief within 1 or 2 days. After 1 or 2 weeks, withdraw drug to determine its continued need. If such disorders recur, reinstitute benztropine.

*BIPERIDEN:*

*Parkinsonism* – 2 mg 3 or 4 times/day, orally. Individualize dosage with dosing titrated to a maximum of 16 mg/24 hours.

*Drug-induced extrapyramidal disorders* –

*Oral:* 2 mg 1 to 3 times/day.

*Parenteral:* 2 mg IM or IV. Repeat every half-hour until symptoms are resolved, but do not give more than 4 consecutive doses per 24 hours.

*ETHOPROPAZINE:*

*Initially* – 50 mg once or twice/day; increase gradually, if necessary.

*Mild to moderate symptoms* – 100 to 400 mg/day.

*Severe cases* – Gradually increase to 500 or 600 mg or more daily.

*DIPHENYDRAMINE:* For complete prescribing information and product availability, see the Antihistamines group monograph.

*Oral* –

*Adults:* 25 to 50 mg 3 to 4 times/day.

*Children more than 20 lbs (9 kg):* 12.5 to 25 mg 3 or 4 times/day or 5 mg/kg/day. Do not exceed 300 mg/day or 150 mg/m$^2$/day.

*Parenteral* – Administer IV or deeply IM.

*Adults:* 10 to 50 mg; 100 mg if required. Maximum daily dosage is 400 mg.

*Children:* 5 mg/kg/day or 150 mg/m$^2$/day.

*PROCYCLIDINE:*

*Parkinsonism (for patients who have received no other therapy)* – Initially, 2.5 mg 3 times/day after meals. If well tolerated, gradually increase dose to 5 mg; administer 3 times/day, and occasionally before retiring, if necessary. In some cases, smaller doses may be effective.

*For drug-induced extrapyramidal symptoms* – Begin with 2.5 mg 3 times/day; increase by 2.5 mg/day increments until the patient obtains relief of symptoms. Individualize dosage. In most cases, results will be obtained with 10 to 20 mg/day.

*TRIHEXYPHENIDYL HCl:*

*Parkinsonism* – Initially, administer 1 to 2 mg the first day; increase by 2 mg increments at intervals of 3 to 5 days, until a total of 6 to 10 mg is given daily. Many patients derive maximum benefit from a total daily dose of 6 to 10 mg; however, postencephalitic patients may require a total daily dose of 12 to 15 mg. Trihexyphenidyl is tolerated best if divided into 3 doses and taken at mealtimes. High doses may be divided into 4 parts, administered at mealtimes and at bedtime.

*Concomitant use with levodopa:* Trihexyphenidyl 3 to 6 mg/day in divided doses is usually adequate.

*Drug-induced extrapyramidal disorders* – Start with a single 1 mg dose. Daily dosage usually ranges between 5 to 15 mg, although reactions have been controlled on as little as 1 mg/day.

*Sustained release* – Do not use for initial therapy. Once patients are stabilized on conventional dosage forms, they may be switched to sustained release capsules on a milligram per milligram of total daily dose basis. Administer as a single dose after breakfast or in 2 divided doses 12 hours apart.

## Actions

*Pharmacology:* Anticholinergic agents reduce the incidence and severity of akinesia, rigidity, and tremor by approximately 20%; secondary symptoms such as drooling are also reduced. In addition to suppressing central cholinergic activity, these agents also may inhibit the reuptake and storage of dopamine at central dopamine receptors, thereby prolonging the action of dopamine.

*Pharmacokinetics:*

| Various Antiparkinson Anticholinergic Pharmacokinetic Parameters | | | | |
| --- | --- | --- | --- | --- |
| Anticholinergic | Time to peak concentration (h) | Peak concentration (mcg/L) | Half-life (h) | Oral bioavailability (%) |
| Benztropine[1] | | | | |
| Biperiden | 1 to 1.5 | 4 to 5 | 18.4 to 24.3 | 29 |
| Diphenhydramine | 2 to 4 | 65 to 90 | 4 to 15 | 50 to 72 |
| Ethopropazine[1] | | | | |
| Procyclidine | 1.1 to 2 | 80 | 11.5 to 12.6 | 52 to 97 |
| Trihexyphenidyl | 1 to 1.3 | 87.2 | 5.6 to 10.2 | $\approx 100$ |

[1] No data available.

## Contraindications

Hypersensitivity to any component; glaucoma, particularly angle-closure glaucoma; pyloric or duodenal obstruction; stenosing peptic ulcers; prostatic hypertrophy or bladder neck obstructions; achalasia (megaesophagus); myasthenia gravis; megacolon.

*Benztropine:* Children younger than 3 years of age; use with caution in older children.

## Warnings

*Ophthalmic:* Incipient narrow-angle glaucoma may be precipitated by these drugs.

*Elderly:* Geriatric patients, particularly older than 60 years of age, frequently develop increased sensitivity to anticholinergic drugs and require strict dosage regulation. Occasionally, mental confusion and disorientation may occur; agitation, hallucinations, and psychotic-like symptoms may develop.

*Pregnancy:* Category C.

*Lactation:* An inhibitory effect on lactation may occur.

*Children:* Safety and efficacy for use in children have not been established.

## Precautions

*Concomitant conditions:* Use caution in patients with tachycardia, cardiac arrhythmias, hypertension, hypotension, prostatic hypertrophy (particularly in the elderly), or any tendency toward urinary retention, liver or kidney disorders, and obstructive disease of the GI or GU tract.

*CNS:* When used to treat extrapyramidal reactions resulting from phenothiazines in psychiatric patients, antiparkinson agents may exacerbate mental symptoms and precipitate a toxic psychosis.

In addition, 19% to 30% of patients given anticholinergics develop depression, confusion, delusions, or hallucinations.

*Tardive dyskinesia* – Tardive dyskinesia may appear in some patients on long-term therapy with phenothiazines and related agents, or may occur after therapy has been discontinued.

*Dry mouth:* If dry mouth is so severe that swallowing or speaking is difficult, or if loss of appetite and weight occurs, reduce dosage or discontinue drug temporarily.

*Abuse potential:* Some patients may use these agents for mood elevations or psychedelic experiences. Cannabinoids, barbiturates, opiates, and alcohol may have additive effects with anticholinergics.

*Hazardous tasks:* May impair mental or physical abilities; patients should observe caution while driving or performing other tasks requiring alertness.

### Drug Interactions
Drugs that may interact with anticholinergic antiparkinson agents include amantadine, digoxin, haloperidol, levodopa, and phenothiazines.

### Adverse Reactions
Adverse reactions include the following: Tachycardia; palpitations; hypotension; disorientation; confusion; memory loss; hallucinations; psychoses; agitation; nervousness; delusions; delirium; paranoia; euphoria; excitement; lightheadedness; dizziness; headache; listlessness; depression; drowsiness; weakness; giddiness; paresthesia; heaviness of the limbs; dry mouth; nausea; vomiting; epigastric distress; constipation; development of duodenal ulcer; skin rash; urticaria; other dermatoses; blurred vision; mydriasis; diplopia; increased intraocular tension; angle-closure glaucoma; dilation of pupils; muscular weakness; muscular cramping; urinary retention; urinary hesitancy; dysuria; elevated temperature; flushing; numbness of fingers; decreased sweating, hyperthermia, heat stroke; difficulty in achieving or maintaining an erection.

## LEVODOPA AND CARBIDOPA

**Tablets**: 10 mg carbidopa and 100 mg levodopa, 25 mg carbidopa and 100 mg levodopa, 25 mg carbidopa and 250 mg levodopa (*Rx*)
Various, *Sinemet* (Bristol-Myers Squibb)

**Tablets, extended-release**: 25 mg carbidopa and 100 mg levodopa, 50 mg carbidopa and 200 mg levodopa (*Rx*)
Various, *Sinemet* CR (Bristol-Myers Squibb)

**Tablets, orally-disintegrating**: 10 mg carbidopa and 100 mg levodopa, 25 mg carbidopa and 100 mg levodopa, 25 mg carbidopa and 250 mg levodopa (*Rx*)
*Parcopa* (Schwarz Pharma)

### Indications
Treatment of symptoms of idiopathic Parkinson's disease (paralysis agitans), postencephalitic parkinsonism, and sympathetic parkinsonism that may follow injury to the nervous system by carbon monoxide and manganese intoxication.

### Administration and Dosage
*Patients not receiving levodopa:*
*Immediate-release tablets* – 1 tablet of carbidopa 25 mg/levodopa 100 mg 3 times/day or carbidopa 10 mg/levodopa 100 mg 3 or 4 times/day. Dosage may be increased by 1 tablet every day or every other day, as necessary, until a dosage of 8 tablets a day is reached.

Tablets of the 2 ratios (eg, 1:4, 25/100 or 1:10, 10/100 and 25/250) may be given separately or combined as needed to provide the optimum dosage.

Provide at least 70 to 100 mg carbidopa per day. When more carbidopa is required, substitute one 25/100 tablet for each 10/100 tablet. When more levodopa is required, substitute the 25/250 tablet for the 25/100 or 10/100 tablet.

*Extended-release tablets* – 1 tablet (usually 50/200 mg tablet) twice/day at intervals of not less than 6 hours. Doses and dosing intervals may be increased or decreased based on response. Most patients have been adequately treated with 2 to 8 tablets (400 to 1600 mg of levodopa) per day (divided doses) at intervals of 4 to 8 hours while awake. Higher doses (12 tablets or more per day, 2400 mg or more levodopa/

day) and intervals of less than 4 hours have been used but are not usually recommended. If an interval of less than 4 hours is used or if the divided doses are not equal, give the smaller doses at the end of the day.

Extended-release tablets may be administered as whole or half tablets which should not be crushed or chewed.

*Patients currently treated with levodopa:* Levodopa must be discontinued at least 12 hours before therapy with levodopa/carbidopa. Substitute the combination drug at a dosage that will provide about 25% of the previous levodopa dosage.

*Immediate-release* – Suggested starting dosage is 1 tablet of carbidopa 25 mg/levodopa 250 mg 3 or 4 times/day for patients taking more than 1500 mg levodopa or carbidopa 25 mg/levodopa 100 mg for patients taking less than 1500 mg levodopa.

*Extended-release* – In patients with mild to moderate disease, the initial dose is usually one 50/200 extended-release tablet twice daily.

*Patients currently treated with conventional carbidopa/levodopa preparations:* Substitute dosage with extended-release tablets at an amount that provides about 10% more levodopa per day, although this may need to be increased to a dosage that provides up to 30% more levodopa per day. Use intervals of 4 to 8 hours while awake.

| Guidelines for Initial Conversion From Immediate-Release to Extended-Release (50/100 mg Tablets) | |
| --- | --- |
| Immediate-release total daily levodopa dose (mg) | Extended-release (50/100 mg tablets) suggested dosage regimen |
| 300 to 400 | 200 mg twice daily |
| 500 to 600 | 300 mg twice daily or 200 mg 3 times/day |
| 700 to 800 | Total of 800 mg in 3 or more divided doses (eg, 300 mg am, 300 mg early pm, and 200 mg later pm) |
| 900 to 1,000 | Total of 1,000 mg in 3 or more divided doses (eg, 400 mg am, 400 mg early pm, and 200 mg later pm) |

*Combination therapy:* Other antiparkinson drugs can be given concurrently; dosage adjustment may be necessary.

*Immediate-release tablets* – Immediate-release tablets (25/100 or 10/100) can be added to the dosage regimen of extended-release tablets in selected patients with advanced disease who need additional levodopa.

*Administration of orally disintegrating tablets:* Just prior to administration, gently remove the tablet from the bottle with dry hands. Immediately place the tablet on top of the tongue where it will dissolve in seconds, then swallow with saliva. Administration with liquid is not necessary.

### Actions

*Pharmacology:* These agents are used in combination because carbidopa inhibits decarboxylation of levodopa and makes more levodopa available for transport to the brain. There is less variation in plasma levodopa levels than with the conventional formulation. However, the extended-release form is less systemically bioavailable (70% to 75%) and may require increased daily doses to achieve the same level of symptomatic relief.

*Pharmacokinetics:* The half-life of levodopa may be prolonged following the extended-release form because of continuous absorption. In elderly subjects, the mean time to peak levodopa concentration was 2 hours for extended-release vs 0.5 hours for conventional. The maximum concentration following the extended-release form was about 35% of the conventional form.

### Warnings

*CNS effects:* Certain adverse CNS effects (eg, dyskinesias) will occur at lower dosages and sooner during therapy with levodopa and carbidopa than with levodopa alone.

#### Drug Interactions

*Drug/Food interactions:* Administration of a single dose of the extended-release form with food increased the extent of levodopa availability by 50% and increased peak levodopa concentrations by 25%.

#### Adverse Reactions

In clinical trials, the adverse reaction profile of the extended-release form did not differ substantially from that of the conventional form.

# ENTACAPONE

| | |
|---|---|
| **Tablets:** 200 mg (*Rx*) | *Comtan* (Novartis) |

#### Indications

*Parkinson's disease:* As an adjunct to levodopa/carbidopa to treat patients with idiopathic Parkinson's disease who experience the signs and symptoms of end-of-dose "wearing-off." The effectiveness of entacapone has not been systematically evaluated in patients with idiopathic Parkinson's disease who do not experience end-of-dose "wearing-off."

#### Administration and Dosage

The recommended dose of entacapone is one 200 mg tablet administered concomitantly with each levodopa/carbidopa dose to a maximum of 8 times/day (200 mg × 8 = 1600 mg/day). Clinical experience with daily doses greater than 1600 mg is limited.

Always administer entacapone in combination with levodopa/carbidopa. Entacapone has no antiparkinsonian effect of its own.

In clinical trials, the majority of patients required a decrease in daily levodopa dose if their daily dose of levodopa had been 800 mg or more, or if they had moderate or severe dyskinesias prior to treatment with entacapone.

Reducing the daily levodopa dose or extending the interval between doses may be necessary to optimize patient response. In clinical trials, the average reduction in the daily levodopa dose was approximately 25% in those patients requiring a levodopa dose reduction. (More than 58% of patients with levodopa doses more than 800 mg daily required such a reduction.)

Entacapone can be combined with the immediate- and sustained-release formulations of levodopa/carbidopa.

Entacapone may be taken with or without food.

*Withdrawing patients from entacapone:* Rapid withdrawal or abrupt reduction in the entacapone dose could lead to emergence of signs and symptoms of Parkinson's disease and may lead to hyperpyrexia and confusion, a symptom complex resembling neuroleptic malignant syndrome (see Precautions). Consider this syndrome in the differential diagnosis for any patient who develops a high fever or severe rigidity. If a decision is made to discontinue treatment with entacapone, monitor patients closely and adjust other dopaminergic agents as needed. Although tapering entacapone has not been evaluated, it seems reasonable to withdraw patients slowly if the decision to discontinue treatment is made.

#### Actions

*Pharmacology:* Entacapone is a selective and reversible inhibitor of catechol-O-methyltransferase (COMT), which alters the plasma pharmacokinetics of levodopa. When entacapone is given in conjunction with levodopa and an aromatic amino acid decarboxylase inhibitor (such as carbidopa), plasma levels of levodopa are greater and more sustained than after administration of levodopa and an aromatic amino acid decarboxylase inhibitor alone.

*Pharmacokinetics:* Entacapone is rapidly absorbed, with a $T_{max}$ of approximately 1 hour. The absolute bioavailability following oral administration is 35%. The plasma protein binding of entacapone is 98%, mainly to serum albumin. Entacapone is almost completely metabolized prior to excretion, with only a small amount (0.2% of dose) excreted in the urine.

### Contraindications
Hypersensitivity to the drug or any of its ingredients.

### Warnings
*Hepatic function impairment:* Treat hepatically impaired patients with caution. The AUC and $C_{max}$ of entacapone approximately doubled in patients with documented liver disease compared with controls.

*Carcinogenesis:* An increased incidence of renal tubular adenomas and carcinomas was found in male rats treated with the highest dose of entacapone.

*Mutagenesis:* Entacapone was mutagenic and clastogenic in the in vitro mouse lymphoma/thymidine kinase assay in the presence and absence of metabolic activation, and was clastogenic in cultured human lymphocytes in the presence of metabolic activation.

*Pregnancy:* Category C.

*Lactation:* It is not known whether entacapone is excreted in human breast milk.

*Children:* There is no identified potential use of entacapone in pediatric patients.

### Precautions
*Hypotension/Syncope:* Dopaminergic therapy in patients with Parkinson's disease has been associated with orthostatic hypotension. Entacapone enhances levodopa bioavailability and, therefore, might be expected to increase the occurrence of orthostatic hypotension. However, in entacapone clinical trials, no differences from placebo were seen for measured orthostasis or symptoms of orthostasis.

*Diarrhea:* In clinical trials, diarrhea developed in 10% and 4% of patients treated with 200 mg entacapone and placebo, respectively, and was regarded as severe in 1.3% of patients.

*Hallucinations:* Dopaminergic therapy in Parkinson's disease patients has been associated with hallucinations. In clinical trials, hallucinations developed in approximately 4% of patients treated with 200 mg entacapone or placebo.

*Dyskinesia:* Entacapone may potentiate the dopaminergic side effects of levodopa and may cause or exacerbate pre-existing dyskinesia.

*Dopaminergic therapy reactions:* The events listed below are rare events known to be associated with the use of drugs that increase dopaminergic activity, although they are most often associated with the use of direct dopamine agonists:

*Rhabdomyolysis* – Cases of severe rhabdomyolysis have been reported with entacapone use. The complicated nature of these cases makes it impossible to determine what role, if any, entacapone played in their pathogenesis.

*Hyperpyrexia and confusion* –
*Tapering of dose:* Cases of a symptom complex resembling neuroleptic malignant syndrome characterized by elevated temperature, muscular rigidity, altered consciousness, and elevated creatine phosphokinase (CPK) have been reported in association with the rapid dose reduction or withdrawal of other dopaminergic drugs.

Prescribers should exercise caution when discontinuing entacapone treatment. When considered necessary, withdrawal should proceed slowly. Consider this syndrome in the differential diagnosis for any patient who develops a high fever or severe rigidity.

*Fibrotic complications* – Cases of retroperitoneal fibrosis, pulmonary infiltrates, pleural effusion, and pleural thickening have been reported in some patients treated with ergot-derived dopaminergic agents. Although these adverse events are believed to be related to the ergoline structure of these compounds, whether other nonergot-derived drugs (eg, entacapone) that increase dopaminergic activity can cause them is unknown.

*Renal toxicity:* In a 1-year toxicity study, entacapone (plasma exposure 20 times that in humans receiving the MRDD of 1600 mg) caused an increased incidence of nephrotoxicity in male rats.

*Biliary excretion:* As most entacapone excretion is via the bile, exercise caution when drugs known to interfere with biliary excretion, glucuronidation, and intestinal beta-glucuronidase are given concurrently with entacapone (see Drug Interactions).

*Lab test abnormalities:* Entacapone is an iron chelator. The impact of entacapone on the body's iron stores is unknown; however, a tendency towards decreasing serum iron concentrations was noted in clinical trials. In a controlled clinical study, serum ferritin levels (as a marker of iron deficiency and subclinical anemia) were not changed with entacapone compared with placebo after 1 year of treatment and there was no difference in rates of anemia or decreased hemoglobin levels.

### Drug Interactions

Entacapone inhibited the CYP isoenzymes 1A2, 2A6, 2C9, 2C19, 2D6, 2E1, and 3A only at very high concentrations and would not be expected to be inhibited in clinical use.

*Monoamine oxidase (MAO) inhibitors:* MAO and COMT are the 2 major enzyme systems involved in the metabolism of catecholamines. Do not treat patients concomitantly with entacapone and a nonselective MAO inhibitor.

Entacapone can be taken concomitantly with a selective MAO-B inhibitor (eg, selegiline).

*Drugs metabolized by COMT:* Administer drugs known to be metabolized by COMT (ie, isoproterenol, epinephrine, norepinephrine, dopamine, dobutamine, methyldopa, apomorphine, isoetherine, bitolterol) with caution in patients receiving entacapone regardless of the route of administration (including inhalation), as their interaction may result in increased heart rates, arrhythmias, and excessive changes in blood pressure.

Drugs that interfere with biliary excretion of glucuronidation (erythromycin, rifampin, cholestyramine) might decrease entacapone elimination.

*Drug/Food interactions:* Food does not affect the pharmacokinetics of entacapone.

### Adverse Reactions

Adverse reactions that occur in 3% or more of patients include the following: Dyskinesias; dizziness; nausea; diarrhea; abdominal pain; urine discoloration; hyper- and hypokinesia; constipation; vomiting; dry mouth; back pain; fatigue; dyspnea.

## AMANTADINE HCl

| | |
|---|---|
| **Capsules:** 100 mg (*Rx*) | Various, *Symadine* (Solvay), *Symmetrel* (DuPont) |
| **Syrup:** 50 mg/5 mL (*Rx*) | *Symmetrel* (DuPont) |

This is an abbreviated monograph. For full prescribing information, refer to the Antiviral Agents monograph.

### Indications

*Parkinson's disease/syndrome and drug-induced extrapyramidal reactions:* Idiopathic Parkinson's disease (paralysis agitans); postencephalitic parkinsonism; arteriosclerotic parkinsonism; drug-induced extrapyramidal reactions; symptomatic parkinsonism following injury to the nervous system by carbon monoxide intoxication.

### Administration and Dosage

*Parkinson's disease:* 100 mg twice/day when used alone. Onset of action is usually within 48 h. Initial dose is 100 mg/day for patients with serious associated medical illnesses or those receiving high doses of other antiparkinson drugs. After one to several weeks at 100 mg once/day, increase to 100 mg twice/day, if necessary. Patients whose responses are not optimal at 200 mg/day may occasionally benefit from an increase up to 400 mg/day in divided doses; supervise closely. Patients initially benefiting from amantadine often experience decreased efficacy after a few months.

Benefit may be regained by increasing to 300 mg/day, or by temporary discontinuation for several weeks. Other antiparkinson drugs may be necessary.

*Concomitant therapy* – When amantadine and levodopa are initiated concurrently, the patient can exhibit rapid therapeutic benefits. Maintain the dose at 100 mg/day or twice/day, while levodopa is gradually increased to optimal benefit.

*Renal function impairment:* The following table is designed to yield steady-state plasma concentrations of 0.7 to 1 mcg/mL.

| Suggested Dosage Guidelines for Amantadine in Impaired Renal Function | | |
|---|---|---|
| Ccr (mL/min/1.73 m$^2$) | Estimated half-life (hours) | Suggested maintenance regimen[1] |
| 100 | 11 | 100 mg twice a day or 200 mg/day |
| 80 | 14 | 100 mg twice a day |
| 60 | 19 | 200 mg alternated with 100 mg/day |
| 50 | 23 | 100 mg/day |
| 40 | 29 | 100 mg/day |
| 30 | 40 | 200 mg twice weekly |
| 20 | 66 | 100 mg 3 times weekly |
| 10 | 178 | 200 mg alternated with 100 mg every 7 days |
| 3 times weekly chronic hemodialysis | 199 | 200 mg alternated with 100 mg every 7 days |

[1] Loading dose on first day of 200 mg. Reproduced with permission from Horadam VW, Sharp JG, Smilack JD, et al. Pharmacokinetics of amantadine HCl in subjects with normal and impaired renal function. *Ann Intern Med.* 1981;94:454-458.

*Drug-induced extrapyramidal reactions:* 100 mg twice/day. Patients with suboptimal responses may benefit from 300 mg/day in divided doses.

### Actions
*Pharmacology:* The exact mechanism of action is unknown, but amantadine is thought to release dopamine from intact dopaminergic terminals that remain in the substantia nigra of parkinson patients.

# BROMOCRIPTINE MESYLATE

| | |
|---|---|
| **Tablets**: 2.5 mg *(Rx)* | *Parlodel SnapTabs* (Sandoz) |
| **Capsules**: 5 mg *(Rx)* | *Parlodel* (Sandoz) |

### Indications
*Parkinson's disease:* Treatment of idiopathic or postencephalitic Parkinson's disease.

### Administration and Dosage
*Parkinson's disease:* Initiate treatment at a low dosage and individualize; increase the daily dosage slowly until a maximum therapeutic response is achieved. If possible, maintain the dosage of levodopa during this introductory period.

Initially, use 1.25 mg (one-half of a 2.5 mg tablet) twice daily with meals. Assess dosage titrations every 2 weeks to ensure that the lowest dosage producing an optimal therapeutic response is not exceeded. If necessary, increase the dosage every 2 to 4 weeks by 2.5 mg/day with meals. If it is necessary to reduce the dose because of adverse reactions, reduce dose gradually in 2.5 mg increments. Usual range is 10 to 40 mg/day.

The safety of bromocriptine has not been demonstrated in dosages exceeding 100 mg/day.

### Actions
*Pharmacology:* Bromocriptine, a dopamine agonist, may relieve akinesia, rigidity, and tremor in patients with Parkinson's disease. It produces its therapeutic effect by directly stimulating the dopamine receptors in the corpus striatum.

# SELEGILINE HCl (L-Deprenyl)

| | |
|---|---|
| **Tablets:** 5 mg (*Rx*) | *Eldepryl* (Somerset) |

## Indications

*Parkinson's disease:* Adjunct in the management of parkinsonian patients being treated with levodopa/carbidopa who exhibit deterioration in the quality of their response to this therapy.

## Administration and Dosage

*Parkinsonian patients receiving levodopa/carbidopa therapy who demonstrate a deteriorating response to this treatment:* 10 mg per day administered as divided doses of 5 mg each taken at breakfast and lunch. There is no evidence that additional benefit will be obtained from the administration of higher doses.

After 2 to 3 days of treatment, attempt to reduce the dose of levodopa/carbidopa. A reduction of 10% to 30% appears typical. Further reductions of levodopa/carbidopa may be possible during continued selegiline therapy.

## Actions

*Pharmacology:* Selegiline HCl is a levorotatory acetylenic derivative of phenethylamine. Although the mechanism of action is not fully understood, inhibition of monoamine oxidase (MAO) type B activity is of primary importance and selegiline may act through other mechanisms to increase dopaminergic activity.

*Pharmacokinetics:*

*Absorption/Distribution* – Selegiline is rapidly absorbed; approximately 73% of a dose is absorbed; maximum plasma concentration occurs 0.5 to 2 hours following administration.

*Metabolism/Excretion* – The drug is rapidly metabolized. Over 48 hours, 45% of the dose appeared in the urine as metabolites. Unchanged selegiline is not detected in urine.

## Contraindications

Hypersensitivity to the drug; use with meperidine.

## Warnings

*Maximum dose:* Do not use at daily doses exceeding those recommended (10 mg/day) because of the risks associated with nonselective inhibition of MAO.

*Pregnancy: Category* C.

*Lactation:* It is not known whether selegiline is excreted in breast milk.

*Children:* The effects of selegiline in children have not been evaluated.

## Precautions

*Hypertensive crisis:* In theory, because MAO-A of the gut is not inhibited, patients treated with selegiline at a dose of 10 mg/day can take medications containing pharmacologically active amines and consume tyramine-containing foods without risk of uncontrolled hypertension.

*Levodopa side effects:* Some patients given selegiline may experience an exacerbation of levodopa-associated side effects, presumably caused by the increased amounts of dopamine reacting with supersensitive postsynaptic receptors.

## Drug Interactions

Drugs that may interact with selegiline include fluoxetine and meperidine.

## Adverse Reactions

Adverse reactions occurring in 3% or more of patients include nausea, dizziness, lightheadedness, fainting, abdominal pain, confusion, hallucinations, depression, loss of balance, insomnia, orthostatic hypotension, increased akinetic involuntary movements, agitation, arrhythmias, bradykinesia, chorea, delusions, hypertension, new or increased angina pectoris, syncope, and dry mouth.

# PERGOLIDE MESYLATE

**Tablets:** 0.05, 0.25, and 1 mg (*Rx*)                    Various, *Permax* (Amarin)

### Indications
*Parkinson disease:* Adjunctive treatment to levodopa/carbidopa in the management of the signs and symptoms of Parkinson disease.

### Administration and Dosage
Initiate with a daily dose of 0.05 mg for the first 2 days. Gradually increase the dosage by 0.1 or 0.15 mg/day every third day over the next 12 days of therapy. The dosage may then be increased by 0.25 mg/day every third day until an optimal therapeutic dosage is achieved.

Pergolide is usually administered in divided doses 3 times/day. During dosage titration, the dosage of concurrent levodopa/carbidopa may be cautiously decreased.

In clinical studies, the mean therapeutic daily dosage of pergolide was 3 mg/day. The average concurrent daily dosage of levodopa/carbidopa (expressed as levodopa) was approximately 650 mg/day. The efficacy of pergolide at doses above 5 mg/day has not been systematically evaluated.

### Actions
*Pharmacology:* Pergolide mesylate is a potent dopamine receptor agonist at both $D_1$ and $D_2$ receptor sites. In Parkinson disease, pergolide is believed to exert its therapeutic effect by directly stimulating postsynaptic dopamine receptors in the nigrostriatal system.

*Pharmacokinetics:* Following oral administration, approximately 55% of the dose can be recovered from the urine. Pergolide is approximately 90% bound to plasma proteins. The major route of excretion is via the kidney.

### Contraindications
Hypersensitivity to pergolide or other ergot derivatives.

### Warnings
*Symptomatic hypotension:* In clinical trials, approximately 10% of patients taking pergolide with levodopa vs 7% taking placebo with levodopa experienced symptomatic orthostatic or sustained hypotension, especially during initial treatment. Increase the dosage in carefully adjusted increments over a period of 3 to 4 weeks.

*Hallucinosis:* Pergolide with levodopa caused hallucinosis in approximately 14% of patients as opposed to 3% taking placebo with levodopa.

*Fatalities:* Of the 2299 patients on pergolide in premarketing studies, 143 died while on the drug or shortly after discontinuing it. The study patients were elderly, ill, and at high risk for death. The possibility that pergolide shortens patient survival cannot be excluded.

*Elderly:* There was an increased incidence of confusion, somnolence, and peripheral edema in patients 65 years of age and older.

*Pregnancy: Category B.*

*Lactation:* It is not known whether this drug is excreted in breast milk.

*Children:* Safety and efficacy for use in children have not been established.

### Precautions
*Monitoring:* There have been rare reports of pleuritis, pleural effusion, pleural fibrosis, pericarditis, pericardial effusion, cardiac valvulopathy, or retroperitoneal fibrosis in patients taking pergolide. Use caution when using pergolide in patients with a history of these conditions, particularly those patients who experienced the events while taking ergot derivatives.

*Cardiac dysrhythmias:* Exercise caution in patients prone to cardiac dysrhythmias. In a study comparing pergolide and placebo, patients on pergolide had significantly more episodes of atrial premature contractions and sinus tachycardia.

The use of pergolide in patients on levodopa may cause or exacerbate preexisting states of confusion and hallucinations or preexisting dyskinesia.

*Discontinuation of therapy:* Abrupt discontinuation of pergolide in patients receiving it chronically as an adjunct to levodopa may precipitate the onset of hallucinations and confusion. Discontinue pergolide gradually whenever possible, even if the patient is to remain on levodopa.

*Neuroleptic malignant syndrome (NMS):* A symptom complex resembling the NMS (characterized by elevated temperature, muscular rigidity, altered consciousness, and autonomic instability), with no other obvious etiology, has been reported in association with rapid dose reduction, withdrawal of, or changes in antiparkinsonian therapy, including pergolide.

**Drug Interactions**

Drugs that may interact with pergolide mesylate include dopamine antagonists, metoclopramide, and drugs known to affect protein binding.

**Adverse Reactions**

Adverse reactions occurring in 3% or more of patients include pain, abdominal pain, injury, accident, headache, asthenia, chest pain, flu syndrome, postural hypotension, vasodilation, nausea, constipation, diarrhea, dyspepsia, anorexia, dry mouth, dyskinesia, dizziness, hallucinations, dystonia, confusion, somnolence, insomnia, anxiety, tremor, depression, rhinitis, dyspnea, rash, abnormal vision, and peripheral edema.

# DOPAMINE RECEPTOR AGONISTS, NON-ERGOT

| **APOMORPHINE HYDROCHLORIDE** | |
| --- | --- |
| **Injection:** 10 mg/mL (*Rx*) | *Apokyn* (Mylan Bertek) |
| **PRAMIPEXOLE** | |
| **Tablets:** 0.125, 0.25, 1, and 1.5 mg (*Rx*) | *Mirapex* (Pharmacia) |
| **ROPINIROLE** | |
| **Tablets:** 0.25, 0.5, 1, 2, and 5 mg (*Rx*) | *Requip* (GlaxoSmithKline) |

**Indications**

*Parkinson disease (PD):* For the treatment of the signs and symptoms of idiopathic PD.

*Apomorphine –* For the acute, intermittent treatment of hypomobility, "off" episodes ("end-of-dose wearing off" and unpredictable "on/off" episodes) associated with advanced PD.

**Administration and Dosage**

APOMORPHINE: Doses greater than 0.6 mL (6 mg) are not recommended.

For subcutaneous administration only.

*Concomitant medication –* Do not initiate apomorphine without the use of a concomitant antiemetic. Start trimethobenzamide (300 mg 3 times daily orally) 3 days prior to the initial dose of apomorphine and continue during at least the first 2 months of therapy.

*Dosage –* Titrate the dose of apomorphine starting at 0.2 mL (2 mg) and up to a maximum recommended dose of 0.6 mL (6 mg) as follows:

Give patients in an "off" state a 0.2 mL (2 mg) test dose where blood pressure can be closely monitored by medical personnel. Check supine and standing blood pressure predose and at 20, 40, and 60 minutes postdose. Do not consider patients who develop clinically significant orthostatic hypotension as candidates for treatment. If the patient tolerates the 0.2 mL (2 mg) dose and responds, use the starting dose of 0.2 mL (2 mg) on an as-needed basis to treat existing "off" episodes. If needed, the dose can be increased in 0.1 mL (1 mg) increments every few days on an outpatient basis.

Generally, the test dose is to determine a dose (0.3 or 0.4 mL) that the patient will tolerate under monitored conditions, and then begin an outpatient dosing trial (periodically assessing efficacy and tolerability) using a dose 0.1 mL (1 mg) lower than the tolerated test dose.

- For patients who tolerate the test dose of 0.2 mL (2 mg) but achieve no response, a dose of 0.4 mL (4 mg) may be administered at the next observed "off" period, but no sooner than 2 hours after the initial test dose. Check supine and standing blood pressure predose and at 20, 40, and 60 minutes postdose.

- If the patient tolerates a test dose of 0.4 mL (4 mg), the starting dose should be 0.3 mL (3 mg) used on an as-needed basis to treat existing "off" episodes. If needed, the dose can be increased in 0.1 mL (1 mg) increments every few days on an outpatient basis.
- If a patient does not tolerate a test dose of 0.4 mL (4 mg), a test dose of 0.3 mL (3 mg) may be administered during a separate "off" period, no sooner than 2 hours after the test dose. Check supine and standing blood pressure predose and at 20, 40, and 60 minutes postdose.
- If the patient tolerates the 0.3 mL (3 mg) test dose, the starting dose should be 0.2 mL (2 mg) used on an as-needed basis to treat existing "off" episodes. If needed, and the 0.2 mL (2 mg) dose is tolerated, the dose can be increased to 0.3 mL (3 mg) after a few days. In such a patient, the dose should ordinarily not be increased to 0.4 mL (4 mg) on an outpatient basis.

Most patients studied in the apomorphine development program responded to 3 to 6 mg. There is no evidence from controlled trials that doses greater than 6 mg give an increased effect, and these doses are not recommended. The average frequency of dosing was 3 times/day in the development program, and there is limited experience with single doses greater than 6 mg, dosing more than 5 times/day, and with total daily doses greater than 20 mg.

If a single dose of apomorphine is ineffective for a particular "off" period, do not give a second dose for that "off" episode. The efficacy of a second dose for a single "off" episode has not been studied and the safety of redosing has not been characterized.

*Interruption of therapy* – Patients who have an interruption in therapy (more than a week) should be restarted on a 0.2 mL (2 mg) dose and gradually titrated to effect.

*Hepatic function impairment* – For patients with mild and moderate hepatic function impairment, exercise caution because of the increased $C_{max}$ and AUC in these patients.

*Renal function impairment* – For patients with mild and moderate renal function impairment, reduce the testing dose and subsequent starting dose to 0.1 mL (1 mg).

PRAMIPEXOLE: May take with food to reduce the occurrence of nausea.

*Initial treatment* – Increase gradually from a starting dose of 0.375 mg/day given in 3 divided doses every 5 to 7 days to 4.5 mg/day in patients with Ccr more than 60 mL/min.

*Maintenance treatment* – Pramipexole is effective and well tolerated over a dosage range of 1.5 to 4.5 mg/day administered in equally divided doses 3 times/day with or without concomitant levodopa (approximately 800 mg/day). When pramipexole is used in combination with levodopa, consider a reduction of the levodopa dosage.

*Discontinuation* – Discontinue over a period of 1 week.

ROPINIROLE: Take 3 times/day, with or without food. Taking ropinirole with food may reduce the occurrence of nausea.

The recommended starting dose is 0.25 mg 3 times/day. Based on individual patient response, dosage should then be titrated in weekly increments as described in the table below. After week 4, if necessary, daily dosage may be increased by 1.5 mg/day on a weekly basis up to a dose of 9 mg/day, and then by 3 mg/day or less weekly to a total dose of 24 mg/day.

| Ascending-Dose Schedule of Ropinirole | | |
|---|---|---|
| Week | Dosage | Total daily dose |
| 1 | 0.25 mg 3 times/day | 0.75 mg |
| 2 | 0.5 mg 3 times/day | 1.5 mg |
| 3 | 0.75 mg 3 times/day | 2.25 mg |
| 4 | 1 mg 3 times/day | 3 mg |

When ropinirole is administered as adjunct therapy to levodopa, the concurrent dose of levodopa may be decreased gradually as tolerated.

Discontinue ropinirole gradually over a 7-day period. Decrease the frequency of administration from 3 times/day to twice/day for 4 days. For the remaining 3 days, decrease the frequency to once/day prior to complete withdrawal of ropinirole.

## Actions

*Pharmacology:* **Apomorphine, pramipexole,** and **ropinirole** are non-ergot dopamine agonists for PD with high specificity at the $D_2$ subfamily of dopamine receptors, binding with higher affinity to $D_3$ than to $D_2$ or $D_4$ receptor subtypes.

The mechanism of action is believed to be related to its ability to stimulate dopamine receptors in the striatum.

*Pharmacokinetics:* Non-ergot dopamine agonists are rapidly absorbed. The absolute bioavailability is more than 90%. Steady-state concentrations are achieved within 2 days of dosing. Terminal half-life is about 8 hours (about 40 minutes for **apomorphine**) in young healthy volunteers and about 12 hours in elderly volunteers. Urinary excretion is the major route of elimination.

## Contraindications

Hypersensitivity to the drug or any components of the product; concomitant use of **apomorphine** with drugs of the $5HT_3$ antagonist class (eg, ondansetron, granisetron, dolasetron, palonosetron, alosetron) due to reports of profound hypotension and loss of consciousness with ondansetron.

## Warnings

*IV administration:* Avoid IV administration with **apomorphine**. Serious adverse events (such as IV crystallization of apomorphine leading to thrombus formation and pulmonary embolism) have followed IV administration.

*Nausea and Vomiting:* At the recommended doses of **apomorphine**, severe nausea and vomiting can be expected. There was no experience with antiemetics other than trimethobenzamide. Some antiemetics with anti-dopaminergic actions have the potential to worsen the clinical state of patients with PD and should be avoided.

*QT prolongation and potential for proarrhythmic effects:* In single dose studies of **apomorphine**, changes in QTc ranging from 0 to 7 msec were reported. Some drugs that prolong the QT/QTc interval have been associated with the occurrence of torsades de pointes and with sudden unexplained death.

*Symptomatic hypotension:* Patients require careful monitoring for signs and symptoms of orthostatic hypotension while being treated with dopaminergic agonists, especially during dose escalation. The effects of **apomorphine** on blood pressure may be increased by the concomitant use of alcohol, antihypertensive medications, and vasodilators (especially nitrates).

*Falls:* Patients with PD are at risk of falling due to the underlying postural instability and concomitant autonomic instability from syncope caused by the blood pressure lowering effects of the drugs used to treat PD. Subcutaneous **apomorphine** might increase the risk of falling by simultaneously lowering blood pressure and altering mobility.

*Hallucinations:* Hallucinations were observed in a greater number of patients receiving dopaminergics than placebo. Age appears to increase the risk of hallucination attributable to dopaminergics.

*Sleepiness during daily activities:* Somnolence is commonly associated with **apomorphine**.

*Coronary events:* Angina, MI, cardiac arrest, and /or sudden death have been reported during clinical trials with **apomorphine**. Use extra caution in prescribing apomorphine for patients with known cardiovascular and cerebrovascular disease.

*Sulfite: Apokyn* (**apomorphine**) contains metabisulfite, a sulfite that may cause allergic-type reactions, including anaphylactic symptoms and life-threatening or less severe asthmatic episodes.

*Injection site reactions:* Injection site reactions, including bruising, granuloma, and pruritus were reported with **apomorphine**.

*Renal function impairment:* Exercise caution when prescribing to patients with renal insufficiency. The starting dose may need to be reduced.

*Hepatic function impairment:* Exercise caution when administrating **apomorphine** to patients with mild and moderate hepatic impairment.

*Elderly:* **Pramipexole** total oral clearance was approximately 30% lower in subjects older than 65 years of age compared with younger subjects, because of a decline in pramipexole renal clearance. The incidence of confusion and hallucinations appears to increase with age. Serious adverse events were more common in older patients (ie, falling, cardiovascular events, respiratory disorders, GI events).

*Pregnancy: Category C.*

*Lactation:* It is not known whether these drugs are excreted in breast milk.

*Children:* Safety and efficacy have not been established.

## Precautions

*Monitoring:* Monitor for signs and symptoms of orthostatic hypotension.

*Dyskinesia:* Dopamine receptor agonists may potentiate the dopaminergic side effects of levodopa and may cause or exacerbate pre-existing dyskinesia. Decreasing the dose of levodopa may ameliorate this side effect.

*CNS effects:* Use concomitant CNS depressants with caution because of the possible additive sedative effects.

*Binding to melanin:* Ropinirole binds to melanin-containing tissues in pigmented rats.

*Priapism:* **Apomorphine** may cause prolonged painful erections in some patients.

*Drug abuse and dependence:* There are rare reports of **apomorphine** abuse by patients with PD. These cases are characterized by increasingly frequent dosing leading to hallucinations, dyskinesia, and abnormal behavior.

## Drug Interactions

$5HT_3$ antagonist use is contraindicated with **apomorphine**. Drugs that may affect dopamine receptors agonists include cimetidine; estrogen; ciprofloxacin; drugs eliminated via renal excretion; inhibitors of CYP1A2 and dopamine antagonists; dopamine agonists, such as neuroleptics (eg, phenothiazines, butyrophenones, thioxanthenes) or metoclopramide. Drugs that may be affected by dopamine receptor agonists include levodopa. Use caution when prescribing apomorphine concomitantly with drugs that prolong the QT/QTc interval.

*Drug/Food interactions:* **Pramipexole** and **ropinirole** $T_{max}$ are increased by approximately 1 and 2.5 hours, respectively, when taken food, although the extent of absorption is not affected.

## Adverse Reactions

Adverse reactions occurring in at least 3% of patients with early PD (without levodopa) included the following: abdominal pain; abnormal vision; amnesia; angina; anorexia; anxiety; arthralgia; asthenia; back pain; bronchitis; chest pain; CHF; confusion; constipation; dehydration; depression; diarrhea; dizziness; drowsiness; dry mouth; dyskinesias; dyspepsia; dyspnea; ecchymosis; edema; eye abnormality; fall; fatigue; flatulence; flushing; hallucinations (see Warnings); headache; hypertension; hypesthesia; impotence; increased alkaline phosphatase; increased sweating; injection site complaint (**apomorphine**); insomnia; limb pain; malaise; nausea; orthostatic symptoms; pain; palpitations; PD aggravated; peripheral edema; peripheral ischemia; pneumonia; postural hypotension; pharyngitis; rhinitis; rhinorrhea; sinusitis; somnolence; syncope; urinary tract infection; viral infection; vomiting; weakness; yawning.

Adverse reactions occurring in at least 3% of patients with advanced PD (with levodopa) included the following: abdominal pain; accidental injury; accommodation abnormalities; akathisia; amnesia; arthritis; asthenia; chest pain; confusion; constipation; diarrhea; dizziness; dream abnormalities; dry mouth; dyskinesia; dyspnea; dystonia; extrapyramidal syndrome; falls; flushing; gait abnormalities/hypokinesia; general edema; hallucinations; headache; hypertonia; increased drug level; increased sweating; insomnia; malaise; nausea; nervousness; pain; pallor; paresis; paresthesia; pneumonia; postural hypotension; rhinitis; rhinorrhea; somnolence; syncope; thinking abnormalities; tremor/twitching; urinary frequency; urinary tract infection; vision abnormalities; vomiting; yawning.

# CARBIDOPA, LEVODOPA, AND ENTACAPONE

| | |
|---|---|
| **Tablets**: 12.5 mg carbidopa, 50 mg levodopa, and 200 mg entacapone | *Stalevo 50* (Novartis) |
| 25 mg carbidopa, 100 mg levodopa, and 200 mg entacapone | *Stalevo 100* (Novartis) |
| 37.5 mg carbidopa, 150 mg levodopa, and 200 mg entacapone | *Stalevo 150* (Novartis) |

### Indications
*Parkinson disease:* To treat patients with idiopathic Parkinson disease; to substitute (with equivalent strength of each of the 3 components) for immediate release carbidopa/levodopa and entacapone previously administered as individual products; to replace immediate release carbidopa/levodopa therapy (without entacapone) when patients experience the signs and symptoms of end-of-dose "wearing-off" (only for patients taking a total daily dose of levodopa of 600 mg or less and not experiencing dyskinesias).

### Administration and Dosage
Do not fractionate individual tablets and administer only 1 tablet at each dosing interval. Individualize therapy and adjust according to the desired therapeutic response.

Use carbidopa, levodopa, and entacapone combination as a substitute for patients already stabilized on equivalent doses of carbidopa/levodopa and entacapone. Some patients who have been stabilized on a given dose of carbidopa/levodopa may be treated with carbidopa, levodopa, and entacapone combination if a decision has been made to add entacapone.

The optimum daily dosage of carbidopa, levodopa, and entacapone combination must be determined by careful titration in each patient. Carbidopa, levodopa, and entacapone combination tablets are available in 3 strengths, each in a 1:4 ratio of carbidopa to levodopa and combined with 200 mg of entacapone in a standard release formulation.

Clinical experience with daily doses above 1600 mg of entacapone is limited. It is recommended that no more than 1 carbidopa, levodopa, and entacapone combination tablet be taken at each dosing administration. Thus, the maximum recommended daily dose of carbidopa, levodopa, and entacapone combination is 8 tablets/day.

*Transferring patients currently treated with carbidopa/levodopa and entacapone to carbidopa, levodopa, and entacapone combination tablet:*
   *Carbidopa/levodopa* – There is no experience in transferring patients currently treated with formulation of carbidopa/levodopa other than immediate release carbidopa/levodopa with a 1:4 ratio (controlled release formulations, or standard release presentations with a 1:10 ratio of carbidopa/levodopa) and entacapone to carbidopa, levodopa, and entacapone combination.

   *Entacapone* – Patients who are currently treated with entacapone 200 mg tablet with each dose of standard release carbidopa/levodopa, can be directly switched to the corresponding strength of carbidopa, levodopa, and entacapone combination containing the same amounts of levodopa and carbidopa.

*Transferring patients not currently treated with entacapone tablets from carbidopa/levodopa to carbidopa, levodopa, and entacapone combination tablets:* In patients with Parkinson disease who experience the signs and symptoms of end-of-dose "wearing-off" on their current standard release carbidopa/levodopa treatment, clinical experience shows that patients with a history of moderate or severe dyskinesias or taking more than 600 mg/day of levodopa are likely to require a reduction in daily levodopa dose when entacapone is added to their treatment.

*Maintenance therapy:* Individualize therapy and adjust for each patient according to the desired therapeutic response.

When less levodopa is required, reduce the total daily dosage of carbidopa/levodopa by decreasing the strength of carbidopa, levodopa, and entacapone combination at each administration or by decreasing the frequency of administration by extending the time between doses.

When more levodopa is required, take the next higher strength of carbidopa, levodopa, and entacapone combination and/or increase the frequency of doses, up to a maximum of 8 times daily and not to exceed the maximum daily dose recommendations as outlined above.

*Addition of other antiparkinsonian medications:* Standard drugs for Parkinson disease may be used concomitantly while carbidopa, levodopa, and entacapone combination is being administered, although dosage adjustments may be required.

*Interruption of therapy:* Sporadic cases of a symptom complex resembling Neuroleptic Malignant Syndrome (NMS) have been associated with dose reductions and withdrawal of levodopa preparations.

*Hepatic function impairment:* Treat patients with hepatic impairment with caution. The AUC and $C_{max}$ of entacapone approximately doubled in patients with documented liver disease, compared with controls.

# DISULFIRAM

| **Tablets**: 250 mg (*Rx*) | Various, *Antabuse* (Odyssey) |

---

**Warning:**
  Never give disulfiram to a patient in a state of alcohol intoxication or without the
  patient's full knowledge. Instruct the patient's relatives accordingly.

---

### Indications
  An aid in the management of selected chronic alcoholics who want to remain in a
    state of enforced sobriety so that supportive and psychotherapeutic treatment may
    be applied to best advantage.

### Administration and Dosage
  Do not administer until the patient has abstained from alcohol for at least 12 hours.

  *Initial dosage schedule:* Administer a maximum of 500 mg/day in a single dose for 1 to
    2 weeks. If a sedative effect is experienced, take at bedtime or decrease dosage.

  *Maintenance regimen:* The average maintenance dose is 250 mg/day (range, 125 to
    500 mg), not to exceed 500 mg/day. Maintenance therapy may be required for
    months or even years.

### Actions
  *Pharmacology:* Disulfiram produces a sensitivity to alcohol that results in a highly
    unpleasant reaction when the patient under treatment ingests even small amounts
    of alcohol. Disulfiram blocks oxidation of alcohol at the acetaldehyde stage by
    inhibiting aldehyde dehydrogenase. Accumulation of acetaldehyde produces the
    disulfiram-alcohol reaction. This reaction persists as long as alcohol is being metabo-
    lized. Disulfiram does not influence alcohol elimination. Prolonged administra-
    tion of disulfiram does not produce tolerance; the longer a patient remains on
    therapy, the more sensitive the patient becomes to alcohol.

  *Pharmacokinetics:* Disulfiram is slowly absorbed from the GI tract and eliminated slowly
    from the body. The average time to reach maximum plasma concentrations were 8
    to 10 hours for disulfiram and its metabolites. Disulfiram is metabolized to dieth-
    yldithiocarbamate, which is oxidized to carbon disulfide and diethylamine. The
    metabolites are primarily excreted in the urine and carbon disulfide is exhaled in the
    breath. Ingestion of alcohol may produce unpleasant symptoms for 1 to 2 weeks
    after the last dose of disulfiram.

### Contraindications
  Severe myocardial disease or coronary occlusion; psychoses; hypersensitivity to
    disulfiram or to other thiuram derivatives used in pesticides and rubber vulcaniza-
    tion; patients receiving or who have recently received metronidazole, paralde-
    hyde, alcohol, or alcohol-containing preparations.

### Warnings
  *Hepatic Toxicity:* Hepatic toxicity including hepatic failure resulting in transplantation
    or death has been reported. Severe and sometimes fatal hepatitis associated with
    disulfiram therapy may develop even after many months of therapy. Hepatic toxic-
    ity has occurred in patients with or without prior history of abnormal liver func-
    tion. Advise patients to immediately notify their physician of any early symptoms of
    hepatitis (eg, fatigue, weakness, malaise, anorexia, nausea, vomiting, jaundice, dark
    urine).

  *Administration:* Never administer to an intoxicated patient or without the patient's
    knowledge (see Warning Box). The patient must be fully informed of the disulfir-
    am-alcohol reaction. The patient must be strongly cautioned against surreptitious
    drinking while taking the drug, and fully aware of the possible consequences.
    Warn patient to avoid alcohol in disguised forms (eg, in sauces, vinegars, cough mix-
    tures, aftershave lotions, back rubs). Also, warn that reactions may occur with
    alcohol up to 14-days after ingesting disulfiram.

*Disulfiram-alcohol reaction:* Disulfiram plus alcohol, even small amounts, produces flushing, throbbing in head and neck, throbbing headaches, respiratory difficulty, nausea, copious vomiting, sweating, thirst, chest pain, palpitations, dyspnea, hyperventilation, tachycardia, hypotension, syncope, marked uneasiness, weakness, vertigo, blurred vision, and confusion. In severe reactions there may be respiratory depression, cardiovascular collapse, arrhythmias, MI, acute CHF, unconsciousness, convulsions, and death. The intensity of the reaction is proportional to the amounts of disulfiram and alcohol ingested. The duration of the reaction varies from 30 to 60 minutes to several hours.

*Concomitant conditions:* Because of the possibility of an accidental reaction, use with caution in patients with diabetes mellitus, hypothyroidism, epilepsy, cerebral damage, chronic and acute nephritis, or hepatic cirrhosis or insufficiency.

*Hypersensitivity reactions:* Evaluate patients with a history of rubber contact dermatitis for hypersensitivity to thiuram derivatives before administering disulfiram.

*Pregnancy:* Category C.

*Lactation:* It is not known whether this drug is excreted in human milk. Do not give disulfiram to breastfeeding mothers.

*Children:* Safety and efficacy in pediatric patients have not been established.

**Precautions**

*Monitoring:* Perform baseline and follow-up LFTs (10 to 14 days) to detect hepatic dysfunction resulting from therapy. Perform a CBC and serum chemistries.

*Dependence and addiction:* Alcoholism may accompany or be followed by dependence on narcotics or sedatives. Barbiturates have been coadministered with disulfiram without untoward effects, but consider the possibility of initiating a new abuse.

*Ethylene dibromide:* Do not expose patients to ethylene dibromide or its vapors. This precaution is based on preliminary results of animal research which suggest a toxic interaction between inhaled ethylene dibromide and ingested disulfiram results in a higher incidence of tumors and mortality in rats.

*Ethylene dibromide:* Patients should not be exposed to ethylene dibromide or its vapors.

**Drug Interactions**

Drugs that may interact with disulfiram include alcohol, benzodiazepines, caffeine, chlorzoxazone, cocaine, hydantoins, isoniazid, metronidazole, theophylline, tricyclic antidepressants, and warfarin.

**Adverse Reactions**

Adverse reactions may include acneiform eruptions; allergic dermatitis; arthropathy; multiple cases of cholestatic and fulminant hepatitis; drowsiness; fatigue; headache; hepatotoxicity resembling viral or alcoholic hepatitis; impotence; metallic or garlic-like aftertaste; peripheral neuropathy; polyneuritis; optic or retrobulbar neuritis; restlessness; occasional skin eruptions.

# ACAMPROSATE CALCIUM

| **Tablets, delayed release:** 333 mg (*Rx*) | *Campral* (Forest) |
|---|---|

**Indications**

For maintenance of abstinence from alcohol in patients with alcohol dependence who are abstinent at treatment initiation. Treatment with acamprosate should be part of a comprehensive management program that includes psychosocial support.

The efficacy of acamprosate in promoting abstinence has not been demonstrated in subjects who have not undergone detoxification and not achieved alcohol abstinence prior to beginning acamprosate treatment. The efficacy of acamprosate in promoting abstinence from alcohol in polysubstance abusers has not been adequately assessed.

## Administration and Dosage

The recommended dose is two 333 mg tablets (total dose, 666 mg) taken 3 times daily. Although dosing may be done without regard to meals, dosing with meals was employed during clinical trials and is suggested as an aid to compliance in those patients who regularly eat 3 meals daily. A lower dose may be effective in some patients.

Initiate treatment with acamprosate as soon as possible after the period of alcohol withdrawal, when the patient has achieved abstinence, and maintain treatment if the patient relapses.

*Renal function impairment:* For patients with moderate renal impairment (Ccr 30 to 50 mL/min), a starting dose of one 333 mg tablet taken 3 times daily is recommended. Do not give acamprosate to patients with severe renal impairment (Ccr 30 mL/min or less).

## Actions

*Pharmacology:* Acamprosate is a synthetic compound with a chemical structure similar to that of the endogenous amino acid homotaurine, which is a structural analogue of the amino acid neurotransmitter γ-aminobutyric acid and the amino acid neuromodulator taurine.

The mechanism of action of acamprosate in the maintenance of alcohol abstinence is not completely understood. Chronic alcohol exposure is hypothesized to alter the normal balance between neuronal excitation and inhibition. Studies suggest acamprosate may interact with glutamate and gamma-aminobutyric acid (GABA) neurotransmitter systems centrally, and have led to the hypothesis that acamprosate restores this balance.

Acamprosate is not known to cause alcohol aversion and does not cause a disulfiram-like reaction as a result of ethanol ingestion.

*Pharmacokinetics:*

*Absorption* – The absolute bioavailability of acamprosate is approximately 11%. Steady-state plasma concentrations are reached within 5 days of dosing. Steady-state peak plasma concentrations after acamprosate doses of two 333 mg tablets 3 times daily average 350 ng/mL and occur at 3 to 8 hours postdose.

*Distribution* – Plasma protein binding of acamprosate is negligible.

*Metabolism* – Acamprosate does not undergo metabolism.

*Excretion* – After oral dosing of two 333 mg acamprosate tablets, the terminal half-life ranges from approximately 20 to 33 hours. The major route of excretion is via the kidneys as acamprosate.

## Contraindications

Patients who have previously exhibited hypersensitivity to acamprosate or any of its components; patients with severe renal impairment (Ccr 30 mL/min or less).

## Warnings

*Renal function impairment:* Treatment with acamprosate in patients with moderate renal impairment (Ccr 30 to 50 mL/min) requires a dose reduction. Do not give acamprosate to patients with severe renal impairment (Ccr 30 mL/min or less).

*Elderly:* Because elderly patients are more likely to have decreased renal function, use care in dose selection.

*Pregnancy: Category C.*

*Lactation:* It is not known whether acamprosate is excreted in human milk. Exercise caution when acamprosate is administered to a woman who is breastfeeding.

*Children:* Safety and efficacy have not been established.

## Precautions

*Withdrawal symptoms:* Use of acamprosate does not eliminate or diminish withdrawal symptoms.

*Suicide:* In controlled clinical trials of acamprosate, adverse events of a suicidal nature (eg, suicidal ideation, suicide attempts, completed suicides) were more common in acamprosate-treated patients than in patients treated with placebo (1.4% vs 0.5%

in studies of 6 months or less; 2.4% vs 0.8% in year-long studies). Completed suicides occurred in 3 of 2,272 (0.13%) patients in the pooled acamprosate group from all controlled studies and 2 of 1,962 patients (0.1%) in the placebo group. Monitor alcohol-dependent patients, including those patients being treated with acamprosate, for the development of symptoms of depression or suicidal thinking. Alert families and caregivers of patients being treated with acamprosate of the need to monitor patients for the emergence of symptoms of depression or suicidality, and to report such symptoms to the patient's health care provider.

**Adverse Reactions**

Adverse reactions occurring in at least 3% of patients include the following: accidental injury, anorexia, anxiety, asthenia, depression, diarrhea, dizziness, dry mouth, flatulence, insomnia, nausea, pain, paresthesia, pruritus, sweating.

# NICOTINE

| | |
|---|---|
| **NICOTINE TRANSDERMAL** | |
| **Transdermal Systems** (*otc*) | Various, *Habitrol* (Basel Pharm.), *Nicoderm CQ* (GlaxoSmithKline Consumer), *Nicotrol* (Pharmacia) |
| **NICOTINE LOZENGE** | |
| **Nicotine lozenge:** 2 and 4 mg nicotine (as polacrilex) | *Commit* (GlaxoSmithKline Consumer) |
| **NICOTINE POLACRILEX** | |
| **Chewing gum:** 2 and 4 mg nicotine (as polacrilex) (*otc*) | Various, *Nicorette* (GlaxoSmithKline Consumer) |
| **NICOTINE INHALATION SYSTEM** | |
| **Inhaler:** 4 mg delivered (10 mg/cartridge) (*Rx*) | *Nicotrol Inhaler* (Pharmacia) |
| **NICOTINE NASAL SPRAY** | |
| **Spray pump:** 0.5 mg nicotine/actuation (10 mg/mL) (*Rx*) | *Nicotrol NS* (Pharmacia) |

### Indications

As an aid to smoking cessation for the relief of nicotine withdrawal symptoms. Use as part of a comprehensive behavioral smoking-cessation program.

### Administration and Dosage

| Nicotine Replacement Pharmacotherapy | | | |
|---|---|---|---|
| Type of therapy | Dosage | Duration | Availability |
| Gum | Less than 24 cigarettes/day: 2 mg gum up to 24 pieces/day | up to 12 weeks | *otc* |
| | More than 25 cigarettes/day: 4 mg gum up to 24 pieces/day | | |
| Inhaler | 6 to 16 cartridges/day | up to 6 months | *Rx* only |
| Transdermal patch | 21 mg/24 h 14 mg/24 h 7 mg/24 h | 4 to 6 weeks then 2 weeks then 2 weeks | *otc* |
| | 15 mg/16 h | 6 weeks | |
| Nasal spray | 8 to 40 doses/day | 3 months | *Rx* only |

*NICOTINE TRANSDERMAL SYSTEM:*

| Recommended Dosing Schedule of Transdermal Nicotine for Healthy Patients | | |
|---|---|---|
| | Duration | |
| Dose | Per strength of patch | Entire course of therapy |
| Nicoderm[1] 21 mg/day 14 mg/day 7 mg/day | First 6 weeks Next 2 weeks Last 2 weeks | 8 to 10 weeks |
| Nicotrol 15 mg/16 h 10 mg/16 h 5 mg/16 h | First 6 weeks Next 2 weeks Last 2 weeks | 10 weeks |

[1] Start with 14 mg/day for 6 weeks for patients who smoke less than 10 cigarettes/day. Decrease dose to 7 mg/day for the final 2 weeks.

*Nicoderm* – After 16 or 24 hours, remove the used system and apply a new system to an alternate skin site. Skin sites should not be reused for at least a week. Caution patients not to continue to use the same system for more than 24 hours.

*Nicotrol* – Each day apply a new system upon waking and remove at bedtime.

*NICOTINE POLACRILEX (GUM):* Advise patient to stop smoking completely when beginning to use the gum. If the patient smokes less than 25 cigarettes/day, start with the 2 mg nicotine gum. If the patient smokes more than 25 cigarettes/day, use according to the following 12-week schedule:

| Nicotine Polacrilex Dosing Schedule | | |
|---|---|---|
| Weeks 1 to 6 | Weeks 7 to 9 | Weeks 10 to 12 |
| 1 piece of gum or lozenge every 1 to 2 hours | 1 piece of gum or lozenge every 2 to 4 hours | 1 piece of gum or lozenge every 4 to 8 hours |

Instruct patient to chew the gum slowly until it tingles, then park it between the cheek and gum. When the tingle is gone, instruct patient to begin chewing again until the tingle returns. Repeat the process until most of the tingle is gone (approximately 30 minutes).

Advise patient not to eat or drink for 15 minutes before chewing the nicotine gum or while chewing a piece. To improve the chances of quitting, chew at least 9 pieces/day for the first 6 weeks. If there are strong and frequent cravings, use a second piece within the hour. However, do not continuously use 1 piece after another since this may cause hiccoughs, heartburn, nausea, or other side effects.

Do not use more than 24 pieces/day. Stop using the nicotine gum at the end of 12 weeks. If there is still a need to use nicotine gum, have the patient contact a physician.

NICOTINE POLACRILEX (LOZENGE): If the patient smokes his/her first cigarette more than 30 minutes after waking up, start with the 2 mg nicotine lozenge. If the patient smokes their first cigarette within 30 minutes of waking up, start with the 4 mg nicotine lozenge. Refer to the dosing schedule in the table above.

Instruct the patient to place the lozenge in the mouth and allow it to slowly dissolve (about 20 to 30 minutes). Minimize swallowing. Advise the patient not to chew or swallow the lozenge. The patient may feel a warm or tingling sensation. Advise the patient to occasionally move the lozenge from one side of the mouth to the other until completely dissolved.

Advise the patient not to eat or drink 15 minutes before using or while the lozenge is in the mouth. To improve the chances of quitting, use at least 9 lozenges/day for the first 6 weeks. Do not use more than 1 lozenge at a time or continuously use 1 lozenge after another because this may cause hiccoughs, heartburn, nausea, or other side effects.

Advise the patient not to use more than 5 lozenges in 6 hours or more than 20 lozenges/day and to stop using the nicotine lozenge at the end of 12 weeks. If there is still a need to use the nicotine lozenge, have the patient contact a physician.

NICOTINE INHALATION SYSTEM: Patients should be encouraged to use at least 6 cartridges/day at least for the first 3 to 6 weeks of treatment. Additional doses may be needed to control the urge to smoke with a maximum of 16 cartridges/day for up to 12 weeks. The safety and efficacy of the continued use of the nicotine inhaler for periods more than 6 months have not been studied and such use is not recommended.

NICOTINE NASAL SPRAY: Instruct patients to stop smoking completely when using the product. Instruct them not to sniff, swallow, or inhale through the nose as the spray is being administered. Advise patients to administer the spray with the head tilted back slightly.

Dosage – Each actuation of the nasal spray delivers a metered 50 mcL spray containing 0.5 mg nicotine. One dose is 1 mg of nicotine (2 sprays, 1 in each nostril). Start patients with 1 or 2 doses per hour, which may be increased up to a maximum recommended dose of 40 mg (80 sprays, somewhat less than ½ of the bottle) per day. For best results, encourage patients to use at least the recommended minimum of 8 doses/day, as less is unlikely to be effective.

| Nicotine Nasal Spray Dosing Recommendations | | | |
|---|---|---|---|
| Maximum recommended duration of treatment | Recommended doses/h | Maximum doses/h | Maximum doses/day |
| 3 months | 1 to 2[1] | 5 | 40 |

[1] One dose = 2 sprays (1 in each nostril). One dose delivers 1 mg of nicotine to the nasal mucosa.

*Individualization of dosage* – The goal of the nasal spray therapy is complete abstinence. If a patient is unable to stop smoking by the fourth week of therapy, discontinue treatment. Regular use of the spray during the first week of treatment may
help patients adapt to the irritant effects of the spray. Patients who are successfully abstinent on the nasal spray should be treated at the selected dosage for up
to 8 weeks, following which use of the spray should be discontinued over the next
4 to 6 weeks. Some patients may not require gradual reduction of dosage and may
abruptly stop treatment successfully. Treatment with the nasal spray for longer periods has not been shown to improve outcome, and the safety of use for periods
longer than 6 months has not been established.

## Actions
*Pharmacology:* Nicotine, the chief alkaloid in tobacco products, binds stereo-selectively
to acetylcholine receptors at the autonomic ganglia, in the adrenal medulla, at neuromuscular junctions, and in the brain.

*Pharmacokinetics:*

| Nicotine Pharmacokinetics | | | | | |
| --- | --- | --- | --- | --- | --- |
| Parameter | Smoking | Gum | Transdermal | Nasal spray | Inhaler |
| Time to peak levels (hours) | ND[1] | 0.25 to 0.5 | 2 to 12 | 0.25 | 0.25 |
| Peak plasma level (ng/mL) | 44 | 5 to 10 | 5 to 17 | 12 | 6 |
| Half-life (hours) | 15 to 20[2] | 3 to 4 | 3 to 4 | 1 to 2 | ND |

[1] No data.
[2] Refers to cotinine, the primary plasma metabolite of nicotine.

## Contraindications
Hypersensitivity to nicotine or any components of the products, including menthol.

## Warnings
*Nicotine risks:* Nicotine from any source can be toxic and addictive. Smoking causes
lung disease, cancer, and heart disease, and may adversely affect pregnant women
or the fetus.

*Renal/Hepatic function impairment:* Anticipate some influence of hepatic impairment on
drug kinetics (reduced clearance). Only severe renal impairment should affect
clearance of nicotine or its metabolites from circulation.

*Elderly:* Nicotine **inhaler** therapy appeared to be as effective in elderly patients 60 years
of age or older as in younger smokers.

*Pregnancy:* Category D (**inhaler, spray, transdermal patch**); Category C (**gum**). Nicotine is contraindicated in women who are or may become pregnant; advise patients
to use contraceptive measures.

*Lactation:* Nicotine passes freely into breast milk and has the potential for serious
adverse reactions in nursing infants.

*Children:* Safety and efficacy in children/adolescents younger than 18 years of age who
smoke are not evaluated.

## Precautions
*General:* Urge the patient to stop smoking completely when initiating nicotine replacement therapy. Inform patients that if they continue to smoke while using the product, they may experience adverse effects because of peak nicotine levels higher
than those experienced from smoking alone. If there is a clinically significant
increase in cardiovascular or other effects attributable to nicotine, the treatment
should be discontinued. Physicians should anticipate that concomitant medications
may need dosage adjustment (see Drug Interactions). Sustained use (older than
6 months) of inhaler or nasal spray by patients who stop smoking has not been studied and is not recommended (see Drug Abuse and Dependence).

*Bronchospastic disease:* The **inhaler** and **nasal spray** have not been specifically studied in asthma or chronic pulmonary disease. Nicotine is an airway irritant and might cause bronchospasm.

Use of the **nasal spray** or **inhaler** in patients with severe reactive airway disease is not recommended.

*Nasal disorders:* Use of the **nasal spray** is not recommended in patients with known chronic nasal disorders (eg, allergy, rhinitis, nasal polyps, sinusitis) because such use has not been adequately studied.

*Cardiovascular:* Specifically, screen and evaluate patients with coronary heart disease, serious cardiac arrhythmias or vasospastic diseases before nicotine is prescribed. There have been occasional reports of tachyarrhythmias associated with nicotine use; therefore, if an increase in cardiovascular symptoms occurs, discontinue the drug.

*Accelerated hypertension* – Nicotine therapy constitutes a risk factor for development of malignant hypertension in patients with accelerated hypertension. **Inhaler** therapy should be used with caution in these patients and only when the benefits of including nicotine replacement in a smoking cessation program outweigh the risks.

*Endocrine:* Because of the action of nicotine on the adrenal medulla, use with caution in patients with hyperthyroidism, pheochromocytoma or insulin-dependent diabetes.

*Oral/GI:* Use caution in patients with oral or pharyngeal inflammation and in those with history of esophagitis or active or inactive peptic ulcer.

*Dental problems:* Dental problems might be exacerbated by chewing nicotine gum.

*Drug abuse and dependence:* Urge patients to stop smoking completely when initiating therapy. If patients smoke while using nicotine, they may experience adverse effects because of peak nicotine levels higher than those caused by smoking alone.

The nicotine **inhaler** is likely to have a low abuse potential based on slower absorption, smaller fluctuations, and lower blood levels of nicotine when compared with cigarettes. Nicotine **nasal spray** has a dependence potential intermediate between other nicotine-based therapies and cigarettes. To minimize risk of dependence, encourage patients to gradually withdraw or stop gum and inhaler usage at 3 months, transdermal nicotine after 4 to 8 weeks. Chronic consumption is toxic and addicting.

## Drug Interactions

Smoking cessation, with or without nicotine substitutes, may alter response to concomitant medication in ex-smokers. Smoking may affect alcohol, benzodiazepines, beta-adrenergic blockers, caffeine, clozapine, fluvoxamine, olanzapine, tacrine, theophylline, clorazepate, lidocaine (oral), estradiol, flecainide, imipramine, heparin, insulin, mexiletine, opioids, propranolol, catecholamines, and cortisol.

*Nasal spray:* The extent of absorption and peak plasma concentration is slightly reduced in patients with the common cold/rhinitis. In addition, the time to peak concentration is prolonged. The use of a nasal vasoconstrictor such as xylometazoline in patients with rhinitis will further prolong the time to peak.

## Adverse Reactions

*Inhaler* – Local irritation (mouth, throat); coughing; rhinitis; dyspepsia; headache; taste complaints; pain in jaw and neck; tooth disorders; sinusitis; influenza-like symptoms; pain; back pain; allergy; paresthesia; flatulence; fever; dizziness; anxiety; sleep disorder; depression; withdrawal syndrome; drug dependence; fatigue; myalgia; nausea; diarrhea; hiccough; chest discomfort; bronchitis; hypertension.

*Nasal spray* – Runny nose; throat irritation; watering eyes; sneezing; cough; nasal congestion; subjective comments related to the taste or usage of the dosage form; sinus irritation; transient epistaxis; eye irritation; transient changes in sense of smell; pharyngitis; paresthesias of the nose, mouth, or head; numbness of the nose or mouth; burning of the nose or eyes; earache; facial flushing; transient changes in sense of taste; hoarseness; nasal ulcer or blister; headache; back pain; dyspnea; nausea; arthralgia; menstrual disorder; palpitation; flatulence; tooth disorder; gum disorder; myalgia; abdominal pain; confusion; acne; dysmenorrhea.

*Gum* – Injury to mouth, teeth, or dental work; belching; increased salivation; mild jaw muscle ache; sore mouth or throat.

*Transdermal* – Erythema, pruritus, and burning at the application site.

# BUPROPION HCI

| | |
|---|---|
| **Tablets, sustained release**: 150 mg (*Rx*) | *Zyban* (GlaxoSmithKline) |

### Indications
*Smoking cessation:* An aid to smoking cessation treatment.

### Administration and Dosage
The recommended and maximum dose of bupropion is 300 mg/day, given as 150 mg twice/day. Begin dosing at 150 mg/day given every day for the first 3 days, followed by a dose increase for most patients to the recommended usual dose of 300 mg/day. There should be an interval of 8 hours or more between successive doses. Do not give doses greater than 300 mg/day.

Initiate treatment with bupropion while the patient is still smoking because approximately 1 week of treatment is required to achieve steady-state blood levels of bupropion. Patients should set a "target quit date" within the first 2 weeks of treatment with bupropion, generally in the second week. Continue treatment for 7 to 12 weeks; base duration of treatment on the relative benefits and risks for individual patients. If a patient has not made significant progress toward abstinence by week 7 of therapy with bupropion, it is unlikely that he or she will quit during that attempt; discontinue treatment. Dose tapering of bupropion is not required when discontinuing treatment. It is important that patients continue to receive counseling and support throughout treatment with bupropion and for a period of time thereafter.

*Maintenance:* Nicotine dependence is a chronic condition. Some patients may need continuous treatment. Systematic evaluation of bupropion 300 mg/day for maintenance therapy demonstrated that treatment for up to 6 months was effective. Whether to continue treatment with bupropion for periods longer than 12 weeks for smoking cessation must be determined for individual patients.

*Combination treatment:* Combination treatment with bupropion and nicotine transdermal system (NTS) may be prescribed for smoking cessation.

*Hepatic function impairment:* Use extreme caution in patients with severe hepatic cirrhosis. The dose should not exceed 150 mg every other day in these patients. Use bupropion with caution in patients with hepatic impairment (including mild to moderate hepatic cirrhosis) and consider a reduced frequency of dosing in patients with mild to moderate hepatic cirrhosis (see Warnings).

*Renal function impairment:* Use caution in patients with renal impairment and consider a reduced frequency of dosing (see Warnings).

### Actions
*Pharmacology:* Bupropion is a nonnicotine aid to smoking cessation. The mechanism by which bupropion enhances the ability of patients to abstain from smoking is unknown. However, it is presumed that this action is mediated by noradrenergic or dopaminergic mechanisms.

*Pharmacokinetics:* Following oral administration to healthy volunteers, mean peak plasma concentrations were achieved within 3 hours. Bupropion is 84% bound to human plasma proteins in vitro. Bupropion is extensively metabolized with a mean elimination half-life of approximately 21 hours.

### Contraindications
Coadministration with a monoamine oxidase (MAO) inhibitor, *Wellbutrin*, *Wellbutrin SR* or any medications that contain bupropion; current or prior diagnosis of bulimia or anorexia nervosa, seizure disorders; patients who have shown an allergic response

to bupropion or other ingredients in the formulation; patients undergoing abrupt discontinuation of alcohol or sedatives (including benzodiazepines).

## Warnings

*Antidepressants:* Bupropion is the active ingredient found in *Wellbutrin* and *Wellbutrin SR* used to treat depression. Do not use in combination with *Wellbutrin*, *Wellbutrin SR* or any other medication that contains bupropion.

*Anorexia nervosa/bulimia:* Do not give with current or prior diagnosis of bulimia or anorexia nervosa because of a higher incidence of seizures noted in patients treated for bulimia with the immediate-release formulation of bupropion.

*Seizures:* Because the use of bupropion is associated with a dose-dependent risk of seizures, do not prescribe doses greater than 300 mg/day for smoking cessation. The seizure rate associated with doses of sustained —release bupropion 300 mg/day or less is approximately 0.1%.

*Concomitant medications* – Many medications (eg, antipsychotics, antidepressants, theophylline, systemic steroids) and treatment regimens (eg, abrupt discontinuation of benzodiazepines) are known to lower seizure threshold.

*Reducing the risk of seizures* – Retrospective analysis suggests that the risk of seizures may be minimized if the total daily dose of bupropion does not exceed 300 mg (the maximum recommended dose) and no single dose exceeds 150 mg.

*Hypersensitivity reactions:* Anaphylactoid reactions characterized by symptoms such as pruritus, urticaria, angioedema, and dyspnea requiring medical treatment have been reported at a rate of approximately 1 to 3 per thousand in clinical trials of bupropion. In addition, there have been rare spontaneous postmarketing reports of erythema multiformes, Stevens-Johnson syndrome, and anaphylactic shock associated with bupropion.

*Renal function impairment:* Use bupropion with caution in patients with renal impairment and consider a reduced frequency of dosing as bupropion and its metabolites may accumulate in such patients to a greater extent than usual.

*Hepatic function impairment:* Use with extreme caution in patients with severe hepatic cirrhosis. In these patients, a reduced frequency of dosing is required, as peak bupropion levels are substantially increased and accumulation is likely to occur in such patients to a greater extent than usual. The dose should not exceed 150 mg every other day.

Use with caution in patients with hepatic impairment (including mild to moderate hepatic cirrhosis) and consider reduced frequency of dosing in patients with mild to moderate hepatic cirrhosis.

*Pregnancy:* Category B.

To monitor fetal outcomes of pregnant women exposed to bupropion, the manufacturer maintains a bupropion pregnancy registry. Health care providers are encouraged to register patients by calling (800) 336-2176.

*Lactation:* Bupropion and its metabolites are secreted in breast milk.

*Children:* Safety and efficacy in patients younger than 18 years of age has not been established.

## Precautions

*Insomnia:* In one trial, 29% of patients treated with 150 mg/day and 35% of patients treated with 300 mg/day experienced insomnia vs 21% with placebo.

*Psychosis or mania:* Antidepressants can precipitate manic episodes in bipolar disorder patients during the depressed phase of their illness and may activate latent psychosis in other susceptible individuals. The sustained-release formulation of bupropion is expected to pose similar risks. There were no reports of activation of psychosis or mania in clinical trials conducted in nondepressed smokers.

*Cardiac effects:* Hypertension, in some cases severe, requiring acute treatment, has been reported in patients receiving bupropion alone and in combination with nicotine replacement therapy. These events have been observed in both patients with and without evidence of pre-existing hypertension.

Use caution in patients with a recent history of MI or unstable heart disease. Bupropion was well tolerated in depressed patients who had previously developed orthostatic hypotension while receiving tricyclic antidepressants and was generally well tolerated in depressed patients with stable CHF. Bupropion was associated with a rise in supine blood pressure in the study of patients with CHF, resulting in discontinuation of treatment in 2 patients for exacerbation of baseline hypertension.

*Drug abuse and dependence:* Bupropion is likely to have a low abuse potential. There have been a few reported cases of drug dependence and withdrawal symptoms associated with the immediate-release formulation of bupropion.

### Drug Interactions

Because bupropion is extensively metabolized, the coadministration of other drugs may affect its clinical activity. In particular, certain drugs may induce the metabolism of bupropion (eg, carbamazepine, phenobarbital, phenytoin) while other drugs may inhibit the metabolism of bupropion (eg, cimetidine, ritonavir).

Drugs that may increase the effects or side effects of bupropion include levodopa, MAOIs, ritonavir, antidepressants, antipsychotics, beta blockers, type IC antiarrhythmics.

*Drugs that lower seizure threshold:* Concurrent administration of bupropion and agents (eg, antipsychotics, antidepressants, theophylline, systemic steroids) or treatment regimens (eg, abrupt discontinuation of benzodiazepines) that lower seizure threshold should be undertaken only with extreme caution.

*Drug/Food interactions:* Food increased the $C_{max}$ by 11%, the extent of absorption (AUC) by 17% and the mean time to peak concentration of bupropion.

### Adverse Reactions

Adverse reactions occurring in 3% or more of patients include: Abdominal pain; insomnia; dream abnormality; anxiety; disturbed concentration; dizziness; nervousness; application site reaction; rash; pruritus; nausea; dry mouth; constipation; diarrhea; anorexia; myalgia; arthralgia; rhinitis; increased cough; pharyngitis; taste perversion.

# BOTULINUM TOXIN TYPE A

**Powder for injection (vacuum-dried):** 100 units of vacuum-dried *Clostridium botulinum* toxin type A neurotoxin complex[1] (*Rx*)

*Botox* (Allergan), *Botox Cosmetic* (Allergan)

[1] One unit corresponds to the calculated median lethal intraperitoneal dose ($LD_{50}$) in mice.

### Indications

*Cervical dystonia (CD) (Botox only):* For the treatment of CD in adults to decrease the severity of abnormal head position and neck pain associated with CD.

*Glabellar lines (Botox Cosmetic only):* For the temporary improvement in the appearance of moderate to severe glabellar lines associated with corrugator or procerus muscle activity in adult patients 65 years of age or younger.

### Administration and Dosage

CD (Botox only):

*Patients with known history of tolerance* – The mean dose administered to patients in the phase 3 study was 236 units (25% to 75%; range, 198 units to 300 units). The dose was divided among the affected muscles. Tailor dosing in initial and sequential treatment sessions to the individual patient based on the patient's head and neck position, localization of pain, muscle hypertrophy, patient response, and adverse event history.

*Patients without prior use* – The initial dose should be lower, with subsequent dosing adjusted based on individual response. Limiting the total dose injected into the sternocleidomastoid muscles to 100 units or less may decrease the occurrence of dysphagia.

A 25-, 27-, or 30-gauge needle may be used for superficial muscles, and a longer 22-gauge needle may be used for deeper musculature. Localization of the involved muscles with electromyographic guidance may be useful.

Clinical improvement generally begins within the first 2 weeks after injection with maximum clinical benefit at approximately 6 weeks postinjection. In the phase 3 study, most subjects were observed to have returned to pretreatment status by 3 months posttreatment.

*Glabellar lines (Botox Cosmetic only):* Inject IM only.

Reconstitute with 0.9% sterile, nonpreserved saline (100 units in 2.5 mL saline) prior to IM injection. The resulting formulation will be 4 units/0.1 mL and a total treatment dose of 20 units in 0.5 mL. The duration of activity of botulinum toxin type A for glabellar lines is approximately 3 to 4 months. Injection intervals should be no more frequent than every 3 months and should be performed using the lowest effective dose. The safety and efficacy of more frequent dosing have not been clinically evaluated; more frequent dosing is not recommended.

### Actions

*Pharmacology:* Botulinum toxin neurotoxin complex is a sterile, vacuum-dried form of purified botulinum toxin type A, produced from a fermentation of the Hall strain of *Clostridium botulinum* type A grown in a medium-containing casein hydrolysate and yeast extract. Botulinum toxin type A blocks neuromuscular conduction by binding to receptor sites on motor nerve terminals, entering the nerve terminals, and inhibiting the release of acetylcholine. When injected IM at therapeutic doses, botulinum toxin type A produces a partial chemical denervation of the muscle, resulting in a localized reduction in muscle activity. In addition, the muscle may atrophy, axonal sprouting may occur, and extrajunctional acetylcholine receptors may develop, thus, slowly reversing muscle denervation produced by botulinum toxin type A.

### Contraindications

Presence of infection at the proposed injection site(s); hypersensitivity to any ingredient in the formulation.

### Warnings

*Neuropathic disorders:* Administer with caution in individuals with peripheral motor neuropathic diseases (eg, amyotrophic lateral sclerosis, motor neuropathy) or neuromuscular junctional disorders (eg, myasthenia gravis, Lambert-Eaton syndrome). Patients with neuromuscular disorders may be at increased risk of clinically significant systemic effects including severe dysphagia and respiratory compromise from typical doses of botulinum toxin type A.

*Dysphagia:* Dysphagia is a commonly reported adverse event following treatment of CD patients with all botulinum toxins. In these patients, there are reports of rare cases of dysphagia severe enough to warrant the insertion of a gastric feeding tube.

*Albumin:* This product contains albumin, a derivative of human blood. Based on effective donor screening and product manufacturing processes, it carries an extremely remote risk for transmission of viral diseases. A theoretical risk for transmission of Creutzfeldt-Jakob disease (CJD) also is considered extremely remote. No cases of transmission of viral diseases or CJD have ever been identified for albumin.

*Dosage, systemic toxicity:* Do not exceed the recommended dosages and frequencies of administration. Risks resulting from administration at higher dosages are not known. Should accidental injection or oral ingestion occur, medically supervise the person for several days on an outpatient basis for signs or symptoms of systemic weakness or muscle paralysis.

*Cardiovascular events:* There have been rare reports following administration of botulinum toxin type A for other indications of adverse events involving the cardiovascular system, including arrhythmia and MI, some with fatal outcomes. Some of these patients had risk factors including pre-existing cardiovascular disease.

*Hypersensitivity reactions:* As with all biologic products, have epinephrine and other precautions available if anaphylactic reaction occurs.

*Elderly:* In general, be cautious in dose selection for an elderly patient, usually starting at the low end of the dosing range, reflecting the greater frequency of decreased hepatic, renal, or cardiac function, and of concomitant disease or other drug therapy.

*Pregnancy:* Category C.

Administration of *Botox Cosmetic* is not recommended during pregnancy.

*Lactation:* It is not known whether this drug is excreted in breast milk. Exercise caution when botulinum toxin type A is administered to a nursing woman.

*Children:* Safety and efficacy in children less than 16 years of age have not been established for CD. Use for glabellar lines is not recommended in children.

## Precautions

*Safe and effective use:* Safe and effective use of botulinum toxin type A depends upon proper storage of the product, selection of the correct dose, and proper reconstitution and administration techniques.

*CD:* Patients with smaller neck muscle mass and patients who require bilateral injections into the sternocleidomastoid muscle have been reported to be at greater risk for dysphagia. Limiting the dose injected into the sternocleidomastoid muscle may reduce the occurrence of dysphagia. Injections into the levator scapulae may be associated with an increased risk of upper respiratory tract infection and dysphagia.

*Injection site:* Use caution when botulinum toxin type A treatment is used in the presence of inflammation at the proposed injection site(s) or when excessive weakness or atrophy is present in the target muscle(s).

*Immunogenicity:* Treatment with botulinum toxin type A may result in the formation of antibodies that may reduce the effectiveness of subsequent treatments with botulinum toxin type A for glabellar lines or other indications.

The results from some studies suggest that botulinum toxin type A injections at more frequent intervals or at higher doses may lead to greater incidence of antibody formation. The potential for antibody formation may be minimized by injecting with the lowest effective dose given at the longest feasible intervals between injections.

*Ophthalmic:* Reduced blinking from injection of the orbicularis muscle can lead to corneal exposure, persistent epithelial defect, and corneal ulceration, especially in patients with VII nerve disorders. Employ careful testing of corneal sensation in eyes previously operated upon, avoidance of injection into the lower lid area to avoid ectropion, and vigorous treatment of any epithelial defect. This may require protective drops, ointment, therapeutic soft contact lenses, or closure of the eye by patching or other means.

Inducing paralysis in 1 or more extraocular muscles may produce spatial disorientation, double vision, or past pointing. Covering the affected eye may alleviate these symptoms.

*Dermatologic:* Use caution in patients who have an inflammatory skin problem at the injection site, marked facial asymmetry, ptosis, excessive dermatochalasis, deep dermal scarring, thick sebaceous skin, or the inability to substantially lessen glabellar lines by physically spreading them apart, as these patients were excluded from safety and efficacy trials.

## Drug Interactions

*Aminoglycosides:* The effect of botulinum toxin may be potentiated by aminoglycoside antibiotics or any other drug that interferes with neuromuscular transmission.

The effect of administering different botulinum neurotoxin serotypes at the same time or within several months of each other is unknown. Excessive neuromuscular weakness may be exacerbated by administration of another botulinum toxin prior to the resolution of the effects of a previously administered botulinum toxin.

## Adverse Reactions

In general, adverse events occur within the first week following injection of botulinum toxin type A and, while generally transient, may have a duration of several months.

CD: Adverse reactions in at least 3% of patients include dysphagia, upper respiratory infection, neck pain, headache, dyspnea, increased cough, flu syndrome, back pain, rhinitis, dizziness, hypertonia, injection site soreness, asthenia, oral dryness, speech disorder, fever, nausea, and drowsiness.

*Glabellar lines:* Adverse reactions in at least 3% of patients include headache, infection, and blepharoptosis.

## Overdosage

An antitoxin is available in the event of immediate knowledge of an overdose or misinjection. In the event of overdosage or injection into the wrong muscle, additional information may be obtained by contacting Allergan at (800) 433-8871 from 8 am to 4 pm Pacific Time, or at (714) 246-5954 for a recorded message at other times. The antitoxin will not reverse any botulinum toxin-induced muscle weakness effects already apparent by the time of antitoxin administration.

# Chapter 8

# GASTROINTESTINAL AGENTS

# ANTACIDS

| | |
|---|---|
| **ALUMINUM CARBONATE GEL, BASIC** | |
| **Tablets**: Equiv. to 608 mg dried aluminum hydroxide gel or 500 mg aluminum hydroxide (*otc*) | *Basaljel* (Wyeth-Ayerst) |
| **Capsules**: Equiv. to 608 mg dried aluminum hydroxide gel or 500 mg aluminum hydroxide (*otc*) | *Basaljel* (Wyeth-Ayerst) |
| **Suspension**: Equiv. to 400 mg aluminum hydroxide/5 mL (*otc*) | *Basaljel* (Wyeth-Ayerst) |
| **ALUMINUM HYDROXIDE GEL** | |
| **Tablets**: 300, 500, 600 mg (*otc*) | *Amphojel* (Wyeth-Ayerst), *Alu-Tab* (3M Pharm) |
| **Capsules**: 400, 500 mg (*otc*) | *Alu-Cap* (3M Pharm), *Dialume* (Aventis) |
| **Suspension**: 320 mg/5 mL, 450 mg/5 mL, 675 mg/5 mL (*otc*) | Various, *Amphojel* (Wyeth-Ayerst) |
| **Liquid**: 600 mg/5 mL (*otc*) | Various, *AlternaGEL* (J & J-Merck) |
| **CALCIUM CARBONATE** | |
| **Tablets, chewable**: 350, 420, 750, 850, 1000 mg (*otc*) | *Extra Strength Tums E-X* (GlaxoSmithKline), *Alka-Mints* (Bayer), *Tums Ultra* (GlaxoSmith-Kline), *Dicarbosil* (BIRA) |
| **Tablets**: 500, 600, 650, 1000, 1250 mg (*otc*) | Various, *Maalox Antacid Caplets* (Aventis) |
| **Gum tablets**: 500 mg (*otc*) | *Chooz* (Schering-Plough) |
| **Suspension**: 1250 mg/5 mL (*otc*) | Various |
| **Lozenges**: 600 mg (*otc*) | *Mylanta* (J & J-Merck) |
| **MAGALDRATE** | |
| **Suspension**: 540 mg/5 mL (*otc*) | *Riopan* (Whitehall) |
| **Liquid**: 540 mg/5 mL (*otc*) | Various, *Iosopan* (Goldline) |
| **MAGNESIA (Magnesium Hydroxide)** | |
| **Tablets, chewable**: 311 mg (*otc*) | *Phillips' Chewable* (Sterling Health) |
| **Liquid**: 400 mg/5 mL, 800 mg/5 mL (*otc*) | Various, *Phillips' Milk of Magnesia* (Sterling Health), *Phillips' Concentrated Milk of Magnesia* (Sterling Health) |
| **MAGNESIUM OXIDE** | |
| **Tablets**: 400, 420, 500 mg (*otc*) | Various, *Mag-Ox 400* (Blaine), *Maox 420* (Kenneth A. Manne) |
| **Capsules**: 140 mg (*otc*) | *Uro-Mag* (Blaine) |
| **SODIUM BICARBONATE** | |
| **Tablets**: 325, 520, 650 mg (*otc*) | Various, *Bellans* (C.S. Dent) |
| **SODIUM CITRATE** | |
| **Solution**: 450 mg (*otc*) | *Citra pH* (ValMed) |

## Indications

*Hyperacidity:* Symptomatic relief of upset stomach associated with hyperacidity (heartburn, gastroesophageal reflux, acid indigestion, and sour stomach); hyperacidity associated with peptic ulcer and gastric hyperacidity.

*Aluminum carbonate:* Treatment, control, or management of hyperphosphatemia, or for use with a low phosphate diet.

*Calcium carbonate:* Treating calcium deficiency states.

*Magnesium oxide:* Treatment of magnesium deficiencies or magnesium depletion.

## Administration and Dosage

ALUMINUM CARBONATE GEL, BASIC:
Antacid – 2 capsules or tablets or 10 mL of regular suspension (in water or fruit juice) as often as every 2 hours, up to 12 times daily.

ALUMINUM HYDROXIDE GEL:
Tablets/Capsules – 500 to 1500 mg 3 to 6 times daily, between meals and at bedtime.
Suspension – 5 to 30 mL as needed between meals and at bedtime or as directed.

CALCIUM CARBONATE: 0.5 to 1.5 g, as needed.

MAGALDRATE (Aluminum Magnesium Hydroxide Sulfate):
Suspension/Liquid – 5 to 10 mL between meals and at bedtime.

MAGNESIA (Magnesium Hydroxide):
  Antacid dose, adults, and children older than 12 years of age –
    Liquid: 5 to 15 mL up to 4 times daily with water.
    Liquid, concentrated: 2.5 to 7.5 mL up to 4 times daily with water.
    Tablets: 622 mg to 1244 mg up to 4 times daily.

MAGNESIUM OXIDE:
  Capsules – 140 mg 3 to 4 times daily.
  Tablets – 400 to 800 mg/day.

SODIUM BICARBONATE: 0.3 to 2 g 1 to 4 times daily.

SODIUM CITRATE: 30 mL daily.

## Actions

*Pharmacology:* Antacids neutralize gastric acidity, resulting in an increase in the pH of the stomach and duodenal bulb. Additionally, by increasing the gastric pH above 4, they inhibit the proteolytic activity of pepsin. Antacids do not "coat" the mucosal lining, but may have a local astringent effect. Antacids also increase the lower esophageal sphincter tone. Aluminum ions inhibit smooth muscle contraction, thus inhibiting gastric emptying.

*Acid neutralizing capacity (ANC) –* ANC is a consideration in selecting an antacid. It varies for commercial antacid preparations and is expressed as mEq/mL. Milliequivalents of ANC is defined by the mEq of HCl required to keep an antacid suspension at pH 3.5 for 10 minutes in vitro. An antacid must neutralize at least 5 mEq/dose. Also, any ingredient must contribute at least 25% of the total ANC of a given product to be considered an antacid.

Aluminum hydroxide and calcium-containing antacids may reduce LDL cholesterol and increase the HDL/LDL ratio.

## Warnings

*Sodium content:* Sodium content of antacids may be significant. Patients with hypertension, CHF, marked renal failure, or those on restricted or low-sodium diets should use a low sodium preparation.

*"Acid rebound":* Antacids may cause dose-related rebound hyperacidity because they may increase gastric secretion or serum gastrin levels.

*Milk-alkali syndrome:* Milk-alkali syndrome, an acute illness with symptoms of headache, nausea, irritability, and weakness, or a chronic illness with alkalosis, hypercalcemia and, possibly, renal impairment, has occurred following the concurrent use of high-dose calcium carbonate and sodium bicarbonate.

*Hypophosphatemia:* Prolonged use of aluminum-containing antacids may result in hypophosphatemia in normophosphatemic patients if phosphate intake is not adequate.

*Renal function impairment:* Use magnesium-containing products with caution, particularly when more than 50 mEq magnesium is given daily. Hypermagnesemia and toxicity may occur because of decreased clearance of the magnesium ion.

Prolonged use of aluminum-containing antacids in patients with renal failure may result in or worsen dialysis osteomalacia.

*Pregnancy:* If pregnant, consult a physician before using.

## Precautions

*GI hemorrhage:* Use aluminum hydroxide with care in patients who have recently suffered massive upper GI hemorrhage.

## Drug Interactions

Drugs that may be affected by antacids include allopurinol, amphetamines, benzodiazepines, captopril, chloroquine, corticosteroids, dicumarol, diflunisal, digoxin, ethambutol, flecainide, fluoroquinolones, histamine $H_2$ antagonists, hydantoins, iron salts, isoniazid, ketoconazole, levodopa, lithium, methenamine, methotrexate, nitrofurantoin, penicillamine, phenothiazines, quinidine, salicylates, sodium polystyrene sulfonate, sulfonylureas, sympathomimetics, tetracyclines, thyroid hormones, ticlopidine, and valproic acid.

**Adverse Reactions**

*Magnesium-containing antacids* – Laxative effect as saline cathartic, may cause diarrhea; hypermagnesemia in renal failure patients.

*Aluminum-containing antacids* – Constipation (may lead to intestinal obstruction); aluminum-intoxication; osteomalacia and hypophosphatemia; accumulation of aluminum in serum, bone, and the CNS (aluminum accumulation may be neurotoxic); encephalopathy.

*Antacids* – Dose-dependent rebound hyperacidity and milk-alkali syndrome.

# SUCRALFATE

| | |
|---|---|
| **Tablets:** 1 g (*Rx*) | Various, *Carafate* (Aventis) |
| **Suspension:** 1 g/10 mL (*Rx*) | *Carafate* (Aventis) |

### Indications
*Duodenal ulcer:* Short-term treatment (up to 8 weeks) of active duodenal ulcer.

*Maintenance therapy (tablets only):* Duodenal ulcer patients at reduced dosage after healing of acute ulcers.

### Administration and Dosage
*Active duodenal ulcer:*

Adults – 1 g 4 times daily on an empty stomach (1 hour before meals and at bedtime).

Take antacids as needed for pain relief but not within ½ hour before or after sucralfate.

While healing with sucralfate may occur within the first 2 weeks, continue treatment for 4 to 8 weeks unless healing is demonstrated by X-ray or endoscopic examination.

*Maintenance therapy (tablets only):*

Adults – 1 g twice daily.

### Actions
*Pharmacology:* Sucralfate does not affect gastric acid output or concentration. It rapidly reacts with hydrochloric acid in the stomach to form a condensed, viscous, adhesive, paste-like substance with the capacity to buffer acid and binds to the surface of gastric and duodenal ulcers.

The barrier formed at the ulcer site protects the ulcer from the potential ulcerogenic properties of pepsin, acid, and bile, thus allowing the ulcer to heal.

*Pharmacokinetics:* Sucralfate is minimally absorbed from the GI tract following an oral dose. The duration of action depends on the time that the drug is in contact with this site. Binding to the ulcer site has been shown for up to 6 hours. Approximately 95% of the dose remains in the GI tract.

### Warnings
*Chronic renal failure/dialysis:* During sucralfate administration, small amounts of aluminum are absorbed. Concomitant use with other aluminum-containing products may increase the total body burden of aluminum. Patients with chronic renal failure or receiving dialysis have impaired excretion of absorbed aluminum, and aluminum is not dialyzed. Aluminum accumulation and toxicity have occurred.

*Pregnancy:* Category B.

*Lactation:* It is not known whether this drug is excreted in breast milk.

*Children:* Safety and efficacy in children have not been established.

### Precautions
*Ulcer recurrence:* Duodenal ulcer is a chronic recurrent disease. While short-term treatment can completely heal the ulcer, do not expect a successful course to alter posthealing frequency or severity of duodenal ulceration.

### Drug Interactions
Drugs that may be affected by sucralfate include aluminum-containing antacids, anticoagulants, diclofenac, digoxin, histamine $H_2$ antagonists (eg, cimetidine, ranitidine), hydantoins, ketoconazole, levothyroxine, penicillamine, quinidine, quinolones, tetracycline, and theophylline.

### Adverse Reactions
Adverse reactions in clinical trials were minor and rarely led to drug discontinuation. Constipation was the most frequent complaint (2%).

# GASTROINTESTINAL ANTICHOLINERGICS/ANTISPASMODICS

**ANISOTROPINE METHYLBROMIDE**

| | |
|---|---|
| **Tablets**: 50 mg (*Rx*) | Various |

**ATROPINE SULFATE**

| | |
|---|---|
| **Injection**: 0.05, 0.1, 0.3, 0.4, 0.5, 0.8, and 1 mg/mL (*Rx*) | Various |
| **Injection**: 0.5, 1, and 2 mg (*Rx*) | Atro-Pen (Meridian) |
| **Tablets**: 0.4 mg (*Rx*) | Atropine Sulfate (Lilly), Sal-Tropine (Hope) |
| **Tablets, soluble**: 0.4 mg (*Rx*) | Atropine Sulfate (Lilly) |

**BELLADONNA**

| | |
|---|---|
| **Liquids**: 27 to 33 mg belladonna alkaloids/100 mL (*Rx*) | Various |

**DICYCLOMINE HCl**

| | |
|---|---|
| **Capsules**: 10 and 20 mg (*Rx*) | Various, Bentyl (Lakeside Pharm.) |
| **Tablets**: 20 mg (*Rx*) | Various, Bentyl (Lakeside Pharm.) |
| **Syrup**: 10 mg/5 mL (*Rx*) | Various, Bentyl (Lakeside Pharm.) |
| **Injection**: 10 mg/mL (*Rx*) | Various, Bentyl (Lakeside Pharm.) |

**GLYCOPYRROLATE**

| | |
|---|---|
| **Tablets**: 1 and 2 mg (*Rx*) | Robinul (Robins) |
| **Injection**: 0.2 mg/mL (*Rx*) | Various, Robinul (Robins) |

**LEVOROTATORY ALKALOIDS OF BELLADONNA**

| | |
|---|---|
| **Tablets**: 0.25 mg (*Rx*) | Bellafoline (Sandoz) |

**L-HYOSCYAMINE SULFATE**

| | |
|---|---|
| **Tablets**: 0.125 and 0.15 mg (*Rx*) | Levsin (Schwarz Pharma), Gastrosed (Roberts/Hauck), Cystospaz (PolyMedica), Donnamar (Marnel), ED-SPAZ (Edwards) |
| **Tablets, sublingual**: 0.125 mg (*Rx*) | Levsin/SL (Schwarz Pharma), A-Spas S/L (Hyrex) |
| **Tablets, extended release**: 0.375 mg (*Rx*) | Levbid (Schwarz Pharma) |
| **Tablets, sustained release**: 0.375 mg (*Rx*) | Symax-SR (Capellon) |
| **Capsules, timed release**: 0.375 mg (*Rx*) | Various, Levsinex Timecaps (Schwarz Pharma) |
| **Capsules, extended release**: 0.375 mg (*Rx*) | Hyoscyamine Sulfate (Ethex) |
| **Solution**: 0.125 mg/mL (*Rx*) | Levsin Drops (Schwarz Pharma), Gastrosed (Roberts Hauck) |
| **Elixir**: 0.125 mg/5 mL (*Rx*) | Levsin (Schwarz Pharma) |
| **Oral spray**: 0.125 mg/mL (0.125 mg/spray) (*Rx*) | IB-Stat (InKine) |
| **Injection**: 0.5 mg/mL (*Rx*) | Levsin (Schwarz Pharma) |

**METHSCOPOLAMINE BROMIDE**

| | |
|---|---|
| **Tablets**: 2.5 and 5 mg (*Rx*) | Pamine (Kenwood/Bradley) |

**MEPENZOLATE BROMIDE**

| | |
|---|---|
| **Tablets**: 25 mg (*Rx*) | Cantil (Aventis) |

**METHANTHELINE BROMIDE**

| | |
|---|---|
| **Tablets**: 50 mg (*Rx*) | Banthine (Schiapparelli Searle) |

**OXYPHENCYCLIMINE HCl**

| | |
|---|---|
| **Tablets**: 10 mg (*Rx*) | Daricon (GlaxoSmithKline) |

**PROPANTHELINE BROMIDE**

| | |
|---|---|
| **Tablets**: 7.5 and 15 mg (*Rx*) | Various, Pro-Banthine (Schiapparelli Searle) |

**SCOPOLAMINE HBr (Hyoscine HBr)**

| | |
|---|---|
| **Injection**: 0.3, 0.4, 0.86, and 1 mg/mL (*Rx*) | Various |
| **Tablets, soluble**: 0.4 mg (*Rx*) | Scopace (Hope Pharm) |

**TRIDIHEXETHYL CHLORIDE**

| | |
|---|---|
| **Tablets**: 25 mg (*Rx*) | Pathilon (Lederle) |

### Indications

*Peptic ulcer:* Adjunctive therapy for peptic ulcer. These agents suppress gastric acid secretion.

*Other GI conditions:* Functional GI disorders (diarrhea, pylorospasm, hypermotility, neurogenic colon), irritable bowel syndrome (spastic colon, mucous colitis), acute enterocolitis, ulcerative colitis, diverticulitis, mild dysenteries, pancreatitis, splenic flexure syndrome, and infant colic.

*Biliary tract:* For spastic disorders of the biliary tract. Given in conjunction with a narcotic analgesic.

*Urogenital tract:* Uninhibited hypertonic neurogenic bladder.

*Bradycardia:* **Atropine** is used in the suppression of vagally mediated bradycardias.

*Preoperative medication:* **Atropine, scopolamine, hyoscyamine,** and **glycopyrrolate** are used as preanesthetic medication to control bronchial, nasal, pharyngeal, and salivary secretions and to block cardiac vagal inhibitory reflexes during induction of anesthesia and intubation. Scopolamine is used for preanesthetic sedation and for obstetric amnesia.

*Antidotes for poisoning by cholinergic drugs:* Atropine is used for poisoning by organophosphorous insecticides, chemical warfare nerve gases, and as an antidote for mushroom poisoning caused by muscarine in certain species, such as *Amanita muscaria.*

*Miscellaneous uses:* Calming delirium: motion sickness (**scopolamine**); parkinsonism.

*Unlabeled uses:*
Bronchial asthma – Atropine and related agents are effective in some patients with cholinergic-mediated bronchospasm.

**Glycopyrrolate** may be effective in the treatment of bronchial asthma.

### Administration and Dosage

ANISOTROPINE METHYLBROMIDE: 50 mg 3 times daily.

ATROPINE SULFATE:
Adults – 0.4 to 0.6 mg.
Children –

| Atropine Dosage Recommendations in Children | | |
|---|---|---|
| Weight | | Dose |
| lb | kg | mg |
| 7 to 16 | 3.2 to 7.3 | 0.1 |
| 16 to 24 | 7.3 to 10.9 | 0.15 |
| 24 to 40 | 10.9 to 18.1 | 0.2 |
| 40 to 65 | 18.1 to 29.5 | 0.3 |
| 65 to 90 | 29.5 to 40.8 | 0.4 |
| > 90 | 40.8 | 0.4 to 0.6 |

*Hypotonic radiography* – 1 mg IM.

*Surgery* – Give subcutaneously, IM, or IV. The average adult dose is 0.5 mg (range, 0.4 to 0.6 mg). In children, it has been suggested to use a dose of 0.01 mg/kg to a maximum of 0.4 mg, repeated every 4 to 6 hours as needed. A recommended infant dose is 0.04 mg/kg (infants less than 5 kg) or 0.03 mg/kg (infants more than 5 kg), repeated every 4 to 6 hours as needed.

*Bradyarrhythmias* – The usual IV adult dosage ranges from 0.4 to 1 mg every 1 to 2 hours as needed; larger doses, up to a maximum of 2 mg, may be required. In children, IV dosage ranges from 0.01 to 0.03 mg/kg.

*Poisoning* – In anticholinesterase poisoning from exposure to insecticides, give large doses of at least 2 to 3 mg parenterally; repeat until signs of atropine intoxication appear.

*Atro-Pen* – Primary protection against exposure to chemical nerve agent and insecticide poisoning is the wearing of protective garments including masks, designed specifically for this use.

The *AtroPen* Auto-injector should be administered as soon as symptoms of organophosphorus. or carbamate poisoning appear (eg, usually tearing, excessive oral secretions, wheezing, muscle fasciculations). In moderate to severe poisoning, the administration of more than 1 *AtroPen* may be required until atropinization is achieved (flushing, mydriasis, tachycardia, dryness of the mouth and nose).

No more than 3 *AtroPen* injections should be used unless the patient is under the supervision of a trained medical provider. Different dose strengths of the *AtroPen* are available depending on the recipient's age and weight.

| AtroPen Dosing | |
|---|---|
| Patient group | Dose strength |
| Adults and children weighing more than 90 lbs (generally over 10 years of age) | 2 mg |
| Children weighing 40 to 90 lbs (generally 4 to 10 years of age) | 1 mg |
| Children weighing 15 to 40 lbs (generally 6 months to 4 years of age)[a] | 0.5 mg |

[a] Children weighing less than 15 lbs (generally younger than 6 months of age) should ordinarily not be treated with the AtroPen auto-injector. Atropine doses for these children should be individualized at doses of 0.05 mg/kg.

BELLADONNA:
    *Belladonna tincture* –
        *Adults:* 0.6 to 1 mL 3 to 4 times daily.
        *Children:* 0.03 mL/kg (0.8 mL/m$^2$) 3 times daily.

DICYCLOMINE HCl:
    *Oral* –
        *Adults:* The only oral dose shown to be effective is 160 mg/day in 4 equally divided doses. However, because of side effects, begin with 80 mg/day (in 4 equally divided doses). Increase dose to 160 mg/day unless side effects limit dosage.
    *Parenteral* – IM only. Not for IV use.
        *Adults:* 80 mg/day in 4 divided doses.

GLYCOPYRROLATE: Not recommended for children younger than 12 years of age for the management of peptic ulcer.
    *Oral* – 1 mg 3 times daily or 2 mg 2 to 3 times daily.
        *Maintenance:* 1 mg 2 times daily.
    *Parenteral* –
        *Peptic ulcer:* 0.1 to 0.2 mg IM or IV 3 or 4 times daily.
        *Preanesthetic medication:* 0.002 mg/lb (0.004 mg/kg) IM, 30 minutes to 1 hour prior to anesthesia. Children younger than 2 years of age may require up to 0.004 mg/lb. Children younger than 12 years of age, give 0.002 to 0.004 mg/lb IM.
        *Intraoperative medication:* Adults, 0.1 mg IV. Repeat as needed at 2- to 3-minute intervals. Children, give 0.002 mg/lb (0.004 mg/kg) IV, not to exceed 0.1 mg in a single dose; may be repeated at 2- to 3-minute intervals.
        *Reversal of neuromuscular blockade:* Adults and children, 0.2 mg for each 1 mg neostigmine or 5 mg pyridostigmine. Administer IV simultaneously.

L-HYOSCYAMINE SULFATE:
    *Oral* –
        *Adults:* 0.125 to 0.25 mg 3 or 4 times/day orally or sublingually; or 0.375 to 0.75 mg in sustained release form every 12 hours.
        *Children:* Individualize dosage according to weight.
    *Parenteral* – 0.25 to 0.5 mg subcutaneously, IM, or IV, 2 to 4 times daily, as needed.

LEVOROTATORY ALKALOIDS OF BELLADONNA:
    *Oral* –
        *Adults:* 0.25 to 0.5 mg 3 times daily.
        *Children (older than 6 years of age):* 0.125 to 0.25 mg 3 times daily.

MEPENZOLATE BROMIDE:
    *Adults* – 25 to 50 mg 4 times daily with meals and at bedtime.
    *Children* – Safety and efficacy have not been established.

METHANTHELINE BROMIDE:
    *Adults* – 50 to 100 mg every 6 hours.
    *Pediatric* –
        *Newborns:* 12.5 mg 2 times daily, then 12.5 mg 3 times daily.
        *Infants (1 to 12 months of age):* 12.5 mg 4 times daily, increased to 25 mg 4 times daily.
        *Children (older than 1 year of age):* 12.5 to 50 mg 4 times daily.

METHSCOPOLAMINE BROMIDE: 2.5 mg 30 minutes before meals and 2.5 to 5 mg at bedtime.

OXPHENCYCLIMINE HCl:
    *Adults* – 5 to 10 mg 2 or 3 times daily, preferably in the morning and at bedtime. Some respond to 5 mg 2 times/day, while some may require higher dosage 3 times/day.
    *Children* – Not for use in children younger than 12 years of age.

*PROPANTHELINE BROMIDE:*
>*Adults* – 15 mg 30 minutes before meals and 30 mg at bedtime. For patients with mild manifestations, geriatric patients, or those of small stature, take 7.5 mg 3 times daily.
>
>*Children* –
>>*Peptic ulcer:* Safety and efficacy have not been established.
>>
>>*Antisecretory:* 1.5 mg/kg/day divided 3 to 4 times daily.
>>
>>*Antispasmodic:* 2 to 3 mg/kg/day divided every 4 to 6 hours and at bedtime.

*SCOPOLAMINE HBr (Hyoscine HBr):* Give subcutaneously or IM; may give IV after dilution with Sterile Water for Injection.
>*Adults* – 0.32 to 0.65 mg.
>
>*Children* – 0.006 mg/kg. Maximum dosage, 0.3 mg.
>
>*Tablets* – 0.4 to 0.8 mg. Dosage may be cautiously increased in parkinsonism and spastic states.

*TRIDIHEXETHYL CHLORIDE:* 25 to 50 mg 3 or 4 times daily before meals and at bedtime. Bedtime dose, 50 mg.

## Actions

*Pharmacology:* GI anticholinergics are used primarily to decrease motility (smooth muscle tone) in GI, biliary, and urinary tracts and for antisecretory effects. Antispasmodics, related compounds, decrease GI motility by acting on smooth muscle.

These agents inhibit the muscarinic actions of acetylcholine at postganglionic parasympathetic neuroeffector sites including smooth muscle, secretory glands, and CNS sites. Large doses may block nicotinic receptors at the autonomic ganglia and at the neuromuscular junction.

*Pharmacokinetics:*
>*Belladonna alkaloids* – Belladonna alkaloids are rapidly absorbed after oral use. They readily cross the blood-brain barrier and affect the CNS.
>
>*Atropine* – Atropine has a half-life of approximately 2.5 hours; 94% of a dose is eliminated through the urine in 24 hours.
>
>*Quaternary anticholinergics* – Synthetic or semisynthetic derivatives structurally related to the belladonna alkaloids, they are poorly and unreliably absorbed orally. Because they do not cross the blood-brain barrier, CNS effects are negligible. Duration of action is more prolonged than alkaloids.

## Contraindications

*Hypersensitivity:* Hypersensitivity to anticholinergic drugs. Patients hypersensitive to belladonna or to barbiturates may be hypersensitive to **scopolamine.**

*Ocular:* Narrow-angle glaucoma; adhesions (synechiae) between the iris and lens.

*Cardiovascular:* Tachycardia; unstable cardiovascular status in acute hemorrhage; myocardial ischemia.

*GI:* Obstructive disease (eg, achalasia, pyloroduodenal stenosis or pyloric obstruction, cardiospasm); paralytic ileus; intestinal atony of the elderly or debilitated; severe ulcerative colitis; toxic megacolon complicating ulcerative colitis; hepatic disease.

*GU:* Obstructive uropathy (eg, bladder neck obstruction caused by prostatic hypertrophy); renal disease.

*Musculoskeletal:* Myasthenia gravis.

*Atropine:* Atropine is contraindicated in asthma patients.

*Dicyclomine:* Dicyclomine is contraindicated in infants younger than 6 months of age.

## Warnings

*Heat prostration:* Heat prostration can occur with anticholinergic drug use (fever and heat stroke caused by decreased sweating) in the presence of a high environmental temperature.

*Diarrhea:* Diarrhea may be an early symptom of incomplete intestinal obstruction, especially in patients with ileostomy or colostomy. Treatment of diarrhea with these drugs is inappropriate and possibly harmful.

*Anticholinergic psychosis:* Anticholinergic psychosis has been reported in sensitive individuals given anticholinergic drugs.

*Gastric ulcer:* Gastric ulcer may produce a delay in gastric emptying time and may complicate therapy (antral stasis).

*Elderly:* Elderly patients may react with excitement, agitation, drowsiness, and other untoward manifestations to even small doses of anticholinergic drugs.

*Pregnancy:* Category B (glycopyrrolate, parenteral); Category C (hyoscyamine, atropine, scopolamine, propantheline, methantheline).

*Lactation:* **Hyoscyamine** is excreted in breast milk; other anticholinergics (especially **atropine**) may be excreted in milk, causing infant toxicity, and may reduce milk production.

*Children:* Safety and efficacy are not established. **Hyoscyamine** has been used in infant colic. Safety and efficacy of **glycopyrrolate** in children younger than 12 years of age are not established for peptic ulcer. **Dicyclomine** is contraindicated in infants younger than 6 months of age.

## Precautions

*Use with caution in the following:*

*Ocular* – Glaucoma; light irides. Use caution in the elderly because of increased incidence of glaucoma.

*GI* – Hepatic disease; early evidence of ileus, as in peritonitis; ulcerative colitis; hiatal hernia associated with reflux esophagitis.

*GU* – Renal disease; prostatic hypertrophy.

*Cardiovascular* – Coronary heart disease; CHF; cardiac arrhythmias; tachycardia; hypertension.

*Pulmonary* – Debilitated patients with chronic lung disease; reduction in bronchial secretions can lead to inspissation and formation of bronchial plugs.

*Miscellaneous* – Autonomic neuropathy; hyperthyroidism.

*Special risk:* Use cautiously in infants, small children, and people with Down syndrome, brain damage, or spastic paralysis.

*Hazardous tasks:* May produce drowsiness, dizziness, or blurred vision; observe caution while driving or performing other tasks requiring alertness.

## Drug Interactions

Drugs that may interact with GI anticholinergics include amantadine, atenolol, digoxin, phenothiazines, and tricyclic antidepressants.

## Adverse Reactions

Xerostomia; altered taste perception; nausea; vomiting; dysphagia; heartburn; constipation; bloated feeling; paralytic ileus; urinary hesitancy and retention; impotence; blurred vision; mydriasis; photophobia; cycloplegia; increased intraocular pressure; dilated pupils; palpitations; tachycardia (after higher doses); headache; flushing; nervousness; drowsiness; weakness; dizziness; confusion; insomnia; fever (especially in children); mental confusion or excitement; CNS stimulation (restlessness, tremor with large doses); severe allergic reactions including anaphylaxis, urticaria and other dermal manifestations; nasal congestion; decreased sweating.

# HISTAMINE H₂ ANTAGONISTS

### CIMETIDINE
**Tablets:** 100 mg (*otc*) — *Tagamet HB* (GlaxoSmithKline)
**Tablets:** 300, 400, and 800 mg (*Rx*) — Various, *Tagamet* (GlaxoSmithKline)
**Liquid:** 300 mg (as HCl)/5 mL (*Rx*) — *Cimetidine Oral Solution* (Barre-National)
**Injection:** 300 mg (as HCl)/2 mL (*Rx*) — *Cimetidine* (Endo)

### FAMOTIDINE
**Tablets:** 10 mg (*otc*) — *Pepcid AC Acid Controller* (J & J Merck)
**Tablets:** 20 and 40 mg (*Rx*) — *Pepcid* (J & J Merck)
**Gelcaps:** 10 mg (*otc*) — *Pepcid AC* (J & J Merck)
**Tablets, chewable:** 10 mg (*otc*) — *Pepcid AC* (J & J Merck)
**Tablets, orally disintegrating:** 20 and 40 mg (*Rx*) — *Pepcid RPD* (J & J Merck)
**Powder for oral suspension:** 40 mg/5 mL when reconstituted (*Rx*) — *Pepcid* (Merck)
**Injection:** 10 mg/mL (*Rx*) — Various, *Pepcid* (Merck)
**Injection, premixed:** 20 mg/50 mL in 0.9% HCl (*Rx*) — *Pepcid* (Merck)

### NIZATIDINE
**Tablets:** 75 mg (*otc*) — *Axid AR* (Whitehall-Robins)
**Capsules:** 150 and 300 mg (*Rx*) — *Axid Pulvules* (Lilly)

### RANITIDINE
**Tablets:** 75 mg (*otc*) — *Zantac 75* (GlaxoSmithKline)
**Tablets:** 150 and 300 mg (as HCl) (*Rx*) — *Zantac* (GlaxoSmithKline)
**Tablets, effervescent:** 150 mg (*Rx*) — *Zantac EFFERdose* (GlaxoSmithKline)
**Capsules:** 150 and 300 mg (*Rx*) — *Zantac GELdose* (GlaxoSmithKline)
**Syrup:** 15 mg (as HCl)/mL (*Rx*) — *Ranitidine HCl* (UDL), *Zantac* (GlaxoSmithKline)
**Granules, effervescent:** 150 mg (*Rx*) — *Zantac EFFERdose* (GlaxoSmithKline)
**Injection:** 0.5 and 25 mg (as HCl)/mL (*Rx*) — *Zantac* (GlaxoSmithKline)

### HISTAMINE H₂ ANTAGONIST COMBINATIONS
**Tablets, chewable:** 10 mg famotidine, 800 mg calcium carbonate, 165 mg magnesium hydroxide (*otc*) — *Pepcid Complete* (J & J Merck)

### Indications

| Histamine H₂ Antagonists: Summary of Indications | | | | | |
|---|---|---|---|---|---|
| | Cimetidine | Famotidine | Nizatidine | Ranitidine | Combinations |
| Duodenal ulcer | | | | | |
|   Treatment | ✔ | ✔ | ✔ | ✔ | |
|   Maintenance | ✔ | ✔ | ✔ | ✔ | |
| Gastroesophageal reflux disease (GERD) (including erosive esophagitis) | ✔ | ✔ | ✔ | ✔ | |
| Gastric ulcer | | | | | |
|   Treatment | ✔ | ✔ | ✔ | ✔ | |
|   Maintenance | | | | ✔ | |
| Pathological hypersecretory conditions | ✔ | ✔ | | ✔ | |
| Heartburn/Acid indigestion/sour stomach | ✔[1,2] | ✔[1,3] | | | ✔ |
| Erosive esophagitis, maintenance | | | | ✔ | |
| Prevent upper GI bleeding | ✔ | | | | |

[1] OTC use only.
[2] Relief of symptoms only.
[3] Relief and prevention of symptoms.

**Administration and Dosage**

CIMETIDINE:

*Duodenal ulcer –*

*Short-term treatment of active duodenal ulcer:* 800 mg at bedtime. Alternate regimens are 300 mg 4 times/day with meals and at bedtime, or 400 mg twice/day.

*Maintenance therapy:* 400 mg at bedtime.

*Active benign gastric ulcer –* For short-term treatment, 800 mg at bedtime or 300 mg 4 times/day with meals and at bedtime.

*Erosive GERD –*

*Adults:* 1600 mg daily in divided doses (800 mg twice daily or 400 mg 4 times/day) for 12 weeks. Use longer than 12 weeks has not been established.

*Pathological hypersecretory conditions –* 300 mg 4 times/day with meals and at bedtime. If necessary, give 300 mg doses more often. Do not exceed 2400 mg/day.

*Prevention of upper GI bleeding –* Continuous IV infusion of 50 mg/h. Patients with Ccr less than 30 mL/min should receive half the recommended dose. Treatment longer than 7 days has not been studied.

*Severely impaired renal function –* Accumulation may occur. Use the lowest dose; 300 mg every 12 hours orally or IV has been recommended. Dosage frequency may be increased to every 8 hours or even further with caution.

*Parenteral –* The usual dose is 300 mg IM or IV every 6 to 8 hours. If it is necessary to increase dosage, do so by more frequent administration of a 300 mg dose, not to exceed 2400 mg/day.

*IM:* Administer undiluted.

*IV:* Dilute to a total volume of 20 mL; inject over at least 2 minutes.

*Intermittent IV infusion:* Dilute 300 mg in at least 50 mL of compatible IV solution; infuse over 15 to 20 minutes.

*Continuous IV infusion:* 37.5 mg/h (900 mg/day).

FAMOTIDINE:

*Duodenal ulcer –*

*Acute therapy:* 40 mg/day at bedtime. 20 mg twice/day is also effective.

*Maintenance therapy:* 20 mg once a day at bedtime.

*Benign gastric ulcer –*

*Acute therapy:* 40 mg orally once a day at bedtime.

*Pathological hypersecretory conditions –* The adult starting dose is 20 mg every 6 hours.

*GERD –* 20 mg twice daily for up to 6 weeks. For esophagitis including erosions and ulcerations and accompanying symptoms caused by GERD, 20 or 40 mg twice daily for up to 12 weeks.

*Severe renal insufficiency –*

*Ccr less than 10 mL/min:* To avoid excess accumulation of the drug, the dose may be reduced to 20 mg at bedtime or the dosing interval may be prolonged to 36 to 48 hours, as indicated.

*Parenteral –*

*IV:* Give famotidine IV 20 mg every 12 hours.

*Children –* Studies suggest the following starting doses in pediatric patients 1 to 16 years of age.

*Peptic ulcer:* 0.5 mg/kg/day orally at bedtime or divided twice daily up to 40 mg/day.

*GERD with or without esophagitis including erosions and ulcerations:* 1 mg/kg/day orally divided twice daily up to 40 mg twice daily.

*Heartburn, acid indigestion, and sour stomach (OTC only) –*

*Acute therapy:* 10 mg (1 tablet) with water.

*Prevention:* 10 mg 15 minutes before eating food or drinking a beverage that is expected to cause symptoms.

*Use:* Can be used up to twice daily (up to 2 tablets in 24 hours). Do not take maximum dose for more than 2 weeks continuously unless otherwise directed by a physician.

*Children:* Do not give to children under 12 years of age unless otherwise directed.

*Moderate (Ccr less than 50 mL/min) or severe renal insufficiency (Ccr less than 10 mL/min) –* To avoid excess accumulation of the drug, the dose may be reduced to half the dose or the dosing interval may be prolonged to 36 to 48 hours, as indicated.

NIZATIDINE:

*Active duodenal ulcer –* 300 mg once daily at bedtime. An alternative dosage regimen is 150 mg twice daily.

*Maintenance of healed duodenal ulcer –* 150 mg once daily at bedtime.

*GERD –* 150 mg twice daily.

*Benign gastric ulcer –* 300 mg given either as 150 mg twice daily or 300 mg once daily at bedtime.

*Heartburn, acid indigestion, and sour stomach (OTC only) –* Can be used up to twice daily (up to 2 tablets in 24 hours).

*Relief:* For relief of symptoms, take 1 tablet with a full glass of water.

*Prevention:* For prevention of symptoms, take 1 tablet with a full glass of water right before eating or up to 60 minutes before consuming food and beverages that cause heartburn.

*Moderate to severe renal insufficiency –*

| Nizatidine Dosage in Renal Insufficiency | | |
|---|---|---|
| | Dosage | |
| Ccr | Active duodenal ulcer | Maintenance therapy |
| 20 to 50 mL/min | 150 mg/day | 150 mg every other day |
| < 20 mL/min | 150 mg every other day | 150 mg every 3 days |

RANITIDINE:

*Duodenal ulcer –*

*Short-term treatment of active duodenal ulcer:* 150 mg orally twice daily. An alternate dosage of 300 mg once daily at bedtime can be used for patients in whom dosing convenience is important.

*Maintenance therapy:* 150 mg at bedtime.

*Pathological hypersecretory conditions –* 150 mg orally twice a day. More frequent doses may be necessary. Doses up to 6 g/day have been used.

*Benign gastric ulcer (oral doseforms only) and GERD –* 150 mg twice daily.

*Gastric ulcer –*

*Treatment:* 150 mg twice daily.

*Maintenance:* 150 mg at bedtime.

*Erosive esophagitis –*

*Treatment:* 150 mg 4 times daily.

*Maintenance:* 150 mg twice daily.

*Heartburn (OTC only) –*

*Treatment:* For relief of symptoms, swallow 1 tablet with a glass of water.

*Prevention:* To prevent symptoms, swallow 1 tablet with a glass of water 30 to 60 minutes before eating food or drinking beverages that cause heartburn.

*Maintenance:* Can be used up to twice daily (up to 2 tablets in 24 hours).

*Children –* The safety and effectiveness of ranitidine have been established in children from 1 month to 16 years of age. There is insufficient information about the pharmacokinetics of ranitidine in neonatal patients under 1 month of age to make dosing recommendations. Do not give OTC ranitidine to children under 12 years of age unless directed by physician.

*Active duodenal and gastric ulcers:*

*Treatment –* 2 to 4 mg/kg/day twice daily to a maximum of 300 mg/day.

*Maintenance –* 2 to 4 mg/kg once daily to a maximum of 150 mg/day.

*GERD and erosive esophagitis:* Although limited data exist for these conditions in pediatric patients, published literature supports a dosage of 5 to 10 mg/kg/day, usually given as 2 divided doses.

*EFFERdose (tablets and granules) –* Dissolve each dose in about 6 to 8 oz. of water before drinking.

*Renal impairment (Ccr less than 50 mL/min)* – 150 mg orally every 24 hours or 50 mg parenterally every 18 to 24 hours. The frequency of dosing may be increased to every 12 hours or further with caution.

*Parenteral* –

IM: 50 mg (2 mL) every 6 to 8 hours (no dilution necessary).

*IV injection:* 50 mg (2 mL) every 6 to 8 hours. Dilute 50 mg to a total volume of 20 mL; inject over at least 5 minutes.

*Intermittent IV infusion:* 50 mg (2 mL) every 6 to 8 hours. Dilute 50 mg and infuse over 15 to 20 minutes; do not exceed 400 mg/day.

*Continuous IV infusion:* Add ranitidine injection to 5% Dextrose Injection or other compatible IV solution. Deliver at a rate of 6.25 mg/h (eg, 150 mg [6 mL] ranitidine injection in 250 mL of 5% Dextrose Injection at 10.7 mL/h).

*Children* – The recommended dose in pediatric patients is for a total daily dose of 2 to 4 mg/kg, to be divided and administered every 6 to 8 hours up to a maximum of 50 mg given every 6 to 8 hours. Limited data in neonatal patients (under 1 month of age) receiving extracorporeal-membrane oxygenation (ECMO) have shown that a dose of 2 mg/kg is usually sufficient to increase gastric pH to greater than 4 for at least 15 hours. Therefore, consider doses of 2 mg/kg given every 12 to 24 hours or as a continuous infusion.

COMBINATIONS:

*12 years of age and older* – To relieve symptoms, chew 1 tablet before swallowing. Do not use more than 2 tablets in 24 hours. Do not swallow tablet whole; chew completely.

## Actions

*Pharmacology:* Histamine H₂ antagonists are reversible competitive blockers of histamine at the H₂ receptors. They also inhibit fasting and nocturnal secretions, and secretions stimulated by food, insulin, caffeine, pentagastrin, and betazole. **Cimetidine, ranitidine,** and **famotidine** have no effect on gastric emptying, and cimetidine and famotidine have no effect on lower esophageal sphincter pressure. Ranitidine, **nizatidine,** and famotidine have little or no effect on fasting or postprandial serum gastrin.

*Pharmacokinetics:*

| Pharmacokinetic Properties of Histamine H₂ Antagonists | | | | | |
|---|---|---|---|---|---|
| H₂ receptor antagonist | Bioavailability (%) | Time to peak plasma concentration (h) | Half-life (h) | Protein binding (%) | Metabolized (%) |
| Cimetidine | 60-70 | 0.75-1.5 | $\approx 2^2$ | 13-25 | 30-40 |
| Famotidine | 40-45 | 1-3 | $2.5\text{-}3.5^3$ | 15-20 | 30-35 |
| Nizatidine | > 90 | 0.5-3 | $1\text{-}2^3$ | $\approx 35$ | < 18 |
| Ranitidine | 50-60 (90-100 IM) | 1-3 (0.25 IM) | $2\text{-}3^3$ | 15 | < 10 |

[1] Dose-dependent.
[2] Increased in renal and hepatic impairment and in the elderly.
[3] Increased in renal impairment.

## Contraindications

Hypersensitivity to individual agents or to other H₂-receptor antagonists.

## Warnings

*Benzyl alcohol:* Benzyl alcohol, contained in some of these products as a preservative, has been associated with a fatal "gasping syndrome" in premature infants.

*Hypersensitivity reactions:* Rare cases of anaphylaxis have occurred as well as rare episodes of hypersensitivity (eg, bronchospasm, laryngeal edema, rash, eosinophilia).

*Renal function impairment:* Because these agents are excreted primarily via the kidneys, decreased clearance may occur; reduced dosage may be necessary.

*Hepatic function impairment:* Observe caution. Decreased clearance may occur; these agents are partly metabolized in the liver.

*Elderly:* Safety and efficacy appear similar to those of younger age; however, the elderly may have reduced renal function. Decreased **cimetidine** clearance may be more common.

*Pregnancy: Category B.*

*Lactation:*
   *Cimetidine* – Do not nurse.
      *Ranitidine/Nizatidine/Famotidine:* Exercise caution when administering to a nursing mother.

*Children:* Safety and efficacy are not established. **Cimetidine** is not recommended for children under 16 years of age, unless anticipated benefits outweigh potential risks. In very limited experience, cimetidine 20 to 40 mg/kg/day has been used. OTC use is not recommended in children under 12 years of age.

### Precautions

*Gastric malignancy:* Symptomatic response to these agents does not preclude gastric malignancy.

*Reversible CNS effects:* Reversible CNS effects (eg, mental confusion, agitation, psychosis, depression, anxiety, hallucinations, disorientation) have occurred with **cimetidine**, predominantly in severely ill patients. Advancing age (at least 50 years) and pre-existing liver or renal disease appear to be contributing factors.

*Hepatocellular injury:* Hepatocellular injury may occur with **nizatidine** as evidenced by elevated liver enzymes (AST, ALT, or alkaline phosphatase).
   Occasionally, reversible hepatitis, hepatocellular, or hepatocanalicular or mixed, with or without jaundice have occurred with oral **ranitidine.**
   *Monitoring* – Laboratory test monitoring for liver abnormalities is appropriate.

*Rapid IV administration:* Rapid IV administration of **cimetidine** has been followed by rare instances of cardiac arrhythmias and hypotension. Bradycardia, tachycardia, and premature ventricular beats in association with rapid administration of IV **ranitidine** may occur rarely, usually in patients predisposed to cardiac rhythm disturbances.

*Antiandrogenic effect:* **Cimetidine** has a weak antiandrogenic effect in animals. Gynecomastia in patients treated for at least 1 month may occur.

*Immunocompromised patients:* Decreased gastric acidity, including that produced by acid-suppressing agents such as H₂ antagonists, may increase the possibility of strongyloidiasis.

### Drug Interactions

**Cimetidine** reduces the hepatic metabolism of drugs metabolized via the cytochrome P450 pathway, delaying elimination and increasing serum levels.

| Cimetidine Drug Interactions (Decreased Hepatic Metabolism) ||
| --- | --- |
| Benzodiazepines[1] | Propafenone |
| Caffeine | Propranolol |
| Calcium channel blockers | Quinidine |
| Carbamazepine | Quinine |
| Chloroquine | Sulfonylureas |
| Labetalol | Tacrine |
| Lidocaine | Theophyllines[2] |
| Metoprolol | Triamterene |
| Metronidazole | Tricyclic antidepressants |
| Moricizine | Valproic acid |
| Pentoxifylline | Warfarin |
| Phenytoin | |

[1] Does not include agents metabolized by glucuronidation (lorazepam, oxazepam, temazepam).
[2] Does not include dyphylline.

**Ranitidine, famotidine,** and **nizatidine** do not inhibit the cytochrome P450-linked oxygenase enzyme system in the liver.

Drugs that may affect histamine H$_2$ antagonists include antacids, anticholinergics, metoclopramide, and cigarette smoking. Drugs that may be affected by histamine H$_2$ antagonists include ferrous salts, indomethacin, ketoconazole, tetracyclines, carmustine, digoxin, flecainide, fluconazole, fluorouracil, narcotic analgesics, procainamide, succinylcholine, tocainide, salicylates, diazepam, sulfonylureas, theophyllines, warfarin, and ethanol.

*Drug/Lab test interactions:* False-positive tests for urobilinogen may occur during **nizatidine** therapy. False-positive tests for urine protein with *Multistix* may occur during **ranitidine** therapy; testing with sulfosalicylic acid is recommended.

*Drug/Food interactions:* Food may increase bioavailability of **famotidine** and **nizatidine**; this is of no clinical consequence. **Cimetidine** and **ranitidine** are not affected.

**Adverse Reactions** Adverse reactions may include headache, somnolence/fatigue, dizziness, confusional states, hallucinations, insomnia, nausea, vomiting, abdominal discomfort, diarrhea, constipation, thrombocytopenia, alopecia, rash, gynecomastia, impotence, loss of libido, and arthralgia.

# MISOPROSTOL

**Tablets:** 100 and 200 mcg *(Rx)*                    Various, *Cytotec* (Pfizer)

---

**Warning:**

Misoprostol administration in pregnant women can cause abortion, premature birth, or birth defects. Uterine rupture has been reported when misoprostol was administered in pregnant women to induce labor or to induce abortion beyond the eighth week of pregnancy. Misoprostol should not be taken by pregnant women to reduce the risk of ulcers induced by nonsteroidal anti-inflammatory drugs (NSAIDs).

Advise patients of the abortifacient property and warn them not to give the drug to others.

Misoprostol should not be used for reducing the risk of NSAID-induced ulcers in women of childbearing potential unless the patient is at high risk of developing complications from gastric ulcers associated with NSAIDs or of developing gastric ulceration. In such patients, misoprostol may be prescribed if the patient:
- Has had a negative serum pregnancy test within 2 weeks prior to beginning therapy;
- is capable of complying with effective contraceptive measures;
- has received both oral and written warnings of the hazards of misoprostol, the risk of possible contraception failure, and the danger to other women of childbearing potential should the drug be taken by mistake; and
- will begin misoprostol only on the second or third day of the next normal menstrual period.

---

### Indications

*Gastric ulcers:* To reduce the risk of NSAID- (including aspirin) induced gastric ulcers in patients at high risk of complications from a gastric ulcer (eg, the elderly, patients with concomitant debilitating disease), as well as patients at high risk of developing gastric ulceration, such as patients with a history of ulcer. Take misoprostol for the duration of NSAID therapy.

*Unlabeled uses:*

*Pregnancy termination* – Misoprostol has been used in combination with mifepristone for pregnancy termination. Patients taking mifepristone must take 400 mcg misoprostol orally 2 days after taking mifepristone unless a complete abortion has already been confirmed before that time.

*Chronic, idiopathic constipation* – Short-term trials have shown an acceleration of intestinal transit in healthy individuals and in those with chronic constipation. Improvement in stool frequency in patients with chronic constipation has been seen with treatment doses of 200 mcg 2 to 4 times/day.

### Administration and Dosage

*Adults:* 200 mcg 4 times daily with food. If this dose cannot be tolerated, 100 mcg may be used. Take misoprostol for the duration of NSAID therapy as prescribed. Take with meals, with the last dose of the day taken at bedtime.

### Actions

*Pharmacology:* Misoprostol, a synthetic prostaglandin $E_1$ analog, inhibits gastric acid secretion. NSAIDs inhibit prostaglandin synthesis; a deficiency of prostaglandins within the gastric mucosa may lead to diminishing bicarbonate and mucous secretion and may contribute to the mucosal damage caused by these agents. Misoprostol can increase bicarbonate and mucus production.

*Pharmacokinetics:* Misoprostol is extensively absorbed, with a time-to-reach peak concentration of misoprostol acid of 12 minutes and a terminal half-life of 20 to 40 minutes. Plasma steady-state was achieved within 2 days. The serum protein binding of misoprostol acid is less than 90%.

**Contraindications**
History of allergy to prostaglandins; pregnancy.

**Warnings**
*Cardiovascular:* Use caution when administering misoprostol to patients with pre-existing cardiovascular disease.

*Duodenal ulcers:* Misoprostol does not prevent duodenal ulcers in patients on NSAIDs.

*Renal function impairment:* No routine dosage adjustment is recommended, but dosage may need to be reduced if usual dose is not tolerated.

*Fertility impairment:* Results of animal studies suggest the possibility of a general adverse effect on fertility in males and females.

*Elderly:* No routine dosage adjustment is recommended. Reduce the dose if the usual dose is not tolerated.

*Pregnancy:* Category X.
    *Labor and delivery* – Misoprostol can induce or augment uterine contractions. A major adverse effect of the obstetrical use of misoprostol is hyperstimulation of the uterus, which may progress to uterine tetany with marked impairment of uteroplacental blood flow, uterine rupture (requiring surgical repair, hysterectomy, and/or salpingo-oophorectomy), or amniotic fluid embolism. Pelvic pain, retained placenta, severe genital bleeding, shock, fetal bradycardia, and fetal and maternal death have been reported.

*Lactation:* It is not known if misoprostol acid is excreted in breast milk. Do not administer to nursing mothers because the potential excretion of misoprostol acid could cause significant diarrhea in nursing infants.

*Children:* Safety and efficacy in children less than 18 years of age have not been established.

**Precautions**
*Women of childbearing potential:* Advise women of childbearing potential that they must not be pregnant when misoprostol therapy is initiated and that they must use an effective contraception method while taking misoprostol.

*Diarrhea:* Diarrhea (13% to 40%) is dose-related, usually develops early in the course of therapy (after 13 days), and usually is self-limiting (often resolving after 8 days), but requires discontinuation of misoprostol in some of patients. The incidence of diarrhea can be minimized by administering after meals and at bedtime and by avoiding coadministration of misoprostol with magnesium-containing antacids.

**Drug Interactions**
*Antacids:* Antacids reduce the total availability of misoprostol acid, but this does not appear clinically important.

*Drug/Food interactions:* Maximum plasma concentrations of misoprostol acid are diminished when taken with food.

**Adverse Reactions**
Adverse reactions associated with misoprostol may include abdominal pain (7% to 20%), diarrhea (13% to 40%), and nausea (3%).

# PROTON PUMP INHIBITORS

**ESOMEPRAZOLE**
**Capsules, delayed-release**: 20 and 40 mg (*Rx*)          *Nexium* (AstraZeneca)
**LANSOPRAZOLE**
**Capsules, delayed-release**: 15 and 30 mg (*Rx*)          *Prevacid* (TAP Pharm)
**Tablets, orally disintegrating, delayed-release**: 15 mg    *Prevacid* (TAP Pharm)
(*Rx*)
**Granules for oral suspension, delayed-release**: 15 mg     *Prevacid* (TAP Pharm)
(*Rx*)
**Powder for injection, lyophilized**: 30 mg/vial (*Rx*)     *Prevacid IV* (TAP Pharm)
**OMEPRAZOLE**
**Capsules, delayed-release**: 10, 20, and 40 mg (*Rx*)      *Prilosec* (AstraZeneca)
**Tablets, delayed-release**: 20 mg (*Rx*)                   *Prilosec OTC* (Proctor and Gamble)
**Powder for oral suspension**: 20 mg (*Rx*)                 *Zegerid* (Santarus)
**PANTOPRAZOLE**
**Tablets, delayed-release**: 20 and 40 mg (*Rx*)            *Protonix* (Wyeth-Ayerst)
**Powder for injection, freeze-dried**: 40 mg/vial (*Rx*)    *Protonix I.V.* (Wyeth-Ayerst)
**RABEPRAZOLE**
**Tablets, delayed-release**: 20 mg (*Rx*)                   *Aciphex* (Eisai/Janssen)

## Indications

| Proton Pump Inhibitors - Summary of Indications[a] | | | | | |
|---|---|---|---|---|---|
| Indication<br>✔ = Labeled | Esomeprazole | Lansoprazole | Omeprazole | Pantoprazole | Rabeprazole |
| Duodenal ulcer | | ✔[b] | ✔ | | ✔ |
| Duodenal ulcer associated with *Helicobacter pylori* (in combination with antibiotics) | ✔ | ✔[b] | ✔[c] | | ✔ |
| Gastric ulcer | | ✔[b] | ✔[c] | | |
| Erosive esophagitis | ✔ | ✔ | ✔ | ✔ | ✔ |
| GERD[d] in adults | ✔ | ✔[b] | ✔ | ✔ | ✔ |
| GERD in children | | | | | |
| *H. pylori* gastritis in children[e] | | | | | |
| Hypersecretory conditions (eg, Zollinger-Ellison syndrome) | | ✔[b] | ✔[c] | ✔ | ✔ |

[a] For more detailed information, see the information below and the individual drug monographs.
[b] Oral only.
[c] Except omeprazole oral suspension.
[d] Gastroesophageal reflux disease.
[e] In combination with amoxicillin and clarithromycin.

*Duodenal ulcer associated with H. pylori infection:* For treatment of patients with *H. pylori* infection and duodenal ulcer to eradicate *H. pylori*.

*Dual therapy* – In combination with clarithromycin (**omeprazole**) or amoxicillin (**lansoprazole**).

*Triple therapy (esomeprazole, lansoprazole, omeprazole, rabeprazole)* – In combination with clarithromycin and amoxicillin.

*NSAID-associated gastric ulcers:* **Lansoprazole** also is indicated for the healing and reducing the risk of nonsteroidal anti-inflammatory agent (NSAID)-associated gastric ulcers in patients who continue NSAID use.

### Administration and Dosage

ESOMEPRAZOLE: Swallow capsules whole. Take at least 1 hour before eating.

*Difficulty swallowing* – For patients who have difficulty swallowing capsules, 1 tablespoon of applesauce can be added to an empty bowl and the esomeprazole capsule opened and the pellets inside carefully emptied onto the applesauce. The pellets should be mixed with the applesauce and swallowed immediately. The applesauce should not be hot and should be soft enough to swallow without chewing. Do not chew or crush the pellets. Do not store the pellet/applesauce mixture for future use.

In vitro, the pellets have been shown to remain intact when exposed to tap water, orange juice, apple juice, and yogurt.

*Erosive esophagitis* –
> *Treatment:* 20 or 40 mg once/day for 4 to 8 weeks.
> *Maintenance:* 20 mg once/day.

*Symptomatic GERD* – 20 mg once/day for 4 weeks.

*Duodenal ulcer associated with Helicobacter pylori* –
> *Esomeprazole:* 40 mg once/day for 10 days.
> *Amoxicillin:* 1000 mg twice/day for 10 days.
> *Clarithromycin:* 500 mg twice/day for 10 days.

*Administration per nasogastric (NG) tube* – For patients who have a NG tube in place, open the esomeprazole capsules and empty the intact granules into a 60 mL syringe. Mix with 50 mL of water. Replace the plunger and shake the syringe vigorously for 15 seconds. Hold the syringe with the tip up and check for granules remaining in the tip. Attach the syringe to a NG tube, and deliver the contents of the syringe through the NG tube into the stomach. After administering the granules, flush the NG tube with additional water. Do no administer the pellets if they have dissolved or disintegrated.

The suspension must be used immediately after preparation.

*Hepatic function impairment* – For patients with severe liver impairment (Child Pugh class C), do not exceed a dose of 20 mg.

LANSOPRAZOLE: Take oral formulations before meals. Do not crush or chew lansoprazole oral products.

*Duodenal ulcer* –
> *Short-term treatment:* 15 mg once/day for 4 weeks.
> *Maintenance:* 15 mg once/day to maintain healing of duodenal ulcers.
> *Associated with H. pylori:*
>> *Dual therapy* – 30 mg lansoprazole plus 1 g amoxicillin both taken 3 times/day for 14 days for patients intolerant or resistant to clarithromycin.
>> *Triple therapy* – 30 mg lansoprazole plus 500 mg clarithromycin and 1 g amoxicillin all taken twice/day for 10 to 14 days.

*Gastric ulcer* –
> *Short-term treatment:* 30 mg once/day for up to 8 weeks.
> *Associated with nonsteroidal anti-inflammatory drugs (NSAIDs):*
>> *Healing* – 30 mg once/day for 8 weeks.
>> *Risk reduction* – 15 mg once/day for up to 12 weeks.

*GERD* –
> *Adults and children 12 to 17 years of age:* 15 mg once/day for up to 8 weeks.
> *Children 1 to 11 years of age (short-term treatment):*
>> *30 kg or less* – 15 mg/day for up to 12 weeks.
>> *Over 30 kg* – 30 mg/day for up to 12 weeks.

*Erosive esophagitis* –
> *Adults and children 12 to 17 years of age:*
>> *Short-term treatment* – 30 mg/day for up to 8 weeks. For patients who do not heal within 8 weeks (5% to 10%), give an additional 8 weeks of treatment. If there is a recurrence of erosive esophagitis, consider an additional 8-week course.
>> *Maintenance (adults)* – 15 mg once/day to maintain healing of erosive esophagitis.
>> *IV formulation* – Administer 30 mg/day by IV infusion over 30 minutes for up to 7 days. Once the patient is able to take medications orally, therapy can be switched to an oral lansoprazole formulation for a total of 6 to 8 weeks.
> *Children 1 to 11 years of age (short-term treatment):*
>> *30 kg or less* – 15 mg/day for up to 12 weeks.
>> *Over 30 kg* – 30 mg/day for up to 12 weeks.

*Hypersecretory conditions including Zollinger-Ellison syndrome* – The recommended starting dose is 60 mg/day. Dosages up to 90 mg twice/day have been administered. Administer daily dosages of greater than 120 mg in divided doses.

*Hepatic function impairment* – Consider dosage adjustment in patients with severe liver disease.

*Difficulty swallowing* – Lansoprazole capsules can be opened and the intact granules contained within can be sprinkled on 1 tablespoon of applesauce, *Ensure* pudding, cottage cheese, yogurt, or strained pears and swallowed immediately. The delayed-release capsules may be emptied into a small volume of either orange juice or tomato juice (60 mL; approximately 2 oz), mixed briefly, and swallowed immediately. To ensure complete delivery of the dose, rinse the glass with 2 or more volumes of juice (apple, cranberry, grape, orange, pineapple, prune, tomato, or V-8 vegetable juice). Do not chew or crush the granules.

*Oral suspension:* Empty packet contents into 2 tablespoons of water. Do not use other liquids or foods. Stir well and drink immediately. If any material remains after drinking, add more water, stir, and drink immediately. Do not give through enteral administration tubes.

*Orally disintegrating tablets:* Place the tablet on the tongue. Allow it to disintegrate with or without water until the particles can be swallowed. The tablet typically disintegrates in less than 1 minute. *SoluTabs* are not designed to be swallowed intact or chewed.

For administration via oral syringe, place a 15 mg tablet in an oral syringe and draw up approximately 4 mL of water, or place a 30 mg tablet in oral syringe and draw up approximately 10 mL of water. Shake gently to allow for a quick dispersal. After the tablet has dispersed, administer the contents within 15 minutes. Refill the syringe with approximately 2 mL (5 mL for the 30 mg tablet) of water, shake gently, and administer any remaining contents.

*IV formulation:* Dilute with 5 mL sterile water for injection. Administer using the in-line filter provided. The filter must be used to remove precipitate that may form when the reconstituted drug product is mixed with IV solutions.

- Inject 5 mL of sterile water for injection into a 30 mg vial of lansoprazole. The resulting solution will contain 6 mg/mL lansoprazole.
- Mix gently until the powder is dissolved.
- Dilute the reconstituted solution in either 50 mL of 0.9% sodium chloride injection, lactated Ringer's injection, or 5% dextrose in water.

*Administration* – An in-line filter must be used. Administer over 30 minutes. A dedicated line is not required; however, flush the IV line before and after administration with 0.9% sodium chloride injection, lactated Ringer's injection, or 5% dextrose injection. Do not administer with other drugs or diluents, as this may cause incompatibilities.

*Nasogastric (NG) tube* –

*Tablets:* Lansoprazole can be opened and the intact granules mixed in 40 mL of apple juice and injected through the NG tube into the stomach. After administering the granules, flush the NG tube with additional apple juice to clear the tube.

*Orally disintegrating tablets:* For administration via NG tube, place a 15 mg tablet in a syringe and draw up 4 mL water, or place a 30 mg tablet in a syringe and draw up 10 mL water. Shake gently to allow for a quick dispersal. After the tablet has dispersed, inject through the NG tube into the stomach within 15 minute. Refill the syringe with approximately 5 mL of water, shake gently, and flush the NG tube.

**OMEPRAZOLE:** Take before eating. Do not open, crush, or chew the capsule; swallow whole. In clinical trials, antacids were used concomitantly with omeprazole.

*Duodenal ulcer* –

*Treatment:* 20 mg/day for 4 to 8 weeks; most patients heal within 4 weeks, although some may require an additional 4 weeks.

*Associated with H. pylori:*

*Triple therapy (omeprazole/clarithromycin/amoxicillin)* – Omeprazole 20 mg plus clarithromycin 500 mg plus amoxicillin 1000 mg each given twice/day for 10 days. If an ulcer is present at the initiation of therapy, continue omeprazole 20 mg for an additional 18 days.

*Dual therapy (omeprazole/clarithromycin)* – Omeprazole 40 mg once/day plus clarithromycin 500 mg 3 times/day for 14 days. If an ulcer is present at the initiation of therapy, continue omeprazole 20 mg for an additional 14 days.

*Gastric ulcer, treatment* – 40 mg once/day for 4 to 8 weeks.

*Erosive esophagitis* –

*Treatment:* 20 mg/day for 4 to 8 weeks.

*Maintenance:* 20 mg/day.

*GERD* –

*GERD without esophageal lesions:* 20 mg/day for 4 weeks.

*GERD with erosive esophagitis:* 20 mg/day for 4 to 8 weeks.

*Pathological hypersecretory conditions* – Initial adult dose is 60 mg/day. Doses up to 120 mg 3 times/day have been administered. Administer daily dosages greater than 80 mg in divided doses.

*Heartburn (OTC)* – Swallow 1 tablet with a glass of water before eating in the morning. Take every day for 14 days. The 14-day course may be repeated every 4 months.

*Pathological hypersecretory conditions* – Individualize dosage. Initial adult dose is 60 mg/ day. Continue for as long as clinically indicated. Doses up to 120 mg 3 times/day have been administered. Administer daily doses greater than 80 mg in divided doses. Some patients with Zollinger-Ellison syndrome have been treated continuously for more than 5 years.

*Children* – For the treatment of GERD or other acid-related disorders, the recommended dose for pediatric patients 2 years of age and older is as follows: 10 mg omeprazole for patients weighing less than 20 kg, and 20 mg omeprazole for patients weighing 20 kg or more. On a per kg basis, the doses of omeprazole required to heal erosive esophagitis are greater than those for adults.

*Difficulty swallowing* – For patients who have difficulty swallowing capsules, add 1 tablespoon of applesauce to an empty bowl, open the omeprazole capsule, and empty the pellets onto the applesauce. Mix the pellets with the applesauce and swallow immediately. Do not heat or chew the applesauce. Do not chew or crush the pellets. Do not store the pellet/applesauce mixture for future use.

*Preparation and administration of oral suspension* – Take on an empty stomach 1 hour before a meal. The powder for oral suspension is supplied as unit-dose packets containing an immediate-release formulation of 20 mg omeprazole.

*Directions for use:* Empty packet contents into a small cup containing 2 tablespoons of water. Do not use other liquids or foods. Stir well and drink immediately. Refill cup with water and drink.

*Hepatic function impairment/race* – Consider dose adjustment, particularly where maintenance of healing of erosive esophagitis is indicated, for hepatically impaired and Asian patients.

No dosage adjustment is necessary for patients with renal impairment, hepatic dysfunction, or for the elderly.

PANTOPRAZOLE: Swallow tablets whole, with or without food. Do not chew, crush, or split.

*Oral* –

*Erosive esophagitis associated with GERD:*

*Treatment* – 40 mg once/day for up to 8 weeks. For those patients who have not healed after 8 weeks, consider an additional 8-week course.

*Maintenance* – 40 mg once/day.

*IV* – Discontinue treatment with IV pantoprazole as soon as the patient is able to resume treatment with pantoprazole delayed-release tablets.

Parenteral routes of administration other than IV are not recommended.

*Pathological hypersecretory conditions including Zollinger-Ellison syndrome* – Individualize dosage. The recommended adult starting dose is 40 mg twice daily. Adjust dosage regimens to individual patient needs and continue for as long as clinically indicated. Doses up to 240 mg/day have been administered. Some patients have been treated continuously for more than 2 years.

*Treatment of GERD associated with a history of erosive esophagitis* – As an alternative to continued oral therapy, administer 40 mg pantoprazole once daily by infusion for 7 to 10 days. Safety and efficacy of IV pantoprazole as a treatment for GERD in patients with a history of erosive esophagitis for more than 10 days have not been demonstrated.

*Reconstitution:*

*15-minute infusion* – Reconstitute IV pantoprazole with 10 mL of 0.9% sodium chloride injection, and further dilute (admix) with 100 mL of 5% dextrose injection, 0.9% sodium chloride injection, or lactated Ringer's injection to a final concentration of approximately 0.4 mg/mL.

*2-minute infusion* – Reconstitute IV pantoprazole with 10 mL of 0.9% sodium chloride injection to a final concentration of approximately 4 mg/mL.

*Administration:*

*15-minute infusion* – Administer IV pantoprazole admixtures over a period of approximately 15 minutes at a rate of approximately 7 mL/min.

*2-minute infusion* – Administer the total volume from vial over at least 2 minutes.

*Pathological hypersecretion associated with Zollinger-Ellison syndrome* – Individualize dosage. The recommended adult dosage is 80 mg every 12 hours. The frequency of dosing can be adjusted to individual patient needs based on acid output measurements. In those patients who need a higher dosage, 80 mg every 8 hours is expected to maintain acid output below 10 mEq/h. Daily doses higher than 240 mg or administered for more than 6 days have not been studied. Perform transition from oral to IV and from IV to oral formulations of gastric acid inhibitors in such a manner to ensure continuity of effect of suppression of acid secretion. Patients with Zollinger-Ellison syndrome may be vulnerable to serious clinical complications of increased acid production even after a short period of loss of effective inhibition.

*Reconstitution:*

*15-minute infusion* – Reconstitute each vial with 10 mL of 0.9% sodium chloride injection. Combine the contents of the 2 vials and further dilute (admix) with 80 mL of 5% dextrose injection, 0.9% sodium chloride injection, or lactated Ringer's injection to a total volume of 100 mL with a final concentration of approximately 0.8 mg/mL.

*2-minute infusion* – Reconstitute with 10 mL of 0.9% sodium chloride injection per vial to a final concentration of approximately 4 mg/mL.

*Administration:*

*15-minute infusion* – Administer IV over a period of approximately 15 minutes at a rate of approximately 7 mL/min.

*2-minute infusion* – The total volume from both vials should be administered IV over a period of at least 2 minutes.

*Incompatibilities* – Midazolam has been shown to be incompatible with Y-site administration of pantoprazole injection and pantoprazole may not be compatible with products containing zinc. Immediately stop use if precipitation or discoloration occurs.

RABEPRAZOLE: Swallow tablets whole, with or without food. Do not chew, crush, or split.

*Duodenal ulcer* – 20 mg once/day after the morning meal for a period of up to 4 weeks. Most patients with duodenal ulcers heal within 4 weeks.

*Erosive or ulcerative GERD* –

*Treatment:* 20 mg once/day for 4 to 8 weeks. For those patients not healed after 8 weeks of treatment, consider an additional 8-week course.

*Maintenance:* 20 mg once/day.

*GERD* – 20 mg once/day for 4 weeks. If symptoms do not resolve completely after 4 weeks, an additional course of treatment may be considered.

*Hypersecretory conditions, including Zollinger-Ellison syndrome* – Start dosing at 60 mg once/day. Dosing may be divided. Doses up to 100 mg/day and 60 mg twice/day have been administered.

*H. pylori eradication to reduce risk of duodenal ulcer recurrence* – Rabeprazole 20 mg, amoxicillin 1,000 mg, and clarithromycin 500 mg twice daily for 7 days with the morning and evening meals.

*Hepatic impairment* – Use caution in patients with mild to moderate hepatic impairment.

## Actions

*Pharmacology:* These agents have been characterized as gastric acid pump inhibitors; they block the final step of acid production. Proton pump inhibitors do not exhibit anticholinergic or $H_2$ histamine antagonistic properties.

*Pharmacokinetics:*

*Absorption/Distribution* – Most of these oral agents contain enteric-coated granules. Absorption of these agents is rapid and begins only after the granules leave the stomach.

*Metabolism/Excretion* – These agents are extensively metabolized by the liver. The plasma elimination half-life is less than 2 hours while the acid inhibitory effect lasts more than 24 hours. When the drug is discontinued, secretory activity returns over 1 to 5 days.

| Proton Pump Inhibitors Pharmacokinetics | | | | | |
|---|---|---|---|---|---|
| Parameter | Esomeprazole | Lansoprazole | Omeprazole[a] | Pantoprazole | Rabeprazole |
| Bioavailability (%) | ≈ 64 (single dose) ≈ 90 (multiple dose) | > 80 | 30 to 40 | ≈ 77 (oral) | ≈ 52 |
| $T_{max}$ (h) | ≈ 1.5 | 1.7 | 0.5 to 3.5 | ≈ 2.5 (oral) | 2 to 5 |
| Protein binding (%) | 97 | 97 | ≈ 95 | ≈ 98 | 96.3 |
| Half-life (h) | ≈ 1 to 1.5 | ≈ 1.5 (oral) ≈ 1.3 (IV) | 0.5 to 1 | ≈ 1 | 1 to 2 |
| Onset (h) | | 1 to 3 | ≤ 1 | | ≤ 1 |
| Duration (h) | | > 24 | 72 | > 24 | |

[a] Capsules.

## Contraindications

Hypersensitivity to any component of the formulation; substituted benzimidazoles (**rabeprazole, esomeprazole**).

## Warnings

*Gastritis:* Atrophic gastritis has been noted occasionally in gastric corpus biopsies from patients treated long-term with **omeprazole** and **esomeprazole**.

Patients with healed GERD were treated for up to 40 months with **rabeprazole** and monitored with serial gastric biopsies. Approximately 4% of patients had intestinal metaplasia at some point during follow-up, but no consistent changes were seen.

*Hepatic effects:* In patients with various degrees/types of hepatic disease, the AUC was prolonged (lansoprazole, esomeprazole, rabeprazole, pantoprazole), half-life was prolonged (lansoprazole, omeprazole, rabeprazole, pantoprazole), increased bioavailability was observed (omeprazole), decreased clearance with rabeprazole and increased maximum pantoprazole concentrations.

*Hypersensitivity reactions:* Anaphylaxis has been reported with the use of IV **pantopra-zole**. This may require emergency medical treatment.

*Elderly:* The elimination rate of **omeprazole** was somewhat decreased in the elderly and the bioavailability increased (see Pharmacokinetics).

The clearance of **lansoprazole** is decreased in the elderly, with an approxi-mately 50% to 100% increase of elimination half-life (see Pharmacokinetics).

AUC values and $C_{max}$ of **esomeprazole, rabeprazole,** and oral **pantoprazole** were increased in elderly subjects compared with healthy controls (see Pharmacokinet-ics), but no dosage adjustment is recommended.

*Pregnancy: Category C* (**omeprazole**); *Category B* (**lansoprazole, rabeprazole, pantopra-zole, esomeprazole**).

*Lactation:* Omeprazole has been measured in the breast milk. Because of the potential for serious adverse reactions in breast-feeding infants, decide whether to discon-tinue breast-feeding or to discontinue the drug, taking into account the importance of the drug to the mother.

*Children:* The safety and efficacy of **esomeprazole, pantoprazole,** and **rabeprazole** in children have not been established. The safety and efficacy of **lansoprazole** in patients younger than 1 year of age have not been established. The safety and effi-cacy of **omeprazole** have not been established for pediatric patients younger than 2 years of age.

## Precautions

*Gastric malignancy:* Symptomatic response to therapy with proton pump inhibitors does not preclude gastric malignancy.

*Vitamin $B_{12}$ deficiency:* Generally, daily treatment with any acid-suppressing medications over a long period of time may lead to malabsorption of cyanocobalamin (vitamin $B_{12}$).

## Drug Interactions

Drugs that may be affected by proton pump inhibitors include azole antifungal agents (eg, itraconazole, ketoconazole), benzodiazepines, cilostazol, clarithromycin, digoxin, phenytoin, salicylates, sulfonylureas, and warfarin. Drugs that may affect proton pump inhibitors include sucralfate and clarithromycin.

Proton pump inhibitors cause a profound and long-lasting inhibition of gastric acid secretion; therefore, proton pump inhibitors may interfere with the absorption of drugs where gastric pH is an important determinant of bioavailability (eg, ketocona-zole, ampicillin, iron salts, digoxin, cyanocobalamin).

*P450 system:* Drugs that may be affected by proton pump inhibitors include benzodiaz-epines, clarithromycin, cyclosporine, disulfiram, digoxin, azole antifungal agents, hydantoins, cilostazol, salicylates, sulfonylureas, and warfarin.

Drugs that affect proton pump inhibitors include clarithromycin and sucralfate.

## Adverse Reactions

The most common adverse effects (greater than 3%) of proton pump inhibitors include headache and diarrhea.

## Patient Information

Take **omeprazole, esomeprazole,** and **lansoprazole** before meals. Take **rabeprazole** and **pantoprazole** without regard to meals.

Do not open, crush or chew omeprazole or esomeprazole capsules; do not chew or crush omeprazole tablets or lansoprazole products; do not chew, crush or split rabeprazole or pantoprazole tablets.

Antacids may be used while taking proton pump inhibitors.

# ORLISTAT

| **Capsules:** 120 mg | *Xenical* (Roche) |
|---|---|

### Indications

*Obesity management:* For management of obesity including weight loss and weight main-tenance when used in conjunction with a reduced-calorie diet. Orlistat also is indi-cated to reduce the risk for weight regain after prior weight loss. Orlistat is indicated for obese patients with an initial body mass index (BMI) greater than or equal to 30 kg/m$^2$, or greater than or equal to 27 kg/m$^2$ in the presence of other risk factors (eg, hypertension, diabetes, dyslipidemia).

### Administration and Dosage

The recommended dose of orlistat is one 120 mg capsule 3 times a day with each main meal containing fat (during or up to 1 hour after the meal).

Place the patient on a nutritionally balanced, reduced-calorie diet that contains approximately 30% of calories from fat. Distribute the daily intake of fat, carbo-hydrate, and protein over 3 main meals. If a meal is occasionally missed or con-tains no fat, the dose of orlistat can be omitted.

Because orlistat reduces the absorption of some fat-soluble vitamins and beta-caro-tene, counsel patients to take a multivitamin containing fat-soluble vitamins to ensure adequate nutrition. Instruct the patient to take the supplement once a day, at least 2 hours before or after the administration of orlistat, such as at bedtime.

Doses greater than 120 mg 3 times a day have not been shown to provide additional benefit.

Based on fecal fat measurements, the effect of orlistat is seen as soon as 24 to 48 hours after dosing. Upon discontinuation of therapy, fecal fat content usually returns to pretreatment levels within 48 to 72 hours.

Safety and effectiveness beyond 2 years have not been determined at this time.

### Actions

*Pharmacology:* Orlistat is a reversible lipase inhibitor for obesity management that acts by inhibiting the absorption of dietary fats. It exerts its therapeutic activity in the lumen of the stomach and small intestine.

*Pharmacokinetics:*

Absorption – Systemic exposure to orlistat is minimal. Peak plasma concentrations occurred at approximately 8 hours following oral dosing with 360 mg orlistat; plasma concentrations of intact orlistat were near the limits of detection (less than 5 ng/mL).

Distribution – In vitro orlistat was greater than 99% bound to plasma proteins (lipo-proteins and albumin were major binding proteins). Orlistat minimally partitioned into erythrocytes.

Metabolism – It is likely that the metabolism of orlistat occurs mainly within the GI wall. In obese patients, 2 metabolites, M1 (4-member lactone ring hydrolyzed) and M3 (M1 with N-formyl leucine moiety cleaved), accounted for approximately 42% in plasma.

Excretion – Fecal excretion was the major route of elimination following a single oral dose of 360 mg orlistat in healthy and obese subjects. Orlistat and its M1 and M3 metabolites also underwent biliary excretion. Approximately 97% was excreted in feces; 83% of that was found to be unchanged orlistat. The cumulative renal excretion was less than 2%. Based on limited data, the half-life of the absorbed drug is in the range of 1 to 2 hours.

### Contraindications

Chronic malabsorption syndrome or cholestasis; hypersensitivity to orlistat or to any component of this product.

### Warnings

*Causes of obesity:* Exclude organic causes of obesity (eg, hypothyroidism) before prescrib-ing orlistat.

*Pregnancy:* Category B.

*Lactation:* It is not known if orlistat is secreted in breast milk.

*Children:* Safety and efficacy in pediatric patients have not been established.

## Precautions

*Diet:* Advise patients to adhere to dietary guidelines. GI events may increase when orlistat is taken with a diet high in fat (greater than 30% total daily calories from fat). The daily intake of fat should be distributed over 3 main meals. If orlistat is taken with any 1 meal that is very high in fat, the possibility of GI effects increases.

*Vitamin supplement:* Counsel patients to take a multivitamin supplement that contains fat-soluble vitamins to ensure adequate nutrition because orlistat reduces the absorption of some fat-soluble vitamins and beta-carotene. Instruct patients to take the supplement once a day at least 2 hours before or after the administration of orlistat, such as at bedtime.

*Urinary oxalate:* Some patients may develop increased levels of urinary oxalate following treatment. Exercise caution in patients with a history of hyperoxaluria or calcium oxalate nephrolithiasis.

*Diabetic patients:* Weight-loss induction by orlistat may be accompanied by improved metabolic control in diabetic patients, which might require a reduction in dose of oral hypoglycemic medication (eg, sulfonylureas, metformin) or insulin.

*Misuse potential:* As with any weight-loss agent, the potential exists for misuse of orlistat in inappropriate patient populations (eg, patients with anorexia nervosa or bulimia).

## Drug Interactions

Drugs that may interact with orlistat include cyclosporine, fat-soluble vitamins, pravastatin, and warfarin.

## Adverse Reactions

Adverse reactions occurring in at least 3% of patients include the following:

*GI:* Oily spotting; flatus with discharge; fecal urgency; fatty/oily stool; oily evacuation; increased defecation; fecal incontinence.

*Miscellaneous:* Anxiety; depression; dizziness; headache; rash; abdominal pain/discomfort; gingival disorder; infectious diarrhea; nausea; rectal pain/discomfort; tooth disorder; vomiting; arthritis; back pain; myalgia; lower extremity pain; menstrual irregularity; vaginitis; influenza; upper/lower respiratory tract infection; fatigue; otitis; sleep disorder; urinary tract infection.

# METOCLOPRAMIDE

| | |
|---|---|
| **Tablets**: 5 and 10 mg (*Rx*) | Various, *Reglan* (Robins), *Maxolon* (GlaxoSmith-Kline) |
| **Syrup**: 5 mg/5 mL (*Rx*) | Various, *Reglan* (Robins) |
| **Concentrated solution**: 10 mg/mL (*Rx*) | *Metoclopramide Intensol* (Roxane) |
| **Injection**: 5 mg/mL (*Rx*) | Various, *Octamide PFS* (Adria), *Reglan* (Robins) |

## Indications

*Diabetic gastroparesis:* Relief of symptoms associated with acute and recurrent diabetic gastroparesis (diabetic gastric stasis). Usual manifestations of delayed gastric emptying (ie, nausea, vomiting, heartburn, persistent fullness after meals, anorexia) respond within different time intervals. Significant relief of nausea occurs early and improves over 3 weeks. Relief of vomiting and anorexia may precede the relief of abdominal fullness by at least 1 week.

*Oral:*

*Symptomatic gastroesophageal reflux* – Short-term (4 to 12 weeks) therapy for adults with symptomatic documented gastroesophageal reflux who fail to respond to conventional therapy.

*Parenteral:* For prevention of nausea and vomiting associated with emetogenic cancer chemotherapy.

Prophylaxis of postoperative nausea and vomiting when nasogastric suction is undesirable.

Single doses may facilitate small bowel intubation when the tube does not pass the pylorus with conventional maneuvers.

Stimulates gastric emptying and intestinal transit of barium in cases where delayed emptying interferes with radiological examination of the stomach or small intestine.

*Unlabeled uses:* Used to improve lactation. Doses of 30 to 45 mg/day have increased milk secretion, possibly by elevating serum prolactin levels (see Warnings). Also for treatment of postoperative gastric bezoars (10 mg 3 or 4 times daily).

## Administration and Dosage

*Diabetic gastroparesis:* 10 mg 30 minutes before each meal and at bedtime for 2 to 8 weeks.

Determine initial route of administration by the severity of symptoms. With only the earliest manifestations of diabetic gastric stasis, initiate oral administration. If symptoms are severe, begin with parenteral therapy. Administer 10 mg IV over 1 to 2 minutes. Parenteral administration up to 10 days may be required before symptoms subside, then oral administration may be instituted. Reinstitute therapy at the earliest manifestation.

*Symptomatic gastroesophageal reflux:* 10 to 15 mg orally up to 4 times daily 30 minutes before each meal and at bedtime. If symptoms occur only intermittently or at specific times of the day, single doses up to 20 mg prior to the provoking situation may be preferred rather than continuous treatment. Occasionally, patients who are more sensitive to the therapeutic or adverse effects of metoclopramide (eg, elderly) will require only 5 mg/dose. Guide therapy directed at esophageal lesions by endoscopy. Therapy longer than 12 weeks has not been evaluated and cannot be recommended.

*Prevention of postoperative nausea and vomiting:* Inject IM near the end of surgery. The usual adult dose is 10 mg; however, doses of 20 mg may be used.

*Prevention of chemotherapy-induced emesis:* Infuse slowly IV over not less than 15 minutes, 30 minutes before beginning cancer chemotherapy; repeat every 2 hours for 2 doses, then every 3 hours for 3 doses.

The initial 2 doses should be 2 mg/kg if highly emetogenic drugs such as cisplatin or dacarbazine are used alone or in combination. For less emetogenic regimens, 1 mg/kg/dose may be adequate.

If extrapyramidal symptoms occur, administer 50 mg diphenhydramine IM.

*IV admixture:* When diluted in a parenteral solution, administer IV slowly over a period of not less than 15 minutes.

*Direct IV injection:* Inject undiluted metoclopramide slowly IV allowing 1 to 2 minutes for 10 mg, because a transient but intense feeling of anxiety and restlessness followed by drowsiness may occur with rapid administration.

*Facilitation of small bowel intubation* – If the tube has not passed the pylorus with conventional maneuvers in 10 minutes, administer a single undiluted dose slowly IV over 1 to 2 minutes.

*Recommended single dose –*

*Adults:* 10 mg (2 mL).

*Children (6 to 14 years of age):* 2.5 to 5 mg (0.5 to 1 mL).

*Children (younger than 6 years of age):* 0.1 mg/kg.

*Radiological examinations* – In patients where delayed gastric emptying interferes with radiological examination of the stomach or small intestine, a single dose may be administered slowly IV over 1 to 2 minutes.

*Rectal administration:* For outpatient treatment when oral dosing is not possible, suppositories containing 25 mg metoclopramide have been extemporaneously compounded (5 pulverized oral tablets in polyethylene glycol). Administer 1 suppository 30 to 60 minutes before each meal and at bedtime.

*Renal/Hepatic function impairment:* Because metoclopramide is excreted principally through the kidneys, in those patients whose Ccr is less than 40 mL/min, initiate therapy at approximately½ the recommended dosage. Depending on clinical efficacy and safety considerations, the dosage may be increased or decreased as appropriate.

Metoclopramide undergoes minimal hepatic metabolism, except for simple conjugation. Its safe use has been described in patients with advanced liver disease whose renal function was normal.

*Admixture compatibilities/incompatibilities:*

*Physically and chemically compatible up to 48 hours* – Cimetidine; mannitol; potassium acetate; potassium chloride; potassium phosphate.

*Physically compatible up to 48 hours* – Ascorbic acid; benztropine; cytarabine; dexamethasone sodium phosphate; diphenhydramine; doxorubicin; heparin sodium; hydrocortisone sodium phosphate; lidocaine; magnesium sulfate; multivitamin infusion (must be refrigerated) vitamin B complex with ascorbic acid.

*Incompatible* – Cephalothin; chloramphenicol; sodium bicarbonate.

## Actions

*Pharmacology:* Metoclopramide stimulates motility of the upper GI tract without stimulating gastric, biliary, or pancreatic secretions. Its mode of action is unclear.

*Pharmacokinetics:*

*Absorption/Distribution* – Metoclopramide is rapidly and well absorbed. Onset of action is 1 to 3 minutes following an IV dose, 10 to 15 minutes following IM administration, and 30 to 60 minutes following an oral dose. Effects persist for 1 to 2 hours.

Relative to an IV dose of 20 mg, the absolute oral bioavailability of metoclopramide is approximately 80%. Peak plasma concentrations occur at approximately 1 to 2 hours after a single oral dose. Similar time to peak is observed after individual doses at steady-state. The area under the drug concentration-time curve increases linearly with doses from 20 to 100 mg; peak concentrations also increase linearly with dose. The whole body volume of distribution is high (approximately 3.5 L/kg), which suggests extensive distribution of drug to the tissues.

*Metabolism/Excretion* – Approximately 85% of an orally administered dose appears in the urine within 72 hours. Of the 85% eliminated in the urine, about one-half is present as free or conjugated metoclopramide. The average elimination half-life in individuals with normal renal function is 5 to 6 hours. The drug is not extensively bound to plasma proteins (about 30%).

### Contraindications

When stimulation of GI motility might be dangerous (eg, in the presence of GI hemorrhage, mechanical obstruction, or perforation); pheochromocytoma (the drug may cause a hypertensive crisis, probably because of release of catecholamines from the tumor; control such crises with phentolamine); sensitivity or intolerance to metoclopramide; epileptics or patients receiving drugs likely to cause extrapyramidal reactions (the frequency and severity of seizures or extrapyramidal reactions may be increased).

### Warnings

*Depression:* Depression has occurred in patients with and without a history of depression. Give metoclopramide to patients with a prior history of depression only if the expected benefits outweigh the potential risks.

*Extrapyramidal symptoms:* Extrapyramidal symptoms, manifested primarily as acute dystonic reactions, occur in approximately 0.2% to 1% of patients treated with the usual adult dosages of 30 to 40 mg/day. These usually are seen during the first 24 to 48 hours of treatment, occur more frequently in children and young adults, and are even more frequent at the higher doses used in prophylaxis of vomiting caused by cancer chemotherapy. If symptoms occur, they usually subside following 50 mg diphenhydramine IM. Benztropine 1 to 2 mg IM may also be used to reverse these reactions.

*Parkinson-like symptoms:* Parkinson-like symptoms have occurred, more commonly within the first 6 months after beginning treatment with metoclopramide but occasionally after longer periods. These symptoms generally subside within 2 to 3 months following discontinuance of metoclopramide. Give metoclopramide cautiously, if at all, to patients with preexisting Parkinson disease, because such patients may experience exacerbation of parkinsonian symptoms when taking metoclopramide.

*Tardive dyskinesia:* Tardive dyskinesia, a syndrome consisting of potentially irreversible, involuntary, dyskinetic movements, may develop in patients treated with metoclopramide. Metoclopramide itself, however, may suppress (or partially suppress) the signs of tardive dyskinesia, thereby masking the underlying disease process. Therefore, the use of metoclopramide for the symptomatic control of tardive dyskinesia is not recommended.

*Hypertension:* In one study of hypertensive patients, IV metoclopramide released catecholamines. Use caution in hypertensive patients.

*Anastomosis or closure of the gut:* Giving a promotility drug such as metoclopramide could theoretically put increased pressure on suture lines following a gut anastomosis or closure.

*Carcinogenesis:* Elevated prolactin levels persist during chronic administration. Approximately one-third of human breast cancers are prolactin-dependent in vitro; use caution if metoclopramide is contemplated in a patient with previously detected breast cancer. Although galactorrhea, amenorrhea, gynecomastia, and impotence have occurred with prolactin-elevating drugs, the clinical significance of elevated serum prolactin levels is unknown.

*Pregnancy: Category B.*

*Lactation:* Metoclopramide is excreted into breast milk and may concentrate at about twice the plasma level at 2 hours postdose. There appears to be no risk to the nursing infant with maternal doses less than or equal to 45 mg/day.

*Children:* Infants and children (21 days to 3.3 years of age) with symptomatic gastroesophageal reflux have been treated with metoclopramide at a dosage of 0.5 mg/kg/day; symptoms improved, the duration of the disease was shortened, and surgery was avoided.

Methemoglobinemia has occurred in premature and full-term neonates given metoclopramide orally, IV or IM, 1 to 4 mg/kg/day for 1 to at least 3 days; this did not occur at 0.5 mg/kg/day. Reverse methemoglobinemia by IV administration of methylene blue.

**Precautions**

   *Hypoglycemia:* Gastroparesis (gastric stasis) may be responsible for poor diabetic control. Exogenously administered insulins may act before food has left the stomach, leading to hypoglycemia.

   *Hazardous tasks:* May cause drowsiness; observe caution while driving or performing other tasks requiring alertness, coordination or physical dexterity.

**Drug Interactions**

Drugs that may affect metoclopramide include levodopa, anticholinergics, and narcotic analgesics. Drugs that may be affected by metoclopramide include alcohol, cimetidine, cyclosporine, digoxin, levodopa, MAO inhibitors, and succinylcholine.

**Adverse Reactions**

Adverse reactions occurring in at least 3% of patients include restlessness; drowsiness; fatigue; lassitude; akathisia; dizziness; anxiety; dystonia; insomnia; headache; myoclonus; confusion; convulsive seizures; hallucinations; nausea; bowel disturbances, primarily diarrhea.

# LAXATIVES

### BISACODYL

**Tablets, enteric-coated**: 5 mg (*otc*)

Various, *Dulcolax* (Boehringer Ingelheim), *Fleet Laxative* (Fleet), *Modane* (Savage), *Women's Gentle Laxative* (Goldline Consumer), *Bisac-Evac* (G & W), *Caroid* (Metholatum Co.), *Correctol* (Schering-Plough), *Feen-a-mint* (Schering-Plough)

**Tablets, enteric-coated, delayed-release**: 5 mg

*Reliable Gentle Laxative* (Goldline Consumer)

**Suppositories**: 10 mg (*otc*)

Various, *Bisacodyl Uniserts* (Upsher-Smith), *Bisac-Evac* (G & W), *Dulcolax* (Novartis Consumer), *Reliable Gentle Laxative* (Goldline Consumer), *Fleet Laxative* (Fleet)

### CASCARA SAGRADA

**Tablets**: 325 mg (*otc*)

Various

**Liquid**: (*otc*)

*Aromatic Cascara Fluid Extract* (Various), *Cascara Aromatic* (Humco)

### CASTOR OIL

**Liquid**: 95% castor oil (*otc*)

Various, *Purge* (Fleming)

**Emulsion**: 95% castor oil with emulsifying agents (*otc*)

*Emulsoil* (Paddock)

36.4% castor oil with 0.1% sodium benzoate, 0.2% potassium sorbate (*sf, otc*)

*Neoloid* (Kenwood)

### CO$_2$ RELEASING SUPPOSITORIES

**Suppositories**: Sodium bicarbonate and potassium bitartrate in a water soluble polyethylene glycol base (*otc*)

*Ceo-Two* (Beutlich)

### DOCUSATE CALCIUM (DIOCTYL CALCIUM SULFOSUCCINATE)

**Capsules**: 240 mg (*otc*)

Various, *DC Softgels* (Goldline), *Stool Softener* (Apothecary), *Stool Softener DC* (Rugby), *Surfak Liquigels* (Pharmacia)

### DOCUSATE SODIUM (DIOCTYL SODIUM SULFOSUCCINATE; DSS)

**Tablets**: 100 mg (*otc*)

*ex-lax Stool Softener* (Novartis Consumer)

**Capsules**: 50 and 100 mg (*otc*)

Various, *Colace* (Roberts), *D-S-S* (Magno-Humphries), *Non-Habit Forming Stool Softener*, *Stool Softener* (Rugby), *Regulax SS* (Republic)

**Capsules**: 250 mg (*otc*)

Various, *Stool Softener* (Rugby)

**Capsules, soft gel**: 50, 100, and 250 mg (*otc*)

Various, *D.O.S.*, *Genasoft* (Goldline Consumer), *Phillip's Liqui-Gels* (Bayer Consumer), *Stool Softener* (Rugby)

**Syrup**: 50, 60, 150 mg/15 mL; 20 mg/5 mL; 100 mg/30 mL (*otc*)

Various, *Colace* (Roberts), *Diocto* (Various), *Docu* (Hi-Tech Pharmacal), *Silace* (Silax)

### GLYCERIN

**Suppositories**: Glycerin (*otc*)

Various, *Sani-Supp* (G & W), *Colace* (Roberts)

**Liquid**: 4 mL/applicator (*otc*)

*Fleet Babylax* (Fleet)

### LACTULOSE

**Syrup**: 10 g lactulose/15 mL (< 1.6 g galactose, < 1.2 g lactose, and ≤ 1.2 g other sugars) (*Rx*)

Various, *Cephulac, Chronulac* (Aventis), *Cholac* (Alra), *Constilac* (Alra), *Constulose, Enulose* (Alpharma), *Duphalac* (Solvay Pharm.)

### MINERAL OIL

**Liquid**: Mineral oil (*otc*)

Various

**Emulsion**: Mineral oil with an emulsifier (*otc*)

*Kondremul Plain* (Heritage Consumer)

### POLYCARBOPHIL

**Tablets**: 500 and 625 mg (*otc*)

*FiberNorm* (G & W), *Konsyl Fiber* (Konsyl)

**Tablets, chewable**: 625 mg (as calcium) (*otc*)

*Equalactin* (Numark), *Mitrolan* (Whitehall-Robins)

**Tablets**: 625 mg (as calcium) (*otc*)

*Bulk Forming Fiber Laxative* (Goldline Consumer), *Fiber-Lax* (Rugby), *FiberCon* (Lederle)

## PSYLLIUM

**Powder**: Psyllium (*otc*)

Various, *Fiberall Tropical Fruit Flavor, Fiberall Orange Flavor* (Heritage Consumer), *Genfiber, Genfiber, Orange Flavor* (Goldline Consumer), *Hydrocil Instant* (Numark), *Konsyl, Konsyl-D, Konsyl-Orange, Konsyl Easy Mix Formula* (Konsyl Pharm.), *Metamucil, Metamucil Sugar Free, Metamucil Orange Flavor* (Procter & Gamble), *Natural Fiber Laxative* (Apothecary), *Reguloid, Reguloid, Orange, Reguloid, Sugar Free Orange* (Rugby), *Syllact* (Wallace)

**Wafers**: Psyllium (*otc*)

*Metamucil* (Procter & Gamble)

**Granules**: Psyllium (*otc*)

*Serutan* (Menley & James)

## SALINE LAXATIVES

**Granules**: Magnesium sulfate (*otc*)

*Epsom Salt* (Various)

**Suspension**: Magnesium hydroxide (*otc*)

*Milk of Magnesia, Milk of Magnesia, Concentrated* (Various), *Phillips' Milk of Magnesia, Phillips' Milk of Magnesia, Concentrated* (Bayer)

**Solution**: Magnesium citrate (*otc*)

*Magnesium Citrate Solution* (Humco)

**Solution**: Sodium phosphates (*otc*)

Various, *Fleet Phospho-soda* (Fleet)

## SENNOSIDES

**Tablets**: 6, 8.6, 15, 17, and 25 mg (*otc*)

*ex•lax, ex•lax, chocolated, Maximum Relief ex•lax* (Novartis Consumer), *Black-Draught* (Monticello), *Senokot* (Purdue Frederick), *Senna-Gen* (Zenith-Goldline), *SenokotXTRA* (Purdue Fredrick)

**Granules**: 15 and 20 mg/5 mL

*Black-Draught* (Monticello), *Senokot* (Purdue Frederick)

**Liquid**: 25 mg sennosides A and B/15 mL and 33.3 mg/mL senna concentrate (*otc*)

*Agoral* (Numark), *Fletcher's Castoria* (Mentholatum)

**Syrup**: 8.8 mg/5 mL sennosides (*otc*)

*Senokot* (Purdue Frederick)

## ENEMAS

**Disposable enemas**

*Fleet, Fleet Bisacodyl, Fleet Mineral Oil* (Fleet), *Therevac-SB, Therevac-Plus* (Jones Medical)

## LAXATIVE COMBINATIONS

**Capsules and tablets**: 50 mg docusate sodium, 8.6 mg senna concentrate (*otc*)

*Senokot-S Tablets* (Purdue Frederick)

100 mg docusate sodium, 30 mg casanthranol (*otc*)

Various, *DSS 100 Plus* (Magno-Humphries), *Peri-Dos Softgels* (Goldline), *Peri-Colace* (Roberts), *Nature's Remedy* (Block Drug)

150 mg cascara sagrada (*otc*)

*Nature's Remedy Tablets* (Block Drug)

**Liquids, syrups, emulsions, suspensions**: 60 mg docusate sodium and 30 mg casanthranol/15 mL (*otc*)

*Diocto C* (Various), *Peri-Colace* (Roberts)

**Mineral oil in emulsifying base** (*otc*)

*Liqui-Doss* (Ferndale)

≈ 900 mg magnesium hydroxide and 3.75 mL mineral oil/ 15 mL (*otc*)

*Haley's M-O* (Bayer)

90 mg/15 mL casanthranol with senna extract, rhubarb, methyl salicylate, and menthol (*otc*)

*Black-Draught* (Monticello)

30 mg casanthranol, 60 mg docusate sodium/15 mL (*otc*)

*Silace-C* (Silarx)

**Granules**: 3.25 g psyllium, 0.74 g senna, 1.8 mg sodium, 35.5 mg potassium/rounded teaspoonful (*otc*)

*Perdiem Overnight Relief* (Novartis Consumer)

## MISCELLANEOUS BOWEL EVACUANTS

**Miscellaneous bowel evacuants** (*otc*)

*Fleet Prep Kit 1, 2, and 3* (Fleet), *X-Prep Liquid, X-Prep Bowel Evacuant Kit-1* (Gray), *Tridate Bowel Cleansing System* (Lafayette)

## MISCELLANEOUS BULK-PRODUCING LAXATIVES

**Powder**: 2 mg methylcellulose per heaping tbsp (*otc*)

*Citrucel, Citrucel Sugar Free* (GlaxoSmithKline)

**Powder**: Powdered cellulose (*otc*)

*Unifiber* (Niche)

**Tablets, coated**: 750 mg malt soup extract (*otc*)

*Maltsupex* (Wallace)

**Powder**: 8 g malt soup extract/scoop (*otc*)

*Maltsupex* (Wallace)

**Liquid**: 16 g malt soup extract/tbsp (*otc*)

*Maltsupex* (Wallace)

### Indications

*Constipation:* Treatment of constipation.

*Rectal/Bowel examinations:* Certain stimulant, lubricant, and saline laxatives are used to evacuate the colon for rectal and bowel examinations.

*Prophylaxis:* Laxatives, generally **fecal softeners** or **mineral oil**, are useful prophylactically in patients who should not strain during defecation (ie, following anorectal surgery, MI).

*Lactulose (certain brands):* Prevention and treatment of portal-systemic encephalopathy, including the stages of hepatic precoma and coma.

*Psyllium:* Useful in patients with irritable bowel syndrome and diverticular disease.

*Polycarbophil:* For constipation or diarrhea associated with conditions such as irritable bowel syndrome and diverticulosis; acute nonspecific diarrhea.

*Mineral oil (enema):* Relief of fecal impaction.

*Docusate sodium:* Prevention of dry, hard stools.

### Administration and Dosage

BISACODYL: Swallow whole; do not chew. Do not take within 1 hour of antacids or milk.

　　*Tablets –*

　　　　*Adults and children 12 years of age and older:* 10 to 15 mg (usually 10 mg) in a single dose once daily.

　　　　*Children (6 to 11 years of age):* 5 mg once daily.

　　*Suppositories –*

　　　　*Adults:* 10 mg once daily.

　　　　*Children (6 to 11 years of age):* 5 mg once daily.

CASCARA SAGRADA:

　　*Tablets –* 1 tablet at bedtime.

　　*Liquid –* 5 mL.

CASTOR OIL:

　　*Liquid –*

　　　　*Adults:* Daily dose range, 15 to 60 mL.

　　　　*Children (2 to 12 years of age):* 5 to 15 mL.

　　　　*Infants:* 2.5 to 7.5 mL.

　　*Emulsion –*

　　　　*Adults:* 67%, 15 to 60 mL; 95%, 45 mL (should be mixed with ½ to 1 glass liquid).

　　　　*Children (2 to 12 years of age):* 67%, 15 mL; 95%, 5 to 10 mL (should be mixed with ½ to 1 glass liquid).

DOCUSATE CALCIUM (Dioctyl Calcium Sulfosuccinate):

　　*Adults and children 12 years of age and older –* 240 mg daily until bowel movements are normal.

DOCUSATE SODIUM (Dioctyl Sodium Sulfosuccinate; DSS): Give in milk, fruit juice, or infant formula to mask taste. In enemas, add 50 to 100 mg (5 to 10 mL liquid) to a retention or flushing enema.

　　*Adults and older children –* 50 to 500 mg.

　　*Children (6 to 12 years of age) –* 40 to 120 mg.

　　*Children (3 to 6 years of age) –* 20 to 60 mg.

　　*Children (younger than 3 years of age) –* 10 to 40 mg.

GLYCERIN:

　　*Suppositories –* Insert 1 suppository high in the rectum and retain 15 to 30 minutes; it need not melt to produce laxative action.

　　*Rectal liquid –* With gentle, steady pressure, insert stem with tip pointing towards navel. Squeeze unit until nearly all the liquid is expelled, then remove. A small amount of liquid will remain in unit.

LACTULOSE:

　　*Chronulac, Constilac, Duphalac, Constulose –*

　　　　*Treatment of constipation:* 15 to 30 mL (10 to 20 g lactulose) daily, increased to 60 mL/day, if necessary.

*Cephulac, Cholac, Enulose* – Prevent and treat portal-systemic encephalopathy
*Oral:*

*Adults* – 30 to 45 mL 3 or 4 times daily. Adjust dosage every day or two to produce 2 or 3 soft stools daily. Hourly doses of 30 to 45 mL may be used to induce rapid laxation in the initial phase of therapy. When the laxative effect has been achieved, reduce dosage to recommended daily dose. Improvement may occur within 24 hours, but may not begin before 48 hours or later. Continuous long-term therapy is indicated to lessen severity and prevent recurrence of portal-systemic encephalopathy.

*Children* – Recommended initial daily oral dose in infants is 2.5 to 10 mL in divided doses. For older children and adolescents, the total daily dose is 40 to 90 mL. If the initial dose causes diarrhea, reduce immediately. If diarrhea persists, discontinue use.

May be more palatable when mixed with fruit juice, water, or milk.

*Rectal:* Administer to adults during impending coma or coma stage of portal-systemic encephalopathy when the danger of aspiration exists or when endoscopic or intubation procedures interfere with oral administration. The goal of treatment is reversal of the coma stage so the patient can take oral medication. Reversal of coma may occur within 2 hours of the first enema. Start recommended oral doses before enema is stopped entirely.

Lactulose may be given as a retention enema via a rectal balloon catheter. Do not use cleansing enemas containing soap suds or other alkaline agents.

Mix 300 mL lactulose with 700 mL water or physiologic saline and retain for 30 to 60 minutes. The enema may be repeated every 4 to 6 hours. If the enema is inadvertently evacuated too promptly, it may be repeated immediately.

MINERAL OIL:
*Dose* –

*Adults and children 12 years of age and older:* 15 to 45 mL, take at bedtime; *Kondremul,* 30 to 75 mL.

*Children 6 to 11 years of age:* 5 to 15 mL; *Kondremul,* 10 to 25 mL.

POLYCARBOPHIL:

*Adults and children 12 years of age and older* – 1 g 1 to 4 times daily or as needed. Do not exceed 4 g in 24 hours.

*Children 6 to 11 years of age* – 500 mg no more than 4 times daily or as needed. Do not exceed 2 g/day.

*Children younger than 6 years of age* – Products vary. Consult product labeling for specific guidelines.

For severe diarrhea, repeat dose every 30 min; do not exceed maximum daily dose.

When using as a laxative, drink 8 oz water or other liquid with each dose.

PSYLLIUM: Refer to respective package inserts for particular dosing.

SALINE LAXATIVES:
*Magnesium sulfate* –

*Adults:* 10 to 15 g in glass of water.

*Children:* 5 to 10 g in glass of water.

*Magnesium hydroxide* –

*Adults:* Recommended dosage varies from product to product, ranging from 10 to 60 mL/day. See individual package labeling for specific dosing information.

*Children (2 years of age and older):* 5 to 30 mL, depending on age (must be at least 2 years of age).

*Magnesium citrate* –

*Adults:* 1 glassful (approximately 240 mL) as needed.

*Children:* ½ the adult dose as needed; repeat if necessary.

*Sodium phosphates* –

*Adults:* 20 to 30 mL mixed with ½ glass cool water.

*Children:* 5 to 15 mL.

SENNOSIDES: The following dosages are for senna concentrate only. For other forms of senna, consult labeling. Dosages are different.

*Tablets (6 and 8.6 mg) –*
    *Adults:* 2 tablets, up to 8/day.
    *Children:* 1 tablet, up to 4/day.
*Tablets (15 mg) –*
    *Adults:* 1 tablet at bedtime, up to 4/day.
*Granules –*
    *Adults:* 1 tsp, up to 4 tsp/day.
    *Children:* ½ tsp, up 2 tsp/day.
*Suppositories –*
    *Adults:* 1 at bedtime; repeat in 2 hours if necessary.
    *Children:* ½ suppository at bedtime.
*Liquid –*
    *Adults:* 15 to 30 mL with or after meals or at bedtime.
    *Children (6 to 15 years of age):* 10 to 15 mL at bedtime.
    *Children (2 to 5 years of age):* 5 to 10 mL at bedtime.
*Syrup –*
    *Adults:* 10 to 15 mL at bedtime (up to 30 mL/day).
    *Children (5 to 15 years of age):* 5 to 10 mL at bedtime (up to 20 mL/day).
    *Children (1 to 5 years of age):* 2.5 to 5 mL at bedtime (up to 10 mL/day).
    *Children (1 month to 1 year of age):* 1.25 to 2.5 mL at bedtime (up to 5 mL/day).
*Miscellaneous BULK-PRODUCING LAXATIVES:*
    *Citrucel –*
    *Adults and children 12 years of age and older:* 1 heaping tbsp (19 g) in 8 oz cold water 1 to 3 times daily.
    *Children (6 to 11 years of age):* ½ the adult dose in 8 oz cold water once daily.
    *Unifiber –* Dose is 1 tbsp in 3 or 4 oz of fruit juice, milk, or water, or mix with soft foods such as applesauce, mashed potatoes, or pudding. Can be taken up to 3 times daily if needed or as recommended by a doctor.
    *Maltsupex –*
    *Tablets:* Adults, 12 to 36 g/day. Initially, 4 tablets 4 times daily (meals and bedtime).
    *Powder:* 16 g equals 1 heaping tablespoon.
        Adults, up to 32 g twice daily for 3 or 4 days, then 16 to 32 g at bedtime. Children 6 to 12 years, up to 16 g twice daily for 3 or 4 days; 2 to 6 years, 8 g twice daily for 3 or 4 days. For infants younger than 2 years of age, consult a doctor.
    *Liquid:* Adults, 2 tbsp twice daily for 3 or 4 days, then 1 to 2 tbsp at bedtime. Children 6 to 12 years, 1 tbsp twice daily for 3 or 4 days; 2 to 6 years, ½ tbsp twice daily for 3 or 4 days. For infants younger than 2 years of age, consult a doctor.

## Actions

*Pharmacology:*

| Pharmacologic Actions of Laxatives | | | | | |
|---|---|---|---|---|---|
| | Laxatives | Onset of action (h) | Site of action | Mechanism of action | Comments |
| Saline | Dibasic sodium phosphate[1,2] Magnesium citrate Magnesium hydroxide Magnesium sulfate Monobasic sodium phosphate[1,2] Sodium biphosphate[1] | 0.5-3 | Small & large intestine | Attract/Retain water in intestinal lumen increasing intraluminal pressure; cholecysto-kinin release | May alter fluid and electrolyte balance. Sulfate salts are considered the most potent. |

| Pharmacologic Actions of Laxatives | | | | |
|---|---|---|---|---|
| Laxatives | Onset of action (h) | Site of action | Mechanism of action | Comments |
| **Stimulant/Irritant** Cascara | 6-8 | Colon | Direct action on intestinal mucosa or nerve plexus, alters water and electrolyte secretion | May prefer castor oil when more complete evacuation is required. |
| Bisacodyl tablets Casanthranol Senna | 6-10 | | | |
| Bisacodyl suppository | 0.25-1 | | | |
| **Bulk-Producing** Methylcellulose Polycarbophil Psyllium | 12-72 | Small & large intestine | Holds water in stool to increase bulk-stimulating peristalsis; forms emollient gel | Safe; minimal side effects. Take with plenty of water (240 mL/dose). |
| **Emollient** Mineral oil | 6-8 | Colon | Retards colonic absorption of fecal water; softens stool | May decrease absorption of fat-soluble vitamins. |
| **Fecal Softeners/ Surfactants** Docusate[3] | 12-72 | Small & large intestine | Facilitates admixture of fat and water to soften stool | Beneficial in anorectal conditions where passage of a firm stool is painful. |
| **Hyperosmotic** Glycerin suppository | 0.25-1 | Colon | Local irritation; hyperosmotic action | Sodium stearate in preparation causes the local irritation. |
| Lactulose | 24-48 | Colon | Osmotic effect retains fluid in the colon, lowering the pH and increasing colonic peristalsis | Also indicated in portal-systemic encephalopathy. |
| **Miscellaneous** Castor oil | 2-6 | Small intestine | Direct action on intestinal mucosa or nerve plexus, alters water and electrolyte secretion | Castor oil is converted to ricinoleic acid (active component) in the gut. |

[1] Onset of action for rectal preparations is 2 to 15 min.
[2] Colon is site of action for rectal preparations.
[3] Site of action for potassium salt is in the colon.

### Contraindications

Hypersensitivity to any ingredient; nausea, vomiting, or other symptoms of appendicitis; fecal impaction; intestinal obstruction; undiagnosed abdominal pain; patients who require a low galactose diet (**lactulose**).

Do not give **docusate sodium** if **mineral oil** is being given.

### Warnings

*Fluid and electrolyte balance:* Excessive laxative use may lead to significant fluid and electrolyte imbalance. Monitor patients periodically.

Preparations containing sodium should be used cautiously by individuals on a sodium-restricted diet, and in the presence of edema, CHF, renal failure, or borderline hypertension.

*Megacolon, bowel obstruction, imperforate anus, or CHF:* Do not use sodium phosphate and sodium biphosphate in these patients; hypernatremic dehydration may occur.

*Abuse/Dependency:* Chronic use of laxatives, particularly stimulants, may lead to laxative dependency, which in turn may result in fluid and electrolyte imbalances, steatorrhea, osteomalacia, vitamin and mineral deficiencies, and a poorly functioning colon. Also known as laxative abuse syndrome (LAS), it is difficult to diagnose.

*Cathartic colon:* Cathartic colon, a poorly functioning colon, results from the chronic abuse of stimulant cathartics.

*Melanosis coli:* Melanosis coli is a darkened pigmentation of the colonic mucosa resulting from chronic use of anthraquinone derivatives (**casanthrol, cascara sagrada, senna**).

*Lipid pneumonitis:* Lipid pneumonitis may result from oral ingestion and aspiration of mineral oil, especially when the patient reclines. The young, elderly, debilitated, and dysphagic are at greatest risk.

*Electrocautery procedures:* A theoretical hazard may exist for patients being treated with **lactulose** who may undergo electrocautery procedures during proctoscopy or colonoscopy. Accumulation of $H_2$ gas in significant concentration in the presence of an electrical spark may result in an explosion. Although this complication has not been reported with lactulose, patients should have a thorough bowel cleansing with a nonfermentable solution.

*Renal function impairment:* Up to 20% of the magnesium in magnesium salts may be absorbed. Do not use products containing phosphate, sodium, magnesium, or potassium salts in the presence of renal dysfunction.

*Pregnancy:* Category B (**Lactulose, magnesium sulfate**). Category C (**Casanthranol, cascara sagrada, danthron, docusate sodium, docusate calcium, docusate potassium, mineral oil, senna**). Do not use **castor oil** during pregnancy; its irritant effect may induce premature labor. Mineral oil may decrease absorption of fat-soluble vitamins. Improper use of saline cathartics can lead to dangerous electrolyte imbalance. If needed, limit use to bulk-forming or surfactant laxatives.

*Lactation:* Anthraquinone derivatives (eg, **casanthranol, cascara sagrada, danthron**) are excreted in breast milk resulting in a potential increased incidence of diarrhea in the nursing infant. Sennosides A and B (eg, **senna**) are not excreted in breast milk. It is not known whether **docusate calcium, docusate potassium, docusate sodium, lactulose**, and **mineral oil** are excreted in breast milk.

*Children:* Physical manipulation of a glycerin suppository in infants often initiates defecation; hence, adverse effects are minimal. Do not administer enemas to children younger than 2 years of age.

## Precautions

*Monitoring:* In the overall management of portal-systemic encephalopathy, there is serious underlying liver disease with complications such as electrolyte disturbance (eg, hypokalemia, hypernatremia), which may require other specific therapy. Elderly, debilitated patients who receive **lactulose** for longer than 6 months should have serum electrolytes (potassium, chloride) and carbon dioxide measured periodically.

*Diabetic patients:* **Lactulose** syrup contains galactose (less than 1.6 g/15 mL) and lactose (less than 1.2 g/15 mL). Use with caution in diabetic patients.

*Concomitant laxative use:* Do not use other laxatives, especially during the initial phase of therapy for portal-systemic encephalopathy; the resulting loose stools may falsely suggest adequate **lactulose** dosage.

*Rectal bleeding or response failure:* Rectal bleeding or failure to respond to therapy may indicate a serious condition that may require further medical attention.

*Discoloration:* Discoloration of acid urine to yellow-brown or black may occur with cascara sagrada or senna. Pink-red, red-violet, or red-brown discoloration of alkaline urine may occur with phenolphthalein, cascara sagrada, or senna.

*Impaction or obstruction:* Impaction or obstruction may be caused by bulk-forming agents if temporarily arrested in their passage through the alimentary canal (eg, patients with esophageal strictures). Administer bulk-forming agents with at least 240 mL fluid.

### Drug Interactions

Drugs that may interact with laxatives include mineral oil, milk or antacids, $H_2$ antagonists, proton pump inhibitors, lipid soluble vitamins (A, D, E, and K), and tetracycline.

### Adverse Reactions

Excessive bowel activity (griping, diarrhea, nausea, vomiting); perianal irritation; weakness; dizziness; fainting; palpitations; sweating; bloating; flatulence; abdominal cramps.

Esophageal, gastric, small intestinal, and rectal obstruction caused by the accumulation of mucilaginous components of bulk laxatives have occurred.

Large doses of mineral oil may cause anal seepage, resulting in itching (pruritus ani), irritation, hemorrhoids, and perianal discomfort.

*Lactulose* – Gaseous distention with flatulence, belching, abdominal discomfort such as cramping (approximately 20%); nausea; vomiting. Excessive dosage can lead to diarrhea.

# POLYETHYLENE GLYCOL-ELECTROLYTE SOLUTION (PEG-ES)

| | |
|---|---|
| **Oral solution**: 146 mg NaCl, 168 mg sodium bicarb, 1.29 g sodium sulfate decahydrate, 75 mg KCl, 6 g PEG 3350, 30 mg polysorbate-80/100 mL (*Rx*) | *OCL* (Abbott) |
| **Powder for oral solution**: 1 gal: 227.1 g PEG 3350, 21.5 g sodium sulfate, 6.36 g sodium bicarb, 5.53 g NaCl, 2.82 g KCl (*Rx*) | *CoLyte* (Schwarz Pharma) |
| **4 L**: 240 g PEG 3350, 22.72 g sodium sulfate, 6.72 g sodium bicarb, 5.84 g NaCl, 2.98 g KCl (*Rx*) | |
| **Powder for oral solution**: 236 g PEG 3350, 22.74 g sodium sulfate, 6.74 g sodium bicarb, 5.86 g NaCl, 2.97 g KCl; 227.1 g PEG 3350, 21.5 g sodium sulfate, 6.36 g sodium bicarb, 5.53 g NaCl, 2.82 g KCl (*Rx*) | *GoLYTELY* (Braintree Labs) |
| **Powder for reconstitution**: 420 g PEG 3350, 5.72 g sodium bicarb, 11.2 g NaCl, 1.48 g KCl (*Rx*) | *NuLytely* (Braintree) |

### Indications

For bowel cleansing prior to GI examination.

*Unlabeled uses:* PEG electrolyte solutions are useful in the management of acute iron overdose in children.

### Administration and Dosage

The patient should fast approximately 3 to 4 hours prior to ingestion of the solution; solid foods should never be given less than 2 hours before solution is administered.

One method is to schedule patients for midmorning exam, allowing 3 hours for drinking and 1 hour to complete bowel evacuation. Another method is to give the solution the evening before the exam, particularly if the patient is to have a barium enema. No foods except clear liquids are permitted after solution administration.

*Adult dosage:* Adult dosage is 4 L orally of solution prior to GI exam. May be given via a nasogastric tube to patients unwilling or unable to drink the preparation. Drink 240 mL every 10 minutes until 4 L are consumed or until the rectal effluent is clear. Rapid drinking of each portion is preferred to drinking small amounts continuously. Nasogastric tube administration is at the rate of 20 to 30 mL/min (1.2 to 1.8 L/hour). The first bowel movement should occur in approximately 1 hour.

## Actions

*Pharmacology:* Oral solution induces diarrhea (onset, 30 to 60 minutes) that rapidly cleanses the bowel, usually within 4 hours. Polyethylene glycol 3350 (PEG 3350), a nonabsorbable solution, acts as an osmotic agent.

## Contraindications

GI obstruction; gastric retention; bowel perforation; toxic colitis, megacolon, or ileus.

## Warnings

*Pregnancy:* Category C.

*Children:* Safety and efficacy for use in children have not been established.

Several studies in infants and children ranging in age from 3 to 14 years of age showed that the use of PEG-electrolyte solutions are safe and effective in bowel evacuation.

## Precautions

*Regurgitation/Aspiration:* Observe unconscious or semiconscious patients with impaired gag reflex and those who are otherwise prone to regurgitation or aspiration during use, especially if given via a nasogastric tube. If GI obstruction or perforation is suspected, rule out these contraindications before administration.

*Severe bloating:* If a patient experiences severe bloating, distention, or abdominal pain, slow or temporarily discontinue administration until symptoms abate.

*Severe ulcerative colitis:* Use with caution.

## Drug Interactions

Oral medication given within 1 hour of start of therapy may be flushed from the GI tract and not absorbed.

## Adverse Reactions

Nausea, abdominal fullness, bloating (50% or less); abdominal cramps, vomiting, anal irritation (less frequent).

# POLYETHYLENE GLYCOL (PEG) SOLUTION

**Powder for Oral Solution:** 255 g PEG 3350, 527 g PEG 3350 (*Rx*)   *MiraLax* (Braintree Labs.)

For complete prescribing information, refer to the Laxatives group monograph.

## Indications

For the treatment of occasional constipation. Do not use for more than 2 weeks.

## Administration and Dosage

The usual dose is 17 g of powder/day in 8 ounces of water. Each bottle is supplied with a measuring cap marked to contain 17 g of laxative powder when filled to the indicated line.

Two to 4 days (48 to 96 hours) may be required to produce a bowel movement.

# DIFENOXIN HCl WITH ATROPINE SULFATE

**Tablets:** 1 mg difenoxin (as HCl) and 0.025 mg atropine     *Motofen* (Carnrick)
sulfate (c-iv)

### Indications
Adjunctive therapy in management of acute nonspecific diarrhea and acute exacerbations of chronic functional diarrhea.

### Administration and Dosage
*Adults:* Recommended starting dose: 2 tablets, then 1 tablet after each loose stool; 1 tablet every 3 to 4 hours as needed. The total dosage during any 24-hour treatment period should not exceed 8 tablets. For diarrhea in which clinical improvement is not observed in 48 hours, continued administration is not recommended. For acute diarrhea and acute exacerbations of functional diarrhea, treatment beyond 48 hours is usually not necessary.

### Actions
*Pharmacology:* Difenoxin is an antidiarrheal agent chemically related to meperidine. Atropine sulfate is present to discourage deliberate overdosage.

Difenoxin manifests its antidiarrheal effect by slowing intestinal motility. The mechanism of action is by a local effect on the GI wall.

Difenoxin is the principal active metabolite of diphenoxylate and is effective at one-fifth the dosage of diphenoxylate.

*Pharmacokinetics:* Difenoxin is rapidly and extensively absorbed orally. Mean peak plasma levels occur within 40 to 60 minutes. Plasma levels decline to less than 10% of their peak values within 24 hours and to less than 1% of their peak values within 72 hours. This decline parallels the appearance of difenoxin and its metabolites in the urine. Difenoxin is metabolized to an inactive hydroxylated metabolite. The drug and its metabolites are excreted, mainly as conjugates, in urine and feces.

### Contraindications
Diarrhea associated with organisms that penetrate the intestinal mucosa (eg, toxigenic *E. coli, Salmonella* sp., *Shigella;*) and pseudomembranous colitis associated with broad-spectrum antibiotics. Antiperistaltic agents may prolong or worsen diarrhea.

*Children:* Children less than 2 years of age because of the decreased margin of safety of drugs in this class in younger age groups.

Hypersensitivity to difenoxin, atropine, or any of the inactive ingredients; jaundice.

### Warnings
Difenoxin HCl with atropine sulfate is not innocuous; strictly adhere to dosage recommendations. Overdosage may result in severe respiratory depression and coma, possibly leading to permanent brain damage or death.

*Fluid and electrolyte balance:* The use of this drug does not preclude the administration of appropriate fluid and electrolyte therapy. Dehydration, particularly in children, may further influence the variability of response and may predispose to delayed difenoxin intoxication. Drug-induced inhibition of peristalsis may result in fluid retention in the colon, and this may further aggravate dehydration and electrolyte imbalance.

*Ulcerative colitis:* Agents that inhibit intestinal motility or delay intestinal transit time have induced toxic megacolon. Consequently, carefully observe patients with acute ulcerative colitis.

*Liver and kidney disease:* Use with extreme caution in patients with advanced hepatorenal disease and in all patients with abnormal liver function tests because hepatic coma may be precipitated.

*Atropine:* A subtherapeutic dose of atropine has been added to difenoxin to discourage deliberate overdosage. A recommended dose is not likely to cause prominent anticholinergic side effects, but avoid in patients in whom anticholinergic drugs are contraindicated. In children, signs of atropinism may occur even with recommended doses, particularly in patients with Down Syndrome.

*Pregnancy:* Category C.

*Lactation:* Decide whether to discontinue nursing or to discontinue the drug, taking into account the importance of the drug to the mother.

*Children:* Contraindicated in children under 2 years of age. Safety and efficacy in children below the age of 12 have not been established.

### Precautions
*Drug abuse and dependence:* Addiction to (dependence on) difenoxin is theoretically possible at high dosage. Therefore, do not exceed recommended dosage.

### Drug Interactions
Drugs that may interact include MAO inhibitors, barbiturates, tranquilizers, narcotics, and alcohol.

### Adverse Reactions
Adverse reactions may include nausea, dry mouth, dizziness, lightheadedness, and drowsiness.

## DIPHENOXYLATE HCl WITH ATROPINE SULFATE

| | |
|---|---|
| **Tablets**: 2.5 mg diphenoxylate HCl and 0.025 mg atropine sulfate (*c-v*) | Various, *Logen* (Goldline), *Lomotil* (Searle), *Lonox* (Geneva) |
| **Liquid**: 2.5 mg diphenoxylate HCl and 0.025 mg atropine sulfate per 5 mL (*c-v*) | Various, *Lomotil* (Searle) |

### Indications
Adjunctive therapy in the management of diarrhea.

### Administration and Dosage
*Adults:* Individualize dosage. Initial dose is 5 mg 4 times/day.

*Children:* In children 2 to 12 years of age, use liquid form only. The recommended initial dosage is 0.3 to 0.4 mg/kg daily, in 4 divided doses.

| Diphenoxylate w/Atropine Pediatric Dosage | | | |
|---|---|---|---|
| | Approximate weight | | Dosage (mL) |
| Age (years) | kg | lb | (4 times daily) |
| 2 | 11-14 | 24-31 | 1.5-3 |
| 3 | 12-16 | 26-35 | 2-3 |
| 4 | 14-20 | 31-44 | 2-4 |
| 5 | 16-23 | 35-51 | 2.5-4.5 |
| 6-8 | 17-32 | 38-71 | 2.5-5 |
| 9-12 | 23-55 | 51-121 | 3.5-5 |

*Reduce dosage:* Reduce dosage as soon as initial control of symptoms is achieved. Maintenance dosage may be as low as ¼ of the initial daily dosage. Do not exceed recommended dosage. Clinical improvement of acute diarrhea is usually observed within 48 hours. If clinical improvement of chronic diarrhea is not seen within 10 days after a maximum daily dose of 20 mg, symptoms are unlikely to be controlled by further use.

### Actions
*Pharmacology:* Diphenoxylate, a constipating meperidine congener, lacks analgesic activity. High doses cause opioid activity.

*Pharmacokinetics:* Bioavailability of tablet vs liquid is approximately 90%. Diphenoxylate is rapidly, extensively metabolized to diphenoxylic acid (difenoxine), the active major metabolite. Elimination half-life is approximately 12 to 14 hours. An average of 14% of drug and metabolites are excreted over 4 days in urine, 49% in feces. Urinary excretion of unmetabolized drug is less than 1%; difenoxine plus its glucuronide conjugate constitutes approximately 6%.

**Contraindications**

Children younger than 2 years of age because of greater variability of response; hypersensitivity to diphenoxylate or atropine; obstructive jaundice; diarrhea associated with pseudomembranous enterocolitis or enterotoxin-producing bacteria.

**Warnings**

*Diarrhea:* Diphenoxylate may prolong or aggravate diarrhea associated with organisms that penetrate intestinal mucosa (ie, toxigenic *Escherichia coli*, *Salmonella*, *Shigella*) or in pseudomembranous enterocolitis associated with broad-spectrum antibiotics. Do not use diphenoxylate in these conditions. In some patients with acute ulcerative colitis, diphenoxylate may induce toxic megacolon.

*Fluid/Electrolyte balance:* Dehydration, particularly in younger children, may influence variability of response and may predispose to delayed diphenoxylate intoxication. Inhibition of peristalsis may result in fluid retention in the intestine, which may further aggravate dehydration and electrolyte imbalance.

*Hepatic function impairment:* Use with extreme caution in patients with advanced hepatorenal disease or abnormal liver function; hepatic coma may be precipitated.

*Pregnancy:* Category C.

*Lactation:* Diphenoxylic acid may be excreted in breast milk and atropine is excreted in breast milk.

*Children:* Use with caution; signs of atropinism may occur with recommended doses, particularly in Down syndrome patients. Use with caution in young children because of variable response. Not recommended in children less than 2 years of age.

**Precautions**

*Drug abuse and dependence:* In recommended doses, diphenoxylate has not produced addiction and is devoid of morphine-like subjective effects. At high doses, it exhibits codeine-like subjective effects; therefore, addiction to diphenoxylate is possible. A subtherapeutic dose of atropine may discourage deliberate abuse.

**Drug Interactions**

Drugs that may interact include MAO inhibitors, barbiturates, tranquilizers, and alcohol.

**Adverse Reactions**

Adverse reactions may include dry skin and mucous membranes, flushing, hyperthermia, tachycardia, urinary retention (especially in children), pruritus, gum swelling, angioneurotic edema, urticaria, anaphylaxis, dizziness, drowsiness, sedation, headache, malaise, lethargy, restlessness, euphoria, depression, numbness of extremities, confusion, anorexia, nausea, vomiting, abdominal discomfort, toxic megacolon, and pancreatitis.

# LOPERAMIDE HCl

| | |
|---|---|
| **Tablets**: 2 mg *(otc)* | *Imodium A-D Caplets* (McNeil-CPC), *Kaopectate II Caplets* (Upjohn), *Maalox Anti-Diarrheal Caplets* (Aventis) |
| **Capsules**: 2 mg *(Rx)* | Various, *Imodium* (Janssen) |
| **Liquid**: 1 mg/5 mL *(otc)* | Various, *Imodium A-D* (McNeil-CPC) |
| 1 mg/mL *(otc)* | *Pepto Diarrhea Control* (Procter & Gamble) |

**Indications**

*Rx:* Control and symptomatic relief of acute nonspecific diarrhea and of chronic diarrhea associated with inflammatory bowel disease.

For reducing the volume of discharge from ileostomies.

*OTC:* Control of symptoms of diarrhea, including traveler's diarrhea.

## Administration and Dosage

Rx:

*Acute diarrhea –*

*Adults:* 4 mg followed by 2 mg after each unformed stool. Do not exceed 16 mg/ day. Clinical improvement is usually observed within 48 hours.

*Children:*

| Loperamide Pediatric Dosage (First Day Schedule) | | | |
| --- | --- | --- | --- |
| Age (years) | Weight (kg) | Doseform | Amount |
| 2-5 | 13-20 | liquid | 1 mg tid |
| 6-8 | 20-30 | liquid or capsule | 2 mg bid |
| 8-12 | > 30 | liquid or capsule | 2 mg tid |

*Subsequent doses:* Administer 1 mg/10 kg only after a loose stool. Total daily dosage should not exceed recommended dosages for the first day.

*Chronic diarrhea –*

*Adults:* 4 mg followed by 2 mg after each unformed stool until diarrhea is controlled. When optimal daily dosage (average, 4 to 8 mg) has been established, administer as a single dose or in divided doses.

If clinical improvement is not observed after treatment with 16 mg/day for at least 10 days, symptoms are unlikely to be controlled by further use.

*Children –* Dose has not been established.

OTC:

*Acute diarrhea, including traveler's diarrhea –*

*Adults:* 4 mg after first loose bowel movement followed by 2 mg after each subsequent loose bowel movement but no more than 8 mg/day for no more than 2 days.

*Children:*

*9 to 11 years of age (60 to 95 lbs) –* 2 mg after first loose bowel movement followed by 1 mg after each subsequent loose bowel movement but no more than 6 mg/day for no more than 2 days.

*6 to 8 years of age (48 to 59 lbs) –* 1 mg after first loose bowel movement followed by 1 mg after each subsequent loose bowel movement but no more than 4 mg/day for no more than 2 days.

*Younger than 6 years of age (up to 47 lbs) –* Consult physician (not for use in children younger than 6 years of age).

## Actions

*Pharmacology:* Loperamide slows intestinal motility and affects water and electrolyte movement through the bowel. It inhibits peristalsis by a direct effect on the circular and longitudinal muscles of the intestinal wall. It reduces daily fecal volume, increases viscosity and bulk density and diminishes the loss of fluid and electrolytes.

*Pharmacokinetics:*

*Absorption/Distribution –* Loperamide is 40% absorbed after oral administration and does not penetrate well into the brain. Peak plasma levels occur approximately 5 hours after capsule administration, 2.5 hours after liquid administration and are similar for both formulations.

*Metabolism/Excretion –* The apparent elimination half-life is 10.8 hours (range, 9.1 to 14.4 hours). Of a 4 mg oral dose, 25% is excreted unchanged in the feces, and 1.3% is excreted in the urine as free drug and glucuronic acid conjugate within 3 days.

## Contraindications

Hypersensitivity to the drug and in patients who must avoid constipation.

*OTC use:* Bloody diarrhea; body temperature greater than 101°F.

## Warnings

*Diarrhea:* Do not use loperamide in acute diarrhea associated with organisms that penetrate the intestinal mucosa (enteroinvasive *Escherichia coli*, *Salmonella*, and *Shigella*) or in pseudomembranous colitis associated with broad-spectrum antibiotics.

*Acute ulcerative colitis:* In some patients with acute ulcerative colitis, agents that inhibit intestinal motility or delay intestinal transit time may induce toxic megacolon.

*Fluid/electrolyte depletion:* Fluid/electrolyte depletion may occur in patients who have diarrhea. Loperamide use does not preclude administration of appropriate fluid and electrolyte therapy.

*Pregnancy:* Category B.

*Lactation:* It is not known whether loperamide is excreted in breast milk.

*Children:* Not recommended for use in children younger than 2 years of age. Use special caution in young children because of the greater variability of response in this age group. Dehydration may further influence variability of response. Dosage has not been established for children in treatment of chronic diarrhea.

**Precautions**

*Acute diarrhea:* If clinical improvement is not observed in 48 hours, discontinue use.

*Hepatic dysfunction:* Monitor patients with hepatic dysfunction closely for signs of CNS toxicity because of the apparent large first-pass biotransformation.

**Adverse Reactions**

Adverse reactions may include abdominal pain, distention, or discomfort; constipation; dry mouth; nausea; vomiting; tiredness, drowsiness, or dizziness; hypersensitivity reactions (including skin rash).

# BISMUTH SUBSALICYLATE (BSS)

| | |
|---|---|
| **Tablets, chewable:** 262 mg *(otc)* | Various, *Pepto-Bismol* (Procter & Gamble) |
| **Caplets:** 262 mg *(otc)* | *Pepto-Bismol* (Procter & Gamble) |
| **Liquid:** 130, 262, 524 mg/15 mL *(otc)* | Various, *Pepto-Bismol* (Procter & Gamble) |

**Indications**

For indigestion without causing constipation; nausea; control of diarrhea, including traveler's diarrhea, within 24 hours. Also relieves abdominal cramps.

**Administration and Dosage**

*Adults:* 2 tablets or 30 mL.

*Children:* 9 to 12 years of age – 1 tablet or 15 mL.
  6 to 9 years of age – ⅔ tablet or 10 mL.
  3 to 6 years of age – ⅓ tablet or 5 mL.
  Younger than 3 years of age – Consult physician.

Repeat dosage every 30 minutes to 1 hour, as needed, up to 8 doses in 24 hours.

**Actions**

*Pharmacology:* BSS appears to have antisecretory and antimicrobial effects in vitro and may have some anti-inflammatory effects. The salicylate moiety provides the antisecretory effect, while the bismuth moiety may exert direct antimicrobial effects against bacterial and viral enteropathogens.

*Pharmacokinetics:* BSS undergoes chemical dissociation in the GI tract. Two BSS tablets yield 204 mg salicylate. Following ingestion, salicylate is absorbed, with greater than 90% recovered in the urine; plasma levels are similar to levels achieved after a comparable dose of aspirin. Absorption of bismuth is negligible.

**Precautions**

*Impaction:* Impaction may occur in infants and debilitated patients.

*Radiologic examinations:* May interfere with radiologic examinations of GI tract. Bismuth is radiopaque.

**Drug Interactions**

Drugs that may be affected by bismuth include aspirin and tetracyclines.

# MESALAMINE (5-aminosalicylic acid, 5-ASA)

| | |
|---|---|
| **Tablets, delayed-release**: 400 mg (*Rx*) | *Asacol* (Procter & Gamble) |
| **Capsules, controlled-release**: 250 and 500 mg (*Rx*) | *Pentasa* (Shire US) |
| **Suppositories**: 500 mg (*Rx*) | *Rowasa* (Solvay) |
| **Rectal suspension**: 4 g/60 mL (*Rx*) | *Rowasa* (Solvay) |

## Indications

*Chronic inflammatory bowel disease:*

*Oral* – Remission and treatment of mildly to moderately active ulcerative colitis.

*Rectal* – Treatment of active mild to moderate distal ulcerative colitis, proctosigmoiditis, or proctitis.

## Administration and Dosage

*Oral:*

*Tablets* – 800 mg 3 times daily for a total dose of 2.4 g/day for 6 weeks.

*Capsules* – 1 g 4 times daily for a total dose of 4 g for up to 8 weeks.

*Suppository:* One suppository (500 mg) 2 times daily. Retain the suppository in the rectum for 1 to 3 hours or more if possible to achieve maximum benefit. While the effect may be seen within 3 to 21 days, the usual course of therapy is 3 to 6 weeks depending on symptoms and sigmoidoscopic findings.

*Suspension:* The usual dosage of mesalamine suspension enema in 60 mL units is 1 rectal instillation (4 g) once a day, preferably at bedtime, and retained for approximately 8 hours. While the effect may be seen within 3 to 21 days, the usual course of therapy is 3 to 6 weeks depending on symptoms and sigmoidoscopic findings.

## Actions

*Pharmacology:* Sulfasalazine is split by bacterial action in the colon into sulfapyridine and mesalamine (5-ASA).

The mechanism of action of mesalamine (and sulfasalazine) is unknown, but appears to be topical rather than systemic, and it is possible that mesalamine diminishes inflammation by blocking cyclooxygenase and inhibiting prostaglandin production in the colon.

*Pharmacokinetics:*

*Absorption/Distribution* –

*Rectal:* Mesalamine administered rectally as a suspension enema is poorly absorbed from the colon and is excreted principally in the feces during subsequent bowel movements. At steady state, approximately 10% to 30% of the daily 4 g dose can be recovered in cumulative 24-hour urine collections.

*Oral:*

*Tablets* – Mesalamine tablets are coated with an acrylic-based resin that delays release of mesalamine until it reaches the terminal ileum and beyond. Approximately 28% is absorbed after oral ingestion, leaving the remainder available for topical action and excretion in the feces. Mesalamine from oral mesalamine tablets appears to be more extensively absorbed than that released from sulfasalazine.

*Capsules* – Mesalamine capsules are designed to release therapeutic quantities of the drug throughout the GI tract; 20% to 30% of mesalamine is absorbed. Plasma mesalamine concentration peaked at approximately 1 mcg/mL 3 hours after administration of a 1 g dose and declined in a biphasic manner. Mean terminal half-life was 42 minutes after IV administration.

*Metabolism/Excretion* –

*Rectal:* Whatever the metabolic site, most absorbed mesalamine is excreted in urine as the N-acetyl-5-ASA metabolite. While the elimination half-life of mesalamine is short (0.5 to 1.5 hours), the acetylated metabolite exhibits a half-life of 5 to 10 hours.

*Oral:*

*Tablets* – Following oral administration, the absorbed mesalamine is rapidly acetylated in the gut mucosal wall and by the liver. It is excreted mainly by the kidneys as N-acetyl-5-ASA. The half-lives of elimination for mesalamine and the metabolite are usually approximately 12 hours, but are variable ranging from 2 to 15 hours.

*Capsules* – Elimination of free mesalamine and salicylates in feces increased proportionately with the dose. N-acetyl-5-ASA was the primary compound excreted in the urine (19% to 30%).

## Contraindications

Hypersensitivity to mesalamine, salicylates, or any component of the formulation.

## Warnings

*Intolerance/Colitis exacerbation:* Mesalamine has been implicated in the production of an acute intolerance syndrome or exacerbation of colitis characterized by cramping, acute abdominal pain and bloody diarrhea, and occasionally fever, headache, malaise, pruritus, conjunctivitis, and rash. Symptoms usually abate when mesalamine is discontinued.

*Pancolitis:* While using mesalamine, some patients have developed pancolitis.

*Hypersensitivity reactions:* Most patients who were hypersensitive to sulfasalazine were able to take mesalamine enemas without evidence of any allergic reaction. Nevertheless, exercise caution when mesalamine is initially used in patients known to be allergic to sulfasalazine.

*Renal function impairment:* Renal impairment, including minimal change nephropathy, and acute and chronic interstitial nephritis, has occurred.

*Pregnancy: Category* B. Mesalamine is known to cross the placental barrier.

*Lactation:* Low concentrations of mesalamine and higher concentrations of N-acetyl-5-ASA have been detected in breast milk.

*Children:* Safety and efficacy for use in children have not been established.

## Precautions

*Pericarditis:* Pericarditis has occurred rarely with mesalamine-containing products including sulfasalazine.

## Adverse Reactions

Adverse reactions may include abdominal pain/cramps/discomfort; colitis exacerbation; constipation; diarrhea; dyspepsia; eructation; flatulence/gas; nausea; vomiting; asthenia; chills; dizziness; fever; headache; malaise/fatigue/weakness; sweating; pharyngitis; rhinitis; pruritus; rash/spots; arthralgia; back pain; hypertonia; myalgia; chest pain; dysmenorrhea; edema; flu syndrome; pain.

# OLSALAZINE SODIUM

| **Capsules:** 250 mg (*Rx*) | *Dipentum* (Pharmacia) |
| --- | --- |

## Indications
Maintenance of remission of ulcerative colitis in patients intolerant of sulfasalazine.

## Administration and Dosage
1 g/day in 2 divided doses.

## Actions
*Pharmacology:* Olsalazine sodium is a sodium salt of a salicylate compound that is effectively bioconverted to 5-aminosalicylic acid (mesalamine; 5-ASA), which has anti-inflammatory activity in ulcerative colitis. Approximately 98% to 99% of an oral dose will reach the colon, where each molecule is rapidly converted into 2 molecules of 5-ASA by colonic bacteria. The liberated 5-ASA is absorbed slowly, resulting in very high local concentrations in the colon.

Mechanism of action of mesalamine is unknown, but appears topical rather than systemic. It may diminish colonic inflammation by blocking cyclooxygenase and inhibiting colon prostaglandin production in bowel mucosa.

*Pharmacokinetics:* After oral administration approximately 2.4% of a single 1 g oral dose is absorbed. Maximum serum concentrations appear after approximately 1 hour, and are low even after a single 1 g dose. Olsalazine has a very short serum half-life of approximately 0.9 hours and is greater than 99% bound to plasma proteins. Urinary recovery is less than 1%. Total oral olsalazine recovery ranges from 90% to 97%.

Serum concentrations of 5-ASA are detected after 4 to 8 hours. Of the total urinary 5-ASA, greater than 90% is in the form of N-acetyl-5-ASA (Ac-5-ASA).

## Contraindications
Hypersensitivity to salicylates.

## Warnings
*Pregnancy: Category C.*

*Lactation:* It is not known whether this drug is excreted in breast milk.

*Children:* Safety and efficacy in children have not been established.

## Precautions
*Diarrhea:* About 17%, resulting in drug withdrawal in 6%; appears dose-related, but may be difficult to distinguish from underlying disease symptoms.

*Colitis symptoms:* Exacerbation of the symptoms of colitis thought to have been caused by mesalamine or sulfasalazine has been noted.

*Renal abnormalities:* Renal abnormalities were not reported in clinical trials with olsalazine; however, the possibility of renal tubular damage caused by absorbed mesalamine or its n-acetylated metabolite must be kept in mind, particularly in pre-existing renal disease.

## Adverse Reactions
Adverse reactions may include headache; diarrhea; pain/cramps; nausea; dyspepsia; arthralgia.

# BALSALAZIDE DISODIUM

**Capsules:** 750 mg *(Rx)*                    *Colazal* (Salix)

### Indications
*Active ulcerative colitis:* Treatment of mildly to moderately active ulcerative colitis.

### Administration and Dosage
*Ulcerative colitis:* Take three 750 mg capsules 3 times a day for a total daily dose of 6.75 g for a duration of 8 weeks. Some patients in clinical trials required treatment for up to 12 weeks. Safety and efficacy of balsalazide disodium beyond 12 weeks have not been established.

### Actions
*Pharmacology:* Balsalazide is delivered intact to the colon where it is cleaved by bacterial azoreduction to release equimolar quantities of mesalamine, which is the therapeutically active portion of the molecule and 4-aminobenzoyl-β-alanine. The recommended dose of 6.75 g/day for the treatment of active disease provides 2.4 g of free 5-aminosalicylic acid (5-ASA) to the colon.

*Pharmacokinetics:*

    *Absorption* – In healthy individuals, the systemic absorption of intact balsalazide was very low and variable. The mean $C_{max}$ occurs approximately 1 to 2 hours after single oral doses of 1.5 or 2.25 g. There was a large intersubject variability in the plasma concentration of balsalazide vs time profiles in all studies, thus its half-life could not be determined.

    *Distribution* – The binding of balsalazide to human plasma proteins was at least 99%.

    *Metabolism* – The products of the azoreduction of this compound, 5-ASA and 4-aminobenzoyl-β-alanine, and their N-acetylated metabolites have been identified in plasma, urine, and feces.

    *Excretion* – Less than 1% of an oral dose was recovered as parent compound, 5-ASA, or 4-aminobenzoyl-β-alanine in the urine of healthy subjects.

### Contraindications
Hypersensitivity to salicylates or any of the components of balsalazide capsules or balsalazide metabolites.

### Warnings
*Renal function impairment:* There have been no reported incidents of renal impairment in patients taking balsalazide. Renal toxicity has been observed in patients given other mesalamine products. Therefore, exercise caution when administering balsalazide to patients with known renal dysfunction or a history of renal disease.

*Pregnancy:* Category B.

*Lactation:* It is not known whether balsalazide is excreted in breast milk. Exercise caution when administering to a nursing woman.

*Children:* Safety and efficacy of balsalazide in pediatric patients have not been established.

### Precautions
*Exacerbation of symptoms:* Exacerbation of the symptoms of colitis, possibly related to drug use, has been reported.

*Pyloric stenosis:* Patients with pyloric stenosis may have prolonged gastric retention of balsalazide capsules.

### Adverse Reactions
Adverse reactions occurring in at least 3% of patients include the following: Headache; abdominal pain; diarrhea and nausea; vomiting; respiratory infection; arthralgia.

# SULFASALAZINE

| | |
|---|---|
| **Tablets:** 500 mg (*Rx*) | Various, *Azulfidine* (Pharmacia) |
| **Tablets, delayed-release:** 500 mg (*Rx*) | *Azulfidine EN-tabs* (Pharmacia) |

Sulfasalazine also is indicated for use in rheumatoid arthritis and juvenile rheumatoid arthritis. Refer to the monograph in the CNS chapter.

### Indications

*Ulcerative colitis:* In the treatment of mild to moderate ulcerative colitis and as adjunctive therapy in severe ulcerative colitis; for the prolongation of the remission period between acute attacks of ulcerative colitis.

*Rheumatoid arthritis (RA; enteric-coated tablets):* In the treatment of patients with RA who have responded inadequately to salicylates or other nonsteroidal anti-inflammatory drugs (NSAIDs).

*Juvenile rheumatoid arthritis (JRA; enteric-coated tablets):* In the treatment of pediatric patients 6 years of age and older with polyarticular-course JRA who have responded inadequately to salicylates or other NSAIDs.

*Unlabeled uses:* Psoriatic arthritis (2 g/day).

### Administration and Dosage

Give the drug in evenly divided doses over each 24-hour period; intervals between nighttime doses should not exceed 8 hours, with administration after meals recommended when feasible. Swallow tablets whole; do not crush or chew. Experience suggests that with daily dosages of at least 4 g, the incidence of adverse effects tends to increase.

Some patients may be sensitive to treatment with sulfasalazine. Various desensitization-like regimens have been reported to be effective. These regimens suggest starting with a total daily dose of 50 to 250 mg initially, and doubling it every 4 to 7 days until the desired therapeutic level has been achieved. If the symptoms of sensitivity recur, discontinue sulfasalazine. Do not attempt desensitization in patients who have a history of agranulocytosis, or who have experienced an anaphylactoid reaction while previously receiving sulfasalazine.

*Ulcerative colitis:*
   Initial therapy –
      Adults: 3 to 4 g daily in evenly divided doses. It may be advisable to initiate therapy with a lower dosage (eg, 1 to 2 g daily), to reduce possible GI intolerance.
      Children 2 years of age and older: 40 to 60 mg/kg in each 24-hour period, divided into 3 to 6 doses.
   Maintenance therapy –
      Adults: 2 g daily.
      Children 2 years of age and older: 30 mg/kg in each 24-hour period, divided into 4 doses.
      It is often necessary to continue medication even when clinical symptoms, including diarrhea, have been controlled. When endoscopic examination confirms satisfactory improvement, reduce dosage to a maintenance level. If diarrhea recurs, increase dosage to previously effective levels.

### Actions

*Pharmacology:* The mode of action of sulfasalazine or its metabolites, 5-aminosalicylic acid (5-ASA) and sulfapyridine (SP), is still under investigation but may be related to the anti-inflammatory or immunomodulatory properties that have been observed in animals and in vitro, to its affinity for connective tissue, or to the relatively high concentration it reaches in serous fluids, the liver, and intestinal walls. In ulcerative colitis, the major therapeutic action may reside in the 5-ASA moiety.

*Pharmacokinetics:*
   Absorption – The absolute bioavailability of oral sulfasalazine is less than 15% for parent drug. In the intestine, sulfasalazine is metabolized by intestinal bacteria to SP and 5-ASA. Of the two, SP is relatively well absorbed from the colon and highly metabolized with an estimated bioavailability of 60%. 5-ASA is much less well

absorbed with an estimated bioavailability of 10% to 30%. Peak plasma levels of both occur approximately 10 hours after dosing.

*Distribution* – Following IV injection, the calculated volume of distribution ($Vd_{ss}$) for sulfasalazine was approximately 7.5 L. Sulfasalazine is highly bound to albumin (greater than 99.3%), while SP is only approximately 70% bound to albumin.

*Metabolism* – The observed plasma half-life for IV sulfasalazine is 7.6 hours. The primary route of metabolism of SP is via acetylation to form AcSP. The rate of metabolism of SP to AcSP is dependent on acetylator phenotype. In fast acetylators, the mean plasma half-life of SP is 10.4 hours, while in slow acetylators it is 14.8 hours.

*Excretion* – Absorbed SP and 5-ASA and their metabolites are primarily eliminated in the urine either as free metabolites or as glucuronide conjugates. The majority of 5-ASA stays within the colonic lumen and is excreted as 5-ASA and acetyl-5-ASA with the feces.

## Contraindications

Pediatric patients younger than 2 years of age; intestinal or urinary obstruction; porphyria, hypersensitivity to sulfasalazine, its metabolites, salicylates, or sulfonamides.

## Warnings

*Porphyria:* Patients with porphyria should not receive sulfonamides as these drugs have been reported to precipitate an acute attack.

*GI intolerance:* Sulfasalazine enteric-coated tablets are particularly indicated in patients with ulcerative colitis who cannot take uncoated sulfasalazine tablets because of GI intolerance, and in whom there is evidence that this intolerance is not primarily the result of high blood levels of sulfapyridine and its metabolites (eg, patients experiencing nausea and vomiting with the first few doses of the drug, or patients in whom a reduction in dosage does not alleviate the adverse GI effects).

*Special risk patients:* The presence of clinical signs such as sore throat, fever, pallor, purpura, or jaundice may be indications of serious blood disorders. Use with caution in patients with severe allergy or bronchial asthma.

*Deaths:* Deaths associated with the administration of sulfasalazine have been reported from hypersensitivity reactions, agranulocytosis, aplastic anemia, other blood dyscrasias, renal and liver damage, irreversible neuromuscular and CNS changes, and fibrosing alveolitis. If toxic or hypersensitivity reactions occur, discontinue sulfasalazine immediately.

*Renal/Hepatic function impairment:* Only after critical appraisal should sulfasalazine be given to patients with hepatic or renal damage or blood dyscrasias.

*Fertility impairment:* Oligospermia and infertility have been observed in men treated with sulfasalazine. Withdrawal of the drug appears to reverse these effects.

*Elderly:* Elderly patients with rheumatoid arthritis showed a prolonged plasma half-life for sulfasalazine, SP, and their metabolites.

*Pregnancy: Category B.*

*Lactation:* Sulfonamides are excreted in breast milk. In newborns, they compete with bilirubin for binding sites on the plasma proteins and may cause kernicterus.

*Children:* The safety and efficacy of sulfasalazine in pediatric patients younger than 2 years of age with ulcerative colitis have not been established.

## Precautions

*Monitoring:* Perform complete blood counts, including differential white cell count and liver function tests before starting sulfasalazine and every second week during the first 3 months of therapy. During the second 3 months, perform the same tests once monthly and, thereafter, once every 3 months and as clinically indicated. Also perform urinalysis and assess renal function periodically during treatment.

The determination of serum sulfapyridine levels may be useful because concentrations greater than 50 mcg/mL appear to be associated with an increased incidence of adverse reactions.

*Ulcerative colitis:* Inform patients with this condition that ulcerative colitis rarely remits completely, and that the risk of relapse can be substantially reduced by continued administration of sulfasalazine at a maintenance dosage.

*Glucose-6-phosphate dehydrogenase deficiency:* Observe patients with glucose-6-phosphate dehydrogenase deficiency closely for signs of hemolytic anemia. This reaction is frequently dose-related.

*Undisintegrated tablets:* Isolated instances have occurred where sulfasalazine enteric-coated tablets have passed undisintegrated. If this is observed, discontinue the administration of the drug immediately.

*Fluid intake:* Adequate fluid intake must be maintained in order to prevent crystalluria and stone formation.

### Drug Interactions

Drugs that may interact with sulfasalazine include digoxin, sulfonylureas, and folic acid.

### Adverse Reactions

Adverse events occurring in at least 3% of patients with ulcerative colitis include the following: Anorexia; headache; nausea; vomiting; gastric distress; reversible oligospermia.

# INFLIXIMAB

| | |
|---|---|
| **Powder for injection, lyophilized:** 100 mg (*Rx*) | *Remicade* (Centocor) |

> **Warning:**
> Tuberculosis (frequently disseminated or extrapulmonary at clinical presentation), invasive fungal infections, and other opportunistic infections have been observed in patients receiving infliximab. Some of these infections have been fatal (see Warnings).
>
> Evaluate patients for latent tuberculosis infection with a tuberculin skin test. Initiate treatment of latent tuberculosis infection prior to therapy with infliximab.

## Indications

*Rheumatoid arthritis (RA; moderate to severe):* In combination with methotrexate for reducing the signs and symptoms and inhibiting the progression of structural damage and improving physical function in patients with moderately to severely active RA who have had an inadequate response to methotrexate.

*Crohn disease, moderate to severe:* For reducing signs and symptoms and inducing and maintaining clinical remission in patients with moderately to severely active Crohn disease who have had an inadequate response to conventional therapy.

*Crohn disease, fistulizing:* For reducing the number of draining enterocutaneous and rectovaginal fistulas and maintaining fistula closure.

## Administration and Dosage

*RA:* 3 mg/kg given as an IV infusion followed with additional similar doses at 2 and 6 weeks after the first infusion, then every 8 weeks thereafter. Give infliximab in combination with methotrexate. For patients who have an incomplete response, consider adjusting the dose up to 10 mg/kg or treating as often as every 4 weeks.

*Crohn disease or fistulizing Crohn disease:* 5 mg/kg given as an induction regimen at 0, 2, and 6 weeks followed by a maintenance regimen of 5 mg/kg every 8 weeks thereafter. For patients who respond and then lose their response, consider treatment with 10 mg/kg. Patients who do not respond by week 14 are unlikely to respond with continued dosing; consider discontinuing infliximab in these patients.

## Actions

*Pharmacology:* Infliximab is a chimeric IgG1κ monoclonal antibody.

Infliximab neutralizes the biological activity of tumor necrosis factor alpha (TNFα) by high-affinity binding to its soluble and transmembrane forms and inhibits TNFα receptor binding. Infliximab does not neutralize TNFβ (lymphotoxin α), a related cytokine that uses the same receptors as TNFα.

Elevated concentrations of TNFα have been found in the joints of RA patients and the stools of Crohn disease patients and correlate with elevated disease activity. In Crohn disease, infliximab reduces infiltration of inflammatory cells and TNFα production in inflamed areas of the intestine and reduces the proportion of mononuclear cells from the lamina propria able to express TNFα and interferon. In RA, treatment with infliximab reduced infiltration of inflammatory cells into inflamed areas of the joint as well as expression of molecules mediating cellular adhesion and vascular cell adhesion molecule-1, chemoattraction, and tissue degradation. After treatment with infliximab, patients with Crohn disease or RA have decreased levels of serum IL-6 and C-reactive protein compared with baseline.

*Pharmacokinetics:* A study of single IV infusions of 3 to 20 mg/kg in Crohn disease or RA patients showed a linear relationship between the dose and the maximum serum concentration. The volume of distribution at steady state was independent of dose and indicated that infliximab was distributed primarily within the vascular compartment. The median terminal half-life of infliximab ranged between 8 to 9.5 days.

No systemic accumulation of infliximab occurred upon continued repeated administration at 4- or 8-week intervals following the initial 0, 2, and 6 week induction regimen. Development of antibodies to infliximab increased infliximab clearance. Infliximab concentrations were not detectable in patients who became positive for antibodies to infliximab.

## Contraindications

Do not administer doses of infliximab greater than 5 mg/kg to patients with moderate to severe heart failure (NYHA Class III/IV) (see Warnings).

Hypersensitivity to any murine proteins or other components of the product.

## Warnings

*Heart failure:* Do not administer doses greater than 5 mg/kg to patients with moderate to severe heart failure. Infliximab has been associated with adverse outcomes in patients with heart failure; use in patients with heart failure only after considering other treatment options. Monitor patients closely; infliximab must not be continued in patients who develop new or worsening symptoms of heart failure.

*Risk of infections:* Serious infections, including sepsis, have been reported in patients receiving TNF-blocking agents. Some of these infections have been fatal. Many of the serious infections in patients treated with infliximab occurred in patients on concomitant immunosuppressive therapy that, in addition to their Crohn disease or RA, could predispose them to infections. Do not give infliximab to patients with a clinically important active infection. Exercise caution when considering the use of infliximab in patients with a chronic infection or a history of recurrent infections.

Cases of histoplasmosis, coccidiomycosis, listeriosis, pneumocystosis, tuberculosis, and other bacterial, mycobacterial, and fungal infections have been observed in patients receiving infliximab. For patients who have resided in regions where histoplasmosis or coccidiomycosis is endemic, carefully consider the benefits and risks of infliximab treatment before initiation of infliximab therapy.

Serious infections were seen in clinical studies with concurrent use of anakinra and another TNFα-blocking agent, etanercept, with no added clinical benefit compared with etanercept alone. The combination of infliximab and anakinra is not recommended.

*Hematologic events:* Cases of leukopenia, neutropenia, thrombocytopenia, and pancytopenia, some with a fatal outcome, have been reported in patients receiving infliximab. The causal relationship to infliximab therapy remains unclear. Advise all patients to seek immediate medical attention if they develop signs and symptoms suggestive of blood dyscrasias or infection (eg, persistent fever) while on infliximab. Consider discontinuation of infliximab therapy in patients who develop significant hematologic abnormalities.

*Autoimmunity:* Treatment with infliximab therapy may result in the formation of autoantibodies and, rarely, in the development of a lupus-like syndrome. Discontinue treatment if a patient develops symptoms suggestive of a lupus-like syndrome following treatment with infliximab.

*Neurologic events:* Infliximab and other agents that inhibit TNF have been associated in rare cases with optic neuritis, seizure, and new onset or exacerbation of clinical symptoms or radiographic evidence of CNS demyelinating disorders, including multiple sclerosis and CNS manifestations of systemic vasculitis. Exercise caution in considering the use of infliximab in patients with pre-existing or recent-onset CNS demyelinating or seizure disorders.

*Malignancy:* Patients with a long duration of Crohn disease or RA and chronic exposure to immunosuppressant therapies are more prone to develop lymphomas.

*Hypersensitivity reactions:* Infliximab has been associated with hypersensitivity reactions that vary in their time of onset and required hospitalization in some cases. Urticaria, dyspnea, and hypotension have occurred during or within 2 hours of infliximab infusion. However, in some cases, serum sickness-like reactions have been observed in Crohn disease patients 3 to 12 days after infliximab therapy was reinstituted following an extended period without infliximab treatment. Symptoms associated with these reactions include the following: Fever, rash, headache, sore throat, myalgias, polyarthralgias, hand and facial edema, dysphagia. These reactions were associated with a marked increase in antibodies to infliximab, loss of detectable serum concentrations of infliximab, and possible loss of drug efficacy. Discontinue infliximab if severe reactions occur.

*Elderly:* Because there is a higher incidence of infections in the elderly population in general, use caution when treating the elderly.

*Pregnancy:* Category B.

*Lactation:* It is not known whether infliximab is excreted in human breast milk or absorbed systemically after ingestion.

*Children:* Safety and efficacy have not been established.

## Precautions

*Monitoring:* Monitor for signs and symptoms of infection during and after treatment with infliximab. Closely monitor new infections. If a serious infection develops, discontinue therapy. Monitor patients closely who develop new or worsening symptoms of heart failure.

*Immunogenicity:* Treatment with infliximab can be associated with the development of antibodies to infliximab. Approximately 10% of patients were antibody-positive. The majority of antibody-positive patients had low titers. Patients who were antibody-positive were more likely to have a higher rate of clearance, reduced efficacy and experience an infusion reaction.

*Vaccinations:* No data are available on the response to vaccination or on the secondary transmission of infection by live vaccines in patients receiving anti-TNF therapy. Do not administer live vaccines concurrently.

## Drug Interactions

Concurrent administration of etanercept (another TNFα-blocking agent) and anakinra (an interleukin-1 antagonist) has been associated with an increased risk of serious infections, and increased risk of neutropenia and no additional benefit compared with these medicinal products alone. Other TNFα-blocking agents (including infliximab) used in combination with anakinra also may result in similar toxicities.

## Adverse Reactions

The most common reasons for discontinuation of treatment were infusion-related reactions (ie, dyspnea, flushing, headache, rash). Adverse events have been reported in a higher proportion of RA patients receiving the 10 mg/kg dose than the 3 mg/kg dose; however, no differences were observed in the frequency of adverse events between the 5 and 10 mg/kg doses in patients with Crohn disease.

Adverse reactions occurring in greater than or equal to 5% of patients receiving 4 or more infusions include the following: Headache, fatigue, insomnia, depression, rash, pruritus, arthralgia, back pain, myalgia, upper respiratory tract infection, pharyngitis, sinusitis, coughing, dyspnea, pain, fever, flu syndrome, chest pain, moniliasis, hypertension, nausea, diarrhea, abdominal pain, vomiting, dyspepsia, urinary tract infection, rhinitis, bronchitis, acute infusion reactions, reactions following readministration.

# TEGASEROD MALEATE

**Tablets:** 2 and 6 mg (*Rx*)                    *Zelnorm* (Novartis)

### Indications

*Irritable bowel syndrome (IBS):* For the short-term treatment of women with IBS whose primary bowel symptom is constipation.

The safety and efficacy of tegaserod in men have not been established.

### Administration and Dosage

*Dose:* The recommended dose is 6 mg taken twice daily orally before meals for 4 to 6 weeks. For those patients who respond to therapy at 4 to 6 weeks, an additional 4- to 6-week course may be considered.

The efficacy of tegaserod beyond 12 weeks has not been studied.

### Actions

*Pharmacology:* Tegaserod, a 5-HT$_4$ receptor partial agonist, triggers the release of further neurotransmitters such as calcitonin gene-related peptide from sensory neurons, stimulates the peristaltic reflex and intestinal secretion, and inhibits visceral sensitivity. It enhances basal motor activity and normalized impaired motility throughout the GI tract. In addition, studies demonstrated that tegaserod moderated visceral sensitivity during colorectal distention in animals.

*Pharmacokinetics:*

*Absorption* – Peak plasma concentrations are reached approximately 1 hour after oral dosing. The absolute bioavailability of tegaserod when administered to fasting subjects is approximately 10%. Pharmacokinetics are dose-proportional.

*Distribution* – Tegaserod is approximately 98% bound to plasma proteins, predominantly alpha-1-acid glycoprotein.

*Metabolism* – Tegaserod is metabolized mainly via 2 pathways. The first is a presystemic acid catalyzed hydrolysis in the stomach followed by oxidation and conjugation that produces the main metabolite of tegaserod, 5-methoxyindole-3-carboxylic acid glucuronide with negligible affinity for 5-HT$_4$ receptors. In humans, systemic exposure to tegaserod was not altered at neutral gastric pH values. The second metabolic pathway of tegaserod is direct glucuronidation that leads to generation of 3 isomeric N-glucuronides.

*Excretion* – The plasma clearance of tegaserod is approximately 77 L/h with an estimated terminal half-life (T½) of approximately 11 hours following IV dosing. Approximately two-thirds of the orally administered dose of tegaserod is excreted unchanged in the feces, with the remaining one-third excreted in the urine, primarily as the main metabolite.

*Special populations –*

*Renal function impairment:* No dosage adjustment is required in patients with mild to moderate renal impairment. Tegaserod is not recommended in patients with severe renal impairment.

*Hepatic function impairment:* No dosage adjustment is required in patients with mild impairment; however, caution is recommended when using tegaserod in this patient population. Tegaserod has not been studied adequately in patients with moderate and severe hepatic impairment and, therefore, is not recommended in these patients.

### Contraindications

Severe renal impairment; moderate or severe hepatic impairment; history of bowel obstruction, symptomatic gallbladder disease, suspected sphincter of Oddi dysfunction, or abdominal adhesions; known hypersensitivity to the drug or any of its excipients.

### Warnings

*Pregnancy: Category B.* Use during pregnancy only if clearly needed.

*Lactation:* It is not known whether tegaserod is excreted in human milk. Many drugs that are excreted in human milk have the potential for serious adverse reactions in nursing infants. Based on the potential for tumorigenicity shown for tegaserod in the mouse carcinogenicity study, decide whether to discontinue nursing or discontinue the drug, taking into account the importance of the drug to the mother.

*Children:* Safety and efficacy have not been established in children under 18 years of age.

## Precautions

*Diarrhea:* Do not initiate tegaserod in patients who are currently experiencing or frequently experience diarrhea. Discontinue tegaserod immediately in patients with new or sudden worsening of abdominal pain. The majority of tegaserod patients reporting diarrhea had a single episode. In most cases, diarrhea occurred within the first week of treatment. Typically, diarrhea resolved with continued therapy. Patients should consult their physician if they experience severe diarrhea or if the diarrhea is accompanied by severe cramping, abdominal pain, or dizziness.

*Abdominal surgeries:* An increase in abdominal surgeries was observed on tegaserod (0.3%) vs placebo (0.2%) in the Phase 3 clinical studies. The increase was primarily because of a numerical imbalance in cholecystectomies reported in patients treated with tegaserod (0.17%) vs placebo (0.06%). A causal relationship between abdominal surgeries and tegaserod has not been established.

## Drug Interactions

Tegaserod may interact with digoxin and oral contraceptives.

*Drug/Food interactions:* When the drug is administered with food, the bioavailability of tegaserod is reduced 40% to 65% and $C_{max}$ approximately 20% to 40%. Similar reductions in plasma concentration occur when tegaserod is administered to subjects within 30 minutes prior to a meal or 2.5 hours after a meal. $T_{max}$ of tegaserod is prolonged from approximately 1 hour to 2 hours when taken following a meal, but decreased to 0.7 hours when taken 30 minutes prior to a meal.

## Adverse Reactions

Adverse reactions occurring in at least 3% of patients include the following: Headache, dizziness, abdominal pain, diarrhea, nausea, flatulence, back pain.

# *HELICOBACTER PYLORI* AGENTS

*Helicobacter pylori:* H. *pylori* is found in approximately 100% of chronic active antral gastritis cases, 90% to 95% of duodenal ulcer patients, and 50% to 80% of gastric ulcer patients. The treatment of documented H. *pylori* infection in patients with confirmed peptic ulcer on first presentation or recurrence has been recommended by the National Institutes for Health in a 1994 Consensus Conference. Once H. *pylori* eradication has been achieved, reinfection rates are less than 0.5% per year, and ulcer recurrence rates are dramatically reduced.

Numerous clinical trials have been done to determine the optimal regimen for H. *pylori* eradication, but there remains no gold standard of therapy to date. When selecting a regimen, take into account efficacy, tolerability, compliance, and cost. H. *pylori* is easily suppressed but, to ensure successful eradication, requires the use of 2 antimicrobial agents with either a bismuth compound, an antisecretory agent, or both. These combinations have been shown to enhance H. *pylori* cure, shorten the duration of treatment and decrease treatment failure caused by antimicrobial resistance.

*Double antimicrobial therapy plus an antisecretory drug:*

| Regimens Used in the Eradication of *H. pylori* [1] | | | |
|---|---|---|---|
| Regimen | Dosing | Duration | Eradication |
| Metronidazole | 500 mg twice daily with meals | 1 week | 87% to 91% |
| Omeprazole | 20 mg twice daily with meals | | |
| Clarithromycin | 500 mg twice daily with meals | | |
| Amoxicillin | 1 g twice daily with meals | 1 to 2 weeks | 77% to 83% |
| Omeprazole | 20 mg twice daily before meals | | |
| Clarithromycin | 500 mg twice daily with meals | | |
| Metronidazole | 500 mg twice daily with meals | 1 to 2 weeks | 77% to 83% |
| Omeprazole | 20 mg twice daily before meals | | |
| Amoxicillin | 1 g twice daily with meals | | |

[1] Extending therapy to 10 to 14 days in the above regimens may provide additional benefit. $H_2$ blockers may be used with 2 antibiotics, but a longer treatment course (10 to 14 days), higher antibiotic doses, and 3 times daily administration are required.

*Triple-therapy regimens:* These regimens have proven to be very effective in eradicating H. *pylori*. The primary disadvantage of these regimens is compliance because of the variety and number of medications used. Likewise, adverse effects are more common in patients taking these regimens compared with alternatives.

| Regimens Used in the Eradication of *H. pylori* [1] | | | |
|---|---|---|---|
| Regimen | Dosing | Duration | Eradication |
| Bismuth subsalicylate | 525 mg 4 times daily with meals and at bedtime | 2 weeks 1 week | 88% to 90% 86% to 90% |
| Metronidazole | 250 mg 4 times daily with meals and at bedtime | | |
| Tetracycline | 500 mg 4 times daily | | |
| Bismuth subsalicylate | 525 mg 4 times daily with meals and at bedtime | 1 week | 94% to 98% |
| Metronidazole | 250 mg 4 times daily with meals and at bedtime | | |
| Tetracycline | 500 mg 4 times daily | | |
| Omeprazole | 20 mg 2 times daily before meals | | |

| Regimen Used in the Eradication of *H. pylori* [1] | | | |
|---|---|---|---|
| Regimen | Dosing | Duration | Eradication |
| Bismuth subsalicylate | 525 mg 4 times daily with meals and at bedtime | 2 weeks 1 week | 80% to 86% 75% to 81% |
| Metronidazole | 250 mg 4 times daily with meals and at bedtime | | |
| Amoxicillin | 500 mg 4 times daily with meals and at bedtime | | |

[1] One week of 4 times daily therapy may be sufficient in the absence of antibiotic resistance. Adding a proton pump inhibitor facilitates shorter treatment periods. Until more data is available, the use of $H_2$ antagonists or proton pump inhibitors with the above regimens is appropriate to enhance ulcer healing and provide symptomatic relief.

*Quadruple therapy regimens (2 antibiotics, bismuth, antisecretory agent):* Like triple therapy regimens, these have proven to be effective in *H. pylori* eradication. The primary disadvantage of these regimens is compliance. In addition, because of the variety and number of medications used, adverse effects are more common in patients taking these regimens compared with alternatives.

| FDA-Approved Regimens for the Eradication of *H. pylori* | | | |
|---|---|---|---|
| Regimen | Dosing | Eradication | Comments |
| Omeprazole | 40 mg once daily followed by a 2-week course of 20 mg once daily | 64% to 74% | The American College of Gastroenterology recommends that either tetracycline or amoxicillin be added to this regimen. |
| Clarithromycin | 500 mg 3 times daily for 2 weeks | | |
| Ranitidine bismuth citrate | 400 mg twice daily for 4 weeks | 82% | The American College of Gastroenterology recommends that either tetracycline or amoxicillin be added to this regimen. |
| Clarithromycin | 500 mg 3 times daily for 2 weeks | | |
| Metronidazole | 250 mg 4 times daily at meals and bedtime | 82% | *Helidac* therapy combines bismuth subsalicylate, metronidazole, and tetracycline in a consumer-tested, patient-friendly kit. |
| Tetracycline HCl | 500 mg 4 times daily at meals and bedtime | | |
| Bismuth subsalicylate | 525 mg 4 times daily at meals and bedtime | | |

*Practice Guidelines from the American College of Gastroenterology:* In the 1996 Consensus Statement on Medical Treatment of Peptic Ulcer Disease, the American College of Gastroenterology does not recommend single-antibiotic combinations of either clarithromycin or amoxicillin with proton pump inhibitors because efficacy is less than 70% (cure), and a high-dose, 2-week treatment period is required. The Consensus Statement recommends a 2-antibiotic combination of clarithromycin, metronidazole, or amoxicillin in regimens that do not employ a bismuth compound. In addition, the American College of Gastroenterology suggests adding either tetracycline or amoxicillin to the recently approved ranitidine-bismuth citrate-clarithromycin combination to enhance successful *H. pylori* eradication. Combining a proton pump inhibitor, either omeprazole or lansoprazole, with 2 antibiotics is thought to enhance effectiveness and allow for a shorter duration of treatment.

There are a number of factors that limit the effectiveness of regimens designed to eradicate *H. pylori*. The first, antibiotic resistance, is seen with metronidazole and clarithromycin but has not been reported with bismuth, amoxicillin, or tetracycline.

Second, mild adverse effects (eg, diarrhea, metallic taste, black stools) do occur in approximately 30% to 50% of patients. Therefore, shorter treatment periods in this group of patients may be better tolerated.

Finally, patient compliance is often a problem because of cumbersome regimens and adverse effects.

*Maintenance therapy with antisecretory agents:* Currently, it is advisable to continue maintenance until *H. pylori* cure has been confirmed in patients with a history of complications, frequent or troublesome recurrences or refractory ulcers.

*Successful eradication:* Confirming successful eradication is important in patients with a
history of complicated or refractory ulcers but is controversial in those with uncomplicated ulcers who remain asymptomatic after therapy.

*Refractory ulcers:* Refractory ulcers in patients receiving antibiotic therapy for *H. pylori*
eradication is often due to failure to successfully eradicate *H. pylori* infection. Resistance patterns, as well as noncompliance, and concurrent NSAID use may play
a role in refractory cases.

# PILOCARPINE HCl

| **Tablets:** 5 mg (Rx) | *Salagen* (MGI Pharma) |

### Indications
Xerostomia: Treatment of symptoms of xerostomia from salivary gland hypofunction caused by radiotherapy for cancer of the head and neck.

### Administration and Dosage
The recommended dose for the initiation of treatment is 5 mg 3 times/day. Titration up to 10 mg 3 times/day may be considered for patients who have not responded adequately and who can tolerate lower doses. The incidence of the most common adverse events increases with dose. Use the lowest dose that is tolerated and effective for maintenance.

### Actions
*Pharmacology:* Pilocarpine is a cholinergic parasympathomimetic agent exerting a broad spectrum of pharmacologic effects with predominant muscarinic action. Pilocarpine can increase secretion by the exocrine glands, can stimulate intestinal tract smooth muscle (dose-related), and may increase bronchial smooth muscle tone. The tone and motility of urinary tract, gallbladder, and biliary duct smooth muscle may be enhanced. Pilocarpine may have paradoxical effects on the cardiovascular system. The expected effect of a muscarinic agonist is vasodepression, but administration of pilocarpine may produce hypertension after a brief episode of hypotension. Bradycardia and tachycardia have been reported with use of pilocarpine.

*Pharmacokinetics:* Following single 5 and 10 mg oral doses, unstimulated salivary flow was time-related with an onset at 20 minutes and a peak at 1 hour with a duration of 3 to 5 hours.

Following 2 days of 5 or 10 mg oral pilocarpine given at 8 am, noon, and 6 pm, the mean elimination half-life was 0.76 and 1.35 hours for the 5 and 10 mg doses, respectively. $T_{max}$ was 1.25 and 0.85 hours and $C_{max}$ was 15 and 41 ng/mL, respectively. The AUC was 33 and 108 h•ng/mL, respectively, following the last 6-hour dose.

Inactivation of pilocarpine is thought to occur at neuronal synapses and probably in plasma. Pilocarpine and its minimally active or inactive degradation products, including pilocarpic acid, are excreted in the urine.

### Contraindications
Uncontrolled asthma; hypersensitivity to pilocarpine; when miosis is undesirable.

### Warnings
*Cardiovascular disease:* Patients with significant cardiovascular disease may be unable to compensate for transient changes in hemodynamics or rhythm induced by pilocarpine. Pulmonary edema has been reported as a complication of pilocarpine toxicity from high ocular doses given for acute angle-closure glaucoma. Administer pilocarpine with caution and under close medical supervision in patients with cardiovascular disease.

The dose-related cardiovascular effects of pilocarpine include hypotension, hypertension, bradycardia, and tachycardia.

*Ocular effects:* Carefully examine the fundus prior to initiating therapy with pilocarpine. An association of ocular pilocarpine use and retinal detachment in patients with preexisting retinal disease has been reported. The systemic blood level that is associated with this finding is not known.

Ocular formulations of pilocarpine have caused visual blurring that may result in decreased visual acuity, especially at night and in patients with central lens changes, and impairment of depth perception. Advise caution while driving at night or performing hazardous activities in reduced lighting.

*Pulmonary disease:* Pilocarpine has been reported to increase airway resistance, bronchial smooth muscle tone, and bronchial secretions. Administer with caution and under close medical supervision in patients with controlled asthma, chronic bronchitis, or chronic obstructive pulmonary disease.

*Elderly:* Adverse events reported by those older than 65 years of age and those 65 years of age and younger were comparable. Elderly women volunteers had a higher $C_{max}$ and AUC than elderly men.

*Pregnancy: Category C.*

*Lactation:* It is not known whether this drug is excreted in breast milk.

*Children:* Safety and efficacy in children have not been established.

### Precautions

*Toxicity:* Toxicity is characterized by an exaggeration of parasympathomimetic effects which may include the following: Headache; visual disturbance; lacrimation; sweating; respiratory distress; GI spasm; nausea; vomiting; diarrhea; AV block; tachycardia; bradycardia; hypotension; hypertension; shock; mental confusion; cardiac arrhythmia; tremors.

*Biliary tract:* Administer with caution to patients with known or suspected cholelithiasis or biliary tract disease. Contractions of the gallbladder or biliary smooth muscle could precipitate complications including cholecystitis, cholangitis, and biliary obstruction.

*Renal colic:* Pilocarpine may increase ureteral smooth muscle tone and could theoretically precipitate renal colic (or "ureteral reflux"), particularly in patients with nephrolithiasis.

*Psychiatric disorder:* Cholinergic agonists may have dose-related CNS effects. Consider this when treating patients with underlying cognitive or psychiatric disturbances.

### Drug Interactions

Drugs that may interact with pilocarpine include beta blockers and anticholinergics.

*Drug/Food interactions:* The rate of absorption of pilocarpine is decreased when taken with a high-fat meal. Maximum concentration is decreased and time to reach maximum concentration is increased.

### Adverse Reactions

The most frequent adverse experiences associated with pilocarpine were a consequence of the expected pharmacologic effects. Adverse reactions occurring in at least 3% of patients include the following: Sweating, nausea, rhinitis, chills, flushing, urinary frequency, dizziness, asthenia, headache, dyspepsia, lacrimation, diarrhea, edema, abdominal pain, amblyopia, vomiting, pharyngitis, and hypertension.

## AMLEXANOX

| Paste: 5% (*Rx*) | *Aphthasol* (Access) |
|---|---|

### Indications

*Aphthous ulcers:* Treatment of aphthous ulcers in people with healthy immune systems.

### Administration and Dosage

Apply 4 times/day beginning as soon as symptoms occur. Use after oral hygiene. With gentle pressure, dab paste onto each ulcer in mouth. Use until ulcer heals. If significant healing or pain reduction has not occurred in 10 days, consult a dentist or physician.

### Actions

*Pharmacology:* The mechanism of action is unknown.

### Contraindications

Hypersensitivity to amlexanox or other ingredients in the formulation.

### Warnings

*Pregnancy: Category B.*

*Lactation:* Exercise caution when administering amlexanox oral paste to a nursing woman.

*Children:* Safety and efficacy in pediatric patients have not been established.

**Precautions**

*Local irritation:* In the event that rash or contact mucositis occurs, discontinue use.

**Adverse Reactions**

Transient pain, stinging, or burning at the site of application (1% to 2%).

# SULFURIC ACID/SULFONATED PHENOLICS

**Liquid**: 30% sulfuric acid and 22% sulfonated phenolics (Rx)   *Debacterol* (Henry Schein/Sullivan-Schein Dental)

**Indications**

*Ulcerating lesions:* Topical treatment of ulcerating lesions of the oral cavity, such as recurrent aphthous stomatitis (canker sores).

Not intended for the treatment of vesicular lesions, such as cold sores or fever blisters.

**Administration and Dosage**

Dry the ulcerated area of oral mucosa using a sterile cotton-tipped applicator or some similar method. After drying the lesion, hold swab with the colored ring end up. Bend the colored ring tip gently to the side until it snaps to release the liquid inside. Then apply the coated applicator directly to the dried ulcer bed. Hold applicator in contact with the ulcer for at least 5 seconds while rolling to thoroughly coat the entire ulcer bed, the ulcer rim, and the surrounding halo of normal mucosa. Do not hold the applicator on the ulcer for more than 10 seconds. Thoroughly rinse out the mouth with water and spit out the rinse water. The stinging sensation and ulcer pain will subside almost immediately after the water rinse.

One application per ulcer treatment is usually sufficient. If the ulcer pain returns shortly after rinsing with water, some part of the ulcer was not covered. Then apply a second application to the ulcer immediately until it remains pain-free after rinsing. It is not recommended that more than 1 treatment session be performed on any individual mucosal ulcer. Do not reapply the product to the same lesion after it is free of pain.

**Actions**

*Pharmacology:* The liquid contains sulfonated phenolics, which are antiseptic agents with topical analgesic properties and sulfuric acid, which is a tissue denaturant and sterilizing agent.

**Contraindications**

Known allergy to sulfonated phenolics.

**Warnings**

Keep out of the reach of children. Do not use if allergic to sulfonated phenolics.

*Prolonged use:* Prolonged use on normal tissue should be avoided. Prolonged use will eventually necrotize and slough all tissue to which it is applied in sufficient volume; apply carefully.

*Pregnancy: Category C.*

*Children:* Safety and efficacy in children under 12 years of age have not been established.

**Precautions**

*External use only:* Avoid eye contact.

**Adverse Reactions**

May cause local irritation upon administration. If excess irritation occurs, a rinse with sodium bicarbonate (baking soda) solution will neutralize the reaction (use 2.5 mL in 120 mL of water).

# Chapter 9

# SYSTEMIC ANTI-INFECTIVE AGENTS

# PENICILLINS

### AMOXICILLIN

**Tablets**: 500 and 875 mg (as trihydrate) (*Rx*)

Various, *Amoxil* (GlaxoSmithKline)

**Tablets, chewable**: 125, 200, 250, and 400 mg (as trihydrate) (*Rx*)

Various, *Amoxil* (GlaxoSmithKline), *Trimox* (Apothecon)

**Capsules**: 250 and 500 mg (as trihydrate) (*Rx*)

Various, *Trimox* (Apothecon)

**Powder for oral suspension**: 50 mg/mL, 125, 200, 250, and 400 mg/5 mL (as trihydrate) when reconstituted (*Rx*)

Various, *Amoxil* (GlaxoSmithKline), *Amoxil Pediatric Drops* (GlaxoSmithKline), *Trimox* (Apothecon)

### AMOXICILLIN AND POTASSIUM CLAVULANATE

**Tablets**: 250, 500, or 875 mg amoxicillin (as trihydrate) and 125 mg clavulanic acid (*Rx*)

Various, *Augmentin* (GlaxoSmithKline)

**Tablets, extended-release**: 1000 mg amoxicillin and 62.5 mg clavulanic acid (*Rx*)

*Augmentin XR* (GlaxoSmithKline)

**Tablets, chewable**: 125 mg amoxicillin (as trihydrate) and 31.25 mg clavulanic acid; 200 mg amoxicillin (as trihydrate) and 28.5 mg clavulanic acid; 250 mg amoxicillin (as trihydrate) and 62.5 mg clavulanic acid; 400 mg amoxicillin (as trihydrate) and 57 mg clavulanic acid (*Rx*)

Various, *Augmentin* (GlaxoSmithKline)

**Powder for oral suspension**: 125 mg amoxicillin and 31.25 mg clavulanic acid/5 mL; 200 mg amoxicillin and 28.5 mg clavulanic acid/5 mL; 250 mg amoxicillin and 62.5 mg clavulanic acid/5 mL; 400 mg amoxicillin and 57 mg clavulanic acid/5 mL; 600 mg amoxicillin and 42.9 mL clavulanic acid/ 5 mL (*Rx*)

Various, *Augmentin*, *Augmentin ES-600* (GlaxoSmithKline)

### AMPICILLIN

**Capsules**: 250 and 500 mg (as trihydrate or anhydrous) (*Rx*)

Various, *Principen* (Geneva)

**Powder for oral suspension**: 125 and 250 mg/5 mL (as trihydrate) when reconstituted (*Rx*)

*Principen* (Geneva)

### AMPICILLIN SODIUM, PARENTERAL

**Powder for injection**: 250 and 500 mg and 1 and 2 g (*Rx*)

Various

### AMPICILLIN SODIUM AND SULBACTAM SODIUM

**Powder for injection**: 1.5 g (1 g ampicillin sodium/0.5 g sulbactam sodium), 3 g (2 g ampicillin sodium/1 g sulbactam sodium), 15 g (10 g ampicillin sodium/5 g sulbactam sodium) (*Rx*)

Various, *Unasyn* (Roerig)

### CARBENICILLIN INDANYL SODIUM

**Tablets, film-coated**: 382 mg carbenicillin (118 mg indanyl sodium ester) (*Rx*)

*Geocillin* (Roerig)

### DICLOXACILLIN SODIUM

**Capsules**: 250 and 500 mg (*Rx*)

Various

### NAFCILLIN SODIUM

**Powder for injection**: 1 and 2 g (*Rx*)

Various

### OXACILLIN SODIUM

**Powder for oral solution**: 250 mg/5 mL when reconstituted (*Rx*)

Various

### OXACILLIN SODIUM, PARENTERAL

**Powder for injection**: 500 mg and 1, 2, and 10 g (*Rx*)

Various

### PENICILLIN G (AQUEOUS)

**Injection, premixed, frozen**: 1, 2, and 3 million units (*Rx*)

*Penicillin G Potassium* (Baxter)

**Powder for injection**: 5 and 20 million units/vial (*Rx*)

*Pfizerpen* (Roerig)

### PENICILLIN G BENZATHINE, IM

**Injection**: 600,000 units, 1,200,000, and 2,400,000 units/ dose (*Rx*)

*Bicillin L-A* (Wyeth-Ayerst), *Permapen* (Roerig)

### PENICILLIN G PROCAINE, IM

**Injection**: 600,000 and 1,200,000 units/vial (*Rx*)

*Wycillin* (Wyeth-Ayerst)

### PENICILLIN G BENZATHINE AND PROCAINE COMBINED, IM

**Injection**: 300,000 units/mL; 600,000, 1,200,000, and 2,400,000 units/dose; 900,000 units penicillin G benzathine and 300,000 units penicillin G procaine/dose (*Rx*)

*Bicillin C-R*, *Bicillin C-R 900/300* (Monarch)

| **PENICILLIN V (PHENOXYMETHYL PENICILLIN)** | |
|---|---|
| **Tablets:** 250 and 500 mg (*Rx*) | Various, *Veetids* (Geneva) |
| **Powder for oral solution:** 125 or 250 mg/5 mL when reconstituted (*Rx*) | Various, *Veetids* (Geneva) |
| **PIPERACILLIN SODIUM** | |
| **Powder for injection:** 2, 3, 4, and 40 g (*Rx*) | *Pipracil* (American Pharmaceutical Partners) |
| **PIPERACILLIN SODIUM AND TAZOBACTAM SODIUM** | |
| **Powder for injection:** 2 g piperacillin/0.25 g tazobactam; 3 g piperacillin/0.375 g tazobactam; 4 g piperacillin/0.5 g tazobactam; 36 g piperacillin/4.5 g tazobactam (*Rx*) | *Zosyn* (Wyeth) |
| **Injection:** 2g piperacillin/0.25 g tazobactam; 3 g piperacillin/0.375 g tazobactam; 4 g piperacillin/0.5 g tazobactam; (*Rx*) | *Zosyn* (Wyeth) |
| **TICARCILLIN DISODIUM** | |
| **Powder for injection:** 3 g (*Rx*) | *Ticar* (GlaxoSmithKline) |
| **TICARCILLIN AND CLAVULANATE POTASSIUM** | |
| **Powder for injection:** 3 g ticarcillin (as disodium) and 0.1 g clavulanic acid (as potassium) (*Rx*) | *Timentin* (GlaxoSmithKline) |
| **Injection solution:** 3 g ticarcillin (as disodium) and 0.1 g clavulanic acid (as potassium)/100 mL (*Rx*) | |

### Indications

*Oral:* Penicillins generally are indicated in the treatment of mild to moderately severe infections caused by penicillin-sensitive microorganisms.

*Penicillinase-resistant penicillins:* The percentage of staphylococcal isolates resistant to **penicillin G** outside the hospital is increasing, approximating the high percentage found in the hospital. Therefore, use a penicillinase-resistant penicillin as initial therapy for any suspected staphylococcal infection until culture and sensitivity results are known.

When treatment is initiated before definitive culture and sensitivity results are known, consider that these agents are only effective in the treatment of infections caused by pneumococci, group A beta-hemolytic streptococci, and penicillin G-resistant and penicillin G-sensitive staphylococci.

*Parenteral:* In patients with severe infection or when there is nausea, vomiting, gastric dilatation, cardiospasm, or intestinal hypermotility.

### Administration and Dosage

Therapy may be initiated prior to obtaining results of bacteriologic studies when there is reason to believe the causative organisms may be susceptible. Once results are known, adjust therapy.

Continue treatment of all infections for a minimum of 48 to 72 hours beyond the time that the patient becomes asymptomatic or evidence of bacterial eradication has been obtained, unless single-dose therapy is employed.

*AMOXICILLIN:* Larger doses may be required for persistent or severe infections. The children's dose should not exceed the maximum adult dose.

| **Amoxicillin Uses and Dosages** | |
|---|---|
| Organisms/Infections | Dosage |
| Ear/Nose/Throat Skin/Skin structure GU tract | *Mild/Moderate:* |
| | *Adults and children ≥ 40 kg:* 500 mg every 12 h or 250 mg every 8 h |
| | *Children > 3 months and < 40 kg:* 25 mg/kg/day in divided doses every 12 h or 20 mg/kg/day in divided doses every 8 h |
| | *Severe:* |
| | *Adults and children ≥ 40 kg:* 875 mg every 12 h or 500 mg every 8 h |
| | *Children > 3 months and < 40 kg:* 45 mg/kg/day in divided doses every 12 h or 40 mg/kg/day in divided doses every 8 h |

| Amoxicillin Uses and Dosages | |
|---|---|
| Organisms/Infections | Dosage |
| Lower respiratory tract | *Adults and children ≥ 40 kg:* 875 mg every 12 h or 500 mg every 8 h |
| | *Children > 3 months and < 40 kg:* 45 mg/kg/day in divided doses every 12 h or 40 mg/kg/day in divided doses every 8 h |
| Gonorrhea:[1] Acute, uncompli- cated anogenital and urethral infections in males and females | *Adults:* 3 g as single oral dose |
| | *Prepubertal children (> 2 years of age):* 50 mg/kg amoxicillin combined with 25 mg/kg probenecid as a single dose |

[1] Evaluate all patients with gonorrhea for syphilis (see Precautions).

AMOXICILLIN AND POTASSIUM CLAVULANATE: May be administered without regard to meals.

To minimize the potential for GI intolerance, take at the start of a meal. Absorption of clavulanate potassium may be enhanced when the drug is administered at the start of a meal.

Because the 250 and 500 mg tablets contain the same amount of clavulanic acid (125 mg as potassium salt), two 250 mg tablets are not equivalent to one 500 mg tablet. The 250 mg tablet and 250 mg chewable tablet do not contain the same amount of potassium clavulanate and should not be substituted for each other.

Usual dose –

Adults: One 250 mg tablet every 8 hours or one 500 mg tablet every 12 hours.

Suspension – Adults who have difficulty swallowing may be given the 125 mg/5 mL or 250 mg/5 mL suspension in place of the 500 mg tablet or give 200 mg/5 mL or 400 mg/5 mL suspension in place of the 875 mg tablet.

Severe infections and respiratory tract infections – One 500 mg tablet every 8 hours or one 875 mg tablet every 12 hours.

Renal function impairment – Renal function impairment generally does not require a dose reduction unless impairment is severe. Severely impaired patients with a glomerular filtration rate (GFR) of less than 30 mL/min should not receive the 875 mg tablet. Give patients with a GFR of 10 to 30 mL/min 500 or 250 mg every 12 hours, depending on the severity of infection. Give patients with a GFR less than 10 mL/min 500 or 250 mg every 24 hours, depending on severity of infection. Give hemodialysis patients 500 or 250 mg every 24 hours and an additional dose during and at the end of dialysis.

Hepatic function impairment – Dose with caution and monitor hepatic function.

Children:

Less than 3 months of age – 30 mg/kg/day divided every 12 hours, based on the amoxicillin component. Use of the 125 mg/5 mL oral suspension is recommended.

3 months of age or older – Children's dose is based on amoxicillin content. Refer to the following table. Because of the different amoxicillin to clavulanic acid ratios in the 250 mg tablets (250/125) vs the 250 mg chewable tablets (250/62.5), do not use the 250 mg tablet until the child weighs 40 kg or more.

40 kg or more – Dose according to adult recommendations.

| Amoxicillin/Potassium Clavulanate Dosing in Children ≥ 3 Months of Age | | |
|---|---|---|
| | Dosing regimen | |
| Infections | 200 mg/5 mL or 400 mg/5 mL (q 12 h)[1,2] | 125 mg/5 mL or 250 mg/5 mL (q 8 h)[2] |
| Otitis media,[3] sinusitis, lower respiratory tract infections, severe infections | 45 mg/kg/day | 40 mg/kg/day |
| Less severe infections | 25 mg/kg/day | 20 mg/kg/day |

[1] The every-12-hour regimen is associated with significantly less diarrhea; however, the 200 and 400 mg formulations (suspension and chewable tablets) contain aspartame and should not be used by phenylketonurics.
[2] Each strength of the suspension is available as a chewable tablet for use by older children.
[3] Recommended duration is 10 days.

Augmentin ES-600 – Augmentin ES-600, 600 mg/5 mL, does not contain the same amount of clavulanic acid (as the potassium salt) as any of the other Augmentin suspensions. Do not substitute Augmentin 200 mg/5 mL and 400 mg/5 mL suspensions for Augmentin ES-600, as they are not interchangeable.

Dosage:

Pediatric patients 3 months and older – Based on the amoxicillin component (600 mg/5 mL), the recommended dose of Augmentin ES-600 is 90 mg/kg/day divided every 12 hours, administered for 10 days (see table below).

| Recommended Dose of Augmentin ES-600 | |
|---|---|
| Body weight (kg) | Volume of Augmentin ES-600 providing 90 mg/kg/day |
| 8 | 3 mL twice daily |
| 12 | 4.5 mL twice daily |
| 16 | 6 mL twice daily |
| 20 | 7.5 mL twice daily |
| 24 | 9 mL twice daily |
| 28 | 10.5 mL twice daily |
| 32 | 12 mL twice daily |
| 36 | 13.5 mL twice daily |

Pediatric patients weighing 40 kg or more – Experience with Augmentin ES-600 in this group is not available.

Adults – Experience with Augmentin ES-600 in adults is not available. Adults who have difficulty swallowing should not be given Augmentin ES-600 in place of the Augmentin 500 mg or 875 mg tablet.

Hepatic impairment – Dose hepatically impaired patients with caution and monitor hepatic function at regular intervals.

Augmentin XR – Take Augmentin XR at the start of a meal to enhance the absorption of amoxicillin and minimize the potential for GI intolerance. Absorption of the amoxicillin component is decreased when Augmentin XR is taken on an empty stomach.

The recommended dose is 4000 mg/250 mg daily according to the following table.

| Augmentin XR Dosing | | |
|---|---|---|
| Indication | Dose | Duration |
| Acute bacterial sinusitis | 2 tablets q 12 h | 10 days |
| Community-acquired pneumonia | 2 tablets q 12 h | 7 to 10 days |

Augmentin tablets (250 or 500 mg) cannot be used to provide the same dosages as Augmentin XR extended-release tablets. This is because Augmentin XR contains 62.5 mg clavulanic acid, while the Augmentin 250 and 500 mg tablets each contain 125 mg clavulanic acid. In addition, the extended-release tablet provides an extended time course of plasma amoxicillin concentrations compared with immediate-release tablets. Thus, 2 *Augmentin* 500 mg tablets are not equivalent to 1 *Augmentin XR* tablet.

The scored *Augmentin XR* tablets are available for greater convenience for adult patients who have difficulty swallowing. The scored *Augmentin XR* tablet may be broken in half at score line. The scored tablet is not intended to reduce the dosage of medication taken; as stated in the table above, the recommended dose of *Augmentin XR* is 2 tablets twice daily every 12 hours.

*Renally impaired patients: Augmentin XR* is contraindicated in severely impaired patients with a Ccr of less than 30 mL/min and in hemodialysis patients.

*Hepatically impaired patients:* Dose hepatically impaired patients with caution and monitor hepatic function at regular intervals.

*Children:* Safety and efficacy in pediatric patients under 16 years of age have not been established.

AMPICILLIN:

| Ampicillin Uses and Dosages | |
|---|---|
| Organisms/Infections | Dosage |
| *Enterococcal endocarditis* | 12 g/day IV either continuously or in equally divided doses every 4 h plus 1 mg/kg IM or IV gentamicin every 8 h for 4 to 6 wk. |
| *Respiratory tract and soft tissue infections* | *Parenteral:* Patients ≥ 40 kg – 250 to 500 mg every 6 h; < 40 kg – 25 to 50 mg/kg/day in equally divided doses at 6- to 8-h intervals |
| | *Oral:* Patients> 20 kg – 250 mg every 6 h; ≤ 20 kg – 50 mg/kg/day in equally divided doses at 6- to 8-h intervals |
| *Bacterial meningitis* | Adults/Children: 150 to 200 mg/kg/day in equally divided doses every 3 to 4 h. Initial treatment is usually by IV, followed by IM injections. |
| *Septicemia* | Adults/Children: 150 to 200 mg/kg/day. Give IV at least 3 days; continue IM every 3 to 4 h. |
| *GI and GU infections:* Other than *N. gonorrhoeae*[1] | *Oral:* Adults/Children> 20 kg - 500 mg orally every 6 h. Use larger doses for severe or chronic infections, if needed. |
| | Children ≤ 20 kg - 100 mg/kg/day every 6 h |
| *N. gonorrhoeae* | *Oral:* Single dose of 3.5 g administered simultaneously with 1 g probenecid |
| | *Parenteral:* Adults/children ≥ 40 kg - 500 mg IV or IM every 6 h |
| | Children < 40 kg - 50 mg/kg/day IV or IM in equally divided doses at 6- to 8-h intervals |
| Urethritis caused by *N. gonorrhoeae* in males | *Parenteral:* Adult males - Two 500 mg doses, IV or IM, at an interval of 8 to 12 h. Treatment may be repeated if necessary or extended if required. In complicated gonorrheal urethritis (eg, prostatitis, epididymitis), prolonged and intensive therapy is recommended. |

[1] Ampicillin is not included in the 2002 CDC recommendations for the treatment of gonorrhea.

*Renal function impairment* – Increase dosing interval to 6 to 12 hours in moderate renal impairment (Ccr 10 to 50 mL/min) and 12 to 24 hours in severe renal impairment (Ccr less than 10 mL/min).

AMPICILLIN SODIUM AND SULBACTAM SODIUM: Give IV or IM. The recommended adult dosage is 1.5 g (1 g ampicillin plus 0.5 g sulbactam) to 3 g (2 g ampicillin plus 1 g sulbactam) every 6 hours. Do not exceed 4 g/day sulbactam.

*Renal function impairment* – In patients with renal impairment, give as follows:

| Ampicillin/Sulbactam Dosage Guide For Patients With Renal Impairment | | |
|---|---|---|
| Ccr (mL/min/1.72 m$^2$) | Half-life (h) | Recommended dosage |
| ≥ 30 | 1 | 1.5 to 3 g q 6 to 8 h |
| 15 to 29 | 5 | 1.5 to 3 g q 12 h |
| 5 to 14 | 9 | 1.5 to 3 g q 24 h |

*Children* – Do not routinely exceed 14 days of IV therapy. Safety and efficacy of IM administration have not been established.

*Children 1 year of age or older (less than 40 kg):* 300 mg/kg/day IV (200 mg ampicillin/ 100 mg sulbactam) in divided doses every 6 hours.

*Children 40 kg or more:* Dose according to adult recommendations; total sulbactam dose should not exceed 4 g/day.

The safety and efficacy of ampicillin/sulbactam sodium has not been established for pediatric patients for intra-abdominal infections.

CARBENICILLIN INDANYL SODIUM:
*Urinary tract infections –*
*Escherichia coli, Proteus species, and Enterobacter:* 382 to 764 mg 4 times daily.
*Pseudomonas and enterococci:* 764 mg 4 times daily.
*Prostatitis caused by E. coli, Proteus mirabilis, Enterobacter, and enterococcus (Streptococcus faecalis)* – 764 mg 4 times daily.

DICLOXACILLIN SODIUM:
*For mild to moderate upper respiratory and localized skin and soft tissue infections –*
*Adults and children (40 kg or more):* 125 mg every 6 hours.
*Children (less than 40 kg):* 12.5 mg/kg/day in equal doses every 6 hours.
*For more severe infections, such as lower respiratory tract or disseminated infections –*
*Adults and children (40 kg or more):* 250 mg every 6 hours.
*Children (less than 40 kg):* 25 mg/kg/day in equally divided doses every 6 hours.
Use in the newborn is not recommended.

NAFCILLIN SODIUM:
*Dose* – The usual IV dosage for adults is 500 mg every 4 hours. For severe infections, 1 g every 4 hours is recommended. Administer slowly over at least 30 to 60 minutes to minimize the risk of vein irritation and extravasation.

*Duration* – Duration of therapy varies with the type and severity of infection as well as the overall condition of the patient; therefore, determine duration by the clinical and bacteriological response of the patient. In severe staphylococcal infections, continue nafcillin therapy for at least 14 days. Continue therapy for at least 48 hours after the patient has become afebrile and asymptomatic and cultures are negative. The treatment of endocarditis and osteomyelitis may require a longer duration of therapy.

OXACILLIN SODIUM:

| Oxacillin Dosage | | |
|---|---|---|
| Indication | Adults | Children (< 40 kg) |
| Oral | | |
| Mild to moderate infection | 500 mg every 4 to 6 h | 50 mg/kg/day every 6 h |
| Severe infection | 1 g every 4 to 6 h (following parenteral therapy) | 100 mg/kg/day every 4 to 6 h (following parenteral therapy) |
| Parenteral (IM or IV) | | |
| Mild to moderate infection | 250 to 500 mg IM or IV every 4 to 6 h | 50 mg/kg/day IM or IV every 6 h |
| Severe infection | 1 g IM or IV every 4 to 6 h | 100 mg/kg/day IM or IV every 4 to 6 h. **Premature/Neonates:** 25 mg/kg/day IM or IV |

PENICILLIN G (AQUEOUS):
*Infants* – Preferably administered IV as 15- to 30-minute infusions.

*Older than 7 days of age:* 75,000 units/kg/day in divided doses every 8 hours (meningitis, 200,000 to 300,000 units/kg/day every 6 hours).

*Younger than 7 days of age:* 50,000 units/kg/day in divided doses every 12 hours (group B streptococcus, 100,000 units/kg/day; meningitis, 100,000 to 150,000 units/kg/day).

Administer penicillin G injection by IV infusion.

| Parenteral Penicillin G Use and Dosages in Adults | |
| --- | --- |
| Indications | Adult dosage |
| *Meningococcal meningitis/septicemia* | 24 million units/day; 1 to 2 million units IM every 2 h; or 20 to 30 million units/day continuous IV drip for 14 days or until afebrile for 7 days; or 200,000 to 300,000 units/kg/day every 2 to 4 h in divided doses for a total of 24 doses |
| *Actinomycosis:* | |
| For cervicofacial cases | 1 to 6 million units/day |
| For thoracic and abdominal disease | 10 to 20 million units/day IV every 4 to 6 h for 6 wk. May be followed by oral penicillin V, 500 mg 4 times daily for 2 to 3 mo |
| *Clostridial infections:* | |
| Botulism (adjunctive therapy to antitoxin), gas gangrene and tetanus (adjunctive therapy to human tetanus immune globulin) | 20 million units/day every 4 to 6 h as adjunct to antitoxin |
| *Fusospirochetal infections:* Severe infections of oropharynx, lower respiratory tract and genital area | 5 to 10 million units/day every 4 to 6 h |
| *Rat-bite fever (Spirillum minus, Streptobacillus moniliformis),* Haverhill fever | 12 to 20 million units/day every 4 to 6 h for 3 to 4 wk |
| *Listeria infections (Listeria monocytogenes):* | |
| Meningitis (adults) | 15 to 20 million units/day every 4 to 6 h for 2 wk |
| Endocarditis (adults) | 15 to 20 million units/day every 4 to 6 h for 4 wk |
| *Pasteurella infections (Pasteurella multocida):* Bacteremia and meningitis | 4 to 6 million units/day every 4 to 6 h for 2 wk |
| *Erysipeloid (Erysipelothrix rhusiopathiae):* Endocarditis | 12 to 20 million units/day every 4 to 6 h for 4 to 6 wk |
| *Diphtheria:* Adjunct to antitoxin to prevent carrier state | 2 to 3 million units/day in divided doses every 4 to 6 h for 10 to 12 days |
| *Anthrax: (Bacillus anthracis* is often resistant) | Minimum 5 million units/day; 12 to 20 million units/day have been used |
| *Serious streptococcal infections (S. pneumoniae):* | |
| Empyema, pneumonia, pericarditis, endocarditis, meningitis | 5 to 24 million units/day in divided doses every 4 to 6 h |
| *Syphilis:* | |
| Neurosyphilis | 18 to 24 million units/day IV (3 to 4 million units every 4 h) for 10 to 14 days. Many recommend benzathine penicillin G 2.4 million units/wk IM for 3 wk following the completion of this regimen |
| *Disseminated gonococcal infections:* (eg, meningitis, endocarditis, arthritis) | 10 million units/day every 4 to 6 h, with the exception of meningococcal meningitis/septicemia (ie, every 2 h) |

*Children –*

| Parenteral Penicillin G Use and Dosages in Children | |
| --- | --- |
| Indications | Pediatric dosage |
| *Serious streptococcal infections,* such as pneumonia and endocarditis (*S. pneumoniae*) and meningococcus | 150,000 units/kg/day divided in equal doses every 4 to 6 h |

| Parenteral Penicillin G Use and Dosages in Children ||
| Indications | Pediatric dosage |
|---|---|
| *Meningitis caused by susceptible strains of pneumococcus and meningococcus* | 250,000 units/kg/day divided in equal doses every 4 h for 7 to 14 days (maximum dose, 12 to 20 million units/day) |
| *Disseminated gonococcal infections (penicillin-susceptible strains):* | *Weight < 45 kg:* |
| Arthritis | 100,000 units/kg/day in 4 equally divided doses for 7 to 10 days |
| Meningitis | 250,000 units/kg/day in equal doses every 4 h for 10 to 14 days |
| Endocarditis | 250,000 units/kg/day in equal doses every 4 h for 4 wk |
| | *Weight ≥ 45 kg:* |
| Arthritis, meningitis, endocarditis | 10 million units/day in 4 equally divided doses |
| *Syphilis (congenital and neurosyphilis) after the newborn period:* | 200,000 to 300,000 units/kg/day (administered as 50,000 units/kg every 4 to 6 h) for 10 to 14 days |
| Congenital syphilis: Symptomatic or asymptomatic infants | *Infants:* 50,000 units/kg/dose IV every 12 h the first 7 days, thereafter every 8 h for total of 10 days. *Children:* 50,000 units/kg every 4 to 6 h for 10 days |
| *Diphtheria (adjunctive therapy to antitoxin and for prevention of carrier state)* | 150,000 to 250,000 units/kg/day every 6 h for 7 to 10 days |
| *Rat-bite fever; Haverhill fever (with endocarditis caused by S. moniliformis)* | 150,000 to 250,000 units/kg/day every 4 h for 4 wk |

PENICILLIN G BENZATHINE, IM: Administer by deep IM injection in the upper outer quadrant of the buttock. In neonates, infants, and small children, the midlateral aspect of the thigh may be preferable. When doses are repeated, rotate the injection site. Do not administer IV.

| Penicillin G Benzathine Uses and Dosages ||
| Organisms/Infections | Dosage |
|---|---|
| *Streptococcal (group A):* Upper respiratory tract infections | *Adults:* 1.2 million units IM as a single injection<br>*Older children:* 900,000 units IM as a single injection<br>*Infants and children (< 60 lbs; 27 kg):* 300,000 to 600,000 units |
| *Syphilis:*[1]<br>Early syphilis - Primary, secondary, or latent syphilis | *Adults:* 2.4 million units IM in single dose<br>*Children:* 50,000 units/kg IM, up to adult dosage |
| *Gummas and cardiovascular syphilis*[1] - Latent | *Adults:* 2.4 million units IM once/wk for 3 wk<br>*Children:* 50,000 units/kg IM, up to adult dosage |
| *Neurosyphilis*[1] | Aqueous penicillin G, 18 to 24 million units/day IV (3 to 4 million units every 4 h) for 10 to 14 days. Many recommend benzathine penicillin G, 2.4 million IM units once/wk for up to 3 wk following completion of this regimen.<br><br>or<br><br>Procaine penicillin G, 2.4 million units/day IM *plus* probenecid 500 mg orally 4 times/day, both for 10 to 14 days. Many recommend benzathine penicillin G, 2.4 million units IM once/wk for up to 3 wk following completion of this regimen. |
| *Syphilis in pregnancy*[1] | Dosage schedule appropriate for stage of syphilis recommended for nonpregnant patients. |
| *Congenital syphilis* | *Children < 2 years of age:* 50,000 units/kg/body weight<br>*Children 2 to 12 years of age:* Adjust dosage based on adult dosage schedule. |
| *Yaws, bejel, and pinta* | 1.2 million units IM in a single dose |

| Penicillin G Benzathine Uses and Dosages | |
|---|---|
| Organisms/Infections | Dosage |
| *Prophylaxis for rheumatic fever and glomerulonephritis* | Following an acute attack, may be given IM in doses of 1.2 million units once/mo or 600,000 units every 2 wk |

[1] CDC 2002 Sexually Transmitted Diseases Treatment Guidelines. MMWR Morbid Mortal Wkly Rept. 2002;51(RR-6):1-82.

*PENICILLIN G PROCAINE, IM:* Administer by deep IM injection only into the upper outer quadrant of the buttock. In infants and small children, the midlateral aspect of the thigh may be preferable. When doses are repeated, rotate the injection site. Do not administer IV.

*Newborns* – Avoid use in these patients because sterile abscesses and procaine toxicity are of much greater concern than in older children.

| Penicillin G Procaine Uses and Dosages | |
|---|---|
| Organisms/Infections | Dosage |
| *Pneumococcal infections:* Moderately severe upper respiratory tract infections | *Adults:* 600,000 to 1 million units/day IM<br>*Children (< 60 lbs, 27 kg):* 300,000 units/day IM |
| *Streptococcal infections* (group A): Moderately severe to severe tonsillitis, erysipelas, scarlet fever, upper respiratory tract, and skin and soft tissue infections | *Adults:* 600,000 to 1 million units/day IM for a minimum of 10 days<br>*Children (< 60 lbs, 27 kg):* 300,000 units/day IM |
| Bacterial endocarditis – Only in extremely sensitive infections (Group A streptococci) | 600,000 to 1 million units/day IM |
| *Staphylococcal infections:* Moderately severe infections of the skin and soft tissue | *Adults:* 600,000 to 1 million units/day IM<br>*Children (< 60 lbs, 27 kg):* 300,000 units/day |
| *Diphtheria:* Adjunctive therapy with antitoxin | 300,000 to 600,000 units/day IM for 14 days. |
| Carrier state | 300,000 units/day IM for 10 days |
| *Anthrax:* Cutaneous | 600,000 to 1 million units/day IM. Continue prophylaxis until exposure to *Bacillus anthracis* has been excluded. If exposure is confirmed and vaccine is available, continue prophylaxis for 4 weeks and until 3 doses of vaccine have been administered, or for 30 to 60 days if vaccine is not available. |
| *Vincent's gingivitis and pharyngitis* (fusospirochetosis) | 600,000 to 1 million units/day IM. Obtain necessary dental care in infections involving gum tissue. |
| *Erysipeloid* | 600,000 to 1 million units/day IM |
| *Rat-bite fever (Streptobacillus moniliformis* and *Spirillum minus)* | 600,000 to 1 million units/day IM |
| *Syphilis:* Primary, secondary, and latent with a negative spinal fluid (adults and children > 12 years of age) | 600,000 units/day IM for 8 days; total, 4.8 million units |
| *Late* (tertiary, neurosyphilis, and latent syphilis with positive spinal fluid examination or no spinal fluid examination) | 600,000 units/day IM for 10 to 15 days; total, 6 to 9 million units |
| *Neurosyphilis*[1] (as an alternative to the recommended regimen of penicillin G aqueous) | 2.4 million units/day IM plus probenecid 500 mg orally 4 times/day, both for 10 to 14 days; many recommend benzathine penicillin G 2.4 million/units IM following the completion of this regimen |
| *Congenital syphilis*[1] | *Children < 70 lb (32 kg):* 50,000 units/kg/day (administered as a single IM dose) for 10 to 14 days. |
| *Yaws, bejel, and pinta* | Treat same as syphilis in corresponding stage of disease |

[1] CDC 2002 Sexually Transmitted Diseases Treatment Guidelines. MMWR Morbid Mortal Wkly Rept. 2002;51(RR-6):1-82.

PENICILLIN G BENZATHINE AND PROCAINE COMBINED, IM: Administer by deep IM injection in the upper outer quadrant of the buttock. In infants, neonates, and small children, the midlateral aspect of the thigh may be preferable. When doses are repeated, rotate the injection site.

*Streptococcal infections* – Treatment with the recommended dosage is usually given in a single session using multiple IM sites when indicated. An alternative dosage schedule may be used, giving half the total dose on day 1 and half on day 3. This will also ensure adequate serum levels over a 10-day period; however, use only when the patient's cooperation can be ensured.

*Adults and children (more than 60 lbs; 27 kg):* 2.4 million units IM.

*Children (30 to 60 lbs; 14 to 27 kg):* 900,000 to 1.2 million units IM.

*Infants and children (less than 30 lbs; 14 kg):* 600,000 units IM.

*Pneumococcal infections (except pneumococcal meningitis)* –

*Children:* 600,000 units IM.

*Adults:* 1.2 million units IM. Repeat every 2 or 3 days until the patient has been afebrile for 48 hours.

PENICILLIN V (PHENOXYMETHYL PENICILLIN): 250 mg equals 400,000 units.

*Adults* – 125 to 500 mg 4 times/day; in renal impairment (Ccr less than or equal to 10 mL/min) - Do not exceed 250 mg every 6 hours.

*Children* – 25 to 50 mg/kg/day in divided doses every 6 to 8 hours.

| Penicillin V Uses and Dosages for Adults and Children > 12 Years of Age | |
| --- | --- |
| Organisms/Infections | Dosage |
| *Streptococcal infections:* Mild to moderately severe infections of the upper respiratory tract, including scarlet fever and mild erysipelas | 125 to 250 mg orally every 6 to 8 h for 10 days |
| Pharyngitis in children | 25 to 50 mg/kg/day divided every 6 h for 10 days |
| *Pneumococcal infections:* Mild to moderately severe respiratory tract infections including otitis media | 250 to 500 mg orally every 6 h until afebrile at least 2 days |
| *Staphylococcal infections:* Mild infections of skin and soft tissue | 250 to 500 mg orally every 6 to 8 h |
| *Fusospirochetosis (Vincent's infection)* of the oropharynx: Mild to moderately severe infections | 250 to 500 mg orally every 6 to 8 h |
| *For prevention of recurrence following rheumatic fever or chorea* | 125 to 250 mg orally 2 times/day on a continuing basis |

PIPERACILLIN SODIUM: Administer IM or IV. For serious infections, give 3 to 4 g every 4 to 6 hours as a 20- to 30-minute IV infusion. Maximum daily dose is 24 g/ day, although higher doses have been used. Limit IM injections to 2 g/site.

*Hemodialysis* – Maximum dose is 6 g/day (2 g every 8 hours). Hemodialysis removes 30% to 50% of piperacillin in 4 hours; administer an additional 1 g after dialysis.

*Renal failure and hepatic insufficiency* – Measure serum levels to provide additional guidance for adjusting dosage; however, this may not be practical.

*Infants and children younger than 12 years of age* – Dosages have not been established; however, the following doses have been suggested:

*Neonates:*

Less than 36 weeks of age – 75 mg/kg IV every 12 hours in the first week of life, then every 8 hours in the second week.

Full-term – 75 mg/kg IV every 8 hours the first week of life, then every 6 hours thereafter.

Other conditions, 200 to 300 mg/kg/day, up to a maximum of 24 g/day divided every 4 to 6 hours.

| Piperacillin Uses and Dosages | |
|---|---|
| Organisms/Infections | Dosage |
| *Serious infections:* Septicemia, nosocomial pneumonia, intra-abdominal infections, aerobic and anaerobic gynecologic infections, and skin and soft tissue infections: | 12 to 18 g/day IV (200 to 300 mg/kg/day) in divided doses every 4 to 6 h |
| Renal impairment – Ccr | |
| 20 to 40 mL/min | 12 g/day; 4 g every 8 h |
| < 20 mL/min | 8 g/day; 4 g every 12 h |
| *Urinary tract infections:* Complicated (normal renal function) | 8 to 16 g/day IV (125 to 200 mg/kg/day) in divided doses every 6 to 8 h |
| Renal impairment – Ccr | |
| 20 to 40 mL/min | 9 g/day; 3 g every 8 h |
| < 20 mL/min | 6 g/day; 3 g every 12 h |
| Uncomplicated UTI and most community-acquired pneumonia (normal renal function) | 6 to 8 g/day IM or IV (100 to 125 mg/kg/day) in divided doses every 6 to 12 h |
| Uncomplicated UTI with renal impairment – Ccr | |
| < 20 mL/min | 6 g/day; 3 g every 12 h |
| *Uncomplicated gonorrhea infections* | 2 g IM in a single dose with 1 g probenecid ½ h prior to injection |
| *Prophylaxis:* Intra-abdominal surgery | 2 g IV just prior to anesthesia; 2 g during surgery; 2 g every 6 h post-op for no more than 24 h |
| Vaginal hysterectomy | 2 g IV just prior to anesthesia; 2 g 6 h after initial dose; 2 g 12 h after first dose |
| Cesarean section | 2 g IV after cord is clamped; 2 g 4 h after initial dose; 2 g 8 h after first dose |
| Abdominal hysterectomy | 2 g IV just prior to anesthesia; 2 g on return to recovery room; 2 g after 6 h |

PIPERACILLIN SODIUM AND TAZOBACTAM SODIUM: Administer by IV infusion over 30 minutes. The usual total daily dose for adults is 12 g/1.5 g, given as 3.375 g every 6 hours.

*Nosocomial pneumonia* – Start with 3.375 g every 4 hours plus an aminoglycoside. Continue the aminoglycoside in patients from whom *Pseudomonas aeruginosa* is isolated.

| Piperacillin Sodium and Tazobactam Sodium Dosage Recommendations | |
|---|---|
| Ccr (mL/min) | Recommended dosage regimen |
| > 40 | 12 g/1.5 g/day in divided doses of 3.375 g every 6 h |
| 20 to 40 | 8 g/1 g/day in divided doses of 2.25 g every 6 h |
| < 20 | 6 g/0.75 g/day in divided doses of 2.25 g every 8 h |

*Hemodialysis* – The maximum dose is 2.25 g every 8 hours. In addition, because hemodialysis removes 30% to 40% of a dose in 4 hours, give 1 additional dose of 0.75 g following each dialysis period.

TICARCILLIN DISODIUM: Use IV therapy in higher doses in serious urinary tract and systemic infections. IM injections should not exceed 2 g/injection. Adjust dose in renal dysfunction.

| Ticarcillin Uses and Dosages | |
|---|---|
| Organisms/Infections | Dosage |
| *Bacterial septicemia, respiratory tract infections, skin and soft tissue infections, intra-abdominal infections and infections of the female pelvis and genital tract* | *Adults:* 200 to 300 mg/kg/day by IV infusion in divided doses every 4 or 6 h (3 g every 4 h or 4 g every 6 h), depending on severity of infection<br>*Children (< 40 kg):* 200 to 300 mg/kg/day by IV infusion in divided doses every 4 or 6 h[1] |

| Ticarcillin Uses and Dosages | |
|---|---|
| Organisms/Infections | Dosage |
| *Urinary tract infections:* Complicated infections | *Adults and children:* 150 to 200 mg/kg/day IV infusion in divided doses every 4 or 6 h. |
| Uncomplicated infections | *Adults:* 1 g IM or direct IV every 6 h<br>*Children (< 40 kg):* 50 to 100 mg/kg/day IM or direct IV in divided doses every 6 or 8 h |
| *Neonates:* Severe infections (sepsis) caused by susceptible strains of *Pseudomonas* sp., *Proteus* sp., and *E. coli* | Give IM or by 10- to 20-min IV infusions. |
| < 2 kg | *< 7 days* – 75 mg/kg/12 h (150 mg/kg/day)<br>*> 7 days* – 75 mg/kg/8 h (225 mg/kg/day) |
| > 2 kg | *< 7 days* – 75 mg/kg/8 h (225 mg/kg/day)<br>*> 7 days* – 100 mg/kg/8 h (300 mg/kg/day) |

[1] Daily dose for children should not exceed adult dosage.

*Renal function impairment –*

| Dosage Adjustments of Ticarcillin in Renal Insufficiency | |
|---|---|
| Organisms/Infections | Dosage |
| *Dosage in renal insufficiency*[1] | Initial loading dose of 3 g IV, then base IV doses on Ccr and type of dialysis |
| Ccr (mL/min) – | |
| > 60 | 3 g every 4 h |
| 30 to 60 | 2 g every 4 h |
| 10 to 30 | 2 g every 8 h |
| < 10 | 2 g every 12 h or 1 g IM every 6 h |
| < 10 with hepatic dysfunction | 2 g every 24 h or 1 g IM every 12 h |
| Patients on peritoneal dialysis | 3 g every 12 h |
| Patients on hemodialysis | 2 g every 12 h and 3 g after each dialysis |

[1] Half-life in patients with renal failure is approximately 13 hours.

*TICARCILLIN AND CLAVULANATE POTASSIUM:* Administer by IV infusion over 30 minutes.

*Adults –*

| Ticarcillin/Clavulanate Potassium Administration in Adults | | | |
|---|---|---|---|
| | Systemic and urinary tract infections | Gynecological infections | |
| | | Moderate | Severe |
| Adults ≥ 60 kg | 3.1 g every 4 to 6 h | 200 mg/kg/day every 6 h | 300 mg/kg/day every 4 h |
| Adults < 60 kg | 200 to 300 mg/kg/day every 4 to 6 h | | |

*Children –*

| Dosage Guidelines for Ticarcillin/Clavulanate Potassium in Children ≥ 3 months of age | | |
|---|---|---|
| | Mild to moderate infections | Severe infections |
| Children ≥ 60 kg | 3.1 g every 6 h | 3.1 g every 4 h |
| Children < 60 kg (dosed at 50 mg/kg/dose) | 200 mg/kg/day every 6 h | 300 mg/kg/day every 4 h |

*Renal function impairment –*

| Dosage of Ticarcillin/Clavulanate Potassium in Renal Insufficiency[1] | |
|---|---|
| Ccr (mL/min) | Dosage |
| > 60 | 3.1 g every 4 h |
| 30 to 60 | 2 g every 4 h |
| 10 to 30 | 2 g every 8 h |
| < 10 | 2 g every 12 h |
| < 10 with hepatic dysfunction | 2 g every 24 h |
| Patients on peritoneal dialysis | 3.1 g every 12 h |

| Dosage of Ticarcillin/Clavulanate Potassium in Renal Insufficiency[1] ||
| Ccr (mL/min) | Dosage |
| --- | --- |
| Patients on hemodialysis | 2 g every 12 h supplemented with 3.1 g after each dialysis |

[1] Initial loading dose is 3.1 g. Follow with doses based on Ccr and type of dialysis.

## Actions

*Pharmacology:* Penicillins inhibit the biosynthesis of cell wall mucopeptide. They are bactericidal against sensitive organisms when adequate concentrations are reached and most effective during the stage of active multiplication. Inadequate concentrations may produce only bacteriostatic effects.

| Penicillins ||||||
| | Routes of administration | Penicillinase-resistant | Acid stable | % Protein bound | May be taken with meals |
| --- | --- | --- | --- | --- | --- |
| *Natural penicillins* ||||||
| Penicillin G | IM-IV | no | †[1] | 60 | †[1] |
| Penicillin V | Oral | no | yes | 80 | yes |
| *Penicillinase-resistant* ||||||
| Dicloxacillin | Oral | yes | yes | 98 | no |
| Nafcillin | IM-IV-Oral | yes | yes | 87 to 90 | no |
| Oxacillin | IM-IV-Oral | yes | yes | 94 | no |
| *Aminopenicillins* ||||||
| Amoxicillin | Oral | no | yes | 20 | yes |
| Amoxicillin/ potassium clavulanate | Oral | yes | yes | 18/25 | yes |
| Ampicillin | IM-IV-Oral | no | yes | 20 | no |
| Ampicillin/ sulbactam | IM-IV | yes | †[1] | 28/38 | †[1] |
| *Extended-spectrum* ||||||
| Carbenicillin | Oral | no | yes | 50 | no |
| Piperacillin | IM-IV | no | †[1] | 16 | †[1] |
| Piperacillin/ Tazobactam sodium | IV | yes | †[1] | 30/30 | †[1] |
| Ticarcillin | IM-IV | no | †[1] | 45 | †[1] |
| Ticarcillin/ Potassium clavulanate | IV | yes | †[1] | 45/9 | †[1] |

[1] Available only for IM or IV use.

*Pharmacokinetics:*

*Absorption* – Peak serum levels occur approximately 1 hour after oral use. Parenteral **penicillin G** (sodium and potassium) gives rapid and high but transient blood levels; derivatives provide prolonged penicillin blood levels with IM use.

*Distribution* – Penicillins are bound to plasma proteins, primarily albumin, in varying degrees. They diffuse readily into most body tissues and fluids.

*Excretion* – Penicillins are excreted largely unchanged in the urine by glomerular filtration and active tubular secretion. Nonrenal elimination includes hepatic inactivation and excretion in bile; this is only a minor route for all penicillins except **nafcillin** and **oxacillin**. Excretion by renal tubular secretion can be delayed by coadministration of probenecid. Elimination half-life of most penicillins is short (no more than 1.5 hours). Impaired renal function prolongs the serum half-life of penicillins eliminated primarily by renal excretion.

## Contraindications

History of hypersensitivity to penicillins, cephalosporins, or imipenem.

Do not treat severe pneumonia, empyema, bacteremia, pericarditis, meningitis, or purulent or septic arthritis with an oral penicillin during the acute stage.

### Warnings

*Bleeding abnormalities:* **Ticarcillin** or **piperacillin** may induce hemorrhagic manifestations associated with abnormalities of coagulation tests.

*Cystic fibrosis:* Cystic fibrosis patients have a higher incidence of side effects (eg, fever, rash) when treated with extended-spectrum penicillins (eg, **piperacillin, carbenicillin**).

*Hypersensitivity reactions:* Serious and occasionally fatal immediate-hypersensitivity reactions have occurred. The incidence of anaphylactic shock is between 0.015% and 0.04%. Anaphylactic shock resulting in death has occurred in approximately 0.002% of the patients treated. These reactions are likely to be immediate and severe in penicillin-sensitive individuals with a history of atopic conditions.

*Hypersensitivity myocarditis* – Hypersensitivity myocarditis is not dose-dependent and may occur at any time during treatment.

An urticarial rash, not representing a true penicillin allergy, occasionally occurs with **ampicillin** (9%). Typically, the rash appears 7 to 10 days after the start of oral ampicillin therapy and remains for a few days to a week after drug discontinuance. In most cases, the rash is maculopapular, pruritic, and generalized.

*Desensitization:* Patients with a positive skin test to one of the penicillin determinants can be desensitized, a relatively safe procedure. This is recommended in instances when penicillin must be given where no proven alternatives exist.

*Cross-allergenicity with cephalosporins:* Individuals with a history of penicillin hypersensitivity have experienced severe reactions when treated with a cephalosporin. The incidence of cross-allergenicity between penicillins and cephalosporins is estimated to range from 5% to 16%; however, it is possible the incidence is much lower, possibly 3% to 7%.

*Renal function impairment:* Because **carbenicillin** is primarily excreted by the kidney, patients with severe renal impairment (Ccr less than 10 mL/min) will not achieve the therapeutic urine levels of carbenicillin. In patients with Ccr 10 to 20 mL/min, it may be necessary to adjust dosage to prevent accumulation of the drug.

*Pregnancy: Category B.* Penicillins cross the placenta.

*Lactation:* Penicillins are excreted in breast milk in low concentrations; use may cause diarrhea, candidiasis, or allergic response in the nursing infant.

*Children:* Safety and efficacy of **carbenicillin, piperacillin**, and the β-lactamase inhibitor/penicillin combinations have not been established in infants and children younger than 12 years of age. Use caution in administering to newborns and evaluate organ system function frequently.

### Precautions

*Monitoring:* Obtain blood cultures, white blood cell, and differential cell counts prior to initiation of therapy and at least weekly during therapy with penicillinase-resistant penicillins. Measure AST and ALT during therapy to monitor for liver function abnormalities.

Perform periodic urinalysis, BUN, and creatinine determinations during therapy with penicillinase-resistant penicillins, and consider dosage alterations if these values become elevated.

Monitoring is particularly important in newborns and infants and when high dosages are used.

*Streptococcal infections:* Therapy must be sufficient to eliminate the organism (minimum, 10 days); otherwise, sequelae (eg, endocarditis, rheumatic fever) may occur.

*Sexually transmitted diseases:* When treating gonococcal infections in which primary and secondary syphilis are suspected, perform proper diagnostic procedures, including darkfield examinations and monthly serological tests for at least 4 months.

*Resistance:* The number of strains of staphylococci resistant to penicillinase-resistant penicillins has been increasing; widespread use of penicillinase-resistant penicillins may result in an increasing number of resistant staphylococcal strains.

*Pseudomembranous colitis:* Pseudomembranous colitis has occurred with the use of broad-spectrum antibiotics caused by overgrowth of clostridia; therefore, it is important to consider its diagnosis in patients who develop diarrhea in association with antibiotic use.

*Procaine sensitivity:* If sensitivity to the procaine in **penicillin G procaine** is suspected, inject 0.1 mL of a 1% to 2% procaine solution intradermally. Development of erythema, wheal, flare, or eruption indicates procaine sensitivity; treat by the usual methods.

*Parenteral administration:* Inadvertent intravascular administration, including direct intra-arterial injection or injection immediately adjacent to arteries, has resulted in severe neurovascular damage, including transverse myelitis with permanent paralysis, gangrene requiring amputation of digits and more proximal portions of extremities, and necrosis and sloughing at and surrounding the injection site.

*Electrolyte imbalance:* Patients given continuous IV therapy with **potassium penicillin G** in high dosage (more than 10 million units daily) may suffer severe or even fatal potassium poisoning particularly if renal insufficiency is present. High dosage of **sodium salts of penicillins** may result in or aggravate CHF caused by high sodium intake. Individuals with liver disease or those receiving cytotoxic therapy or diuretics rarely demonstrated a decrease in serum potassium concentrations with high doses of **piperacillin**. **Sodium penicillin G** contains 2 mEq sodium per million units, **potassium penicillin G** contains 1.7 mEq potassium and 0.3 mEq sodium per million units. The sodium content of other IV penicillin derivatives is listed below:

| Sodium Content of IV Penicillins | | | |
| --- | --- | --- | --- |
| Penicillin | Maximum recommended daily dose (g) | Sodium content (mEq/g)[1] | Sodium (mEq/day)[1,2] |
| Ampicillin sodium | 14 | 2.9 to 3.1 | 40.6 to 43.4 |
| Nafcillin sodium | 6 | 2.9 | 17.4 |
| Oxacillin sodium | 6 | 2.5 to 3.1 | 15 to 18.6 |
| Piperacillin sodium | 24 | 1.85 | 44.4 |
| Piperacillin/Tazobactam sodium | 12 | 2.35 | 28.2 |
| Ticarcillin disodium | 18 | 5.2 to 6.5 | 93.6 to 117 |

[1] 1 mEq sodium equals 23 mg.
[2] Based on maximum daily dose.

*Hypokalemia* – Hypokalemia has occurred in a few patients receiving **ticarcillin** and **piperacillin**.

**Drug Interactions**
Drugs that may affect penicillins include allopurinol, aminoglycosides (parenteral), aspirin, beta blockers, chloramphenicol, erythromycin, ethacrynic acid, furosemide, indomethacin, phenylbutazone, probenecid, sulfonamides, tetracycline, and thiazide diuretics. Drugs that may be affected by penicillins include aminoglycosides (parenteral), anticoagulants, beta blockers, chloramphenicol, cyclosporine, oral contraceptives, erythromycin, heparin, and vecuronium.

*Drug/Lab test interactions:* False-positive **urine glucose** reactions may occur with penicillin therapy if *Clinitest, Benedict's Solution,* or *Fehling's Solution* are used. It is recommended that enzymatic glucose oxidase tests (such as *Clinistix* or *Tes-Tape*) be used. Positive Coombs' tests have occurred. High urine concentrations of some penicillins may produce false-positive protein reactions (pseudoproteinuria) with the following methods: Sulfosalicylic acid and boiling test, acetic acid test, biuret reaction, and nitric acid test. The bromphenol blue (*Multi-Stix*) reagent strip test has been reported to be reliable.

*Drug/Food interactions:* Absorption of most penicillins is affected by food; these medications are best taken on an empty stomach, 1 hour before or 2 hours after meals. **Penicillin V** may be given with meals; however, blood levels may be slightly higher when taken on an empty stomach. **Amoxicillin** and **amoxicillin/potassium clavulanate** tablets may be given without regard to meals.

## Adverse Reactions

*CNS:* Penicillins have caused neurotoxicity (manifested as lethargy, neuromuscular irritability, hallucinations, convulsions, and seizures) when given in large IV doses, especially in patients with renal failure.

*GI:* Glossitis; stomatitis; gastritis; sore mouth or tongue; dry mouth; furry tongue; black "hairy" tongue; abnormal taste sensation; nausea; vomiting; abdominal pain or cramp; epigastric distress; diarrhea or bloody diarrhea; rectal bleeding; flatulence; enterocolitis; pseudomembranous colitis.

*Hematologic/Lymphatic:* Anemia; hemolytic anemia; thrombocytopenia; thrombocytopenic purpura; eosinophilia; leukopenia; granulocytopenia; neutropenia; bone marrow depression; agranulocytosis; reduction of hemoglobin or hematocrit; prolongation of bleeding and prothrombin time; decrease in WBC and lymphocyte counts; increase in lymphocytes, monocytes, basophils, and platelets.

*Hypersensitivity:* Adverse reactions (estimated incidence, 1% to 10%) are more likely to occur in individuals with previously demonstrated hypersensitivity. In penicillin-sensitive individuals with a history of allergy, asthma, or hay fever, the reactions may be immediate and severe.

Allergic symptoms include urticaria; angioneurotic edema; laryngospasm; bronchospasm; hypotension; vascular collapse; death; maculopapular to exfoliative dermatitis; vesicular eruptions; erythema multiforme; reactions resembling serum sickness (eg, chills, fever, edema, arthralgia, arthritis, malaise); laryngeal edema; skin rashes; prostration.

*Lab test abnormalities:* Elevations of AST, ALT, bilirubin, and LDH have been noted in patients receiving semisynthetic penicillins (particularly **oxacillin**); such reactions are more common in infants. Elevations of serum alkaline phosphatase and hypernatremia and reduction in serum potassium, albumin, total proteins, and uric acid may occur.

*Local:* Pain (accompanied by induration) at the site of injection; ecchymosis; deep vein thrombosis; hematomas.

*Miscellaneous:* Vaginitis and anorexia.

# CEPHALOSPORINS AND RELATED ANTIBIOTICS

**CEFACLOR**
**Capsules**: 250 and 500 mg (*Rx*) — Various, *Ceclor Pulvules* (Eli Lilly)
**Powder for oral suspension**: 125, 187, 250, and 375 mg/5 mL (*Rx*) — Various, *Ceclor* (Eli Lilly)

**CEFADROXIL**
**Capsules**: 500 mg (as monohydrate) (*Rx*) — Various, *Duricef* (Bristol-Myers Squibb)
**Tablets**: 1 g (as monohydrate) (*Rx*) — Various, *Duricef* (Bristol-Myers Squibb)
**Powder for oral suspension**: 125, 250, and 500 mg/5 mL (*Rx*) — Various, *Duricef* (Bristol-Myers Squibb)

**CEFAZOLIN SODIUM**
**Powder for injection**: 250 and 500 mg, 1, 5, 10, and 20 g (*Rx*) — Various, *Ancef* (SmithKline Beecham), *Zolicef* (Apothecon)
**Injection**: 500 mg or 1 g (*Rx*) — *Ancef* (GlaxoSmithKline), *Kefzol* (Eli Lilly)

**CEFDINIR**
**Capsules**: 300 mg (*Rx*) — *Omnicef* (Abbott)
**Oral suspension**: 125 mg and 5 mL, 250 mg per 5 mL (*Rx*) — *Omnicef* (Abbott)

**CEFDITOREN PIVOXIL**
**Tablets**: 200 mg (*Rx*) — *Spectracef* (TAP Pharm.)

**CEFEPIME HCl**
**Powder for injection**: 500 mg, 1 and 2 g (*Rx*) — *Maxipime* (Dura)

**CEFMETAZOLE SODIUM**
**Powder for injection**: 1 and 2 g (*Rx*) — *Zefazone* (Pharmacia)
**Injection**: 1 and 2 g/50 mL (*Rx*) — *Zefazone* (Pharmacia)

**CEFOPERAZONE SODIUM**
**Powder for injection**: 1 and 2 g (*Rx*) — *Cefobid* (Roerig)
**Injection**: 1, 2, and 10 g (*Rx*) — *Cefobid* (Roerig)

**CEFOTAXIME SODIUM**
**Powder for injection**: 500 mg, 1, 2, and 10 g (*Rx*) — *Claforan* (Aventis)
**Injection**: 1 and 2 g (*Rx*) — *Claforan* (Aventis)

**CEFOTETAN DISODIUM**
**Powder for injection**: 1, 2, and 10 g (*Rx*) — *Cefotan* (AstraZeneca)
**Injection**: 1 and 2 g/50 mL (*Rx*) — *Cefotan* (AstraZeneca)

**CEFOXITIN SODIUM**
**Powder for injection**: 1, 2, and 10 g (*Rx*) — *Mefoxin* (Merck)
**Injection**: 1 and 2 g (*Rx*) — *Mefoxin* (Merck)

**CEFPODOXIME PROXETIL**
**Tablets**: 100 and 200 mg (*Rx*) — *Vantin* (Pharmacia)
**Granules for suspension**: 50 and 100 mg/5 mL (*Rx*) — *Vantin* (Pharmacia)

**CEFPROZIL**
**Tablets**: 250 and 500 mg (as anhydrous) (*Rx*) — *Cefzil* (Bristol-Myers Squibb)
**Powder for oral suspension**: 125 and 250 mg (as anhydrous)/5 mL (*Rx*) — *Cefzil* (Bristol-Myers Squibb)

**CEFTAZIDIME**
**Powder for injection**: 500 mg, 1, 2, and 6 g (*Rx*) — *Fortaz* (GlaxoSmithKline), *Tazidime* (Eli Lilly), *Ceptaz* (GlaxoSmithKline), *Tazicef* (GlaxoSmithKline/Bristol-Myers Squibb)
**Injection**: 1 and 2 g (*Rx*) — *Fortaz* (GlaxoSmithKline), *Tazicef* (GlaxoSmithKline/Bristol-Myers Squibb)

**CEFTIBUTEN**
**Capsules**: 400 mg (*Rx*) — *Cedax* (Schering-Plough)
**Powder for oral suspension**: 90 mg per 5 mL (*Rx*) — *Cedax* (Schering-Plough)

**CEFTIZOXIME SODIUM**
**Powder for injection**: 500 mg, 1, 2, and 10 g (as sodium) (*Rx*) — *Cefizox* (Fujisawa)
**Injection**: 1 and 2 g (as sodium) (*Rx*) — *Cefizox* (Fujisawa)

**CEFTRIAXONE SODIUM**
**Powder for injection**: 250 and 500 mg, 1, 2, and 10 g (*Rx*) — *Rocephin* (Roche)
**Injection**: 1 and 2 g (*Rx*) — *Rocephin* (Roche)

| | |
|---|---|
| **CEFUROXIME** | |
| **Tablets**: 125, 250, and 500 mg (*Rx*) | *Ceftin* (GlaxoSmithKline) |
| **Suspension**: 125 and 250 mg (as axetil)/5 mL (when reconstituted) (*Rx*) | *Ceftin* (GlaxoSmithKline) |
| **Powder for injection**: 750 mg, 1.5 and 7.5 g (as sodium)/vial (*Rx*) | Various, *Zinacef* (GlaxoSmithKline), *Kefurox* (Lilly) |
| **Injection**: 750 mg and 1.5 g (as sodium) (*Rx*) | *Zinacef* (GlaxoSmithKline) |
| **CEPHALEXIN** | |
| **Capsules**: 250 and 500 mg (*Rx*) | Various, *Keflex* (Dista), *Biocef* (Inter Ethical Labs) |
| **Tablets**: 250 and 500 mg and 1 g (*Rx*) | Various |
| **Powder for oral suspension**: 125 and 250 mg/5 mL (*Rx*) | Various, *Biocef* (Inter. Ethical Labs), *Keflex* (Dista) |
| **CEPHALEXIN HCl MONOHYDRATE** | |
| **Tablets**: 500 mg (*Rx*) | *Keftab* (Dista) |
| **CEPHRADINE** | |
| **Capsules**: 250 and 500 mg (*Rx*) | Various, *Velosef* (Bristol-Myers Squibb) |
| **Powder for oral suspension**: 125 and 250 mg/5 mL (when reconstituted) (*Rx*) | Various, *Velosef* (Bristol-Myers Squibb) |
| **LORACARBEF** | |
| **Pulvules (capsules)**: 200 and 400 mg (*Rx*) | *Lorabid* (Eli Lilly) |
| **Powder for oral suspension**: 100 and 200 mg/5 mL (*Rx*) | *Lorabid* (Eli Lilly) |

### Indications
For approved indications, refer to the Administration and Dosage section.

### Administration and Dosage
*Duration of therapy:* Continue administration for a minimum of 48 to 72 hours after fever abates or after evidence of bacterial eradication has been obtained.

*Perioperative prophylaxis:* Discontinue prophylactic use within 24 hours after the surgical procedure. In surgery where infection may be particularly devastating, prophylactic use may be continued for 3 to 5 days following surgery completion.

CEFACLOR:

    *Adults* – Usual dosage is 250 mg every 8 hours. In severe infections or those caused by less susceptible organisms, dosage may be doubled.

        *Capsules:* Food does not affect the extent of absorption.

        *Tablets, extended release:* Administer with food to enhance absorption. Do not cut, crush, or chew.

            *Acute bacterial exacerbations of chronic bronchitis* – 500 mg/12 hours for 7 days.
            *Secondary bacterial infection of acute bronchitis* – 500 mg/12 hours for 7 days.
            *Pharyngitis or tonsillitis* – 375 mg/12 hours for 10 days.
            *Uncomplicated skin and skin structure infections* – 375 mg/12 hours for 7 to 10 days.

    *Children* – Give 20 mg/kg/day in divided doses, every 8 hours. In more serious infections, otitis media, and infections caused by less susceptible organisms, administer 40 mg/kg/day, with a maximum dosage of 1 g/day.

    *Twice-daily treatment option:* For otitis media and pharyngitis, the total daily dosage may be divided and administered every 12 hours.

CEFADROXIL: Can be given without regard to meals.

    *Urinary tract infections* – For uncomplicated lower urinary tract infection (eg, cystitis), the usual dosage is 1 or 2 g/day in single or 2 divided doses. For all other urinary tract infections, the usual dosage is 2 g/day in 2 divided doses.

    *Skin and skin structure infections* – 1 g/day in single or 2 divided doses.

    *Pharyngitis and tonsillitis* –

        *Group A β-hemolytic streptococci:* 1 g/day in single or 2 divided doses for 10 days.

    *Children* –

        *Urinary tract infections, skin and skin structure infections:* 30 mg/kg/day in divided doses every 12 hours.

        *Pharyngitis, tonsillitis:* 30 mg/kg/day in single or 2 divided doses. For β-hemolytic streptococcal infections, continue treatment for at least 10 days.

*Renal impairment* – Adjust dosage according to Ccr rates to prevent drug accumulation.

*Initial adult dose:* 1 g: The maintenance dose (based on Ccr rate, mL/min/1.73 m$^2$) is 500 mg at the intervals below:

| Cefadroxil Dosage in Renal Impairment | |
|---|---|
| Ccr (mL/min) | Dosage interval (hours) |
| 0 to 10 | 36 |
| 10 to 25 | 24 |
| 25 to 50 | 12 |
| > 50 | No adjustment |

CEFAZOLIN SODIUM: Total daily dosages are the same for IM and IV administration.

*Mild infections caused by susceptible gram-positive cocci* – 250 to 500 mg every 8 hours.

*Moderate-to-severe infections* – 500 mg to 1 g every 6 to 8 hours.

*Pneumococcal pneumonia* – 500 mg every 12 hours.

*Severe, life-threatening infections (eg, endocarditis, septicemia)* – 1 to 1.5 g every 6 hours. Rarely, 12 g/day have been used.

*Acute uncomplicated urinary tract infections* – 1 g every 12 hours.

*Perioperative prophylaxis* –

*Preoperative:* 1 g IV or IM, ½ to 1 hour prior to surgery.

*Intraoperative (at least 2 h):* 0.5 to 1 g IV or IM during surgery at appropriate intervals.

*Postoperative:* 0.5 to 1 g IV or IM every 6 to 8 hours for 24 hours after surgery.

*Renal function impairment* – All reduced dosage recommendations apply after an initial loading dose appropriate to the severity of the infection.

| Cefazolin Dosage in Renal Impairment | | Dose | | Dosage interval (h) |
|---|---|---|---|---|
| Serum Creatinine (mg %) | Ccr (mL/min) | ≤ 1.5 | ≥ 55 | |
| ≤ 1.5 | ≥ 55 | 250 to 500 | 500 to 1000 | 6 to 8 |
| 1.6 to 3 | 35 to 54 | 250 to 500 | 500 to 1000 | ≥ 8 |
| 3.1 to 4.5 | 11 to 34 | 125 to 250 | 250 to 500 | 12 |
| ≥ 4.6 | ≤ 10 | 125 to 250 | 250 to 500 | 18 to 24 |

*Children* –

*Mild to moderately severe infections:* A total daily dosage of 25 to 50 mg/kg (approximately 10 to 20 mg/lb) in 3 or 4 equal doses.

*Severe infections:* Total daily dosage may be increased to 100 mg/kg (45 mg/lb).

CEFDINIR:

*Adults/Adolescents* – Capsules may be taken without regard to meals.

| Cefdinir Dosage in Adults and Adolescents (≥ 13 years of age) | | |
|---|---|---|
| Type of infection | Dosage | Duration |
| Community-acquired pneumonia | 300 mg q 12 h | 10 days |
| Acute exacerbations of chronic bronchitis | 300 mg q 12 h *or* 600 mg q 24 h | 5 to 10 days / 10 days |
| Acute maxillary sinusitis | 300 mg q 12 h *or* 600 mg q 24 h | 10 days / 10 days |
| Pharyngitis/Tonsillitis | 300 mg q 12 h *or* 600 mg q 24 h | 5 to 10 days / 10 days |
| Uncomplicated skin and skin structure infections | 300 mg q 12 h | 10 days |

*Children (6 months to 12 years of age)* –

*Powder for oral suspension:* The recommended dosage in pediatric patients is 14 mg/kg, up to a maximum dose of 600 mg/day. Once daily dosing for 10 days is as effective as twice-daily dosing. Once-daily dosing has not been studied in skin infections; therefore, administer oral suspension twice daily in this infection. Oral suspension may be administered without regard to meals.

| Cefdinir Dosage in Pediatric Patients (6 Months Through 12 Years of Age) | | |
|---|---|---|
| Type of infection | Dosage | Duration |
| Acute bacterial otitis media | 7 mg/kg q 12 h<br>or<br>14 mg/kg q 24 h | 5 to 10 days<br><br>10 days |
| Acute maxillary sinusitis | 7 mg/kg q 12 h<br>or<br>14 mg/kg q 24 h | 10 days<br><br>10 days |
| Pharyngitis/Tonsillitis | 7 mg/kg q 12 h<br>or<br>14 mg/kg q 24 h | 5 to 10 days<br><br>10 days |
| Uncomplicated skin and skin structure infections | 7 mg/kg q 12 h | 10 days |

| Cefdinir for Oral Suspension Pediatric Dosage Chart | | | | |
|---|---|---|---|---|
| Weight | | 125 mg per 5 mL | 250 mg per 5 mL | |
| kg | lb | | | |
| 9 | 20 | 2.5 mL (½ tsp) q 12 h<br>or 5 mL (1 tsp) q 24 h | use 125 mg per 5 mL product | |
| 18 | 40 | 5 mL (1 tsp) q 12 h<br>or 10 mL (2 tsp) q 24 h | 2.5 mL q 12 h or<br>5 mL q 24 h | |
| 27 | 60 | 7.5 mL (1½ tsp) q 12 h<br>or 15 mL (3 tsp) q 24 h | 3.75 mL q 12 h or<br>7.5 mL q 24 h | |
| 36 | 80 | 10 mL (2 tsp) q 12 h<br>or 20 mL (4 tsp) q 24 h | 5 mL q 12 h or<br>10 mL q 24 h | |
| ≥ 43[a] | 95 | 12 mL (2½ tsp) q 12 h<br>or 24 mL (5 tsp) q 24 h | 6 mL q 12 h or<br>12 mL q 24 h | |

[a] Pediatric patients who weigh at least 43 kg should receive the maximum daily dose of 600 mg.

*Renal function impairment* – For adult patients with Ccr less than 30 mL/min, the dose of cefdinir should be 300 mg given once daily.

For pediatric patients with a Ccr of less than 30 mL/min/1.73 $m^2$, the dose of cefdinir should be 7 mg/kg (less than or equal to 300 mg) given once daily.

*Hemodialysis* – Hemodialysis removes cefdinir from the body. In patients maintained on chronic hemodialysis, the recommended initial dosage regimen is a 300 mg or 7 mg/kg dose every other day. At the conclusion of each hemodialysis session, give 300 mg (or 7 mg/kg). Subsequent doses (300 mg or 7 mg/kg) are then administered every other day.

CEFDITOREN PIVOXIL:

| Cefditoren Dosage and Administration<br>in Adults and Adolescents ≥ 12 Years of Age[1] | | |
|---|---|---|
| Type of infection | Dosage | Duration (days) |
| Acute bacterial exacerbation of chronic bronchitis | 400 mg BID | 10 |
| Pharyngitis/Tonsillitis | 200 mg BID | |
| Uncomplicated skin and skin structure infections | | |

[1] Take with meals.

*Renal impairment* – It is recommended that 200 mg or less twice daily be administered to patients with moderate renal impairment (Ccr 30 to 49 mL/min/1.73 $m^2$) and 200 mg every day be administered to patients with severe renal impairment (Ccr < 30 mL/min/1.73 $m^2$).

CEFEPIME:

| Recommended Dosage Schedule for Cefepime | | | |
|---|---|---|---|
| Site and type of infection | Dose | Frequency | Duration (days) |
| Mild to moderate uncomplicated or complicated urinary tract infections, including pyelonephritis, caused by *Escherichia coli, Klebsiella pneumoniae*, or *Proteus mirabilis*.[1] | 0.5 to 1 g IV/IM[2] | q 12 h | 7 to 10 |
| Severe uncomplicated or complicated urinary tract infections, including pyelonephritis, caused by *E. coli* or *K. pneumoniae*.[1] | 2 g IV | q 12 h | 10 |
| Moderate to severe pneumonia caused by *Streptococcus pneumoniae*,[1] *Pseudomonas aeruginosa, K. pneumoniae*, or *Enterobacter* sp. | 1 to 2 g IV | q 12 h | 10 |
| Moderate to severe uncomplicated skin and skin structure infections caused by *Staphylococcus aureus* or *Streptococcus pyogenes*. | 2 g IV | q 12 h | 10 |
| Empiric therapy for febrile neutropenic patients. | 2 g IV | q 8 h | 7[3] |
| Complicated intra-abdominal infections (used in combination with metronidazole) caused by *E. coli*, viridans group streptococci, *P. aeruginosa, K. pneumoniae, Enterobacter* species, or *Bacteroides fragilis*. | 2 g IV | q 12 h | 7 to 10 |

[1] Including cases associated with concurrent bacteremia.
[2] IM route of administration is indicated only for mild to moderate, uncomplicated, or complicated UTIs caused by *E. coli* when the IM route is a more appropriate route of drug administration.
[3] Or until resolution of neutropenia. In patients whose fever resolves but who remain neutropenic for more than 7 days, frequently re-evaluate the need for continued antimicrobial therapy.

*Empiric therapy for febrile neutropenic patients* – As monotherapy for empiric treatment of febrile neutropenic patients. In patients at high risk for severe infection (including patients with a history of recent bone marrow transplantation, with hypotension at presentation, with an underlying hematologic malignancy, or with severe or prolonged neutropenia), antimicrobial monotherapy may not be appropriate. Insufficient data exist to support the efficacy of cefepime monotherapy in such patients.

*Complicated intra-abdominal infections* – In combination with metronidazole for complicated intra-abdominal infections caused by *E. coli*, viridans group streptococci, *P. aeruginosa, K. pneumoniae, Enterobacter* sp., or *B. fragilis*.

*Pediatric patients (2 months to 16 years of age)* – Treatment of uncomplicated and complicated urinary tract infections (including pyelonephritis), uncomplicated skin and skin structure infections, pneumonia, and as empiric therapy for febrile neutropenic patients.

*Renal function impairment* – In patients with impaired renal function (Ccr less than 60 mL/min), adjust the dose of cefepime to compensate for the slower rate of renal elimination. The recommended initial dose should be the same as in patients with normal renal function.

In patients undergoing hemodialysis, approximately 68% of the total amount of cefepime present in the body at the start of dialysis will be removed during a 3-hour dialysis period. Give a repeat dose, equivalent to the initial dose, at the completion of each dialysis session.

In elderly patients with renal insufficiency, adjust dosage and administration.

In patients undergoing continuous ambulatory peritoneal dialysis, administer cefepime at normal recommended doses at a dosage interval of every 48 hours.

| Recommended Cefepime Maintenance Schedule in Patients with Renal Impairment | | | | |
|---|---|---|---|---|
| Ccr (mL/min) | Recommended maintenance schedule | | | |
| > 60 | 500 mg q 12 h [1] | 1 g q 12 h | 2 g q 12 h | 2 g q 8 h |
| 30 to 60 | 500 mg q 24 h | 1 g q 24 h | 2 g q 24 h | 2 g q 12 h |
| 11 to 29 | | 500 mg q 24 h | 1 g q 24 h | 2 g q 24 h |
| ≤ 11 | 250 mg q 24 h | 250 mg q 24 h | 500 mg q 24 h | 1 g q 24 h |

[1] Normal recommended dosing schedule.

*IV administration* – Administer over approximately 30 minutes. Reconstitute with 50 or 100 mL of a compatible IV fluid. Cefepime is compatible at concentrations of 1 to 40 mg/mL with 0.9% Sodium Chloride Injection, 5% and 10% Dextrose Injection, M/6 Sodium Lactate Injection, 5% Dextrose and 0.9% Sodium Chloride Injection, Lactated Ringers and 5% Dextrose Injection, *Normosol-R* or *Normosol-M* in 5% Dextrose injection.

| Cefepime Admixture Stability | | | | |
|---|---|---|---|---|
| Cefepime concentration (mg/mL) | Admixture and concentration | IV Infusion solutions | Stability time for RT/L[1] (20° to 25°C) (hours) | Stability time for refrigeration (2° to 8°C) |
| 40 | Amikacin 6 mg/mL | NS[2] or D5W[3] | 24 | 7 days |
| 40 | Ampicillin 1 mg/mL | D5W[3] | 8 | 8 h |
| 40 | Ampicillin 10 mg/mL | D5W[3] | 2 | 8 h |
| 40 | Ampicillin 1 mg/mL | NS[2] | 24 | 48 h |
| 40 | Ampicillin 10 mg/mL | NS[2] | 8 | 48 h |
| 4 | Ampicillin 40 mg/mL | NS[2] | 8 | 8 h |
| 4 to 40 | Clindamycin phosphate 0.25 to 6 mg/mL | NS[2] or D5W[3] | 24 | 7 days |
| 4 | Heparin 10 to 50 units/mL | NS[2] or D5W[3] | 24 | 7 days |
| 4 | Potassium chloride 10 to 40 mEq/L | NS[2] or D5W[3] | 24 | 7 days |
| 4 | Theophylline 0.8 mg/mL | D5W[3] | 24 | 7 days |
| 1 to 4 | na | *Aminosyn II* 4.25% with electrolytes and calcium | 8 | 3 days |
| 0.125 to 0.25 | na | *Inpersol* with 4.25% dextrose | 24 | 7 days |

[1] Ambient room temperature and light.
[2] 0.9% sodium chloride injection.
[3] 5% dextrose injection.

*Admixture compatibility/incompatibility:* Intermittent IV infusion with a Y-type administration set can be accomplished with compatible solutions; however, during infusion of a solution containing cefepime, it is desirable to discontinue the other solution.

Solutions of cefepime, like those of most β-lactam antibiotics, should not be added to solutions of ampicillin at a concentration greater than 40 mg/mL, and should not be added to metronidazole, vancomycin, gentamicin, tobramycin, netilmicin sulfate, or aminophylline because of potential interaction. However, if concurrent therapy with cefepime is indicated, each of these antibiotics can be administered separately.

*IM administration:* Reconstitute cefepime with the following diluents: Sterile Water for Injection, 0.9% Sodium Chloride, 5% Dextrose Injection, 0.5% or 1% lidocaine HCl, or Sterile Bacteriostatic Water for Injection with parabens or benzyl alcohol.

*Pediatric dosing:* The usual recommended daily dosage in pediatric patients up to 40 kg in weight is 50 mg/kg/dose administered every 12 hours (every 8 hours for febrile neutropenic patients), for 7 to 10 days, depending on the indication and severity of infection. The maximum dose for pediatric patients (2 months to 16 years of age) should not exceed the recommended adult dose.

*Renal impairment* – Data in pediatric patients with impaired renal function are not available; however, because cefepime pharmacokinetics are similar in adult and pediatric patients, changes in dosing regimen similar to those in adults are recommended for pediatric patients.

*CEFMETAZOLE SODIUM:*
*Adults* –
*General guidelines:* 2 g IV every 6 to 12 hours for 5 to 14 days.
*Prophylaxis* –

| Cefmetazole Dosing Regimen for Prophylaxis ||
| --- | --- |
| Surgery | Dosing Regimen |
| Vaginal hysterectomy | 2 g single dose 30 to 90 min before surgery or 1 g doses 30 to 90 min before surgery and repeated 8 and 16 h later. |
| Abdominal hysterectomy | 1 g doses 30 to 90 min before surgery and repeated 8 and 16 h later. |
| Cesarean section | 2 g single dose after clamping cord or 1 g doses after clamping cord; repeated at 8 and 16 h. |
| Colorectal surgery | 2 g single dose 30 to 90 min before surgery or 2 g doses 30 to 90 min before surgery and repeated 8 to 16 h later. |
| Cholecystectomy (high risk) | 1 g doses 30 to 90 min before surgery and repeated 8 and 16 h later. |

*Renal function impairment* –

| Cefmetazole Dosage Guidelines in Renal Function Impairment ||||
| --- | --- | --- | --- |
| Renal function | Ccr (mL/min/1.73 m$^2$) | Dose (g) | Frequency (h) |
| Mild impairment | 50 to 90 | 1 to 2 | q 12 |
| Moderate impairment | 30 to 49 | 1 to 2 | q 16 |
| Severe impairment | 10 to 29 | 1 to 2 | q 24 |
| Essentially no function | < 10 | 1 to 2 | q 48[1] |

[1] Administered after hemodialysis.

*CEFOPERAZONE SODIUM:* Administer IM or IV.

Usual adult dose is 2 to 4 g/day administered in equally divided doses every 12 hours.

In severe infections or infections caused by less sensitive organisms, the total daily dose or frequency may be increased. Patients have been successfully treated with a total daily dosage of 6 to 12 g divided into 2, 3, or 4 administrations ranging from 1.5 to 4 g/dose. A total daily dose of 16 g by constant infusion has been given without complications.

*Hepatic disease or biliary obstruction* – In general, total daily dosage greater than 4 g should not be necessary.

*Renal function impairment* –

*Hemodialysis:* The half-life is reduced slightly during hemodialysis. Thus, schedule dosing to follow a dialysis period.

CEFOTAXIME SODIUM:

*Adults* – Administer IV or IM. Maximum daily dosage should not exceed 12 g.

| Cefotaxime Dosage Guidelines for Adults | | |
|---|---|---|
| Type of infection | Daily dosage (g) | Frequency and route |
| Gonococcal urethritis/cervicitis in males and females | 0.5 | 0.5 g IM (single dose) |
| Rectal gonorrhea in females | 0.5 | 0.5 g IM (single dose) |
| Rectal gonorrhea in males | 1 | 1 g IM (single dose) |
| Uncomplicated infections | 2 | 1 g every 12 h IM or IV |
| Moderate to severe infections | 3 to 6 | 1 to 2 g every 8 h IM or IV |
| Infections commonly needing higher dosage (eg, septicemia) | 6 to 8 | 2 g every 6 to 8 h IV |
| Life-threatening infections | ≤ 12 | 2 g every 4 h IV |

*Perioperative prophylaxis:* 1 g IV or IM, 30 to 90 minutes prior to surgery.

*Cesarean section:* Administer the first 1 g dose IV as soon as the umbilical cord is clamped. Administer the second and third doses as 1 g IV or IM at 6- and 12-hour intervals after the first dose.

*Children* –

| Cefotaxime Dosage Guidelines in Pediatrics | | | |
|---|---|---|---|
| Age | Weight (kg) | Dosage schedule | Route |
| 0 to 1 week | - | 50 mg/kg every 12 h | IV |
| 1 to 4 weeks | - | 50 mg/kg every 8 h | IV |
| 1 month to 12 years | < 50[1] | 50 to 180 mg/kg/day in 4 to 6 divided doses[2] | IV or IM |

[1] For children at least 50 kg, use adult dosage.
[2] Use higher doses for more severe or serious infections including meningitis.

*Renal function impairment* – In patients with estimated Ccr less than 20 mL/min/ 1.73 m$^2$, reduce dosage by 50%.

When only serum creatinine is available, the following formula may be used to convert this value into Ccr. The serum creatinine should represent steady-state renal function.

*CDC-recommended treatment schedules for gonorrhea* –

*Disseminated gonococcal infection:* Give 1 g IV every 8 hours.

*Gonococcal ophthalmia in adults:* For penicillinase-producing *Neisseria gonorrhoeae* (PPNG), give 500 mg IV 4 times/day.

CEFOTETAN DISODIUM:

*Adults* – The usual dosage is 1 or 2 g IV or IM every 12 hours for 5 to 10 days. Determine proper dosage and route of administration by the condition of the patient, severity of the infection and susceptibility of the causative organism.

| General Cefotetan Dosage Guidelines | | |
|---|---|---|
| Type of Infection | Daily Dose | Frequency and Route |
| Urinary tract | 1 to 4 g | 500 mg every 12 h IV or IM |
| | | 1 or 2 g every 24 h IV or IM |
| | | 1 or 2 g every 12 h IV or IM |
| Skin/Skin structure Mild to moderate[1] | 2 g | 2 g q 24 h IV |
| | | 1 g q 12 h IV or IM |
| Severe | 4 g | 2 g q 12 h IV |
| Other sites | 2 to 4 g | 1 or 2 g every 12 h IV or IM |
| Severe | 4 g | 2 g every 12 h IV |
| Life-threatening | 6 g[2] | 3 g every 12 h IV |

[1] Treat *K. pneumoniae* skin and skin structure infections with 1 or 2 g every 12 hours IV or IM.
[2] Maximum daily dosage should not exceed 6 g.

*Prophylaxis* – To prevent postoperative infection in clean contaminated or potentially contaminated surgery in adults, give a single 1 or 2 g IV dose 30 to 60 minutes prior to surgery. In patients undergoing cesarean section, give the dose as soon as the umbilical cord is clamped.

*Renal function impairment* – Reduce the dosage schedule using the following guidelines:

| Cefotetan Dosage in Renal Impairment | | |
| --- | --- | --- |
| Ccr (mL/min) | Dose | Frequency |
| > 30 | Usual recommended dose[1] | Every 12 h |
| 10 to 30 | Usual recommended dose[1] | Every 24 h |
| < 10 | Usual recommended dose[1] | Every 48 h |

[1] Dose determined by the type and severity of infection and susceptibility of the causative organism.

Alternatively, the dosing interval may remain constant at 12-hour intervals, but reduce dose by ½ for patients with a Ccr of 10 to 30 mL/min, and by ¼ for patients with a Ccr less than 10 mL/min.

*Dialysis* – Cefotetan is dialyzable; for patients undergoing intermittent hemodialysis, give ¼ of the usual recommended dose every 24 hours on days between dialysis and ½ of the usual recommended dose on the day of dialysis.

CEFOXITIN SODIUM:

*Adult* – Adult dosage range is 1 to 2 g every 6 to 8 hours.

| Cefoxitin Dosage Guidelines | | |
| --- | --- | --- |
| Type of infection | Daily dosage | Frequency and route |
| Uncomplicated (pneumonia, urinary tract, cutaneous)[1] | 3 to 4 g | 1 g every 6 to 8 h IV or IM |
| Moderately severe or severe | 6 to 8 g | 1 g every 4 h or 2 g every 6 to 8 h IV |
| Infections commonly requiring higher dosage (eg, gas gangrene) | 12 g | 2 g every 4 h or 3 g every 6 h IV |

[1] Including patients in whom bacteremia is absent or unlikely.

*Uncomplicated gonorrhea* – 2 g IM with 1 g oral probenecid given concurrently or up to 30 minutes before cefoxitin.

*Prophylactic use, surgery* – Administer 2 g IV or IM 30 to 60 minutes prior to surgery followed by 2 g every 6 hours after the first dose for no more than 24 hours.

*Prophylactic use, cesarean section* – Administer 2 g IV as soon as the umbilical cord is clamped. If a 3-dose regimen is used, give the second and third 2 g dose IV, 4 and 8 hours after the first dose.

*Prophylactic use, transurethral prostatectomy* – Administer 1 g prior to surgery; 1 g every 8 hours for up to 5 days.

*Renal function impairment* –

*Adults:* Initial loading dose is 1 to 2 g. Maintenance doses:

| Maintenance Cefoxitin Dosage in Renal Impairment | | | |
| --- | --- | --- | --- |
| Renal function | Ccr (mL/min/1.73 m$^2$) | Dose (g) | Frequency (h) |
| Mild impairment | 30 to 50 | 1 to 2 | 8 to 12 |
| Moderate impairment | 10 to 29 | 1 to 2 | 12 to 24 |
| Severe impairment | 5 to 9 | 0.5 to 1 | 12 to 24 |
| Essentially no function | < 5 | 0.5 to 1 | 24 to 48 |

*Hemodialysis* – Administer a loading dose of 1 to 2 g after each hemodialysis. Give the maintenance dose as indicated in the table above.

*Infants and children 3 months of age and older:* 80 to 160 mg/kg/day divided every 4 to 6 hours. Use higher dosages for more severe or serious infections. Do not exceed 12 g/day.

*Prophylactic use (at least 3 months)* – 30 to 40 mg/kg/dose every 6 hours

*Renal function impairment* – Modify consistent with recommendation for adults.

*CDC recommended treatment schedules for acute pelvic inflammatory disease (PID)* – 2 g IV every 6 hours plus 100 mg doxycycline IV or orally every 12 hours.

CEFPODOXIME PROXETIL: Administer with food to enhance absorption.

| Dosage/Duration of Cefpodoxime | | | |
|---|---|---|---|
| Type of infection | Total daily dose | Dose frequency | Duration |
| *Adults ≥ 13 years of age* | | | |
| Acute community-acquired pneumonia | 400 mg | 200 mg every 12 h | 14 days |
| Acute bacterial exacerbations of chronic bronchitis (tablets) | 400 mg | 200 mg every 12 h | 10 days |
| Uncomplicated gonorrhea (men and women) and rectal gonococcal infections (women) | 200 mg | single dose | |
| Skin and skin structure | 800 mg | 400 mg every 12 h | 7 to 14 days |
| Pharyngitis/Tonsillitis | 200 mg | 100 mg every 12 h | 5 to 10 days |
| Uncomplicated urinary tract infection | 200 mg | 100 mg every 12 h | 7 days |
| *Children (5 months through 12 years of age):*[1] | | | |
| Acute otitis media | 10 mg/kg/day (max 400 mg/day) | 10 mg/kg every 24 h (max 400 mg/dose) or 5 mg/kg every 12 h (max 200 mg/dose) | 10 days |
| Pharyngitis/Tonsillitis | 10 mg/kg/day (max 200 mg/day) | 5 mg/kg every 12 h (max 100 mg/dose) | 5 to 10 days |

[1] Do not exceed adult recommended doses.

*Renal dysfunction* – For patients with severe renal impairment (Ccr less than 30 mL/min), increase the dosing intervals to every 24 hours. In patients maintained on hemodialysis, use a frequency of 3 times/week after hemodialysis.

CEFPROZIL:

| Cefprozil Dosage and Duration | | |
|---|---|---|
| Population/Infection | Dosage (mg) | Duration (days) |
| *Adults ( ≥ 13 years of age)* | | |
| Pharyngitis/Tonsillitis | 500 q 24 h | 10[1] |
| Acute sinusitis (use higher dose for moderate to severe infections) | 250 q 12 h or 500 q 12 h | 10 |
| Secondary bacterial infection of acute bronchitis and acute bacterial exacerbation of chronic bronchitis | 500 q 12 h | 10 |
| Uncomplicated skin and skin structure infections | 250 q 12 h, 500 q 24 h, or 500 q 12 h | 10 |
| *Children (2 to 12 years of age)*[2] | | |
| Pharyngitis/Tonsillitis | 7.5 mg/kg q 12 h | 10[1] |
| Uncomplicated skin and skin structure infections | 20 mg/kg q 24 h | 10 |
| *Infants and children (6 months to 12 years of age)*[2] | | |
| Otitis media | 15 mg/kg q 12 h | 10 |
| Acute sinusitis (use higher dose for moderate to severe infections) | 7.5 mg/kg q 12 h or 15 mg/kg q 12 h | 10 |

[1] For infections caused by S. pyogenes, administer for at least 10 days.
[2] Not to exceed adult recommended doses.

*Renal function impairment* – For Ccr of 30 to 120 mL/min, use standard dosage and dosing interval. For Ccr less than 30 mL/min, use a dosage 50% of standard at the standard dosing interval.

Cefprozil is in part removed by hemodialysis; therefore, administer after the completion of hemodialysis.

CEFTAZIDIME:

| Ceftazidime Dosage Guidelines | | |
|---|---|---|
| Patient/Infection site | Dose | Frequency |
| *Adults*<br>Usual recommended dose | 1 g IV or IM | q 8 to 12 h |
| Uncomplicated urinary tract infections | 250 mg IV or IM | q 12 h |
| Complicated urinary tract infections | 500 mg IV or IM | q 8 to 12 h |
| Uncomplicated pneumonia; mild skin and skin structure infections | 500 mg to 1 g IV or IM | q 8 h |
| Bone and joint infections | 2 g IV | q 12 h |
| Serious gynecological and intra-abdominal infections | 2 g IV | q 8 h |
| Meningitis | | |
| Very severe life-threatening infections, especially in immunocompromised patients | | |
| Pseudomonal lung infections in cystic fibrosis patients w/normal renal function[1] | 30 to 50 mg/kg IV up to 6 g/day | q 8 h |
| *Neonates* (0 to 4 weeks) | 30 mg/kg IV | q 12 h |
| *Infants and children* (1 month to 12 years of age) | 30 to 50 mg/kg IV up to 6 g/day[2] | q 8 h |

[1] Although clinical improvement has been shown, bacteriological cures cannot be expected in patients with chronic respiratory disease and cystic fibrosis.
[2] Reserve the higher dose for immunocompromised children or children with cystic fibrosis or meningitis.

*Renal function impairment* – Ceftazidime is excreted by the kidneys, almost exclusively by glomerular filtration. In patients with impaired renal function (glomerular filtration rate (GFR) less than 50 mL/min), reduce dosage to compensate for slower excretion. In patients with suspected renal insufficiency, give an initial loading dose of 1 g. Estimate GFR to determine the appropriate maintenance dose.

| Ceftazidime Dosage in Renal Impairment | | |
|---|---|---|
| Ccr (mL/min) | Recommended unit dose of ceftazidime | Frequency of dosing |
| 31 to 50 | 1 g | q 12 h |
| 16 to 30 | 1 g | q 24 h |
| 6 to 15 | 500 mg | q 24 h |
| ≤ 5 | 500 mg | q 48 h |

In patients with severe infections who normally receive 6 g ceftazidime daily were it not for renal insufficiency, the unit dose given in the table above may be increased by 50% or the dosing frequency increased appropriately.

*Dialysis* – Give a 1 g loading dose, followed by 1 g after each hemodialysis period.

Ceftazidime also can be used in patients undergoing intraperitoneal dialysis (IPD) and continuous ambulatory peritoneal dialysis (CAPD). Give a loading dose of 1 g, followed by 500 mg every 24 hours. In addition to IV use, ceftazidime can be incorporated in the dialysis fluid at a concentration of 250 mg per 2 L of dialysis fluid.

CEFTIBUTEN: Ceftibuten suspension must be administered at least 2 hours before or 1 hour after a meal.

| Ceftibutin Dosage and Duration | | | |
|---|---|---|---|
| Type of infection | Daily maximum dose | Dose and frequency | Duration |
| *Adults ≥ 12 years of age* | | | |
| Acute bacterial exacerbations of chronic bronchitis caused by H. influenzae, M. catarrhalis, or Streptococcus pneumoniae | 400 mg | 400 mg/day | 10 days |
| Pharyngitis and tonsillitis caused by S. pyogenes | | | |
| Acute bacterial otitis media caused by H. influenzae, M. catarrhalis, or S. pyogenes | | | |
| *Children* | | | |
| Pharyngitis and tonsillitis caused by S. pyogenes | 400 mg | 9 mg/kg/day | 10 days |
| Acute bacterial otitis media caused by H. influenzae, M. catarrhalis, or S. pyogenes | | | |

| Ceftibuten Oral Suspension Pediatric Dosage Chart[1] | | | |
|---|---|---|---|
| Weight | | 90 mg/5 mL | 180 mg/5 mL |
| kg | lb | | |
| 10 | 22 | 5 mL (1 tsp)/day | 2.5 mL (½ tsp)/day |
| 20 | 44 | 10 mL (2 tsp)/day | 5 mL (1 tsp)/day |
| 40 | 88 | 20 mL (4 tsp)/day | 10 mL (2 tsp)/day |

[1] Children greater than 45 kg should receive the maximum daily dose of 400 mg.

*Renal function impairment* – Ceftibuten may be given at normal doses in impaired renal function with creatinine clearance of at least 50 mL/min. Dosing recommendations for patients with varying degrees of renal insufficiency are presented in the following table.

| Ceftibuten Dosage in Renal Impairment | |
|---|---|
| Ccr (mL/min) | Recommended dosing schedules |
| > 50 | 9 mg/kg or 400 mg q 24 h (normal dosing schedule) |
| 30 to 49 | 4.5 mg/kg or 200 mg q 24 h |
| 5 to 29 | 2.25 mg/kg or 100 mg q 24 h |

*Hemodialysis patients* – In patients undergoing hemodialysis 2 or 3 times weekly, a single 400 mg dose of ceftibuten capsules or a single dose of 9 mg/kg (maximum of 400 mg) oral suspension may be given at the end of each hemodialysis session.

CEFTIZOXIME SODIUM:

*Adults* – Usual dosage is 1 or 2 g every 8 to 12 hours.

| Ceftizoxime Dosage Guidelines in Adults | | |
|---|---|---|
| Type of infection | Daily dose (g) | Frequency and route |
| Uncomplicated urinary tract | 1 | 500 mg every 12 h IM or IV |
| Pelvic inflammatory disease (PID)[1] | 6 | 2 g every 8 h IV |
| Other sites | 2 to 3 | 1 g every 8 to 12 h IV or IM |
| Severe or refractory | 3 to 6 | 1 g every 8 hours IM or IV 2 g every 8 to 12 h IM[1] or IV |
| Life-threatening[2] | 9 to 12 | 3 to 4 g every 8 h IV |

[1] Dosages up to 2 g every 4 hours have been given.
[2] Divide 2 g IM doses and give in different large muscle masses.

*Urinary tract infections* – Higher dosage is recommended.

*Gonorrhea, uncomplicated* – A single 1 g IM injection is the usual dose.

*Life-threatening infections* – The IV route may be preferable for patients with bacterial septicemia, localized parenchymal abscesses (such as intra-abdominal abscess), peritonitis or other severe or life-threatening infections.

In those patients with normal renal function, the IV dosage is 2 to 12 g daily. In conditions such as bacterial septicemia, 6 to 12 g/day IV may be given initially for several days, and the dosage gradually reduced according to clinical response and laboratory findings.

*Pediatric* –

*Children (6 months of age and older):* 50 mg/kg every 6 to 8 hours. Dosage may be increased to 200 mg/kg/day. Do not exceed the maximum adult dose for serious infection.

*Renal function impairment:* Renal function impairment requires modification of dosage. Following an initial loading dose of 500 mg to 1 g IM or IV, use the maintenance dosing schedule in the following table.

*Hemodialysis* – No additional supplemental dosing is required following hemodialysis; give the dose (according to the table below) at the end of dialysis.

| Ceftizoxime Dosage in Adults with Renal Impairment | | | |
|---|---|---|---|
| Renal function | Ccr (mL/min) | Less severe infections | Life-threatening infections |
| Mild impairment | 50 to 79 | 500 mg q 8 h | 750 mg to 1.5 g q 8 h |
| Moderate to severe impairment | 5 to 49 | 250 to 500 mg q 12 h | 500 mg to 1 g q 12 h |
| Dialysis patients | 0 to 4 | 500 mg q 48 h or 250 mg q 24 h | 500 mg to 1 g q 48 h or 500 mg q 24 h |

*CEFTRIAXONE SODIUM:* Administer IV or IM.

*Adults* – Usual daily dosage is 1 to 2 g once a day (or in equally divided doses twice a day) depending on type and severity of infection. Do not exceed a total daily dose of 4 g.

*Uncomplicated gonococcal infections:* Give a single IM dose of 250 mg.

*Surgical prophylaxis:* Give a single 1 g dose ½ to 2 hours before surgery.

*Children* – To treat serious infections other than meningitis, administer 50 to 75 mg/kg/day (not to exceed 2 g) in divided doses every 12 hours.

*Meningitis:* 100 mg/kg/day (not to exceed 4 g). Thereafter, a total daily dose of 100 mg/kg/day (not to exceed 4 g/day) is recommended. May give daily dose once per day or in equally divided doses every 12 hours. Usual duration is 7 to 14 days.

*Skin and skin structure infections:* Give 50 to 75 mg/kg once daily (or in equally divided doses twice daily), not to exceed 2 g.

*CDC-recommended treatment schedules for chancroid, gonorrhea, and acute PID* –

*Chancroid (Haemophilus ducreyi infection):* 250 mg IM as a single dose.

*Gonococcal infections:*

*Uncomplicated* – 125 mg IM in a single dose plus 1 g azithromycin in single oral dose or 100 mg doxycycline twice a day for 7 days.

*Conjunctivitis* – 1 g IM single dose.

*Disseminated* – 1 g IM or IV every 24 hours.

*Meningitis/Endocarditis* – 1 to 2 g IV every 12 hours for 10 to 14 days (meningitis) or for at least 4 weeks (endocarditis).

*Children (less than 45 kg)* – With bacteremia or arthritis, use 50 mg/kg (maximum, 1 g) IM or IV in a single dose for 7 days. For meningitis, increase duration to 10 to 14 days and maximum dose to 2 g.

*Infants* – 25 to 50 mg/kg/day IV or IM in a single daily dose, not to exceed 125 mg. For disseminated infection, continue for 7 days, with a duration of 7 to 14 days with documented meningitis.

*Acute PID (ambulatory):* 250 mg IM plus doxycycline.

*CEFUROXIME:*

*Oral* – Tablets and suspension are not bioequivalent and not substitutable on a mg/mg basis.

*Tablets:* The tablets may be given without regard to meals.

*Suspension:* Administer with food.

| Dosage for Cefuroxime Axetil Tablets | | |
|---|---|---|
| Population/Infection | Dosage | Duration (days) |
| *Adults (≥ 13 years of age)* | | |
| Pharyngitis/Tonsillitis | 250 mg bid | 10 |
| Acute bacterial exacerbations of chronic bronchitis[1] | 250 or 500 mg bid | 10 |
| Secondary bacterial infections of acute bronchitis | | 5 to 10 |
| Uncomplicated skin and skin structure infections | 250 or 500 mg bid | 10 |
| Uncomplicated urinary tract infections | 125 or 250 mg bid | 7 to 10 |
| Uncomplicated gonorrhea | 1000 mg once | single dose |
| Early Lyme disease | 500 mg bid | 20 |
| *Children who can swallow tablets whole*[2] | | |
| Pharyngitis/Tonsillitis | 125 mg bid | 10 |
| Acute otitis media | 250 mg bid | 10 |

[1] Safety and efficacy of drug administered less than 10 days in patients with acute exacerbations of chronic bronchitis have not been established.
[2] Do not exceed adult recommended doses.

| Dosage for Cefuroxime Axetil Suspension | | | |
|---|---|---|---|
| Population/Infection | Dosage | Daily maximum dose | Duration (days) |
| *Infants and children (3 months to 12 years of age)* | | | |
| Pharyngitis/Tonsillitis | 20 mg/kg/day divided bid | 500 mg | 10 |
| Acute otitis media | 30 mg/kg/day divided bid | 1000 mg | 10 |
| Impetigo | 30 mg/kg/day divided bid | 1000 mg | 10 |

*Renal failure:* Because cefuroxime is renally eliminated, its half-life will be prolonged in patients with renal failure.

*Parenteral –*

   *Dosage:*

   Adults – 750 mg to 1.5 g IM or IV every 8 hours, usually for 5 to 10 days.

| Cefuroxime Dosage Guidelines | | |
|---|---|---|
| Type of infection | Daily dosage (g) | Frequency |
| Uncomplicated urinary tract, skin and skin structure, disseminated gonococcal, uncomplicated pneumonia | 2.25 | 750 mg every 8 h |
| Severe or complicated | 4.5 | 1.5 g every 8 h |
| Bone and joint | 4.5 | 1.5 g every 8 h |
| Life-threatening or caused by less susceptible organisms | 6 | 1.5 g every 6 h |
| Bacterial meningitis | 9 | ≤ 3 g every 8 h |
| Uncomplicated gonococcal | 1.5 g IM[1] | single dose |

[1] Administered at 2 different sites together with 1 g oral probenecid.

   *Preoperative prophylaxis:* For clean-contaminated or potentially contaminated surgical procedures, administer 1.5 g IV prior to surgery (approximately ½ to 1 hour before). Thereafter, give 750 mg IV or IM every 8 hours when the procedure is prolonged.

   For preventative use during open heart surgery, give 1.5 g IV at the induction of anesthesia and every 12 hours thereafter for a total of 6 g.

   *Renal function impairment:* Reduce dosage.

| Parenteral Cefuroxime Dosage in Renal Impairment (Adults) | |
|---|---|
| Ccr (mL/min) | Dose and frequency |
| > 20 | 750 mg to 1.5 g every 8 h |
| 10 to 20 | 750 mg every 12 h |
| < 10 | 750 mg every 24 h [1] |

[1] Because cefuroxime is dialyzable, give patients on hemodialysis a further dose at the end of the dialysis.

*Infants and children (3 months of age and older)* – 50 to 100 mg/kg/day in equally divided doses every 6 to 8 hours. Use 100 mg/kg/day (not to exceed maximum adult dose) for more severe or serious infections.

*Bone and joint infections:* 150 mg/kg/day (not to exceed maximum adult dose) in equally divided doses every 8 hours.

*Bacterial meningitis:* Initially, 200 to 240 mg/kg/day IV in divided doses every 6 to 8 hours.

In renal insufficiency, modify dosage frequency per adult guidelines.

CEPHALEXIN:
*Adults* – 1 to 4 g/day in divided doses.

*Usual dose:* 250 mg every 6 hours.

*Streptococcal pharyngitis, skin and skin structure infections, uncomplicated cystitis in patients older than 15 years of age:* 500 mg every 12 hours.

May need larger doses for more severe infections or less susceptible organisms. If dose is greater than 4 g/day, use parenteral drugs.

*Children* – Do not exceed adult recommended doses.

*Monohydrate:* 25 to 50 mg/kg/day in divided doses. For streptococcal pharyngitis in patients older than 1 year of age and for skin and skin structure infections, divide total daily dose and give every 12 hours. In severe infections, double the dose.

*Otitis media* – 75 to 100 mg/kg/day in 4 divided doses.

β-*hemolytic streptococcal infections* – Continue treatment for at least 10 days.

*HCl monohydrate* – Safety and efficacy not established for use in children.

CEPHRADINE:
*Oral* – May be given without regard to meals.

*Adults:*

*Skin, skin structure, and respiratory tract infections (other than lobar pneumonia)* – Usual dose is 250 mg every 6 hours or 500 mg every 12 hours.

*Lobar pneumonia* – 500 mg every 6 hours or 1 g every 12 hours.

*Uncomplicated urinary tract infections* – The usual dose is 500 mg every 12 hours. In more serious infections and prostatitis, 500 mg every 6 hours or 1 g every 12 hours. Severe or chronic infections may require larger doses (up to 1 g every 6 hours).

*Children:* No adequate information is available on the efficacy of twice a day regimens in children younger than 9 months of age. For children older than 9 months, the usual dose is 25 to 50 mg/kg/day, in equally divided doses every 6 or 12 hours. For otitis media caused by *H. influenzae*, 75 to 100 mg/kg/day in equally divided doses every 6 or 12 hours is recommended; do not exceed 4 g/day.

*All patients regardless of age and weight:* Larger doses (up to 1 g 4 times/day) may be given for severe or chronic infections.

*Parenteral* – Parenteral therapy may be followed by oral. To minimize pain and induration, inject IM deep into a large muscle mass.

*Adults:* Daily dose is 2 to 4 g in equally divided doses 4 times/day, IM or IV. In bone infections, the usual dosage is 1 g IV 4 times/day. A dose of 500 mg 4 times/day is adequate in uncomplicated pneumonia, skin and skin structure infections, and most urinary tract infections. In severe infections, dose may be increased by giving every 4 hours or by increasing dose up to a maximum of 8 g/day.

*Perioperative prophylaxis* – Recommended doses are 1 g IV or IM administered 30 to 90 minutes prior to the start of surgery, followed by 1 g every 4 to 6 hours after the first dose for 1 or 2 doses, or for up to 24 hours postoperatively.

*Cesarean section* – Give 1 g IV as soon as the umbilical cord is clamped. Give the second and third doses as 1 g IM or IV at 6 to 12 hours after the first dose.

*Infants and children* – 50 to 100 mg/kg/day in 4 equally divided doses; determine by age, weight, and infection severity.

*Renal impairment dosage –*

*Patients not on dialysis:*

| Cephradine Dosage in Renal Impairment | | |
|---|---|---|
| Ccr (mL/min) | Dose (mg) | Time interval (hours) |
| > 20 | 500 | 6 |
| 5 to 20 | 250 | 6 |
| < 5 | 250 | 12 |

*Patients on chronic, intermittent dialysis:* 250 mg initially; repeat at 12 hours and after 36 to 48 hours.

LORACARBEF: Administer at least 1 hour before or 2 hours after a meal.

| Dosage/Duration of Loracarbef | | |
|---|---|---|
| Population/Infection | Dosage (mg) | Duration (days) |
| *Adults ≥ 13 years of age* | | |
| *Lower respiratory tract* | | |
| Secondary bacterial infection of acute bronchitis | 200 to 400 q 12 h | 7 |
| Acute bacterial exacerbation of chronic bronchitis | 400 q 12 h | 7 |
| Pneumonia | 400 q 12 h | 14 |
| *Upper respiratory tract* | | |
| Pharyngitis/Tonsillitis | 200 q 12 h | 10[1] |
| Sinusitis | 400 q 12 h | 10 |
| *Skin and skin structure* | | |
| Uncomplicated | 200 q 12 h | 7 |
| *Urinary tract* | | |
| Uncomplicated cystitis | 200 q 24 h | 7 |
| Uncomplicated pyelonephritis | 400 q 12 h | 14 |
| *Infants and children (6 months to 12 years)[2]* | | |
| *Upper respiratory tract* | | |
| Acute otitis media[3] | 30 mg/kg/day in divided doses q 12 h | 10 |
| Acute maxillary sinusitis | | |
| Pharyngitis/Tonsillitis | 15 mg/kg/day in divided doses q 12 h | 10[1] |
| *Skin and skin structure* | | |
| Impetigo | 15 mg/kg/day in divided doses q 12 h | 7 |

[1] In treatment of infections caused by *S. pyogenes*, administer for at least 10 days.

[2] Do not exceed adult recommended doses.

[3] Use suspension; it is more rapidly absorbed than capsules, resulting in higher peak plasma concentrations when given at the same dose.

*Renal function impairment* – Use usual dose and schedule in patients with Ccr levels at least 50 mL/min. Patients with Ccr between 10 and 49 mL/min may be given half the recommended dose at the usual dosage interval. Patients with Ccr levels less than 10 mL/min may receive recommended dose given every 3 to 5 days; patients on hemodialysis should receive another dose following dialysis.

## Actions

*Pharmacology:* Cephalosporins are structurally and pharmacologically related to penicillins. **Cefoxitin** and **cefotetan** (cephamycins) and **loracarbef** (a carbacephem) are included because of their similarity.

Cephalosporins inhibit mucopeptide synthesis in the bacterial cell wall, making it defective and osmotically unstable. The drugs are usually bactericidal, depending on organism susceptibility, dose, tissue concentrations, and the rate at which organisms are multiplying. They are more effective against rapidly growing organisms forming cell walls.

*Pharmacokinetics:*

| | Drug | Routes | Normal renal function (minutes) | ESRD[1] (hours) | Hemodialysis (hours) | Protein bound (%) | Recovered unchanged in urine (%) | Peak serum level 1 g IV dose (mcg/mL) | Sodium (mEq/g) |
|---|---|---|---|---|---|---|---|---|---|
| | | | | Half-Life | | | | | |
| **First** | Cefadroxil | Oral | 78-96 | 20-25 | 3-4 | 20 | > 90 | — | — |
| | Cefazolin | IM-IV | 90–120 | 3-7 | 9-14 | 80-86 | 60-80 | 185 | 2-2.1 |
| | Cephalexin | Oral | 50-80 | 19-22 | 4-6 | 10 | > 90 | — | — |
| | Cephradine | Oral/IM-IV | 48-80 | 8-15 | — | 8-17 | > 90 | 86 | 6[2] |
| **Second** | Cefaclor | Oral | 35-54 | 2-3 | 1.6-2.1 | 25 | 60-85 | — | — |
| | Cefmetazole | IM-IV | 72-90 | — | — | 65 | 85 | — | 2 |
| | Cefotetan | IM-IV | 180-276 | 13-35 | 5 | 88-90 | 51-81 | 158 | 3.5 |
| | Cefoxitin | IV | 40-60 | 20 | 4 | 73 | 85 | 110 | 2.3 |
| | Cefprozil | Oral | 78 | 5.2-5.9 | decreased | 36 | 60 | — | — |
| | Cefuroxime | Oral/IM-IV | 80 | 16-22[3] | 3.5 | 50 | 66-100 | 100[4] | 2.4[3] |
| | Loracarbef | Oral | 60 | 32 | 4 | 25 | > 90 | — | — |
| **Third** | Cefdinir | Oral | 100 | 16 | 3.2 | 60-70 | 12-18 | — | — |
| | Cefepime | IM-IV | 102-138 | 17-21 | 11-16 | 20 | 85 | 79 | — |
| | Cefoperazone | IM-IV | 120 | 1.3-2.9 | 2 | 82-93 | 20-30 | 73-153 | 1.5 |
| | Cefotaxime | IM-IV | 60 | 3-11 | 2.5 | 30-40 | 60 | 42-102 | 2.2 |
| | Cefpodoxime[5] | Oral | 120-180 | 9.8 | | 21-29 | 29-33 | — | — |
| | Ceftazidime | IM-IV | 114-120 | 14-30 | — | < 10 | 80-90 | 69-90 | 2.3 |
| | Ceftibuten | Oral | 144 | 13.4-22.3 | 2-4 | 65 | 56 | — | — |
| | Ceftizoxime | IM-IV | 102 | 25-30 | 6 | 30 | 80 | 60-87 | 2.6 |
| | Ceftriaxone | IM-IV | 348-522 | 15.7 | 14.7 | 85-95 | 33-67 | 151 | 3.6 |

[1] ESRD = End stage renal disease (Ccr < 10 mL/min/1.73 m$^2$).
[2] Also available in sodium-free form.
[3] Injection only.
[4] Following 1.5 g IV dose.
[5] Extended spectrum agent.

**Cephalexin, cephradine, cefaclor, cefprozil, cefadroxil, ceftibuten,** and **loracarbef** are well absorbed from the GI tract. Cephalosporins are widely distributed to most tissues and fluids. First and second generation agents do not readily enter cerebrospinal fluid (CSF), except **cefuroxime,** even when meninges are inflamed. Third generation compounds readily diffuse into the CSF of patients with inflamed meninges. However, CSF levels of **cefoperazone** are relatively low. Most cephalosporins and metabolites are primarily excreted renally.

*Microbiology:*

## Organisms Generally Susceptible to Cephalosporins

✓ = generally susceptible
+ = demonstrated in vitro activity

**Gram-positive**

| Organisms | First Generation | | | | Second Generation | | | | | | | Third Generation | | | | | | | | |
|---|---|---|---|---|---|---|---|---|---|---|---|---|---|---|---|---|---|---|---|---|
| | Cefadroxil | Cefazolin | Cephalexin | Cephradine | Cefaclor | Cefoxitin | Cefuroxime | Cefmetazole | Cefotetan | Cefprozil | Loracarbef | Cefdinir | Cefepime[1] | Cefoperazone | Cefotaxime | Cefpodoxime[2] | Ceftazidime | Ceftibuten | Ceftizoxime | Ceftriaxone |
| Staphylococci[3] | ✓ | ✓ | ✓[4] | ✓ | ✓[4] | ✓ | ✓ | ✓ | ✓ | ✓ | ✓ | ✓[5] | ✓[6] | ✓ | ✓[5] | ✓[4] | ✓ | | ✓ | ✓ |
| Staphylococcus aureus | | | | | | | | | | | | ✓[5] | ✓[6] | | | | | | | |
| Staphylococcus epidermidis | | | | | | | + | | | | + | +[6] | | | | | | | | |
| Staphylococcus saprophyticus | | | | | | | + | | | | ✓ | | | | | | | | | |
| Streptococci, beta-hemolytic | ✓ | ✓ | ✓ | ✓ | ✓ | ✓ | ✓ | ✓ | ✓ | ✓ | ✓ | | ++ | ✓ | ✓ | ✓ | ✓ | | ✓ | ✓ |
| Streptococcus agalactiae | | | | | | | ++ | | | | + | + | | | | | | | | |
| Streptococcus bovis | | | | | | | | | | | ++ | | | | | | | | | |
| Streptococcus pneumoniae | ✓ | ✓ | ✓ | ✓ | ✓ | ✓ | ✓ | ✓ | ✓ | ✓ | ✓ | ✓[7] | ✓ | ✓ | ✓ | ✓ | ✓ | ✓[7] | ✓ | ✓ |
| Streptococcus pyogenes | | ✓ | | | ✓ | ✓ | ✓ | ✓ | ✓ | ✓ | ✓ | ✓ | ✓[8] | ✓ | ✓ | ✓ | ✓ | ✓ | ✓ | ✓ |
| Streptococcus viridans | | | | | | | | | | | ++ | ++ | | | ++ | | | | | |

## Organisms Generally Susceptible to Cephalosporins

✓ = generally susceptible
+ = demonstrated in vitro activity

| Organism (Gram-negative) | Cefadroxil | Cefazolin | Cephalexin | Cephradine | Cefaclor | Cefoxitin | Cefuroxime | Cefmetazole | Cefotetan | Cefprozil | Loracarbef | Cefdinir | Cefepime[1] | Cefoperazone | Cefotaxime | Cefpodoxime[2] | Ceftazidime | Ceftibuten | Ceftizoxime | Ceftriaxone |
|---|---|---|---|---|---|---|---|---|---|---|---|---|---|---|---|---|---|---|---|---|
| Acinetobacter sp. | | | | | | | | | | | | | ++ | ✓[4] | ✓ | | ++ | | ✓ | ++ |
| Citrobacter sp. | | | | | | | ✓[4] | ++ | ++ | ++ | ++ | ++ | ++ | ✓ | ✓ | ++ | ✓ | | ++ | ++ |
| Enterobacter sp. | | ✓[4] | | | | | ✓[4] | ++ | ✓ | | ++ | | ✓ | ✓ | ✓ | | ✓ | | ✓ | ✓ |
| Escherichia coli | ✓ | ✓ | ✓ | ✓ | ✓ | | ✓ | ✓ | ✓ | ++ | ✓ | ++ | +[5] | ✓[5] | ✓[5] | ✓ | ✓ | | ✓ | ✓ |
| Haemophilus influenzae | | ✓ | ✓ | ✓ | ✓[5] | ✓[5] | ✓[5] | ✓[5] | ✓[5] | ✓[5] | ✓[5] | ✓[5] | +[5] | | ✓[5] | ✓[5] | ✓[5] | ✓[5] | ✓[5] | ✓[5] |
| Haemophilus parainfluenzae | | | | | ++ | | ++ | | | | ++ | ✓[5] | | | ✓ | ++ | ++ | | | ✓ |
| Hafnia alvei | | | | | | | | | | | ++ | | ++ | | | | | | | |
| Klebsiella sp. | ✓ | ✓ | ✓ | ✓ | ✓ | | ✓ | ✓ | ✓ | ++ | ++ | ++ | ✓ | ✓ | ✓ | ✓ | ✓ | | ✓ | ✓ |
| Klebsiella pneumoniae | | | ++ | | ++ | | | | | | ++ | | +[5] | | | | | | | |
| Moraxella (Branhamella) catarrhalis | ++ | | ++ | | ✓[5] | | ++ | ++ | ++ | ✓[5] | ✓[5] | ✓[5] | +[5] | ✓ | ✓ | ✓ | ✓ | ✓[5] | ++ | |
| Morganella (Proteus) morganii | | | | | | ✓ | ✓[4] | | ✓ | | | | ++ | ✓ | ✓ | | ++ | | ✓ | ✓ |

**Organisms Generally Susceptible to Cephalosporins**

✓ = generally susceptible
‡ = demonstrated in vitro activity

| Organisms (Gram-negative, con't) | First Generation | | | | Second Generation | | | | | | | | Third Generation | | | | | | | |
|---|---|---|---|---|---|---|---|---|---|---|---|---|---|---|---|---|---|---|---|---|
| | Cefadroxil | Cefazolin | Cephalexin | Cephradine | Cefaclor | Cefoxitin | Cefuroxime | Cefmetazole | Cefotetan | Cefprozil | Loracarbef | Cefdinir | Cefepime[1] | Cefoperazone | Cefotaxime | Cefpodoxime[2] | Ceftazidime | Ceftibuten | Cefizoxime | Ceftriaxone |
| Neisseria catarrhalis | ✓ | | ✓ | | | | | | | | | | | | | | | | ✓ | ✓ |
| Neisseria gonorrhoeae | | | | | ‡ | ✓ | ✓ | ‡ | ‡ | ‡ | ‡[3] | | | ✓[5] | ✓ | ✓[4] | ‡ | | ‡ | ✓ |
| Neisseria meningitidis | | | | | | | ✓ | | | | | | | ‡ | ✓ | | ✓ | | | ✓ |
| Pasteurella multocida | | | | | | | | | | | ‡ | | | | | | | | | |
| Proteus inconstans | | | | | | | ‡ | | | | | ‡ | ✓ | | | | | | | |
| Proteus mirabilis | ✓ | ✓ | ✓ | ✓ | ✓ | ✓ | ✓ | ✓ | ✓ | ‡ | ‡ | | ‡ | ✓ | ✓ | ✓ | ✓ | | ✓ | ✓ |
| Proteus vulgaris | | | | | | ✓ | ✓ | ✓ | ✓ | | | | ‡ | ✓ | ✓ | ‡ | ✓ | | ✓ | ✓ |
| Providencia sp. | | | | | | ✓ | | ✓ | ✓ | | | | ‡ | ✓ | ‡ | | ‡ | | ‡ | ‡ |
| Providencia rettgeri | | | | | | ✓ | ✓ | ‡ | ✓ | | | | ‡ | ✓ | ✓ | ‡ | ‡ | | ✓ | ‡ |
| Pseudomonas aeruginosa | | | | | | | | | ‡ | ‡ | ‡ | | ✓ | ‡ | ✓[4] | | ✓ | | ✓[4] | ✓[4] |
| Salmonella sp. | | | | | | | ✓ | | ‡ | | | | | | ‡ | | ‡ | | ‡ | ‡ |
| Salmonella typhi | | | | | | | | | ‡ | | | | ‡ | ✓ | ‡ | | | | ‡ | ‡ |
| Serratia sp. | | | | | | | | | ‡ | | | | ‡ | ‡ | ✓ | | ✓ | | ✓ | ✓ |
| Shigella sp. | | | | | | | ✓ | ‡ | ‡ | ‡ | ‡ | | ✓ | ✓ | ‡ | | ‡ | | ‡ | ‡ |
| Yersinia enterocolitica | | | | | | | | | ✓ | | ‡ | | | | | | | | | |

## Organisms Generally Susceptible to Cephalosporins

✓ = generally susceptible
+ = demonstrated in vitro activity

| Organisms | First Generation | | | | Second Generation | | | | | | | Third Generation | | | | | | | | |
|---|---|---|---|---|---|---|---|---|---|---|---|---|---|---|---|---|---|---|---|---|
| | Cefadroxil | Cefazolin | Cephalexin | Cephradine | Cefaclor | Cefoxitin | Cefuroxime | Cefmetazole | Cefotetan | Cefprozil | Loracarbef | Cefdinir | Cefepime[1] | Cefoperazone | Cefotaxime | Cefpodoxime[2] | Ceftazidime | Ceftibuten | Ceftizoxime | Ceftriaxone |
| **Anaerobes** | | | | | | | | | | | | | | | | | | | | |
| Bacteroides sp. | | | | | ✓ | ✓ | ✓ | ✓ | ✓[4] | + | | | | ✓ | ✓ | | | | + | ✓ |
| Bacteroides fragilis | | | | | | ✓ | ✓ | ✓ | ✓ | | | | | ✓ | ✓ | | | | ✓ | + |
| Clostridium sp. | | | | | | ✓ | ✓ | ✓ | ✓ | + | + | | | ✓ | ✓ | | + | | + | + |
| Clostridium difficile | | | | | | | | | + | + | + | | | + | | | | | | + |
| Eubacterium sp. | | | | | | | | | | | | | | + | | | | | | + |
| Fusobacterium sp. | | | | | | ✓ | ✓ | ✓ | ✓ | + | + | | | + | ✓ | | | | + | + |
| Peptococcus sp. | | | | | + | ✓ | ✓ | + | ✓ | | + | | | ✓ | ✓ | | | | ✓ | + |
| Peptococcus niger | | | | | + | | | | | | + | | | | | | + | | | |
| Peptostreptococcus sp. | | | | | + | ✓ | ✓ | + | ✓ | + | + | | | ✓ | + | + | + | | ✓ | + |
| Porphyromonas asaccharolytica | | | | | | | | | | | | | | | | | | | | |
| Prevotella bivia | | | | | | | | | ✓ | | | | | | | | | | | |
| Prevotella disiens | | | | | | | | | ✓ | | | | | | | | | | | |
| Prevotella melaninogenica | | | | | | | | | + | | | | | | | | | | | |
| Prevotella oralis | | | | | | | | | + | | + | | | | | | | | | |
| Propionibacterium acnes | | | | | + | | | | + | | | | | | | | | | | |
| Propionibacterium sp. | | | | | | | | | + | | | | | | | | | | | |
| Veillonella sp. | | | | | | | | | + | | | | | | | | | | | |
| **Other** | | | | | | | | | | | | | | | | | | | | |
| Borrelia burgdorferi | | | | | | | ✓ | | | | | | | | | | | | | |

[1] Extended spectrum agent.
[2] Some other references consider this fourth generation.
[3] Coagulase-positive, coagulase-negative and penicillinase-producing.
[4] Some strains are resistant.
[5] Including some β-lactamase-producing strains.
[6] Methicillin-susceptible strains only.
[7] Penicillin-susceptible strains only.
[8] Lancefield's Group A streptococci.

**Contraindications**

Hypersensitivity to cephalosporins or related antibiotics.

*Cefditoren:* Cefditoren is contraindicated in patients with carnitine deficiency or inborn errors of metabolism that may result in clinically significant carnitine deficiency because use of cefditoren causes renal excretion of carnitine.

Cefditoren contains sodium caseinate, a milk protein. Do not administer cefditoren to patients with milk protein hypersensitivity (not lactose intolerance).

**Warnings**

*Cross-allergenicity with penicillin:* Administer cautiously to penicillin-sensitive patients. There is evidence of partial cross-allergenicity; cephalosporins cannot be assumed to be an absolutely safe alternative to penicillin in the penicillin-allergic patient. The estimated incidence of cross-sensitivity is 5% to 16%; however, it is possibly as low as 3% to 7%.

*Serum sickness-like reactions:* (erythema multiforme or skin rashes accompanied by polyarthritis, arthralgia and, frequently, fever) have been reported; these reactions usually occurred following a second course of therapy. Signs and symptoms occur after a few days of therapy and resolve a few days after drug discontinuation with no serious sequelae.

*Seizures:* Several cephalosporins have been implicated in triggering seizures, particularly in patients with renal impairment when the dosage was not reduced.

*Coagulation abnormalities:* **Cefmetazole, cefoperazone, cefotetan,** and **ceftriaxone** may be associated with a fall in prothrombin activity. Those at risk include patients with renal impairment, cancer, impaired vitamin K synthesis, or low vitamin K stores (eg, chronic hepatic disease or malnutrition), as well as patients receiving a protracted course of antimicrobial therapy. Monitor prothrombin time for patients at risk and administer exogenous vitamin K as indicated. Vitamin K administration may be necessary if the prothrombin time is prolonged before therapy.

*Predisposing factors* – Predisposing factors to cephalosporin bleeding abnormalities include hepatic and renal dysfunction, thrombocytopenia and the concomitant use of "high dose" heparin (greater than 20,000 units/day), oral anticoagulants, or other drugs that affect hemostasis (eg, aspirin). Elderly, malnourished or debilitated patients are more likely to experience bleeding abnormalities than other patients.

*Pseudomembranous colitis:* Pseudomembranous colitis occurs with the use of cephalosporins (and other broad spectrum antibiotics); therefore, consider its diagnosis in patients who develop diarrhea with antibiotic use.

*Immune hemolytic anemia:* Immune hemolytic anemia has been observed in patients receiving cephalosporin class antibiotics.

*Hypersensitivity reactions:* Reactions range from mild to life-threatening. Before therapy is instituted, inquire about previous hypersensitivity reactions to cephalosporins and penicillins.

*Renal function impairment:* Cephalosporins may be nephrotoxic; use with caution in the presence of markedly impaired renal function (Ccr less than 50 mL/min/1.73 m$^2$).

*Hepatic function impairment:* Cefoperazone is extensively excreted in bile. Serum half-life increases 2-fold to 4-fold in patients with hepatic disease or biliary obstruction.

*Pregnancy: Category B.* These agents cross the placenta.

*Lactation:* Most of these agents are excreted in breast milk in small quantities.

*Children:* When using cephalosporins in infants, consider the relative benefit to risk. In neonates, accumulation of cephalosporin antibiotics (with resulting prolongation of drug half-life) has occurred.

Safety and efficacy in children younger than 1 month (**cefazolin** and **cefaclor** capsule and suspension), younger than 3 months (**cefuroxime,** and **cefoxitin**), younger than 5 months (**cefpodoxime**), younger than 6 months (**cefdinir, loracarbef, cef-**

tozoxime, and **cefprozil**), younger than 9 months (**oral cephradine**) and younger than 1 year of age (**cefepime** and **parenteral cephradine**) have not been established.

Safety and efficacy of **cefaclor** extended-release tablets in children younger than 16 years of age have not been established.

Safety and efficacy of **cefmetazole, cefoperazone, cephalexin,** and **cefotetan** in children have not been established.

### Precautions

*Parenteral use:* Inject IM preparations deep into musculature; properly dilute IV preparations and administer over an appropriate time interval.

*Gonorrhea:* In the treatment of gonorrhea, all patients should have a serologic test for syphilis. Patients with incubating syphilis (seronegative without clinical signs of syphilis) are likely to be cured by the regimens used for gonorrhea.

*Superinfection:* Use of antibiotics (especially prolonged or repeated therapy) may result in bacterial or fungal overgrowth of nonsusceptible organisms. Such overgrowth may lead to a secondary infection. Take appropriate measures if superinfection occurs.

### Drug Interactions

Agents that may interact with cephalosporins include ethanol, aminoglycosides, anticoagulants, polypeptide antibiotics, probenecid, antacids, $H_2$ antagonists, iron supplements, and loop diuretics.

*Drug/Lab test interactions:* A false-positive reaction for **urine glucose** may occur with *Benedict's* solution, *Fehling's* solution, or with *Clinitest* tablets, but not with enzyme-based tests such as *Clinistix* and *Tes-Tape*.

**Cephradine** may cause false-positive reactions in urinary protein tests that use sulfosalicylic acid.

**Cefuroxime** may cause a false-negative reaction in the ferricyanide test for blood glucose.

**Cefdinir** may cause a false-positive reaction for ketones in urine when measured using nitroprusside but not nitroferricynide.

A false-positive direct *Coombs' test* has occurred in some patients receiving cephalosporins.

Cephalosporins may falsely elevate *urinary 17-ketosteroid* values.

High concentrations of **cefoxitin** (greater than 100 mcg/mL) may interfere with measurement of *creatinine levels* by the Jaffe reaction and produce false results. **Cefotetan** may also affect these measurements.

*Drug/Food interactions:* Food increases absorption of **cefpodoxime** and oral **cefuroxime**.

### Adverse Reactions

*Most common –* GI disturbances (nausea, vomiting, diarrhea); hypersensitivity phenomena (most common); hypotension; fever; dyspnea; candidal overgrowth consisting of oral candidiasis, vaginitis, genital moniliasis, vaginal discharge and genitoanal pruritus; nervousness; insomnia; confusion; hypertonia; dizziness; somnolence.

*CNS:* Headache; dizziness; lethargy; fatigue; paresthesia; confusion; diaphoresis; flushing.

*Hematologic:* Eosinophilia; transient neutropenia; leukocytosis; leukopenia; thrombocythemia; thrombocytopenia; agranulocytosis; granulocytopenia; hemolytic anemia; bone marrow depression; pancytopenia; decreased platelet function; anemia; aplastic anemia; hemorrhage.

*Hepatic:* Elevated AST, ALT, GGTP, total bilirubin, alkaline phosphatase, LDH; hepatitis.

*Local:* IM administration commonly results in pain, induration, temperature elevation, and tenderness.

*Renal:* Transitory elevations in BUN with and without elevated serum creatinine (frequency increases in patients older than 50 years of age and in children younger than 3 years of age).

# MEROPENEM

| Powder for injection: 500 mg and 1 g (Rx) | Merrem IV (AstraZeneca) |
|---|---|

### Indications
For the treatment of the following infections when caused by susceptible strains of the designated microorganisms:

Intra-abdominal infections: Complicated appendicitis and peritonitis caused by viridans group streptococci, Escherichia coli, Klebsiella pneumoniae, Pseudomonas aeruginosa, Bacterioides fragilis, Bacterioides thetaiotaomicron, and Peptostreptococcus sp.

Bacterial meningitis (pediatric patients 3 months of age or older only): Bacterial meningitis caused by Streptococcus pneumoniae, Haemophilus influenzae (β-lactamase and non-β-lactamase-producing strains), and Neisseria meningitidis.

### Administration and Dosage
Adults: 1 g IV every 8 hours. Give over approximately 15 to 30 minutes or as an IV bolus injection (5 to 20 mL) over approximately 3 to 5 minutes.

Renal function impairment: Reduce dosage in patients with Ccr less than 50 mL/min.

| Recommended Meropenem IV Dosage Schedule for Adults with Impaired Renal Function | | |
|---|---|---|
| Ccr (mL/min) | Dose (dependent on type of infection) | Dosing interval |
| 26 to 50 | recommended dose (100 mg) | every 12 hours |
| 10 to 25 | ½ recommended dose | every 12 hours |
| < 10 | ½ recommended dose | every 24 hours |

Use in pediatric patients: For pediatric patients 3 months of age and older, the meropenem dose is 20 or 40 mg/kg every 8 hours (maximum dose, 2 g every 8 hours), depending on the type of infection (intra-abdominal or meningitis). Administer pediatric patients weighing more than 50 kg 1 g every 8 hours for intra-abdominal infections and 2 g every 8 hours for meningitis. Give over approximately 15 to 30 minutes or as an IV bolus injection (5 to 20 mL) over approximately 3 to 5 minutes.

| Recommended Meropenem IV Dosage Schedule for Pediatric Patients with Normal Renal Function | | |
|---|---|---|
| Type of infection | Dose (mg/kg) | Dosing interval |
| Intra-abdominal | 20 | every 8 hours |
| Meningitis | 40 | every 8 hours |

### Actions
Pharmacology: Meropenem is a broad-spectrum carbapenem antibiotic. The bactericidal activity of meropenem results from the inhibition of cell-wall synthesis. Meropenem readily penetrates the cell wall of most gram-positive and gram-negative bacteria to reach penicillin-binding-protein (PBP) targets.

Pharmacokinetics: Meropenem has dose-dependent kinetics.

In subjects with normal renal function, the elimination half-life of meropenem is approximately 1 hour. Meropenem is excreted by the kidney with a half-life of 0.8 to 1.24 hours; 65% to 83% of the dose is recovered in the urine as meropenem and 20% to 28% as the inactive open β-lactam metabolite.

Plasma protein binding of meropenem is approximately 2%. The volume of meropenem distribution is 15.7 to 26.68 L. Meropenem penetrates well into most body fluids and tissues, including cerebrospinal fluid, achieving concentrations matching or exceeding those required to inhibit most susceptible bacteria.

The pharmacokinetics of meropenem in pediatric patients 2 years of age and older are essentially similar to those in adults. In infants and children 2 months to 12 years of age, no age- or dose-dependent effects on pharmacokinetic parameters were observed. Mean half-life was 1.13 hours, mean volume of distribution at steady state was 0.43 L/kg, mean residence time was 1.57 hours, clearance was 5.63 mL/min/kg and renal clearance was 2.53 mL/min/kg. The elimination half-life is slightly prolonged (1.5 hours) in pediatric patients 3 months to 2 years of age.

*Microbiology:* Meropenem has significant stability to hydrolysis by β-lactamases of most categories, both penicillinases and cephalosporinases produced by gram-positive and gram-negative bacteria, with the exception of matallo-β-lactamases. Do not use to treat methicillin-resistant staphylococci. Cross-resistance is sometimes observed with strains resistant to other carbapenems. In vitro tests show meropenem to act synergistically with aminoglycoside antibiotics against some isolates of *P. aeruginosa*.

## Contraindications

Hypersensitivity to any component of this product or to other drugs in the same class or in patients who have demonstrated anaphylactic reactions to β-lactams.

## Warnings

*Pseudomembranous colitis:* Pseudomembranous colitis has been reported with nearly all antibacterial agents, including meropenem and may range in severity from mild to life-threatening. Therefore, it is important to consider this diagnosis in patients who develop diarrhea subsequent to the administration of antibacterial agents.

*Hypersensitivity reactions:* Serious and occasionally fatal hypersensitivity (anaphylactic) reactions have been reported in patients receiving therapy with β-lactams. These reactions are more likely to occur with a history of sensitivity to multiple allergens.

There have been reports of individuals with a history of penicillin hypersensitivity who have experienced severe hypersensitivity reactions when treated with other β-lactams.

*Renal function impairment:* Plasma clearance of meropenem correlates with Ccr. In moderate renal dysfunction (Ccr 30 to 80 mL/min), mean half-life has been prolonged to 1.93 to 3.36 hours. In patients with greater dysfunction (Ccr 2 to 30 mg/min), mean half-life has been further prolonged to 3.82 to 5.73 hours. Patients undergoing hemodialysis (patients with end-stage renal disease) had mean predialysis half-lives of 7 to 10 hours. Hemodialysis shortened elimination half-life to 1.4 to 2.9 hours during the dialysis period.

*Elderly:* Elderly patients with renal insufficiency have shown a reduction in plasma clearance of meropenem that correlates with age-associated reduction in creatinine clearance. The mean terminal half-life is prolonged slightly to 1.27 hours.

*Pregnancy:* Category B.

*Lactation:* It is not known whether this drug is excreted in breast milk.

*Children:* The safety and efficacy of meropenem have not been established for children younger than 3 months of age (see Administration and Dosage).

## Precautions

*Monitoring:* Periodic assessment of organ system functions, including renal, hepatic, and hematopoietic is advisable during prolonged therapy.

*Seizures:* Seizures and other CNS adverse experiences have been reported during treatment with meropenem. These adverse experiences have occurred most commonly in patients with CNS disorders (eg, brain lesions or history of seizures) or with bacterial meningitis or compromised renal function.

*Superinfection:* As with other broad-spectrum antibiotics, prolonged use of meropenem may result in overgrowth of nonsusceptible organisms.

## Drug Interactions

*Probenecid:* Probenecid may interact with meropenem.

## Adverse Reactions

Adverse reactions occurring in at least 3% of patients include inflammation at the injection site, diarrhea, nausea, and vomiting.

Adverse reactions occuring in at least 3% of pediatric patients include diarrhea, vomiting, and rash (mostly diaper-area moniliasis).

# IMIPENEM-CILASTATIN

**Powder for injection:** 250, 500, and 750 mg imipenem equivalent and cilastatin equivalent (*Rx*)    *Primaxin I.V.* (Merck), *Primaxin I.M.* (Merck)

## Indications

IV: Treatment of serious infections caused by susceptible strains of the designated microorganisms in the conditions listed below:

*Lower respiratory tract infections* – Staphylococcus aureus (penicillinase-producing), Escherichia coli, Klebsiella sp., Enterobacter sp., Haemophilus influenzae, Haemophilus parainfluenzae, Acinetobacter sp., Serratia marcescens.

*Urinary tract infections (complicated and uncomplicated)* – Enterococcus faecalis, S. aureus (penicillinase-producing), E. coli, Klebsiella sp., Enterobacter sp., Proteus vulgaris, Providencia rettgeri, Morganella morganii, Pseudomonas aeruginosa.

*Intra-abdominal infections* – Enterococcus faecalis, S. aureus (penicillinase-producing), Staphylococcus epidermidis, E. coli, Klebsiella sp., Enterobacter sp., Proteus sp., M. morganii, P. aeruginosa, Citrobacter sp., Clostridium sp., Bacteroides sp. including Bacteroides fragilis, Fusobacterium sp.; Peptococcus sp., Peptostreptococcus sp., Eubacterium sp., Propionibacterium sp., Bifidobacterium sp.

*Gynecologic infections* – E. faecalis, S. aureus (penicillinase-producing), S. epidermidis, Streptococcus agalactiae (group B streptococcus), E. coli, Klebsiella sp., Proteus sp., Enterobacter sp., Bifidobacterium sp., Bacteroides sp. including B. fragilis, Gardnerella vaginalis; Peptococcus sp., Peptostreptococcus sp., Propionibacterium sp.

*Bacterial septicemia* – E. faecalis, S. aureus (penicillinase-producing), E. coli, Klebsiella sp., P. aeruginosa, Serratia sp., Enterobacter sp., Bacteroides sp.

*Bone and joint infections* – E. faecalis; S. aureus (penicillinase-producing), S. epidermidis, Enterobacter sp., P. aeruginosa.

*Skin and skin structure infections* – E. faecalis, S. aureus (penicillinase-producing), S. epidermidis, E. coli, Klebsiella sp., Enterobacter sp., P. vulgaris, P. rettgeri, M. morganii, P. aeruginosa, Serratia sp., Citrobacter sp., Acinetobacter sp., Bacteroides sp., Fusobacterium sp.; Peptococcus sp., Peptostreptococcus sp.

*Endocarditis* – S. aureus (penicillinase-producing).

*Polymicrobic infections* – Polymicrobic infections, including those in which S. pneumoniae (pneumonia, septicemia), S. pyogenes (skin and skin structure) or nonpenicillinase-producing S. aureus is one of the causative organisms. However, these monobacterial infections usually are treated with narrower spectrum antibiotics (eg, penicillin G). Although clinical improvement has been observed in patients with cystic fibrosis, chronic pulmonary disease, and lower respiratory tract infections caused by P. aeruginosa, bacterial eradication may not be achieved.

IM: Treatment of serious infections of mild to moderate severity where IM therapy is appropriate. Not intended for severe or life-threatening infections, including bacterial sepsis or endocarditis, or in major physiological impairments (eg, shock).

*Lower respiratory tract infections* – Lower respiratory tract infections, including pneumonia and bronchitis as an exacerbation of COPD, caused by S. pneumoniae and H. influenzae.

*Intra-abdominal infections* – Intra-abdominal infections, including acute gangrenous or perforated appendicitis and appendicitis with peritonitis, caused by group D streptococcus including E. faecalis; Streptococcus (viridans group); E. coli; Klebsiella pneumoniae; P. aeruginosa; Bacteroides sp. including B. fragilis, B. distasonis, B. intermedius, and B. thetaiotaomicron; Fusobacterium sp.; Peptostreptococcus sp.

*Skin and skin structure infections* – Skin and skin structure infections, including abscesses, cellulitis, infected skin ulcers, and wound infections caused by S. aureus (including penicillinase-producing strains); Streptococcus pyogenes; group D streptococcus including E. faecalis; Acinetobacter sp. including A. calcoaceticus; Citrobacter sp.; E. coli; Enterobacter cloacae; K. pneumoniae; P. aeruginosa; Bacteroides sp. including B. fragilis.

*Gynecologic infections* – Gynecologic infections, including postpartum endomyometritis, caused by group D streptococcus such as *E. faecalis; E. coli; K. pneumoniae; B. intermedius; Peptostreptococcus* sp.

Infections resistant to other antibiotics (eg, cephalosporins, penicillins, aminoglycosides) have responded to treatment with imipenem.

### Administration and Dosage

Dosage recommendations represent the quantity of imipenem to be administered. An equivalent amount of cilastatin is also present in the solution.

*IV:*

*Adults* – Give a 125, 250, or 500 mg dose by IV infusion over 20 to 30 minutes. Infuse a 750 or 1 g dose over 40 to 60 minutes. In patients who develop nausea, slow the infusion rate.

Because of high antimicrobial activity, do not exceed 50 mg/kg/day or 4 g/day, whichever is lower.

| Imipenem-Cilastatin IV Dosing Schedule for Adults with Normal Renal Function | | | | |
|---|---|---|---|---|
| Type or severity of infection | Fully susceptible organisms[1] | Total daily dose | Moderately susceptible organisms, primarily some strains of P. aeruginosa | Total daily dose |
| Mild | 250 mg q 6 h | 1 g | 500 mg q 6 h | 2 g |
| Moderate | 500 mg q 8 h or 500 mg q 6 h | 1.5 or 2 g | 500 mg q 6 h or 1 g q 8 h | 2 or 3 g |
| Severe, life-threatening | 500 mg q 6 h | 2 g | 1 g q 8 h or 1 g q 6 h | 3 or 4 g |
| Uncomplicated UTI | 250 mg q 6 h | 1 g | 250 mg q 6 h | 1 g |
| Complicated UTI | 500 mg q 6 h | 2 g | 500 mg q 6 h | 2 g |

[1] Including gram-positive and -negative aerobes and anaerobes

*Children –*

| Pediatric Dosing Guidelines (≥ 3 months old) |
|---|
| ≥ 3 months old (non-CNS infections) |
| 15 to 25 mg/kg/dose every 6 hours |
| Maximum daily dose for fully susceptible organisms is 2 g/day, and for infections with moderately susceptible organisms (primarily some strains of P. aeruginosa) is 4 g/day (based on adults studies). |
| Higher doses (≤ 90 mg/kg/day in older children) have been used in cystic fibrosis patients. |

| Pediatric Dosing Guidelines (≤ 3 months old) |
|---|
| ≤ 3 months old (weighing ≥ 1500 g; non-CNS infections) |
| < 1 week old: 25 mg/kg every 12 hours |
| 1 to 4 weeks old: 25 mg/kg every 8 hours |
| 4 weeks to 3 months old: 25 mg/kg every 6 hours |

Give doses less than or equal to 500 mg by IV infusion over 15 to 30 minutes. Give doses greater than 500 mg by IV infusion over 40 to 60 minutes.

Imipenem-cilastatin IV is not recommended in pediatric patients with CNS infections because of the risk of seizures and in pediatric patients less than 30 kg with impaired renal function, as no data are available.

*Renal function impairment –*

| Reduced IV Dosage in Adult Patients with Impaired Renal Function or Body Weight < 70 kg | | | | | |
|---|---|---|---|---|---|
| Body weight | ≥ 70 kg | 60 kg | 50 kg | 40 kg | 30 kg |
| Ccr (mL/min/1.73 m²) | If total daily dose for normal renal function is 1 g/day, use: | | | | |
| ≥ 71 | 250 q 6 h | 250 q 8 h | 125 q 6 h | 125 q 6 h | 125 q 8 h |
| 41 to 70 | 250 q 8 h | 125 q 6 h | 125 q 6 h | 125 q 8 h | 125 q 8 h |
| 21 to 40 | 250 q 12 h | 250 q 12 h | 125 q 8 h | 125 q 12 h | 125 q 12 h |
| 6 to 20 | 250 q 12 h | 125 q 12 h | 125 q 12 h | 125 q 12 h | 125 q 12 h |
| | If total daily dose for normal renal function is 1.5 g/day, use: | | | | |
| ≥ 71 | 500 q 8 h | 250 q 6 h | 250 q 6 h | 250 q 8 h | 125 q 6 h |
| 41 to 70 | 250 q 6 h | 250 q 8 h | 250 q 8 h | 125 q 6 h | 125 q 8 h |
| 21 to 40 | 250 q 8 h | 250 q 8 h | 250 q 12 h | 125 q 8 h | 125 q 8 h |
| 6 to 20 | 250 q 12 h | 250 q 12 h | 250 q 12 h | 125 q 12 h | 125 q 12 h |
| | If total daily dose for normal renal function is 2 g/day, use: | | | | |
| ≥ 71 | 500 q 6 h | 500 q 8 h | 250 q 6 h | 250 q 6 h | 250 q 8 h |
| 41 to 70 | 500 q 8 h | 250 q 6 h | 250 q 6 h | 250 q 8 h | 125 q 6 h |
| 21 to 40 | 250 q 6 h | 250 q 8 h | 250 q 8 h | 250 q 12 h | 125 q 8 h |
| 6 to 20 | 250 q 12 h | 250 q 12 h | 250 q 12 h | 250 q 12 h | 125 q 12 h |
| | If total daily dose for normal renal function is 3 g/day, use: | | | | |
| ≥ 71 | 1000 q 8 h | 750 q 8 h | 500 q 6 h | 500 q 8 h | 250 q 6 h |
| 41 to 70 | 500 q 6 h | 500 q 8 h | 500 q 8 h | 250 q 6 h | 250 q 8 h |
| 21 to 40 | 500 q 8 h | 500 q 8 h | 250 q 6 h | 250 q 8 h | 250 q 8 h |
| 6 to 20 | 500 q 12 h | 500 q 12 h | 250 q 12 h | 250 q 12 h | 250 q 12 h |
| | If total daily dose for normal renal function is 4 g/day, use: | | | | |
| ≥ 71 | 1000 q 6 h | 1000 q 8 h | 750 q 8 h | 500 q 6 h | 500 q 8 h |
| 41 to 70 | 750 q 8 h | 750 q 8 h | 500 q 6 h | 500 q 8 h | 250 q 6 h |
| 21 to 40 | 500 q 6 h | 500 q 8 h | 500 q 8 h | 250 q 6 h | 250 q 8 h |
| 6 to 20 | 500 q 12 h | 500 q 12 h | 500 q 12 h | 250 q 12 h | 250 q 12 h |

IM: Total daily IM dosages greater than 1500 mg/day are not recommended. Administer by deep IM injection into a large muscle mass (such as the gluteal muscles or lateral part of the thigh) with a 21-gauge 2″ needle.

| Imipenem-Cilastatin IM Dosage Guidelines | | |
|---|---|---|
| Type/Location of infection | Severity | Dosage regimen |
| Lower respiratory tract Skin and skin structure Gynecologic | Mild/Moderate | 500 or 750 mg q 12 h depending on the severity of infection |
| Intra-abdominal | Mild/Moderate | 750 mg q 12 h |

*Hemodialysis* – Imipenem-cilastatin is cleared by hemodialysis. The patient should receive imipenem-cilastatin after hemodialysis and at 12-hour intervals timed from the end of that dialysis session.

## Actions

*Pharmacology:* This product is a formulation of imipenem, a thienamycin antibiotic, and cilastatin sodium, the inhibitor of the renal dipeptidase, dehydropeptidase-1, which is responsible for the extensive metabolism of imipenem when it is administered alone. Cilastatin prevents the metabolism of imipenem, increasing urinary recovery and decreasing possible renal toxicity. The bactericidal activity of imipenem results from the inhibition of cell-wall synthesis, related to binding to penicillin-binding proteins (PBP).

*Pharmacokinetics:*
   *Absorption/Distribution –*
      *IV:* IV infusion over 20 minutes results in peak plasma levels of imipenem antimicrobial activity that range from 14 to 83 mcg/mL, depending on the dose. Plasma levels declined to 1 mcg/mL or less in 4 to 6 hours. Peak plasma levels of cilastatin following a 20-minute IV infusion range from 15 to 88 mcg/mL, depending on the dose. The plasma half-life of each component is approximately 1 hour. Protein binding is 20% for imipenem and 40% for cilastatin.

      *IM:* Following IM administration of 500 or 750 mg doses, peak plasma levels of imipenem antimicrobial activity occur within 2 hours and average 10 and 12 mcg/mL, respectively. When compared with IV administration, imipenem is approximately 75% bioavailable following IM administration, while cilastatin is approximately 95% bioavailable. The prolonged absorption of imipenem following IM use results in an effective plasma half-life of approximately 2 to 3 hours and plasma levels that remain greater than 2 mcg/mL for at least 6 or 8 hours following a 500 or 750 mg dose, respectively. This plasma profile for imipenem permits IM administration every 12 hours with no accumulation of cilastatin and only slight accumulation of imipenem.

      Imipenem urine levels remain above 10 mcg/mL for the 12-hour dosing interval following IM administration of 500 or 750 mg doses. Total urinary excretion of imipenem and cilastatin averages 50% and 75%, respectively, following either dose.

   *Metabolism/Excretion –* Cilastatin prevents renal metabolism of imipenem. The protein binding of imipenem and cilastatin is approximately 20% and 40%, respectively. Approximately 70% of imipenem and cilastatin is recovered in urine within 10 hours of administration.

*Microbiology:* Imipenem-cilastatin has a high degree of stability in the presence of β-lactamases, including penicillinases and cephalosporinases produced by gram-negative and gram-positive bacteria.

## Contraindications
Hypersensitivity to any component of this product.

*IM:* Hypersensitivity to local anesthetics of the amide type and in patients with severe shock or heart block due to the use of lidocaine HCl diluent.

*IV:* Patients with meningitis (safety and efficacy have not been established).

## Warnings
*Resistance:* As with other β-lactam antibiotics, some strains of *P. aeruginosa* may develop resistance fairly rapidly during treatment with imipenem-cilastatin.

*Pseudomembranous colitis:* Pseudomembranous colitis has occurred with virtually all antibiotics.

*Hypersensitivity reactions:* Serious and occasionally fatal hypersensitivity reactions have occurred in patients receiving therapy with β-lactams. They are more apt to occur in people with a history of sensitivity to multiple allergens. Patients with a history of penicillin hypersensitivity have experienced severe reactions when treated with another β-lactam.

*Renal function impairment:* Do not give imipenem-cilastatin IV to patients with Ccr less than or equal to 5 mL/min/1.73 m$^2$, unless hemodialysis is instituted within 48 hours. For patients on hemodialysis, imipenem-cilastatin IV is recommended only when the benefit outweighs the potential risk of seizures.

*Pregnancy:* Category C.

*Lactation:* It is not known whether this drug is excreted in breast milk.

*Children:*
      *IM –* Safety and efficacy for use in children younger than 12 years of age are not established for IM use.

      *IV –* Use of IV in neonates to 16 years of age (with non-CNS infections) is supported by evidence from adequate and well-controlled studies. IV use is not recommended in pediatric patients with CNS infections because of the risk of seizures, or in pediatric patients less than 30 kg with impaired renal function as no data are available.

### Precautions

*Monitoring:* Periodically assess organ system function during prolonged therapy.

*CNS adverse experiences:* CNS adverse experiences have occurred with the IV formulation, especially when recommended dosages were exceeded. They are most common in patients with CNS disorders who also have compromised renal function and are rare when no underlying CNS disorder exists. (Continue anticonvulsants in patients with a known seizure disorder.) If focal tremors, myoclonus, or seizures occur, neurologically evaluate the patient, institute anticonvulsants, re-examine the dose, and determine whether to decrease dosage or discontinue the drug. If these effects occur with the IM formulation, discontinue the drug.

### Drug Interactions

Drugs that may interact with imipenem-cilastatin include ganciclovir, probenecid, and cyclosporine.

### Adverse Reactions

Adverse reactions occurring in at least 3% of patients include phlebitis and thrombophlebitis; in newborn patients to 3 months of age and older, diarrhea and convulsions have occurred.

# ERTAPENEM

| | |
|---|---|
| **Powder, lyophilized:** 1.046 g ertapenem sodium (equivalent to 1 g ertapenem) (*Rx*) | *Invanz* (Merck) |

### Indications

For the treatment of adult patients with the following moderate to severe infections caused by susceptible strains of the designated microorganisms.

*Complicated intra-abdominal infections:* Caused by *Escherichia coli*, *Clostridium clostridioforme*, *Eubacterium lentum*, *Peptostreptococcus* sp., *Bacteroides fragilis*, *B. distasonis*, *B. ovatus*, *B. thetaiotaomicron*, or *B. uniformis*.

*Complicated skin and skin structure infections:* Caused by *Staphylococcus aureus* (methicillin-susceptible strains only), *Streptococcus pyogenes*, *E. coli*, or *Peptostreptococcus* sp.

*Community-acquired pneumonia:* Caused by *Streptococcus pneumoniae* (penicillin-susceptible strains only), including cases with concurrent bacteremia, *Haemophilus influenzae* (beta-lactamase-negative strains only), or *Moraxella catarrhalis*.

*Complicated urinary tract infections, including pyelonephritis:* Caused by *E. coli*, including cases with concurrent bacteremia, or *Klebsiella pneumoniae*.

*Acute pelvic infections, including postpartum endomyometritis, septic abortion, and postsurgical gynecologic infections:* Caused by *Streptococcus agalactiae*, *E. coli*, *B. fragilis*, *Porphyromonas asaccharolytica*, *Peptostreptococcus* sp., or *Prevotella bivia*.

### Administration and Dosage

1 g given once a day.

Ertapenem may be administered by IV infusion for up to 14 days or IM injection for up to 7 days. When administered IV, infuse ertapenem over a period of 30 minutes.

IM administration of ertapenem may be used as an alternative to IV administration in the treatment of those infections for which IM therapy is appropriate.

Do not mix or co-infuse ertapenem with other medications. Do not use diluents containing dextrose ($\alpha$-D-glucose).

| Ertapenem Dosage Guidelines for Adults with Normal Renal Function[1] and Body Weight | | |
|---|---|---|
| Infection[2] | Daily dose (IV or IM) | Recommended duration of total antimicrobial treatment |
| Complicated intra-abdominal infections | 1 g | 5 to 14 days |
| Complicated skin and skin-structure infections | 1 g | 7 to 14 days |
| Community-acquired pneumonia | 1 g | 10 to 14 days[3] |
| Complicated urinary tract infections, including pyelonephritis | 1 g | 10 to 14 days[3] |
| Acute pelvic infections, including post-partum endomyometritis, septic abortion, and postsurgical gynecologic infections | 1 g | 3 to 10 days |

[1] Defined as Ccr greater than 90 mL/min/1.73 m$^2$.
[2] Caused by the designated pathogens (see Indications).
[3] Duration includes a possible switch to an appropriate oral therapy after at least 3 days of parenteral therapy once clinical improvement has been demonstrated.

*Renal insufficiency:* Patients with advanced renal insufficiency (Ccr less than or equal to 30 mL/min/1.73 m$^2$) and end-stage renal insufficiency (Ccr less than or equal to 10 mL/min/1.73 m$^2$) should receive 500 mg daily.

*Hemodialysis:* When patients on hemodialysis are given the recommended daily dose of 500 mg of ertapenem within 6 hours prior to hemodialysis, a supplementary dose of 150 mg is recommended following the hemodialysis session. If ertapenem is given at least 6 hours prior to hemodialysis, no supplementary dose is needed. There are no data in patients undergoing peritoneal dialysis or hemofiltration.

### Actions
*Pharmacokinetics:*

*Absorption* – The mean bioavailability is approximately 90%. Following 1 g daily IM administration, mean peak plasma concentrations ($C_{max}$) are achieved in approximately 2.3 hours ($T_{max}$).

*Distribution* – Ertapenem is highly bound to human plasma proteins, primarily albumin.

The apparent volume of distribution at steady state of ertapenem is approximately 8.2 L.

*Metabolism* – In vitro studies in human liver microsomes indicate that ertapenem does not inhibit metabolism mediated by any of the following cytochrome P450 (CYP) isoforms: 1A2, 2C9, 2C19, 2D6, 2E1, and 3A4.

*Excretion* – Ertapenem is eliminated primarily by the kidneys. The mean plasma half-life in healthy young adults is approximately 4 hours, and the plasma clearance is approximately 1.8 L/hour.

Following the administration of 1 g IV radiolabeled ertapenem to healthy young adults, approximately 80% is recovered in urine and 10% in feces. Of the 80% recovered in urine, approximately 38% is excreted as unchanged drug and approximately 37% as the ring-opened metabolite.

### Contraindications
Ertapenem is contraindicated in patients with known hypersensitivity to any component of this product or to other drugs in the same class or in patients who have demonstrated anaphylactic reactions to beta-lactams.

### Warnings
*Seizures:* Seizures and other CNS adverse experiences have been reported during treatment with ertapenem.

*Pseudomembranous colitis:* Pseudomembranous colitis has been reported and may range in severity from mild to life-threatening.

*Hypersensitivity reactions:* Serious and occasionally fatal hypersensitivity (anaphylactic) reactions have been reported in patients receiving therapy with beta-lactams. These reactions are more likely to occur in individuals with a history of sensitivity to multiple allergens. There have been reports of individuals with a history of penicillin hypersensitivity who have experienced severe hypersensitivity reactions when treated with another beta-lactam.

*Elderly:* This drug is known to be substantially excreted by the kidney, and the risk of toxic reactions to this drug may be greater in patients with impaired renal function. Because elderly patients are more likely to have decreased renal function, take care in dose selection; it may be useful to monitor renal function.

*Pregnancy:* Category B.

*Lactation:* Ertapenem is excreted in breast milk. Exercise caution when ertapenem is administered to a nursing woman. Administer ertapenem to nursing mothers only when the expected benefit outweighs the risk.

*Children:* Safety and effectiveness in pediatric patients have not been established.

## Precautions

*Monitoring:* As with other antibiotics, prolonged use of ertapenem may result in overgrowth of nonsusceptible organisms.

While ertapenem possesses toxicity similar to the beta-lactam group of antibiotics, periodic assessment of organ system function, including renal, hepatic, and hematopoietic, is advisable during prolonged therapy.

*Special risk:* Seizures, irrespective of drug relationship, occurred in 0.5% of patients during study therapy plus 14-day follow-up period. These experiences have occurred most commonly in patients with CNS disorders (eg, brain lesions or history of seizures) or compromised renal function.

## Drug Interactions

Ertapenem interacts with probenecid.

## Adverse Reactions

The most common drug-related adverse experiences in patients treated with ertapenem, including those who were switched to therapy with an oral antimicrobial, were diarrhea, infused vein complication, nausea, headache, vaginitis, phlebitis/thrombophlebitis, and vomiting.

Adverse reactions occurring in at least 3% of patients included the following: Altered mental status, headache, insomnia, infused vein complication, abdominal pain, constipation, diarrhea, nausea, vomiting, edema/swelling, fever, and vaginitis.

Drug-related laboratory adverse experiences that were reported during therapy in at least 1% of patients treated with ertapenem in clinical studies were ALT increased, AST increased, serum alkaline phosphatase increased, platelet count increased, and eosinophils increased.

# AZTREONAM

**Powder for injection (lyophilized cake):** 500 mg, 1 g, and  *Azactam* (Squibb)
2 g (*Rx*)

### Indications

*Urinary tract infections:* Urinary tract infections (complicated and uncomplicated), including pyelonephritis and cystitis (initial and recurrent) caused by *Escherichia coli, Klebsiella pneumoniae, Proteus mirabilis, Pseudomonas aeruginosa, Enterobacter cloacae,
Klebsiella oxytoca, Citrobacter* sp., and *Serratia marcescens.*

*Lower respiratory tract infections:* Lower respiratory tract infections, including pneumonia
and bronchitis caused by *E. coli, K. pneumoniae, P. aeruginosa, Haemophilus influenzae, P. mirabilis, Enterobacter* sp. and *S. marcescens.*

*Septicemia:* Septicemia caused by *E. coli, K. pneumoniae, P. aeruginosa, P. mirabilis, S.
marcescens,* and *Enterobacter* sp.

*Skin and skin structure infections:* Skin and skin structure infections, including those associated with postoperative wounds, ulcers, and burns caused by *E. coli, P. mirabilis, S.
marcescens, Enterobacter* sp., *P. aeruginosa, K. pneumoniae,* and *Citrobacter* sp.

*Intra-abdominal infections:* Intra-abdominal infections, including peritonitis caused by *E.
coli, Klebsiella* sp. including *K. pneumoniae, Enterobacter* sp. including *E. cloacae, P.
aeruginosa, Citrobacter* sp. including *C. freundii* and *Serratia* sp. including *S. marcescens.*

*Gynecologic infections:* Gynecologic infections, including endometritis and pelvic cellulitis caused by *E. coli, K. pneumoniae, Enterobacter* sp. including *E. cloacae,* and *P.
mirabilis.*

*Surgery:* For adjunctive therapy to surgery to manage infections caused by susceptible
organisms.

*Concurrent initial therapy:* Concurrent initial therapy with other antimicrobials and aztreonam is recommended before the causative organism(s) is known in seriously ill
patients who also are at risk of having an infection caused by gram-positive aerobic pathogens. If anaerobic organisms are also suspected, initiate therapy concurrently with aztreonam.

*Unlabeled uses:* 1 g IM may be beneficial for acute uncomplicated gonorrhea in patients
with penicillin-resistant gonococci, as an alternative to spectinomycin.

### Administration and Dosage

Give IM or IV.

| Aztreonam Dosage Guide (Adults) | | |
|---|---|---|
| Type of infection | Dose[1] | Frequency (hours) |
| Urinary tract infection | 500 mg or 1 g | 8 or 12 |
| Moderately severe systemic infections | 1 or 2 g | 8 or 12 |
| Severe systemic or life-threatening infections | 2 g | 6 or 8 |

[1] Maximum recommended dose is 8 g/day.

| Aztreonam Dosage Guide (Children) | | |
|---|---|---|
| Type of infection | Dose[1] | Frequency (hours) |
| Mild to moderate infections | 30 mg/kg | 8 |
| Moderate to severe infections | 30 mg/kg | 6 or 8 |

[1] Maximum recommended dose is 120 mg/kg/day.

*IV route:* IV route is recommended for patients requiring single doses greater than 1 g
or those with bacterial septicemia, localized parenchymal abscess (eg, intra-abdominal abscess), peritonitis, or other severe systemic or life-threatening infections. For
infections due to *P. aeruginosa,* a dosage of 2 g every 6 or 8 hours is recommended, at
least upon initiation of therapy.

*Duration:* Duration of therapy depends on the severity of infection. Generally, continue aztreonam for at least 48 hours after the patient becomes asymptomatic or

evidence of bacterial eradication has been obtained. Persistent infections may require treatment for several weeks.

*Children:* Administer aztreonam IV to pediatric patients with normal renal function. There are insufficient data regarding IM administration to pediatric patients or dosing in pediatric patients with renal impairment.

*Renal function impairment:* Reduce dosage by 50% in patients with estimated Ccr between 10 and 30 mL/min/1.73 m$^2$ after an initial loading dose of 1 or 2 g.

In patients with severe renal failure, give 500 mg, 1 or 2 g initially. The maintenance dose should be 25% of the usual initial dose given at the usual fixed interval of 6, 8, or 12 hours. For serious or life-threatening infections, in addition to the maintenance doses, give 12.5% of the initial dose after each hemodialysis session.

*Elderly:* Obtain estimates of Ccr and make appropriate dosage modifications.

*IV:* Bolus injection may be used to initiate therapy. Slowly inject directly into a vein, or into the tubing of a suitable administration set, over 3 to 5 minutes.

*IM:* Inject deeply in large muscle mass.

### Actions

*Pharmacology:* Aztreonam, a synthetic bactericidal antibiotic, is the first of a class identified as monobactams. The monobactams have a monocyclic β-lactam nucleus. Aztreonam's bactericidal action results from the inhibition of bacterial cell wall synthesis because of a high affinity of aztreonam for penicillin-binding protein 3 (PBP3).

*Pharmacokinetics:*

*Absorption/Distribution* – Following single IM injections of 500 mg and 1 g, maximum serum concentrations occur at about 1 hour.

The serum half-life averaged 1.7 hours in subjects with normal renal function. In healthy subjects, the serum clearance was 91 mL/min and renal clearance was 56 mL/min; the apparent mean volume of distribution at steady state averaged 12.6 L.

*Metabolism/Excretion* – In healthy subjects, aztreonam is excreted in the urine about equally by active tubular secretion and glomerular filtration. Approximately 60% to 70% of an IV or IM dose was recovered in the urine by 8 hours; recovery was complete by 12 hours.

Administration IV or IM of a single 500 mg or 1 g dose every 8 hours for 7 days to healthy subjects produced no apparent accumulation; serum protein binding averaged 56% and was independent of dose.

### Contraindications

Hypersensitivity to aztreonam or any other component in the formulation.

### Warnings

*Pseudomembranous colitis:* Pseudomembranous colitis has been reported with nearly all antibacterial agents, including aztreonam, and may range in severity from mild to life-threatening.

*Epidermal necrolysis:* Epidermal necrolysis rarely has been reported in association with aztreonam in patients undergoing bone marrow transplant with multiple risk factors.

*Hypersensitivity reactions:* Make careful inquiry for a history of hypersensitivity reactions. Monitor patients who have had immediate hypersensitivity reactions to penicillins or cephalosporins. If an allergic reaction occurs, discontinue the drug and institute supportive treatment. Cross-sensitivity with other penicillins or β-lactam antibiotics is rare.

*Renal/Hepatic function impairment:* Appropriate monitoring is recommended.

In patients with impaired renal function, the serum half-life is prolonged.

*Pregnancy: Category B.* Aztreonam crosses the placenta and enters fetal circulation.

*Lactation:* Aztreonam is excreted in breast milk in concentrations that are less than 1% of maternal serum. Consider temporary discontinuation of nursing.

*Children:* Safety and efficacy of IV aztreonam have been established children 9 months to 16 years of age. Sufficient data are not available for pediatric patients younger than 9 months of age or for treatment of the following indications/pathogens: Septicemia and skin and skin-structure infections (where the skin infection is caused by *H. influenzae* type b). In pediatric patients with cystic fibrosis, higher doses of aztreonam may be warranted.

### Drug Interactions

Drugs that may interact with aztreonam include other β-lactamase-inducing antibiotics and aminoglycosides.

### Adverse Reactions

*Adults:* No adverse reactions have been reported in at least 3% of adult patients.

*Children:* Of patients younger than 2 years of age receiving 30 mg/kg every 6 hours, 11.6% experienced neutropenia; of patients older than 2 years of age receiving 50 mg/kg every 6 hours, 15% to 20% had elevations of AST and ALT more than 3 times the upper limit of normal. The increased frequency of these reported laboratory adverse events may be caused by increased severity of illness treated or higher doses of aztreonam administered.

# CHLORAMPHENICOL

| | |
|---|---|
| **Powder for injection**: 100 mg/mL (as sodium succinate) when reconstituted (*Rx*) | Various, *Chloromycetin Sodium Succinate* (Parke-Davis) |

---

> **Warning:**
> Serious and fatal blood dyscrasias occur after short-term and prolonged therapy with chloramphenicol. Aplastic anemia, which later terminated in leukemia, has been reported. Chloramphenicol must not be used when less potentially dangerous agents are effective. It must not be used to treat trivial infections or infections other than indicated, or as prophylaxis for bacterial infections.

### Indications

*Serious infections:* Serious infections for which less potentially dangerous drugs are ineffective or contraindicated caused by susceptible strains of *Salmonella* sp.; *Haemophilus influenzae*, specifically, meningeal infections; rickettsiae; lymphogranuloma-psittacosis group; various gram-negative bacteria causing bacteremia, meningitis or other serious gram-negative infections; infections involving anaerobic organisms, when *Bacteroides fragilis* is suspected; or other susceptible organisms that have been demonstrated to be resistant to all other appropriate antimicrobial agents.

If presumptive therapy is initiated, perform in vitro sensitivity tests concurrently, so that the drug may be discontinued if less potentially dangerous agents are indicated.

*Acute infections:* In acute infections caused by *Salmonella typhi*, chloramphenicol is a drug of choice.

*Cystic fibrosis regimens:* In cystic fibrosis regimens.

### Administration and Dosage

*Therapeutic concentrations:* Therapeutic concentrations generally should be maintained as follows: Peak 10 to 20 mcg/mL; trough 5 to 10 mcg/mL.

*Monitoring:* Monitoring serum levels is important because of the variability of chloramphenicol's pharmacokinetics. Monitor serum concentrations weekly; monitor more often in patients with hepatic dysfunction, in therapy more than 2 weeks, or with potentially interacting drugs.

*Adults:* 50 mg/kg/day in divided doses every 6 hours for typhoid fever and rickettsial infections. Exceptional infections (ie, meningitis, brain abscess) caused by moderately resistant organisms may require dosage up to 100 mg/kg/day to achieve blood levels inhibiting the pathogen; decrease high doses as soon as possible.

*Renal/Hepatic function impairment* – An initial loading dose of 1 g followed by 500 mg every 6 hours has been recommended in impaired hepatic function.

*Children:* 50 to 75 mg/kg/day in divided doses every 6 hours has been recommended for most indications. For meningitis, 50 to 100 mg/kg/day in divided doses every 6 hours has been recommended.

*Newborns:* 25 mg/kg/day in 4 doses every 6 hours usually produces and maintains adequate concentrations in blood and tissues. Give increased dosage demanded by severe infections only to maintain the blood concentration within an effective range. After the first 2 weeks of life, full-term infants ordinarily may receive up to 50 mg/kg/day in 4 doses every 6 hours.

*Neonates (less than 2 kg)* – 25 mg/kg once daily.

*Neonates from birth to 7 days (greater than 2 kg)* – 25 mg/kg once daily.

*Neonates over 7 days (greater than 2 kg)* – 50 mg/kg/day in divided doses every 12 hours.

These dosage recommendations are extremely important because blood concentration in all premature and full-term infants younger than 2 weeks of age differs from that of other infants because of variations in the maturity of the metabolic functions of the liver and kidneys.

*Infants and children with immature metabolic processes:* 25 mg/kg/day usually produces therapeutic concentrations. In this group particularly, carefully monitor the concentration of drug in the blood.

*IV administration:* Chloramphenicol sodium succinate is intended for IV use only; it is ineffective when given IM. Administer IV as a 10% solution injected over at least 1 minute. Substitute oral dosage as soon as feasible.

## Actions

*Pharmacology:* Chloramphenicol binds to 50 S ribosomal subunits of bacteria and interferes with or inhibits protein synthesis.

*Pharmacokinetics:*

    *Absorption* – Chloramphenicol base is absorbed rapidly from the intestinal tract and is 75% to 90% bioavailable. The inactive prodrug, chloramphenicol palmitate, is rapidly hydrolyzed to active chloramphenicol base. Bioavailability is approximately 80% for the palmitate ester. The bioavailability of the IV succinate is approximately 70%. Approximately 30% is eliminated in the urine as unhydrolyzed ester.

    *Distribution* – The therapeutic range for total serum chloramphenicol concentration is: Peak, 10 to 20 mcg/mL; trough, 5 to 10 mcg/mL. The drug is ≈ 60% bound to plasma proteins. Chloramphenicol enters the cerebrospinal fluid (CSF), even in the absence of meningeal inflammation.

    *Metabolism/Excretion* – Total urinary excretion of chloramphenicol ranges from 68% to 99% over 3 days. Most chloramphenicol detected in the blood is in the active free form. The elimination half-life of chloramphenicol is approximately 4 hours.

## Contraindications

History of hypersensitivity to, or toxicity from, chloramphenicol.

Chloramphenicol must not be used to treat trivial infections or infections other than those indicated, or as prophylaxis for bacterial infections.

## Warnings

*Blood dyscrasias:* An irreversible type of marrow depression leading to aplastic anemia with a high rate of mortality is characterized by appearance of bone marrow aplasia or hypoplasia weeks or months after therapy. Peripherally, pancytopenia is most often observed, but only 1 or 2 of the 3 major cell types may be depressed.

    A dose-related reversible type of bone marrow depression may occur and is associated with sustained serum levels at peak greater than or equal to 25 mcg/mL, trough greater than or equal to 10 mcg/mL.

*Renal/Hepatic function impairment:* Excessive blood levels may result in patients with impaired liver or kidney function, including that caused by immature metabolic processes in the infant.

*Pregnancy:* Chloramphenicol readily crosses the placental barrier; cautious use is particularly important during pregnancy at term or during labor because of potential toxic effects on the fetus.

*Lactation:* Chloramphenicol appears in breast milk with a milk:plasma ratio of 0.5. Use with caution, if at all, during lactation.

*Children:* Use with caution and in reduced dosages in premature and full-term infants to avoid gray syndrome toxicity. Monitor drug serum levels carefully during therapy of the newborn.

## Precautions

*Hematology:* Evaluate baseline and periodic blood studies approximately every 2 days during therapy. Discontinue the drug upon appearance of reticulocytopenia, leukopenia, thrombocytopenia, anemia, or any other findings attributable to chloramphenicol. Avoid concurrent therapy with other drugs that may cause bone marrow depression.

    Avoid repeated courses if at all possible. Do not continue treatment longer than required to produce a cure.

*Acute intermittent porphyria or glucose-6-phosphate dehydrogenase deficiency:* Use with caution in patients with acute intermittent porphyria or glucose-6-phosphate dehydrogenase deficiency.

### Drug Interactions

Drugs that may affect chloramphenicol include barbiturates, rifampin, and hydantoins. Drugs that may be affected by chloramphenicol include barbiturates, anticoagulants, cyclophosphamide, hydantoins, iron salts, penicillins, sulfonylureas, and vitamin $B_{12}$.

### Adverse Reactions

Adverse reactions may include nausea; vomiting; glossitis; stomatitis; diarrhea; headache; mild depression; mental confusion; fever; macular/vesicular rashes; angioedema; urticaria; anaphylaxis; optic and peripheral neuritis.

Toxic reactions including fatalities (approximately 40%) have occurred in the premature infant and newborn; the signs and symptoms associated with these reactions have been referred to as the "gray syndrome."

# FLUOROQUINOLONES

| | |
|---|---|
| **CIPROFLOXACIN** | |
| **Tablets**: 100, 250, 500, and 750 mg (*Rx*) | Various, *Cipro* (Bayer) |
| **Tablets, extended-release**: 500 and 1000 mg (*Rx*) | *Cipro XR* (Bayer) |
| **Powder for oral suspension**: 250 mg/5 mL (5%) and 500 mg/5 mL (10%) (when reconstituted) (*Rx*) | Various, *Cipro* (Bayer) |
| **Injection**: 200 and 400 mg (*Rx*) | *Cipro IV* (Bayer) |
| **GATIFLOXACIN** | |
| **Tablets**: 200 and 400 mg (*Rx*) | *Tequin* (Bristol-Myers Squibb) |
| **Injection (concentrate) (single-use vials)**: 400 mg (*Rx*) | |
| **Injection (premix)**: 200 and 400 mg (*Rx*) | |
| **GEMIFLOXACIN MESYLATE** | |
| **Tablets**: 320 mg (as base) (*Rx*) | *Factive* (Oscient) |
| **LEVOFLOXACIN** | |
| **Tablets**: 250, 500, and 750 mg (*Rx*) | *Levaquin* (Ortho-McNeil) |
| **Injection (concentrate) (single-use vials)**: 500 mg (25 mg/mL) and 750 mg (25 mg/mL) (*Rx*) | |
| **Injection (premix)**: 250 (5 mg/mL), 500 mg (5 mg/mL), and 750 mg (5 mg/mL) (*Rx*) | |
| **LOMEFLOXACIN HCl** | |
| **Tablets**: 400 mg (*Rx*) | *Maxaquin* (Biovail) |
| **MOXIFLOXACIN HCl** | |
| **Tablets**: 400 mg (*Rx*) | *Avelox* (Bayer) |
| **Injection (premix)**: 400 mg (*Rx*) | *Avelox I.V.* (Bayer) |
| **NORFLOXACIN** | |
| **Tablets**: 400 mg (*Rx*) | *Noroxin* (Merck) |
| **OFLOXACIN** | |
| **Tablets**: 200, 300, and 400 mg (*Rx*) | *Floxin* (Ortho-McNeil) |
| **SPARFLOXACIN** | |
| **Tablets**: 200 mg (*Rx*) | *Zagam* (Bertek) |

**Indications**
For specific approved indications, refer to the Administration and Dosage section.

**Administration and Dosage**
*CIPROFLOXACIN:*

### Ciprofloxacin Dosage Guidelines

| Location of infection | Type or severity | Unit dose | Frequency | Daily dose | Usual durations[1] (oral doseforms only) |
|---|---|---|---|---|---|
| Urinary tract | acute uncomplicated | 100 or 250 mg (500 mg XR) | q 12 h (q 24 h XR) | 200 or 500 mg (500 mg XR) | 3 days |
| | mild/moderate | 250 mg (200 mg IV) | q 12 h | 500 mg (400 mg IV) | 7 to 14 days |
| | severe/complicated[2] | 500 mg (400 mg IV) (1000 mg XR) | q 12 h | 1000 mg (800 mg IV) (1000 mg XR) | 7 to 14 days |
| Pyelonephritis | acute uncomplicated | 1000 mg XR | q 24 h | 1000 mg XR | 7 to 14 days |
| Lower respiratory tract Bone and joint Skin and skin structure | mild/moderate | 500 mg (400 mg IV) | q 12 h | 1000 mg (800 mg IV) | 7 to 14 days ≥ 4 to 6 weeks (bone and joint only) |
| | severe/complicated | 750 mg (400 mg IV) | q 12 h (q 8 h) | 1500 mg (1200 mg) | 7 to 14 days ≥ 4 to 6 weeks (bone and joint only) |
| Nosocomial pneumonia | mild/moderate/severe | 400 mg IV | q 8 h | 1200 mg IV | 10 to 14 days |
| Intra-abdominal[3] | complicated | 500 mg (400 mg IV) | q 12 h | 1000 mg (800 mg IV) | 7 to 14 days |
| Acute sinusitis | mild/moderate | 500 mg (400 mg IV) | q 12 h | 1000 mg (800 mg IV) | 10 days |
| Chronic bacterial prostatitis | mild/moderate | 500 mg (400 mg IV) | q 12 h | 1000 mg (800 mg IV) | 28 days |
| Empirical therapy in febrile neutropenic patients | severe: ciprofloxacin + piperacillin | 400 mg IV 50 mg/kg IV | q 8 h q 4 h | 1200 mg IV not to exceed 24 g/day | 7 to 14 days |
| Infectious diarrhea | mild/moderate/severe | 500 mg | q 12 h | 1000 mg | 5 to 7 days |
| Typhoid fever | mild/moderate | 500 mg | q 12 h | 1000 mg | 10 days |
| Urethral/Cervical gonococcal infections | uncomplicated | 250 mg | single dose | 250 mg | single dose |

| Ciprofloxacin Dosage Guidelines | | | | | |
|---|---|---|---|---|---|
| Location of infection | Type or severity | Unit dose | Frequency | Daily dose | Usual durations[1] (oral doseforms only) |
| Inhalational anthrax (postexposure)[4] | adult | 500 mg (400 mg IV) | q 12 h | 1000 mg (800 mg IV) | 60 days |
| | pediatric | 15 mg/kg/dose, not to exceed 500 mg/dose (10 mg/kg/IV dose, not to exceed 400 mg/IV dose) | q 12 h | not to exceed 1000 mg (not to exceed 800 mg IV) | 60 days |

[1] Generally, ciprofloxacin should be continued for ≥ 2 days after the signs and symptoms of infection have disappeared, except for inhalational anthrax (postexposure).

[2] Including secondary bacteremia from *Escherichia coli* (IV only).

[3] Used in conjunction with metronidazole.

[4] Begin drug administration as soon as possible after suspected or confirmed exposure. This indication is based on a surrogate endpoint, ciprofloxacin serum concentrations achieved in humans, reasonably likely to predict clinical benefit. Total duration of ciprofloxacin administration (IV, IR, or oral) for inhalational anthrax (postexposure) is 60 days.

XR and IR tablets are not interchangeable.

XR tablets may be taken with meals that include milk; however, avoid coadministration with dairy products alone or with calcium-fortified products because decreased absorption is possible. A 2-hour window between substantial calcium intake (more than 800 mg) and dosing with XR tablets is recommended. Swallow the XR tablet whole; do not split, crush, or chew.

The duration of treatment depends upon the severity of infection. Generally, continue ciprofloxacin for at least 2 days after the signs and symptoms of infection have disappeared. The usual duration is 7 to 14 days; however, for severe and complicated infections, more prolonged therapy may be required.

*IR tablets* – Administer ciprofloxacin at least 2 hours before or 6 hours after magnesium/aluminum antacids, sucralfate, didanosine chewable/buffered tablets or pediatric powder for oral solution, or other products containing calcium, iron, or zinc.

*Renal function impairment* –

| Ciprofloxacin Dosage in Impaired Renal Function | |
| --- | --- |
| Ccr (mL/min) | Dose |
| > 50 (IR, suspension); > 30 (IV) | See usual dosage |
| 30 to 50 (IR, suspension) | 250 to 500 mg q 12 h |
| 5 to 29 | 250 to 500 mg q 18 h (IR, suspension); 200 to 400 mg q 18 to 24 h (IV) |
| Hemodialysis or peritoneal dialysis (IR, suspension) | 250 to 500 mg q 24 h (after dialysis) |

In patients with severe infections and severe renal impairment, 750 mg may be administered orally at the intervals noted in the table.

*XR tablets:* No dosage adjustment is required for patients with uncomplicated urinary tract infections receiving 500 mg ciprofloxacin XR. In patients with complicated urinary tract infections and acute uncomplicated pyelonephritis who have a Ccr of less than 30 mL/min, reduce the dose of XR tablets from 1000 to 500 mg/day. For patients on hemodialysis or peritoneal dialysis, administer XR tablets after the dialysis procedure is completed.

*CDC recommended treatment schedules for uncomplicated gonorrhea* – 500 mg orally in a single dose plus 1 g azithromycin orally in a single dose or 100 mg doxycycline orally twice daily for 7 days, if chlamydial infection is not ruled out.

*IV* – Administer by IV infusion over 60 minutes. Slow infusion of a dilute solution into a large vein will minimize patient discomfort and reduce the risk of venous irritation.

*IV to oral switch* – Patients whose therapy is started with ciprofloxacin IV may be switched to ciprofloxacin tablets or oral suspension when clinically indicated. Equivalent dosing regimens are indicated in the table below:

| Equivalent AUC Dosing Regimens | |
| --- | --- |
| Ciprofloxacin oral dosage[1] | Equivalent ciprofloxacin IV dosage |
| 250 mg tablet q 12 h | 200 mg IV q 12 h |
| 500 mg tablet q 12 h | 400 mg IV q 12 h |
| 750 mg tablet q 12 h | 400 mg IV q 8 h |

[1] IR tablets and oral suspension only.

GATIFLOXACIN: Gatifloxacin may be administered without regard to food, including milk and dietary supplements containing calcium, and without regard to age (18 years of age and older) or gender.

*Oral* – Administer oral gatifloxacin at least 4 hours before the administration of ferrous sulfate; dietary supplements containing zinc, magnesium, or iron (such as multivitamins); aluminum/magnesium-containing antacids; or didanosine (buffered tablets, buffered solution, or buffered powder for oral suspension).

*IV* – Administer injection by IV infusion only. It is not intended for IM, intrathecal, intraperitoneal, or subcutaneous administration.

| Gatifloxacin Dosage Guidelines | | |
|---|---|---|
| Infection[1] | Daily dose (mg)[2] | Duration |
| Acute bacterial exacerbation of chronic bronchitis | 400 | 5 days |
| Acute sinusitis | 400 | 10 days |
| Community-acquired pneumonia | 400 | 7 to 14 days |
| Uncomplicated skin and skin structure infections | 400 | 7 to 10 days |
| Uncomplicated UTIs (cystitis) | 400 | Single dose |
| | or 200 | 3 days |
| Complicated UTIs | 400 | 7 to 10 days |
| Acute pyelonephritis | 400 | 7 to 10 days |
| Uncomplicated urethral gonorrhea in men; endocervical and rectal gonorrhea in women | 400 | Single dose |

[1] Caused by the designated pathogens (see Indications).
[2] For either the oral and IV routes of administration.

*Renal function impairment* – The recommended dosage of gatifloxacin follows:

| Recommended Dosage of Gatifloxacin in Adult Patients with Renal Impairment | | |
|---|---|---|
| Ccr | Initial dose (mg) | Subsequent dose[1] |
| ≥ 40 mL/min | 400 | 400 mg daily |
| < 40 mL/min | 400 | 200 mg daily |
| Hemodialysis | 400 | 200 mg daily |
| Continuous peritoneal dialysis | 400 | 200 mg daily |

[1] Start of subsequent dose on day 2 of dosing.

Administer gatifloxacin after a dialysis session for patients on hemodialysis.

*Uncomplicated UTIs and gonorrhea* – Single 400 mg dose regimen (for the treatment of uncomplicated UTIs and gonorrhea) and 200 mg once daily for 3 days regimen (for the treatment of uncomplicated UTIs) require no dosage adjustment in patients with impaired renal function.

GEMIFLOXACIN: Gemifloxacin can be taken with or without food and should be swallowed whole with a liberal amount of liquid. The recommended dose of gemifloxacin is 320 mg/day, according to the following table.

*Acute bacterial exacerbation of chronic bronchitis and community acquired pneumonia (of mild to moderate severity)* –

| Gemifloxacin Dosage Guidelines | | |
|---|---|---|
| Indication | Dose (mg) | Duration (days) |
| Acute bacterial exacerbation of chronic bronchitis | 320 once daily | 5 |
| Community-acquired pneumonia (of mild to moderate severity) | 320 once daily | 7 |

*Renal function impairment* –

| Recommended Doses for Patients with Impaired Renal Function | |
|---|---|
| Creatinine clearance (mL/min) | Dose |
| > 40 | See usual dosage |
| ≤ 40, hemodialysis, CAPD[1] | 160 mg q 24 h |

[1] CAPD = continuous ambulatory peritoneal dialysis.

LEVOFLOXACIN: Administer oral doses at least 2 hours before or 2 hours after antacids containing magnesium or aluminum, as well as sucralfate, metal cations such as iron and multivitamin preparations with zinc, or didanosine (chewable/buffered tablets or pediatric powder for oral solution).

| Levofloxacin Dosing with Normal Renal Function (Ccr > 80 mL/min) | | | | |
|---|---|---|---|---|
| Infection[1] | Unit dose | Frequency | Duration[2] | Daily dose |
| Acute bacterial exacerbation of chronic bronchitis | 500 mg | q 24 h | 7 days | 500 mg |
| Acute maxillary sinusitis | 500 mg | q 24 h | 10 to 14 days | 500 mg |
| Acute pyelonephritis | 250 mg | q 24 h | 10 days | 250 mg |
| Chronic bacterial prostatitis | 500 mg | q 24 h | 28 days | 500 mg |
| Pneumonia, community-acquired | 500 mg | q 24 h | 7 to 14 days | 500 mg |
|  | 750 mg[3] | q 24 h | 5 days | 750 mg |
| Pneumonia, nosocomial | 750 mg | q 24 h | 7 to 14 days | 750 mg |
| SSSI, complicated | 750 mg | q 24 h | 7 to 14 days | 750 mg |
| SSSI, uncomplicated | 500 mg | q 24 h | 7 to 10 days | 500 mg |
| UTI, complicated | 250 mg | q 24 h | 10 days | 250 mg |
| UTI, uncomplicated | 250 mg | q 24 h | 3 days | 250 mg |

[1] Caused by the designated pathogens (see Indications).
[2] Sequential therapy (IV to oral) may be instituted at the discretion of the physician.
[3] Efficacy of this alternative regimen has only been documented for infections caused by penicillin-susceptible S. pneumoniae, H. influenzae, H. parainfluenzae, M. pneumoniae, and C. pneumoniae.

| Levofloxacin Dosing with Renal Function Impairment | | |
|---|---|---|
| Renal status | Initial dose | Subsequent dose |
| Acute bacterial exacerbation of chronic bronchitis/community-acquired pneumonia/acute maxillary sinusitis/uncomplicated SSSI/chronic bacterial prostatitis | | |
| Ccr from 50 to 80 mL/min | No dosage adjustment required | |
| Ccr from 20 to 49 mL/min | 500 mg | 250 mg q 24 h |
| Ccr from 10 to 19 mL/min | 500 mg | 250 mg q 48 h |
| Hemodialysis/CAPD[1] | 500 mg | 250 mg q 48 h |
| Complicated SSSI/nosocomial pneumonia | | |
| Ccr from 50 to 80 mL/min | No dosage adjustment required | |
| Ccr from 20 to 49 mL/min | 750 mg | 750 mg q 48 h |
| Ccr from 10 to 19 mL/min | 750 mg | 500 mg q 48 h |
| Hemodialysis/CAPD[1] | 750 mg | 500 mg q 48 h |
| Complicated UTI/acute pyelonephritis | | |
| Ccr ≥ 20 mL/min | No dosage adjustment required | |
| Ccr from 10 to 19 mL/min | 250 mg | 250 mg q 48 h |
| Uncomplicated UTI | No dosage adjustment required | |

[1] CAPD = chronic ambulatory peritoneal dialysis.

*IV administration* – Administer by IV infusion only, slowly over a period of 60 minutes or more (750 mg over 90 minutes). Avoid rapid or bolus IV infusion. Do not administer by IM, intrathecal, intraperitoneal, or subcutaneous routes.

LOMEFLOXACIN HCl: Risk of reaction to solar UVA light may be reduced by taking lomefloxacin at least 12 hours before exposure to the sun (eg, in the evening). Lomefloxacin may be taken without regard to meals. Sucralfate and antacids containing magnesium or aluminum, or didanosine chewable/buffered tablets or the pediatric powder for oral solution should not be taken within 4 hours before or 2 hours after taking lomefloxacin.

| Recommended Daily Dose of Lomefloxacin | | | | |
|---|---|---|---|---|
| Body system | Infection | Dose | Frequency | Duration |
| Lower respiratory tract | Acute bacterial exacerbation of chronic bronchitis | 400 mg | once daily | 10 days |
| Urinary tract | Uncomplicated cystitis caused by K. pneumoniae, P. mirabilis, or Staphylococcus saprophyticus | 400 mg | once daily | 10 days |
| | Uncomplicated cystitis in females caused by E. coli | 400 mg | once daily | 3 days |
| | Complicated UTI | 400 mg | once daily | 14 days |

*Renal function impairment* – Lomefloxacin primarily is eliminated by renal excretion. Modification of dosage is recommended in patients with renal dysfunction. In patients with a Ccr greater than 10 but less than 40 mL/min/1.73 m$^2$, the recommended dosage is an initial loading dose of 400 mg followed by daily maintenance doses of 200 mg once daily for the duration of the treatment.

*Dialysis patients* – Hemodialysis removes only a negligible amount of lomefloxacin (3% in 4 hours). Give hemodialysis patients an initial loading dose of 400 mg followed by maintenance dose of 200 mg once daily for duration of treatment.

*Preoperative prevention* –

*Transrectal prostate biopsy:* The recommended dose for transrectal prostate biopsy is a single 400 mg dose 1 to 6 hours prior to the procedure.

*Transurethral surgical procedures:* A single 400 mg dose 2 to 6 hours prior to surgery when oral preoperative prophylaxis for transurethral surgical procedures is considered appropriate.

MOXIFLOXACIN HCl: The dose of moxifloxacin is 400 mg (orally or as an IV infusion) once every 24 hours.

| Moxifloxacin Dosage Guidelines (IV and Oral) | | | |
|---|---|---|---|
| Infection[1] | Daily dose (mg) | Frequency | Duration (days) |
| Acute bacterial sinusitis | 400 | q 24 h | 10 |
| Acute bacterial exacerbation of chronic bronchitis | 400 | q 24 h | 5 |
| Community-acquired pneumonia | 400 | q 24 h | 7 to 14 |
| Uncomplicated skin and skin structure infections | 400 | q 24 h | 7 |

[1] Caused by the designated pathogens (see Indications).

Administer oral doses of moxifloxacin at least 4 hours before or 8 hours after antacids containing magnesium or aluminum, sucralfate, metal cations such as iron, multivitamin preparations with zinc, or didanosine (chewable/buffered tablets or pediatric powder for oral solution).

Moxifloxacin may be administered without regard to food.

*Switching from IV to oral dosing* – When switching from IV to oral dosage administration, no dosage adjustment is necessary.

*IV* – Administer IV moxifloxacin by IV infusion only. It is not intended for IM, intrathecal, intra-arterial, intraperitoneal, or subcutaneous administration.

Administer by IV infusion over a period of 60 minutes by direct infusion or through a Y-type IV infusion set that may already be in place. Rapid or bolus IV infusion must be avoided.

Do not add additives or other medications to IV moxifloxacin or infuse simultaneously through the same IV line. If the same IV line is used for sequential infusion of other drugs, or if the "piggyback" method of administration is used, flush the line before and after infusion of moxifloxacin IV with a compatible solution.

Moxifloxacin IV is compatible with the following IV solutions at ratios from 1:10 to 10:1: 0.9% sodium chloride injection, 1M sodium chloride injection, 5% dextrose injection, sterile water for injection, 10% dextrose for injection, Lactated Ringer's for injection.

*NORFLOXACIN:* Take 1 hour before or 2 hours after meals or dairy products and with a glass of water. Patients should be well hydrated.

| Recommended Norfloxacin Dosage | | | | | |
|---|---|---|---|---|---|
| Infection | Description | Dose | Frequency | Duration | Daily dose |
| Urinary tract infections (UTI) | Uncomplicated (cystitis) caused by *E. coli*, *Klebsiella pneumoniae*, or *Proteus mirabilis* | 400 mg | q 12 h | 3 days | 800 mg |
| | Uncomplicated caused by other organisms | 400 mg | q 12 h | 7 to 10 days | 800 mg |
| | Complicated | 400 mg | q 12 h | 10 to 21 days | 800 mg |
| Sexually transmitted diseases | Uncomplicated gonorrhea | 800 mg | single dose | 1 day | 800 mg |
| Prostatitis | Acute or chronic | 400 mg | q 12 h | 28 days | 800 mg |

*Renal function impairment* – In patients with Ccr less than or equal to 30 mL/min/ 1.73 m², administer 400 mg once daily for the duration given above.

*CDC-recommended treatment schedules for gonorrhea* –

*Gonococcal infections, uncomplicated:* 800 mg as a single dose (alternative regimen to **ciprofloxacin** or **ofloxacin**).

*OFLOXACIN:* Usual daily dose is 200 to 400 mg every 12 hours as described in the following table:

| Ofloxacin Dosage Guidelines (Oral and IV)[1] | | | | | |
|---|---|---|---|---|---|
| Infection | Description | Dose | Frequency | Duration | Daily dose |
| Lower respiratory tract | Exacerbation of chronic bronchitis | 400 mg | q 12 h | 10 days | 800 mg |
| | Community acquired pneumonia | 400 mg | q 12 h | 10 days | 800 mg |
| Sexually transmitted diseases | Acute, uncomplicated urethral and cervical gonorrhea | 400 mg | single dose | 1 day | 400 mg |
| | Cervicitis/Urethritis caused by *Chlamydia trachomatis* | 300 mg | q 12 h | 7 days | 600 mg |
| | Cervicitis/Urethritis caused by *C. trachomatis* and *Neisseria gonorrhoeae* | 300 mg | q 12 h | 7 days | 600 mg |
| | Acute pelvic inflammatory disease | 400 mg | q 12 h | 10 to 14 days | 800 mg |
| Skin and skin structure | Uncomplicated | 400 mg | q 12 h | 10 days | 800 mg |
| Urinary tract | Uncomplicated cystitis caused by *E. coli* or *K. pneumoniae* | 200 mg | q 12 h | 3 days | 400 mg |
| | Uncomplicated cystitis caused by other organisms | 200 mg | q 12 h | 7 days | 400 mg |
| | Complicated UTIs | 200 mg | q 12 h | 10 days | 400 mg |
| Prostatitis | Caused by *E. coli* | 300 mg | q 12 h | 6 weeks[2] | 600 mg |

[1] Caused by the designated pathogens (see Indications).
[2] Because there are no safety data presently available to support the use of the IV formulation for greater than 10 days, switch to oral or other appropriate therapy after 10 days.

Do not take antacids containing calcium, magnesium, or aluminum; sucralfate; divalent or trivalent cations such as iron; multivitamins containing zinc; or didanosine (chewable/buffered tablets or pediatric powder for oral solution) 2 hours before or 2 hours after taking ofloxacin.

*Renal function impairment* – Adjust dosage in patients with Ccr less than or equal to 50 mL/min. After a normal initial dose, adjust the dosing interval as follows:

| Ofloxacin Dosage in Impaired Renal Function | | |
|---|---|---|
| Ccr (mL/min) | Maintenance dose | Frequency |
| 20 to 50 | usual dose | q 24 h |
| < 20 | ½ usual dose | q 24 h |

*Chronic hepatic impairment (cirrhosis)* – The excretion of ofloxacin may be reduced in patients with severe liver function disorders (eg, cirrhosis with or without ascites). Do not exceed a maximum dose of 400 mg/day.

*CDC-recommended treatment schedules for chlamydia, epididymitis, pelvic inflammatory disease (PID), and gonorrhea†* –

> *Chlamydia:* 300 mg orally 2 times/day for 7 days (alternative regimen).
>
> *Epididymitis:* 300 mg orally 2 times/day for 10 days.
>
> *PID, outpatient:* 400 mg orally 2 times/day for 14 days plus metronidazole.
>
> *Gonococcal infections, uncomplicated:* 400 mg orally in a single dose plus doxycycline or azithromycin.

SPARFLOXACIN: Sparfloxacin may be taken with or without food.

> *Community-acquired pneumonia; acute bacterial exacerbations of chronic bronchitis* – The recommended daily dose of sparfloxacin in patients with normal renal function is two 200 mg tablets taken on the first day as a loading dose. Thereafter, take one 200 mg tablet every 24 hours for a total of 10 days of therapy.
>
> *Renal function impairment* – The recommended daily dose of sparfloxacin in patients with renal impairment (Ccr less than 50 mL/min) is two 200 mg tablets taken on the first day as a loading dose. Thereafter, take one 200 mg tablet every 48 hours for a total of 9 days of therapy.

## Actions

*Pharmacology:* The fluoroquinolones are synthetic, broad-spectrum antibacterial agents that inhibit DNA gyrase and topoisomerase IV. DNA gyrase is an essential enzyme that is involved in the replication, transcription, and repair of bacterial DNA. Topoisomerase IV is an enzyme known to play a key role in the partitioning of the chromosomal DNA during bacterial cell division.

*Pharmacokinetics:*

| Pharmacokinetics of Fluoroquinolones | | | | | |
|---|---|---|---|---|---|
| Fluoroquinolone | Bio-availability (%) | Mean peak plasma concentration (mcg/mL) (dose) | Area under curve (AUC) (mcg • h/mL) (dose) | Protein binding (%) | $t\frac{1}{2}$ (h) |
| Ciprofloxacin Oral | ≈ 70-80 | 1.2 (250 mg) 2.4 (500 mg) 4.3 (750 mg) 5.4 (1000 mg) | 4.8 (250 mg) 11.6 (500 mg) 20.2 (750 mg) 30.8 (1000 mg) | 20 to 40 | ≈ 4 |
| IV | | 4.4 (400 mg) | 4.8 (200 mg) 11.6 (400 mg) | | ≈ 5 to 6 |
| Gatifloxacin[1] Oral | ≈ 96 | ≈ 2 (200 mg single dose) ≈ 3.8 (400 mg single dose) ≈ 4.2 (400 mg multiple dose) | ≈ 14.2 (200 mg single dose) ≈ 33 (400 mg single dose) ≈ 34.4 (400 mg multiple dose) | ≈ 20 | ≈ 7.8 (400 mg single dose) ≈7.1 (400 mg multiple dose) |
| IV | | ≈ 2.2 (200 mg single dose) ≈ 2.4 (200 mg multiple dose) ≈ 5.5 (400 mg single dose) ≈ 4.6 (400 mg multiple dose) | ≈ 15.9 (200 mg single dose) ≈ 16.8 (200 mg multiple dose) ≈ 35.1 (400 mg single dose) ≈ 35.4 (400 mg multiple dose) | | ≈ 11.1 (200 mg single dose) ≈ 12.3 (200 mg multiple dose) ≈ 7.4 (400 mg single dose) ≈ 13.9 (400 mg multiple dose) |
| Levofloxacin | ≈ 99 | ≈ 2.8 to 11.5 (single dose oral or IV) ≈ 5.7 to 12.1 (multiple dose oral or IV) | ≈ 27.2 to 110 (single dose oral or IV) ≈ 47.5 to 108 (multiple dose oral or IV) | ≈ 24-38 | ≈ 6.3 to 7.5 (single dose oral or IV) ≈ 7 to 8.8 (multiple dose oral or IV) |
| Lomefloxacin | ≈ 95-98 | 0.8 (100 mg) 1.4 (200 mg) 3.2 (400 mg) | 5.6 (100 mg) 10.9 (200 mg) 26.1 (400 mg) | ≈ 10 | ≈ 8 |
| Moxifloxacin | ≈ 90 | 4.5 (400 mg) | ≈ 48 (400 mg) | ≈ 50 | ≈ 12 |
| Norfloxacin | 30 to 40 | 0.8 (200 mg) 1.5 (400 mg) 2.4 (800 mg) | | 10 to 15 | 3 to 4 |

† CDC 1998 Sexually Transmitted Diseases Treatment Guidelines. *MMWR.* 1998 ;47(RR-1):1-118.

| Pharmacokinetics of Fluoroquinolones | | | | | |
|---|---|---|---|---|---|
| Fluoroquinolone | Bio-avail-ability (%) | Mean peak plasma concentration (mcg/mL) (dose) | Area under curve (AUC) (mcg • h/mL) (dose) | Protein binding (%) | t½ (h) |
| Ofloxacin Oral | ≈ 98 | 1.5 (200 mg) 2.4 (300 mg) 2.9 (400 mg) 4.6 (400 mg steady-state) | 14.1 (200 mg) 21.2 (300 mg) 31.4 (400 mg) 61 (400 mg steady-state) | ≈ 32 | ≈ 9 |
| IV | | 2.7 (200 mg) 4 (400 mg) | 43.5 (400 mg) | ≈ 32 | 5 to 10 |
| Sparfloxacin | 92 | ≈ 1.3 (400 mg) | ≈ 34 (400 mg) | ≈ 45 | ≈ 20 |

[1] Single dose: AUC (0-∞); Multiple dose: AUC (0-24).

*Ciprofloxacin* – Ciprofloxacin is rapidly and well absorbed from the GI tract after oral administration with no substantial loss by first-pass metabolism. When given concomitantly with food, there is a delay in the absorption of the drug; however, the overall absorption is not substantially affected. Maximum serum concentrations are attained 1 to 2 hours after oral dosing. The drug diffuses into the cerebrospinal fluid (CSF); however, CSF concentrations are generally less than 10% of peak serum concentrations. Active tubular secretion plays a significant role in clearance; only a small amount is recovered from the bile. In patients with reduced renal function, the half-life is slightly prolonged; dosage adjustments may be required.

*Gatifloxacin* – Gatifloxacin is well absorbed from the GI tract after oral administration and can be given without regard to food. Peak plasma concentrations usually occur 1 to 2 hours after oral dosing. The oral and IV routes of administration can be considered interchangeable. Steady-state concentrations are achieved by the third daily oral or IV dose. The mean volume of distribution of gatifloxacin ranged from 1.5 to 2 L/kg. Gatifloxacin was widely distributed throughout the body into many body tissues and fluids. Gatifloxacin undergoes limited biotransformation. It does not inhibit cytochrome P450. Gatifloxacin is excreted as unchanged drug primarily by the kidney. The mean elimination half-life ranges from 7 to 14 hours. Gatifloxacin undergoes glomerular filtration and tubular secretion.

*Levofloxacin* – Levofloxacin is rapidly and completely absorbed after oral administration. Peak plasma concentrations are usually attained 1 to 2 hours after oral dosing. Steady-state is reached within 48 hours following a 500 or 750 mg once-daily dosage regimen. Levofloxacin tablets can be administered without regard to food. The oral and IV routes of administration can be considered interchangeable. The mean volume of distribution of levofloxacin generally ranges from 74 to 112 L after single and multiple doses, indication widespread distribution into body tissues. It reaches peak levels in skin tissues and in blister fluid at about 3 hours after dosing. Levofloxacin also penetrates well into the lung tissues. Levofloxacin undergoes limited metabolism and is primarily excreted as unchanged drug in the urine. Renal clearance in excess of the glomerular filtration rate suggest the tubular secretion of levofloxacin occurs in addition to glomerular filtration.

*Lomefloxacin* – Absorption is rapid. Following coadministration with food, rate of absorption is delayed, and the extent of absorption (AUC) is decreased by 12%. Steady-state concentrations are achieved within 48 hours of initiating once daily dosing. Mean renal clearance is 145 mL/min in subjects with normal renal function, which may indicate tubular secretion. In healthy elderly volunteers, plasma clearance was reduced by about 25% and the AUC was increased by about 33%. Adjustment of dosage is necessary.

*Moxifloxacin* – Moxifloxacin is well absorbed from the GI tract. Coadministration with a high-fat meal or yogurt does not affect the absorption of moxifloxacin. The $C_{max}$ is attained 1 to 3 hours after oral dosing. Steady state is achieved after 3 days or more with a 400 mg once daily regimen. The volume of distribution ranges from 1.7 to 2.7 L/kg. Moxifloxacin is widely distributed throughout the body. Moxifloxacin is metabolized via glucuronide and sulfate conjugation. The cytochrome P450 system is not involved and is not affected by moxifloxacin.

*Norfloxacin* – Absorption is rapid. Food or dairy products may decrease absorption. Steady-state norfloxacin levels will be attained within 2 days of dosing. Norfloxacin is eliminated through metabolism, biliary excretion, and renal excretion. Renal excretion occurs by glomerular filtration and tubular secretion. In healthy elderly volunteers, norfloxacin is eliminated more slowly because of decreased renal function. In patients with Ccr rates 30 mL/min/1.73 $m^2$ or less, the renal elimination decreases so that the effective serum half-life is 6.5 hours; dosage alteration is necessary.

*Ofloxacin* – Maximum serum concentrations are achieved 1 to 2 hours after an oral dose. Elimination is biphasic; half-lives are about 4 to 5 hours and 20 to 25 hours, although accumulation at steady state can be estimated using a half-life of 9 hours. Steady-state concentrations are achieved after 4 doses. Ofloxacin is widely distributed to body tissues and fluids. Elimination is mainly by renal excretion; 4% to 8% is excreted in the feces. A longer plasma half-life of about 6.4 to 7.4 hours was observed in elderly subjects, compared with 4 to 5 hours for young subjects. Dosage adjustment is necessary for patients with impaired renal function (Ccr 50 mL/min or less).

*Sparfloxacin* – Sparfloxacin is well absorbed following oral administration. Steady-state concentration was achieved on the first day by giving a loading dose that was double the daily dose. Oral absorption of sparfloxacin is unaffected by administration with milk or food, including high-fat meals. Sparfloxacin distributed well into the body. The volume of distribution is 3.9 L/kg. It has low plasma protein binding. It penetrates well into body fluids and tissues. Sparfloxacin is metabolized by the liver. It does not utilize or interfere with cytochrome P450. It is excreted in the feces (50%) and urine (50%).

Microbiology:

### Organisms Generally Susceptible to Fluoroquinolones In Vitro

| | Organism | Ciprofloxacin | Gatifloxacin | Levofloxacin | Lomefloxacin | Moxifloxacin | Norfloxacin | Ofloxacin | Sparfloxacin |
|---|---|---|---|---|---|---|---|---|---|
| Gram-negative | Acinetobacter anitratus | | | | | | | | ✓[1] |
| | Acinetobacter iwoffi | ✓[1] | ✓[1] | ✓[1] | | | | | ✓[1] |
| | Acinetobacter calcoaceticus | | | | | | | ✓[1] | |
| | Aeromonas hydrophilia | ✓[1] | | | ✓[1] | | | | |
| | Bacteroides distasonis | | | | | | | | |
| | Bacteroides ovatus | | | | | | | | |
| | Bordetella pertussis | | | | | | | ✓[1] | |
| | Campylobacter jejuni | ✓[2] | | ✓[1] | | | | ✓[1] | |
| | Chlamydia trachomatis | | | | | | | | |
| | Citrobacter diversus | ✓ | ✓[1] | ✓[1] | ✓ | | ✓[1] | ✓ | ✓[1] |
| | Citrobacter freundii | ✓ | ✓[1] | | ✓[1] | ✓[1] | ✓ | ✓ | |
| | Citrobacter koseri | | ✓[1] | | | | | ✓[1] | |
| | Enterobacter cloacae | ✓ | ✓[1] | ✓ | ✓ | ✓[1] | ✓ | ✓[1] | ✓ |
| | Enterobacter aerogenes | ✓[1] | ✓[1] | ✓[1] | ✓[1] | | ✓ | ✓ | ✓[1] |
| | Enterobacter agglomerans | | | ✓[1] | ✓[1] | | ✓[1] | | |
| | Enterobacter sakazakii | | | ✓[1] | | | | | |
| | Escherichia coli | ✓ | ✓ | ✓ | ✓ | ✓[1] | ✓ | ✓ | ✓ |
| | Edwardsiella tarda | ✓[1] | | | | | ✓[1] | | |
| | Fusobacterium sp. | | | | | ✓[1] | | | |
| | Gardenella vaginalis | | | | | | | | |
| | Haemophilus ducreyi | | | | | | ✓[1] | ✓ | |
| | Haemophilus influenzae | ✓ | ✓ | ✓ | ✓ | ✓ | | ✓[1] | ✓ |
| | Haemophilus parainfluenzae | ✓ | ✓ | ✓ | ✓[1] | ✓ | | ✓ | ✓ |
| | Hafnia alvei | | | | ✓[1] | | | | |

**Organisms Generally Susceptible to Fluoroquinolones In Vitro**

| Organism | Ciprofloxacin | Gatifloxacin | Levofloxacin | Lomefloxacin | Moxifloxacin | Norfloxacin | Ofloxacin | Sparfloxacin |
|---|---|---|---|---|---|---|---|---|
| *Klebsiella pneumoniae* | ✓ | ✓ | ✓ | ✓ | ✓ | ✓ | ✓ | ✓ |
| *Klebsiella oxytoca* | ✓[1] | ✓[1] | ✓[1] | ✓[1] | ✓[1] | ✓[1] | ✓[1] | ✓[1] |
| *Klebsiella ozaenae* | | | | ✓[1] | | | | |
| *Moraxella-catarrhalis* | ✓[2] | ✓ | ✓ | ✓ | ✓ | | ✓[1] | ✓ |
| *Morganella morganii* | ✓ | ✓[1] | ✓[1] | ✓[1] | ✓ | ✓[1] | ✓[1] | ✓[1] |
| *Mycoplasma hominis* | | | | | | | ✓[1] | |
| *Neisseria gonorrhoeae* | ✓[2] | ✓ | | | | ✓ | ✓ | |
| *Pasteurella multocida* | ✓[1] | | | | | | | |
| *Prevotella sp.* | | | | | ✓[1] | | | |
| *Proteus mirabilis* | ✓ | ✓ | ✓ | ✓ | ✓[1] | ✓ | ✓ | ✓[1] |
| *Proteus vulgaris* | ✓ | ✓[1] | ✓[1] | ✓[1] | ✓[1] | ✓ | ✓[1] | ✓[1] |
| *Providencia alcalifaciens* | | | | ✓[1] | | ✓[1] | | |
| *Providencia rettgeri* | ✓ | | ✓[1] | ✓[1] | | ✓[1] | ✓[1] | |
| *Providencia stuartii* | ✓ | | ✓[1] | | | ✓[1] | ✓[1] | |
| *Pseudomonas aeruginosa* | ✓ | | ✓[3] | ✓[4] | | ✓ | ✓[3] | |
| *Pseudomonas fluorescens* | | | ✓[1] | | | ✓[1] | | |
| *Pseudomonas stutzeri* | | | | | | ✓[1] | | |
| *Salmonella sp.* | ✓[5] | ✓ | ✓ | | ✓ | | ✓ | ✓ |
| *Salmonella typhi* | ✓ | | | | | | | |
| *Salmonella enteritidis* | ✓[1] | | | | | | | |
| *Serratia marcescens* | ✓ | | ✓[1] | ✓[1] | | ✓ | ✓[1] | |
| *Serratia proteomaculans* | | | | ✓[1] | | | | |
| *Shigella sp.* | ✓[5] | ✓ | ✓ | | ✓ | | ✓ | ✓ |
| *Shigella boydii* | ✓[2] | | | | | | | |
| *Shigella dysenteriae* | ✓[2] | | | | | | | |
| *Shigella flexneri* | ✓[2] | | | | | | | |
| *Shigella sonnei* | ✓[2] | | | | | | | |

*Gram-negative con't*

**Organisms Generally Susceptible to Fluoroquinolones In Vitro**

| | Organism | Ciprofloxacin | Gatifloxacin | Levofloxacin | Lomefloxacin | Moxifloxacin | Norfloxacin | Ofloxacin | Sparfloxacin |
|---|---|---|---|---|---|---|---|---|---|
| *Gram-negative con't* | Ureaplasma urealyticum | ✓[1] | | | | | | ✓[1] | |
| | Vibrio parahemolyticus | ✓[1] | | | | | | | |
| | Vibrio vulnificus | ✓[1] | | | | | | | |
| | Vibrio cholerae | ✓[1] | | | | | | | |
| | Yersinia enterocolitica | ✓[1] | | | | | | | |
| *Gram-positive* | Staphylococcus aureus methicillin susceptible | ✓ | ✓ | ✓ | ✓[1] | ✓ | ✓[6] | ✓ | ✓[6] |
| | Staphylococcus aureus methicillin resistant | | | | ✓[1] | | | | |
| | Staphylococcus epidermidis methicillin susceptible | ✓[6] | ✓ | ✓[1] | ✓[1] | ✓ | ✓[6] | ✓[1] | ✓ |
| | Staphylococcus epidermidis methicillin resistant | | ✓ | | ✓[1] | ✓ | | | |
| | Staphylococcus hemolyticus | ✓ | | | | | | | |
| | Staphylococcus hominis | ✓ | | | | | ✓ | | |
| | Staphylococcus saprophyticus | ✓ | ✓[1] | ✓ | ✓ | | ✓ | ✓[1] | |
| | Streptococci pyogenes | ✓ | ✓[1] | ✓ | | ✓[1] | | ✓ | ✓[1] |
| | Streptococcus viridans | | | ✓[1] | | | | | ✓[1] |
| | Streptococcus group c/f, g | | | ✓[1] | | | | | |
| | Streptococcus milleri | | | ✓[1] | | | | | |
| | Streptococcus agalactiae | | | ✓[1] | | ✓ | ✓ | | ✓[1] |
| | Enterococcus faecalis | ✓[7] | | ✓[7] | | | ✓ | | |
| | Penicillin susceptible | | ✓ | ✓ | | ✓ | | ✓ | ✓ |
| | Penicillin resistant | | ✓[1] | ✓ | | ✓[1] | | ✓[1] | ✓[1] |

## Organisms Generally Susceptible to Fluoroquinolones In Vitro

| | Organism | Ciprofloxacin | Gatifloxacin | Levofloxacin | Lomefloxacin | Moxifloxacin | Norfloxacin | Ofloxacin | Sparfloxacin |
|---|---|---|---|---|---|---|---|---|---|
| Atypical bacteria | Legionella pneumophila | ✓[1] | ✓ | ✓ | ✓[1] | ✓[1] | | ✓[1] | ✓[1] |
| | Mycoplasma pneumoniae | | ✓ | ✓ | | ✓ | | ✓[1] | ✓[1] |
| | Chlamydia pneumoniae | | ✓ | ✓ | ✓ | ✓ | | ✓[1] | ✓[1] |
| Anaerobe bacteria | Bacteroides fragilis | | | | | | | | |
| | Peptostreptococcus sp. | | ✓[1] | | | ✓[1] | | | |
| | Clostridium perfringes | | | ✓[1] | | | ✓ | ✓[1] | |

[1] Exhibits in vitro MIC of 1 mcg/mL or less (ciprofloxacin, sparfloxacin); 2 mcg/mL or less (gatifloxacin, levofloxacin, lomefloxacin, moxifloxacin, and ofloxacin); 4 mcg/mL or less norfloxacin against most (90% or more) strains of microorganisms; however, the safety and effectiveness in treating clinical infections caused by these microorganisms have not been established in adequate and well-controlled clinical trials.

[2] Oral ciprofloxacin.

[3] As with other drugs in this class, some strains of P. aeruginosa may develop resistance fairly rapidly during treatment.

[4] Urinary tract only.

[5] See following text for individual microorganisms.

[6] Does not specify susceptible or resistant.

[7] Many strains are moderately susceptible.

## Contraindications

Hypersensitivity to fluoroquinolones or the quinolone group; tendinitis or tendon rupture associated with quinolone use; patients receiving disopyramide and amiodarone or other $QT_c$-prolonging antiarrhythmic drugs reported to cause torsade de pointes, such as class IA antiarrhythmic agents (eg, quinidine, procainamide), class III antiarrhythmic agents (eg, sotalol), and bepridil (**sparfloxacin**); patients with known $QT_c$ prolongation or patients being treated concomitantly with medications known to produce an increase in the $QT_c$ interval or torsades de pointes (**sparfloxacin**); patients whose lifestyle or employment will not permit compliance with required safety precautions concerning phototoxicity (**sparfloxacin**).

## Warnings

*Phototoxicity:* Moderate-to-severe phototoxic reactions have occurred in patients exposed to direct or indirect sunlight or to artificial ultraviolet light (eg, sunlamps) during or following treatment with **lomefloxacin, sparfloxacin,** or **ofloxacin**.

*Cardiac toxicity:* **Moxifloxacin** and **gatifloxacin** have been shown to prolong the QT interval of the electrocardiogram in some patients. Avoid in patients with known prolongation of the QT interval, patients with uncorrected hypokalemia, and patients receiving class IA (eg, quinidine, procainamide) or class III (eg, amiodarone, sotalol) antiarrhythmic agents.

Increases in the $QT_c$ interval have been observed in healthy volunteers treated with **sparfloxacin**.

Avoid the concomitant prescription of medications known to prolong the $QT_c$ interval (eg, erythromycin, cisapride, pentamidine, tricyclic antidepressants, some antipsychotics including phenothiazines). **Sparfloxacin** is not recommended for use in patients with proarrhythmic conditions (eg, hypokalemia, significant bradycardia, CHF, myocardial ischemia, atrial fibrillation).

*Tendon rupture/Tendinitis:* Ruptures of the shoulder, hand, and Achilles tendons that required surgical repair or resulted in prolonged disability have been reported with fluoroquinolone antimicrobials. Discontinue therapy if the patient experiences pain, inflammation, or rupture of a tendon. Tendon rupture can occur at any time during or after therapy.

*Seizures:* Increased intracranial pressure, convulsions, and toxic psychosis have occurred. CNS stimulation also may occur and may lead to tremor, restlessness, lightheadedness, confusion, dizziness, depression, hallucinations, and rarely, suicidal thoughts or acts. Use with caution in patients with known or suspected CNS disorders or in the presence of other risk factors that may predispose to seizures or lower the seizure threshold.

*Syphilis:* **Ciprofloxacin, gatifloxacin, norfloxacin,** and **ofloxacin** are not effective for syphilis. High doses of antimicrobial agents for short periods of time to treat gonorrhea may mask or delay symptoms of incubating syphilis. All patients should have a serologic test for syphilis at the time of gonorrhea diagnosis. Patients treated with ciprofloxacin, gatifloxacin, norfloxacin, and ofloxacin should have a follow-up serologic test after 3 months.

*Chronic bronchitis due to S. pneumoniae:* **Lomefloxacin** is not indicated for the empiric treatment of acute bacterial exacerbation of chronic bronchitis when it is probable that *S. pneumoniae* is a causative pathogen.

*P. aeruginosa:* Serum levels of lomefloxacin do not reliably exceed the MIC of *Pseudomonas* isolates. The safety and efficacy of lomefloxacin in treating patients with *Pseudomonas* bacteremia have not been established.

*Pseudomembranous colitis:* Pseudomembranous colitis has been reported with nearly all antibacterial agents, including fluoroquinolones, and may range from mild to life-threatening in severity.

*Hypersensitivity reactions:* Hypersensitivity reactions, serious and occasionally fatal, have occurred in patients receiving quinolone therapy, some following the first dose. Refer to Management of Acute Hypersensitivity Reactions.

*Renal function impairment:* Alteration in dosage regimen is necessary. See Administration and Dosage.

*Hepatic function impairment:* There are no data in patients with severe cirrhosis. Dosage adjustment is recommended in patients with mild-to-moderate cirrhosis.

*Elderly:* **Norfloxacin** is eliminated more slowly because of decreased renal function. The apparent half-life of **ofloxacin** is 6 to 8 hours, compared to approximately 5 hours in younger adults. **Lomefloxacin** plasma clearance was reduced by ≈ 25% and the AUC was increased by approximately 33% in the elderly.

*Pregnancy: Category C.*

*Lactation:* Because of the potential for serious adverse reactions in nursing infants, decide whether to discontinue nursing or to discontinue the drug, taking into account the importance of the drug to the mother.

*Children:* Safety and efficacy of **gatifloxacin, levofloxacin, lomefloxacin, moxifloxacin, norfloxacin, ofloxacin,** and **sparfloxacin** in children younger than 18 years of age have not been established.

## Precautions

*Monitoring:* Periodic assessment of organ system functions, including renal, hepatic, and hematopoietic, is advisable during prolonged therapy.

*Crystalluria:* Needle-shaped crystals were found in the urine of some volunteers who received either placebo or **norfloxacin.** Do not exceed the daily recommended dosage. The patient should drink sufficient fluids to ensure proper hydration and adequate urinary output.

*Hemolytic reactions:* Rarely, hemolytic reactions have been reported in patients with latent or actual defects in glucose-6-phosphate dehydrogenase activity who take quinolone antibacterial agents, including **norfloxacin.**

*Myasthenia gravis:* Quinolones may exacerbate the signs of myasthenia gravis and lead to life-threatening weakness of the respiratory muscles. Exercise caution when using quinolones in patients with myasthenia gravis.

*Blood glucose abnormalities:* As with other quinolones, disturbances of blood glucose, including symptomatic hyper- and hypoglycemia, have been reported, usually in diabetic patients receiving concomitant treatment with an oral hypoglycemic agent or with insulin. In these patients, careful monitoring of blood glucose is recommended.

## Drug Interactions

Drugs that may affect fluoroquinolones include antacids, didanosine, iron salts, sucralfate, azlocillin, bismuth subsalicylate, cimetidine, nitrofurantoin, cisapride, nonsteroidal anti-inflammatory drugs (NSAIDs), morphine, and probenecid.

Drugs that may be affected by fluoroquinolones include caffeine, cyclosporine, digoxin, antiarrhythmic agents, bepridil, erythromycin, phenothiazine, tricyclic antidepressants, procainamide, anticoagulants, and theophylline.

*Drug/Food interactions:* Refer to the Administration and Dosage section.

**Adverse Reactions**

Adverse reactions occurring in at least 3% of patients are in the following table.

| | Adverse reaction | Ciprofloxacin[1] | Gatifloxacin | Levofloxacin | Lomefloxacin | Moxifloxacin | Norfloxacin[2] | Ofloxacin[1] | Sparfloxacin |
|---|---|---|---|---|---|---|---|---|---|
| CNS | Headache | 1.2 | 3 | 0.1-6.4 | 3.6 | 2 | 2-2.8 | 1-9 | 4.2-8.1 |
| | Dizziness | < 1 | 3 | 0.3-2.7 | 2.1 | 3 | 1.7-2.6 | 1-5 | 2-3.8 |
| | Insomnia | < 1 | ≥ 0.1-< 3 | 0.5-4.6 | < 1 | > 0.05-< 1 | 0.3-1 | 3-7 | 1.9 |
| GI | Nausea | 5.2 | 8 | 1.3-7.2 | 3.5 | 8 | 2.6-4.2 | 3-10 | 4.3-7.6 |
| | Diarrhea | 2.3 | 4 | 1-5.6 | 1.4 | 6 | 0.3-1 | 1-4 | 3.2-4.6 |
| | Vomiting | ≤ 1-2 | ≥ 0.1-< 3 | 0.2-2.3 | < 1 | 2 | 0.3-1 | 1-4 | < 1-1.3 |
| | Constipation | < 1 | ≥ 0.1-< 3 | 0.1-3.2 | < 1 | > 0.05-< 1 | 0.3-1 | 1-3 | < 1 |
| | Flatulence | < 1 | < 0.1 | 0.4-1.5 | < 1 | < 0.1 | 0.3-1 | 1-3 | < 1-1.1 |
| Miscellaneous | Visual disturbances | < 1 | | | < 1 | | 0.1-0.2 | 1-3 | |
| | Vaginitis | < 1 | 6 | 0.7-1.8 | < 1 | > 0.05-< 1 | | 1-5 | < 1 |
| | Pruritus | < 1 | < 0.1 | 0.4-1.3 | < 1 | > 0.05-< 1 | 0.3-1 | 1-3 | 1.8-3.3 |

[1] Includes data for oral and IV formulations.
[2] From single- and multiple-dose studies.

# TETRACYCLINES

| | |
|---|---|
| **DEMECLOCYCLINE HCl** | |
| **Tablets:** 150 and 300 mg (*Rx*) | *Declomycin* (Lederle) |
| **DOXYCYCLINE** | |
| **Tablets:** 100 mg (as hyclate) (*Rx*) | Various, *Vibra-Tabs* (Pfizer) |
| **Capsules:** 50 and 100 mg (as hyclate) (*Rx*) | Various, *Vibramycin* (Pfizer) |
| **Capsules, coated pellets:** 75 and 100 mg (as hyclate) (*Rx*) | *Doryx* (Warner Chilcott) |
| **Tablets:** 50, 75, and 100 mg (as monohydrate) (*Rx*) | *Adoxa* (Bioglan) |
| **Capsules:** 50 and 100 mg (as monohydrate) (*Rx*) | *Monodox* (Oclassen) |
| **Powder for oral suspension:** 25 mg (as monohydrate)/5 mL when reconstituted (*Rx*) | *Vibramycin* (Pfizer) |
| **Syrup:** 50 mg (as calcium)/5 mL (*Rx*) | *Vibramycin* (Pfizer) |
| **Powder for injection, lyophilized:** 100 and 200 mg (as hyclate) (*Rx*) | Various, *Doxy 100, Doxy 200* (APP) |
| **MINOCYCLINE** | |
| **Capsules:** 50, 75, and 100 mg (*Rx*) | Various, *Dynacin* (Medicis) |
| **Capsules, pellet filled:** 50 and 100 mg (*Rx*) | *Minocin* (Lederle) |
| **Oral suspension:** 50 mg/5 mL (*Rx*) | *Minocin* (Lederle) |
| **Powder for injection, cryodesiccated:** 100 mg (*Rx*) | *Minocin* (Lederle) |
| **OXYTETRACYCLINE** | |
| **Injection:** 50 and 125 mg/mL with 2% lidocaine (*Rx*) | *Terramycin* (Roerig/Pfizer) |
| **TETRACYCLINE HCl** | |
| **Capsules:** 250 and 500 mg (*Rx*) | Various, *Sumycin 250, Sumycin 500* (Par) |
| **Oral suspension:** 125 mg/5 mL (*Rx*) | Various, *Sumycin Syrup* (Par) |

## Indications

*Gram-negative organisms:* Haemophilus ducreyi (chancroid); *Francisella tularensis* (tularemia); *Yersinia pestis* (plague); *Bartonella bacilliformis* (bartonellosis); *Campylobacter fetus*; *Vibrio cholerae* (cholera); *Brucella* sp. (brucellosis, may be in conjunction with streptomycin); *Calymmatobacterium granulomatis* (granuloma inguinale).

*Infections caused by the following miscellaneous microorganisms:* Rickettsiae (Rocky Mountain spotted fever, typhus fever and the typhus group, Q fever, rickettsialpox, and tick fevers); *Mycoplasma pneumoniae* (PPLO, Eaton agent, respiratory tract infections); *Chlamydia trachomatis* (lymphogranuloma venereum, trachoma [infectious agent not always eliminated], inclusion conjunctivitis, uncomplicated urethral, endocervical, or rectal infections); *Chlamydia psittaci* (psittacosis [ornithosis]); *Borrelia* sp. (relapsing fever); *Ureaplasma urealyticum* (nongonococcal urethritis).

*Following susceptibility testing (resistance has been documented):* Escherichia coli; *Enterobacter aerogenes*; *Acinetobacter* sp.; *Haemophilus influenzae* (respiratory tract infections); *Klebsiella* sp. (respiratory and urinary infections); *Streptococcus pneumoniae* (upper respiratory tract infections); *S. pyogenes, S. pneumoniae, Mycoplasma pneumoniae* (Eaton agent), and *Klebsiella* sp. (lower respiratory tract infections); *Staphylococcus aureus, S. pyogenes* (skin and skin structure infections); *Bacteroides* and *Shigella* sp.

*Alternative therapy for the following infections when penicillin is contraindicated:* Uncomplicated gonorrhea due to *Neisseria gonorrhoeae*; syphilis due to *Treponema pallidum*; yaws due to *T. pertenue*; *Listeria monocytogenes*; anthrax due to *Bacillus anthracis*; Vincent's infection due to *Fusobacterium fusiforme*; actinomycosis due to *Actinomyces* sp.; *Clostridium* sp.

*Acute intestinal amebiasis:* Due to *Entamoeba histolytica* as adjunct to amebicides.

*Severe acne (tetracycline, doxycycline, minocycline only):* As adjunctive therapy.

*Anthrax, including inhalational anthrax (doxycycline only):* To reduce the incidence or progression of disease following exposure to aerosolized *Bacillus anthracis*.

*Malaria (doxycycline only):* Prophylaxis of malaria due to *Plasmodium falciparum* in short-term travelers (less than 4 months) to areas with chloroquine and/or pyrimethamine-sulfadoxine resistant strains.

*Neisseria meningitidis (minocycline only):* Treatment of asymptomatic meningococcal carriers of *N. meningitidis*.

*Note:* Do not use tetracyclines for streptococcal disease unless organism has been shown to be susceptible. Tetracyclines are not the drugs of choice in treatment of any type of staphylococcal infection.

*Unlabeled uses:*

*Tetracycline* – Adjunctive therapy for peptic ulcers due to *Helicobacter pylori* (500 mg 4 times/day).

*Doxycycline* – Treatment of malaria (100 mg twice daily for 7 days in combination with other antimalarial agents).

*Lyme disease:*

*Tick bite from endemic area* – 200 mg once.

*Early Lyme disease* – 100 mg twice daily for 14 to 21 days.

*Carditis (first degree AV block)* – 100 mg twice daily for 14 to 21 days.

*Facial nerve paralysis* – 100 mg twice daily for 14 to 21 days.

*Arthritis* – 100 mg twice daily for 30 to 60 days.

*CDC recommended treatment schedules for sexually transmitted diseases:*

*Granuloma inguinale (donovanosis)* – 100 mg twice daily for at least 3 weeks.

*Early syphilis* – 100 mg twice daily for 14 days.

*Latent syphilis* – 100 mg twice daily for 28 days.

*Chlamydial infections* –

*Adults and children (8 years of age and older):* 100 mg twice daily for 7 days.

*Pelvic inflammatory disease* – 100 mg orally or IV every 12 hours plus cefotetan 2 g IV every 12 hours or cefoxitin 2 g IV every 6 hours. May discontinue parenteral therapy after 24 hours; continue oral therapy with doxycycline for a total of 14 days.

*Epididymitis most likely caused by gonococcal or chlamydial infection* – 100 mg twice daily for 10 days plus a single dose of ceftriaxone 250 mg IM.

*Sexual assault prophylaxis* – 100 mg twice daily for 7 days plus ceftriaxone and metronidazole.

## Administration and Dosage

Avoid rapid IV administration. Thrombophlebitis may result from prolonged IV therapy.

Continue therapy at least 24 to 48 hours after symptoms and fever subside. Treat all infections caused by group A β-hemolytic streptococci for at least 10 days.

Take on an empty stomach, at least 2 hours before or after meals. Absorption and peak plasma levels may be reduced when administered with meals or with dairy products, including milk.

*DEMECLOCYCLINE HCl:*

*Adults* –

*Daily dose:* 4 divided doses of 150 mg each or 2 divided doses of 300 mg each.

*Children (over 8 years of age)* –

*Usual daily dose:* 3 to 6 mg/lb (6.6 to 13.2 mg/kg), depending upon the severity of the disease, divided into 2 or 4 doses.

*Gonorrhea patients sensitive to penicillin* – Initially, 600 mg; follow with 300 mg every 12 hours for 4 days to a total of 3 g.

*Streptococcal infections* – Treat streptococcal infections for at least 10 days.

*Concomitant therapy* – Absorption is impaired by antacids containing aluminum, calcium, or magnesium, and by preparations containing iron. Take demeclocycline at least 1 hour before or 2 hours after these products.

*DOXYCYCLINE:*

*Oral* – When used in streptococcal infections, continue therapy for 10 days. Take with plenty of fluids.

*Adults:*

*Usual dose* – 200 mg on the first day of treatment (100 mg every 12 hours); follow with a maintenance dose of 100 mg/day. The maintenance dose may be administered as a single dose or as 50 mg every 12 hours.

*More severe infections (particularly chronic urinary tract infections)* – 100 mg every 12 hours.

*Children (over 8 years of age):*

*100 lbs or less (less than 45 kg)* – 2 mg/lb (4.4 mg/kg) divided into 2 doses on the first day of treatment; follow with 1 mg/lb (2.2 mg/kg) given as a single daily dose or divided into 2 doses on subsequent days.

*More severe infections* – Up to 2 mg/lb (4.4 mg/kg) may be used.

*More than 100 lbs (45 kg)* – Use the usual adult dose.

*Uncomplicated gonococcal infection in adults (except anorectal infections in men):* 100 mg twice daily for at least 7 days.

*Single visit dose* – Immediately give 300 mg; follow with 300 mg in 1 hour, which should be administered with plenty of water.

*Nongonococcal urethritis:* 100 mg twice daily for 7 days.

*Syphilis:*

*Early (except Adoxa, Doryx, Monodox)* – 100 mg twice daily for 2 weeks.

*More than 1 year duration (except Adoxa, Doryx, Monodox)* – 100 mg twice daily for 4 weeks.

*Primary and secondary (Adoxa, Doryx, Monodox only)* – 300 mg/day in divided doses for at least 10 days.

*Uncomplicated urethral, endocervical or rectal infections in adults caused by C. trachomatis:* 100 mg twice daily for at least 7 days.

*Acute epididymo-orchitis caused by N. gonorrhoeae or C. trachomatis:* 100 mg twice daily for at least 10 days.

*Malaria prophylaxis (except Adoxa, Doryx, Monodox):* Begin prophylaxis 1 to 2 days prior to travel to an endemic area, continue during travel and for 4 weeks after returning from travel.

*Adults* – 100 mg/day.

*Children (older than 8 years of age)* – 2 mg/kg once daily up to 100 mg/day.

*Inhalation anthrax (post-exposure)* –

*Adults and children (100 lb [45 kg] or more):* 100 mg twice daily for 60 days.

*Children (less than 100 lb [45 kg]):* 1 mg/lb (2.2 mg/kg) twice daily for 60 days.

*Parenteral* – Do not inject IM or SC. Avoid rapid administration. Switch to oral therapy as soon as possible. The duration of IV infusion may vary with the dose (100 to 200 mg/day), but is usually 1 to 4 hours. A recommended minimum infusion time for 100 mg of a 0.5 mg/mL solution is 1 hour.

*Adults:* The usual dosage is 200 mg IV on the first day of treatment, administered in 1 or 2 infusions. Subsequent daily dosage is 100 to 200 mg, depending upon the severity of infection, with 200 mg administered in 1 or 2 infusions.

*Primary and secondary syphilis* – 300 mg/day for at least 10 days.

*Children (older than 8 years of age):*

*Up to 100 lb (45 kg)* – Give 2 mg/lb (4.4 mg/kg) on the first day of treatment, in 1 or 2 infusions. Subsequent daily dosage is 1 to 2 mg/lb (2.2 to 4.4 mg/kg) given as 1 or 2 infusions, depending on the severity of the infection.

*Over 100 lb (45 kg)* – Use the usual adult dose.

*CDC recommended treatment schedules for sexually transmitted diseases†* –

*Granuloma inguinale (donovanosis):* 100 mg twice daily for at least 3 weeks.

*Syphilis in patients allergic to penicillins:*

*Early syphilis* – 100 mg twice daily for 14 days.

*Latent syphilis* – 100 mg twice daily for 28 days.

*Chlamydial infections:*

*Adults and children (8 years of age or older)* – 100 mg twice daily for 7 days.

*Pelvic inflammatory disease:* 100 mg orally or IV every 12 hours plus 2 g cefotetan IV every 12 hours or 2 g cefoxitin IV every 6 hours. May discontinue parenteral therapy after 24 hours; continue oral therapy with doxycycline for a total of 14 days.

*Epididymitis most likely caused by gonococcal or chlamydial infection:* 100 mg twice daily for 10 days plus a single dose of 250 mg ceftriaxone IM.

*Sexual assault prophylaxis:* 100 mg twice daily for 7 days plus ceftriaxone and metronidazole.

*Lymphogranuloma venereum:* 100 mg twice daily for at least 21 days.

*Nongonococcal urethritis:* 100 mg twice daily for 7 days.

MINOCYCLINE:

*Oral* – May be taken with or without food. Take with plenty of fluids.

*Usual dosage:*

*Adults* – 200 mg initially, followed by 100 mg every 12 hours. If more frequent doses are preferred, give 100 or 200 mg initially; follow with 50 mg 4 times/day.

*Children (older than 8 years of age)* – Initially, 4 mg/kg; follow with 2 mg/kg every 12 hours.

*Syphilis:* Administer usual dose over a period of 10 to 15 days. Close follow-up, including laboratory tests, is recommended.

*Uncomplicated urethral infections in adults caused by C. trachomatis or Ureaplasma urealyticum:* 100 mg every 12 hours for at least 7 days.

*Uncomplicated gonococcal urethritis in men:* 100 mg every 12 hours for 5 days.

*Uncomplicated gonococcal infections except urethritis and anorectal infections in men:* 200 mg initially, followed by 100 mg every 12 hours for at least 4 days, with posttherapy cultures within 2 to 3 days.

*Meningococcal carrier state:* 100 mg every 12 hours for 5 days.

*Parenteral* – Administer diluted injections immediately. Avoid rapid administration. Switch to oral therapy as soon as possible.

*Adults:* 200 mg followed by 100 mg every 12 hours; do not exceed 400 mg in 24 hours.

*Children (older than 8 years of age):* Initially, usual pediatric dose is 4 mg/kg, followed by 2 mg/kg every 12 hours, not to exceed the usual adult dose.

*Incompatibilities:* Do not mix IV minocycline before or during administration with any solutions containing the following: Adrenocorticotropic hormone (ACTH), aminophylline, amobarbital sodium, amphotericin B, bicarbonate infusion mixtures, calcium gluconate or chloride, carbenicillin, cephalothin sodium, cefazolin sodium, chloramphenicol succinate, colistin sulfate, heparin sodium, hydrocortisone sodium succinate, iodine sodium, methicillin sodium, novobiocin, penicillin, pentobarbital, phenytoin sodium, polymyxin, prochlorperazine, sodium ascorbate, sulfadiazine, sulfisoxazole, thiopental sodium, vitamin K (sodium bisulfate or sodium salt), whole blood.

*Renal function impairment* – Decrease the recommended dosage and/or increase the dosing intervals in patients with renal impairment. Do not exceed 200 mg Minocin in 24 hours in patients with renal impairment.

OXYTETRACYCLINE: Reserve IM therapy for situations where oral therapy is not feasible. IM administration produces lower blood levels than oral administration. Switch to oral therapy as soon as possible. If rapid, high blood levels are needed, administer oxytetracycline IV.

The preferred sites of IM injection are the upper outer quadrant of the buttock or mid-lateral thigh in adults and mid-lateral thigh in children.

Treat Group A beta-hemolytic streptococci infections for at least 10 days.

*Adults* – The usual daily dose is 250 mg administered IM once every 24 hours or 300 mg given in divided doses at 8- to 12-hour intervals.

*Children (older than 8 years of age)* – 15 to 25 mg/kg, up to a maximum of 250 mg/single daily IM injection. Dosage may be divided and given at 8 to 12 hour intervals.

*Renal function impairment* – Decrease recommended dosage and/or extend dosing intervals in patients with renal impairment.

TETRACYCLINE HCl:

*Adults* –

*Usual dose:* 1 to 2 g/day in 2 or 4 equal doses.

*Mild to moderate infections:* 500 mg 2 times/day or 250 mg 4 times/day.

*Severe infections:* 500 mg 4 times/day.

*Children (older than 8 years of age)* – Daily dose is 10 to 20 mg/lb (25 to 50 mg/kg) in 4 equal doses.

*Brucellosis* – 500 mg 4 times/day for 3 weeks, accompanied by 1 g streptomycin IM twice/day the first week, and once daily the second week.

*Syphilis –*

*Sumycin only:* A total of 30 to 40 g in equally divided doses over 10 to 15 days. Perform close follow-up and laboratory tests.

*All except Sumycin:*

*Early (less than 1 year)* – 500 mg 4 times/day for 15 days.

*More than 1 year duration* – 500 mg 4 times/day for 30 days.

*CDC recommended treatment schedules for syphilis (penicillin-allergic patients)†:*

*Early* – 500 mg 4 times/day for 14 days.

*More than 1 year's duration* – 500 mg 4 times/day for 28 days.

*Uncomplicated gonorrhea* – 500 mg every 6 hours for 7 days.

*Uncomplicated urethral, endocervical, or rectal infections caused by Chlamydia trachomatis* – 500 mg 4 times/day for at least 7 days.

*Severe acne (long-term therapy)* – Initially, 1 g/day in divided doses. For maintenance, give 125 to 500 mg/day.

*Streptococcal infections* – Treat streptococcal infections for at least 10 days.

*Concomitant therapy* – Absorption is impaired by antacids containing aluminum, calcium, or magnesium, and preparations containing iron, zinc, or sodium bicarbonate.

## Actions

*Pharmacology:* The tetracyclines are bacteriostatic. They exert their antimicrobial effect by inhibition of protein synthesis. Tetracyclines are active against a wide range of gram-positive and gram-negative organisms.

*Pharmacokinetics:*

| Tetracycline Pharmacokinetics | | | | | |
|---|---|---|---|---|---|
| Tetracyclines | Absorption (%) | $C_{max}$ (mcg/mL) | $T_{max}$ (h) | Protein binding (%) | Serum half-life (h) |
| Demeclocycline | 60 to 80 | 1.5 to 1.7[1] | 3 to 4[1] | 35 to 90 | 16 |
| Doxycycline | 90 to 100 | 2.6 (hyclate)[2] 3.61 (monohydrate)[2] 3.6 (IV)[3] | 2 (hyclate)[2] 2.6 (monohydrate)[2] | 80 to 95 | 18 to 22 |
| Minocycline | 90 to 100 | 2.1 to 5.1[4] | 1 to 4 | 75 | 11 to 22 (oral) 15 to 23 (IV) |
| Oxytetracycline | 60 to 80 | nd | 2 to 4 | 20 to 40 | 6 to 12 |
| Tetracycline | 60 to 80 | nd | 2 to 4 | 20 to 65 | 6 to 12 |

* nd = no data
[1] 300 mg single oral dose.
[2] 200 mg single oral dose.
[3] 200 mg administered IV over 2 hours.
[4] Single oral dose of two 100 mg pellet-filled capsules.

## Contraindications

Hypersensitivity to any of the tetracyclines.

## Warnings

*Malaria prophylaxis (doxycycline only):* **Doxycycline** offers substantial but not complete suppression of the asexual stages of *Plasmodium* strains. Advise patients taking doxycycline for malaria prophylaxis of when prophylaxis should begin and end; that no present-day antimalarial, including doxycycline, guarantees protection against malaria; and to avoid being bitten by mosquitos by wearing protective clothing, using effective insect-repellent, mosquito nets, etc.

*Pseudomembranous colitis:* Treatment with antibacterial agents alters the normal flora of the colon and may permit overgrowth of clostridia. Pseudomembranous colitis has been reported with nearly all antibacterial agents.

† MMWR. 2002 May 10;51 (No. RR-6):1-84.

*Parenteral therapy:* Reserve for situations in which oral therapy is not indicated. Institute oral therapy as soon as possible. If given IV over prolonged periods, thrombophlebitis may result. IM use produces lower blood levels than recommended oral dosages.

*Nephrogenic diabetes insipidus:* Administration of **demeclocycline** has resulted in appearance of the diabetes insipidus syndrome (polyuria, polydipsia, and weakness) in some patients on long-term therapy.

*Hypersensitivity reactions:* Sensitivity reactions are more likely to occur on patients with a history of allergy, asthma, hay fever, or urticaria.

*Renal function impairment:* If renal impairment exists, even usual doses may lead to excessive systemic accumulation of the tetracyclines (with the exception of doxycycline and minocycline) and possible liver toxicity. Use lower than usual doses and/or extend the dosing interval.

*Hepatic function impairment:* Doses more than 2 g/day IV can be extremely dangerous. In the presence of renal dysfunction, and particularly in pregnancy, IV tetracycline more than 2 g/day has been associated with death secondary to liver failure. Hepatotoxicity has been reported with **minocycline**. Administer with caution; reduce the recommended dosage and/or extend the dosing interval.

*Carcinogenesis:* There has been evidence of oncogenic activity in studies with **oxytetracycline** (adrenal and pituitary tumors) in rats and **minocycline** (thyroid tumors) in rats and dogs.

*Mutagenesis:* **Tetracycline** and **oxytetracycline** have produced positive mutagenic results in mammalian cell assays in vitro.

*Fertility impairment:* **Minocycline** has been shown to impair fertility in male rats.

*Pregnancy: Category D.*

*Lactation:* Tetracyclines are excreted in breast milk.

*Children:* Tetracyclines generally should not be used in children less than 8 years of age (except for anthrax, including inhalational) unless other drugs are not likely to be effective or are contraindicated.

    *Teeth* – The use of tetracyclines during the period of tooth development may cause permanent discoloration of deciduous and permanent teeth.

    *Bone* – Tetracycline forms a stable calcium complex in any bone-forming tissue. Decreased fibula growth rate occurred in premature infants given 25 mg/kg oral tetracycline every 6 hours.

**Precautions**

*Monitoring:* In sexually transmitted diseases when coexistent syphilis is suspected, perform darkfield examination before starting treatment and repeat the blood serology monthly for at least 4 months.

    In long-term therapy, perform periodic laboratory evaluation of organ systems, including hematopoietic, renal, and hepatic studies.

*Pseudotumor cerebri:* Pseudotumor cerebri (benign intracranial hypertension) in adults has been associated with tetracycline use.

*Outdated products:* Under no circumstances should outdated tetracyclines be administered; the degradation products of tetracyclines are highly nephrotoxic and have, on occasion, produced a Fanconi-like syndrome.

*Hazardous tasks:* Lightheadedness, dizziness or vertigo may occur with tetracyclines. Patients should observe caution while driving or performing other tasks requiring alertness.

*Superinfection:* Use of antibiotics (especially prolonged or repeated therapy) may result in bacterial or fungal overgrowth of nonsusceptible organisms.

*Photosensitivity:* Photosensitivity manifested by an exaggerated sunburn reaction has been observed in some individuals taking tetracyclines. Advise patients who are apt to be exposed to direct sunlight or ultraviolet light that this reaction can occur with tetracycline drugs, and discontinue treatment at the first evidence of skin erythema.

Phototoxic reactions are most frequent with demeclocycline, and occur less frequently with the other tetracyclines; minocycline is least likely to cause phototoxic reactions.

### Drug Interactions

Drugs that may affect tetracyclines include antacids containing aluminum, calcium, or magnesium; iron salts; zinc salts; barbiturates; bismuth salts; carbamazepine; cholestyramine; colestipol; phenytoin; rifamycins; urinary alkalinizers (eg, sodium lactate, potassium citrate).

Drugs that may be affected by tetracyclines include oral anticoagulants, digoxin, insulin, isotretinoin, methoxyflurane, oral contraceptives, penicillins, and theophyllines.

*Drug/Lab test interactions:* The antianabolic action of tetracyclines may cause an increase in blood urea nitrogen. During **doxycycline** or **minocycline** therapy, false elevations of urinary catecholamine levels may occur

*Drug/Food interactions:* The administration of **demeclocycline, oxytetracycline**, and **tetracycline** with milk and dairy products forms poorly absorbed chelates. Administer the interacting tetracyclines at least 2 hours before or after meals. The inhibitory effect of food and milk on the absorption of **doxycycline** and **minocycline** is considerably less than that observed with the other tetracycline derivatives. These 2 drugs are often administered without regard to meals; but the potential risk of decreased drug efficacy must be weighed against the benefit of treating the infection.

### Adverse Reactions

The following adverse reactions have been reported with the tetracyclines.

*CNS:* Bulging fontanel, convulsions, dizziness, headache, hypesthesia, paresthesia, pseudotumor cerebri, sedation, vertigo.

*Dermatologic:* Alopecia, balanitis, erythema multiforme, erythema nodosum, fixed drug eruptions, hyperpigmentation of the nails, injection site erythema and injection site pain, maculopapular and erythematous rashes, photosensitivity, pruritus, skin and mucus membrane pigmentation, Stevens-Johnson syndrome, toxic epidermal necrolysis, vasculitis.

*GI:* Anorexia, diarrhea, dyspepsia, dysphagia, enamel hypoplasia, enterocolitis, esophageal ulcerations, esophagitis, glossitis, inflammatory lesions (with monilial overgrowth) in the anogenital region, nausea, pancreatitis, pseudomembranous colitis, stomatitis, vomiting; black hairy tongue, bulky loose stools, hoarseness, sore throat **(tetracycline)**.

*Hematologic:* Agranulocytosis, anemia, eosinophilia, hemolytic anemia, leukopenia, neutropenia, pancytopenia, thrombocytopenia.

*Hepatic:* Hepatic cholestasis, hepatic toxicity, hepatitis, hyperbilirubinemia, increased liver enzymes, jaundice, liver failure.

*Hypersensitivity:* Anaphylactoid purpura, anaphylaxis, angioneurotic edema, myocarditis, pericarditis, polyarthralgia, pulmonary infiltrates with eosinophilia, systemic lupus erythematous exacerbation, urticaria; hypersensitivity syndrome (cutaneous reaction, eosinophilia, and one or more of the following: Hepatitis, pneumonitis, nephritis, myocarditis, pericarditis, fever, lymphadenopathy).

*Musculoskeletal:* Arthralgia, arthritis, bone discoloration, joint stiffness and swelling, myalgia, polyarthralgia.

*Renal:* Acute renal failure, dose-related increase in BUN, interstitial nephritis; nephrogenic diabetes insipidus **(demeclocycline)**.

*Respiratory:* Asthma exacerbation, bronchospasm, cough, dyspnea.

*Miscellaneous:* Brown-black microscopic discoloration of thyroid glands (prolonged therapy), decreased hearing, fever, lupus-like syndrome, secretion discoloration, serum sickness-like syndrome, tinnitus, tooth discoloration, vulvovaginitis.

# MACROLIDES

| | |
|---|---|
| **AZITHROMYCIN** | |
| **Tablets**: 250, 500, and 600 mg (as dihydrate) (*Rx*) | *Zithromax* (Pfizer) |
| **Powder for oral suspension**: 100 and 200 mg/5 mL, 1 g/packet (*Rx*) | |
| **Powder for injection**: 500 mg (*Rx*) | |
| **CLARITHROMYCIN** | |
| **Tablets**: 250 and 500 mg (*Rx*) | *Biaxin* (Abbott) |
| **Tablets, extended-release**: 500 mg (*Rx*) | *Biaxin XL* (Abbott) |
| **Granules for oral suspension**: 125 and 250 mg/5 mL (*Rx*) | *Biaxin* (Abbott) |
| **DIRITHROMYCIN** | |
| **Tablets, enteric-coated**: 250 mg (*Rx*) | *Dynabac* (Sanofi) |
| **ERYTHROMYCIN BASE** | |
| **Tablets, enteric-coated**: 250, 333, and 500 mg (*Rx*) | *E-Mycin* (Knoll), *Ery-Tab* (Abbott), *E-Base* (Barr) |
| **Tablets with polymer-coated particles**: 333 and 500 mg (*Rx*) | *PCE Dispertab* (Abbott) |
| **Tablets, film-coated**: 250 and 500 mg (*Rx*) | *Erythromycin Filmtabs* (Abbott) |
| **Capsules, delayed-release**: 250 mg (*Rx*) | Various, *Eryc* (Warner Chilcott) |
| **ERYTHROMYCIN ESTOLATE** | |
| **Tablets**: 500 mg (as estolate) | *Ilosone* (Lilly) |
| **Capsules**: 250 mg (as estolate) | Various, *Ilosone Pulvules* (Lilly) |
| **Suspension**: 235 and 250 mg (as estolate)/5 mL | Various, *Ilosone* (Lilly) |
| **ERYTHROMYCIN LACTOBIONATE** | |
| **Powder for injection**: 500 mg and 1 g (as lactobionate) (*Rx*) | Various, *Erythrocin* (Abbott) |
| **ERYTHROMYCIN GLUCEPTATE** | |
| **Injection**: 1 g (as gluceptate) (*Rx*) | *Ilotycin Gluceptate* (Lilly) |
| **ERYTHROMYCIN ETHYLSUCCINATE** | |
| **Tablets**: 400 mg (as ethylsuccinate) (*Rx*) | Various, *E.E.S. 400* (Abbott) |
| **Suspension**: 200 and 400 mg (as ethylsuccinate)/5 mL (*Rx*) | Various, *E.E.S. 200* (Abbott), *E.E.S. 400* (Abbott), *EryPed 200* (Abbott), *EryPed 400* (Abbott) |
| **Drops, suspension**: 100 mg (as ethylsuccinate)/2.5 mL (*Rx*) | *EryPed Drops* (Abbott) |
| **Powder for oral suspension**: 200 mg (as ethylsuccinate)/5 mL when reconstituted (*Rx*) | *E.E.S. Granules* (Abbott) |
| **ERYTHROMYCIN STEARATE** | |
| **Tablets, film-coated**: 250 and 500 mg (*Rx*) | Various, *Erythrocin Stearate* (Abbott) |
| **TROLEANDOMYCIN** | |
| **Capsules**: 250 mg (*Rx*) | *Tao* (Pfizer) |

## Indications

For specific approved indications, refer to the Administration and Dosage sections.

## Administration and Dosage

AZITHROMYCIN: Azithromycin tablets and oral suspension can be taken with or without food; however, increased tolerability has been observed when tablets are taken with food. Single-dose 1 g packets are not for pediatric use.

*Adults –*

*Mild to moderate acute bacterial exacerbations of chronic obstructive pulmonary disease (COPD):* 500 mg/day for 3 days or 500 mg as a single dose on the first day followed by 250 mg once daily on days 2 through 5.

*Community-acquired pneumonia of mild severity, pharyngitis/tonsillitis (as second-line therapy), and uncomplicated skin and skin structure infections:* 500 mg as a single dose on the first day followed by 250 mg once daily on days 2 through 5.

*Acute bacterial sinusitis:* 500 mg/day for 3 days.

*Genital ulcer disease caused by Haemophilus ducreyi (chancroid):* Single 1 g dose.

*Nongonococcal urethritis/cervicitis caused by Chlamydia trachomatis:* Single 1 g dose.

*Gonococcal urethritis/cervicitis caused by Neisseria gonorrhoeae:* Single 2 g dose.

*Prevention of disseminated Mycobacterium avium (MAC) infections:* 1200 mg taken once weekly. This dose may be combined with the approved dosage regimen of rifabutin.

*Treatment of disseminated MAC infections:* Take 600 mg/day in combination with ethambutol at the recommended daily dose of 15 mg/kg. Other antimycobacterial drugs that have shown in vitro activity against MAC may be added to the regimen of azithromycin plus ethambutol at the discretion of the physician or health care provider.

*Children (6 months of age and older) –*

*Acute otitis media:* The recommended dose of azithromycin for oral suspension for the treatment of children with acute otitis media is 30 mg/kg given as a single dose or 10 mg/kg once daily for 3 days or 10 mg/kg as a single dose on the first day (not to exceed 500 mg/day), followed by 5 mg/kg on days 2 through 5 (not to exceed 250 mg/day).

*Acute bacterial sinusitis:* 10 mg/kg oral suspension once daily for 3 days.

*Community-acquired pneumonia:* The recommended dose of azithromycin for oral suspension for the treatment of children with community-acquired pneumonia is 10 mg/kg as a single dose on the first day followed by 5 mg/kg on days 2 through 5.

| Azithromycin Pediatric Dosage Guidelines for Otitis Media and Community-Acquired Pneumonia (≥ 6 months of age) 5-Day Regimen[1,2] | | | | | | | |
|---|---|---|---|---|---|---|---|
| Weight | | Amount of 100 mg/5 mL suspension | | Amount of 200 mg/5 mL suspension | | Total mL per treatment course | Total mg per treatment course |
| kg | lbs | Day 1 | Days 2 to 5 | Day 1 | Days 2 to 5 | | |
| 5 | 11 | 2.5 mL | 1.25 mL | | | 7.5 mL | 150 mg |
| 10 | 22 | 5 mL | 2.5 mL | | | 15 mL | 300 mg |
| 20 | 44 | | | 5 mL | 2.5 mL | 15 mL | 600 mg |
| 30 | 66 | | | 7.5 mL | 3.75 mL | 22.5 mL | 900 mg |
| 40 | 88 | | | 10 mL | 5 mL | 30 mL | 1200 mg |
| ≥ 50 | ≥ 110 | | | 12.5 mL | 6.25 mL | 37.5 mL | 1500 mg |

[1] Dosing calculated on 10 mg/kg on day 1, followed by 5 mg/kg on days 2 to 5.
[2] Effectiveness of the 1- or 3-day regimen in children with community-acquired pneumonia has not been established.

| Azithromycin Pediatric Dosage Guidelines for Otitis Media and Acute Bacterial Sinusitis: 3-Day Regimen[1] | | | | | |
|---|---|---|---|---|---|
| Weight | | Amount of 100 mg/5 mL suspension | Amount of 200 mg/5 mL suspension | Total mL per treatment course | Total mg per treatment course |
| kg | lbs | Day 1 to 3 | Day 1 to 3 | | |
| 5 | 11 | 2.5 mL | | 7.5 mL | 150 mg |
| 10 | 22 | 5 mL | | 15 mL | 300 mg |
| 20 | 44 | | 5 mL | 15 mL | 600 mg |
| 30 | 66 | | 7.5 mL | 22.5 mL | 900 mg |
| 40 | 88 | | 10 mL | 30 mL | 1200 mg |
| ≥ 50 | ≥ 110 | | 12.5 mL | 37.5 mL | 1500 mg |

[1] Dosing calculated on 10 mg/kg/day.

| Azithromycin Pediatric Dosage Guidelines for Otitis Media: 1-Day Regimen[1] | | | | |
|---|---|---|---|---|
| Weight | | Amount of 200 mg/5 mL suspension | Total mL per treatment course | Total mg per treatment course |
| kg | lbs | Day 1 | | |
| 5 | 11 | 3.75 mL | 3.75 mL | 150 mg |
| 10 | 22 | 7.5 mL | 7.5 mL | 300 mg |
| 20 | 44 | 15 mL | 15 mL | 600 mg |
| 30 | 66 | 22.5 mL | 22.5 mL | 900 mg |
| 40 | 88 | 30 mL | 30 mL | 1200 mg |
| ≥ 50 | ≥ 110 | 37.5 mL | 37.5 mL | 1500 mg |

[1] Dosing calculated on 30 mg/kg as a single dose.

*Pharyngitis/Tonsillitis:* The recommended dose for children with pharyngitis/tonsillitis is 12 mg/kg once daily for 5 days (not to exceed 500 mg/day). See the following.

| Pediatric Dosage Guidelines for Pharyngitis/Tonsillitis (≥ 2 years of age) | | | | |
|---|---|---|---|---|
| Dosing calculated on 12 mg/kg once daily on days 1 through 5 | | | | |
| Weight | | Amount of 200 mg/5 mL suspension | Total mL per treatment course | Total mg per treatment course |
| kg | lbs | Days 1 to 5 | | |
| 8 | 18 | 2.5 mL | 12.5 mL | 500 mg |
| 17 | 37 | 5 mL | 25 mL | 1,000 mg |
| 25 | 55 | 7.5 mL | 37.5 mL | 1,500 mg |
| 33 | 73 | 10 mL | 50 mL | 2,000 mg |
| 40 | 88 | 12.5 | 62.5 mL | 2,500 mg |

*Parenteral* – Infuse injections over a period of longer than 60 minutes. Do not administer azithromycin for injection as a bolus or IM injection.

*Community-acquired pneumonia:* 500 mg as a single daily dose IV for at least 2 days. Follow IV therapy by the oral route at a single daily dose of 500 mg to complete a 7- to 10-day course of therapy.

*Pelvic inflammatory disease (PID):* 500 mg as a single daily dose for 1 or 2 days. Follow IV therapy by the oral route at a single daily dose of 250 mg to complete a 7-day course of therapy. If anaerobic microorganisms are suspected of contributing to the infection, administer an antimicrobial agent with anaerobic activity in combination with azithromycin.

The infusate concentration and rate of infusion for azithromycin for injection should be either 1 mg/mL over 3 hours or 2 mg/mL over 1 hour.

CLARITHROMYCIN: Clarithromycin may be given with or without meals.

*Helicobacter pylori* –

| Clarithromycin and Omeprazole Dosage Regimens for Active Duodenal Ulcer Associated with *H. pylori* Infection (28-Day Therapy) | |
|---|---|
| Days 1 to 14 | Days 15 to 28 |
| 500 mg clarithromycin tablet 3 times daily plus omeprazole 2 × 20 mg every morning | Omeprazole 20 mg every morning |

| Clarithromycin and Ranitidine Bismuth Citrate Dosage Regimens for Active Duodenal Ulcer Associated with *H. pylori* Infection (28-Day Therapy) | |
|---|---|
| Days 1 to 14 | Days 15 to 28 |
| 500 mg clarithromycin tablet 3 times daily plus ranitidine bismuth citrate 400 mg tablet twice daily | Ranitidine bismuth citrate 400 mg tablet twice daily |

*H. pylori eradication to reduce the risk of duodenal ulcer recurrence triple therapy:*

*Clarithromycin/Lansoprazole/Amoxicillin* – 500 mg clarithromycin, 30 mg lansoprazole, and 1 g amoxicillin every 12 hours for 14 days.

*Clarithromycin/Omeprazole/Amoxicillin* – 500 mg clarithromycin, 20 mg omeprazole, and 1 g amoxicillin every 12 hours for 10 days. In patients with an ulcer present at the time of initiation of therapy, an additional 18 days of omeprazole 20 mg once daily is recommended for ulcer healing and symptom relief.

*Adults* –

| Clarithromycin Dosage Guidelines | | | | |
|---|---|---|---|---|
| | Tablets | | Extended-release tablets | |
| Infection | Dosage (q 12 h) | Duration (days) | Dosage (q 24 h) | Duration (days) |
| Pharyngitis/Tonsillitis | 250 mg | 10 | - | - |
| Acute maxillary sinusitis | 500 mg | 14 | 2 × 500 mg | 14 |
| Acute exacerbation of chronic bronchitis caused by: | | | | |
|    *Haemophilus parainfluenzae* | 500 mg | 7 | 2 × 500 mg | 7 |

| Clarithromycin Dosage Guidelines | | | | |
|---|---|---|---|---|
| | Tablets | | Extended-release tablets | |
| Infection | Dosage (q 12 h) | Duration (days) | Dosage (q 24 h) | Duration (days) |
| Streptococcus pneumoniae | 250 mg | 7 to 14 | 2 × 500 mg | 7 |
| Moraxella catarrhalis | 250 mg | 7 to 14 | 2 × 500 mg | 7 |
| Haemophilus influenzae | 500 mg | 7 to 14 | 2 × 500 mg | 7 |
| Community-acquired pneumonia caused by: | | | | |
| S. pneumoniae | 250 mg | 7 to 14 | 2 × 500 mg | 7 |
| Mycoplasma pneumoniae | 250 mg | 7 to 14 | 2 × 500 mg | 7 |
| H. influenzae | 250 mg | 7 | 2 × 500 mg | 7 |
| H. parainfluenzae | - | - | 2 × 500 mg | 7 |
| M. catarrhalis | - | - | 2 × 500 mg | 7 |
| Chlamydia pneumoniae | 250 mg | 7 to 14 | 2 × 500 mg | 7 |
| Uncomplicated skin and skin structure infection | 250 mg | 7 to 14 | - | - |

*Mycobacterial infections* – Recommended as the primary agent for the treatment of disseminated *Mycobacterium avium* complex (MAC). Use in combination with other antimycobacterial drugs that have shown an in vitro activity against MAC. Continue therapy for life if clinical and mycobacterial improvements are observed.

*Dosage for mycobacterial infection:*

*Adults* – 500 mg twice daily.

*Children* – 7.5 mg/kg twice daily up to 500 mg twice daily. Refer to the Pediatric Dosing table.

*Children* – Usual recommended daily dosage is 15 mg/kg/day divided every 12 hours for 10 days.

| Pediatric Dosage Guidelines (based on body weight) | | | | |
|---|---|---|---|---|
| Dosing calculated on 7.5 mg/kg q 12 h | | | | |
| Weight kg | Weight lb | Dose (q 12 h) | 125 mg/5 mL (q 12 h) | 250 mg/5 mL (q 12 h) |
| 9 | 20 | 62.5 mg | 2.5 mL | 1.25 mL |
| 17 | 37 | 125 mg | 5 mL | 2.5 mL |
| 25 | 55 | 187.5 mg | 7.5 mL | 3.75 mL |
| 33 | 73 | 250 mg | 10 mL | 5 mL |

*Renal/Hepatic function impairment* – In the presence of severe renal impairment (Ccr less than 30 mL/min) with or without co-existing hepatic impairment, halved doses or prolongation of dosing intervals may be needed.

DIRITHROMYCIN: Administer with food or within 1 hour of eating. Do not cut, crush, or chew the tablets.

| Recommended Dosage Schedule for Dirithromycin (≥ 12 years of age) | | | |
|---|---|---|---|
| Infection (mild to moderate severity) | Dose | Frequency | Duration (days) |
| Acute bacterial exacerbations of chronic bronchitis caused by *H. influenzae*, *M. catarrhalis*, or *S. pneumoniae*. | 500 mg | once a day | 5 to 7 |
| Secondary bacterial infection of acute bronchitis caused by *M. catarrhalis* or *S. pneumoniae*. | 500 mg | once a day | 7 |
| Community-acquired pneumonia caused by *Legionella pneumophila*, *M. pneumoniae*, or *S. pneumoniae*. | 500 mg | once a day | 14 |
| Pharyngitis/Tonsillitis caused by *Streptococcus pyogenes*. | 500 mg | once a day | 10 |

| Recommended Dosage Schedule for Dirithromycin (≥ 12 years of age) | | | |
|---|---|---|---|
| Infection (mild to moderate severity) | Dose | Frequency | Duration (days) |
| Uncomplicated skin and skin structure infections caused by *Staphylococcus aureus* (methicillin-susceptible) or *S. pyogenes*. | 500 mg | once a day | 5 to 7 |

*ERYTHROMYCIN, IV:*

*Erythromycin IV* – Erythromycin IV is indicated when oral use is impossible, or when severity of the infection requires immediate high serum levels. Replace IV therapy with oral as soon as possible.

*Continuous infusion:* Continuous infusion is preferable, but intermittent infusion in 20- to 60-minute periods at intervals of up to 6 hours is also effective. Because of irritative properties of erythromycin, IV push is unacceptable.

*Severe infections* – 15 to 20 mg/kg/day. Up to 4 g/day in very severe infections.

ERYTHROMYCIN, ORAL: Dosages and product strengths are expressed as erythromycin base equivalents.

Optimal serum levels of erythromycin are reached when erythromycin base or stearate is taken in the fasting state or immediately before meals. Erythromycin ethylsuccinate, estolate, and enteric-coated erythromycin may be administered without regard to meals.

*Usual dosage –*

*Adults:* 250 mg (or 400 mg ethylsuccinate) every 6 hours, or 500 mg every 12 hours, or 333 mg every 8 hours. May increase up to at least 4 g/day, according to severity of infection. If twice-daily dosage is desired, the recommended dose is 500 mg every 12 hours. Twice-daily dosing is not recommended when doses larger than 1 g daily are administered.

*Children:* 30 to 50 mg/kg/day in divided doses.

| Erythromycin Uses and Dosages | |
|---|---|
| Indication (Organism) | Dosage (Stated as erythromycin base) |
| **Labeled uses:** | |
| Upper respiratory tract infections of mild to moderate severity | |
| S. pyogenes (group A beta-hemolytic streptococcus) | 250 to 500 mg 4 times/day or 20 to 50 mg/kg/day for children (not to exceed the adult dose) in divided doses for 10 days. |
| S. pneumoniae | 250 to 500 mg every 6 hours. |
| H. influenzae (used concomitantly with a sulfonamide) | Erythromycin ethylsuccinate: 50 mg/kg/day for children (not to exceed 6 g/day). Sulfisoxazole: 150 mg/kg/day. Combination given for 10 days. |
| Lower respiratory tract infections of mild to moderate severity | |
| S. pyogenes (group A beta-hemolytic streptococcus) | 250 to 500 mg 4 times/day or 20 to 50 mg/kg/day for children (not to exceed the adult dose) in divided doses for 10 days. |
| S. pneumoniae | 250 to 500 mg every 6 hours. |
| Respiratory tract infections | |
| M. pneumoniae (Eaton agent, PPLO) | 500 mg every 6 hours for 5 to 10 days. Treat severe infections for up to 3 weeks. |
| Skin and skin structure infections of mild to moderate severity | |
| S. pyogenes | 250 to 500 mg 4 times/day or 20 to 50 mg/kg/day for children (not to exceed the adult dose) in divided doses for 10 days. |
| S. aureus (resistant organisms may emerge) | 250 mg every 6 hours or 500 mg every 12 hours, maximum 4 g/day. |

## Erythromycin Uses and Dosages

| Indication (Organism) | Dosage (Stated as erythromycin base) |
|---|---|
| Pertussis (whooping cough)<br>*Bordetella pertussis*: Effective in eliminating the organism from the nasopharynx of infected patients. May be helpful in prophylaxis of pertussis in exposed individuals. | 40 to 50 mg/kg/day for children (not to exceed the adult dose) in divided doses for 5 to 14 days, or 500 mg 4 times/day for 10 days. |
| Diphtheria<br>*Corynebacterium diphtheriae*: Adjunct to antitoxin to prevent establishment of carriers and to eradicate organism in carriers. | 500 mg every 6 hours for 10 days. |
| Erythrasma<br>*Corynebacterium minutissiumum* | 250 mg 3 times daily for 21 days. |
| Intestinal amebiasis<br>*Entamoeba histolyticia*: Oral erythromycin only. | *Adults:* 250 mg 4 times daily for 10 to 14 days.<br>*Children:* 30 to 50 mg/kg/day in divided doses for 10 to 14 days. |
| Pelvic inflammatory disease (PID), acute<br>*N. gonorrhoeae*: Erythromycin lactobionate IV followed by oral erythromycin.[1] | 500 mg IV every 6 hours for 3 days, then 250 mg orally every 6 hours for 7 days. |
| Conjunctivitis of the newborn, pneumonia of infancy, urogenital infections during pregnancy<br><br>*C. trachomatis* | 50 mg/kg/day for children (not to exceed the adult dose) in 4 divided doses for 10 to ≥ 14 days (conjunctivitis) or ≥ 21 days (pneumonia)<br>500 mg 4 times daily for 7 days or 250 mg 4 times daily on an empty stomach for ≥ 14 days (urogenital infections). |
| Urethral, endocervical, or rectal infections, uncomplicated<br>*C. trachomatis*[1] | 500 mg ≥ 4 times daily for 7 days or 250 mg 4 times daily for 14 days if patient cannot tolerate high-dose erythromycin.[2] |
| Nongonococcal urethritis<br>*Ureaplasma urealyticum*[1] | 500 mg 4 times daily for at least 7 days or 250 mg orally 4 times daily for 14 days if patient cannot tolerate high-dose erythromycin.[2] |
| Primary syphilis<br>*Treponema pallidum*: Oral erythromycin only[1] | 20 to 40 g in divided doses over 10 to 15 days. |
| Legionnaire's disease<br>*Legionella pneumophila*: No controlled clinical efficacy studies have been conducted, but data suggest effectiveness | 1 to 4 g daily in divided doses for 10 to 14 days. |
| Rheumatic fever<br>*S. pyogenes* (group A beta-hemolytic streptococci): Prevention of initial or recurrent attacks.[1] | 250 mg 2 times daily. |
| Bacterial endocarditis (in penicillin-allergic patients with valvular heart disease who are to undergo dental procedures or surgical procedures of the upper respiratory tract).<br><br>*Alpha-hemolytic streptococcus* (viridans)[1] | Adults: 1 g 1 to 2 hours prior to procedure, then 500 mg 6 hours after initial dose.[3]<br>Children: 20 mg/kg 2 hours prior to procedure, then 10 mg/kg 6 hours after initial dose.[3] |
| *Listeria monocytogenes* | *Adults:* 250 mg every 6 hours or 500 mg every 12 hours, maximum 4 g/day. |
| **Unlabeled uses:**<br>*Campylobacter jejuni*: Has been successful in severe or prolonged diarrhea associated with *Campylobacter enteritis* or enterocolitis.[2] | 500 mg 4 times a day for 7 days. |
| *Lymphogranuloma venereum*: Genital, inguinal, or anorectal.[2] | 500 mg 4 times a day for 21 days. |
| *Haemophilus ducreyi* (chancroid): Treat until ulcers or lymph nodes are healed.[2] | 500 mg 4 times a day for 7 days. |

| Erythromycin Uses and Dosages | |
|---|---|
| Indication (Organism) | Dosage (Stated as erythromycin base) |
| *T. pallidum:* Early syphilis (primary or secondary) | 500 mg 4 times a day for 14 days. |
| Prior to elective colorectal surgery, to reduce wound complications | Combination of erythromycin base and neomycin is a popular preoperative preparation. |
| *Clostridium tetani:* Tetanus[1] | 500 mg every 6 hours for 10 days. |
| Granuloma inguinale *Calymmatobacterium granulomatis*[2,4] | 500 mg orally 4 times daily for ≥ 21 days. |

[1] Use as alternative drug in penicillin or tetracycline hypersensitivity or when penicillin or tetracycline are contraindicated or not tolerated.
[2] CDC 1998 Guidelines for Sexually Transmitted Diseases Treatment. MMWR. 1998;47:1-117.
[3] American Heart Association statement. JAMA. 1990;264:2919-2922.
[4] Use as alternate therapy to trimethoprim-sulfamethoxazole or doxycycline.

ERYTHROMYCIN ETHYLSUCCINATE: Expressed in base equivalents, 400 mg erythromycin ethylsuccinate produces the same free erythromycin serum levels as 250 mg of erythromycin base, stearate, or estolate.

TROLEANDOMYCIN: Continue therapy for 10 days when used for streptococcal infection.

Adults – 250 to 500 mg 4 times a day.

Children – 125 to 250 mg (6.6 to 11 mg/kg) every 6 hours.

**Actions**

Pharmacology: Macrolide antibiotics reversibly bind to the P site of the 50S ribosomal subunit of susceptible organisms and inhibit RNA-dependent protein synthesis. They may be bacteriostatic or bactericidal, depending on such factors as drug concentration.

Macrolides are weak bases; their activity increases in alkaline pH. Macrolides enter pleural fluid, ascitic fluid, middle-ear exudates, and sputum. When meninges are inflamed, macrolides may enter the CSF. They are used for respiratory, genital, GI tract, and skin and soft tissue infections, especially when beta-lactam antibiotics or tetracyclines are contraindicated.

Pharmacokinetics:

| Various Pharmacokinetic Parameters of Macrolides | | | | | | | | |
|---|---|---|---|---|---|---|---|---|
| Macrolide | Route of administration | Protein binding (%) | Bioavailability (%) | Effect of food | $C_{max}$* (mcg/mL) | $T_{max}$* (h) | Half-life (h) | Metabolism | Elimination |
| Azithromycin | Oral IV | 51 (0.02 mcg/L) 7 (2 mcg/L) | ≈ 40 | Food increases absorption, $C_{max}$ by 23% and suspension by 56%; take on empty stomach. | 0.5 1.14[2] 3.63[3] | 2.2 | 68[1] | Some hepatic but mainly excreted unchanged | 6% excreted unchanged in urine; primarily excreted unchanged in bile |
| Clarithromycin | Oral | 40-70 | ≈ 50 | Food delays onset of absorption and formation of metabolite. Take without regard to meals. | 1-3 | 2-3 | 3-7 | Metabolized to active metabolite (14-OH clarithromycin) | Primarily renal; rate approximates normal GFR |
| Dirithromycin | Oral | 15-30[4] | ≈ 10 | Take with food or within an hour of eating. | 0.3 - 0.4[4] | 3.9 - 4.1[4] | 2-36 | Nonenzymatic conversion to erythromycylamine | 81%-97% fecal/hepatic[2] |

| Various Pharmacokinetic Parameters of Macrolides | | | | | | | | | |
|---|---|---|---|---|---|---|---|---|---|
| Macrolide | Route of administration | Protein binding (%) | Bioavailability (%) | Effect of food | $C_{max}^*$ (mcg/mL) | $T_{max}^*$ (h) | Half-life[1] (h) | Metabolism | Elimination |
| Erythromycin | Oral IV | 70-80 (96 estolate) | > 35 | Base or stearate: Take on an empty stomach. Estolate, ethylsuccinate, delayed release base: Take without regard to meals. | 0.3-2 | 1.5 | 1.6 | Hepatic; demethylation | < 5% (oral) and 12% to 15% (IV) excreted unchanged in urine; significant quantity excreted in bile |
| Troleandomycin | Oral | | | | 2 | 2 | | | 20% excreted in urine; significant quantity excreted in bile |

* $C_{max}$ = Maximum concentration; $T_{max}$ = Time to reach maximum concentration.
[1] Average terminal half-life.
[2] At a concentration of 1 mg/mL.
[3] At a concentration of 2 mg/mL.
[4] Value listed for erythromycylamine, the active moiety.

Microbiology:

| | Organisms Generally Susceptible to Macrolides In Vitro | | | | | |
|---|---|---|---|---|---|---|
| | Organisms (✔ = generally susceptible) | Azithromycin | Clarithromycin | Dirithromycin | Erythromycin | Troleandomycin[1] |
| Gram-positive aerobes | Staphylococcus aureus | ✔ | ✔ | ✔ | ✔ | |
| | Streptococcus pyogenes | ✔ | ✔ | ✔ | ✔ | ✔ |
| | Streptococcus pneumoniae | ✔ | ✔ | ✔ | ✔ | ✔ |
| | Streptococcus agalactiae | ✔ | ✔ | ✔ | ✔ | |
| | Streptococcus sp. | ✔ | ✔ | ✔ | | |
| | Streptococcus viridans | ✔ | ✔ | ✔ | ✔ | |
| | Listeria monocytogenes | | | ✔ | ✔ | |
| | Corynebacterium diphtheriae | | | | ✔ | |
| | Corynebacterium minutissimum | | | | ✔ | |
| Gram-negative aerobes | Haemophilus influenzae | ✔ | ✔ | ✔ | †[2] | |
| | Haemophilus ducreyi | ✔ | | | | |
| | Moraxella catarrhalis | ✔ | ✔ | ✔ | ✔ | |
| | Bordetella pertussis | ✔ | ✔ | ✔ | ✔ | |
| | Legionella pneumophila | ✔ | ✔ | ✔ | ✔ | |
| | Neisseria gonorrhoeae | ✔ | ✔ | | ✔ | |
| | Pasteurella multocida | | ✔ | | | |
| Anaerobes | Prevotella (formerly Bacteroides) bivius | ✔ | | | | |
| | Prevotella (formerly Bacteroides) melaninogenicus | | ✔ | | | |
| | Clostridium perfringens | | ✔ | | | |
| | Propionibacterium acnes | | ✔ | ✔ | | |
| | Peptococcus niger | | ✔ | | | |
| | Peptostreptococcus sp. | ✔ | | | | |

| Organisms Generally Susceptible to Macrolides In Vitro | | | | | | |
|---|---|---|---|---|---|---|
| | Organisms (✔ = generally susceptible) | Azithromycin | Clarithromycin | Dirithromycin | Erythromycin | Troleandomycin[1] |
| Other | *Borrelia burgdorferi* | ✔ | | | | |
| | *Chlamydia trachomatis* | ✔ | ✔ | | ✔ | |
| | *Mycobacterium kansasii* | | ✔ | | | |
| | *Mycoplasma pneumoniae* | ✔ | ✔ | ✔ | ✔ | |
| | *Treponema pallidum* | ✔ | | | ✔ | |
| | *Ureaplasma urealyticum* | ✔ | | | ✔ | |
| | *Entamoeba histolytica* | | | | ✔ | |
| | *Chlamydia pneumoniae* (TWAR strain) | ✔ | ✔ | | | |
| | *Mycoplasma hominis* | ✔ | | | | |
| | *Mycobacterium avium* | | ✔ | | | |
| | *Mycobacterium intracellulare* | | ✔ | | | |
| | *Helicobacter pylori* | | ✔ | | | |
| | *Clostridium tetani* | | | | ✔ | |

[1] Data is limited for troleandomycin.

[2] Many strains resistant to erythromycin alone; may be susceptible to erythromycin plus a sulfonamide.

The in vitro spectrum of erythromycin covers primarily gram-positive microorganisms and gram-negative cocci.

**Azithromycin** is less active than **erythromycin** against most *Staphylococcus* and *Streptococcus* sp, but it is more potent against other organisms, including many gram-negative bacteria considered resistant to erythromycin. Azithromycin may expand the therapeutic range traditionally assigned to macrolides.

**Clarithromycin** exhibits the same spectrum of in vitro activity as erythromycin, but appears to have significantly increased potency against those organisms.

**Troleandomycin**, an acetylated ester of oleandomycin, is less active than erythromycin and offers no advantage. It also can cause hepatotoxicity.

### Contraindications

Hypersensitivity to any of the macrolide antibiotics; patients receiving cisapride, or pimozide; known, suspected, or potential bacteremias (**dirithromycin**); pre-existing liver disease (**erythromycin estolate**).

### Warnings

*Pseudomembranous colitis:* Pseudomembranous colitis has occurred with nearly all antibacterial agents and may range in severity from mild to life-threatening. Consider this diagnosis in patients who present with diarrhea subsequent to the administration of antibacterial agents.

*Cardiac effects:* Ventricular arrhythmias in individuals with prolonged QT intervals have occurred with macrolide products.

*Acute porphyria:* Do not use **clarithromycin** in combination with ranitidine bismuth citrate in patients with a history of acute porphyria.

*Azithromycin:*

*Pneumonia* – Do not use oral **azithromycin** in patients with pneumonia who are judged to be inappropriate for oral therapy because of moderate to severe illness or risk factors such as any of the following: Nosocomially acquired infections; known or suspected bacteremia; conditions requiring hospitalization; cystic fibrosis; significant underlying health problems that may compromise patients' ability to respond to their illness (including immunodeficiency or functional asplenia); elderly or debilitated patients.

*Hypersensitivity* – Rare serious allergic reactions, including angioedema, anaphylaxis, and dermatologic reactions including Stevens-Johnson syndrome and toxic epidermal necrolysis have occurred in patients on **azithromycin** therapy.

*Dirithromycin:*

*Bacteremias* – Dirithromycin should not be used in patients with known, suspected or potential bacteremias as serum levels are inadequate to provide antibacterial coverage of the blood stream.

*Erythromycin:*

*Hepatotoxicity* – Erythromycin administration has been associated with the infrequent occurrence of cholestatic hepatitis. This effect is most common with erythromycin estolate; however, it has also occurred with other erythromycin salts.

Although initial symptoms have developed after a few days of treatment, they generally have followed 1 or 2 weeks of continuous therapy. Symptoms reappear promptly, usually within 48 hours after the drug is readministered to sensitive patients. The syndrome seems to result from a form of sensitization, occurs chiefly in adults, and is reversible when medication is discontinued.

*Myasthenia gravis* – **Erythromycin** may aggravate the weakness of patients with myasthenia gravis.

*Troleandomycin:*

*Hepatic effects* – Troleandomycin has been associated with allergic cholestatic hepatitis. Some patients receiving troleandomycin for more than 2 weeks or in repeated courses have developed jaundice accompanied by right upper quadrant pain, fever, nausea, vomiting, eosinophilia, and leukocytosis. These have reversed on drug discontinuance. Readministration reproduces hepatotoxicity, often within 24 to 48 hours.

*Renal/Hepatic function impairment:*

*Clarithromycin* – In the presence of severe renal impairment (Ccr less than 30 mL/min) with or without co-existing hepatic impairment, decreased dosage or prolonged dosing intervals may be appropriate.

*Azithromycin and troleandomycin* – Exercise caution when administering to patients with impaired renal or hepatic function.

*Erythromycin* – Erythromycin is principally excreted by the liver. Exercise caution in administering to patients with impaired hepatic function.

*Dirithromycin* – No dosage adjustment should be necessary in patients with impaired renal function, including dialysis patients. In patients with mild hepatic impairment, mean peak serum concentration, AUC and volume of distribution increased somewhat with multiple-dose administration; however, no dosage adjustment should be necessary in patients with mildly impaired hepatic function.

*Elderly:*

*Clarithromycin* – Studies show age-related decreases in renal function. Consider dosage adjustment in elderly patients with severe renal impairment.

*Pregnancy: Category B* (azithromycin, erythromycin); *Category C* (clarithromycin, dirithromycin, troleandomycin).

*Lactation:*

*Clarithromycin, dirithromycin, and azithromycin* – It is not known whether these agents are excreted in breast milk.

*Erythromycin* – Erythromycin is excreted in breast milk, and may concentrate (observed milk:plasma ratio of 0.5 to 3). Erythromycin is considered compatible with breastfeeding by the American Academy of Pediatrics.

*Children:*

*Dirithromycin* – Safety and efficacy in children under 12 years of age have not been established.

*Clarithromycin* – Safety and efficacy in children under 6 months of age have not been established.

*Azithromycin* – Safety and efficacy in children under 6 months of age (acute otitis media, community-acquired pneumonia) or under 2 years of age (pharyngitis/tonsillitis) have not been established.

*IV use:* Safety and efficacy of azithromycin for IV injection in children or adolescents under 16 years of age have not been established.

**Precautions**

*Azithromycin:*

*Local IV site reactions* – Local IV site reactions have been reported with the IV administration of azithromycin. The incidence and severity of these reactions were the same when 500 mg was given over 1 hour (2 mg/mL as 250 mL infusion) or over 3 hours (1 mg/mL as 500 mL infusion). All volunteers who received infusate concentrations greater than 2 mg/mL experienced local IV site reactions; therefore, avoid higher concentrations.

**Drug Interactions**

*Clarithromycin:* Drugs that may be affected by clarithromycin include anticoagulants, benzodiazepines, buspirone, carbamazepine, cisapride, cyclosporine, digoxin, disopyramide, ergot alkaloids, HMG-CoA reductase inhibitors, omeprazole, ranitidine bismuth citrate, tacrolimus, theophylline, and zidovudine. Also consider all drug interactions with erythromycin. Drugs that may affect clarithromycin include fluconazole, ranitidine bismuth citrate, pimozide, rifamycins, and omeprazole.

*Azithromycin:* Drugs that may interact with azithromycin include antacids, cyclosporine, HMG-CoA reductase inhibitors, pimozide, tacrolimus, theophyllines, and warfarin. Also consider all drug interactions with erythromycin.

*Dirithromycin:* Drugs that may be affected by dirithromycin include antacids. Drugs that may affect dirithromycin include antacids, pimozide, and $H_2$ antagonists. Also consider all drug interactions with erythromycin.

*Erythromycin:* Drugs that may be affected by erythromycin include alfentanil, anticoagulants, benzodiazepines, buspirone, carbamazepine, cisapride, cyclosporine, digoxin, disopyramide, ergot alkaloids, felodipine, fluoroquinolones, HMG-CoA reductase inhibitors, lincosamides, methylprednisolone, penicillins, and theophyllines. Drugs that may affect erythromycin include antacids, pimozide, rifamycins, and theophyllines.

*Troleandomycin:* Drugs that may be affected by troleandomycin include benzodiazepines, buspirone, carbamazepine, cisapride, oral contraceptives, cyclosporine, ergot alkaloids, methylprednisolone, tacrolimus, and theophyllines. Drugs that may affect troleandomycin include rifamycins.

*Drug/Food interactions:*

*Clarithromycin* – Following tablet administration, food delays both the onset of clarithromycin absorption and the formulation of 14 OH clarithromycin, but does not affect bioavailability. Following administration of the oral suspension, food decreases mean peak clarithromycin levels and extent of absorption.

*Dirithromycin* – Dirithromycin should be administered with food or within an hour of eating. After administration of two 250 mg tablets 1 or 4 hours before food and immediately after a standard breakfast indicated an increase in absorption of erythromycylamine when dirithromycin was administered after food, while a significant decrease in $C_{max}$ (33%) and AUC (31%) occurred when administered 1 hour before food.

*Erythromycin* – Antimicrobial effectiveness of erythromycin stearate and certain formulations of erythromycin base may be reduced. Take at least 2 hours before or after a meal. Erythromycin estolate and ethylsuccinate and the base in a delayed release form may be administered without regard to meals.

**Adverse Reactions**

*Clarithromycin* – Adverse reactions occurring in at least 3% of patients include diarrhea, nausea, abdominal pain, rash, increased BUN, and abnormal taste.

*Azithromycin* – Adverse reactions occurring in at least 3% of patients include diarrhea/loose stools, vomiting, nausea, abdominal pain, increased ALT and AST, increased serum creatinine, and increased bilirubin.

*Dirithromycin* – Adverse reactions occurring in at least 3% of patients include abdominal pain/discomfort, diarrhea/loose stools, nausea, vomiting, increased platelet count, and headache.

*Erythromycin* – Adverse reactions occurring in at least 3% of patients include abdominal pain/discomfort, diarrhea/loose stools, nausea, increased platelet count, and headache.

*Hepatic:* Hepatotoxicity is most commonly associated with erythromycin estolate.

*Local* – Venous irritation and phlebitis have occurred with parenteral administration, but the risk of such reactions may be reduced if the infusion is given slowly, in dilute solution, by continuous IV infusion or intermittent infusion over 20 to 60 minutes.

# TELITHROMYCIN

| | |
|---|---|
| **Tablets**: 400 mg | *Ketek* (Aventis) |

## Indications

For the treatment of the following infections for patients 18 years of age and older:

*Acute bacterial exacerbation of chronic bronchitis:* Caused by *Streptococcus pneumoniae*, *Haemophilus influenzae*, or *Moraxella catarrhalis*.

*Acute bacterial sinusitis:* Caused by *S. pneumoniae*, *H. influenzae*, *M. catarrhalis*, or *Staphylococcus aureus*.

*Community-acquired pneumonia:* Of mild to moderate severity caused by *S. pneumoniae* (including multidrug resistant isolates (MDRSP), *H. influenzae*, *M. catarrhalis*, *Chlamydophila pneumoniae*, or *Mycoplasma pneumoniae*.

## Administration and Dosage

*Approved by the FDA:* April 1, 2004.

The dose of telithromycin tablets is 800 mg taken orally once every 24 hours. Telithromycin can be administered with or without food.

| Telithromycin Dosage | | | |
|---|---|---|---|
| Infection | Daily dose | Frequency of administration | Duration of treatment |
| Acute bacterial exacerbation of chronic bronchitis | 800 mg oral (2 tablets of 400 mg) | Once daily | 5 days |
| Acute bacterial sinusitis | 800 mg oral (2 tablets of 400 mg) | Once daily | 5 days |
| Community-acquired pneumonia | 800 mg oral (2 tablets of 400 mg) | Once daily | 7 to 10 days |

## Actions

*Pharmacology:* Telithromycin belongs to the ketolide class of antibacterials and is structurally related to the macrolide family of antibiotics. Telithromycin blocks protein synthesis by binding to domains II and V of 23S rRNA of the 50S ribosomal subunit.

*Pharmacokinetics:*

*Absorption/Distribution* – Following oral administration, telithromycin reached maximal concentration at about 1 hour.

| Mean Telithromycin Pharmacokinetic Parameters | | |
|---|---|---|
| Parameter | Single dose (n = 18) | Multiple dose (n = 18) |
| $C_{max}$ (mcg/mL) | 1.9 | 2.27 |
| $T_{max}$ (hr; median value) | 1 | 1 |
| $AUC_{(0\ to\ 24)}$ (mcg•h/mL) | 8.25 | 12.5 |
| Terminal $t_{1/2}$ (h/ | 7.16 | 9.81 |
| $C_{24h}$[1] (mcg/mL) | 0.03 | 0.07 |

[1] $C_{24h}$ = Plasma concentration at 24 hours postdose

In a patient population, mean peak and trough plasma concentrations were 2.9 mcg/mL (n = 219) and 0.2 mcg/mL (n = 204), respectively, after 3 to 5 days of 800 mg telithromycin once daily.

Total in vitro protein binding is approximately 60% to 70% and is primarily caused by human serum albumin. The volume of distribution of telithromycin after IV infusion is 2.9 L/kg.

*Metabolism/Excretion* – Metabolism accounts for approximately 70% of the dose. It is estimated that approximately 50% of its metabolism is mediated by CYP450 3A4 and the remaining 50% is CYP450-independent. Seven percent of the dose is excreted unchanged in feces; 13% is excreted unchanged in urine; and 37% of the dose is metabolized by the liver. The mean terminal elimination half-life is 10 hours.

## Contraindications

A history of hypersensitivity to telithromycin and/or any components of the product or any macrolide antibiotic. Coadministration of telithromycin with cisapride or pimozide is contraindicated.

## Warnings

*Pseudomembranous colitis:* Pseudomembranous colitis has been reported with nearly all antibacterial agents, including telithromycin.

*Cardiac effects:* Telithromycin has the potential to prolong the QTc interval in some patients. QTc prolongation may lead to an increased risk for ventricular arrhythmias, including torsades de pointes.

*Myasthenia gravis:* Exacerbations of myasthenia gravis have been reported in patients with myasthenia gravis treated with telithromycin. This has sometimes occurred within a few hours after intake of the first dose of telithromycin. Reports have included life-threatening acute respiratory failure with a rapid onset. Telithromycin is not recommended in patients with myasthenia gravis unless no other therapeutic alternatives are available.

*Renal/Hepatic function impairment:* Hepatic dysfunction, including increased liver enzymes and hepatitis, with or without jaundice, has been reported with the use of telithromycin. In the presence of severe renal impairment (Ccr less than 30 mL/min), including patients who need dialysis, the dose of telithromycin has not been established.

Telithromycin is principally excreted via the liver and kidney. Telithromycin may be administered without dosage adjustment in the presence of hepatic impairment.

*Pregnancy:* Category C.

*Lactation:* Exercise caution when telithromycin is given to a nursing mother.

*Children:* The safety and effectiveness of telithromycin in pediatric patients has not been established.

## Precautions

Prescribing telithromycin in the absence of a proven or strongly suspected bacterial infection or a prophylactic indication is unlikely to benefit the patient and increases the risk of the development of drug-resistant bacteria.

*Visual disturbances:* Telithromycin may cause visual disturbances particularly in slowing the ability to accommodate and the ability to release accommodation. Most visual adverse events (65%) occurred following the first or second dose. Visual disturbances included blurred vision, difficulty focusing, and diplopia. Caution patients about the potential effects of these visual disturbances on driving a vehicle, operating machinery, or engaging in other potentially hazardous activities (see Adverse Reactions).

## Drug Interactions

Drugs that may affect telithromycin include itraconazole, ketoconazole, rifampin, phenytoin, phenobarbital, carbamazepine.

Drugs that may be affected by telithromycin include cisapride, digoxin, ergot alkaloids, metoprolol, midazolam, pimozide, HMG-CoA reductase inhibitors, sotalol, and theophylline.

*Cytochrome P450:* Telithromycin is a strong inhibitor of the cytochrome P450 3A4 system.

## Adverse Reactions

Adverse reactions occurring in at least 3% of patients include the following: diarrhea, dizziness (excluding vertigo), headache, nausea, vomiting.

*Lab test abnormalities:* Increased platelet count; increased transaminases and increased liver enzymes (eg, ALT, AST) were usually asymptomatic and reversible.

*Special senses:* Visual adverse events most often included blurred vision, diplopia, or difficulty focusing.

# DAPTOMYCIN

Powder for injection, lyophilized: 250 and 500 mg (Rx)    Cubicin (Cubist)

## Indications

Complicated skin and skin structure infections: For the treatment of complicated skin and skin structure infections caused by susceptible strains of the following gram-positive microorganisms: Staphylococcus aureus (including methicillin-resistant strains), Streptococcus pyogenes, Streptococcus agalactiae, Streptococcus dysgalactiae subsp. equisimilis, and Enterococcus faecalis (vancomycin-susceptible strains only). Combination therapy may be clinically indicated if the documented or presumed pathogens include gram-negative or anaerobic organisms.

## Administration and Dosage

Complicated skin and skin structure infections: Administer daptomycin 4 mg/kg over a 30-minute period by IV infusion in 0.9% sodium chloride injection once every 24 hours for 7 to 14 days. In phase 1 and 2 clinical studies, creatine phosphokinase (CPK) elevations appeared to be more frequent when daptomycin was dosed more frequently than once daily. Therefore, do not dose daptomycin more frequently than once a day.

Renal function impairment: Because daptomycin is eliminated primarily by the kidney, a dosage modification is recommended for patients with creatinine clearance (Ccr) less than 30 mL/min, including patients receiving hemodialysis or continuous ambulatory peritoneal dialysis (CAPD). When possible, administer daptomycin following hemodialysis on hemodialysis days.

| Daptomycin Dosage in Adult Patients with Renal Impairment | |
|---|---|
| Creatinine clearance | Dosage regimen |
| ≥ 30 mL/min | 4 mg/kg once every 24 h |
| < 30 mL/min, including hemodialysis or CAPD | 4 mg/kg once every 48 h |

Incompatibilities: Daptomycin is not compatible with dextrose-containing diluents. Do not add additives or other medications to daptomycin single-use vials or infuse simultaneously through the same IV line.

## Actions

Pharmacology: Daptomycin is an antibacterial agent of a new class of antibiotics, the cyclic lipopeptides. The mechanism of action of daptomycin is distinct from any other antibiotic. Daptomycin binds to bacterial membranes and causes a rapid depolarization of membrane potential. The loss of membrane potential leads to inhibition of protein, DNA, and RNA synthesis, which results in bacterial cell death. Daptomycin is a natural product that has clinical utility in the treatment of infections caused by aerobic gram-positive bacteria. Daptomycin exhibits rapid, concentration-dependent bactericidal activity against gram-positive organisms in vitro. Daptomycin retains potency against antibiotic-resistant gram-positive bacteria, including isolates resistant to methicillin, vancomycin, and linezolid.

Pharmacokinetics:

Absorption – The mean pharmacokinetic parameters of daptomycin on day 7 following the IV administration of 4, 6, and 8 mg/kg once daily to healthy young adults (mean age, 35.8 years) are summarized in the following table.

| Mean Daptomycin Pharmacokinetic Parameters in Healthy Volunteers on Day 7 | | | | | | | | |
|---|---|---|---|---|---|---|---|---|
| Dose mg/kg | $C_{max}$ (mcg/mL) | $T_{max}$[1] (h) | $AUC_{0-24}$ (mcg•h/ mL) | $t_{1/2}$ (h) | $V_d$ (L/kg) | $CL_T$ (mL/h/ kg) | $CL_R$ (mL/h/ kg) | $Ae_{24}$ % |
| 4 (n = 6) | 57.8 | 0.8 | 494 | 8.1 | 0.096 | 8.3 | 4.8 | 53 |
| 6 (n = 6) | 98.6 | 0.5 | 747 | 8.9 | 0.104 | 8.1 | 4.4 | 47.4 |

| Mean Daptomycin Pharmacokinetic Parameters in Healthy Volunteers on Day 7 | | | | | | | | |
|---|---|---|---|---|---|---|---|---|
| Dose mg/kg | $C_{max}$ (mcg/mL) | $T_{max}$[1] (h) | $AUC_{0-24}$ (mcg•h/ mL) | $t_{1/2}$ (h) | $V_d$ (L/kg) | $CL_T$ (mL/h/ kg) | $CL_R$ (mL/h/ kg) | $Ae_{24}$ % |
| 8 (n = 6) | 133 | 0.5 | 1130 | 9 | 0.092 | 7.2 | 3.7 | 52.1 |

[1] Median (minimum, maximum).
$CL_T$ = Systemic clearance.
$CL_R$ = Renal clearance.
$Ae_{24}$ = Percent of dose recovered in urine over 24 hours as unchanged daptomycin following the first dose.

Daptomycin pharmacokinetics are nearly linear and time-independent at doses up to 6 mg/kg administered once daily for 7 days. Steady-state concentrations are achieved by the third daily dose.

*Distribution* – Daptomycin is reversibly bound to human plasma proteins, primarily to serum albumin, in a concentration-independent manner. The mean serum protein binding of daptomycin was approximately 92% in healthy adults.

*Metabolism* – It is unlikely that daptomycin will inhibit or induce the metabolism of drugs metabolized by the CYP 450 system. It is unknown whether daptomycin is a substrate of the CYP 450 system.

*Excretion* – Daptomycin is excreted primarily by the kidney.

### Contraindications
Known hypersensitivity to daptomycin.

### Warnings
*Pseudomembranous colitis:* Pseudomembranous colitis has been reported with nearly all antibacterial agents, including daptomycin, and may range in severity from mild to life-threatening. Therefore, it is important to consider this diagnosis in patients who present with diarrhea subsequent to the administration of any antibacterial agent.

*Elderly:* In the two phase 3 clinical studies in patients with complicated skin and skin structure infections (cSSSI), lower clinical success rates were seen in patients 65 years of age and older compared with those younger than 65 years of age. In addition, treatment-emergent adverse events were more common in patients 65 years of age and older than in patients younger than 65 years of age in both cSSSI studies.

*Pregnancy: Category B.*

*Lactation:* It is not known if daptomycin is excreted in human milk. Exercise caution when administering daptomycin to nursing women.

*Children:* Safety and efficacy of daptomycin in patients younger than 18 years of age have not been established.

### Precautions
*Monitoring:* Monitor CPK levels weekly in patients who receive daptomycin. Monitor patients who develop unexplained elevations in CPK while receiving daptomycin more frequently.

*Skeletal muscle effects:* Monitor patients receiving daptomycin for the development of muscle pain or weakness, particularly of the distal extremities. Monitor CPK levels weekly in patients who receive daptomycin. Monitor patients who develop unexplained elevations in CPK while receiving daptomycin more frequently.

Discontinue daptomycin in patients with unexplained signs and symptoms of myopathy in conjunction with CPK elevation greater than 1000 units/L (approximately $5 \times$ ULN), or in patients without reported symptoms who have marked elevations in CPK ($10 \times$ ULN or greater). In addition, consider temporarily suspending agents associated with rhabdomyolysis, such as HMG-CoA reductase inhibitors, in patients receiving daptomycin.

*Neuropathy:* Administration of daptomycin was associated with decreases in nerve con-duction velocity and with adverse events (eg, paresthesias, Bell palsy), possibly reflective of peripheral or cranial neuropathy. Nerve conduction deficits were also detected in a similar number of comparator subjects in these studies.

*Superinfection:* The use of antibiotics may promote the overgrowth of nonsusceptible organisms. Should superinfection occur during therapy, take appropriate measures.

**Drug Interactions**

Although no specific drug-drug interactions have been documented, exercise caution when using daptomycin in patients receiving warfarin (monitor INR) or HMG-CoA reductase inhibitors (may cause myopathy and increase CPK levels).

**Adverse Reactions**

Adverse drug reactions occurring in at least 3% of patients receiving daptomycin include abnormal liver function tests, constipation, diarrhea, headache, injection-site reactions, insomnia, nausea, rash, and vomiting.

# VANCOMYCIN

| | |
|---|---|
| **Pulvules:** 125 mg and 250 mg (Rx) | *Vancocin* (Lilly) |
| **Powder for oral solution:** 1 and 10 g (Rx) | *Vancomycin HCl* (ESI Lederle) |
| **Powder for injection:** 500 mg, 1, 5, and 10 g (Rx) | Various, *Vancocin* (Lilly), *Vancoled* (Lederle) |

### Indications

*Parenteral:* Serious or severe infections not treatable with other antimicrobials, including the penicillins and cephalosporins.

*Severe staphylococcal infections* – Severe staphylococcal infections (including methicillin-resistant staphylococci) in patients who cannot receive or who have failed to respond to penicillins and cephalosporins, or who have infections with resistant staphylococci. Infections may include endocarditis, bone infections, lower respiratory tract infections, septicemia, and skin and skin structure infections.

*Endocarditis* –

*Staphylococcal:* Vancomycin is effective alone.

*Streptococcal:* Vancomycin is effective alone or in combination with an aminoglycoside for endocarditis caused by S. *viridans* or S. *bovis*. It is only effective in combination with an aminoglycoside for endocarditis caused by enterococci (eg, S. *faecalis*).

*Diphtheroid:* Vancomycin is effective for diphtheroid endocarditis, and has been used successfully with rifampin, an aminoglycoside, or both in early onset prosthetic valve endocarditis caused by *Staphylococcus epidermidis* or diphtheroids.

*Prophylactic:* Although no controlled clinical efficacy studies have been conducted, IV vancomycin has been suggested for prophylaxis against bacterial endocarditis in penicillin-allergic patients who have congenital heart disease or rheumatic or other acquired or valvular heart disease when these patients undergo dental procedures or surgical procedures of the upper respiratory tract.

*Pseudomembranous colitis/staphylococcal enterocolitis caused by Clostridium difficile* – The parenteral form may be administered orally; parenteral use alone is unproven. The oral use of parenteral vancomycin is not effective for other infections.

*Oral:* Staphylococcal enterocolitis and antibiotic-associated pseudomembranous colitis produced by C. *difficile*. The parenteral product may also be given orally for these infections. Oral vancomycin is *not* effective for other types of infection.

### Administration and Dosage

Complete full course of therapy; do not discontinue therapy without notifying physician.

*Oral:*

*Adults* – 500 mg to 2 g/day given in 3 or 4 divided doses for 7 to 10 days.

Alternatively, dosages of 125 mg 3 or 4 times daily for C. *difficile* colitis may be as effective as the 500 mg dose regimen.

*Children* – 40 mg/kg/day in 3 or 4 divided doses for 7 to 10 days. Do not exceed 2 g/day.

*Neonates* – 10 mg/kg/day in divided doses.

*Parenteral:* Administer each dose over at least 60 minutes. Intermittent infusion is the preferred administration method.

*Adults* – 500 mg IV every 6 hours or 1 g every 12 hours.

*Children* – 10 mg/kg/dose given every 6 hours.

*Infants and neonates* – Initial dose of 15 mg/kg, followed by 10 mg/kg every 12 hours for neonates in the first week of life and every 8 hours thereafter up to the age of 1 month.

*Prevention of bacterial endocarditis:*

*GU/GI procedures (high-risk, penicillin-allergic patients)* – 1 g IV over 1 to 2 hours (children, 20 mg/kg) plus gentamicin 1.5 mg/kg IV or IM for both adult (not to exceed 120 mg) and children. Complete injection or infusion within 30 minutes of starting procedure.

*(Moderate-risk, penicillin-allergic patients)* – 1 g IV over 1 to 2 hours (children 20 mg/kg). Complete infusion within 30 minutes of starting procedure.

*Renal function impairment:* Adjust dosage; check serum levels regularly. In premature infants and the elderly, dosage reduction may be necessary caused by decreasing renal function.

For most patients, if Ccr can be measured or estimated accurately, the dosage may be calculated by using the following table.

| Vancomycin Dosage in Impaired Renal Function | |
|---|---|
| Ccr (mL/min) | Dose (mg/24 h) |
| 100 | 1545 |
| 90 | 1390 |
| 80 | 1235 |
| 70 | 1080 |
| 60 | 925 |
| 50 | 770 |
| 40 | 620 |
| 30 | 465 |
| 20 | 310 |
| 10 | 155 |

The table is not valid for functionally anephric patients on dialysis. For such patients, give a loading dose of 15 mg/kg to achieve therapeutic serum levels promptly and a maintenance dose of 1.9 mg/kg/24 h. In patients with marked renal impairment, it may be more convenient to give maintenance doses of 250 to 1000 mg once every several days rather than administering the drug on a daily basis. In anuria a dose of 1000 mg every 7 to 10 days has been recommended.

### Actions
*Pharmacology:* Vancomycin is a tricyclic glycopeptide antibiotic that inhibits cell-wall biosynthesis. It also alters bacterial-cell-membrane permeability and RNA synthesis.

*Pharmacokinetics:*

*Absorption/Distribution* – Systemic absorption of oral vancomycin is generally poor.

*Metabolism/Excretion* – In the first 24 hours, approximately 75% of a dose is excreted in urine by glomerular filtration. Elimination half-life is 4 to 6 hours in adults and 2 to 3 hours in children. About 60% of an intraperitoneal dose administered during peritoneal dialysis is absorbed systemically in 6 hours. Accumulation occurs in renal failure. Serum half-life in anephric patients is approximately 7.5 days. Vancomycin is not significantly removed by hemodialysis or continuous ambulatory peritoneal dialysis, although there have been reports of increased clearance with hemoperfusion and hemofiltration.

### Contraindications
Hypersensitivity to vancomycin.

### Warnings
*Ototoxicity:* Ototoxicity has occurred in patients receiving vancomycin. It may be transient or permanent. It has occurred mostly in patients who have been given excessive doses, who have an underlying hearing loss, or who are receiving concomitant therapy with another ototoxic agent.

*Hypotension:* Rapid bolus administration may be associated with exaggerated hypotension, including shock, and rarely, cardiac arrest. To avoid hypotension, administer in a dilute solution over 60 minutes or more. Stopping the infusion usually results in prompt cessation of these reactions. Frequently monitor blood pressure and heart rate.

*Pseudomembranous colitis:* In rare instances, pseudomembranous colitis has occurred because of *C. difficile* developing in patients who received IV vancomycin.

*Reversible neutropenia:* Reversible neutropenia has occurred in patients receiving vancomycin.

*Tissue irritation:* Vancomycin is irritating to tissue and must be given by a secure IV route of administration. Pain, tenderness, and necrosis occur with IM injection or inadvertent extravasation.

Reports have revealed that administration of sterile vancomycin by the intraperitoneal route during continuous ambulatory peritoneal dialysis (CAPD) has resulted in a syndrome of chemical peritonitis. This syndrome has ranged from a cloudy dialysate alone to a cloudy dialysate accompanied by variable degrees of abdominal pain and fever. This syndrome appears to be short-lived after discontinuation of intraperitoneal vancomycin.

*Nephrotoxicity:* The risk of toxicity may be appreciably increased by high serum concentrations or prolonged therapy. Factors that may increase the risk of nephrotoxicity include use in elderly and neonatal patients and concomitant use with other nephrotoxic drugs.

*Renal function impairment:* Because of its nephrotoxicity, use carefully in renal insufficiency.

*Pregnancy:* Category C; Category B (pulvules only).

*Lactation:* Vancomycin is excreted in breast milk.

*Children:* In premature and full-term neonates it may be appropriate to confirm desired vancomycin serum concentrations.

## Precautions

*Monitoring:* Perform auditory function serial tests and monitor serum levels. When monitoring vancomycin serum levels, draw a peak concentration 1.5 to 2.5 hours after the completion of a 1-hour infusion and a trough concentration within 1 hour of the next scheduled dose. Peak levels are generally expected to be in the 30 to 40 mg/mL range and trough levels in the 10 to 15 mg/mL range.

*Systemic absorption:* Clinically significant serum concentrations may occur in some patients who have taken multiple oral doses for active C. *difficile*-induced pseudomembranous colitis or who have inflammatory disorders of the intestinal mucosa; the risk is greater with the presence of renal impairment.

*Red Man (or Redneck) syndrome:* Red Man (or Redneck) syndrome is usually stimulated by a too-rapid IV infusion (dose given over a few minutes), but it has been reported rarely when given as recommended and following oral or intraperitoneal administration. The onset may occur anytime within a few minutes of starting an IV infusion to a short time after infusion completion. The rash generally resolves several hours after termination of administration.

## Drug Interactions

Drugs that may interact with vancomycin include aminoglycosides, anesthetics, neurotoxic/nephrotoxic agents, and nondepolarizing muscle relaxants.

## Adverse Reactions

Adverse reactions may include renal impairment; hearing loss; neutropenia; vertigo; dizziness; anaphylaxis; drug fever; nausea; chills; eosinophilia; rashes; hypotension; wheezing; dyspnea; urticaria; inflammation at injection site; Red Man (or Redneck) syndrome; chemical peritonitis has been reported following intraperitoneal administration of vancomycin.

# LINEZOLID

**Tablets**: 400[1] and 600 mg[2] (*Rx*)                    *Zyvox* (Pharmacia)
**Powder for reconstitution**:[3] 100 mg/5 mL (*Rx*)
**Injection**:[4] 2 mg/mL (*Rx*)

[1] Sodium content is 1.95 mg/400 mg tablet (0.1 mEq/tablet).
[2] Sodium content is 2.92 mg/600 mg tablet (0.1 mEq/tablet).
[3] Sodium content is 8.52 mg/5 mL (0.4 mEq/5 mL).
[4] Sodium content 0.38 mg/mL (5 mEq/300 mL bag, 3.3 mEq/200 mL bag, 1.7 mEq/100 mL bag).

## Indications

*Vancomycin-resistant Enterococcus faecium infections:* For the treatment of vancomycin-resistant *E. faecium* infections including cases with concurrent bacteremia.

*Nosocomial pneumonia:* For the treatment of nosocomial pneumonia caused by *Staphylococcus aureus* (methicillin-susceptible and -resistant strains), or *Streptococcus pneumoniae* (penicillin-susceptible strains only). Combination therapy may be indicated if the documented or presumptive pathogens include gram-negative organisms.

*Complicated skin and skin structure infections:* For the treatment of complicated skin and skin structure infections caused by *S. aureus* (methicillin-susceptible and -resistant strains), *Streptococcus pyogenes*, or *Streptococcus agalactiae*. It has not been studied in the treatment of diabetic foot and decubitus ulcers. Combination therapy may be clinically indicated if the documented or presumptive pathogens include gram-negative organisms.

*Uncomplicated skin and skin structure infections:* For the treatment of uncomplicated skin and skin structure infections caused by *S. aureus* (methicillin-susceptible strains only) or *S. pyogenes*.

*Community-acquired pneumonia:* For the treatment of community-acquired pneumonia caused by *S. pneumoniae* (penicillin-susceptible strains only), including cases with concurrent bacteremia, or *S. aureus* (methicillin-susceptible strains only).

Because of concerns about inappropriate use of antibiotics leading to increase in resistant organisms, carefully consider alternatives before initiating treatment with linezolid in the outpatient setting.

## Administration and Dosage

Administer without regard to meals.

| Linezolid Dosage Guidelines | | | |
|---|---|---|---|
| Infection[1] | Dosage and route of administration | | Recommended duration of treatment (consecutive days) |
| | Pediatric patients[2] (birth through 11 years of age) | Adults and adolescents (12 years and older) | |
| Complicated skin and skin-structure infections | 10 mg/kg IV or oral[3] q 8 h | 600 mg IV or oral[3] q 12 h | 10 to 14 |
| Community-acquired pneumonia, including concurrent bacteremia | | | |
| Nosocomial pneumonia | | | |
| Vancomycin-resistant Enterococcus faecium infections, including concurrent bacteremia | 10 mg/kg IV or oral[3] q 8 h | 600 mg IV or oral[3] q 12 h | 14 to 28 |

| Linezolid Dosage Guidelines | | | |
|---|---|---|---|
| | Dosage and route of administration | | Recommended duration of treatment (consecutive days) |
| Infection[1] | Pediatric patients[2] (birth through 11 years of age) | Adults and adolescents (12 years and older) | |
| Uncomplicated skin and skin-structure infections | < 5 yrs: 10 mg/kg oral[3] q 8 h 5 to 11 yrs: 10 mg/kg oral[3] q 12 h | *Adults:* 400 mg oral[3] q 12 h *Adolescents:* 600 mg oral[3] q 12 h | 10 to 14 |

[1] Due to the designated pathogens.
[2] Neonates younger than 7 days: Most preterm neonates younger than 7 days of age (gestational age less than 34 weeks) have lower systemic linezolid clearance values and larger AUC values than many full-term neonates and older infants. Initiate these neonates with a dosing regimen of 10 mg/kg twice daily. Consider the use of 10 mg/kg 3 times daily regimen in neonates with a suboptimal clinical response. Give all neonatal patients 10 mg/kg 3 times daily by 7 days of life.
[3] Oral dosing using either linezolid tablets or linezolid for oral suspension.

Treat patients with methicillin-resistant *S. aureus* (MRSA) infection with linezolid 600 mg/12 hours.

No dose adjustment is necessary when switching from IV to oral administration. Patients who are started on IV therapy may be switched to tablets or oral suspension when clinically indicated.

*IV administration:* Administer over a period of 30 to 120 minutes. Do not use IV infusion bag in series connections. Do not introduce additives into this solution. Do not administer concomitantly with another drug; administer each drug separately.

*Compatible IV solutions:* 5% Dextrose Injection, 0.9% NaCl Injection; Lactated Ringer's Injection.

*Admixture incompatibilities:* Physical incompatibilities resulted when linezolid IV injection was combined with the following drugs during simulated Y-site administration: Amphotericin B, chlorpromazine HCl, diazepam, pentamidine isothionate, erythromycin lactobionate, phenytoin sodium, and trimethoprim-sulfamethoxazole. Additionally, chemical incompatibility resulted when linezolid IV injection was combined with ceftriaxone sodium.

If the same IV line is used for sequential infusion of several drugs, the line should be flushed before and after infusion of IV injection with an infusion solution compatible with linezolid IV injection and with any other drug(s) administered via this common line.

### Actions
*Pharmacology:* Linezolid binds to a site on the bacterial 23S ribosomal RNA of the 50S subunit and prevents the formation of a functional 70S initiation complex, which is an essential component of the bacterial translation process. The results of time-kill studies have shown linezolid to be bacteriostatic against *Enterococci* and *Staphylococci*. For *Streptococci*, linezolid was found to be bactericidal for the majority of strains.

*Pharmacokinetics:*
  *Absorption* – Linezolid is rapidly and extensively absorbed after oral dosing with an absolute bioavailability of approximately 100%.
  *Distribution* – The plasma protein binding of linezolid is approximately 31% and is concentration-independent. The volume of distribution of linezolid at steady-state averaged 40 to 50 L in healthy adult volunteers.
  *Metabolism* – Linezolid is primarily metabolized by oxidation of the morpholine ring, which results in 2 inactive ring-opened carboxylic acid metabolites.

*Excretion* – Nonrenal clearance accounts for approximately 65% of the total clearance of linezolid. Under steady-state conditions, approximately 30% of the dose appears in the urine as linezolid, 40% as metabolite B, and 10% as metabolite A. The renal clearance of linezolid is low (average, 40 mL/min) and suggests net tubular reabsorption. Virtually, no linezolid appears in the feces, while approximately 6% of the dose appears in the feces as metabolite B and 3% as metabolite A.

*Special populations* –

*Children:* The $C_{max}$ and the volume of distribution ($V_{ss}$) of linezolid are similar regardless of age in pediatric patients. However, clearance of linezolid varies as a function of age. With the exclusion of preterm neonates less than 1 week of age, clearance is most rapid in the youngest age groups ranging from older than 1 week old to 11 years of age, resulting in lower single-dose AUC and shorter half-life as compared with adults. As age of pediatric patients increases, the clearance of linezolid gradually decreases, and by adolescence mean clearance values approach those observed for the adult population.

Recommendations for the dosage regimen for preterm neonates younger than 7 days of age (gestational age less than 34 weeks) are based on pharmacokinetic data from 9 preterm neonates. Most of these preterm neonates have lower systemic linezolid clearance values and larger AUC values than many full-term neonates and older infants. Therefore, initiate these preterm neonates with a dosing regimen of 10 mg/kg twice daily. Consideration may be given to the use of a 10 mg/kg 3 times daily regimen in neonates with a suboptimal clinical response. Give all neonatal patients 10 mg/kg 3 times daily by 7 days of life.

*Gender:* Females have a slightly lower volume of distribution of linezolid than males. Plasma concentrations are higher in females than in males, which is partly due to body weight differences. After a 600 mg dose, mean oral clearance is approximately 38% lower in females than in males. However, there are no significant gender differences in mean apparent elimination-rate constant or half-life. Thus, drug exposure in females is not expected to substantially increase beyond levels known to be well tolerated. Therefore, dose adjustment by gender does not appear to be necessary.

*Renal function impairment:* The pharmacokinetics of the parent drug, linezolid, are not altered in patients with any degree of renal insufficiency; however, the 2 primary metabolites of linezolid may accumulate in patients with renal insufficiency, with the amount of accumulation increasing with the severity of renal dysfunction. The clinical significance of accumulation of these 2 metabolites has not been determined in patients with severe renal insufficiency. Given the absence of information on the clinical significance of accumulation of the primary metabolites, weigh the use of linezolid in patients with renal insufficiency against the potential risks of accumulation of these metabolites. Linezolid and the 2 metabolites are eliminated by dialysis. No information is available on the effect of peritoneal dialysis on the pharmacokinetics of linezolid. Approximately 30% of a dose was eliminated in a 3-hour dialysis session beginning 3 hours after the dose of linezolid was administered; therefore, give linezolid after hemodialysis.

## Contraindications

Hypersensitivity to linezolid or any of the other product components.

## Warnings

*Myelosuppression:* Myelosuppression (including anemia, leukopenia, pancytopenia, and thrombocytopenia) has been reported in patients receiving linezolid. In cases where the outcome is known, when linezolid was discontinued, the affected hematologic parameters rose toward pretreatment levels. Monitor complete blood counts weekly in patients who receive linezolid, particularly in those who receive linezolid for more than 2 weeks, those with preexisting myelosuppression, those receiving concomitant drugs that produce bone marrow suppression, or those with a chronic infection who have received previous or concomitant antibiotic therapy. Consider discontinuation of therapy with linezolid in patients who develop or have worsening myelosuppression.

*Pseudomembranous colitis:* Pseudomembranous colitis has been reported with nearly all antibacterial agents, including linezolid, and may range in severity from mild to life-threatening.

*Pregnancy: Category C.*

*Lactation:* Linezolid and its metabolites are excreted in the milk of lactating rats. Concentrations in milk were similar to those in maternal plasma. It is not known whether linezolid is excreted in human breast milk.

*Children:* Safety and efficacy in children have been established in pediatric patients from birth to 11 years of age.

### Precautions

*Duration of therapy:* The safety and efficacy of linezolid formulations given for more than 28 days have not been evaluated in controlled clinical trials.

*Phenylketonurics:* Each 5 mL of the 100 mg/5 mL oral suspension contains 20 mg phenylalanine. The other linezolid formulations do not contain phenylalanine. Advise patients to contact their physician or pharmacist.

*Lactic acidosis:* Lactic acidosis has been reported with the use of linezolid. In reported cases, patients experienced repeated episodes of nausea and vomiting. Patients who develop recurrent nausea or vomiting, unexplained acidosis, or a low bicarbonate level while receiving linezolid should receive immediate medical evaluation.

### Drug Interactions

Drugs that may interact with linezolid include monoamine oxidase inhibitors, SSRIs, and adrenergic agents (eg, dopamine and epinephrine).

*Drug/Food interactions:* Large quantities of foods or beverages with high tyramine content should be avoided while taking linezolid. Quantities of tyramine consumed should be less than 100 mg/meal.

### Adverse Reactions

*Thrombocytopenia* – Linezolid has been associated with thrombocytopenia when used in doses of 600 mg or less every 12 hours for up to 28 days. Thrombocytopenia associated with the use of linezolid appears to be dependent on duration of therapy (generally more than 2 weeks of treatment). The platelet counts for most patients returned to the normal range/baseline during the follow-up period.

During clinical trials, 2% to 3% of linezolid patients discontinued therapy because of adverse effects. Adverse reactions occurring in at least 3% of patients include diarrhea, headache, lab test abnormalities (hemoglobin, ALT, alkaline phosphatase, and lipase), nausea, upper respiratory infection, and vomiting.

# LINCOSAMIDES

**CLINDAMYCIN**
**Capsules:** 75, 150, and 300 mg (as HCl) (*Rx*)          Various, *Cleocin* (Pharmacia)
**Granules for oral solution:** 75 mg (as palmitate)/5 mL (*Rx*)   *Cleocin Pediatric* (Pharmacia)
**Injection:** 150 mg (as phosphate)/mL (*Rx*)          Various, *Cleocin Phosphate* (Pharmacia)

**LINCOMYCIN**
**Capsules:** 500 mg (as HCl) (*Rx*)          *Lincocin* (Pharmacia)
**Injection:** 300 mg/mL (as HCl) (*Rx*)          *Lincomycin HCl* (Steris), *Lincocin* (Pharmacia), *Lincorex* (Hyrex)

---

**Warning:**
These agents can cause severe and possibly fatal colitis, characterized by severe persistent diarrhea, severe abdominal cramps, and possibly, the passage of blood and mucus.

Reserve for serious infections where less toxic antimicrobial agents are inappropriate. Do not use in patients with nonbacterial infections (ie, most upper respiratory tract infections).

---

**Indications**

*Anaerobes:* Serious respiratory tract infections such as empyema, anaerobic pneumonitis, and lung abscess; serious skin and soft tissue infections; septicemia, intra-abdominal infections such as peritonitis and intra-abdominal abscess (typically resulting from anaerobic organisms resident in the normal GI tract); infections of the female pelvis and genital tract such as endometritis, nongonococcal tubo-ovarian abscess, pelvic cellulitis, and postsurgical vaginal cuff infection.

*Streptococci and staphylococci:* Serious respiratory tract infections; serious skin and soft tissue infections; septicemia (parenteral only); acute staphylococcal hematogenous osteomyelitis (parenteral only).

*Pneumococci:* Serious respiratory tract infections.

**Administration and Dosage**

CLINDAMYCIN:

*Oral* – Take with a full glass of water or with food to avoid esophageal irritation. Clindamycin absorption is not affected by food.

   *Adults:*
      *Serious infections* – 150 to 300 mg every 6 hours.
      *More severe infections* – 300 to 450 mg every 6 hours.
   *Children:*
      Clindamycin HCl –
         *Serious infections:* 8 to 16 mg/kg/day divided into 3 or 4 equal doses.
         *More severe infections:* 16 to 20 mg/kg/day divided into 3 or 4 equal doses.
      Clindamycin palmitate HCl –
         *Serious infections:* 8 to 12 mg/kg/day divided into 3 or 4 equal doses.
         *Severe infections:* 13 to 25 mg/kg/day divided into 3 or 4 equal doses. In children weighing no more than 10 kg, administer 37.5 mg 3 times daily as the minimum dose.
   *Parenteral* –
      *Adults:*
         *Serious infections* – Serious infections due to aerobic gram-positive cocci and the more sensitive anaerobes: 600 to 1200 mg/day in 2 to 4 equal doses.
         *More severe infections* – More severe infections, particularly those caused by *Bacteroides fragilis*, *Peptococcus* sp. or *Clostridium* sp. other than *C. perfringens*: 1.2 to 2.7 g/day in 2 to 4 equal doses.
            *In life-threatening situations* – In life-threatening situations caused by aerobes or anaerobes, doses of 4.8 g/day have been given IV to adults. Single IM injections greater than 600 mg are not recommended.

*Children (older than 1 month of age):* 20 to 40 mg/kg/day in 3 or 4 equal doses, depending on the severity of infection.

Alternatively, children may be dosed based on body surface area:

*Serious infections* – 350 mg/m²/day; *more serious infections* – 450 mg/m²/day.

*Neonates (younger than 1 month of age):* 15 to 20 mg/kg/day in 3 to 4 equal doses.

*CDC recommendation for acute pelvic inflammatory disease* – 900 mg IV every 8 hours plus gentamicin loading dose 2 mg/kg IV or IM, followed by 1.5 mg/kg every 8 hours.

After discharge from hospital, continue with oral doxycycline 100 mg 2 times/day for 10 to 14 days total. Alternatively, continue with oral clindamycin 450 mg 4 times daily for 10 to 14 days.

LINCOMYCIN:

*Oral* – Take at least 1 to 2 hours before or after eating to ensure optimum absorption.

*Adults:*

*Serious infections* – 500 mg every 8 hours.

*More severe infections* – At least 500 mg every 6 hours.

*Children older than 1 month of age:*

*Serious infections* – 30 mg/kg/day (15 mg/lb/day) divided into 3 or 4 equal doses.

*More severe infections* – 60 mg/kg/day (30 mg/lb/day) divided into 3 or 4 equal

doses.

*IM* –

*Adults:*

*Serious infections* – 600 mg every 24 hours.

*More severe infections* – 600 mg every 12 hours or more often.

*Children older than 1 month of age:*

*Serious infections* – 10 mg/kg (5 mg/lb) every 24 hours.

*More severe infections* – 10 mg/kg (5 mg/lb) every 12 hours or more often.

*IV* – Dilute to 1 g/100 mL (minimum) and infuse over 1 hour/1 g dose. Severe cardiopulmonary reactions have occurred when given at greater than the recommended concentration and rate.

*Adults:*

*Serious infections* – 600 mg to 1 g every 8 to 12 hours.

*Severe to life-threatening situations* – Doses of 8 g/day have been given.

*Maximum recommended dose* – 8 g/day.

*Children older than 1 month of age:* Infuse 10 to 20 mg/kg/day (5 to 10 mg/lb/day), depending on severity of infection, in divided doses as described above for adults.

*Subconjunctival injection* – 75 mg/0.25 mL injected subconjunctivally results in ocular fluid levels of antibiotic (lasting for 5 hours or more) with MICs sufficient for most susceptible pathogens.

*Renal function impairment* – When required, an appropriate dose is 25% to 30% of that recommended for patients with normal renal function.

## Actions

*Pharmacology:* **Lincomycin** and **clindamycin**, known collectively as lincosamides, bind exclusively to the 50 S subunit of bacterial ribosomes and suppress protein synthesis. Cross-resistance has been demonstrated between these 2 agents. Clindamycin is preferred because it is better absorbed and more potent.

*Pharmacokinetics:* Administration with food markedly impairs **lincomycin** (but not **clindamycin**) oral absorption.

*Dialysis –*

| Select Pharmacokinetic Parameters of Lincosamides | | | | | | | | |
|---|---|---|---|---|---|---|---|---|
| | | | | | | Elimination (%) | | |
| Lincosamides | Bioavailability (%) | Mean peak serum level (mcg/mL) | Time to peak serum level (h) | Protein binding (%) | Half-life (h) | Hepatic | Unchanged in urine (range) | Feces |
| *Clindamycin[1]* | | | | | | | | |
| Oral | 90 | 2.5 | 0.75 | ≈ 90 | 2.4 to 3[3] | > 90 | 10 | 3.6 |
| IM | | 6 to 9 | 1 to 3 | | | | | |
| IV | | 7 to 14 | 0[2] | | | | | |
| *Lincomycin* | | | | | | | | |
| Oral | 20 to 30 | 1.8 to 5.3 | 2 to 4 | 57 to 72 | 4.4 to 6.4 | > 90 | 4 (1 to 31) | 40 |
| IM | | 9.3 to 18.5 | 0.5 | | | | 17.3 (2 to 25) | |
| IV | | 15.9 to 20.9 | 0 | | | | 13.8 (5 to 30) | |

[1] Clindamycin palmitate and phosphate are rapidly hydrolyzed to the base.
[2] By end of infusion, peak levels are reached.
[3] Increased slightly in patients with markedly reduced renal or hepatic function.

*Microbiology:*

| Organisms Generally Susceptible to Lincosamides | | | |
|---|---|---|---|
| ✔ = generally susceptible | | Lincosamides | |
| | Microorganism | Lincomycin | Clindamycin |
| Gram-positive | *Staphylococcus aureus* | ✔ | ✔ |
| | *Staphylococcus epidermidis[1]* | ✔ | ✔ |
| | *Staphylococcus albus* | ✔ | |
| | *Streptococcus pneumoniae* | ✔ | ✔ |
| | *Streptococcus pyogenes* | ✔ | ✔ |
| | *β-hemolytic streptococci* | ✔ | |
| | *Streptococcus viridans* | ✔ | ✔ |
| | *Pneumococci* | | ✔ |
| | *Corynebacterium diphtheriae* | ✔ | ✔ |
| | *Diplococcus pneumoniae* | ✔ | |
| | *Corynebacterium acnes* | ✔ | |
| | *Nocardia asteroides* | ✔ | ✔ |
| Anaerobes | *Bacteroides* sp. | ✔ | ✔[2] |
| | *Fusobacterium* sp. | | ✔ |
| | *Propionibacterium* (same as *C. acnes*) | ✔ | ✔ |
| | *Eubacterium* sp. | ✔ | ✔ |
| | *Actinomyces* sp. | ✔ | ✔ |
| | *Peptococcus* sp. | ✔ | ✔ |
| | *Peptostreptococcus* | ✔ | ✔ |
| | *Microaerophilic streptococci* | | ✔ |
| | *Clostridium perfringens* | ✔ | ✔ |
| | *Clostridium tetani* | ✔ | ✔ |
| | *Veillonella* sp. | | ✔ |

[1] Penicillinase and nonpenicillinase.
[2] Including *B. fragilis* and *B. melaninogenicus*.

### Contraindications
Hypersensitivity to lincosamides; treatment of minor bacterial or viral infections.

### Warnings
*Meningitis:* **Clindamycin** does not diffuse adequately into CSF; do not use for meningitis.

*Diarrhea:* If significant diarrhea occurs during therapy with **lincomycin** or **clindamycin**, discontinue therapy.

*Hypersensitivity reactions:* Use with caution in patients with a history of asthma or significant allergies. Refer to Management of Acute Hypersensitivity Reactions.

*Renal function impairment:* Cautiously give **clindamycin** to patients with severe renal or hepatic disease accompanied by severe metabolic aberrations. Use of **lincomycin** in pre-existing liver disease is not recommended unless special clinical circumstances so indicate.

*Elderly:* Older patients with associated severe illness may not tolerate diarrhea well.

*Pregnancy:* Category B **(clindamycin)**.

*Lactation:* **Clindamycin** and **lincomycin** appear in breast milk. The American Academy of Pediatrics considers clindamycin to be compatible with breastfeeding.

*Children:* **Lincomycin** is not indicated for use in the newborn. When **clindamycin** is administered to newborns and infants, monitor organ system functions.

### Precautions
*Monitoring:* In prolonged therapy, perform liver/kidney function tests and blood counts.

### Drug Interactions
Drugs that may interact with lincosamides include erythromycin, kaolin-pectin, and neuromuscular blockers (nondepolarizing).

*Drug/Food interactions:* Food impairs the absorption of **lincomycin**; do not take anything by mouth (except water) for 1 to 2 hours before and after lincomycin. **Clindamycin** absorption is not affected by food.

### Adverse Reactions
Nausea; vomiting; diarrhea (**clindamycin** 3.4% to 30%); pseudomembranous colitis (clindamycin 0.01% to 10%; 3 to 4 times more frequent with oral administration); neutropenia (sometimes transient); leukopenia; agranulocytosis; thrombocytopenic purpura; skin rashes, urticaria, erythema multiforme; anaphylaxis; jaundice; liver function test abnormalities (serum transaminase elevations).

# AMINOGLYCOSIDES, PARENTERAL

| | |
|---|---|
| **AMIKACIN SULFATE** | |
| **Injection:** 250 mg/mL *(Rx)* | Various, *Amikin* (Apothecon) |
| **Pediatric injection:** 50 mg/mL *(Rx)* | Various, *Amikin* (Apothecon) |
| **GENTAMICIN** | |
| **Injection:** 2, 10, and 40 mg/mL *(Rx)* | Various, *Garamycin* (Schering) |
| **KANAMYCIN SULFATE** | |
| **Injection:** 500 mg and 1 g *(Rx)* | Various, *Kantrex* (Apothecon) |
| **Pediatric injection:** 75 mg *(Rx)* | Various, *Kantrex* (Apothecon) |
| **STREPTOMYCIN SULFATE** | |
| **Injection:** 400 mg/mL *(Rx)* | *Streptomycin Sulfate* (Pfizer) |
| **TOBRAMYCIN SULFATE** | |
| **Injection:** 10 and 40 mg/mL *(Rx)* | Various |
| **Pediatric injection:** 10 mg/mL *(Rx)* | Various |
| **Powder for injection:** 1.2 g (after reconstitution) *(Rx)* | Various |
| **Nebulizer solution:** 300 mg/5 mL *(Rx)* | *TOBI* (PathoGenesis) |

## Indications

Reserve these drugs for treatment of infections caused by organisms not sensitive to less toxic agents. Safety for treatment periods longer than 14 days has not been established.

For approved indications, refer to the Administration and Dosage section.

*Unlabeled uses:*

*Gentamicin* – An alternative regimen for pelvic inflammatory disease is gentamicin plus clindamycin. Continue for at least 4 days and at least 48 hours after patient improves; then continue clindamycin 450 mg orally 4 times daily for 10 to 14 days total therapy.

*Amikacin sulfate* – Intrathecal/intraventricular administration has been suggested at 8 mg/24 hours.

## Administration and Dosage

*Synergism:* In vitro studies indicate that aminoglycosides combined with penicillins or cephalosporins act synergistically against some strains of gram-negative organisms and enterococci (*Streptococcus faecalis*). Aminoglycosides may exhibit a synergistic effect when combined with carbenicillin or ticarcillin for *Pseudomonas* infections.

AMIKACIN SULFATE:

*Adults and children* – Use the patient's ideal body weight for dosage calculation. Administer IM or IV. Administer 15 mg/kg/day divided into 2 or 3 equal doses at equally divided intervals. Treatment of heavier patients should not exceed 1.5 g/day. In uncomplicated UTIs, use 250 mg twice daily.

*Neonates:* A loading dose of 10 mg/kg is recommended, followed by 7.5 mg/kg every 12 hours. Lower dosages may be safer during the first 2 weeks of life.

*Renal function impairment* – Adjust doses in patients with impaired renal function by administering normal doses at prolonged intervals or by administering reduced doses at a fixed interval.

*Normal dosage at prolonged intervals:* If the Ccr is not available and the patient's condition is stable, calculate a dosage interval (in hours) for the normal dose by multiplying the patient's serum creatinine by 9.

*Reduced dosage at fixed time intervals:* Measure serum concentration to ensure accurate administration and to avoid concentrations greater than 35 mcg/mL. Initiate therapy by administering a normal dose, 7.5 mg/kg, as a loading dose.

To determine maintenance doses administered every 12 hours, reduce the loading dose in proportion to the reduction in the patient's Ccr:

$$\frac{\text{Maintenance dose}}{\text{every 12 hours}} = \frac{\text{observed Ccr (mL/min)}}{\text{normal Ccr (mL/min)}} \times \frac{\text{calculated loading}}{\text{dose (mg)}}$$

*Dialysis:* Approximately half the normal mg/kg dose can be given after hemodialysis; in peritoneal dialysis, a parenteral dose of 7.5 mg/kg is given, and then amikacin is instilled in peritoneal dialysate at a concentration desired in serum.

GENTAMICIN:

*Dosage* – May be given IM or IV. For patients with serious infections and normal renal function, give 3 mg/kg/day in 3 equal doses every 8 hours. For patients with life-threatening infections, administer up to 5 mg/kg/day in 3 or 4 equal doses. Reduce dosage to 3 mg/kg/day as soon as clinically indicated.

*Obese patients:* Base dosage on an estimate of lean body mass.

*Children:* 6 to 7.5 mg/kg/day (2 to 2.5 mg/kg every 8 hours).

*Infants and neonates:* 7.5 mg/kg/day (2.5 mg/kg every 8 hours).

*Premature or full term neonates (1 week of age or younger):* 5 mg/kg/day (2.5 mg every 12 hours). A regimen of either 2.5 mg/kg every 18 hours or 3 mg/kg every 24 hours may also provide satisfactory peak and trough levels in preterm infants younger than 32 weeks gestational age.

*Prevention of bacterial endocarditis* –

*In dental, oral, or upper respiratory tract procedures (alternate regimen):* 1 to 2 g (50 mg/kg for children) ampicillin plus 1.5 mg/kg (2 mg/kg for children) gentamicin not to exceed 80 mg, both IM or IV ½ hour prior to procedure, followed by 1.5 g (25 mg/kg for children) amoxicillin 6 hours after initial dose or repeat parenteral dose 8 hours after initial dose.

*GU or GI procedures (standard regimen):* 2 g (50 mg/kg for children) ampicillin plus 1.5 mg/kg (2 mg/kg for children) gentamicin not to exceed 80 mg, both IM or IV ½ hour prior to procedure followed by 1.5 mg (25 mg/kg for children) amoxicillin.

*Renal function impairment* –

*Rule of eights:* Approximate the interval between doses (in hours) by multiplying the serum creatinine level (mg/dL) by 8. For example, a patient weighing 60 kg with a serum creatinine level of 2 mg/dL could be given 60 mg (1 mg/kg) every 16 hours (2 × 8).

*IV* – A 1 to 2 mg/kg loading dose may be used, followed by a maintenance dose.

*Intrathecal* – In general, the recommended dose for infants and children 3 months of age and older is 1 to 2 mg once a day. For adults, administer 4 to 8 mg once a day.

KANAMYCIN SULFATE: Do not exceed total 1.5 g/day by any route.

*IM* – For adults or children, 7.5 mg/kg every 12 hours (15 mg/kg/day). If continuously high blood levels are desired, give daily dose of 15 mg/kg in equally divided doses every 6 or 8 hours. Usual treatment duration is 7 to 10 days. Doses of 7.5 mg/kg give mean peak levels of 22 mcg/mL. At 8 hours after a 7.5 mg/kg dose, mean serum levels are 3.2 mcg/mL.

*IV* –

*Adults:* Do not exceed 15 mg/kg/day. Give slowly over 30 to 60 minutes. Divide daily doses into 2 to 3 equal doses.

*Children:* Use sufficient diluent to infuse drug over 30 to 60 minutes.

*Renal failure* – Calculate the dosage interval with the following formula: Serum creatinine (mg/dL) × 9 equals dosage interval (in hours).

*Intraperitoneal (following exploration for peritonitis or after peritoneal contamination caused by fecal spill during surgery)* – 500 mg in 20 mL sterile distilled water instilled through a polyethylene catheter into wound.

*Aerosol treatment* – 250 mg 2 to 4 times/day.

*Other routes* – Concentrations of 0.25% have been used as irrigating solutions in abscess cavities, pleural space, peritoneal and ventricular cavities.

STREPTOMYCIN SULFATE: Administer IM only.

*Tuberculosis (TB)* – The standard regimen for the treatment of drug-susceptible TB has been 2 months of INH, rifampin, and pyrazinamide followed by 4 months of

INH and rifampin. When streptomycin is added to this regimen because of suspected or proven drug resistance, the recommended dosing for streptomycin is as follows:

| Streptomycin Dosing for TB | | | |
| --- | --- | --- | --- |
| | Daily | Twice weekly | Three times weekly |
| Children | 20 to 40 mg/kg max 1 g | 25 to 30 mg/kg max 1.5 g | 25 to 30 mg/kg max 1.5 g |
| Adults | 15 mg/kg max 1 g | 25 to 30 mg/kg max 1.5 g | 25 to 30 mg/kg max 1.5 g |

Streptomycin usually is administered daily as a single IM injection. Give a total dose of less than 120 g over the course of therapy unless there are no other therapeutic options. In patients older than 60 years of age, use a reduced dosage. The total period of drug treatment for TB is a minimum of 1 year.

*Tularemia* – 1 to 2 g/day in divided doses for 7 to 14 days, or until afebrile 5 to 7 days.

*Plague* – 2 g daily in 2 divided doses for a minimum of 10 days.

*Bacterial endocarditis* –

*Streptococcal:* In penicillin-sensitive alpha and nonhemolytic streptococci, use streptomycin for 2 weeks with penicillin: 1 g twice daily for 1 week, 0.5 g twice daily for the second week. If patient is older than 60 years of age, give 0.5 g twice daily for the entire 2-week period.

*Enterococcal:* 1 g twice daily for 2 weeks and 0.5 g twice daily for 4 weeks in combination with penicillin.

*Adults* – 1 to 2 g in divided doses every 6 to 12 hours for moderate-to-severe infections. Doses should generally not exceed 2 g/day.

*Children* – 20 to 40 mg/kg/day in divided doses every 6 to 12 hours.

TOBRAMYCIN SULFATE:

*Dosage* – Use the patient's ideal body weight for dosage calculation. Peak and trough serum concentrations should be measured. Avoid prolonged peak concentrations greater than 12 mcg/mL or troughs greater than 2 mcg/mL.

*Adults with serious infections* – Administer 3 mg/kg/day in 3 equal doses every 8 hours.

*Life-threatening infections:* Administer up to 5 mg/kg/day in 3 or 4 equal doses. Reduce dosage to 3 mg/kg/day as soon as clinically indicated.

*Children* – Administer 6 to 7.5 mg/kg/day in 3 or 4 equally divided doses (2 to 2.5 mg/kg every 8 hours or 1.5 to 1.9 mg/kg every 6 hours).

*Premature or full-term infants (1 year of age or younger)* – Administer up to 4 mg/kg/day in 2 equal doses every 12 hours. Preliminary data suggest that 2.5 mg/kg every 18 hours or 3 mg/kg every 24 hours may achieve safe and effective peak and trough serum concentrations in newborn infants weighing less than 1 kg at birth.

*Renal function impairment* – Following a loading dose of 1 mg/kg, adjust subsequent dosage, either with reduced doses administered at 8-hour intervals or with normal doses given at prolonged levels.

An alternative guide for determining reduced dosage at 8-hour intervals (for patients whose steady-state serum creatinine values are known) is to divide the normally recommended dose by the patient's serum creatinine.

*Hemodialysis* – Hemodialysis removes approximately 50% of a dose in 6 hours. In patients maintained by regular dialysis, the usual dose of 1.5 to 2 mg/kg given after every dialysis usually maintains therapeutic, nontoxic serum levels. In patients receiving intermittent peritoneal dialysis, patients dialyzed twice weekly should receive a 1.5 to 2 mg/kg loading dose followed by 1 mg/kg every 3 days. Where dialysis occurs every 2 days, a 1.5 mg/kg loading dose is given after the first dialysis and 0.75 mg/kg after each subsequent dialysis.

*IV administration* – The IV dose is the same as the IM dose. Infuse the diluted solution over a period of 20 to 60 minutes. Infusion periods of less than 20 minutes are not recommended because peak serum levels may exceed 20 mcg/mL.

*Cystic fibrosis (nebulizer solution)* – Recommended dosage for adults and children 6 years of age and older is 300 mg twice a day in repeating cycles of 28 days on drug/28 days off drug. Do not adjust dosage by age or weight. Take as close to 12 hours apart as possible; do not take less than 6 hours apart. Administer by inhalation over a 10- to 15-minute period, using a hand-held *PARI LC PLUS* reusable nebulizer with a *DeVilbiss Pulmo-Aide* compressor. Do not dilute or mix with dornase alfa in the nebulizer. Instruct patients on multiple therapies to take them first, followed by tobramycin. Bronchospasm, which can occur with inhalation of tobramycin, may be reduced if inhalation of tobramycin nebulization solution follows bronchodilator therapy.

*Monitoring:* In patients with normal renal function, serum tobramycin concentrations are approximately 1 mcg/mL 1 hour after dose administration. Monitoring of serum concentrations in patients with renal dysfunction or patients treated with concomitant parenteral tobramycin may reduce the risk of toxicity.

**Actions**

*Pharmacology:* The aminoglycosides are bactericidal antibiotics used primarily in the treatment of gram-negative infections.

*Pharmacokinetics:*

*Absorption/Distribution* – Absorption from IM injection is rapid, with peak blood levels achieved within 1 hour.

Excretion is by glomerular filtration, largely as unchanged drug; thus, high urine levels are attained. Aminoglycosides are removed by hemodialysis (4 to 6 hours removes approximately 50%) and peritoneal dialysis (range, removal of 23% in 8 hours to only 4% in 22 hours).

*Serum levels* – Because of the narrow range between therapeutic and toxic serum levels, careful attention to dosage calculations is essential, especially in patients with renal impairment, geriatric and female patients, those requiring high peak serum levels, patients on prolonged therapy (longer than 10 days), patients with unstable renal function or those undergoing dialysis, those with abnormal extracellular fluid volume, or with prior exposure to ototoxic or nephrotoxic drugs. Age markedly affects peak concentration in children; it is generally lower in young children and infants. Monitor drug serum levels. Peak levels indicate therapeutic levels. Trough serum level determinations (just before next dose) best indicate drug accumulation. Obtain serum levels within 48 hours of start of therapy and every 3 to 4 days assuming stable renal function; also, levels are indicated when dose is changed or in changing renal function. Generally, to measure peak levels, draw a serum sample about 30 minutes after IV infusion or 1 hour after an IM dose. For trough levels, obtain serum samples at 8 hours or just prior to the next dose.

| Various Pharmacokinetic Parameters of the Aminoglycosides | | | | | | |
|---|---|---|---|---|---|---|
| | Half-life (h) | | Therapeutic serum levels (peak) (mcg/mL) | Toxic serum levels (mcg/mL) | | Dose (mg/kg/day) (normal Ccr) |
| Aminoglycoside | Normal | ESRD | | Peak[1] | Trough[2] | |
| Amikacin | 2 to 3 | 24 to 60 | 16 to 32 | > 35 | > 10 | 15 |
| Gentamicin | 2 | 24 to 60 | 4 to 8 | > 12 | > 2 | 3 to 5 |
| Kanamycin | 2 to 3 | 24 to 60 | 15 to 40 | > 35 | > 10 | 15 |
| Streptomycin | 2.5 | 100 | 20 to 30 | > 50 | — | 15 |
| Tobramycin | 2 to 2.5 | 24 to 60 | 4 to 8 | > 12 | > 2 | 3 to 5 |

[1] Measured 1 hour after IM administration.
[2] Measured immediately prior to next dose.

*Microbiology:*

| | Organisms | Amikacin | Gentamicin | Kanamycin | Streptomycin | Tobramycin |
|---|---|---|---|---|---|---|
| **Organisms Generally Susceptible to Aminoglycosides** | | | | | | |
| Gram-positive | Mycobacterium tuberculosis | ✔[1] | | | ✔[2] | |
| | Staphylococci | ✔[3] | ✔[3] | | | ✔ |
| | Staphylococcus aureus | ✔ | ✔ | ✔[3] | | ✔ |
| | Staphylococcus epidermidis | ✔ | | ✔ | | |
| | Streptococci | | | | ✔[2] | |
| | Streptococcus faecalis | | ✔[2] | | ✔[2] | ✔[2] |
| Gram-negative | Acinetobacter sp. | ✔ | | ✔ | | |
| | Brucella sp. | | | | ✔ | |
| | Citrobacter sp. | ✔ | ✔ | ✔ | ✔ | ✔ |
| | Enterobacter sp. | ✔ | ✔ | ✔ | ✔ | ✔ |
| | Escherichia coli | ✔ | ✔ | ✔ | ✔ | ✔ |
| | Haemophilus influenzae | ✔ | | ✔ | ✔[2] | |
| | Haemophilus ducreyi | | | | ✔ | |
| | Klebsiella sp. | ✔ | ✔ | ✔ | ✔[2] | ✔ |
| | Morganella morganii | | | | | ✔ |
| | Neisseria sp. | ✔ | | ✔ | ✔ | |
| | Proteus sp. | ✔[4] | ✔[4] | ✔[4] | ✔ | ✔[4] |
| | Providencia sp. | ✔ | ✔ | ✔ | ✔ | ✔ |
| | Pseudomonas sp. | ✔ | | | | |
| | P. aeruginosa | ✔ | ✔[2] | | ✔ | ✔ |
| | Salmonella sp. | ✔ | ✔ | ✔ | ✔ | ✔ |
| | Serratia sp. | ✔ | ✔ | ✔ | ✔ | ✔ |
| | Shigella sp. | ✔ | ✔ | ✔ | ✔ | ✔ |
| | Yersinia (Pasteurella) pestis | ✔ | ✔ | ✔ | ✔ | ✔ |

[1] ✔ = generally susceptible
[2] Usually used concomitantly with other anti-infectives.
[3] Penicillinase-producing and nonpenicillinase-producing.
[4] Indole-positive and indole-negative.

### Contraindications

Previous reactions to these agents. With the exception of the use of streptomycin in tuberculosis, these agents generally are not indicated in long-term therapy because of the ototoxic and nephrotoxic hazards of extended administration.

### Warnings

*Toxicity:* Aminoglycosides are associated with significant nephrotoxicity or ototoxicity. These agents are excreted primarily by glomerular filtration; thus, the serum half-life will be prolonged and significant accumulation will occur in patients with impaired renal function. Toxicity may develop even with conventional doses, particularly in prerenal azotemia or impaired renal function.

*Ototoxicity* – Neurotoxicity, manifested as auditory (cochlear) and vestibular ototoxicity, can occur with any of these agents. Auditory changes are irreversible, usually bilateral, and may be partial or total. Risk of hearing loss increases with degree of exposure to either high peak or high trough serum concentrations and continues to progress after drug withdrawal. Risk is greater with renal impairment and with pre-existing hearing loss. High frequency deafness usually occurs first and can be detected by audiometric testing. Relative ototoxicity is: **Streptomycin = Kanamycin > Amikacin = Gentamicin = Tobramycin.**

*Renal toxicity* – Renal toxicity may be characterized by decreased creatinine clearance, cells or casts in the urine, decreased urine specific gravity, oliguria, proteinuria, or evidence of nitrogen retention. Renal damage is usually reversible. The relative nephrotoxicity of these agents is estimated to be: **Kanamycin = Amikacin = Gentamicin = Tobramycin > Streptomycin**.

*Monitoring* – Closely observe all patients treated with aminoglycosides. Monitoring renal and eighth cranial nerve function at onset of therapy is essential for patients with known or suspected renal impairment and also in those whose renal function is initially normal but who develop signs of renal dysfunction.

*Burn patients:* In patients with extensive burns, altered pharmacokinetics may result in reduced serum concentrations of aminoglycosides.

*Hypomagnesemia:* Hypomagnesemia may occur in more than⅓ of patients whose oral diet is restricted or who are eating poorly.

*Neuromuscular blockade:* Neurotoxicity can occur. Aminoglycosides may aggravate muscle weakness because of a potential curare-like effect on the neuromuscular junction.

Neuromuscular blockade resulting in respiratory paralysis has occurred with these agents, especially if given with or soon after anesthesia or muscle relaxants.

*Nephrotoxicity:* Nephrotoxicity may occur. Risk factors include the elderly, patients with a history of renal impairment who are treated for longer periods or with higher doses than those recommended, a recent course of aminoglycosides (within 6 weeks), concurrent use of other nephrotoxic agents, frequent dosing, potassium depletion, and decreased intravascular volume. Adverse renal effects can occur in patients with initially normal renal function. Of patients receiving an aminoglycoside for several days or more, approximately 8% to 26% will develop mild renal impairment that is generally reversible.

*Hydration* – These drugs reach high concentrations in the renal system; keep patients well hydrated to minimize chemical irritation of tubules.

*Dosing interval:* Preliminary evidence indicates that aminoglycosides may be administered on a once-daily basis without compromising efficacy and without increasing the potential for nephrotoxicity and ototoxicity. It is possible that the incidence of nephrotoxicity may even be decreased.

*Elderly:* Elderly patients may have reduced renal function that is not evident in the results of routine screening tests, such as BUN or serum creatinine. A Ccr determination may be more useful.

*Pregnancy: Category* D (amikacin, gentamicin, kanamycin, tobramycin).

*Lactation:* Small amounts of **streptomycin** and **kanamycin**are excreted in breast milk.

*Children:* Use with caution in premature infants and neonates because of their renal immaturity and the resulting prolongation of serum half-life of these drugs.

**Precautions**

*Intrathecal gentamicin:* Use of excessive (40 to 160 mg) doses of intrathecal **gentamicin** has produced neuromuscular disturbances (eg, ataxia, paresis, incontinence).

*Cross-allergenicity:* Cross-allergenicity among the aminoglycosides has been demonstrated.

*Monitoring:* Monitor peak and trough serum concentrations periodically to ensure adequate levels and to avoid potentially toxic levels. Also monitor serum calcium, magnesium and sodium (see Adverse Reactions).

*Eighth cranial nerve function testing* – Serial audiometric tests are suggested, particularly when renal function is impaired or prolonged aminoglycoside therapy is required; also repeat such tests periodically after treatment if there is evidence of a hearing deficit or vestibular abnormality before or during therapy, or when consecutive or concomitant use of other potentially ototoxic drugs is unavoidable.

*Syphilis:* In the treatment of sexually transmitted disease, if concomitant syphilis is suspected, perform a darkfield examination before treatment is started. Perform monthly serologic tests for 4 months or more.

*Topical use:* Aminoglycosides are quickly and almost totally absorbed when applied topically in association with surgical procedures, except to the urinary bladder.

### Drug Interactions

Drugs that may affect aminoglycosides include cephalosporins, enflurane, methoxyflurane, vancomycin, indomethacin IV, loop diuretics, and penicillins.

Drugs that may be affected by aminoglycosides include depolarizing and nondepolarizing neuromuscular blockers and polypeptide antibiotics.

### Adverse Reactions

| Aminoglycoside Adverse Reactions (%) | | | | | | |
|---|---|---|---|---|---|---|
| | Adverse Reaction | Amikacin | Gentamicin | Kanamycin | Streptomycin | Tobramycin |
| Central/Peripheral nervous system | Headache | rare | ✓[1] | rare | | ✓ |
| | Confusion | | ✓ | | | ✓ |
| | Fever | | ✓ | | ✓ | ✓ |
| | Lethargy | | ✓ | | | ✓ |
| | Disorientation | | | | | ✓ |
| | Neuromuscular blockade[2] | ✓ | | ✓ | ✓ | |
| | Paresthesia | rare | | rare | | |
| GI | Vomiting | rare | ✓ | rare | ✓ | ✓ |
| | Nausea | rare | ✓ | rare | ✓ | ✓ |
| | Diarrhea | | | rare | | ✓ |
| Hematologic | Anemia | rare | ✓ | | | ✓ |
| | Eosinophilia | rare | ✓ | | ✓ | ✓ |
| | Leukopenia | | ✓ | | ✓ | ✓ |
| | Thrombocytopenia | | ✓ | | ✓ | ✓ |
| Hypersensitivity | Rash | rare | ✓ | rare | ✓ | ✓ |
| | Urticaria | | ✓ | | ✓ | ✓ |
| | Itching | | ✓ | | | ✓ |
| Special senses | Dizziness | | ✓ | | | ✓ |
| | Tinnitus | | ✓ | | | ✓ |
| | Vertigo | | ✓ | | ✓ | ✓ |
| | Hearing loss/deafness | ✓ | ✓ | ✓[3] | ✓ | ✓ |
| Renal[1] | Oliguria | ✓ | ✓ | ✓ | | ✓ |
| | Proteinuria | ✓ | ✓ | ✓ | | ✓ |
| | Rising serum creatinine[2] | ✓ | ✓ | ✓ | | |
| | Casts | ✓ | ✓ | | | |
| | Rising BUN[2] | | ✓ | | ✓ | ✓ |
| | Red and white cells in urine | ✓ | | ✓ | | |
| | Azotemia | ✓ | | | ✓ | |
| Lab test abnormalities | Increased AST/ALT | | ✓ | | | ✓ |
| | Increased bilirubin | | ✓ | | | ✓ |
| Other | Apnea | ✓ | ✓ | ✓ | ✓ | ✓ |
| | Pain/Irritation at injection site | | ✓ | ✓ | | ✓ |
| | Hypotension | rare | ✓ | | | |

[1] ✓ = Reported; no incidence given
[2] See Warnings
[3] Partially reversible to irreversible bilateral hearing loss.

# AMINOGLYCOSIDES, ORAL

| | |
|---|---|
| **KANAMYCIN SULFATE** | |
| **Capsules**: 500 mg (*Rx*) | *Kantrex* (Apothecon) |
| **NEOMYCIN SULFATE** | |
| **Tablets**: 500 mg (*Rx*) | Various, *Neo-Tabs* (Pharma-Tek) |
| **Oral solution**: 125 mg/5 mL (*Rx*) | *Mycifradin* (Pharmacia), *Neo-Fradin* (Pharma-Tek) |
| **PAROMOMYCIN SULFATE** | |
| **Capsules**: 250 mg (*Rx*) | *Humatin* (Parke-Davis) |

For complete information on the aminoglycosides, refer to the Aminoglycosides, Parenteral monograph.

### Indications

Suppression of intestinal bacteria.

Hepatic coma.

*Neomycin sulfate:* Many studies have documented lipid-lowering efficacy of neomycin. Alone, it reduced LDL cholesterol levels by 24%. Combined with niacin, it reduced LDL cholesterol levels to below the 90th percentile in 92% of patients.

### Administration and Dosage

KANAMYCIN SULFATE:

> *Suppression of intestinal bacteria* – As an adjunct to mechanical cleansing of the large bowel in short-term therapy — 1 g for every hour for 4 hours, followed by 1 g every 6 hours for 36 to 72 hours.
>
> *Hepatic coma* – 8 to 12 g/day in divided doses.

NEOMYCIN SULFATE:

> *Preoperative prophylaxis for elective colorectal surgery* –

| Recommended Bowel Preparation Regimen (Proposed Surgery Time 8 am)[1] | | | |
|---|---|---|---|
| Therapy | Day 3 before surgery | Day 2 before surgery | Day 1 before surgery |
| Diet | Minimum residue or clear liquid | Minimum residue or clear liquid | Clear liquid |
| Bisacodyl, 1 oral cap | 6 pm (-62 h) | | |
| Magnesium sulfate, 30 mL of a 50% solution orally | | 10 am (-46 h). Repeat at 2 pm (-42 h) and 6 pm (-38 h) | 10 am (-22 h). Repeat at 2 pm (-18 h). |
| Enema | | 7 pm (-37 h) & 8 pm (-36 h). Repeat hourly until no solid feces return with last enema | None |
| Supplemental IV fluids | | | As needed |
| Neomycin and erythromycin tablets, 1 g each, orally | | | 1 pm (-19 h). Repeat at 2 pm (-18 h) and 11 pm (-9 h) |

[1] On day of surgery, patient should evacuate rectum at 6:30 am (-1½ h) for 8 am procedure.

> *Hepatic coma (as adjunct)* –
> > *Adults:* 4 to 12 g/day in divided doses.
> > *Children:* 50 to 100 mg/kg/day in divided doses. Continue treatment over a period of 5 to 6 days; during this time, return protein to the diet incrementally. Chronic hepatic insufficiency may require up to 4 g/day over an indefinite period.

PAROMOMYCIN SULFATE:

> *Intestinal amebiasis* –
> > *Adults and children:* Usual dose is 25 to 35 mg/kg/day, in 3 doses with meals for 5 to 10 days.
> > *Management of hepatic coma* –
> > *Adults:* Usual dose: 4 g/day in divided doses at regular intervals for 5 to 6 days.
> Paromomycin sulfate has been recommended for other parasitic infections — *Dientamoeba fragilis* (25 to 30 mg/kg/day in 3 doses for 7 days); *Diphyllobothrium latum, Taenia saginata, Taenia solium, Dipylidium caninum* (adults: 1 g every 15 min-

utes for 4 doses; *pediatric:* 11 mg/kg every 15 minutes for 4 doses); *Hymenolepis nana* (45 mg/kg/day for 5 to 7 days).

### Actions
*Pharmacokinetics:* Oral aminoglycosides are poorly absorbed; therefore, use only for suppression of GI bacterial flora.

### Contraindications
Presence of intestinal obstruction; hypersensitivity to aminoglycosides.

### Warnings
*Increased absorption:* Although negligible amounts are absorbed through intact mucosa, consider the possibility of increased absorption from ulcerated or denuded areas.

*Nephrotoxicity/Ototoxicity:* Because of reported cases of deafness and potential nephrotoxic effects, closely observe patients. Refer to the Warning Box in the Aminoglycosides, Parenteral monograph concerning aminoglycoside toxicity.

*Pregnancy:*
  Neomycin – *Category D.*

*Lactation:* It is not known whether **neomycin** is excreted in breast milk. Other aminoglycosides are excreted in breast milk.

*Children:* The safety and efficacy of oral **neomycin** in patients younger than 18 years of age have not been established. If treatment is necessary, use with caution; do not exceed a treatment period of 3 weeks because of absorption from the GI tract.

### Precautions
*Muscular disorders:* Use with caution in patients with muscular disorders such as myasthenia gravis or parkinsonism.

*GI effects:*
  Neomycin – Orally administered neomycin increases fecal bile acid excretion and reduces intestinal lactase activity.
  Paromomycin – Use with caution in individuals with ulcerative lesions of the bowel to avoid renal toxicity through inadvertent absorption.

### Drug Interactions
Drugs that may be affected by aminoglycosides include anticoagulants, digoxin, methotrexate, neuromuscular blockers (depolarizing and nondepolarizing).

### Adverse Reactions
Nausea, vomiting, diarrhea (most common); "malabsorption syndrome" characterized by increased fecal fat, decreased serum carotene, and fall in xylose absorption. *Clostridium difficile*-associated colitis (following **neomycin** therapy); nephrotoxicity and ototoxicity (following prolonged and high-dosage therapy in hepatic coma).

# METRONIDAZOLE

| | |
|---|---|
| **Tablets**: 250 mg and 500 mg (*Rx*) | Various, *Flagyl* (Pharmacia) |
| **Tablets, extended-release**: 750 mg (*Rx*) | *Flagyl ER* (Pharmacia) |
| **Capsules**: 375 mg (*Rx*) | *Flagyl 375* (Pharmacia) |
| **Powder for injection, lyophilized**: 500 mg (as HCl) (*Rx*) | *Flagyl IV* (Pharmacia) |
| **Injection, ready-to-use**: 500 mg/100 mL (*Rx*) | Various, *Metronidazole* (B. Braun), *Flagyl IV RTU* (Pharmacia) |

Metronidazole also is available for topical and intravaginal use and also is used orally as an amebicide.

> **Warning:**
> Metronidazole is carcinogenic in rodents. Avoid unnecessary use.

## Indications

*Anaerobic infections:* Treatment of serious infections caused by susceptible anaerobic bacteria. Effective in *Bacteroides fragilis* infections resistant to clindamycin, chloramphenicol, and penicillin.

*Intra-abdominal infections* – Peritonitis, intra-abdominal abscess, and liver abscess caused by *Bacteroides* sp. (*B. fragilis*, *B. distasonis*, *B. ovatus*, *B. thetaiotaomicron*, *B. vulgatus*), *Clostridium* sp., *Eubacterium* sp., *Peptostreptococcus* sp., and *Peptococcus* sp.

*Skin and skin structure infections* – Caused by *Bacteroides* sp. including the *B. fragilis* group, *Clostridium* sp., *Peptococcus* sp., *Peptostreptococcus niger*, and *Fusobacterium* sp.

*Gynecologic infections* – Endometritis, endomyometritis, tubo-ovarian abscess, and postsurgical vaginal cuff infection caused by *Bacteroides* sp. including the *B. fragilis* group, *Clostridium* sp., *Peptococcus niger*, and *Peptostreptococcus* sp.; bacterial vaginosis (*Flagyl ER* only).

*Bacterial septicemia* – Caused by *Bacteroides* sp. including the *B. fragilis* group and *Clostridium* sp.

*Bone and joint infections* – Caused by *Bacteroides* sp. including the *B. fragilis* group, as adjunctive therapy.

*CNS infections* – Meningitis and brain abscess caused by *Bacteroides* sp. including the *B. fragilis* group.

*Lower respiratory tract infections* – Pneumonia, empyema, and lung abscess caused by *Bacteroides* sp. including the *B. fragilis* group.

*Endocarditis* – Caused by *Bacteroides* sp. including the *B. fragilis* group.

*Prophylaxis:* Preoperative, intraoperative, and postoperative IV metronidazole may reduce the incidence of postoperative infection in patients undergoing elective colorectal surgery which is classified as contaminated or potentially contaminated.

Discontinue within 12 hours after surgery. If there are signs of infection, obtain specimens for cultures to identify the causative organisms.

Metronidazole also is indicated for amebiasis and trichomoniasis, intravaginally for bacterial vaginosis, and topically for acne rosacea.

*Unlabeled uses:* The CDC has recommended the use of oral metronidazole for bacterial vaginosis (500 mg twice daily for 7 days). Single-dose therapy for bacterial vaginosis (2 g) also appears to be as effective as multiple-dose therapy.

## Administration and Dosage

*Anaerobic bacterial infections:* In the treatment of most serious anaerobic infections, metronidazole is usually administered IV initially.

IV –

*Loading dose:* 15 mg/kg infused over 1 hour (about 1 g for a 70 kg adult).

*Maintenance dose:* 7.5 mg/kg infused over 1 hour every 6 hours (about 500 mg for a 70 kg adult). Administer the first maintenance dose 6 hours following the initiation of loading dose. Do not exceed a maximum of 4 g in 24 hours.

Administer by slow IV drip infusion only, either as continuous or intermittent infusion. Do not use equipment containing aluminum (eg, needles, cannulae). If used with a primary IV fluid system, discontinue the primary solution during infusion. Do not give by direct IV bolus injection because of the low pH (0.5 to 2) of the reconstituted product. The drug must be further diluted and neutralized for infusion. Do not introduce additives into the solution.

*Oral:* Following IV therapy, use oral metronidazole when conditions warrant. The usual adult oral dosage is 7.5 mg/kg every 6 hours (about 500 mg for a 70 kg adult). Do not exceed a maximum of 4 g in 24 hours.

*Duration:* The usual duration of therapy is 7 to 10 days; however, infections of the bone and joints, lower respiratory tract, and endocardium may require longer treatment.

*Bacterial vaginosis:*
    *7-day course of treatment –* 750 mg ER once daily by mouth for 7 consecutive days.
    Take *Flagyl ER* tablets under fasting conditions, at least 1 hour before or 2 hours after meals.

*Prophylaxis:* To prevent postoperative infection in contaminated or potentially contaminated colorectal surgery, the recommended adult dosage is 15 mg/kg infused over 30 to 60 minutes and completed about 1 hour before surgery; followed by 7.5 mg/kg infused over 30 to 60 minutes at 6 and 12 hours after the initial dose.

Complete administration of the initial preoperative dose about 1 hour before surgery so that adequate drug levels are present in the serum and tissues at the time of initial incision, and administer, if necessary, at 6-hour intervals to maintain effective drug levels. Limit prophylactic use to the day of surgery only.

*Elderly:* Dosage adjustment may be necessary; monitor serum levels.

## Actions
*Pharmacology:* Metronidazole, a nitroimidazole, is active against various anaerobic bacteria and protozoa. It is believed to invoke cytotoxicity on the reduced nitro group in the bacterium cell. The liberated inactive end products are believed to target the RNA, DNA, or cellular proteins of the organisms.

*Pharmacokinetics:*
    *Absorption/Distribution –* Metronidazole is well absorbed after oral administration. Peak serum levels occur at about 1 to 2 hours. Metronidazole appears in CSF, saliva, and breast milk in concentrations similar to those found in plasma. Less than 20% of the circulating metronidazole is bound to plasma proteins.
    *Metabolism –* Unchanged metronidazole accounts for about 20% of the total.
    *Excretion –* The major route of elimination of metronidazole and its metabolites is via the urine (60% to 80% of the dose); fecal excretion accounts for 6% to 15% of the dose. Metronidazole has an average elimination half-life in healthy subjects of 8 hours. Metronidazole and its metabolites are removed by hemodialysis.

## Contraindications
Hypersensitivity to metronidazole or other nitroimidazole derivatives; pregnancy (first trimester in patients with trichomoniasis).

## Warnings
*Neurologic effects:* Seizures and peripheral neuropathy have occurred. Appearance of abnormal neurologic signs demands prompt discontinuation of therapy. Administer metronidazole with caution to patients with CNS diseases.

*Renal function impairment:* Do not specifically reduce the dose in anuric patients; accumulated metabolites may be rapidly removed by dialysis.

*Hepatic function impairment:* Patients with severe hepatic disease metabolize metronidazole slowly. Accumulation of the drug and its metabolites may occur.

*Carcinogenesis:* Metronidazole has shown evidence of carcinogenic activity with chronic oral administration in rodents.

*Elderly:* Because the pharmacokinetics of metronidazole may be altered in the elderly, monitoring of serum levels may be necessary to adjust the dosage accordingly.

*Pregnancy: Category B.* Do not administer to pregnant women during the first trimester. Restrict metronidazole for trichomoniasis in the second and third trimesters to those in whom local palliative treatment has been inadequate to control symptoms.

*Lactation:* Because of the potential for tumorigenicity, decide whether to discontinue nursing or to discontinue the drug, taking into account the importance of the drug to the mother. Metronidazole is secreted in breast milk in concentrations similar to those found in plasma.

*Children:* Safety and efficacy in children have not been established, except for the treatment of amebiasis. Newborns demonstrate a diminished capacity to eliminate metronidazole; half-life may be as high as 22 hours.

### Precautions

*Crohn's disease:* Crohn's disease patients are known to have an increased incidence of GI and certain extraintestinal cancers. There have been some reports in the medical literature of breast and colon cancer in Crohn's disease patients who have been treated with metronidazole at high doses for extended periods of time.

*Candidiasis:* Candidiasis may present more prominent symptoms during therapy and requires treatment with a candicidal agent.

*Hematologic effects:* Use with care in patients with evidence or history of blood dyscrasia. Mild leukopenia has been seen during administration. Perform total and differential leukocyte counts before and after therapy.

### Drug Interactions

Drugs that may affect metronidazole include barbiturates and cimetidine. Drugs that may be affected by metronidazole include anticoagulants, disulfiram, ethanol, hydantoins, and lithium.

*Drug/Lab test interactions:* The drug may interfere with chemical analyses for AST, ALT, LDH, triglycerides, and hexokinase glucose.

### Adverse Reactions

Adverse reactions may include dysuria; cystitis; polyuria; incontinence; proliferation of *Candida* in the vagina; dyspareunia; darkened urine; seizures and peripheral neuropathy; dizziness; vertigo; incoordination; ataxia; confusion; irritability; depression; weakness; insomnia; headache; syncope; nausea; diarrhea; epigastric distress; constipation; proctitis; glossitis; stomatitis; sharp, unpleasant metallic taste; urticaria; erythematous rash; flushing; nasal congestion; vaginitis; genital pruritus; abnormal urine; dysmenorrhea; upper respiratory tract infection; rhinitis; sinusitis; pharyngitis; bacterial infection; influenza-like symptoms; moniliasis; abnormal cramping; furry tongue; decreased libido; neutropenia; thrombocytopenia (rare); dryness of the mouth, vagina, or vulva; fever; thrombophlebitis (after IV infusion); abdominal pain. Flattening of the T-wave may be seen in ECG tracings.

# NYSTATIN, ORAL

**Tablets:** 500,000 units (*Rx*)        Various, *Nystatin* (Major), *Mycostatin* (Apothecon)

### Indications
*Nonesophageal membrane GI candidiasis:* Treatment of nonesophageal membrane GI candidiasis

### Administration and Dosage
500,000 to 1,000,000 units 3 times daily. Continue treatment for at least 48 hours after clinical cure to prevent relapse.

### Actions
*Pharmacology:* A polyene antibiotic with antifungal activity. Nystatin probably acts by binding to sterols in the cell membrane of the fungus, with a resultant change in membrane permeability allowing leakage of intracellular components.

*Pharmacokinetics:* Sparingly absorbed after oral use.

### Contraindications
Hypersensitivity to nystatin.

### Adverse Reactions
Nystatin is virtually nontoxic and nonsensitizing and is well tolerated by all age groups including debilitated infants, even on prolonged administration.

# MICONAZOLE

**Injection:** 10 mg/mL (*Rx*)        *Monistat i.v.* (Janssen)

### Indications
Use only to treat severe systemic fungal disease: Coccidioidomycosis, candidiasis, cryptococcosis, pseudoallescheriosis (petriellidiosis, allescheriosis), paracoccidioidomycosis, and for the treatment of chronic mucocutaneous candidiasis.

In the treatment of fungal meningitis or *Candida* urinary bladder infections, IV infusion alone is inadequate. It must be supplemented with intrathecal administration or bladder irrigation.

### Administration and Dosage
*Adults:* The following daily doses are recommended:

| Recommended Miconazole Daily Doses | | |
| --- | --- | --- |
| Organism | Total daily dosage range[1] (mg) | Duration of therapy (weeks) |
| Coccidioidomycosis | 1800 to 3600 | 3 to > 20 |
| Cryptococcosis | 1200 to 2400 | 3 to > 12 |
| Pseudoallescheriosis | 1600 to 3000 | 5 to > 20 |
| Candidiasis | 1600 to 1800 | 1 to > 20 |
| Paracoccidioidomycosis | 1200 to 1200 | 2 to > 16 |

[1] May be divided over 3 infusions.

Repeated courses may be necessitated by relapse or reinfection.

*Children:*
    *Younger than 1 year of age* – 15 to 30 mg/kg/day.
    *1 to 12 years of age* – 20 to 40 mg/kg/day. Do not exceed 15 mg/kg/dose.

*IV:* For doses less than or equal to 2400 mg/day, infuse at a rate of approximately 2 hours/amp. For doses greater than 2400 mg/day, adjust infusion rate and diluent according to patient tolerability.

*Intrathecal:* Administer undiluted solution by various intrathecal routes (20 mg/dose) as an adjunct to IV treatment in fungal meningitis. Succeeding intrathecal injections may be alternated between lumbar, cervical, and cisternal punctures every 3 to 7 days.

*Bladder instillation:* 200 mg diluted solution for *Candida* of the urinary bladder.

## Actions

*Pharmacology:* Miconazole, an imidazole derivative, exerts a fungicidal effect by altering the permeability of the fungal cell membrane.

*Pharmacokinetics:*

*Absorption/Distribution* – CSF levels following IV administration are undetectable. Penetration of the drug into inflamed joints, the vitreous body of the eye, and the peritoneal cavity is good. Greater than 90% is bound to serum protein.

*Metabolism/Excretion* – Miconazole is rapidly metabolized in the liver. About 14% to 22% of the administered dose is excreted in the urine, mainly as inactive metabolites. The terminal elimination half-life is 20 to 25 hours.

## Contraindications

Hypersensitivity to miconazole.

## Warnings

*Cardiac effects:* Cardiorespiratory arrest or anaphylaxis has occurred, possibly because of excessively rapid administration in some cases. Rapid injection of undiluted miconazole may produce transient tachycardia or arrhythmia.

*Pregnancy:* Category C.

*Children:* Safety for use in children younger than 1 year of age has not been extensively studied.

## Precautions

**Give by IV infusion.** Start treatment under stringent conditions of hospitalization. Subsequently, it may be given to suitable patients under ambulatory conditions with close clinical monitoring. Monitor hemoglobin, hematocrit, electrolytes, and lipids.

*Systemic fungal mycoses:* Systemic fungal mycoses may be complications of chronic underlying conditions which, in themselves, may require appropriate measures.

## Drug Interactions

Drugs that may interact with miconazole include amphotericin B, astemizole, cisapride, oral anticoagulants, phenytoin, and terfenadine.

## Adverse Reactions

Adverse reactions occurring in at least 3% of patients include phlebitis at infusion site, pruritus/rash (if severe, discontinuation may be necessary), nausea, vomiting, fever, and chills.

# KETOCONAZOLE

| **Tablets:** 200 mg (*Rx*) | Various, *Nizoral* (Janssen) |
| --- | --- |

---

**Warning:**
Ketoconazole has been associated with hepatic toxicity, including some fatalities. Closely monitor patients and inform them of the risk.

---

## Indications

*Systemic fungal infections:* Candidiasis, chronic mucocutaneous candidiasis, oral thrush, candiduria, blastomycosis, coccidioidomycosis, histoplasmosis, chromomycosis, and paracoccidioidomycosis.

Treatment of severe recalcitrant cutaneous dermatophyte infections not responding to topical therapy or oral griseofulvin or in patients unable to take griseofulvin.

Do not use ketoconazole for fungal meningitis because it penetrates poorly into the CSF.

## Administration and Dosage

If antacids, anticholinergics, or $H_2$ blockers are needed, give at least 2 hours after administration. Take with food to alleviate GI disturbance.

*Adults:* Initially, 200 mg once daily. In very serious infections, or if clinical response is insufficient, increase dose to 400 mg once daily.

*Children:*
  *(Older than 2 years of age)* – 3.3 to 6.6 mg/kg/day as a single daily dose.
  *(Younger than 2 years of age)* – Daily dosage has not been established.

Minimum treatment is 1 or 2 weeks for candidiasis and 6 months for the other indicated systemic mycoses. Chronic mucocutaneous candidiasis usually requires maintenance therapy.

Minimum treatment of recalcitrant dermatophyte infections is 4 weeks in cases involving glabrous skin. Palmar and plantar infections may respond more slowly.

## Actions

*Pharmacology:* Ketoconazole, an imidazole broad-spectrum antifungal agent, impairs the synthesis of ergosterol, the main sterol of fungal cell membranes, allowing increased permeability and leakage of cellular components.

*Pharmacokinetics:*
  *Absorption/Distribution* – Bioavailability depends on an acidic pH for dissolution and absorption. In vitro, plasma protein binding is approximately 95% to 99%, mainly to albumin.
  *Metabolism/Excretion* – The drug undergoes extensive hepatic metabolism to inactive metabolites. Plasma elimination is biphasic; half-life is 2 hours during the first 10 hours, and 8 hours thereafter. The major excretory route is enterohepatic. From 85% to 90% is excreted in bile and feces and 13% in urine.

## Contraindications

Hypersensitivity to ketoconazole. Do not use ketoconazole for the treatment of fungal meningitis because it penetrates poorly into the CSF. Concomitant administration of ketoconazole with oral triazolam is contraindicated.

## Warnings

*Hepatotoxicity:* Hepatotoxicity, primarily of the hepatocellular type, has been associated with ketoconazole, including rare fatalities. Measure liver function before starting treatment and frequently during treatment. Monitor patients receiving ketoconazole concurrently with other potentially hepatotoxic drugs, particularly those patients requiring prolonged therapy or those with a history of liver disease. Transient minor elevations in liver enzymes have occurred.

*Prostatic cancer:* In clinical trials involving 350 patients with metastatic prostatic cancer, 11 deaths were reported within 2 weeks of starting high-dose ketoconazole (1200 mg/day). It is not known whether death was related to therapy. High ketoconazole doses are known to suppress adrenal corticosteroid secretion.

*Hypersensitivity reactions:* Anaphylaxis occurs rarely after the first dose. Hypersensitivity reactions, including urticaria, have been reported.

*Pregnancy:* Category C.

*Lactation:* Ketoconazole is excreted in breast milk. Administer to nursing mothers only if the potential benefits outweigh the potential risks to the infant.

*Children:* Safety for use in children younger than 2 years of age has not been established.

## Precautions

*Hormone levels:* Testosterone levels are impaired with doses of 800 mg/day and abolished by 1600 mg/day. It also decreases ACTH-induced corticosteroid serum levels at similar high doses.

*Gastric acidity:* Ketoconazole requires acidity for dissolution and absorption. In achlorhydria, dissolve each tablet in 4 mL aqueous solution of 0.2 N HCl. Use a glass or plastic straw to avoid contact with teeth. Follow with a glass of water.

## Drug Interactions

Ketoconazole is a potent inhibitor of the cytochrome P450 3A4 enzyme system. Coadministration of ketoconazole with other drugs metabolized by the same enzyme system may result in increased plasma concentrations of the drugs that could increase or prolong both therapeutic and adverse effects. Unless otherwise specified, dosage adjustment may be necessary.

Drugs that may affect ketoconazole include antacids, didanosine, histamine $H_2$ antagonists, isoniazid, sucralfate, proton pump inhibitors, and rifampin. Drugs that may be affected by ketoconazole include oral anticoagulants, corticosteroids, cyclosporine, protease inhibitors, tricyclic antidepressants, carbamazepine, quinidine, sulfonylureas, benzodiazepines, buspirone, oral contraceptives, donepezil, nisoldipine, tacrolimus, vinca alkaloids, zolpidem, and theophylline.

### Adverse Reactions

Adverse reactions occurring in at least 3% of patients include nausea and vomiting.

# AMPHOTERICIN B

| | |
|---|---|
| **Powder for injection**: 50 mg (as deoxycholate) (*Rx*) | Amphotericin B (PharmaTek), *Fungizone Intravenous* (Apothecon), *Amphocin* (Pharmacia) |
| **Suspension for injection**: 100 mg/20 mL (as lipid complex) (*Rx*) | *Abelcet* (Liposome Co.) |
| **Powder for injection**: 50 mg and 100 mg (as cholesteryl) (*Rx*) | *Amphotec* (Sequus Pharmaceuticals) |
| 50 mg (as liposomal) (*Rx*) | *AmBisome* (Fujisawa) |

---

**Warning:**
Use primarily for treatment of patients with progressive and potentially fatal fungal infections. Do not use to treat noninvasive forms of fungal disease such as oral thrush, vaginal candidiasis, and esophageal candidiasis in patients with normal neutrophil counts.

---

### Indications

*Fungal infections, systemic:*

*Amphotericin B deoxycholate* – Intended to treat the following potentially life-threatening invasive fungal infections: Aspergillosis; cryptococcosis (torulosis); North American blastomycosis; candidiasis; coccidioidomycosis; histoplasmosis; zygomycosis including mucormycosis caused by *Mucor*, *Rhizopus*, and *Absidia* sp.; infections caused by related susceptible species of *Conidiobolus* and *Basidiobolus*; sporotrichosis.

*Lipid-based formulations* – For use in patients refractory to conventional amphotericin B deoxycholate therapy or where renal impairment or unacceptable toxicity precludes the use of the deoxycholate formulation for the treatment of invasive fungal infections (lipid complex); for the treatment of invasive aspergillosis (cholesteryl); for the treatment of infections caused by *Aspergillus*, *Candida*, or *Cryptococcus* sp. (liposomal).

*Fungal infections, empirical:* For empirical treatment in febrile, neutropenic patients with presumed fungal infection (liposomal only).

*Cryptococcal meningitis in HIV:* Treatment of cryptococcal meningitis in HIV-infected patients (*AmBisome* only).

*Leishmaniasis:* For treatment of visceral leishmaniasis (liposomal only); treatment of American mucocutaneous leishmaniasis but not as primary therapy (deoxycholate).

*Unlabeled uses:* Prophylaxis for fungal infection in patients with bone marrow transplantation (0.1 mg/kg/day).

### Administration and Dosage

*Fungal infection, empirical:* Administer 3 mg/kg/day of liposomal amphotericin B using a controlled infusion device over ≈ 120 minutes; infusion time may be reduced to 60 minutes if well tolerated or increased if patient experiences discomfort.

*Fungal infection, systemic:*
  *Amphotericin B deoxycholate (eg, Fungizone)* –

| Suggested Indication-Specific Dosage Regimens for Amphotericin B Deoxycholate | | |
|---|---|---|
| Fungal infection, systemic | Treatment regimen | Dose[1] (mg/kg/day) |
| *Aspergillosis* | up to 3.6 g total dose | 1 to 1.5 |
| *Blastomyces* | 4 to 12 weeks | 0.5 to 0.6 |
| *Candidiasis* | 4 to 12 weeks | 0.5 to 1 |
| *Coccidioidomycosis* | 4 to 12 weeks | 0.5 to 1 |
| *Cryptococcus* | 4 to 12 weeks | 0.5 to 0.7 |
| *Histoplasmosis* | 4 to 12 weeks | 0.5 to 0.6 |
| *Mucormycosis* | 4 to 12 weeks | 1 to 1.5 |
| *Rhinocerebral phycomycosis* | 3 to 4 g total dose | 0.25 to 0.3 up to 1 to 1.5 |
| *Sporotrichosis* | up to 2.5 g total dose | 0.5 |

[1] Some of these dosages are not FDA-approved.

Because patient tolerance varies greatly, a test dose may be preferred; 1 mg in 20 mL of 5% Dextrose delivered IV over 20 to 30 minutes. Record patient's temperature, pulse, respiration, and blood pressure every 30 minutes for 2 to 4 hours.

The recommended initial dose is 0.25 to 0.3 mg/kg/day prepared as 0.1 mg/mL infusion and delivered slowly over 2 to 6 hours. Depending on the patient's cardio-renal status, dosage may be gradually increased by 5 to 10 mg/day up to a total dose of 0.5 to 0.7 mg/kg/day. Some mycoses may require total doses up to 1 to 1.5 mg/kg/day. Do not exceed a total daily dose of 1.5 mg/kg; overdoses can result in cardio-respiratory arrest. Alternate daily dosing is recommended for total daily doses of 1.5 mg/kg.

In patients with impaired cardio-renal function or a severe reaction to the test dose, initiate therapy with smaller daily doses (eg, 5 to 10 mg).

An in-line membrane filter of greater than or equal to 1 micron mean pore diameter may be used.

  *Amphotericin B cholesteryl (Amphotec)* – A test dose is advisable (eg, 10 mL of final preparation containing between 1.6 to 8.3 mg infused over 15 to 30 min). The recommended dose is 3 to 4 mg/kg/day prepared as a 0.6 mg/mL (range, 0.16 to 0.83 mg/mL) infusion delivered at a rate of 1 mg/kg/hr. Do not use an in-line filter.

  *Amphotericin B lipid complex (Abelcet)* – The recommended dose is 5 mg/kg/day prepared as a 1 mg/mL infusion and delivered at a rate of 2.5 mg/kg/hr. For pediatric patients and patients with cardiovascular disease, the drug may be diluted to a final concentration of 2 mg/mL. If the infusion exceeds 2 hours, mix the contents by shaking the infusion bag every 2 hours. Do not use an in-line filter.

  *Liposomal amphotericin B (AmBisome)* – The recommended dose is 3 to 5 mg/kg/day prepared as a 1 to 2 mg/mL infusion delivered initially over 120 minutes; infusion time may be reduced to 60 minutes if well tolerated or increased if patient experiences discomfort. Lower infusion concentrations of 0.2 to 0.5 mg/mL may be appropriate for infants and small children to provide sufficient volume for infusion. An in-line membrane filter of greater than or equal to 1 micron mean pore diameter may be used.

*Cryptococcal meningitis in HIV:*
  *AmBisome* – Administer 6 mg/kg/day using a controlled infusion device over approximately 120 minutes; infusion time may be reduced to 60 minutes if well tolerated or increased if patient experiences discomfort.

*Leishmaniasis:*
  *Liposomal amphotericin B (AmBisome)* – Administer 3 mg/kg/day on days 1 through 5, 14 and 21 to immunocompetent patients; a repeat course of therapy may be useful if parasitic clearance is not achieved. Administer 4 mg/kg/day on days 1 through 5, 10, 17, 24, 31, and 38 to immunosuppressed patients; seek expert advice regarding further therapy if parasitic clearance is not achieved.

Amphotericin B deoxycholate (eg, Fungizone) – 0.5 mg/kg/day administered on alternate days for 14 doses has been effective but is not recommended as primary therapy.

Rhinocerebral phycomycosis: A cumulative dose of at least 3 g amphotericin B is recommended. Although a total dose of 3 to 4 g will infrequently cause lasting renal impairment, it is a reasonable minimum where there is clinical evidence of deep tissue invasion. Rhinocerebral phycomycosis usually follows a rapidly fatal course; therapy must be more aggressive than that for more indolent mycoses.

Unlabeled:

Cystitis, candidal – Irrigate bladder with a 50 mcg/mL solution, instilled periodically or continuously for 5 to 10 days.

Meningitis, coccidioidal or cryptococcal – Administer amphotericin B deoxycholate intrathecally at initial doses of 0.025 mg, gradually increased to the maximum tolerable dose. The usual dose is 0.25 to 1 mg every 48 to 72 hours. A maximum total dose of 15 mg has been suggested.

Paracoccidioidomycosis – Administer 0.4 to 0.5 mg/kg/day slow IV infusion, treat for 4 to 12 weeks.

## Actions

Pharmacology: Amphotericin B is fungistatic or fungicidal, depending on the concentration obtained in body fluids and on the susceptibility of the fungus. It acts by binding to sterols in the fungal cell membrane with a resultant change in membrane permeability, allowing leakage of a variety of intracellular components.

Liposomal encapsulation or incorporation in a lipid complex can substantially affect a drug's functional properties relative to those of the unencapsulated or non-lipid-associated drug. Lipid-based formulations increase the circulation time and alter the biodistribution of associated amphotericin. Increasing drug levels at site of action and reducing levels in normal tissues offers 2 distinct clinical advantages: An increased therapeutic index and altered toxicity profile relative to free drug.

Different lipid-based formulations with a common active ingredient may vary from one another in the chemical composition (eg, phospholipid and cholesterol content) and physical form of the lipid component (eg, sphere, disc, or ribbon). Such differences may affect functional properties of these drug products.

Pharmacokinetics:

Absorption/Distribution – Amphotericin B is highly protein bound (greater than 90%) and is poorly dialyzable.

Metabolism/Excretion – Amphotericin B has a relatively short initial serum half-life of 24 hours, followed by a second elimination phase with a half-life of approximately 15 days. The drug is slowly excreted by the kidneys with 2% to 5% as the biologically active form.

The following table presents pharmacokinetic parameters at steady-state for lipid-based formulations of amphotericin B; the assay used to measure serum levels did not distinguish between free and complex amphotericin B.

| Pharmacokinetic Parameters of Lipid-Based Amphotericin B Formulations[1] | | | | | |
|---|---|---|---|---|---|
| Parameter | AmBisome 1 mg/kg/day (n = 7) | AmBisome 2.5 mg/kg/day (n = 7) | AmBisome 5 mg/kg/day (n = 9) | Amphotec 3 mg/kg/day (predicted)[2] | Amphotec 4 mg/kg/day (predicted)[2] | Abelcet 5 mg/kg/day (n = varied)[3] |
| Cmax (mcg/mL) | ≈ 12.2 | ≈ 31.4 | ≈ 83 | 2.6 | 2.9 | ≈ 1.7 |
| AUC (mcg/mL•h) | ≈ 60 | ≈ 197 | ≈ 555 | 29 | 36 | ≈ 14 |
| t½ (h) | ≈ 7 | ≈ 6.3 | ≈ 6.8 | 27.5 (100 to 153)[4] | 28.2 (100 to 153)[4] | ≈ 173.4 |
| Vss (L/kg) | ≈ 0.14 | ≈ 0.16 | ≈ 0.1 | 3.8 | 4.1 | ≈ 131 |
| CL (mL/h/kg) | ≈ 17 | ≈ 22 | ≈ 11 | 105 | 112 | ≈ 436 |

[1] Data are pooled from separate studies and are not necessarily comparable.
[2] Values based on the population model developed from 51 bone marrow transplant patients with systemic fungal infections given Amphotec 0.5 to 8 mg/kg/day.
[3] Data obtained from various studies in patients with mucocutaneous leishmaniasis or cancer with presumed or proven fungal infections.
[4] Based on total amphotericin B levels measured within a 24-hour dosing interval (or up to 49 days after dosing).

**Contraindications**

Hypersensitivity to amphotericin B, unless the condition requiring treatment is life-threatening and amenable only to amphotericin B therapy.

**Warnings**

*Fatal fungal diseases:* Amphotericin B is frequently the only effective treatment for potentially fatal fungal diseases. Balance its possible lifesaving effect against its dangerous side effects.

*Nephrotoxicity:* Renal damage is a limiting factor for the use of amphotericin B. Renal dysfunction usually improves upon interruption of therapy, dose reduction or increased dosing interval; however, some permanent impairment often occurs, especially in patients receiving large doses (greater than 5 g) or receiving other nephrotoxic agents. Decreased glomerular filtration rate and renal blood flow, increased serum creatinine and renal tubular dysfunction are prominent. In some patients, hydration and sodium repletion prior to amphotericin B administration may reduce the risk of developing nephrotoxicity.

Lipid formulations of amphotericin B have been shown to reduce the severe kidney toxicity of amphotericin B and are indicated in patients with renal impairment or when unacceptable toxicity precludes the use of amphotericin B deoxycholate in effective doses.

*Infusion reactions:* Acute reactions including fever, shaking chills, hypotension, anorexia, vomiting, nausea, headache, and tachypnea are common 1 to 3 hours after starting an IV infusion. These reactions usually are more severe with the first few doses of amphotericin B and usually diminish with subsequent doses. Avoid rapid IV infusion because it has been associated with hypotension, hypokalemia, arrhythmias, bronchospasm, and shock.

*Leukoencephalopathy:* This has been reported following use of amphotericin B. The literature has suggested that total body irradiation may be a predisposition.

*Rhinocerebral phycomycosis:* A fulminating disease, this generally occurs in association with diabetic ketoacidosis. Diabetic control must be instituted before successful treatment with amphotericin B can be accomplished. Pulmonary phycomycosis, which is more common in association with hematologic malignancies, is often an incidental finding at autopsy.

*Hypersensitivity reactions:* Anaphylaxis has been reported with amphotericin B. If severe respiratory distress occurs, discontinue the infusion immediately. Do not give further infusions. Have cardiopulmonary resuscitation facilities available during administration.

*Renal function impairment:* Use amphotericin B desoxycholate with care in patients with reduced renal function; frequent monitoring is recommended (see Precautions). Lipid formulations have been reported to overcome most problems of chronic nephrotoxicity, even in patients with impaired renal function following previous treatment with amphotericin B desoxycholate.

*Pregnancy: Category B.*

*Lactation:* It is not known whether amphotericin B is excreted in breast milk; however, consider discontinuing nursing.

*Children:* Safety and efficacy of amphotericin B desoxycholate in children have not been established. Systemic fungal infections have been successfully treated in children without reports of unusual side effects. Limit administration to the least amount compatible with an effective therapeutic regimen.

Pediatric patients younger than 16 years of age (n = 97) with systemic fungal infections have been treated with amphotericin B cholesteryl at daily mg/kg doses similar to those given in adults and had significantly less renal toxicity than the desoxycholate formulation (12% vs 52%); 273 pediatric patients age 1 month to 16 years with presumed fungal infections, confirmed systemic fungal infections or with visceral leishmaniasis have been successfully treated with liposomal amphotericin B (*AmBisome*); 111 children younger than 16 years of age, including 11 patients younger than 1 year of age, have been treated with amphotericin B lipid complex (*Abelcet*) at 5 mg/kg/day and 5 children with hepatosplenic candidiasis were effectively treated with 2.5 mg/kg/day. Safety and efficacy in patients younger than 1 month of age have not been established.

## Precautions

*Monitoring:* Monitor renal function frequently during amphotericin B therapy. It is also advisable to monitor liver function, serum electrolytes (particularly magnesium and potassium), blood counts, and hemoglobin concentrations on a regular basis. Use laboratory test results as a guide to subsequent dose adjustments. Monitor complete blood count and prothrombin time as medically indicated.

Record the patient's temperature, pulse, respiration, and blood pressure every 30 minutes for 2 to 4 hours after administration.

*Resistance:* Variants with reduced susceptibility to amphotericin B have been isolated from several fungal species after serial passage in cell culture media containing the drug and from some patients receiving prolonged therapy with amphotericin B desoxycholate. The relevance of drug resistance to clinical outcome has not been established.

*Therapy interruption:* Whenever medication is interrupted for more than 7 days, resume therapy with the lowest dosage level; increase gradually.

*Pulmonary reactions:* Pulmonary reactions characterized by acute dyspnea, hypoxemia, and interstitial infiltrates have been observed in neutropenic patients receiving amphotericin B and leukocyte transfusions. Separate the infusion as far as possible from the time of a leukocyte transfusion.

*Lab test abnormalities:*

*Serum electrolyte abnormalities* – Hypomagnesemia, hyperkalemia, hypokalemia, hypercalcemia, hypocalcemia, hypophosphatemia.

*Liver function test abnormalities* – Increased AST, ALT, GGT, bilirubin, alkaline phosphatase, and LDH.

*Renal function impairment* – Increased BUN and serum creatinine.

*Other test abnormalities* – Acidosis, hyperamylasemia, hypoglycemia, hyperglycemia, hyperuricemia.

## Drug Interactions

Drugs that may interact with amphotericin B include antineoplastic agents, corticosteroids, zidovudine, other nephrotoxic agents, digitalis glycosides, flucytocine, skeletal muscle relaxants, cyclosporine, azole antifungal agents, and thiazides.

## Adverse Reactions

*Prevention of adverse reactions* – Most patients will exhibit some intolerance, often at less than full therapeutic dosage. Severe reactions may be lessened by giving aspirin, antipyretics (eg, acetaminophen), antihistamines, and antiemetics before the infusion and by maintaining sodium balance. Administration on alternate days may decrease anorexia and phlebitis. Small doses of IV adrenal corticosteroids given prior to or during the infusion may decrease febrile reactions. Meperidine (25 to 50 mg IV) has been shown in some patients to decrease the duration of shaking chills and fever that may accompany infusion of amphotericin B.

Adverse reactions may include abdominal pain; acidosis; anemia; anorexia; anxiety; apnea; asthenia; asthma; arrhythmias; azotemia; bilirubinemia; blood product transfusion reaction; chest/back pain; coagulation disorder; confusion; cough increased; cramping; decreased prothrombin time; depression; diarrhea; dizziness; dry mouth; dyspepsia; dyspnea; edema; epigastric pain; epistaxis; eye hemorrhage; face edema; fever (sometimes with shaking chills); generalized pain, including muscle and joint pains; GI hemorrhage; headache; heart arrest; hematemesis; hematuria; hemoptysis; hemorrhage; hypernatremia; hypertension; hyperventilation; hypokalemia; hypovolemia; hyposthenuria; hypotension; hypoxia; increased serum creatinine; infection; insomnia; jaundice; leukopenia; lung disorder; maculopapular rash; malaise; mucous membrane disorder; multiple organ failure; nausea; normochromic, normocytic anemia; pain; peripheral edema; pleural effusion; pneumonia;

pruritus; rash; renal tubular acidosis and nephrocalcinosis; respiratory disorder; respiratory failure; rhinitis; sepsis; somnolence; stomatitis; sweating; tachycardia; tachypnea; thinking abnormal; thrombocytopenia; tremor; vomiting; venous pain at the injection site with phlebitis and thrombophlebitis; weight loss/gain.

# VORICONAZOLE

**Tablets**: 50 and 200 mg                          Vfend (Roerig)
**Powder for oral suspension**: 45 g (40 mg/mL after reconstitution)
**Powder for injection, lyophilized**: 200 mg

### Indications

*Esophageal candidiasis:* For the treatment of esophageal candidiasis.

*Invasive aspergillosis:* For the treatment of invasive aspergillosis. In clinical trials, the majority of isolates recovered were *Aspergillus fumigatus*. There were a small number of cases of culture-proven disease caused by species of *Aspergillus* other than *A. fumigatus*.

*Serious fungal infections:* For the treatment of serious fungal infections caused by *Scedosporium apiospermum* (asexual form of *Pseudallescheria boydii*) and *Fusarium* sp. including *Fusarium solani*, in patients intolerant of, or refractory to, other therapy.

### Administration and Dosage

Correct electrolyte disturbances (eg, hypokalemia, hypomagnesemia, hypocalcemia) prior to initiation of voriconazole therapy.

*Invasive aspergillosis and serious fungal infections:* Initiate therapy with the specified loading dose regimen of IV voriconazole to achieve plasma concentrations on day 1 that are close to steady state. On the basis of high oral bioavailability, switching between IV and oral administration is appropriate when clinically indicated.

For the treatment of adults with invasive aspergillosis and infections caused by *Fusarium* sp. and *S. apiospermum*, the recommended dosing regimen of voriconazole is as follows: Loading dose of 6 mg/kg IV every 12 hours for 2 doses, followed by a maintenance dose of 4 mg/kg IV every 12 hours.

*Dosage adjustment* – If patient response is inadequate, the oral maintenance dose may be increased from 200 mg every 12 hours to 300 mg every 12 hours. For adult patients weighing less than 40 kg, the oral maintenance dose may be increased from 100 mg every 12 hours to 150 mg every 12 hours.

If patients are unable to tolerate treatment, reduce the IV maintenance dose to 3 mg/kg every 12 hours and the oral maintenance dose by 50 mg steps to a minimum of 200 mg every 12 hours (or to 100 mg every 12 hours for adult patients weighing less than 40 kg).

*Esophageal candidiasis (oral only):* Recommended dosing regimen is an oral dose of 200 mg every 12 hours for patients who weigh 40 kg or more. Adult patients who weigh less than 40 kg should receive an oral dose of 100 mg every 12 hours. Treat patients for a minimum of 14 days and for at least 7 days following resolution of symptoms.

*Hepatic function impairment:* No dose adjustment is necessary in patients with this degree of abnormal liver function, but continued monitoring of liver function tests for further elevations is recommended (see Warnings).

It is recommended that the standard loading dose regimens be used but that the maintenance dose be halved in patients with mild to moderate hepatic cirrhosis (Child-Pugh class A and B).

*Renal function impairment:*
*Oral* – No adjustment is necessary for oral dosing in patients with mild to severe renal impairment.

*IV* – In patients with moderate or severe renal insufficiency (Ccr below 50 mL/min), accumulation of the IV vehicle, SBECD, occurs. Administer oral voriconazole to these patients, unless an assessment of the benefit/risk to the patient justifies the use of IV voriconazole. Closely monitor serum creatinine levels in these patients, and, if increases occur, consider changing to oral voriconazole therapy.

*IV administration:* Voriconazole IV for injection requires reconstitution to 10 mg/mL and subsequent dilution to 5 mg/mL or less prior to administration as an infusion. Infuse at a maximum rate of 3 mg/kg/h over 1 to 2 hours. Not for IV bolus injection.

*Oral administration:* Take voriconazole tablets or oral suspension at least 1 hour before or 1 hour following a meal.

*Instructions for use* – Shake the closed bottle of reconstituted suspension for approximately 10 seconds before each use. Administer the reconstituted oral suspension only using the oral dispenser supplied with each pack.

### Actions

*Pharmacology:* Voriconazole is a triazole antifungal agent. The primary mode of action of voriconazole is the inhibition of fungal cytochrome P450-mediated 14 alpha-lanosterol demethylation, an essential step in fungal ergosterol biosynthesis. The accumulation of 14 alpha-methyl sterols correlates with the subsequent loss of ergosterol in the fungal cell wall and may be responsible for the antifungal activity of voriconazole. Voriconazole has been shown to be more selective for fungal cytochrome P450 enzymes than for various mammalian cytochrome P450 enzyme systems.

*Pharmacokinetics:*

*Absorption* – The pharmacokinetic properties of voriconazole are similar following administration by the IV and oral routes. The oral bioavailability of voriconazole is estimated to be 96% (CV 13%). Bioequivalence was established between the 200 mg tablet and the 40 mg/mL oral suspension when administered as a 400 mg loading dose every 12 hours followed by a 200 mg maintenance dose every 12 hours. Maximum plasma concentration ($C_{max}$) is achieved 1 to 2 hours after dosing.

The pharmacokinetics of voriconazole are nonlinear because of the saturation of its metabolism. The interindividual variability of voriconazole pharmacokinetics is high.

Steady-state trough plasma concentrations with voriconazole are achieved after approximately 5 days of oral or IV dosing without a loading dose regimen. However, when an IV loading dose regimen is used, steady-state trough plasma concentrations are achieved within 1 day.

*Distribution* – The volume of distribution at steady state for voriconazole is estimated to be 4.6 L/kg, suggesting extensive distribution into tissues. Plasma protein binding is estimated to be 58% and was shown to be independent of plasma concentrations achieved following single and multiple oral doses. Varying degrees of hepatic and renal insufficiency do not affect the protein binding of voriconazole.

*Metabolism* – In vitro studies showed that voriconazole is metabolized by the human hepatic cytochrome P450 enzymes CYP2C19, CYP2C9, and CYP3A4.

*Excretion* – Voriconazole is eliminated via hepatic metabolism with less than 2% of the dose excreted unchanged in the urine.

*Special populations* –

*Race:* CYP2C19 exhibits genetic polymorphism. For Caucasians and Blacks, the prevalence of poor metabolizers is 3% to 5%. Studies conducted in healthy Caucasian and Japanese subjects have shown that poor metabolizers have, on average, a 4-fold higher voriconazole exposure (AUC) than their homozygous extensive metabolizer counterparts. Subjects who are heterozygous extensive metabolizers have, on average, a 2-fold higher voriconazole exposure than their homozygous extensive metabolizer counterparts.

*Renal function impairment:* A pharmacokinetic study in subjects with renal failure undergoing hemodialysis showed that voriconazole is dialyzed with clearance of 121 mL/min. The IV vehicle, SBECD, is hemodialyzed with clearance of 55 mL/min. A 4-hour hemodialysis session does not remove a sufficient amount of voriconazole to warrant dose adjustment.

*Microbiology:* Voriconazole has demonstrated in vitro activity against *Aspergillus* sp. (*A. fumigatus, A. flavus, A. niger, A. terreus*), *Candida* sp. (*C. albicans, C. glabrata, C. krusei*), *Scedosporium apiospermum*, and *Fusarium* sp., including *F. solani*.

*Cross-resistance* – Fungal isolates exhibiting reduced susceptibility to fluconazole or itraconazole also may show reduced susceptibility to voriconazole, suggesting that cross-resistance can occur among these azoles.

## Contraindications

Known hypersensitivity to voriconazole or its excipients. Use caution when prescribing voriconazole to patients with hypersensitivity to other azoles.

Coadministration of the CYP3A4 substrates, cisapride, pimozide, or quinidine with voriconazole is contraindicated because increased plasma concentrations of these drugs can lead to QT prolongation and rare occurrences of torsades de pointes.

Coadministration of voriconazole with sirolimus, rifampin, carbamazepine, long-acting barbiturates, rifabutin, ergot alkaloids (ergotamine and dihydroergotamine), ritonavir (400 mg every 12 hours), or efavirenz.

## Warnings

*Visual disturbances:* If treatment continues beyond 28 days, the effect of voriconazole on visual function is not known. If treatment continues beyond 28 days, monitor visual function including visual acuity, visual field, and color perception.

*Hepatic toxicity:* There have been uncommon cases of serious hepatic reactions during treatment with voriconazole (eg, clinical hepatitis, cholestasis, and fulminant hepatic failure, including fatalities). Liver dysfunction usually has been reversible on discontinuation of therapy.

Evaluate liver function tests at the start of and during the course of voriconazole therapy. Monitor patients who develop abnormal liver function tests during voriconazole therapy for the development of more severe hepatic injury. Discontinuation of voriconazole must be considered if clinical signs and symptoms consistent with liver disease develop that may be attributable to voriconazole.

*Hepatic function impairment:* It is recommended that the standard loading dose regimens be used but that the maintenance dose be halved in patients with mild to moderate hepatic cirrhosis (Child-Pugh class A and B) receiving voriconazole.

*Renal function impairment:* In patients with moderate to severe renal dysfunction (Ccr below 50 mL/min), accumulation of the IV vehicle, SBECD, occurs.

*Galactose intolerance:* Voriconazole tablets contain lactose and should not be given to patients with rare hereditary problems of galactose intolerance, Lapp lactase deficiency, or glucose-galactose malabsorption.

*Pregnancy: Category D.*

*Lactation:* Voriconazole should not be used by nursing mothers unless the benefit clearly outweighs the risk.

*Children:* Safety and effectiveness in pediatric patients younger than 12 years of age have not been established.

## Precautions

*Monitoring:* Patient management should include laboratory evaluation of renal (particularly serum creatinine) and hepatic function (particularly liver function tests and bilirubin).

*Cardiovascular:* Some azoles, including voriconazole, have been associated with prolongation of the QT interval on the electrocardiogram.

*Infusion-related reactions:* Anaphylactoid-type reactions, including flushing, fever, sweating, tachycardia, chest tightness, dyspnea, faintness, nausea, pruritus, and rash, have occurred uncommonly. Symptoms appeared immediately upon initiating the infusion.

*Renal toxicity:* Acute renal failure has been observed in severely ill patients undergoing treatment with voriconazole.

*Dermatological reactions:* Patients have rarely developed serious cutaneous reactions, such as Stevens-Johnson syndrome, during treatment with voriconazole.

**Drug Interactions**

*CYP450:* Voriconazole is metabolized by CYP2C19, CYP2C9, and CYP3A4. The affinity of voriconazole is highest for CYP2C19, followed by CYP2C9, and is appreciably lower for CYP3A4. Inhibitors or inducers of these 3 enzymes may increase or decrease voriconazole systemic exposure (plasma concentrations), respectively.

Voriconazole inhibits the metabolic activity of CYP2C19, CYP2C9, and CYP3A4. The inhibition potency of voriconazole for CYP3A4 was significantly less than that of 2 other azoles, ketoconazole and itraconazole. The major metabolite of voriconazole, the voriconazole N-oxide, inhibits the metabolic activity of CYP2C9 and CYP3A4 to a greater extent than that of CYP2C19. There is potential for voriconazole and its major metabolite to increase the systemic exposure (plasma concentration) of other drugs metabolized by these CYP450 enzymes.

Drugs that affect voriconazole include the following: barbiturates (long acting), cimetidine, nonnucleoside reverse transcriptase inhibitors (NNRIs), phenytoin, protease inhibitors, proton pump inhibitors, rifampin, rifabutin.

Drugs affected by voriconazole include the following: benzodiazepines, calcium channel blockers, cisapride, coumarin anticoagulants, cyclosporine, ergot alkaloids, HMG-CoA reductase inhibitors, NNRTIs, phenytoin, protease inhibitors, pimozide, quinidine, prednisolone, rifabutin, sirolimus, sulfonylureas, tacrolimus, vinca alkaloids.

**Adverse Reactions**

The most frequently reported adverse events (all causalities) in the therapeutic trials were visual disturbances, fever, rash, vomiting, nausea, diarrhea, headache, sepsis, peripheral edema, abdominal pain, and respiratory disorder. The treatment-related adverse events that most often led to discontinuation of voriconazole therapy were elevated liver function tests, rash, and visual disturbances.

Adverse reactions occurring in at least 3% of patients included the following: abnormal vision, alkaline phosphatase increased, ALT/AST increased, chills, fever, hallucinations, headache, hepatic enzymes increased, liver function test abnormal, nausea, peripheral edema, photophobia, rash, vomiting.

# FLUCONAZOLE

**Tablets:** 50, 100, 150, and 200 mg *(Rx)*  
**Powder for oral suspension:** 10 and 40 mg/mL when reconstituted *(Rx)*  
**Injection:** 2 mg/mL *(Rx)*

*Diflucan* (Roerig)

### Indications

*Candidiasis:* Oropharyngeal and esophageal candidiasis.

Candidal urinary tract infections, peritonitis, and systemic candidal infections including candidemia, disseminated candidiasis and pneumonia.

*Cryptococcal meningitis:* Treatment of cryptococcal meningitis.

*Prophylaxis:* To decrease the incidence of candidiasis in patients undergoing bone marrow transplantation who receive cytotoxic chemotherapy or radiation therapy.

*Vaginal candidiasis:* Vaginal candidiasis (vaginal yeast infections caused by *Candida*).

### Administration and Dosage

*Single dose:*

Vaginal candidiasis – 150 mg as a single oral dose.

*Multiple dose:* The daily dose of fluconazole is the same for oral and IV administration. In general, a loading dose of twice the daily dose is recommended on the first day of therapy to result in plasma levels close to steady state by the second day of therapy.

Patients with AIDS and cryptococcal meningitis or recurrent oropharyngeal candidiasis usually require maintenance therapy to prevent relapse.

*Adults* –

*Oropharyngeal candidiasis:* 200 mg on the first day, followed by 100 mg once daily. Continue treatment for at least 2 weeks to decrease the likelihood of relapse.

*Esophageal candidiasis:* 200 mg on the first day, followed by 100 mg once daily. Doses up to 400 mg/day may be used, based on the patient's response. Treat patients with esophageal candidiasis for a minimum of 3 weeks and for at least 2 weeks following resolution of symptoms.

*Candidiasis, other:* For candidal UTIs and peritonitis, 50 to 200 mg/day has been used. For systemic candidal infections (including candidemia, disseminated candidiasis, and pneumonia), optimal dosage and duration have not been determined, although doses up to 400 mg/day have been used.

*Prevention of candidiasis in bone marrow transplant:* 400 mg once daily. In patients who are anticipated to have severe granulocytopenia (less than 500 neutrophils/mm$^3$), start fluconazole prophylaxis several days before the anticipated onset of neutropenia, and continue for 7 days after the neutrophil count rises above 1000 cells/mm$^3$.

*Cryptococcal meningitis:* 400 mg on the first day, followed by 200 mg once daily. A dosage of 400 mg once daily may be used, based on the patient's response to therapy. The duration of treatment for initial therapy of cryptococcal meningitis is 10 to 12 weeks after the cerebrospinal fluid becomes culture negative. The dosage of fluconazole for suppression of relapse of cryptococcal meningitis in patients with AIDS is 200 mg once daily.

*Children* –

| Fluconazole Dosage in Children | |
| --- | --- |
| Pediatric Patients | Adults |
| 3 mg/kg | 100 mg |
| 6 mg/kg | 200 mg |
| 12 mg/kg[1] | 400 mg |

[1] Some older children may have clearances similar to that of adults. Absolute doses greater than 600 mg/day are not recommended.

*Neonates:* Based on the prolonged half-life seen in premature newborns (gestational age 26 to 29 weeks), these children, in the first 2 weeks of life, should receive the same dosage (mg/kg) as older children, but administered every 72 hours. After the first 2 weeks, dose neonates once daily.

*Oropharyngeal candidiasis:* The recommended dosage is 6 mg/kg on the first day, followed by 3 mg/kg once daily. Administer treatment for at least 2 weeks.

*Esophageal candidiasis:* The recommended dosage is 6 mg/kg on the first day followed by 3 mg/kg once daily. Doses up to 12 mg/kg/day may be used based on medical judgment of the patient's response to therapy. Treat patients with esophageal candidiasis for a minimum of 3 weeks and for at least 2 weeks following the resolution of symptoms.

*Systemic Candida infections:* For the treatment of candidemia and disseminated *Candida* infections, daily doses of 6 to 12 mg/kg/day have been used.

*Cryptococcal meningitis:* The recommended dosage is 12 mg/kg on the first day, followed by 6 mg/kg once daily. A dosage of 12 mg/kg once daily may be used. The recommended duration of treatment for initial therapy of cryptococcal meningitis is 10 to 12 weeks after the CSF becomes culture negative. For suppression of relapse of cryptococcal meningitis in children with AIDS, the recommended dose is 6 mg/kg once daily.

*Renal function impairment:* There is no need to adjust single dose therapy for vaginal candidiasis in patients with impaired renal function. In patients with impaired renal function who will receive multiple doses, give an initial loading dose of 50 to 400 mg. After the loading dose, base the daily dose on the following table:

| Fluconazole Dose in Impaired Renal Function | |
|---|---|
| Ccr (mL/min) | Percent of recommended dose |
| > 50 | 100% |
| ≤ 50 | 50% |
| Patients receiving regular hemodialysis | One recommended dose after each dialysis |

*Injection:* Fluconazole injection has been used safely for up to 14 days of IV therapy. Administer the IV infusion of fluconazole at a maximum rate of approximately 200 mg/h, given as a continuous infusion. Fluconazole injections are intended only for IV administration.

### Actions

*Pharmacology:* Fluconazole, a synthetic broad spectrum bis-triazole antifungal agent, is a highly selective inhibitor of fungal cytochrome P450 and sterol C-14 alpha-demethylation.

*Pharmacokinetics:*

    *Absorption/Distribution* – The pharmacokinetic properties of fluconazole are similar following administration by the IV or oral routes. In healthy volunteers, the bioavailability of oral fluconazole is more than 90% compared with IV administration.

    Peak plasma concentrations ($C_{max}$) in fasted healthy volunteers occur between 1 and 2 hours with a terminal plasma elimination half-life of approximately 30 hours (range, 20 to 50 hours) after oral administration.

    Steady-state concentrations are reached within 5 to 10 days following oral doses of 50 to 400 mg given once daily. The apparent volume of distribution approximates that of total body water. Plasma protein binding is low (11% to 12%).

    *Metabolism/Excretion* – Fluconazole is cleared primarily by renal excretion, with approximately 80% of the dose appearing in the urine unchanged, approximately 11% as metabolites. The dose may need to be reduced in patients with impaired renal function. A 3-hour hemodialysis session decreases plasma concentrations by approximately 50%.

### Contraindications

Hypersensitivity to fluconazole or to any excipients in the product. There is no information regarding cross-hypersensitivity between fluconazole and other azole antifungal agents; use with caution in patients with hypersensitivity to other azoles.

### Warnings

*Hepatic injury:* Fluconazole has been associated with rare cases of serious hepatic toxicity. Instances of fatal hepatic reactions occurred primarily in patients with serious underlying medical conditions (predominantly AIDS or malignancy) and often while taking multiple concomitant medications.

*Anaphylaxis:* In rare cases, anaphylaxis has occurred.

*Dermatologic changes:* Patients have rarely developed exfoliative skin disorders during treatment with fluconazole.

*Pregnancy: Category C.*

*Lactation:* The use of fluconazole in nursing mothers is not recommended.

*Children:* Efficacy has not been established in children younger than 6 months of age, although a small number of patients ranging from day 1 to 6 months of age have been treated safely with fluconazole.

### Precautions

*Vaginal candidiasis:* Weigh the convenience and efficacy of the single-dose regimen for treatment of vaginal yeast infections against the acceptability of a higher incidence of adverse reactions with fluconazole (26%) vs intravaginal agents (16%).

### Drug Interactions

Fluconazole is an inhibitor of the cytochrome P450 3A4 and 2C9 enzyme systems. Coadministration of fluconazole with other drugs metabolized by the same enzyme system may result in increased plasma concentrations of the drugs, which could increase or prolong therapeutic and adverse effects. Unless otherwise specified, dosage adjustment may be necessary.

Drugs that may affect fluconazole include cimetidine, hydrochlorothiazide, and rifampin. Drugs that may be affected by fluconazole include alfentanil, benzodiazepines, buspirone, carbamazepine, cisapride, oral contraceptives, corticosteroids, cyclosporine, haloperidol, HMG-CoA reductase inhibitors, losartan, nisoldipine, phenytoin, protease inhibitors, rifabutin, sirolimus, sulfonylureas, tacrolimus, theophylline, tolterodine, tricyclic antidepressants, vinca alkaloids, warfarin, zidovudine, and zolpidem.

### Adverse Reactions

Adverse reactions occurring in at least 3% of patients include headache, nausea, abdominal pain, and diarrhea.

## ITRACONAZOLE

| | |
|---|---|
| **Capsules**: 100 mg (*Rx*) | *Sporanox* (Janssen-Ortho) |
| **Oral solution**: 10 mg/mL (*Rx*) | *Sporanox* (Ortho Biotech) |
| **Injection**: 10 mg/mL (*Rx*) | *Sporanox* (Ortho Biotech) |

> **Warning:**
>
> *CHF:* Do not administer itraconazole for the treatment of onychomycosis in patients with evidence of ventricular dysfunction, such as CHF or a history of CHF. Discontinue if signs and symptoms of CHF occur during treatment. If signs and symptoms of CHF occur during treatment, reassess the continued use of itraconazole. When itraconazole was administered IV to dogs and healthy human volunteers, negative inotropic effects were seen.
>
> *Drug interactions:* Coadministration of cisapride, pimozide, dofetilide, or quinidine with itraconazole is contraindicated. Itraconazole is a potent inhibitor of the cytochrome P450 3A4 isoenzyme system and may raise plasma concentrations of drugs metabolized by this pathway. Serious cardiovascular events, including QT prolongation, torsades de pointes, ventricular tachycardia, cardiac arrest, and/or sudden death have occurred in patients taking itraconazole concomitantly with cisapride, pimozide, or quinidine, which are inhibitors of the cytochrome P450 3A4 system.

### Indications

*Aspergillosis (capsules and injection):* Treatment of pulmonary and extrapulmonary aspergillosis in nonimmunocompromised or immunocompromised patients who are intolerant of or who are refractory to amphotericin B therapy.

*Blastomycosis (capsules and injection):* Treatment of pulmonary and extrapulmonary blastomycosis in nonimmunocompromised or immunocompromised patients.

*Febrile neutropenia, empiric (oral solution and injection):* For empiric therapy of febrile neutropenic (ETFN) patients with suspected fungal infections.

*Histoplasmosis (capsules and injection):* Treatment of histoplasmosis, including chronic cavitary pulmonary disease and disseminated, nonmeningeal histoplasmosis in nonimmunocompromised or immunocompromised patients.

*Onychomycosis (capsules only):* Treatment of onychomycosis of the toenail with or without fingernail involvement and onychomycosis of the fingernail because of dermatophytes (*Tinea unguium*) in nonimmunocompromised patients.

*Oropharyngeal/esophageal candidiasis (oral solution only):* Treatment of oropharyngeal or esophageal candidiasis.

*Unlabeled uses:* Itraconazole solution (200 mg/day) is recommended as an alternative to fluconazole as secondary prevention of oropharyngeal, vaginal, or esophageal candidiasis in HIV-infected patients who have severe or frequent recurrences; itraconazole capsules (200 mg/day) have been used as an alternative to fluconazole for primary prevention of cryptococcosis in adults with advanced HIV disease (CD4 counts less than 50 cells/mcL) and are recommended as an alternate to fluconazole for lifelong secondary prevention of cryptococcal disease in HIV-infected adults; itraconazole capsules (200 mg/day) are recommended as first-line agent in the primary prevention of histoplasmosis in adults with advanced HIV disease (CD4 counts less than 100 cells/mcL) and live in endemic areas (rate greater than or equal to 10 cases per 100 patient-years) and also as first-line agent for lifelong secondary prophylaxis (200 mg twice daily); itraconazole capsules (200 mg twice daily) are recommended as an alternate agent to fluconazole for lifelong secondary prevention of coccidioidomycosis in HIV-infected adults; oral itraconazole also is recommended for secondary prevention of histoplasmosis (first line; 2 to 5 mg/kg every 12 to 48 hours), cryptococcal disease (alternate therapy; 2 to 5 mg/kg every 12 to 24 hours), and coccidioidomycosis (alternate therapy; 2 to 5 mg/kg every 12 to 48 hours) in children with HIV; oral itraconazole (2 to 5 mg/kg every 12 to 24 hours) is recommended for primary prevention of histoplasmosis (first-line agent) and cryptococcal disease (alternate therapy) in children with HIV, severe immunosuppression, and live in endemic areas (histoplasmosis).

### Administration and Dosage

When itraconazole therapy may be indicated, isolate and identify the type of organism responsible for the infection; however, therapy may be initiated prior to obtaining these results when clinically warranted.

Do not use capsules and oral solution interchangeably.

*Capsules:* Take with a full meal to ensure maximal absorption.

*Aspergillosis* – A daily dose of 200 to 400 mg is recommended.

*Blastomycosis/histoplasmosis* – 200 mg once daily. If there is no obvious improvement or there is evidence of progressive fungal disease, increase the dose in 100 mg increments to a maximum of 400 mg/day. Give doses above 200 mg/day in 2 divided doses.

*Life-threatening situations* – Although clinical studies did not provide for a loading dose, it is recommended, based on pharmacokinetic data, that a loading dose of 200 mg 3 times/day be given for the first 3 days of treatment.

Continue treatment for a minimum of 3 months and until clinical parameters and laboratory tests indicate that the active fungal infection has subsided. An inadequate period of treatment may lead to recurrence of active infection.

*Treatment of onychomycosis (fingernails only)* – Two treatment pulses, each consisting of 200 mg twice daily for 1 week. The pulses are separated by a 3-week period without itraconazole.

*Treatment of onychomycosis (toenails with or without fingernail involvement)* – 200 mg/day for 12 weeks.

*Oral solution:* Take without food, if possible.

*Esophageal candidiasis* – 100 mg/day for a minimum treatment of 3 weeks. Continue treatment for 2 weeks following resolution of symptoms. Doses up to 200 mg/day may be used based on medical judgment of the patient's response to therapy. Vigorously swish the solution in the mouth (10 mL at a time) for several seconds and swallow.

*ETFN patients with suspected fungal infections* – After approximately 14 days of IV therapy, continue treatment with oral solution 200 mg twice daily until resolution of clinically significant neutropenia. The safety and efficacy of itraconazole use exceeding 28 days in ETFN is not known.

*Oropharyngeal candidiasis* – 200 mg/day for 1 to 2 weeks. Vigorously swish the solution in the mouth (10 mL at a time) for several seconds and swallow. For patients with oropharyngeal candidiasis unresponsive/refractory to treatment with fluconazole tablets, the recommended dose of itraconazole is 100 mg twice daily. Expect clinical response in 2 to 4 weeks. Patients may be expected to relapse shortly after discontinuing therapy. Limited data on the safety of long-term use (more than 6 months) of the oral solution are available at this time.

*Injection:* Use only the components provided in the kit. Do not substitute.

*Blastomycosis, histoplasmosis, and aspergillosis* – 200 mg IV twice daily for 4 doses, followed by 200 mg/day. Infuse each IV dose over 1 hour.

For the treatment of blastomycosis, histoplasmosis, and aspergillosis, itraconazole can be given as oral capsules or IV. The safety and efficacy of the injection administered for more than 14 days are not known.

Continue total itraconazole therapy (injection followed by capsules) for a minimum of 3 months and until clinical parameters and laboratory tests indicate that the active fungal infection has subsided. An inadequate period of treatment may lead to recurrence of active infection.

*Renal function impairment:* Do not use in patients with Ccr below 30 mL/min.

*ETFN patients with suspected fungal infections* – 200 mg twice daily for 4 doses, followed by 200 mg once daily for up to 14 days. Infuse each IV dose over 1 hour. Continue treatment with 200 mg itraconazole oral solution (20 mL) twice daily until resolution of clinically significant neutropenia. The safety and efficacy of itraconazole use exceeding 28 days in ETFN is not known.

## Actions

*Pharmacology:* Itraconazole is a synthetic triazole antifungal agent. In vitro, itraconazole inhibits the cytochrome P450-dependent synthesis of ergosterol, which is a vital component of fungal cell membranes.

*Pharmacokinetics:*

*Absorption/Distribution –*

*Oral solution/injection:* The oral bioavailability is maximal when itraconazole oral solution is taken without food. Steady state is reached after 1 to 2 weeks during chronic administration. Peak plasma levels are observed 2 hours (fasting) to 5 hours (with food) following oral administration. Steady-state plasma concentrations are approximately 25% lower when the oral solution is taken with food.

*Capsules:* The oral bioavailability of itraconazole is maximal when itraconazole capsules are taken with a full meal. Peak plasma levels are observed 3.3 hours (fasting) and 4 hours (with food) following capsule administration.

Plasma protein binding is 99.8%. It is extensively distributed into tissues that are prone to fungal invasion. Concentrations in the lung, kidney, liver, bone, stomach, spleen, and muscle were found to be 2 to 3 times higher than the corresponding plasma concentration. Following IV administration, the volume of distribution averaged 796 ± 185 L.

*Metabolism/Excretion –* Itraconazole is extensively metabolized by the cytochrome P450 3A4 to several metabolites including the major metabolite hydroxyitraconazole. Fecal excretion of the parent drug varies between 3% and 18% of the dose. Renal excretion of the parent drug is less than 0.03% of the dose. Itraconazole is not removed by hemodialysis.

The estimated mean half-life at steady-state of itraconazole after IV infusion was 35.4 hours.

## Contraindications

*CHF:* Do not administer itraconazole capsules for the treatment of onychomycosis or dermatomycoses in patients with evidence of ventricular dysfunction, such as CHF or a history of CHF.

Coadministration of pimozide, quinidine, dofetilide, cisapride, triazolam, or oral midazolam; HMG-CoA reductase inhibitors metabolized by the CYP3A4 enzyme system (eg, lovastatin, simvastatin) (see Warning Box and Drug Interactions); hypersensitivity to the drug or its excipients (there is no information regarding cross-hypersensitivity between itraconazole and other azole antifungal agents; use caution in prescribing to patients with hypersensitivity to other azoles); treatment of onychomycosis in pregnant women or in women contemplating pregnancy.

## Warnings

*Cystic fibrosis:* If a patient with cystic fibrosis does not respond to itraconazole oral solution, consider switching to alternative therapy.

*HIV infection:* Because hypochlorhydria has been reported in HIV-infected patients, the absorption of itraconazole may be decreased in these patients. Administration with a cola beverage has been shown to increase itraconazole absorption in these patients.

*Cardiac dysrhythmias:* Life-threatening cardiac dysrhythmias or sudden death have occurred in patients using pimozide or quinidine concomitantly with itraconazole or other CYP3A4 inhibitors. Concomitant administration of these drugs with itraconazole is contraindicated.

*CHF:* Do not administer itraconazole for the treatment of onychomycosis in patients with evidence of ventricular dysfunction such as CHF or a history of CHF. Do not use itraconazole capsules for other indications in patients with evidence of ventricular dysfunction unless the benefit clearly outweighs the risk.

Itraconazole has been shown to have a negative inotropic effect, and has been associated with reports of CHF. Do not use itraconazole in patients with CHF or with a history of CHF unless the benefit clearly outweighs the risk. This individual benefit/risk assessment should take into consideration factors such as the severity of the indication, the dosing regimen, and the individual risk factors for CHF.

*Hepatotoxicity:* Itraconazole has been associated with rare cases of serious hepatotoxicity, including liver failure and death. Some of these cases had neither pre-existing liver disease, nor a serious underlying medical condition. If liver function tests are abnormal, discontinue treatment. In patients with raised liver enzymes or an active liver disease or who have experienced liver toxicity with other drugs, do not start treatment unless the expected benefit exceeds the risk of hepatic injury. In such cases, liver enzyme monitoring is necessary.

*Bioequivalency:* Do not use itraconazole capsules and oral solution interchangeably. Drug exposure is greater with the oral solution than with the capsules when the same dose of drug is given. Additionally, the topical effects of mucosal exposure may be different between the two formulations.

*Renal function impairment:* Do not use itraconazole injection in patients with severe renal dysfunction (Ccr less than 30 mL/min) because of prolonged elimination of hydroxypropyl-β-cyclodextrin.

*Elderly:* In general, use caution in dose selection for an elderly patient, reflecting the greater frequency of decreased hepatic, renal, or cardiac function, and of concomitant disease or other drug therapy.

*Pregnancy:* Category C.

*Lactation:* Itraconazole is excreted in breast milk.

*Children:* Safety and efficacy have not been established. A small number of patients from 3 to 16 years of age have been treated with 100 mg/day for systemic fungal infections and no serious adverse effects have been reported.

### Precautions

*Monitoring:* Monitor liver function in patients with pre-existing hepatic function abnormalities or those who have experienced liver toxicity with other medications; consider monitoring in all patients. Stop treatment immediately and conduct liver function testing in patients who develop signs and symptoms suggestive of liver dysfunction.

*Neuropathy:* Discontinue if neuropathy occurs that may be attributable to itraconazole capsules or oral solution.

*Decreased gastric acidity:* Under fasted conditions, itraconazole absorption was decreased in the presence of decreased gastric acidity. The absorption of itraconazole may be decreased with coadministration of antacids or gastric acid secretion suppressors. Studies conducted under fasted conditions demonstrated that administration with 8 oz of a cola beverage resulted in increased absorption of itraconazole in AIDS patients with relative or absolute achlorhydria. This increase relative to the effects of a full meal is unknown.

**Drug Interactions**
Both itraconazole and its major metabolite, hydroxyitraconazole, are inhibitors of the cytochrome P450 3A4 enzyme system. Coadministration of itraconazole and drugs primarily metabolized by the cytochrome P450 3A4 enzyme system may result in increased plasma concentrations of the drugs that could increase or prolong therapeutic and adverse effects.

Drugs that may affect itraconazole include antacids, carbamazepine, didanosine, $H_2$ antagonists, hydantoins, macrolide antibiotics, nevirapine, phenobarbital, phenytoin, protease inhibitors, proton pump inhibitors, and rifamycins.

Drugs that may be affected by itraconazole include benzodiazepines, busulfan, buspirone, calcium blockers, cisapride, cyclosporine, digoxin, docetaxel, tacrolimus, sirolimus, warfarin, alfentanil, zolpidem, vinca alkaloids, corticosteroids, protease inhibitors, HMG-CoA reductase inhibitors, triazolam, oral midazolam, alprazolam, carbamazepine, dofetilide, haloperidol, hydantoins (phenytoin), pimozide, polyenes, amphotericin B, quinidine, tolterodine, hypoglycemic agents, and rifamycins.

**Adverse Reactions**
Adverse reactions occurring in at least 3% of patients include the following: Nausea, vomiting, diarrhea, rash, hypokalemia, bilirubinemia, increased ALT.

# TERBINAFINE HCl

| Tablets: 250 mg (*Rx*) | *Lamisil* (Novartis) |
|---|---|

**Warning:**
Rare cases of hepatic failure, some leading to death or liver transplant, have occurred with the use of terbinafine for the treatment of onychomycosis in individuals with and without pre-existing liver disease. In the majority of liver cases reported in association with terbinafine use, the patients had serious underlying systemic conditions and an uncertain causal relationship with terbinafine. Terbinafine is not recommended for patients with chronic or active liver disease. Before prescribing terbinafine, assess pre-existing liver disease. Hepatotoxicity may occur in patients with and without preexisting liver disease. Pretreatment serum transaminase (ALT and AST) tests are advised for all patients before taking terbinafine.

**Indications**
*Onychomycosis:* Treatment of onychomycosis of the toenail or fingernail caused by dermatopytes.

**Administration and Dosage**
*Onychomycosis:*
  *Fingernail* – 250 mg/day for 6 weeks.
  *Toenail* – 250 mg/day for 12 weeks.
  The optimal clinical effect is seen some months after mycological cure and cessation of treatment. This is related to the period required for outgrowth of healthy nail.

**Actions**
*Pharmacology:* Terbinafine is a synthetic allylamine derivative that exerts its antifungal effect by inhibiting squalene epoxidase, a key enzyme in sterol biosynthesis in fungi. This action results in a deficiency in ergosterol and a corresponding accumulation of squalene within the fungal cell and causes fungal cell death.

*Pharmacokinetics:* Terbinafine is well absorbed (more than 70%). Bioavailability is approximately 40%. Peak plasma concentrations of 1 mcg/mL appear up to 2 hours after a single 250 mg dose. The AUC is approximately 4.56 mcg•h/mL.

Prior to excretion, terbinafine is extensively metabolized. No metabolites have been identified that have antifungal activity similar to terbinafine. Approximately 70% of the administered dose is eliminated in the urine.

### Contraindications
Hypersensitivity to terbinafine or any component of the product.

### Warnings
*Hepatic failure:* Rare cases of liver failure, some leading to death or liver transplant, have occurred with the use of terbinafine for the treatment of onychomycosis in individuals with and without pre-existing liver disease.

The severity of hepatic events or their outcome may be worse in patients with active or chronic liver disease. Discontinue treatment with terbinafine if biochemical or clinical evidence of liver injury develops.

*Ophthalmic:* Changes in the ocular lens and retina have been reported following the use of terbinafine.

*Neutropenia:* Isolated cases of severe neutropenia have been reported but were reversible with discontinuation of treatment with or without supportive therapy. If the neutrophil count is 1000 cells/mm$^3$ or less, discontinue treatment and start supportive management.

*Dermatologic:* There have been isolated reports of serious skin reactions (eg, Stevens-Johnson syndrome, toxic epidermal necrolysis).

*Renal/Hepatic function impairment:* In patients with renal impairment (Ccr 50 mL/min or less) or chronic or active liver disease, the use of terbinafine is not recommended

*Pregnancy:* Category B.

*Lactation:* After oral administration, terbinafine is present in the breast milk of nursing mothers. Use of terbinafine tablets is not recommended in nursing mothers.

*Children:* Safety and efficacy have not been established.

### Precautions
*Monitoring:*

*Immunodeficiency* – Monitor CBC in patients receiving treatment for longer than 6 weeks.

*Hepatic* – Pretreatment serum transaminase (ALT and AST) tests are advised for all patients before taking terbinafine. Warn patients to immediately report to their physician any symptoms of persistent nausea, anorexia, fatigue, vomiting, right upper abdominal pain or jaundice, dark urine, or pale stools. Discontinue treatment in patients with these symptoms taking oral terbinafine, and immediately evaluate the patient's liver function.

### Drug Interactions
Drugs that may interact with terbinafine include the following: Cimetidine, rifampin, terfenadine, caffeine, dextromethorphan, cyclosporine.

### Adverse Reactions
Adverse reactions occurring in at least 3% of patients include the following: Diarrhea, dyspepsia, rash, liver enzyme abnormalities, headache.

# SULFONAMIDES

| | |
|---|---|
| **SULFADIAZINE** | |
| **Tablets**: 500 mg (*Rx*) | Various, *Sulfadiazine* (Stanley) |
| **SULFAMETHIZOLE** | |
| **Tablets**: 500 mg (*Rx*) | *Thiosulfil Forte* (Wyeth-Ayerst) |
| **SULFAMETHOXAZOLE** | |
| **Tablets**: 500 mg (*Rx*) | Various, *Gantanol* (Roche), *Urobak* (Shionogi) |
| **Oral suspension**: 500 mg/5 mL (*Rx*) | *Gantanol* (Roche) |
| **SULFISOXAZOLE** | |
| **Tablets**: 500 mg (*Rx*) | Various, *Gantrisin* (Roche) |

### Indications

| Sulfonamide Indications | | | | | |
|---|---|---|---|---|---|
| ✔ – Labeled Indications | Multiple sulfas | Sulfadiazine | Sulfamethizole | Sulfamethoxazole | Sulfisoxazole |
| Chancroid | ✔ | ✔ | | ✔ | ✔ |
| Inclusion conjunctivitis | ✔ | ✔ | | ✔ | ✔ |
| Malaria[1] | ✔ | ✔ | | ✔ | ✔ |
| Meningitis, *Haemophilus influenzae*[2] | ✔ | ✔ | | | ✔ |
| Meningitis, meningococcal[3] | ✔ | ✔ | | ✔ | ✔ |
| Nocardiosis | ✔ | ✔ | | ✔ | ✔ |
| Otitis media, acute[4] | ✔ | ✔ | | ✔ | ✔ |
| Rheumatic fever | | ✔ | | | |
| Rheumatoid arthritis | | | | | |
| Toxoplasmosis[5] | ✔ | ✔ | | ✔ | ✔ |
| Trachoma | ✔ | ✔ | | ✔ | ✔ |
| Urinary tract infections[6] (pyelonephritis, cystitis) | ✔ | ✔ | ✔ | ✔ | ✔ |

[1] As adjunctive therapy because of chloroquine-resistant strains of *Plasmodium falciparum*.
[2] As adjunctive therapy with parenteral streptomycin.
[3] When the organism is susceptible and for prophylaxis when sulfonamide-sensitive group A strains prevail.
[4] Caused by *H. influenzae* when used with penicillin or erythromycin.
[5] As adjunctive therapy with pyrimethamine.
[6] In the absence of obstructive uropathy or foreign bodies, when caused by *Escherichia coli*, *Klebsiella-Enterobacter*, *Staphylococcus aureus*, *Proteus mirabilis*, and *Proteus vulgaris*.

### Administration and Dosage

*CDC-recommended treatment schedules for sexually transmitted diseases:*

*Lymphogranuloma venereum* – As an alternative regimen to doxycycline, sulfisoxazole 500 mg 4 times/day for 21 days or equivalent sulfonamide course.

*Treatment of uncomplicated urethral, endocervical, or rectal Chlamydia trachomatic infections* – As an alternative regimen to doxycycline or tetracycline (or if erythromycin is not tolerated), sulfisoxazole 500 mg 4 times/day for 10 days or equivalent sulfonamide course.

*SULFADIAZINE:*

*Adults* – *Loading dose* - 2 to 4 g. *Maintenance dose* - 4 to 8 g/day in 4 to 6 divided doses.

*Children (older than 2 months of age)* –

*Loading dose:* 75 mg/kg (or 2 g/m$^2$).

*Maintenance dose:* 120 to 150 mg/kg/day (4 g/m$^2$/day) in 4 to 6 divided doses.

*Maximum dose:* 6 g/day.

*Infants (younger than 2 months of age)* – Contraindicated, except as adjunctive therapy with pyrimethamine in the treatment of congenital toxoplasmosis.

*Loading dose* – 75 to 100 mg/kg.

*Maintenance dose* – 100 to 150 mg/kg/day in 4 divided doses.

*Other recommended doses for toxoplasmosis (for 3 to 4 weeks) include* –

*Infants (younger than 2 months of age):* 25 mg/kg/dose 4 times daily.

*Children (older than 2 months of age):* 25 to 50 mg/kg/dose 4 times daily.

*Prevention of recurrent attacks of rheumatic fever* – Prevention of recurrent attacks of rheumatic fever (not for initial treatment of streptococcal infections): Patients greater than 30 kg (greater than 66 lbs) - 1 g/day; less than 30 kg (less than 66 lbs) - 0.5 g/day.

SULFAMETHIZOLE:

*Adults* – 0.5 to 1 g 3 or 4 times daily.

*Children and infants (older than 2 months of age )* – 30 to 45 mg/kg/day in 4 divided doses.

SULFAMETHOXAZOLE:

*Adults* –

*Mild to moderate infections:* 2 g initially; maintenance dose is 1 g morning and evening thereafter.

*Severe infections:* 2 g initially, then 1 g 3 times daily.

*Children and infants (older than 2 months of age )* – Initially, 50 to 60 mg/kg; maintenance dose is 25 to 30 mg/kg morning and evening. Do not exceed 75 mg/kg/day.

Another recommended dose is 50 to 60 mg/kg/day divided every 12 hours, not to exceed 3 g/24 hours.

SULFISOXAZOLE:

*Loading dose* – 2 to 4 g.

*Maintenance dose:* 4 to 8 g/day in 4 to 6 divided doses. Although recommended, a loading dose is unnecessary because sulfisoxazole is rapidly absorbed and appears in high concentrations in the urine.

*Children and infants (older than 2 months of age )* –

*Initial dose:* 75 mg/kg.

*Maintenance dose:* 120 to 150 mg/kg/day (4 g/m$^2$/day) in 4 to 6 divided doses (max, 6 g/day).

## Actions

*Pharmacology:* Sulfonamides exert their bacteriostatic action by competitive antagonism of para-aminobenzoic acid (PABA), an essential component in folic acid synthesis.

*Pharmacokinetics:*

*Absorption/Distribution* – The oral sulfonamides are readily absorbed from the GI tract. Approximately 70% to 100% of an oral dose is absorbed. Sulfonamides are bound to plasma proteins in varying degrees.

*Metabolism* – Metabolism occurs in the liver by conjugation, acetylation, and other metabolic pathways to inactive metabolites.

*Excretion* – Renal excretion is mainly by glomerular filtration; tubular reabsorption occurs in varying degrees.

*Microbiology:* Sulfonamides have a broad antibacterial spectrum that includes grampositive and gram-negative organisms.

## Contraindications

Hypersensitivity to sulfonamides or chemically related drugs (eg, sulfonylureas, thiazide and loop diuretics, carbonic anhydrase inhibitors, sunscreens with PABA, local anesthetics); pregnancy at term; lactation; infants less than 2 months of age (except in congenital toxoplasmosis as adjunct with pyrimethamine); porphyria; salicylate hypersensitivity.

## Warnings

*Group A beta-hemolytic streptococcal infections:* Do not use for treatment of these infections.

*Severe reactions:* Severe reactions including deaths caused by sulfonamides have been associated with hypersensitivity reactions, agranulocytosis, aplastic anemia, other blood dyscrasias, and renal and hepatic damage. Irreversible neuromuscular and CNS changes and fibrosing alveolitis may occur.

*Porphyria:* In patients with porphyria, these drugs have precipitated an acute attack.

*Photosensitivity:* Photosensitization (photoallergy or phototoxicity) may occur.

*Renal/Hepatic function impairment:* Use with caution. The frequency of renal complications is considerably lower in patients receiving the more soluble sulfonamides (sulfisoxazole and sulfamethizole).

*Pregnancy:* Category B; Category D near term. Significant levels may persist in the neonate if these drugs are given near term; jaundice, hemolytic anemia, and kernicterus may occur. Do not use at term.

*Lactation:* According to the American Academy of Pediatrics, breastfeeding and sulfonamide use are compatible. However, do not nurse premature infants or those with hyperbilirubinemia or G-6-PD deficiency.

*Children:* Do not use in infants less than 2 months of age (except for congenital toxoplasmosis as adjunctive therapy with pyrimethamine).

## Precautions

*Allergy or asthma:* Give with caution to patients with severe allergy or bronchial asthma.

*Hemolytic anemia:* Hemolytic anemia, frequently dose-related, may occur in G-6-PD deficient individuals.

## Drug Interactions

Drugs that may interact with sulfonamides include oral anticoagulants, cyclosporine, hydantoins, methotrexate, and sulfonylureas.

Drugs that may interact with sulfisoxazole include barbiturate anesthetics.

*Drug/Lab test interactions:* Sulfonamides may produce false-positive **urinary glucose tests** when performed by Benedict's method. Sulfisoxazole may interfere with the **Urobilistix test** and may produce false-positive results with sulfosalicylic acid tests for urinary protein.

## Adverse Reactions

Agranulocytosis; aplastic anemia; thrombocytopenia; leukopenia; hemolytic anemia; purpura; hypoprothrombinemia; cyanosis; methemoglobinemia; megaloblastic (macrocytic) anemia; Stevens-Johnson type erythema multiforme; generalized skin eruptions; epidermal necrolysis; urticaria; serum sickness; pruritus; exfoliative dermatitis; anaphylactoid reactions; periorbital edema; nausea; emesis; abdominal pains; diarrhea; bloody diarrhea; anorexia; pancreatitis; stomatitis; hepatitis; pseudomembranous enterocolitis; glossitis; headache; peripheral neuropathy; mental depression; convulsions; ataxia; hallucinations; tinnitus; vertigo; insomnia; hearing loss; drowsiness; apathy; crystalluria; hematuria; proteinuria; elevated creatinine; drug fever; chills; pyrexia; alopecia; arthralgia; myalgia.

# ANTITUBERCULOSIS DRUGS

Antituberculosis drugs have been described in terms of the following 3 areas of activity: Bactericidal activity, sterilizing activity, and drug resistance prevention.

Standard treatment regimens are divided into the following 2 phases: An initial phase, during which agents are used to kill rapidly multiplying populations of *Mycobacterium tuberculosis* and to prevent the emergence of drug resistance, followed by a continuation phase, during which sterilizing drugs kill the intermittently dividing populations.

The initial phase of the regimen must contain at least 3 of the following drugs: Isoniazid, rifampin, and pyrazinamide, along with either ethambutol or streptomycin if the local resistance pattern to isoniazid is not documented or is greater than 4%.

*Directly observed therapy (DOT):* Adherence to the treatment regimen can be achieved by DOT, the "gold standard." The health care provider watches the patient swallow each dose of medication. This allows for monitoring of the number of doses that an individual has taken. DOT may be given intermittently (2 to 3 times/week) or daily.

| Recommended Drugs for the Treatment of Tuberculosis in Children and Adults[1] | | | | | | | |
|---|---|---|---|---|---|---|---|
| | Daily dose[2] | | Maximum daily dose in children and adults | Twice weekly dose | | 3 times/week dose | |
| Drug | Children | Adults | | Children | Adults | Children | Adults |
| *Initial treatment* | | | | | | | |
| Isoniazid | 10 to 20 mg/kg PO or IM | 5 mg/kg PO or IM | 300 mg | 20 to 40 mg/kg max 900 mg | 15 mg/kg max 900 mg | 20 to 40 mg/kg max 900 mg | 15 mg/kg max 900 mg |
| Rifampin | 10 to 20 mg/kg PO | 10 mg/kg PO | 600 mg | 10 to 20 mg/kg max 600 mg | 10 mg/kg max 600 mg | 10 to 20 mg/kg max 600 mg | 10 mg/kg max 600 mg |
| Pyrazin-amide | 15 to 30 mg/kg PO | 15 to 30 mg/kg PO | 2 g | 50 to 70 mg/kg max 4 g | 50 to 70 mg/kg max 4 g | 50 to 70 mg/kg max 3 g | 50 to 70 mg/kg max 3 g |
| Strepto-mycin | 20 to 40 mg/kg IM | 15 mg/kg IM | 1 g[3] | 25 to 30 mg/kg IM max 1.5 g | 25 to 30 mg/kg IM max 1.5 g | 25 to 30 mg/kg max 1.5 g | 25 to 30 mg/kg max 1.5 g |
| Etham-butol | 15 to 25 mg/kg PO | 15 to 25 mg/kg PO | — | 50 mg/kg | 50 mg/kg | 25 to 30 mg/kg | 25 to 30 mg/kg |
| Rifapen-tine | — | — | — | — | 600 mg PO | — | — |
| *Second-line treatment* | | | | | | | |
| Cyclo-serine | 15 to 20 mg/kg PO | 15 to 20 mg/kg PO | 1 g | — | — | — | — |
| Ethiona-mide | 15 to 20 mg/kg PO | 15 to 20 mg/kg PO | 1 g | — | — | — | — |
| Capreo-mycin | 15 to 30 mg/kg IM | 15 to 30 mg/kg IM | 1 g | — | — | — | — |
| Kana-mycin | 15 to 30 mg/kg IM or IV | 15 to 30 mg/kg IM or IV | 1 g | — | — | — | — |
| Cipro-floxacin | — | 1000 to 1500 mg PO | 1500 mg | — | — | — | — |
| Ofloxacin | — | 800 mg PO | 800 mg | — | — | — | — |
| Levoflox-acin | — | 500 to 750 mg PO | 750 mg | — | — | — | — |
| Sparflox-acin | — | 200 mg PO | 200 mg | — | — | — | — |

| Recommended Drugs for the Treatment of Tuberculosis in Children and Adults[1] | | | | | | |
|---|---|---|---|---|---|---|
| Drug | Daily dose[2] | | Maximum daily dose in children and adults | Twice weekly dose | | 3 times/week dose | |
| | Children | Adults | | Children | Adults | Children | Adults |
| P-amino-salicy-clic acid | 150 mg/kg PO | 150 mg/kg PO | 12 g | — | — | — | — |
| Rifabutin | — | 300 to 450 mg PO | — | — | — | — | — |

[1] For detailed dosing information and frequency, see individual monographs.
[2] Doses based on weight. Adjust as weight changes.
[3] In people ≥ 60 years of age, limit the daily dose of streptomycin to 0.5 g IM.

*Treatment regimens:* The CDC recommends at least a 3-drug regimen with rifampin, isoniazid, and pyrazinamide for a minimum of 2 months, followed by rifampin and isoniazid for 4 months in areas with a low incidence of tuberculosis. Administer
streptomycin or ethambutol for the first 2 months in areas with a high incidence of
tuberculosis.

*Retreatment:* Retreatment is necessary when treatment fails because of noncompliance
or inadequate drug treatment. Retreatment regimens include at least 4 drugs; however, depending on disease progression and the bacteriostatic or bactericidal activity of the drug, no more than 7 drugs can be used. Retreatment drug regimens most
commonly include the second-line agents of ethionamide, aminosalicylic acid,
cycloserine, and capreomycin, as well as ofloxacin and ciprofloxacin.

Individualize treatment on the basis of the susceptibility pattern of the infecting
organism when retreating patients known to be infected with drug-resistant isolates.
Include in this regimen at least 3 new drugs to which the organism is susceptible. Continue therapy until sputum cultures convert to negative, and then continue therapy for an additional 12 months with 2 drugs. Treatment may be
continued for 24 months after sputum culture conversion.

*HIV:* The initial phase of a 6-month tuberculosis regimen consists of isoniazid, rifabutin, pyrazinamide, and ethambutol for patients receiving therapy with protease
inhibitors or nonnucleoside reverse transcriptase inhibitors. These drugs are administered a) daily for at least the first 2 weeks, followed by twice weekly dosing for
6 weeks or b) daily for 8 weeks to complete the 2-month induction phase. The second phase of treatment consists of rifabutin and isoniazid administered twice
weekly or daily for 4 months.

Do not use tuberculosis regimens consisting of isoniazid, ethambutol, and pyrazinamide (ie, 3-drug regimens that do not contain a rifamycin, an aminoglycoside [eg,
streptomycin, amikacin, kanamycin], or capreomycin) for the treatment of patients
with HIV-related tuberculosis. The minimum duration of therapy is 18 months
(or 12 months after documented culture conversion) if these regimens are used for
the treatment of tuberculosis.

Administer pyridoxine (vitamin $B_6$) 25 to 50 mg daily or 50 to 100 mg twice
weekly to all HIV-infected patients who are undergoing tuberculosis treatment with
isoniazid to reduce the occurrence of isoniazid-induced side effects in the central
and peripheral nervous system.

Because the MMWR's most recent recommendations for the use of antiretroviral therapy strongly advise against interruptions of therapy, and because alternative tuberculosis treatments that do not contain rifampin are available, previous
antituberculosis therapy options that involved stopping protease inhibitor therapy
to allow the use of rifampin are no longer recommended.

*Pregnancy:* Do not delay treatment for suspected or confirmed tuberculosis during pregnancy. The best therapeutic choices with the least danger to the fetus appear to
be combinations of isoniazid, ethambutol, and rifampin. Pyrazinamide and streptomycin are not recommended during pregnancy because of possible teratogenic
effects. Administer pyridoxine to all pregnant women receiving tuberculosis treat-

ment to prevent peripheral neuropathy as a result of taking isoniazid. In pregnant women, delay prophylaxis until after delivery.

*Multidrug resistance:* The most recent cultures should undergo susceptibility testing to all antituberculosis drugs if cultures remain positive after 3 to 4 months of treatment.

*Chemoprophylaxis:* Administer isoniazid to adults in a daily dose of 300 mg for 1 year. Administer 10 mg/kg to a maximum daily dose of 300 mg for 1 year to children.

# ISONIAZID (Isonicotinic acid hydrazide; INH)

| | |
|---|---|
| **Tablets:** 100 and 300 mg (*Rx*) | Various, *Isoniazid* (Barr) |
| **Syrup:** 50 mg/5 mL (*Rx*) | *Isoniazid* (Carolina Medical) |
| **Injection:** 100 mg/mL (*Rx*) | *Nydrazid* (Apothecon) |

**Warning:**

Severe and sometimes fatal hepatitis associated with isoniazid therapy may occur or develop even after many months of treatment. The risk of developing hepatitis is age-related. Risk of hepatitis increases with daily alcohol consumption.

Carefully monitor and interview patients at monthly intervals. For people older than 35 years of age, in addition to a monthly symptom review, measure hepatic enzymes (specifically AST and ALT) prior to starting isoniazid therapy and periodically throughout treatment. Isoniazid-associated hepatitis usually occurs during the first 3 months of treatment. Enzyme levels generally return to normal despite continuance of the drug, but in some cases, progressive liver dysfunction occurs. Other factors associated with an increased risk of hepatitis include daily use of alcohol, chronic liver disease, and injection drug use. A report suggests an increased risk of fatal hepatitis associated with isoniazid among women, particularly black and Hispanic women. The risk also may be increased during the postpartum period. Consider more careful monitoring in these groups, possibly including more frequent laboratory monitoring. If abnormalities of liver function exceed 3 to 5 times the upper limit of normal, consider discontinuation of isoniazid. Liver function tests are not a substitute for a clinical evaluation at monthly intervals or for the prompt assessment of signs or symptoms of adverse reactions occurring between regularly scheduled evaluations. Instruct patients to report immediately signs or symptoms consistent with liver damage or other adverse effects. If these symptoms appear, or if signs suggestive of hepatic damage are detected, discontinue isoniazid promptly because continued use of the drug in such cases may cause a more severe form of liver damage.

Treat patients with tuberculosis who have hepatitis attributed to isoniazid with appropriate alternative drugs. Reinstitute isoniazid after symptoms and laboratory abnormalities have become normal. Restart the drug in very small doses; gradually increase doses and withdraw immediately if there is any indication of recurrent liver involvement.

Defer preventive treatment in people with acute hepatic diseases.

**Indications**

Used for all forms of tuberculosis in which organisms are susceptible.

Also recommended as preventive therapy (chemoprophylaxis) for specific situations.

IM administration is intended for use whenever oral is not possible.

**Administration and Dosage**

*Treatment of tuberculosis:* Use in conjunction with other effective antituberculosis agents.

Adults – 5 mg/kg/day (up to 300 mg total) in a single dose, or 15 mg/kg (less than or equal to 900 mg daily) 2 to 3 times weekly.

*Children* – 10 to 15 mg/kg (less than or equal to 300 mg daily) in a single dose, or 20 to 40 mg/kg (less than or equal to 900 mg/day) 2 to 3 times weekly.

*Preventive treatment:*
 *Adults (greater than 30 kg)* – 300 mg/day in a single dose.
 *Infants and children* – 10 mg/kg/day (up to 300 mg total) in a single dose.

## Actions

*Pharmacology:* Isoniazid inhibits the synthesis of mycoloic acids, an essential component of the bacterial cell wall. At therapeutic levels, isoniazid is bacteriocidal against actively growing intracellular and extracellular *Mycobacterium tuberculosis* organisms.

Pyridoxine (vitamin B$_6$) deficiency sometimes is observed in adults taking high doses of INH and is probably caused by the drug's competition with pyridoxal phosphate for the enzyme apotryptophanase.

*Pharmacokinetics:*
 *Absorption* – INH is rapidly and completely absorbed orally and parenterally and produces peak blood levels within 1 to 2 hours. However, the rate and extent of absorption is decreased by food.

 *Distribution* – INH readily diffuses into all body fluids (including cerebrospinal, pleural, and ascitic), tissues, organs, and excreta (saliva, sputum, feces). It also passes through the placental barrier and into breast milk in concentrations comparable to those in plasma.

 *Metabolism* – The half-life of INH is widely variable and dependent on acetylator status. Isoniazid is primarily acetylated by the liver; this process is genetically controlled. Fast acetylators metabolize the drug about 5 to 6 times faster than slow acetylators. Several minor metabolites have been identified, one or more of which may be "reactive" (monoacetylhydrazine is suspected), and responsible for liver damage. The rate of acetylation does not significantly alter the effectiveness of INH. However, slow acetylation may lead to higher blood levels of the drug, and thus to an increase in toxic reactions.

 *Excretion* – Approximately 50% to 70% of a dose of isoniazid is excreted as unchanged drug and metabolites by the kidneys in 24 hours.

## Contraindications

Previous isoniazid-associated hepatic injury or other severe adverse reactions.

## Warnings

*Hypersensitivity reactions:* Stop all drugs and evaluate at the first sign of a hypersensitivity reaction. If isoniazid must be reinstituted, give only after symptoms have cleared. Restart the drug in very small and gradually increasing doses and withdraw immediately if there is any indication of recurrent hypersensitivity reaction.

*Renal/Hepatic function impairment:* Monitor patients with active chronic liver disease or severe renal dysfunction.

*Carcinogenesis:* Isoniazid induces pulmonary tumors in a number of strains of mice.

*Pregnancy: Category C.*

*Lactation:* The small concentrations of isoniazid in breast milk do not produce toxicity in the nursing newborn; therefore, do not discourage breastfeeding. However, because levels of isoniazid are so low in breast milk, they cannot be relied upon for prophylaxis or therapy in nursing infants.

## Precautions

*Laboratory tests:* Because there is a higher frequency of isoniazid-associated hepatitis among certain patient groups, obtain transaminase measurements prior to starting and monthly during preventative therapy, or more frequently as needed. If any of the values exceed 3 to 5 times the upper limit of normal, temporarily discontinue isoniazid and consider restarting therapy.

*Periodic ophthalmologic examinations:* Periodic ophthalmologic examinations during isoniazid therapy are recommended even when visual symptoms do not occur.

*Pyridoxine administration:* Pyridoxine administration is recommended in individuals likely to develop peripheral neuropathies secondary to INH therapy. Prophylactic doses of 10 to 25 mg of pyridoxine daily have been recommended.

### Drug Interactions

Drugs that may interact with isoniazid include acetaminophen, carbamazepine, chlorzoxazone, disulfiram, enflurane, hydantoins, ketoconazole, rifampin, and theophylline.

*Drug/Food interactions:* Rate and extent of INH absorption is decreased by food.

### Adverse Reactions

Toxic effects are usually encountered with higher doses of isoniazid; the most frequent are those affecting the nervous system and the liver.

Adverse reactions include pyridoxine deficiency; hyperglycemia; gynecomastia; peripheral neuropathy; convulsions; optic neuritis and atrophy; memory impairment; toxic psychosis; nausea; vomiting; epigastric distress; elevated AST, ALT; bilirubinemia; jaundice; anorexia; fatigue; malaise; weakness; agranulocytosis; hemolytic, sideroblastic, or aplastic anemia; thrombocytopenia; eosinophilia; fever; skin eruptions; lymphadenopathy; vasculitis.

# RIFAMPIN

| | |
|---|---|
| **Capsules:** 150 and 300 mg (*Rx*) | Various, *Rifadin* (Aventis), *Rimactane* (Novartis) |
| **Powder for injection:** 600 mg (*Rx*) | *Rifadin* (Aventis) |

### Indications

*Tuberculosis:*

   *Oral* – Oral treatment is for all forms of tuberculosis. A 3-drug regimen consisting of rifampin, isoniazid, and pyrazinamide is recommended in the initial phase of short-course therapy that is usually continued for 2 months.

   *IV* – Initial treatment and retreatment of tuberculosis when the drug cannot be taken by mouth.

*Neisseria meningitidis carriers:* Treatment of asymptomatic carriers of *N. meningitidis* to eliminate meningococci from the nasopharynx. Not indicated for treatment of meningococcal infection.

### Administration and Dosage

*Oral:* Administer once daily, either 1 hour before or 2 hours after meals.

   Data is not available to determine dosage for children younger than 5 years of age.

*Oral and IV:*

   *Tuberculosis: Adults* – 10 mg/kg in a single daily administration not to exceed 600 mg once daily.

   *Children* – 10 to 20 mg/kg, not to exceed 600 mg/day.

*The 2-month regimen:* According to the MMWR, the 2-month daily regimen of rifampin and pyrazinamide is recommended in HIV-infected people. However, the drug toxicities may be increased.

*The 4-month regimen:* According to the MMWR, rifampin given daily for 3 months has resulted in better protection than placebo in treatment of LTBI in non-HIV patients with silicosis in a randomized prospective trial. However, because the patients receiving rifampin had a high rate of active tuberculosis (4%), experts have concluded that a 4-month regimen would be more prudent when using rifampin alone. This option may be useful for patients who cannot tolerate isoniazid or pyrazinamide.

*The 6-month regimen:* Ordinarily this consists of an initial 2-month phase of rifampin, isoniazid, and pyrazinamide and, if clinically indicated, streptomycin or ethambutol, followed by 4 months of rifampin and isoniazid. Reassess the need for a fourth drug when the results of susceptibility testing are known. If community rates of INH resistance are currently less than 4%, an initial treatment regimen with less than 4 drugs may be considered. Continue treatment for more than 6 months if the patient is still sputum- or culture-positive, if resistant organisms are present, or if the patient is HIV positive.

*Meningococcal carriers:* Once daily for 4 consecutive days in the following doses:

*Adults* – 600 mg.

*Children* – 10 to 20 mg/kg, not to exceed 600 mg/day.

*The following dosage has also been recommended –*

*Adults:* 600 mg every 12 hours for 2 days.

*Children (1 month of age and older):* 10 mg/kg every 12 hours for 2 days.

*Children (younger than 1 month of age):* 5 mg/kg every 12 hours for 2 days.

## Actions

*Pharmacology:* Rifampin inhibits DNA-dependent RNA polymerase activity in susceptible cells. Specifically, it interacts with bacterial RNA polymerase, but does not inhibit the mammalian enzyme. Cross-resistance has only been shown with other rifamycins. Rifampin at therapeutic levels has demonstrated bactericidal activity against intracellular and extracellular *Mycobacterium tuberculosis* organisms.

*Pharmacokinetics:*

Oral –

*Absorption/Distribution:* Rifampin is almost completely absorbed and achieves mean peak plasma levels within 1 to 4 hours. Absorption of rifampin is reduced by approximately 30% when the drug is ingested with food.

*Metabolism:* Rifampin is metabolized in the liver by deacetylation; the metabolite is still active against *Mycobacterium tuberculosis.* About 40% is excreted in bile and undergoes enterohepatic circulation; however, the deacetylated metabolite is poorly absorbed. The half-life is approximately 3 hours after a 600 mg oral dose, up to 5.1 after a 900 mg oral dose. With repeated administration, the half-life decreases and averages approximately 2 to 3 hours.

*Excretion:* Elimination occurs mainly through the bile and, to a much lesser extent, the urine. Dosage adjustment is not necessary in renal failure, but is with hepatic dysfunction. Rifampin is not significantly removed by hemodialysis.

## Contraindications

Hypersensitivity to any rifamycin.

## Warnings

*Hepatotoxicity:* There have been fatalities associated with jaundice in patients with liver disease or patients receiving rifampin concomitantly with other hepatotoxic agents. Carefully monitor liver function, especially AST and ALT, prior to therapy and then every 2 to 4 weeks during therapy.

*Hyperbilirubinemia:* Hyperbilirubinemia, resulting from competition between rifampin and bilirubin for excretory pathways of the liver at the cell level, can occur in early days of treatment.

*Porphyria:* Isolated reports have associated porphyria exacerbation with rifampin administration.

*Meningococci resistance:* The possibility of rapid emergence of resistant meningococci restricts use to short-term treatment of asymptomatic carrier state. Not for treatment of meningococcal disease.

*Hypersensitivity reactions:* Hypersensitivity reactions have occurred during intermittent therapy or when treatment was resumed following accidental or intentional interruption and were reversible with rifampin discontinuation and appropriate therapy.

*Hepatic function impairment:* Dosage adjustment is necessary.

*Pregnancy: Category* C.

*Lactation:* Rifampin is excreted in breast milk.

## Precautions

*Monitoring:* Perform baseline measurements of hepatic enzymes, bilirubin, serum creatinine, CBC, and platelet count (or estimate) in adults treated for tuberculosis with rifampin. Baseline tests are unnecessary in pediatric patients unless a complicating condition is known or clinically suspected.

*Intermittent therapy:* Intermittent therapy may be used if the patient cannot or will not self-administer drugs on a daily basis. Closely monitor patients on intermittent therapy for compliance, and caution against intentional or accidental interruption of prescribed therapy because of increased risk of serious adverse reactions.

Urine, feces, saliva, sputum, sweat, and tears may be colored red-orange. Soft contact lenses may be permanently stained. Advise patients of these possibilities.

*IV:* For IV infusion only. Must not be administered by IM or subcutaneous route.

*Thrombocytopenia:* Thrombocytopenia has occurred, primarily with high dose intermittent therapy, but has also been noted after resumption of interrupted treatment. Cerebral hemorrhage and fatalities have occurred when rifampin administration has continued or resumed after appearance of purpura.

### Drug Interactions

Rifampin is known to induce the hepatic microsomal enzymes that metabolize various drugs such as acetaminophen, oral anticoagulants, barbiturates, benzodiazepines, beta blockers, chloramphenicol, clofibrate, oral contraceptives, corticosteroids, cyclosporine, disopyramide, estrogens, hydantoins, mexiletine, quinidine, sulfones, sulfonylureas, theophyllines, tocainide, verapamil, digoxin, enalapril, morphine, nifedipine, ondansetron, progestins, protease inhibitors, buspirone, delavirdine, doxycycline, fluoroquinolones, losartan, macrolides, sulfonylureas, tacrolimus, thyroid hormones, TCAs, zolpidem, zidovudine, and ketoconazole. The therapeutic effects of these drugs may be decreased.

*Enzyme induction properties:* Rifampin has enzyme induction properties that can enhance the metabolism of endogenous substrates including adrenal hormones, thyroid hormones, and vitamin D. Rifampin and isoniazid have been reported to alter vitamin D metabolism. In some cases, reduced levels of circulating 25-hydroxy vitamin D and 1,25-dihydroxy vitamin D have been accompanied by reduced serum calcium and phosphate, and elevated parathyroid hormone.

*Drug/Lab test interactions:* Therapeutic levels of rifampin inhibit standard assays for serum folate and vitamin $B_{12}$.

Transient abnormalities in liver function tests (eg, elevation in serum bilirubin, alkaline phosphatase, serum transaminases), and reduced biliary excretion of contrast media used for visualization of the gallbladder have also been observed.

*Drug/Food interactions:* Food interferes with the absorption of rifampin, possibly resulting in decreased peak plasma concentrations. Take on an empty stomach with a full glass of water.

### Adverse Reactions

High doses of rifampin (greater than 600 mg) given once or twice weekly have resulted in a high incidence of adverse reactions including the following: "Flu-like" syndrome; hematopoietic reactions; cutaneous, GI, and hepatic reactions; shortness of breath; shock; renal failure; asymptomatic elevations of liver enzymes; rash.

# RIFABUTIN

**Capsules:** 150 mg (*Rx*)                    Mycobutin (Pharmacia)

### Indications

Prevention of disseminated *Mycobacterium avium* complex (MAC) disease in patients with advanced HIV infection.

### Administration and Dosage

*Usual dose:* 300 mg once daily. For those patients with propensity to nausea, vomiting, or other GI upset, administration of rifabutin at doses of 150 mg twice daily taken with food may be useful.

## Actions

*Pharmacology:* Rifabutin, an antimycobacterial agent, is a semisynthetic ansamycin antibiotic derived from rifamycin S. It is not known whether rifabutin inhibits DNA-dependent RNA polymerase in *Mycobacterium avium* or in *Mycobacterium intracellulare* that comprise MAC.

*Pharmacokinetics:* Following a single oral dose of 300 mg to healthy adult volunteers, rifabutin was readily absorbed from the GI tract with mean peak plasma levels attained in 3.3 hours. Plasma concentrations post-$C_{max}$ declined in an apparent biphasic manner. Rifabutin was slowly eliminated from plasma in healthy adult volunteers, presumably because of distribution-limited elimination, with a mean terminal half-life of 45 hours. Although the systemic levels of rifabutin following multiple dosing decreased by 38%, its terminal half-life remained unchanged. Estimates of apparent steady-state distribution volume (9.3 L/kg) in HIV-positive patients, following IV dosing, exceed total body water by approximately 15-fold. About 85% of the drug is bound in a concentration-independent manner to plasma proteins over a concentration range of 0.05 to 1 mcg/mL.

Mean systemic clearance in healthy adult volunteers following a single oral dose was 0.69 L/h/kg; renal and biliary clearance of unchanged drug each contribute approximately 5%. About 30% of the dose is excreted in the feces; 53% of the oral dose is excreted in the urine, primarily as metabolites. Of the five metabolites that have been identified, 25-O-desacetyl and 31-hydroxy are the most predominant, and show a plasma metabolite:parent AUC ratio of 0.1 and 0.07, respectively. The 25-O-desacetyl metabolite has an activity equal to the parent drug and contributes less than or equal to 10% to the total antimicrobial activity.

Absolute bioavailability assessed in HIV-positive patients averaged 20%. Somewhat reduced drug distribution and faster drug elimination in compromised renal function may result in decreased drug concentrations.

## Contraindications

Hypersensitivity to this drug or to any other rifamycins.

## Warnings

*Active tuberculosis:* Rifabutin prophylaxis must not be administered to patients with active tuberculosis. HIV-positive patients are likely to have a nonreactive purified protein derivative (PPD) despite active disease. Chest X-ray, sputum culture, blood culture, urine culture, or biopsy of a suspicious lymph node may be useful in the diagnosis of tuberculosis in the HIV-positive patient.

There is no evidence that rifabutin is effective prophylaxis against M. *tuberculosis.* Patients requiring prophylaxis against both M. *tuberculosis* and M. *avium* complex may be given isoniazid and rifabutin concurrently.

*Pregnancy: Category B.*

*Lactation:* It is not known whether rifabutin is excreted in breast milk. Because of the potential for serious adverse reactions in nursing infants, decide whether to discontinue nursing or discontinue the drug, taking into account the importance of the drug to the mother.

*Children:* Safety and efficacy in children have not been established. Limited safety data are available from treatment use in 22 HIV-positive children with MAC who received rifabutin in combination with at least 2 other antimycobacterials for periods from 1 to 183 weeks. Mean doses (mg/kg) for these children were: 18.5 for infants 1 year of age; 8.6 for children 2 to 10 years of age; and 4 for adolescents 14 to 16 years of age. There is no evidence that doses greater than 5 mg/kg/day are useful.

## Precautions

*Monitoring:* Because rifabutin may be associated with neutropenia, and, more rarely, thrombocytopenia, consider obtaining hematologic studies periodically in patients receiving prophylaxis.

### Drug Interactions

*CYP450:* Rifabutin has liver enzyme-inducing properties. The related drug, rifampin, is known to reduce the activity of a number of other drugs. Because of the structural similarity of rifabutin and rifampin, rifabutin may be expected to have similar interactions. However, unlike rifampin, rifabutin appears not to affect the acetylation of isoniazid. Rifabutin appears to be a less potent enzyme inducer than rifampin. The significance of this finding for clinical drug interactions is not known.

Drugs that may interact with rifabutin include the following: Anticoagulants, azole antifungal agents, benzodiazepines, beta blockers, buspirone, corticosteroids, cyclosporine, delavirdine, doxycycline, hydantoins, indinavir, rifamycins, losartan, macrolide antibiotics, methadone, morphine, nelfinavir, quinine, quinidine, theophylline, aminophylline, tricyclic antidepressants, and zolpidem.

*Drug/Food interactions:* High-fat meals slow the rate of absorption without influencing the extent.

### Adverse Reactions

Rifabutin is generally well tolerated. Discontinuation of therapy because of an adverse event was required in 16% of patients receiving rifabutin vs 8% with placebo.

Adverse reactions occurring in at least 3% of patients include the following: Abdominal pain, headache, diarrhea, dyspepsia, eructation, nausea, vomiting, rash, taste perversion, discolored urine, increased AST and ALT, anemia, leukopenia, neutropenia, and thrombocytopenia.

# ETHAMBUTOL HCl

| **Tablets:** 100 and 400 mg (*Rx*) | *Myambutol* (X-Gen) |
|---|---|

### Indications

*Pulmonary tuberculosis:* Use in conjunction with at least 1 other antituberculosis drug(s). In patients who have received previous therapy, mycobacterial resistance to other drugs used in initial therapy is frequent. In retreatment patients, combine ethambutol with at least 1 of the second-line drug(s) not previously administered to the patient, and to which bacterial susceptibility has been indicated.

### Administration and Dosage

Do not use ethambutol alone. Administer once every 24 hours only. Absorption is not significantly altered by administration with food. Continue therapy until bacteriological conversion has become permanent and maximal clinical improvement has occurred.

*Initial treatment:* In patients who have not received previous antituberculosis therapy, administer 15 mg/kg (7 mg/lb) as a single oral dose once every 24 hours. Isoniazid has been administered concurrently in a single, daily oral dose.

*Retreatment:* In patients who have received previous antituberculosis therapy, administer 25 mg/kg (11 mg/lb) as a single oral dose once every 24 hours. Concurrently administer at least 1 other antituberculosis drug(s) to which the organisms have been demonstrated to be susceptible by in vitro tests. Suitable drugs usually include those not previously used in the treatment of the patient. After 60 days of administration, decrease the dose to 15 mg/kg and administer as a single oral dose once every 24 hours.

*Children:* Not recommended for use in children younger than 13 years of age.

### Actions

*Pharmacology:* Ethambutol diffuses into actively growing mycobacterium cells such as tubercle bacilli. It inhibits the synthesis of at least 1 metabolite, thus causing impairment of cell metabolism, arrest of multiplication, and cell death. No cross-resistance with other agents has been demonstrated.

*Pharmacokinetics:*

*Absorption/Distribution* – Ethambutol absorption is not influenced by food. Following a single oral dose of 15 to 25 mg/kg, ethambutol attains a peak of 2 to 5 mcg/mL in serum 2 to 4 hours after administration. Serum levels are similar after prolonged dosing. The serum level is undetectable 24 hours after the last dose except in some patients with abnormal renal function.

*Metabolism* – During the 24 hours following oral administration, approximately 20% of ethambutol is metabolized by the liver.

*Excretion* – Unchanged drug is excreted (approximately 50%) in the urine, 8% to 15% as metabolites and 20% to 22% unchanged in the feces. Marked accumulation may occur with renal insufficiency. Ethambutol is not significantly removed by hemodialysis.

## Contraindications

Hypersensitivity to ethambutol; known optic neuritis, unless clinical judgment determines that it may be used.

## Warnings

*Renal function impairment:* Patients with decreased renal function require reduced dosage (as determined by serum levels) because this drug is excreted by the kidneys.

*Pregnancy: Category B.*

*Children:* Not recommended for use in children younger than 13 years of age.

## Precautions

*Monitoring:* Perform periodic assessment of renal, hepatic, and hematopoietic systems during long-term therapy.

*Visual effects:* This drug may have adverse effects on vision. The effects are generally reversible when the drug is discontinued promptly. Perform testing before beginning therapy and periodically during drug administration (monthly when a patient is receiving more than 15 mg/kg/day).

Advise patients to report promptly any change in visual acuity. If evaluation confirms visual change and fails to reveal other causes, discontinue drug and reevaluate patient at frequent intervals.

## Drug Interactions

*Aluminum salts:* Aluminum salts may delay and reduce the absorption of ethambutol. Separate their administration by several hours.

## Adverse Reactions

Adverse reactions may include anaphylactoid reactions, dermatitis, pruritus, decreases in visual acuity, anorexia, nausea, vomiting, GI upset, abdominal pain, fever, malaise, headache, dizziness, mental confusion, disorientation, possible hallucinations, peripheral neuritis, elevated serum uric acid levels, precipitation of acute gout, transient impairment of liver function, and joint pain.

# PYRAZINAMIDE

**Tablets:** 500 mg *(Rx)*                    *Pyrazinamide (UDL, ESI)*

## Indications

*Tuberculosis:* Initial treatment of active tuberculosis in adults and children when combined with other antituberculosis agents.

The current CDC recommendation for drug-susceptible initial treatment of active tuberculosis disease is a 6-month regimen consisting of isoniazid, rifampin, and pyrazinamide given for 2 months, followed by isoniazid and rifampin for 4 months.

*Treatment failure:* After treatment failure with other primary drugs in any form of active tuberculosis.

## Administration and Dosage

Administer pyrazinamide with other effective antituberculosis drugs. It is administered for the initial 2 months of a 6-month or longer treatment regimen for drug susceptible patients. Treat patients who are known or suspected to have drug-resistant disease with regimens individualized to their situation. Pyrazinamide frequently will be an important component of such therapy.

*HIV infection:* Patients with concomitant HIV infection may require longer courses of therapy. Be alert to any revised recommendations from CDC for this group of patients.

*Usual dose:* 15 to 30 mg/kg once daily. Do not exceed 2 g/day.

*Alternative dosing:* Alternatively, a twice weekly dosing regimen (50 to 70 mg/kg twice weekly based on lean body weight) has been developed to promote patient compliance on an outpatient basis. In studies evaluating the twice weekly regimen, doses of pyrazinamide in excess of 3 g twice weekly have been administered without an increased incidence of adverse reactions.

### Actions
*Pharmacology:* Pyrazinamide, the pyrazine analog of nicotinamide, may be bacteriostatic or bactericidal against *Mycobacterium tuberculosis* depending on the concentration of the drug attained at the site of infection. The mechanism of action is unknown.

*Pharmacokinetics:*

*Absorption/Distribution* – Pyrazinamide is well absorbed from the GI tract and attains peak plasma concentrations within 2 hours. It is widely distributed in body tissues and fluids including the liver, lungs, and cerebrospinal fluid. Pyrizinamide is approximately 10% bound to plasma proteins.

*Metabolism/Excretion* – The half-life is 9 to 10 hours; it may be prolonged in patients with impaired renal or hepatic function.

Approximately 70% of an oral dose is excreted in urine, mainly by glomerular filtration, within 24 hours. Pyrazinamide is significantly dialyzed and should be dosed after hemodialysis.

### Contraindications
Severe hepatic damage; hypersensitivity; acute gout.

### Warnings
*Combination therapy:* Use only in conjunction with other effective antituberculosis agents.

*Hyperuricemia:* Pyrazinamide inhibits renal excretion of urates, frequently resulting in hyperuricemia that is usually asymptomatic. Patients started on pyrazinamide should have baseline serum uric acid determinations. Discontinue the drug and do not resume if signs of hyperuricemia accompanied by acute gouty arthritis appear.

*Renal function impairment:* It does not appear that patients with impaired renal function require a reduction in dose. It may be prudent to select doses at the low end of the dosing range, however.

*Hepatic function impairment:* Patients started on pyrazinamide should have baseline liver function determinations. Closely follow those patients with pre-existing liver disease or those at increased risk for drug-related hepatitis. Discontinue pyrazinamide and do not resume if signs of hepatocellular damage appear.

*Elderly:* In general, dose selection for an elderly patient should be cautious, usually starting at the low end of the dosing range, reflecting the greater frequency of decreased hepatic or renal function, and of concomitant disease or other drug therapy.

*Pregnancy: Category* C.

*Lactation:* Pyrazinamide has been found in small amounts in breast milk. Therefore, it is advised that pyrazinamide be used with caution in nursing mothers, taking into account the risk-benefit of this therapy.

*Children:* Pyrazinamide appears to be well tolerated in children.

### Precautions
*Monitoring:* Determine baseline liver function studies and uric acid levels prior to therapy. Perform appropriate laboratory testing at periodic intervals and if any clinical signs or symptoms occur during therapy.

*HIV infection:* In patients with concomitant HIV infection, be aware of current recommendations of CDC. It is possible these patients may require a longer course of treatment.

*Diabetes mellitus:* Use with caution in patients with a history of diabetes mellitus, as management may be more difficult.

*Primary resistance of M. tuberculosis:* Primary resistance of M. *tuberculosis* to pyrazinamide is uncommon. In cases with known or suspected drug resistance, perform in vitro susceptibility tests with recent cultures of M. *tuberculosis* against pyrazinamide and the usual primary drugs.

### Drug Interactions
*Drug/Lab test interactions:* Pyrazinamide has been reported to interfere with *Acetest* and *Ketostix* urine tests to produce a pink-brown color.

### Adverse Reactions
Adverse reactions may include the following: Fever; porphyria; dysuria; gout; hepatic reaction; nausea; vomiting; anorexia; thrombocytopenia and sideroblastic anemia with erythroid hyperplasia; vacuolation of erythrocytes; increased serum iron concentration; adverse effects on blood clotting mechanisms; mild arthralgia and myalgia; hypersensitivity reactions including rashes, urticaria, pruritus; fever; acne; photosensitivity; porphyria; dysuria; interstitial nephritis.

# AMINOSALICYLATE SODIUM (Para-Aminosalicylate Sodium)

| **Granules, delayed-release:** 4 g (*Rx*) | *Paser* (Jacobus Pharm.) |
| --- | --- |

Refer to the general discussion in the Antituberculosal Agents introduction.

### Indications
*Tuberculosis:* Treatment of tuberculosis in combination with other active agents. It is most commonly used in patients with multi-drug resistant tuberculosis (MDR-TB) or in situations when therapy with isoniazid and rifampin is not possible because of a combination of resistance and intolerance.

### Administration and Dosage
*Tuberculosis:* The adult dosage of 4 g (1 packet) 3 times/day, or correspondingly smaller doses in children, is to be taken without chewing by sprinkling on applesauce or yogurt or by swirling in the glass to suspend the granules in an acidic drink such as tomato or orange juice or food such as applesauce or yogurt. The coating will last at least 2 hours.

Do not use if packet is swollen or the granules have lost their tan color, turning dark brown or purple.

### Actions
*Pharmacology:* Aminosalicylic acid is bacteriostatic against *Mycobacterium tuberculosis*. It inhibits the onset of bacterial resistance to streptomycin and isoniazid. The mechanism of action has been postulated to be inhibition of folic acid synthesis (but without potentiation with antifolic compounds) or inhibition of synthesis of the cell wall component, mycobactin, thus reducing iron uptake by M. *tuberculosis*.

*Pharmacokinetics:*
    *Absorption/Distribution* – In a single 4 g pharmacokinetic study with food in normal volunteers, the initial time to a 2 mcg/mL serum level of aminosalicylic acid was 2 hours; the median time to peak was 6 hours; the mean peak level was 20 mcg/mL; a level of 2 mcg/mL was maintained for an average of 7.9 hours; a level of 1 mcg/mL was maintained for an average of 6.8 hours. Approximately 50% to 60% of aminosalicylic acid is protein-bound; binding is reported to be reduced 50% in kwashiorkor.
    *Excretion* – 80% of aminosalicylic acid is excreted in the urine by glomerular filtration, with at least 50% of the dosage excreted in acetylated form.

**Contraindications**
Hypersensitivity to any component of this medication; severe renal disease.

**Warnings**
*Hepatitis:* In 1 retrospective study of 7492 patients on rapidly absorbed aminosalicylic acid preparations, drug-induced hepatitis occurred in 38 patients (0.5%); in these 38, the first symptom usually appeared within 3 months of the start of therapy with a rash as the most common event followed by fever and much less frequently by GI disturbances of anorexia, nausea, or diarrhea.

*Hypersensitivity reactions:* Stop all drugs at the first sign suggesting a hypersensitivity reaction. They may be restarted one at a time in very small but gradually increasing doses to determine whether the manifestations are drug-induced and, if so, which drug is responsible.

Desensitization has been accomplished successfully.

*Renal function impairment:* Patients with severe renal disease will accumulate amino-salicylic acid and its acetyl metabolite but will continue to acetylate, thus leading exclusively to the inactive acetylated form; deacetylation, if any, is not significant. Patients with end-stage renal disease should not receive aminosalicylic acid.

*Hepatic function impairment:* Use with caution.

*Pregnancy:* Category C.

*Lactation:* Aminosalicylic acid is excreted in breast milk.

**Precautions**
*Malabsorption syndrome:* A malabsorption syndrome can develop in patients on amino-salicylic acid but usually is not complete.

*Lab test abnormalities:* Aminosalicylic acid has been reported to interfere technically with the serum determinations of albumin by dye-binding AST by the azoene dye method and with qualitative urine tests for ketones, bilirubin, urobilinogen, or porphobilinogen.

Crystalluria may develop and can be prevented by the maintenance of urine at a neutral or alkaline pH.

**Drug Interactions**
Aminosalicylic acid may affect isoniazid, digoxin, and vitamin $B_{12}$.

**Adverse Reactions**
*GI:* The most common side effect is GI intolerance manifested by nausea, vomiting, diarrhea, and abdominal pain.

*Hypersensitivity:* Fever, skin eruptions of various types, including exfoliative dermatitis, infectious mononucleosis-like, or lymphoma-like syndrome, leukopenia, agranulocytosis, thrombocytopenia, Coombs' positive hemolytic anemia, jaundice, hepatitis, pericarditis, hypoglycemia, optic neuritis, encephalopathy, Leoffler's syndrome, vasculitis, and a reduction in prothrombin.

# ETHIONAMIDE

| **Tablets:** 250 mg (Rx) | *Trecator-SC* (Wyeth-Ayerst) |
|---|---|

**Indications**
Recommended for any form of active tuberculosis when treatment with first-line drugs (isoniazid, rifampin) has failed. Use only with other effective antituberculosis agents.

**Administration and Dosage**
Administer with at least 1 other effective antituberculosis drug(s).

*Average adult dose:* 15 to 20 mg/kg/day taken once daily up to a maximum of 1 g/day.

*Children:* A dose of 10 to 20 mg/kg/day in 2 to 3 divided doses given after meals or 15 mg/kg/24 hours as a single daily dose has been recommended.

Concomitant administration of pyridoxine is recommended.

## Actions

*Pharmacology:* Ethionamide may be bacteriostatic or bactericidal in action, depending on the concentration of the drug attained at the site of infection and the susceptibility of the infecting organism. The exact mechanism of action of ethionamide has not been fully elucidated, but the drug appears to inhibit peptide synthesis in susceptible organisms.

*Pharmacokinetics:*

*Absorption/Distribution* – Ethionamide is essentially completely absorbed following oral administration and is not subjected to any appreciable first pass metabolism.

The drug is approximately 30% bound to plasma proteins. Ethionamide is rapidly and widely distributed into body tissues and fluids, with concentrations in plasma and various organs being approximately equal. Significant concentrations also are present in cerebrospinal fluid.

*Metabolism/Excretion* – Ethionamide is extensively metabolized to active and inactive metabolites with less than 1% excreted as the free form in urine. Ethionamide has a plasma elimination half-life of approximately 2 hours after oral dosing.

*Monitoring* – Normal serum concentrations of 1 to 5 mcg/mL are usually seen 2 hours following doses of 250 to 500 mg and approximate the therapeutic range for this drug.

## Contraindications

Severe hypersensitivity to ethionamide; severe hepatic damage.

## Warnings

*Resistance:* The use of ethionamide alone in the treatment of tuberculosis results in rapid development of resistance.

*Compliance:* It is recommended that directly observed therapy be practiced when patients are receiving antituberculosis medication.

*Pregnancy: Category C.*

*Lactation:* Because no information is available on the excretion of ethionamide in breast milk, administer to nursing mothers only if the benefits outweigh the risks.

*Children:* Investigations have been limited; do not use in pediatric patients younger than 12 years of age except when the organisms are definitely resistant to primary therapy and systemic dissemination of the disease, or other life-threatening complications of tuberculosis, is judged to be imminent.

## Precautions

*Monitoring:* Make determinations of serum transaminase (AST, ALT) prior to and monthly during therapy. Monitor blood glucose and thyroid function tests periodically.

## Drug Interactions

Ethionamide may interact with isoniazid and cycloserine.

## Adverse Reactions

Adverse reactions may include the following: Depression; drowsiness and asthenia; convulsions; peripheral neuritis and neuropathy; olfactory disturbances; blurred vision; diplopia; optic neuritis; dizziness; headache; restlessness; tremors; psychosis; anorexia; nausea and vomiting; diarrhea; metallic taste; hepatitis; jaundice; stomatitis; postural hypotension; skin rash; acne; alopecia; thrombocytopenia; pellagra-like syndrome; gynecomastia; impotence; menorrhagia; and increased difficulty managing diabetes mellitus.

# CYCLOSERINE

**Capsules**: 250 mg *(Rx)*                    *Seromycin Pulvules* (Dura)

## Indications

Treatment of active pulmonary and extrapulmonary tuberculosis (including renal disease) when organisms are susceptible, after failure of adequate treatment with the primary medications. Use in conjunction with other effective chemotherapy.

May be effective in the treatment of acute urinary tract infections caused by susceptible strains of gram-positive and gram-negative bacteria, especially *Enterobacter* sp. and *Escherichia coli.* It usually is less effective than other antimicrobial agents in the treatment of urinary tract infections caused by bacteria other than mycobacteria. Consider using only when the more conventional therapy has failed and when the organism has demonstrated sensitivity.

### Administration and Dosage

Administer 500 mg to 1 g daily in divided doses monitored by blood levels. The usual initial dosage is 250 mg twice daily at 12-hour intervals for the first 2 weeks. Do not exceed 1 g/day.

Pyridoxine 200 to 300 mg/day may prevent the neurotoxic effects.

### Actions

*Pharmacology:* Inhibits cell-wall synthesis in susceptible strains of gram-positive and gram-negative bacteria and in *Mycobacterium tuberculosis.*

*Pharmacokinetics:*

*Absorption/Distribution* – When given orally, cycloserine is rapidly absorbed, reaching peak plasma concentrations in 4 to 8 hours. It is widely distributed throughout body fluids and tissues; cerebrospinal fluid levels are similar to plasma.

*Metabolism/Excretion* – Approximately 35% of the drug is metabolized; 50% of a parenteral dose is excreted unchanged in the urine in the first 12 hours. About 65% of the drug is recoverable in 72 hours.

### Contraindications

Hypersensitivity to cycloserine; epilepsy; depression; severe anxiety; psychosis; severe renal insufficiency; excessive concurrent use of alcohol.

### Warnings

*CNS toxicity:* Discontinue or reduce dosage if patient develops symptoms of CNS toxicity, such as convulsions, psychosis, somnolence, depression, confusion, hyperreflexia, headache, tremor, vertigo, paresis, or dysarthria. The risk of convulsions is increased in chronic alcoholics.

*Allergic dermatitis:* Discontinue the drug or reduce dosage if patient develops allergic dermatitis.

*Toxicity:* Toxicity is closely related to excessive blood levels (more than 30 mcg/mL) that are caused by high dosage or inadequate renal clearance. The therapeutic index in tuberculosis is small.

*Renal function impairment:* Patients will accumulate cycloserine and may develop toxicity if the dosage regimen is not modified. Patients with severe impairment should not receive the drug.

*Pregnancy:* Category C.

*Lactation:* Because of the potential for serious adverse reactions in nursing infants, decide whether to discontinue nursing or to discontinue the drug.

*Children:* Safety and dosage not established for pediatric use.

### Precautions

*Monitoring:* Monitor patients by hematologic, renal excretion, blood level, and liver function studies.

*Obtain cultures:* Obtain cultures and determine susceptibility before treatment.

*Determine blood levels:* Determine blood levels weekly for patients having reduced renal function, for individuals receiving more than 500 mg/day, and for those with symptoms of toxicity. Adjust dosage to maintain blood level less than 30 mcg/mL.

*Anticonvulsant drugs or sedatives:* Anticonvulsant drugs or sedatives may be effective in controlling symptoms of CNS toxicity, such as convulsions, anxiety, and tremor. Closely observe patients receiving more than 500 mg/day for such symptoms. Pyridoxine may prevent CNS toxicity, but its efficacy has not been proven.

*Anemia:* Administration has been associated in a few cases with vitamin $B_{12}$ or folic acid deficiency, megaloblastic anemia, and sideroblastic anemia. If evidence of anemia develops, institute appropriate studies and therapy.

### Drug Interactions

Drugs that may interact with cycloserine include alcohol, ethionamide, and isoniazid.

### Adverse Reactions

Adverse reactions related to more than 500 mg/day may include the following: Convulsions; drowsiness and somnolence; headache; tremor; dysarthria; vertigo; confusion and disorientation with loss of memory; psychoses, possibly with suicidal tendencies, character changes, hyperirritability, aggression; paresis; hyperreflexia; paresthesias; major and minor (localized) clonic seizures; coma; sudden development of CHF; skin rash; and elevated transaminase.

# STREPTOMYCIN SULFATE

| **Cake, lyophilized**: 1 g | *Streptomycin Sulfate* (Pharma-Tek) |
|---|---|

Also refer to the streptomycin sulfate monograph in the Aminoglycosides, Parenteral section.

---

**Warning:**

The risk of severe neurotoxic reactions is sharply increased in patients with impaired renal function or prerenal azotemia. These include disturbances of vestibular and cochlear function, optic nerve dysfunction, peripheral neuritis, arachnoiditis, and encephalopathy. The incidence of clinically detectable, irreversible vestibular damage is particularly high in patients treated with streptomycin.

Monitor renal function carefully; patients with renal impairment and/or nitrogen retention should receive reduced doses. Do not exceed peak serum concentrations of 20 to 25 mcg/mL in individuals with kidney damage.

Avoid concurrent or sequential use of other neurotoxic and/or nephrotoxic drugs with streptomycin sulfate, including neomycin, kanamycin, gentamicin, cephaloridine, paromomycin, viomycin, polymyxin B, colistin, tobramycin, and cyclosporine.

The neurotoxicity of streptomycin can result in respiratory paralysis from neuromuscular blockage, especially when the drug is given soon after the use of anesthesia or muscle relaxants. Reserve the administration of streptomycin in parenteral form for patients where adequate laboratory and audiometric testing facilities are available during therapy.

---

### Indications

*Mycobacterium tuberculosis:* Add streptomycin or ethambutol as a fourth drug in a regimen containing isoniazid (INH), rifampin, and pyrazinamide for initial treatment of tuberculosis unless the likelihood of INH or rifampin resistance is very low.

Streptomycin also is indicated for therapy of tuberculosis when one or more of the above drugs is contraindicated because of toxicity or intolerance.

For more indications, see individual monograph in Aminoglycosides, Parenteral section.

### Administration and Dosage

*Skin sensitivity:* Take care handling streptomycin for injection to avoid skin sensitivity reactions. As with all IM preparations, inject streptomycin sulfate injection well within the body of a relatively large muscle and take care to minimize the possibility of damage to peripheral nerves.

Administer by the IM route only.

*Adults:* The preferred IM injection site is the upper outer quadrant of the buttock (ie, gluteus maximus) or the mid-lateral thigh.

*Children:* It is recommended that IM injections be given preferably in the mid-lateral muscles of the thigh. In infants and small children, use the periphery of the upper outer quadrant of the gluteal region only when necessary, such as in burn patients, in order to minimize the possibility of damage to the sciatic nerve.

*Tuberculosis:* The standard regimen for the treatment of drug-susceptible tuberculosis has been 2 months of INH, rifampin, and pyrazinamide followed by 4 months of INH and rifampin (patients with concomitant infection with tuberculosis and HIV may require treatment for a longer period). When streptomycin is added to this regimen because of suspected or proven drug resistance, the recommended dosing for streptomycin is as follows:

| Streptomycin Recommended Dosing | | | |
| --- | --- | --- | --- |
| Patient | Daily | Twice daily | 3 times/wk |
| Children | 20 to 40 mg/kg; max, 1 g | 25 to 30 mg/kg; max, 1.5 g | 25 to 30 mg/kg; max, 1.5 g |
| Adults | 15 mg/kg; max, 1 g | 25 to 30 mg/kg; max, 1.5 g | 25 to 30 mg/kg; max, 1.5 g |

Streptomycin usually is administered daily as a single IM injection. Give a total dose of not more than 120 g over the course of therapy unless there are no other therapeutic options. In patients older than 60 years of age, reduce dosage because of the risk of increased toxicity (see Warning Box).

As with other aminoglycosides, reduce dosage in impaired renal function.

### Actions

*Pharmacology:* Streptomycin sulfate is a bactericidal antibiotic that interferes with normal protein synthesis.

*Pharmacokinetics:* Following IM injection of 1 g of streptomycin as the sulfate, a peak serum level of 25 to 50 mcg/mL is reached within 1 hour, diminishing slowly to about 50% after 5 to 6 hours. Appreciable concentrations are found in all organ tissues except the brain. Streptomycin is excreted by glomerular filtration.

### Contraindications

Hypersensitivity to streptomycin sulfate or any other aminoglycoside.

### Warnings

*Ototoxicity:* Vestibular and auditory dysfunction can follow the administration of streptomycin. The degree of impairment is directly proportional to the dose and duration of streptomycin administration, the age of the patient, the level of renal function, and the amount of underlying existing auditory dysfunction.

*Renal function impairment:* Exercise extreme caution in patients with pre-existing renal insufficiency.

*Pregnancy: Category D.*

*Lactation:* Because of the potential for serious adverse reactions in nursing infants from streptomycin, decide whether to discontinue nursing or to discontinue the drug, taking into account the importance of the drug to the mother.

*Children:*
   Infants – A syndrome of apparent CNS depression, characterized by stupor and flaccidity, occasionally coma, and deep respiratory depression, has been reported in young infants in whom streptomycin dosage had exceed the recommended limits. Do not give infants streptomycin in excess of the recommended dosage.

### Precautions

*Monitoring:* Baseline and periodic caloric stimulation tests and audiometric tests are advisable with extended streptomycin therapy. Tinnitus, roaring noises, or a sense of fullness in the ears indicates need for audiometric examination, termination of streptomycin therapy, or both.

*Superinfection:* Use of this drug may result in overgrowth of nonsusceptible organisms, including fungi.

**Drug Interactions**

The ototoxic effects of streptomycin are potentiated by the coadministration of ethacrynic acid, furosemide, mannitol, and possibly other diuretics.

**Adverse Reactions**

The following reactions are common: Vestibular ototoxicity (eg, nausea, vomiting, vertigo); paresthesia of face; rash; fever; urticaria; angioneurotic edema; eosinophilia.

The following reactions are less frequent: Cochlear ototoxicity (deafness); exfoliative dermatitis; anaphylaxis; azotemia; leukopenia; thrombocytopenia; pancytopenia; hemolytic anemia; muscular weakness; amblyopia; nephrotoxicity (rare).

*Vestibular dysfunction* – Vestibular dysfunction resulting from the parenteral administration of streptomycin is cumulatively related to the total daily dose.

# CAPREOMYCIN

**Powder for injection:** 1 g (as sulfate)/10 mL vial (*Rx*)          *Capastat Sulfate* (Dura)

---

**Warning:**

Undertake the use of capreomycin in patients with renal insufficiency or preexisting auditory impairment with great caution. Weigh the risk of additional eighth nerve impairment or renal injury against benefits to be derived from therapy.

Because other parenteral antituberculosis agents (eg, streptomycin, viomycin) also have similar and sometimes irreversible toxic effects, particularly on eighth cranial nerve and renal function, simultaneous administration of these agents with capreomycin is not recommended. Use concurrent nonantituberculosis drugs (eg, polymyxin A sulfate, colistin sulfate, amikacin, gentamicin, tobramycin, vancomycin, kanamycin, neomycin) having ototoxic or nephrotoxic potential only with great caution.

---

**Indications**

Intended for use concomitantly with other antituberculosis agents in pulmonary infections caused by capreomycin-susceptible strains of *Mycobacterium tuberculosis*, when the primary agents (eg, isoniazid, rifampin) have been ineffective or cannot be used because of toxicity or the presence of resistant tubercle bacilli.

**Administration and Dosage**

May be administered IM or IV following reconstitution.

*IV:* For IV infusion, further dilute reconstituted capreomycin solution in 100 mL of 0.9% Sodium Chloride Injection and administer over 60 minutes.

*IM:* Give reconstituted capreomycin by deep IM injection into a large muscle mass; superficial injections may be associated with increased pain and sterile abscesses.

*Usual dose:* 1 g daily (not to exceed 20 mg/kg/day) given IM or IV for 60 to 120 days, followed by 1 g by either route 2 or 3 times weekly.

*Renal function impairment:* Reduce the dosage based on Ccr using the guidelines in the table. These dosages are designed to achieve a mean steady-state capreomycin level of 10 mcg/L.

| Capreomycin Dosage in Renal Function Impairment | | | | | |
|---|---|---|---|---|---|
| Ccr (mL/min) | Capreomycin clearance (L/kg/h×10⁻²) | Half-life (hours) | Dose[1] (mg/kg) for the following dosing intervals | | |
| | | | 24 h | 48 h | 72 h |
| 0 | 0.54 | 55.5 | 1.29 | 2.58 | 3.87 |
| 10 | 1.01 | 29.4 | 2.43 | 4.87 | 7.30 |

| Capreomycin Dosage in Renal Function Impairment | | | | | |
|---|---|---|---|---|---|
| Ccr (mL/min) | Capreomycin clearance (L/kg/h×10$^{-2}$) | Half-life (hours) | Dose[1] (mg/kg) for the following dosing intervals | | |
| | | | 24 h | 48 h | 72 h |
| 20 | 1.49 | 20.0 | 3.58 | 7.16 | 10.7 |
| 30 | 1.97 | 15.1 | 4.72 | 9.45 | 14.2 |
| 40 | 2.45 | 12.2 | 5.87 | 11.7 | |
| 50 | 2.92 | 10.2 | 7.01 | 14 | |
| 60 | 3.40 | 8.8 | 8.16 | | |
| 80 | 4.35 | 6.8 | 10.4[2] | | |
| 100 | 5.31 | 5.6 | 12.7[2] | | |
| 110 | 5.78 | 5.2 | 13.9[2] | | |

[1] Initial maintenance dose estimates are given for optional dosing intervals; longer dosing intervals are expected to provide greater peak and lower trough serum capreomycin levels than shorter dosing intervals.

[2] The usual dosage for patients with normal renal function is 1 g daily, not to exceed 20 mg/kg/day, for 60 to 120 days, then 1 g 2 to 3 times weekly.

## Actions

*Pharmacology:* A polypeptide antibiotic isolated from *Streptomyces capreolus*.

*Pharmacokinetics:*

*Absorption* – Capreomycin sulfate is not absorbed in significant quantities from the GI tract and must be administered parenterally. The AUC is similar for single-dose capreomycin (1 g) administered IM and by IV (over 1 hour) routes of administration. Capreomycin peak concentrations after IV infusion were approximately 30% higher than after IM administration.

*Distribution* – Peak serum concentrations following IM administration of 1 g are achieved in 1 to 2 hours. Low serum concentrations are present at 24 hours. Doses of 1 g daily for 30 days or longer produce no significant accumulation in subjects with normal renal function.

*Excretion* – Capreomycin is excreted essentially unaltered; 52% is excreted in the urine within 12 hours.

## Contraindications

Hypersensitivity to capreomycin.

## Warnings

*Hypersensitivity reactions:* Has occurred when capreomycin and other antituberculosis drugs were given concomitantly.

*Renal function impairment:* Dosage reduction is necessary. See Administration and Dosage.

*Pregnancy:* Category C.

*Lactation:* It is not known whether this drug is excreted in breast milk.

*Children:* Safety for use in infants and children has not been established.

## Precautions

*Neuromuscular blockade:* A partial neuromuscular blockade was demonstrated after large IV doses of capreomycin. This action was enhanced by ether anesthesia (as has been reported for neomycin) and was antagonized by neostigmine.

*Ototoxicity:* Perform audiometric measurements and assessment of vestibular function prior to initiation of therapy and at regular intervals during treatment.

*Nephrotoxicity:* Perform regular tests of renal function throughout treatment, and reduce dose in patients with renal impairment. Renal injury with tubular necrosis, elevation of BUN or serum creatinine, and abnormal sediment have been noted. Reduce the dosage or withdraw the drug.

*Hypokalemia:* Hypokalemia may occur during therapy; therefore, determine serum potassium levels frequently.

**Drug Interactions**

Drugs that may interact with capreomycin include aminoglycosides and nondepolarizing neuromuscular blocking agents.

**Adverse Reactions**

Adverse reactions may include the following: Ototoxicity; tinnitus; vertigo; pain, induration, and excessive bleeding at the injection sites; sterile abscesses; leukocytosis; leukopenia; eosinophilia; abnormal results in liver function tests; urticaria; and maculopapular skin rashes.

# RIFAPENTINE

**Tablets:** 150 mg *(Rx)*                                      *Priftin* (Aventis)

**Indications**

*Tuberculosis:* For the treatment of pulmonary tuberculosis (TB). Rifapentine must always be used in conjunction with at least 1 other antituberculosis drug(s) to which the isolate is susceptible.

**Administration and Dosage**

Do not use rifapentine alone. Concomitant administration of pyridoxine (vitamin $B_6$) is recommended in the malnourished, in those predisposed to neuropathy (eg, alcoholics, diabetics), and in adolescents.

*Tuberculosis:*

*Intensive phase* – 600 mg (four 150 mg tablets twice weekly) with an interval of 3 days or more (72 hours) between doses continued for 2 months. May be given with food if stomach upset, nausea, or vomiting occurs.

*Continuation phase* – Continue treatment with rifapentine once weekly for 4 months in combination with isoniazid or an appropriate agent for susceptible organisms. If the patient is still sputum-smear- or culture-positive, if resistant organisms are present, or if the patient is HIV-positive, follow ATS/CDC treatment guidelines.

The above recommendations apply to patients with drug-susceptible organisms. Patients with drug-resistant organisms may require longer duration treatment with other drug regimens.

*CDC recommendations:* Rifapentine may be used once weekly with isoniazid in the continuation phase of treatment for HIV-seronegative patients with noncavitary, drug-susceptible pulmonary tuberculosis who have negative sputum smears at completion of the initial phase of treatment. Continue this regimen for 4 months (total of 6 months of TB treatment). Have treatment for patients receiving isoniazid and rifapentine, and whose 2–month cultures are positive, extended by an additional 3 months (total of 9 months).

For adults, the maximum recommended dose is 10 mg/kg (600 mg), once weekly during the continuation phase. Data have suggested that a dose of 900 mg is well tolerated, but the clinical efficacy of this dose has not been established.

**Actions**

*Pharmacology:* Rifapentine is a rifamycin-derivative antibiotic and has a similar profile of microbiological activity to rifampin.

*Pharmacokinetics:*

*Absorption/Distribution* – The absolute bioavailability of rifapentine has not been determined. $C_{max}$ is 15.05 mcg/mL and half-life is 13.19 hours. The estimated apparent volume of distribution is approximately 70 L. In healthy volunteers, rifapentine and 25-desacetyl rifapentine (active metabolite) were 97.7% and 93.2% bound to plasma proteins, respectively, mainly to albumin.

*Metabolism/Excretion* – Rifapentine is hydrolyzed by an esterase enzyme to form a microbiologically active 25-desacetyl rifapentine. Rifapentine and 25-desacetyl rifapentine account for 99% of total drug in plasma. Plasma AUC and $C_{max}$ values of the 25-desacetyl rifapentine metabolite are 50% and 33% those of rifapentine, respectively. Eighty-seven percent of the total dose was recovered in the urine (17%) and feces (70%); more than 80% was excreted within 7 days.

*Special populations –*

*Gender:* The estimated apparent oral clearance of rifapentine for males and females was approximately 2.51 and 1.69 L/h, respectively. The clinical significance of the difference in the estimated apparent oral clearance is not known.

## Contraindications

Hypersensitivity to any of the rifamycins (rifampin and rifabutin).

## Warnings

*Compliance:* Poor compliance with the dosage regimen, particularly daily administered nonrifamycin drugs in the intensive phase, was associated with late sputum conversion and a high relapse rate.

*Hyperbilirubinemia:* An isolated report showing a moderate rise in bilirubin or transaminase level is not an indication to interrupt treatment; rather, repeat tests, noting trends in the levels, and consider them in conjunction with the patient's clinical condition.

*Pseudomembranous colitis:* If suspected, stop rifapentine immediately and treat the patient with supportive and specific treatment without delay (eg, oral vancomycin). Products inhibiting peristalsis are contraindicated in this clinical situation.

*HIV-infected patients:* As with other antituberculosis treatments, when rifapentine is used in HIV-infected patients, employ a more aggressive regimen (eg, more frequent dosing). Once-weekly dosing during the continuation phase of treatment is not recommended at this time.

*Hepatic function impairment:* Only give patients with abnormal liver tests or liver disease rifapentine in cases of necessity and then with caution and under strict medical supervision. In these patients, carefully monitor liver tests (especially serum transaminases) prior to therapy and then every 2 to 4 weeks during therapy. If signs of liver disease occur or worsen, discontinue rifapentine.

*Elderly:* In general, use caution in dose selection for elderly patients, usually starting at the low end of the dosing range, reflecting the greater frequency of decreased hepatic, renal, or cardiac function and of concomitant disease or other drug therapy.

*Pregnancy: Category* C.

*Lactation:* Because of the potential for serious adverse reactions in nursing infants, decide whether to discontinue nursing or discontinue the drug, taking into account the importance of the drug to the mother.

*Children:* Safety and efficacy in children younger than 12 years of age have not been established.

## Precautions

*Monitoring:* Obtain baseline measurements of hepatic enzymes, bilirubin, a CBC, and a platelet count (or estimate). Assess patients at least monthly during therapy. Routine laboratory monitoring for toxicity in people with normal baseline measurements is generally not necessary.

*Porphyria:* Do not use rifapentine in patients with porphyria.

*Resistance:* M. *tuberculosis* organisms resistant to other rifamycins are likely to be resistant to rifapentine. Cross-resistance does not appear between rifapentine and nonrifamycin antimycobacterial agents such as isoniazid and streptomycin.

*Red discoloration of body fluids:* Rifapentine may produce a predominately red-orange discoloration of body tissues or fluids (eg, skin, teeth, tongue, urine, feces, saliva, sputum, tears, sweat, cerebrospinal fluid). Contact lenses may become permanently stained.

## Drug Interactions

Use rifapentine with extreme caution, if at all, in patients who are also taking protease inhibitors (eg, indinavir).

*Cytochrome P450:* Rifapentine is an inducer of cytochromes P450 3A4 and P450 2C8/9 and may increase the metabolism of other coadministered drugs that are metabolized by these enzymes.

*Note:* Advise patients using oral or other systemic hormonal contraceptives to change to nonhormonal methods of birth control.

Antiarrhythmics (eg, disopyramide, mexiletine, quinidine, tocainide).

Antibiotics (eg, chloramphenicol, clarithromycin, dapsone, doxycycline, fluoroquinolones [such as ciprofloxacin]).

Anticonvulsants (eg, phenytoin).

Antifungals (eg, fluconazole, itraconazole, ketoconazole).

Barbiturates.

Benzodiazepines (eg, diazepam).

Beta blockers.

Buspirone.

Calcium channel blockers (eg, diltiazem, nifedipine, verapamil).

Cardiac glycoside preparations.

Clofibrate.

Corticosteroids.

Estrogens.

Haloperidol.

HIV protease inhibitors (eg, indinavir, ritonavir, nelfinavir, saquinavir [see Rifapentine-indinavir interaction above]).

HMG-CoA reductase inhibitors (eg, simvastatin).

Immunosuppressants (eg, cyclosporine, tacrolimus).

Lamotrigine.

Levothyroxine.

Meglitinides (eg, repaglinide).

Narcotic analgesics (eg, methadone).

Oral anticoagulants (eg, warfarin).

Oral hypoglycemic agents (eg, sulfonylureas).

Oral or other systemic hormonal contraceptives.

Progestins.

Quinine.

Reverse transcriptase inhibitors (eg, delavirdine, zidovudine).

Sildenafil.

Tamoxifen.

Theophylline.

Toremifene.

Tricyclic antidepressants (eg, amitriptyline, nortriptyline).

*Drug/Lab test interactions:* Therapeutic concentrations of rifampin have been shown to inhibit standard microbiological assays for serum folate and vitamin $B_{12}$.

*Drug/Food interactions:* Food (850 total calories: 33 g protein, 55 g fat, and 58 g carbohydrate) increased AUC and $C_{max}$ in healthy volunteers by 43% and 44%, respectively, and in asymptomatic HIV-infected volunteers by 51% and 53%, respectively.

**Adverse Reactions**

Adverse reactions occurring in 3% or more of patients receiving rifapentine combination therapy include the following: Rash; pyuria; proteinuria; hematuria; urinary casts; neutropenia; lymphopenia; hyperuricemia; and an increase in ALT and AST.

# FOSCARNET SODIUM (Phosphonoformic acid)

| **Injection:** 24 mg/mL (Rx) | Foscavir (Astra) |
|---|---|

---

**Warning:**

Renal impairment, the major toxicity, occurs to some degree in most patients. Continual assessment of a patient's risk and frequent monitoring of serum creatinine with dose adjustment for changes in renal function are imperative.

Seizures related to alterations in plasma minerals and electrolytes have been associated with foscarnet treatment. Therefore, patients must be carefully monitored for such changes and their potential sequelae. Mineral and electrolyte supplementation may be required.

Foscarnet causes alterations in plasma minerals and electrolytes that have led to seizures. Monitor patients frequently for such changes and their potential sequelae.

---

## Indications

*Cytomegalovirus (CMV) retinitis:* Treatment of CMV retinitis in patients with AIDS.

*Combination:* Combination therapy with ganciclovir for patients who have relapsed after monotherapy with either drug.

*Herpes simplex virus (HSV) infections:* Treatment of acyclovir-resistant mucocutaneous HSV infections in immunocompromised patients.

## Administration and Dosage

*HSV infections:* Foscarnet is not a cure for HSV infections. While complete healing may occur, relapse occurs in most patients.

*Caution:* Do not administer by rapid or bolus IV injection. Toxicity may be increased as a result of excessive plasma levels. An infusion pump must be used.

It is recommended that 750 to 1000 mL of normal saline or 5% dextrose solution be given prior to the first infusion of foscarnet to establish diuresis. With subsequent infusions, 750 to 1000 mL of hydration fluid should be given with 90 to 120 mg/kg of foscarnet, and 500 mL with 40 to 60 mg/kg of foscarnet. Hydration fluid may need to be decreased if clinically warranted. After the first dose, administer the hydration fluid concurrently with each infusion of foscarnet.

*Induction treatment:* The recommended initial dose for patients with normal renal function is 60 mg/kg, adjusted for individual patients' renal function, given IV at a constant rate over a minimum of 1 hour every 8 hours for 2 to 3 weeks, depending on clinical response.

*Maintenance treatment:* 90 to 120 mg/kg/day (individualized for renal function) as an IV infusion over 2 hours. It is recommended that most patients be started on maintenance treatment with 90 mg/kg/day. Escalation to 120 mg/kg/day may be considered should early reinduction be required because of retinitis progression.

Patients who experience progression of retinitis while receiving maintenance therapy may be retreated with the induction and maintenance regimens above.

*Dose adjustment in renal impairment:*

| Foscarnet Dosing Guide Based on Ccr for Induction | | | |
|---|---|---|---|
| | HSV: Equivalent to | | CMV: Equivalent to |
| Ccr (mL/min/kg) | 80 mg/kg/day | 120 mg/kg/day | 180 mg/kg/day |
| > 1.4 | 40 q 12 h | 40 q 8 h | 60 q 8 h |
| > 1 to 1.4 | 30 q 12 h | 30 q 8 h | 45 q 8 h |
| > 0.8 to 1 | 20 q 12 h | 35 q 12 h | 50 q 12 h |
| > 0.6 to 0.8 | 35 q 24 h | 25 q 12 h | 40 q 12 h |
| > 0.5 to 0.6 | 25 q 24 h | 40 q 24 h | 60 q 24 h |
| ≥ 0.4 to 0.5 | 20 q 24 h | 35 q 24 h | 50 q 24 h |
| < 0.4 | Not recommended | Not recommended | Not recommended |

| Foscarnet Dosing Guide Based on Ccr for Maintenance | | |
|---|---|---|
| Ccr (mL/min/kg) | CMV: Equivalent to | |
| | 90 mg/kg/day | 120 mg/kg/day |
| > 1.4 | 90 q 24 h | 120 q 24 h |
| > 1 to 2.4 | 70 q 24 h | 90 q 24 h |
| > 0.8 to 1 | 50 q 24 h | 65 q 24 h |
| > 0.6 to 0.8 | 80 q 48 h | 105 q 48 h |
| > 0.5 to 0.6 | 60 q 48 h | 30 q 48 h |
| ≥ 0.4 to 0.5 | 50 q 48 h | 65 q 48 h |
| < 0.4 | Not recommended | Not recommended |

**Actions**

*Pharmacology:* Foscarnet exerts its antiviral activity by a selective inhibition at the pyrophosphate binding site on virus-specific DNA polymerases and reverse transcriptases at concentrations that do not affect cellular DNA polymerases. CMV strains resistant to ganciclovir may be sensitive to foscarnet. Acyclovir- or ganciclovir-resistant mutants may be resistant to foscarnet.

*Pharmacokinetics:* Foscarnet is 14% to 17% bound to plasma protein at plasma drug concentrations of 1 to 1000 mcM.

Approximately 80% to 90% of IV foscarnet is excreted unchanged in the urine of patients with normal renal function. Both tubular secretion and glomerular filtration account for urinary elimination of foscarnet.

Plasma half-life increases with the severity of renal impairment. Half-lives of 2 to 8 hours occurred in patients having estimated or measured 24-hour Ccr of 44 to 90 mL/min.

The foscarnet terminal half-life determined by urinary excretion was 87.5 ± 41.8 hours, possibly because of release of foscarnet from bone. Postmortem data provide evidence that foscarnet does accumulate in bone in humans.

Variable penetration into cerebrospinal fluid (CSF) has been observed. Disease-related defects in the blood-brain barrier may be responsible for the variations seen.

**Contraindications**

Hypersensitivity to foscarnet.

**Warnings**

*Mineral and electrolyte imbalances:* Foscarnet has been associated with changes in serum electrolytes including hypocalcemia (15%), hypophosphatemia (8%) and hyperphosphatemia (6%), hypomagnesemia (15%), and hypokalemia (16%). Foscarnet is associated with a transient, dose-related decrease in ionized serum calcium, which may not be reflected in total serum calcium.

*Accidental exposure:* Accidental skin and eye contact with foscarnet sodium solution may cause local irritation and burning sensation. Flush the exposed area with water.

*Other CMV infections:* Safety and efficacy have not been established for the treatment of other CMV infections (eg, pneumonitis, gastroenteritis); congenital or neonatal CMV disease; nonimmunocompromised individuals.

*Neurotoxicity and seizures:* Foscarnet was associated with seizures in AIDS patients. Statistically significant risk factors associated with seizures were low baseline absolute neutrophil count (ANC), impaired baseline renal function, and low total serum calcium. Several cases of seizures were associated with death.

*Renal function impairment:* The major toxicity of foscarnet is renal impairment, which occurs to some degree in most patients. Approximately 33% of 189 patients with AIDS and CMV retinitis who received IV foscarnet in clinical studies developed significant impairment of renal function, manifested by a rise in serum creatinine concentration to 2 mg/dL or more.

*Elderly:* Because these individuals frequently have reduced glomerular filtration, pay particular attention to assessing renal function before and during administration.

*Pregnancy: Category C.*

*Lactation:* It is not known whether foscarnet is excreted in breast milk.

*Children:* The safety and efficacy of foscarnet in children have not been studied.

**Precautions**

*Monitoring:* The majority of patients will experience some decrease in renal function due to foscarnet administration. Therefore, it is recommended that Ccr be determined at baseline, 2 to 3 times/week during induction therapy, and at least once every 1 to 2 weeks during maintenance therapy, with foscarnet dose adjusted accordingly. More frequent monitoring may be required for some patients. It also is recommended that a 24-hour Ccr be determined at baseline and periodically thereafter to ensure correct dosing. Discontinue if Ccr drops to less than 0.4 mL/min/kg.

Because of foscarnet's propensity to chelate divalent metal ions and alter levels of serum electrolytes, closely monitor patients for such changes. It is recommended that a schedule similar to that recommended for serum creatinine be used to monitor serum calcium, magnesium, potassium, and phosphorus.

Careful monitoring and appropriate management of creatinine are of particular importance in patients with conditions that may predispose them to seizures.

*Diagnosis of CMV retinitis:* Diagnosis of CMV retinitis should be established by an ophthalmologist familiar with the retinal presentation of these conditions.

*Toxicity/Local irritation:* The maximum single-dose administered was 120 mg/kg by IV infusion over 2 hours. It is likely that larger doses, or more rapid infusions, would result in increased toxicity. Infuse solutions containing foscarnet only into veins with adequate blood flow to permit rapid dilution and distribution, and avoid local irritation. Local irritation and ulcerations of penile epithelium have occurred in patients receiving foscarnet, possibly because of drug in urine. Adequate hydration with close attention to personal hygiene may minimize the occurrence of such events.

*Anemia:* Anemia occurred in 33% of patients. Granulocytopenia occurred in 17% of patients.

**Drug Interactions**

Drugs that may interact with foscarnet include nephrotoxic drugs (eg, aminoglycosides, amphotericin B, IV pentamidine), pentamidine, and zidovudine.

Foscarnet decreases serum levels of ionized calcium. Exercise particular caution when other drugs known to influence serum calcium levels are used concurrently.

**Adverse Reactions**

Adverse reactions occurring in at least 3% of patients include fever; nausea; anemia; diarrhea; abnormal renal function including acute renal failure, decreased Ccr and increased serum creatinine; vomiting; headache; seizure; death; marrow suppression; injection site pain or inflammation; paresthesia; dizziness; involuntary muscle contractions; hypoesthesia; neuropathy; sensory disturbances; influenza-like symptoms; bacterial/fungal infections; rectal hemorrhage; dry mouth; melena; flatulence; ulcerative stomatitis; pancreatitis; granulocytopenia; leukopenia; thrombocytopenia; platelet abnormalities; thrombosis; WBC abnormalities; lymphadenopathy; electrolyte abnormalities; neurotoxicity; renal impairment; decreased weight; increased alkaline phosphatase, LDH and BUN; acidosis; cachexia; thirst; depression; confusion; anxiety; aggressive reaction; hallucination; coughing; dyspnea; pneumonia; sinusitis; pharyngitis; rhinitis; respiratory disorders or insufficiency; pulmonary infiltration; stridor; pneumothorax; hemoptysis; bronchospasm; rash; increased sweating; pruritus; skin ulceration; seborrhea; erythematous rash; maculopapular rash; vision abnormalities; taste perversions; eye abnormalities; eye pain; conjunctivitis; hypertension; palpitations; ECG abnormalities.

# GANCICLOVIR (DHPG)

**Capsules:** 250 and 500 mg (*Rx*)                                *Cytovene* (Roche)
**Powder for injection, lyophilized:** 500 mg/vial ganciclovir
(*Rx*)

**Warning:**
   The clinical toxicity of ganciclovir includes granulocytopenia, anemia, and thrombocytopenia. In animal studies, ganciclovir was carcinogenic, teratogenic, and
   caused aspermatogenesis.

   Ganciclovir IV is indicated for use only in the treatment of cytomegalovirus (CMV)
   retinitis in immunocompromised patients and for the prevention of CMV disease in transplant patients at risk for CMV disease.

   Ganciclovir capsules are indicated only for prevention of CMV disease in patients
   with advanced HIV infection at risk for CMV disease and for maintenance treatment of CMV retinitis in immunocompromised patients.

   Because oral ganciclovir is associated with a risk of more rapid rate of CMV retinitis progression, use only in those patients for whom this risk is balanced by the
   benefit associated with avoiding daily IV infusions.

## Indications

*IV:*
   *CMV retinitis* – Treatment of CMV retinitis in immunocompromised patients,
   including patients with AIDS.
   *CMV disease* – Prevention of CMV disease in transplant recipients at risk for CMV
   disease.

*Oral:*
   *CMV retinitis* – Alternative to the IV formulation for maintenance treatment of
   CMV retinitis in immunocompromised patients, including patients with AIDS, in
   whom retinitis is stable following appropriate induction therapy and for whom the
   risk of more rapid progression is balanced by the benefit associated with avoiding
   daily IV infusions.
   *CMV disease* – Prevention of CMV disease in individuals with advanced HIV infection at risk for developing CMV disease.

## Administration and Dosage

*IV:* Do not administer by rapid or bolus IV injection. The toxicity may be increased
   as a result of excessive plasma levels. Do not exceed the recommended infusion
   rate. IM or subcutaneous injection of reconstituted ganciclovir may result in severe
   tissue irritation because of high pH.

*CMV retinitis treatment (normal renal function):*
   *Induction* – Recommended initial dose is 5 mg/kg (given IV at a constant rate of
   1 hour) every 12 hours for 14 to 21 days. Do not use oral ganciclovir for induction.
   *Maintenance* –
      *IV:* Following induction, the recommended maintenance dose is 5 mg/kg given
   as a constant rate IV infusion over 1 hour once per day 7 days per week, or 6 mg/kg
   once per day 5 days/week.
      *Oral:* Following induction, the recommended maintenance dose of oral gan-
   ciclovir is 1000 mg 3 times daily with food. Alternatively, the dosing regimen of
   500 mg 6 times daily every 3 hours with food during waking hours may be used.
      For patients who experience progression of CMV retinitis while receiving
   maintenance treatment with either formulation of ganciclovir, reinduction treatment is recommended.

*Prevention of CMV disease in transplant recipients with normal renal function:*
IV – The recommended initial dose of IV ganciclovir for patients with normal renal function is 5 mg/kg (given IV at a constant rate over 1 hour) every 12 hours for 7 to 14 days, followed by 5 mg/kg once daily 7 days/week or 6 mg/kg once daily 5 days/week.

*Oral* – The recommended prophylactic dosage is 1000 mg 3 times daily with food.

The duration of treatment with ganciclovir in transplant recipients is dependent on the duration and degree of immunosuppression. In controlled clinical trials in bone marrow allograft recipients, IV ganciclovir treatment was continued until day 100 to 120 posttransplantation. CMV disease occurred in several patients who discontinued treatment with IV ganciclovir prematurely. In heart allograft recipients, the onset of newly diagnosed CMV disease occurred after treatment with IV ganciclovir was stopped at day 28 post-transplant, suggesting that continued dosing may be necessary to prevent late occurrence of CMV disease in this patient population.

*Prevention of CMV disease in patients with advanced HIV infection and normal renal function:* The recommended dose of ganciclovir capsules is 1000 mg 3 times daily with food.

*Renal function impairment:*
IV – Refer to the table for recommended doses and adjust the dosing interval as indicated.

| IV Ganciclovir Dose in Renal Impairment | | | | |
|---|---|---|---|---|
| Ccr (mL/min) | Ganciclovir induction dose (mg/kg) | Dosing interval (hours) | Ganciclovir maintenance dose (mg/kg) | Dosing interval (hours) |
| ≥ 70 | 5 | 12 | 5 | 24 |
| 50 to 69 | 2.5 | 12 | 2.5 | 24 |
| 25 to 49 | 2.5 | 24 | 1.25 | 24 |
| 10 to 24 | 1.25 | 24 | 0.625 | 24 |
| < 10 | 1.25 | 3 times/week following hemodialysis | 0.625 | 3 times/week following hemodialysis |

*Hemodialysis:* Dosing for patients undergoing hemodialysis should not exceed 1.25 mg/kg 3 times/week, following each hemodialysis session. Give shortly after completion of the hemodialysis session, since hemodialysis reduces plasma levels by approximately 50%.

*Oral:* In renal impairment, modify the dose of oral ganciclovir as follows:

| Oral Ganciclovir Dose in Renal Impairment | |
|---|---|
| Ccr (mL/min) | Ganciclovir doses |
| ≥ 70 | 1000 mg TID or 500 mg q3h, 6 times/day |
| 50 to 69 | 1500 mg QD or 500 mg TID |
| 25 to 49 | 1000 mg QD or 500 mg BID |
| 10 to 24 | 500 mg QD |
| < 10 | 500 mg 3 times/week, following hemodialysis |

*Patient monitoring:* Because of the frequency of granulocytopenia, anemia, and thrombocytopenia, it is recommended that CBCs and platelet counts be performed frequently, especially in patients in whom ganciclovir or other nucleoside analogs have previously resulted in cytopenia, or in whom neutrophil counts are less than 1000/mcL at the beginning of treatment. Patients should have serum creatinine or Ccr values followed carefully to allow for dosage adjustment in renally impaired patients.

*Reduction of dose:* Dose reductions are required with IV therapy and should be considered with oral therapy for patients with renal impairment and for those with neutropenia, anemia, or thrombocytopenia. Do not administer in severe neutropenia (ANC less than 500/mcL) or severe thrombocytopenia (platelets less than 25,000/mcL).

## Actions

*Pharmacology:* Ganciclovir, a synthetic guanine derivative active against CMV, is an acyclic nucleoside analog of 2'-deoxyguanosine that inhibits replication of herpes viruses both in vitro and in vivo. Sensitive human viruses include CMV, herpes simplex virus (HSV)-1 and -2, herpes virus type 6, Epstein-Barr virus, varicella-zoster virus, and hepatitis B virus.

*Pharmacokinetics:*

*Absorption* – Absolute bioavailability of oral ganciclovir under fasting conditions was approximately 5%; following food it was 6% to 9%. When given with a high-fat meal, steady-state AUC increased and there was a significant prolongation of time to peak serum concentrations.

At the end of a 1-hour IV infusion of 5 mg/kg, total AUC and $C_{max}$ ranged between 22.1 and 26.8 mcg•h/mL and 8.27 and 9 mcg/mL, respectively.

*Distribution* – The steady-state volume of distribution after IV administration was 0.74 L/kg. Cerebrospinal fluid concentrations obtained 0.25 and 5.67 hours postdose in 3 patients who received 2.5 mg/kg ganciclovir IV every 8 or 12 hours ranged from 0.31 to 0.68 mcg/mL, representing 24% to 70% of the respective plasma concentrations. Binding to plasma proteins was 1% to 2% over ganciclovir concentrations of 0.5 and 51 mcg/mL.

*Metabolism* – Following oral administration of a single 1000 mg dose, 86% of the administered dose was recovered in the feces and 5% was recovered in the urine.

*Excretion* – When administered IV, ganciclovir exhibits linear pharmacokinetics over the range of 1.6 to 5 mg/kg and when administered orally, it exhibits linear kinetics up to a total daily dose of 4 g/day. Renal excretion of unchanged drug by glomerular filtration and active tubular secretion is the major route of elimination. In patients with normal renal function, 91.3% of IV ganciclovir was recovered unmetabolized in the urine. After oral administration, steady state is achieved within 24 hours. Renal clearance following oral administration was 3.1 mL/min/kg. Half-life was 3.5 hours following IV administration and 4.8 following oral use.

*Children:* At an IV dose of 4 or 6 mg/kg in 27 neonates (2 to 49 days of age), the pharmacokinetic parameters were, respectively, $C_{max}$ of 5.5 and 7 mcg/mL, systemic clearance of 3.14 and 3.56 mL/min/kg and half-life of 2.4 hours for both.

## Contraindications

Hypersensitivity to ganciclovir or acyclovir.

## Warnings

*CMV disease:* Safety and efficacy have not been established for congenital or neonatal CMV disease, nor for the treatment of established CMV disease other than retinitis, nor for use in nonimmunocompromised individuals. The safety and efficacy of oral ganciclovir have not been established for treating any manifestation of CMV disease other than maintenance treatment of CMV retinitis.

*Diagnosis of CMV retinitis:* The diagnosis should be made by indirect ophthalmoscopy. Other conditions in the differential diagnosis of CMV retinitis include candidiasis, toxoplasmosis, histoplasmosis, retinal scars, and cotton wool spots, any of which may produce a retinal appearance similar to CMV. The diagnosis may be supported by a culture of CMV from urine, blood, or throat, but a negative CMV culture does not rule out CMV retinitis.

*Retinal detachment:* Retinal detachment has been observed in subjects with CMV retinitis both before and after initiation of therapy with ganciclovir. Its relationship to therapy is unknown. Patients with CMV retinitis should have frequent ophthalmologic evaluations to monitor the status of their retinitis and to detect any other retinal pathology.

*Hematologic:* Do not administer if the absolute neutrophil count is less than 500/mm³ or the platelet count is less than 25,000/mm³. Granulocytopenia (neutropenia), anemia, and thrombocytopenia have been observed in patients treated with ganciclovir. The frequency and severity of these events vary widely in different patient populations. Therefore, use with caution in patients with pre-existing cytopenias or with a history of cytopenic reactions to other drugs, chemicals, or irradiation. Granulocytopenia usually occurs during the first or second week of treatment, but may occur at any time during treatment. Cell counts usually begin to recover within 3 to 7 days of discontinuing the drug. Colony-stimulating factors have increased neutrophil and WBC counts in patients receiving IV ganciclovir for CMV retinitis.

*Renal function impairment:* Use ganciclovir with caution. Half-life and plasma/serum concentrations of ganciclovir will be increased because of reduced renal clearance (see Administration and Dosage).

If renal function is impaired, dosage adjustments are required for ganciclovir IV and should be considered for oral ganciclovir. Base such adjustments on measured or estimated Ccr values.

Hemodialysis reduces plasma levels of ganciclovir by approximately 50%.

*Carcinogenesis:* Consider ganciclovir a potential carcinogen.

*Mutagenesis:* Because of the mutagenic and teratogenic potential of ganciclovir, advise women of childbearing potential to use effective contraception during treatment. Similarly, advise men to practice barrier contraception during and for at least 90 days following treatment with ganciclovir.

*Fertility impairment:* Although data in humans have not been obtained regarding this effect, it is considered probable that ganciclovir, at recommended doses, causes temporary or permanent inhibition of spermatogenesis.

*Elderly:* Pharmacokinetic profile in elderly patients is not established. Because elderly individuals frequently have a reduced glomerular filtration rate, pay particular attention to assessing renal function before and during ganciclovir therapy.

*Pregnancy: Category C.*

*Lactation:* It is not known whether ganciclovir is excreted in breast milk. The possibility of serious adverse reactions from ganciclovir in nursing infants is considered likely. Instruct mothers to discontinue nursing if they are receiving ganciclovir. The minimum interval before nursing can safely be resumed after the last dose of ganciclovir is unknown.

*Children:* Safety and efficacy in children have not been established. The use of ganciclovir in children warrants extreme caution to the probability of long-term carcinogenicity and reproductive toxicity. Administer to children only after careful evaluation and only if the potential benefits of treatment outweigh the risks. Oral ganciclovir has not been studied in children younger than 13 years of age.

There has been very limited clinical experience using ganciclovir for the treatment of CMV retinitis in patients younger than 12 years of age.

The spectrum of adverse reactions reported in 120 immunocompromised pediatric clinical trial participants with serious CMV infections receiving IV ganciclovir were similar to those reported in adults. Granulocytopenia (17%) and thrombocytopenia (10%) were most commonly reported.

## Precautions

*Monitoring:* Because of the frequency of neutropenia, anemia, and thrombocytopenia in patients receiving ganciclovir, it is recommended that CBCs and platelet counts be performed frequently, especially in patients in whom ganciclovir or other nucleoside analogs have previously resulted in leukopenia, or in whom neutrophil counts are less than 1000/mm$^3$ at the beginning of treatment. Patients should also have serum creatinine or Ccr values followed carefully.

*Large doses/rapid infusion:* The maximum single dose administered was 6 mg/kg by IV infusion over 1 hour. Larger doses have resulted in increased toxicity. It is likely that more rapid infusions would also result in increased toxicity.

*Phlebitis/Pain at injection site:* Initially, reconstituted ganciclovir solutions have a high pH (pH 11). Despite further dilution in IV fluids, phlebitis or pain may occur at the site of IV infusion. Take care to infuse solutions containing ganciclovir only into veins with adequate blood flow to permit rapid dilution and distribution.

*Hydration:* Because ganciclovir is excreted by the kidneys and normal clearance depends on adequate renal function, administration of ganciclovir should be accompanied by adequate hydration.

### Drug Interactions

Drugs that may affect ganciclovir include imipenem-cilastatin, nephrotoxic drugs, probenecid, didanosine, and zidovudine. Drugs that may be affected by ganciclovir include cytotoxic drugs, didanosine, and zidovudine.

### Adverse Reactions

Adverse reactions occurring in at least 3% of AIDS patients include fever; infection; chills; sepsis; diarrhea; anorexia; vomiting; leukopenia; anemia; thrombocytopenia; neuropathy; sweating; pruritus.

# VALGANCICLOVIR

| | | |
|---|---|---|
| **Tablets:** 450 mg *(Rx)* | | *Valcyte* (Roche) |

> **Warning:**
> The clinical toxicity of valganciclovir, which is metabolized to ganciclovir, includes granulocytopenia, anemia, and thrombocytopenia. In animal studies, ganciclovir was carcinogenic, teratogenic, and caused aspermatogenesis.

### Indications

*Cytomegalovirus (CMV) retinitis:* For the treatment of CMV retinitis in patients with acquired immunodeficiency syndrome (AIDS).

*CMV disease:* For the prevention of CMV disease in kidney, heart, and kidney-pancreas transplant patients at high risk (Donor CMV seropositive/Recipient CMV seronegative [(D+/R−)]).

### Administration and Dosage

Strict adherence to dosage recommendations is essential to avoid overdose. Valganciclovir tablets cannot be substituted for ganciclovir capsules on a one-to-one basis.

*CMV retinitis (normal renal function):*
Induction – 900 mg (two 450 mg tablets) twice daily for 21 days with food.
Maintenance – Following induction treatment, or in patients with inactive CMV retinitis, the recommended dosage is 900 mg (two 450 mg tablets) once daily with food.

*Prevention of CMV disease:* 900 mg (two 450 mg tablets) once daily with food starting within 10 days of transplantation until 100 days posttransplantation.

*Renal impairment:* Monitor serum creatinine or Ccr levels carefully. Dosage adjustment is required according to Ccr, as shown in the table below. Increased monitoring for cytopenias may be warranted in patients with renal impairment.

| Oral Valganciclovir in Renal Impairment | | |
|---|---|---|
| Ccr[1] (mL/min) | Induction dose | Maintenance/prevention dose |
| ≥ 60 | 900 mg twice daily | 900 mg once daily |
| 40 to 59 | 450 mg twice daily | 450 mg once daily |
| 25 to 39 | 450 mg once daily | 450 mg every 2 days |
| 10 to 24 | 450 mg every 2 days | 450 mg twice weekly |

[1] Estimated creatinine clearance.

*Hemodialysis patients:* Do not prescribe valganciclovir to patients receiving hemodialysis.

*Handling and disposal:* Exercise caution in the handling of valganciclovir tablets. Do not break or crush tablets. Because valganciclovir is considered a potential teratogen and carcinogen in humans, observe caution in handling broken tablets. Avoid direct contact of broken or crushed tablets with skin or mucous membranes. If such contact occurs, wash thoroughly with soap and water, and rinse eyes thoroughly with plain water.

Because ganciclovir shares some of the properties of antitumor agents (ie, carcinogenicity and mutagenicity), consider handling and disposing according to guidelines issued for antineoplastic drugs.

### Actions

*Pharmacology:* Valganciclovir is an L-valyl ester (prodrug) of ganciclovir that exists as a mixture of 2 diastereomers. After oral administration, both diastereomers are rapidly converted to ganciclovir by intestinal and hepatic esterases.

*Drug resistance* – Viruses resistant to ganciclovir can arise after prolonged treatment with valganciclovir.

*Pharmacokinetics:*

*Absorption* – Valganciclovir is well absorbed from the GI tract and rapidly metabolized in the intestinal wall and liver to ganciclovir. The absolute bioavailability of ganciclovir from valganciclovir tablets following administration with food was about 60%. Ganciclovir median $T_{max}$ following administration of 450 to 2625 mg valganciclovir tablets ranged from 1 to 3 hours. Systemic exposure to the prodrug, valganciclovir, is transient and low, and the $AUC_{24}$ and $C_{max}$ values are about 1% and 3% of those of ganciclovir, respectively.

*Distribution* – Plasma protein binding of ganciclovir is 1% to 2%. When ganciclovir was administered IV, the steady-state volume of distribution of ganciclovir was about 0.703 L/kg (n = 69).

*Metabolism* – Valganciclovir is rapidly hydrolyzed to ganciclovir; no other metabolites have been detected.

*Excretion* – The major route of elimination of valganciclovir is by renal excretion as ganciclovir through glomerular filtration and active tubular secretion. Systemic clearance of IV administered ganciclovir was about 3.07 mL/min (n = 68) while renal clearance was about 2.99 mL/min/kg (n = 16).

The terminal half-life of ganciclovir following oral administration of valganciclovir tablets to either healthy or HIV-positive/CMV-positive subjects was about 4.08 hours (n = 73), and that following administration of IV ganciclovir was about 3.81 hours (n = 69).

### Contraindications

Hypersensitivity to valganciclovir or ganciclovir.

### Warnings

*Liver transplant patients:* In liver transplant patients, there was a significantly higher incidence of tissue-invasive CMV disease in the valganciclovir-treated group compared with the oral ganciclovir group. Valganciclovir is not indicated for use in liver transplant patients.

*Toxicity:* The clinical toxicity of valganciclovir, which is metabolized to ganciclovir, includes granulocytopenia, anemia, and thrombocytopenia. In animal studies, ganciclovir was carcinogenic, teratogenic, and caused aspermatogenesis.

*Hematologic:* Valganciclovir tablets should not be administered if the absolute neutrophil count is less than 500 cells/mm$^3$, the platelet count is less than 25,000/mm$^3$, or the hemoglobin is less than 8 g/dL.

Severe leukopenia, neutropenia, anemia, thrombocytopenia, pancytopenia, bone marrow depression, and aplastic anemia have been observed in patients treated with valganciclovir tablets (and ganciclovir) (see Precautions and Adverse Reactions).

Cytopenia may occur at any time during treatment and may increase with continued dosing. Cell counts usually begin to recover within 3 to 7 days of discontinuing drug.

*Renal function impairment:* If renal function is impaired, dosage adjustments are required for valganciclovir.

*Fertility impairment:* It is considered probable that in humans, valganciclovir at the recommended doses may cause temporary or permanent inhibition of spermatogenesis. Animal data also indicate that suppression of fertility in females may occur.

Because of the mutagenic and teratogenic potential of ganciclovir, advise women of childbearing potential to use effective contraception during treatment. Similarly, advise men to practice barrier contraception during and for at least 90 days following treatment with valganciclovir.

*Elderly:* The pharmacokinetic characteristics of valganciclovir in elderly patients have not been established. Since elderly individuals frequently have a reduced glomerular filtration rate, pay particular attention to assessing renal function before and during administration of valganciclovir.

*Pregnancy: Category* C.

*Lactation:* It is not known whether ganciclovir or valganciclovir is excreted in human milk. Because of potential for serious adverse events in nursing infants, mothers should be instructed not to breastfeed if they are receiving valganciclovir tablets. In addition, the Centers for Disease Control and Prevention recommend that HIV-infected mothers not breastfeed their infants to avoid risking postnatal transmission of HIV.

*Children:* Safety and efficacy of valganciclovir in pediatric patients have not been established.

## Precautions

*Monitoring:* Because of the frequency of neutropenia, anemia, and thrombocytopenia in patients receiving valganciclovir tablets, it is recommended that complete blood counts and platelet counts be performed frequently, especially in patients in whom ganciclovir or other nucleoside analogs have previously resulted in leukopenia, or in whom neutrophil counts are less than 1000 cells/mm$^3$ at the beginning of treatment. Increased monitoring for cytopenias may be warranted if therapy with oral ganciclovir is changed to oral valganciclovir, because of increased plasma concentrations of ganciclovir after valganciclovir administration.

Increased serum creatinine levels have been observed in trials evaluating valganciclovir tablets. Patients should have serum creatinine or Ccr values monitored carefully to allow for dosage adjustments in renally impaired patients. The mechanism of impairment of renal function is not known.

## Drug Interactions

No in vivo drug interaction studies were conducted with valganciclovir. However, because valganciclovir is rapidly and extensively converted to ganciclovir, interactions associated with ganciclovir will be expected for valganciclovir tablets (see Ganciclovir monograph).

Drugs that may affect valganciclovir include didanosine, imipenem-cilastin, nephrotoxic drugs, probenecid, trimethoprim, zalcitabine, and zidovudine. Drugs that may be affected by valganciclovir include cytotoxic drugs, didanosine, and zidovudine.

*Drug/Food interactions:* When valganciclovir tablets were administered with a high-fat meal containing about 600 total calories (31.1 g fat, 51.6 g carbohydrates, and 22.2 g protein) at a dose of 875 mg once daily to 16 HIV-positive subjects, the steady-state ganciclovir AUC increased by 30% (95% CI 12% to 51%), and the $C_{max}$ increased by 14% (95% CI −5% to 36%), without any prolongation in time to peak plasma concentrations ($T_{max}$). Administer valganciclovir tablets with food.

## Adverse Reactions

Adverse reactions occurring in at least 3% of patients include the following: Abdominal pain, anemia, diarrhea, graft rejection, headache, hypertension, insomnia, leukopenia, nausea, neutropenia, paresthesia, peripheral neuropathy, pyrexia, retinal detachment, thrombocytopenia, tremors, vomiting.

# ACYCLOVIR (Acycloguanosine)

**Tablets**: 400 and 800 mg (*Rx*)                              Various, *Zovirax* (GlaxoWellcome)
**Capsules**: 200 mg (*Rx*)
**Suspension**: 200 mg/5 mL (*Rx*)
**Injection**: 50 mg/mL (*Rx*)
**Powder for injection**: 500 and 1000 mg/vial (as sodium)
(*Rx*)

## Indications

*Neonatal herpes simplex virus infection:* Treatment of neonatal herpes infections.

*Parenteral:* Treatment of initial and recurrent mucosal and cutaneous herpes simplex virus (HSV)-1 and -2 and varicella-zoster virus (VZV/shingles) infections in immunocompromised patients.

Herpes simplex encephalitis.

Severe initial clinical episodes of genital herpes in patients who are not immunocompromised.

*Oral:* Treatment of initial episodes and management of recurrent episodes of genital herpes.

## Administration and Dosage

*Parenteral:* For IV infusion only. Avoid rapid or bolus IV, IM, or subcutaneous injection. Administer over at least 1 hour to prevent renal tubular damage. Initiate therapy as soon as possible following onset of signs and symptoms.

| IV Acyclovir Dosage/Management Guidelines | | |
|---|---|---|
| | Dosage | |
| Indication | Adults | Children (< 12 years) |
| Mucosal and cutaneous HSV infections in immuno-compromised patients | 5 mg/kg infused at a constant rate over 1 hour every 8 hours (15 mg/kg/day) for 7 days[1] | 10 mg/kg[2] infused at a constant rate over 1 hour every 8 hours for 7 days |
| Varicella-zoster infections (shingles) in immuno-compromised patients[2] | 10 mg/kg infused at a constant rate over 1 hour every 8 hours for 7 days[3] | 20 mg/kg infused at a constant rate over at least 1 hour every 8 hours for 7 days |
| Herpes simplex encephalitis | 10 mg/kg infused at a constant rate over at least 1 hour every 8 hours for 10 days | 20 mg/kg infused at a constant rate over at least 1 hour every 8 hours for 10 days[3] |
| Neonatal HSV infections | NA | 10 mg/kg infused at a constant rate over 1 hour every 8 hours for 10 days[4] |

[1] For severe initial clinical episodes of herpes genitalis, use the same dose for 5 days.
[2] Base dosage for obese patients on ideal body weight (10 mg/kg).
[3] Children 3 months to 12 years of age.
[4] Children birth to 3 months. Doses of 15 or 20 mg/kg infused at a constant rate over 1 hour every 8 hours have been used; however, safety and efficacy of these doses are unknown.

CDC *recommendations for neonatal herpes infections* –
*Disseminated and CNS disease:* 20 mg/kg IV every 8 hours for 21 days.
*Mucocutaneous disease:* 20 mg/kg IV every 8 hours for 14 days.
*Renal function impairment, acute or chronic* –

| Parenteral Acyclovir Dosage in Renal Function Impairment | | |
|---|---|---|
| Ccr (mL/min/1.73 m²) | Percent of recommended dose | Dosing interval (hours) |
| > 50 | 100% | 8 |
| 25 to 50 | 100% | 12 |
| 10 to 25 | 100% | 24 |
| 0 to 10 | 50% | 24 |

*Hemodialysis* – The mean plasma half-life of acyclovir during hemodialysis is approximately 5 hours; a 60% decrease in plasma concentrations follows a 6-hour dialysis period. Therefore, administer a dose after each dialysis.

*Oral:*

*Herpes simplex* – For severe disease that requires hospitalization (eg, disseminated infection, pneumonitis, hepatitis, meningitis, encephalitis) IV acyclovir therapy is recommended.

*Initial genital herpes:* 200 mg every 4 hours 5 times/day for 10 days.

*Chronic suppressive therapy for recurrent disease:* 400 mg 2 times/day for up to 12 months, followed by reevaluation. Reevaluate the frequency and severity of the patient's HSV after 1 year of therapy to assess the need for continuation of therapy.

*Intermittent therapy:* 200 mg every 4 hours 5 times daily for 5 days. Initiate therapy at the earliest sign or symptom (prodrome) of recurrence.

*CDC guidelines recommend the following oral regimens* –

*First initial clinical episode of genital herpes:* 400 mg 3 times/day for 7 to 10 days or 200 mg 5 times/day for 7 to 10 days.

*Episodic therapy for recurrent genital herpes:* 400 mg 3 times/day or 200 mg 5 times/day for 5 days.

*Herpes zoster, acute treatment* – 800 mg every 4 hours 5 times/day for 7 to 10 days.

*Chickenpox* – Initiate treatment at earliest sign or symptom. There are no data about the efficacy of therapy initiated more than 24 hours after onset of signs and symptoms.

*Adults and children (greater than 40 kg):* 800 mg 4 times daily for 5 days.

*Children (2 years and older; 40 kg or less):* 20 mg/kg 4 times daily for 5 days.

*Renal impairment, acute or chronic* –

| Oral Acyclovir Dosage in Renal Function Impairment | | | |
|---|---|---|---|
| Normal dosage regimen (5× daily) | Ccr (mL/min/1.73 m²) | Adjusted dosage regimen | |
| | | Dose (mg) | Dosing interval |
| 200 mg every 4 hours | > 10<br>0 to 10 | 200<br>200 | Every 4 hours, 5× daily<br>Every 12 hours |
| 400 mg every 12 hours | > 10<br>0 to 10 | 400<br>200 | Every 12 hours<br>Every 12 hours |
| 800 mg every 4 hours | > 25<br>10 to 25<br>0 to 10 | 800<br>800<br>800 | Every 4 hours, 5× daily<br>Every 8 hours<br>Every 12 hours |

*Hemodialysis* – For patients that require hemodialysis, adjust dosing schedule so that a dose is administered after each dialysis. No supplemental dose is necessary after peritoneal dialysis.

*Bioequivalence:* Acyclovir suspension was shown to be bioequivalent to acyclovir capsules, and one 800 mg acyclovir tablet was shown to be bioequivalent to four 200 mg acyclovir capsules.

**Actions**

*Pharmacology:* A synthetic purine nucleoside analog, acyclovir has in vitro and in vivo inhibitory activity against HSV-1, HSV-2, and VZV (shingles).

In vitro, acyclovir triphosphate stops replication of herpes viral DNA.

*Drug resistance* – Consider the possibility of viral resistance to acyclovir in patients who show poor clinical response during therapy.

*Pharmacokinetics:*

*Absorption/Distribution* – When acyclovir was administered to adults at 5 mg/kg by 1 hour infusions every 8 hours, mean steady-state peak and trough concentrations were 9.8 mcg/mL and 0.7 mcg/mL, respectively. When acyclovir was administered to adults at 10 mg/kg by 1 hour infusions every 8 hours, mean steady-state peak and trough concentrations were 22.9 mcg/mL and 1.9 mcg/mL, respectively. Absorption is unaffected by food. Bioavailability is between 10% and 20% and decreases with increasing doses. Concentrations achieved in CSF are approximately 50% of plasma values. Plasma protein binding is 9% to 33%. Acyclovir distributes widely in body fluids including vesicular fluid, aqueous humor, and cerebrospinal fluid. Acyclovir is concentrated in breast milk, amniotic fluid, and placenta.

*Metabolism/Excretion* – Renal excretion of unchanged drug following IV use accounts for 62% to 91% of the dose.

Half-life and total body clearance depend on renal function:

| Acyclovir Half-Life and Total Body Clearance Based on Renal Function | | |
| --- | --- | --- |
| Ccr (mL/min/1.73 m$^2$) | Half-life (h) | Total body clearance (mL/min/1.73 m$^2$) |
| > 80 | 2.5 | 327 |
| 50 to 80 | 3 | 248 |
| 15 to 50 | 3.5 | 190 |
| 0 (Anuric) | 19.5 | 29 |

*Special populations* –

*Elderly:* Acyclovir plasma concentrations are higher in elderly patients compared with younger adults. This may be in part because of age-related renal function changes.

## Contraindications

Hypersensitivity to acyclovir or any component of the formulation.

## Warnings

*Pregnancy: Category B.*

*Lactation:* Acyclovir concentrates in breast milk. Exercise caution when administering to a breastfeeding woman.

*Children:* Safety and efficacy of oral acyclovir in children younger than 2 years of age have not been established.

## Precautions

*Genital herpes:* Acyclovir is not a cure for genital herpes. There are no data evaluating whether acyclovir will prevent transmission of infection to others. Avoid contact with lesions, or avoid intercourse when lesions and/or symptoms are present to prevent infecting partners. Genital herpes can also be transmitted in the absence of symptoms. Initiate therapy at the first sign or symptom of an episode.

*Herpes zoster infections:* There are no data on treatment initiated more than 72 hours after the onset of the rash. Initiate treatment as soon as possible after diagnosis. In clinical trials, treatment was most effective when started within the first 48 hours of rash onset.

*Chickenpox:* Although chickenpox in otherwise healthy children is usually a self-limited disease of mild to moderate severity, adolescents and adults tend to have more severe disease. Treatment was initiated within 24 hours of the typical chickenpox rash in the controlled studies, and there is no information regarding the effects of treatment begun later in the disease course. IV acyclovir is indicated for the treatment of varicella-zoster infections in immunocompromised patients.

*Do not exceed:* Do not exceed the recommended dosage, frequency, or length of treatment. Base dosage adjustments on estimated Ccr.

*Renal function impairment:* Renal failure, sometimes fatal, has been observed with acyclovir therapy. Dosage adjustment is recommended in patients with renal impairment (see Administration and Dosage). Use caution when coadministering acyclovir with other potentially nephrotoxic agents.

Precipitation of acyclovir crystals in renal tubules can occur if the drug is administered by bolus injection. Ensuing renal tubular damage can produce acute renal failure.

Occurrence of renal failure depends also on the patient's state of hydration, other treatments, and the rate of drug administration. Concomitant use of other nephrotoxic agents, pre-existing renal disease, and dehydration make further renal impairment with acyclovir more likely.

*Thrombotic thrombocytopenic purpura/hemolytic uremic syndrome (TTP/HUS):* TTP/HUS which has resulted in death, has occurred in immunocompromised patients receiving acyclovir therapy.

*Hydration:* Accompany IV infusion by adequate hydration.

*Encephalopathic changes:* Approximately 1% of patients receiving acyclovir IV have manifested encephalopathic changes characterized by either lethargy, obtundation, tremors, confusion, hallucinations, agitation, seizures, or coma. Use with caution in those patients who have underlying neurologic abnormalities; those with serious renal, hepatic, or electrolyte abnormalities or significant hypoxia.

*Photosensitivity:* Photosensitive rash may occur; therefore, caution patients to take protective measures (ie, sunscreens, protective clothing) against exposure to ultraviolet light or sunlight until tolerance is determined.

### Drug Interactions
Drugs that may interact with acyclovir include hydantoins, probenecid, theophylline, valproic acid, and zidovudine.

### Adverse Reactions
Adverse reactions (parenteral) occurring in at least 3% of patients include inflammation or phlebitis at injection site, transient elevations of serum creatinine or BUN, and nausea or vomiting.

Adverse reactions (oral) occurring in at least 3% of patients include diarrhea, malaise, and nausea.

## FAMCICLOVIR

| Tablets: 125, 250, and 500 mg (*Rx*) | *Famvir* (Novartis) |
|---|---|

### Indications
*Acute herpes zoster:* Management of acute herpes zoster (shingles).

*Genital herpes:* Treatment or suppression of recurrent episodes of genital herpes.

*Herpes simplex:* Treatment of recurrent mucocutaneous herpes simplex infections in HIV-infected patients.

### Administration and Dosage
May be taken without regard to meals.

*Herpes zoster:* 500 mg every 8 hours for 7 days. Initiate therapy promptly as soon as herpes zoster is diagnosed.

*Genital herpes (recurrent episodes):* 125 mg twice daily for 5 days. Initiate therapy at the first sign or symptom if medical management of a genital herpes recurrence is indicated.

*Suppression of recurrent genital herpes:* 250 mg twice/day for up to 1 year. The safety and efficacy of famciclovir therapy beyond 1 year of treatment have not been established.

*HIV-infected patients:* 500 mg twice daily for 7 days for recurrent orolabial or genital herpes simplex infection.

*Renal function impairment:*

| Famciclovir Dosage in Renal Function Impairment | |
|---|---|
| Creatinine clearance (mL/min) | Dose regimen |
| Herpes zoster | |
| ≥ 60 | 500 mg every 8 hours |
| 40 to 59 | 500 mg every 12 hours |
| 20 to 39 | 500 mg every 24 hours |
| < 20 | 250 mg every 24 hours |
| Recurrent genital herpes | |
| ≥ 40 | 125 mg every 12 hours |

| Famciclovir Dosage in Renal Function Impairment | |
|---|---|
| Creatinine clearance (mL/min) | Dose regimen |
| 20 to 39 | 125 mg every 24 hours |
| < 20 | 125 mg every 24 hours |
| Suppression of recurrent genital herpes | |
| ≥ 40 | 250 mg every 12 hours |
| 20 to 39 | 125 mg every 12 hours |
| < 20 | 125 mg every 24 hours |
| Recurrent orolabial and genital herpes simplex infection in HIV-infected patients | |
| ≥ 40 | 500 mg every 12 hours |
| 20 to 39 | 500 mg every 24 hours |
| < 20 | 250 mg every 24 hours |

| Recommended Dosage Following Dialysis Treatment | |
|---|---|
| Herpes zoster | 250 mg |
| Recurrent genital herpes | 125 mg |
| Suppression of recurrent genital herpes | 125 mg |
| Recurrent orolabial and genital herpes simplex infection in HIV-infected patients | 250 mg |

## Actions

*Pharmacology:* Famciclovir undergoes rapid biotransformation to the active antiviral compound penciclovir, which is converted to penciclovir triphosphate. Penciclovir triphosphate inhibits HSV-2 polymerase. Consequently, herpes viral DNA synthesis and, therefore, replication are selectively inhibited.

*Pharmacokinetics:*

*Absorption* – The absolute bioavailability of famciclovir is 77%. The area under the plasma concentration-time curve (AUC) was 8.6 mcg•h/mL. The maximum concentration ($C_{max}$) was 3.3 mcg/mL and the time to $C_{max}$ ($T_{max}$) was 0.9 hours.

Penciclovir is less than 20% bound to plasma proteins. The blood/plasma ratio of penciclovir is approximately 1.

*Metabolism* – Famciclovir given orally is deacetylated and oxidized to form penciclovir. Cytochrome P450 does not play an important role in famciclovir metabolism.

*Excretion* – The plasma elimination half-life of penciclovir was 2 hours after IV penciclovir and 2.3 hours after 500 mg oral famciclovir.

## Contraindications

Hypersensitivity to famciclovir.

## Warnings

*Renal function impairment:* Dosage adjustment is recommended in renal insufficiency (see Administration and Dosage).

*Elderly:* Mean penciclovir AUC was 40% larger and penciclovir renal clearance was 22% lower after the oral administration of famciclovir in elderly volunteers compared with younger volunteers.

*Pregnancy: Category B.*

*Lactation:* It is not known whether famciclovir is excreted in breast milk. Decide whether to discontinue breastfeeding or to discontinue the drug, taking into account the importance of the drug to the mother.

*Children:* Safety and efficacy in children younger than 18 years of age have not been established.

#### Drug Interactions

The conversion of 6-deoxy penciclovir to penciclovir is catalyzed by aldehyde oxidase. Interactions with other drugs metabolized by this enzyme could occur.

Concurrent use with probenecid or other drugs significantly eliminated by active renal tubular secretion may result in increased plasma concentrations of penciclovir.

*Drug/Food interactions:* When famciclovir was administered with food, penciclovir $C_{max}$ decreased approximately 50%. Because the systemic availability of penciclovir (AUC) was not altered, it appears that famciclovir may be taken without regard to meals.

#### Adverse Reactions

Adverse reactions occurring in 3% or more of patients include dizziness, diarrhea, abdominal pain, dysmenorrhea, fatigue, fever, flatulence, headache, migraine, nausea, pruritus, rash, and vomiting.

*Drug/Lab:* Neutropenia (less than $0.8 \times$ normal range low), ALT (more than $2 \times$ normal range high), lipase (more than $1.5 \times$ normal range high).

# VALACYCLOVIR HCl

| **Caplets:** 500 mg, 1 g (*Rx*) | *Valtrex* (GlaxoSmithKline) |
|---|---|

#### Indications

*Herpes zoster:* Treatment of herpes zoster (shingles).

*Genital herpes:* Treatment or suppression of genital herpes in immunocompetent individuals and for the suppression of recurrent genital herpes in HIV-infected individuals.

When valacyclovir is used as suppressive therapy in immunocompetent individuals with genital herpes, the risk of heterosexual transmission to susceptible partners is reduced. Instruct patients to use safer sex practices with suppressive therapy (see current Centers for Disease Control and Prevention *Sexually Transmitted Disease Treatment Guidelines*).

*Herpes labialis:* For the treatment of herpes labialis (cold sores).

#### Administration and Dosage

Valacyclovir may be given without regard to meals.

*Herpes zoster:* The recommended dosage is 1 g 3 times daily for 7 days. Initiate therapy at the earliest sign or symptom of herpes zoster; it is most effective when started within 48 hours of the onset of zoster rash. No data are available on efficacy of treatment started more than 72 hours after rash onset.

*Genital herpes:*

    *Initial episodes* – The recommended dosage is 1 g twice daily for 10 days. There are no data on the effectiveness of treatment when initiated more than 72 hours after the onset of signs and symptoms. Therapy was most effective when administered within 48 hours of the onset of signs and symptoms.

    *Recurrent episodes* – The recommended dosage is 500 mg twice daily for 3 days. Advise patients to initiate therapy at the first sign or symptom of an episode. There are no data on the efficacy of treatment started more than 24 hours after the onset of signs or symptoms.

    *Suppressive therapy* – The recommended dosage for chronic suppressive therapy of recurrent genital herpes is 1 g once daily in immunocompetent patients. In patients with a history of 9 or fewer recurrences per year, an alternative dose is 500 mg once daily. The safety and efficacy of therapy with valacyclovir beyond 1 year have not been established.

    *Transmission* – The recommended dosage of valacyclovir for reduction of transmission of genital herpes in patients with a history of 9 or fewer recurrences per year is 500 mg once daily for the source partner. Counsel patients to use safer sex practices in combination with suppressive therapy with valacyclovir. The efficacy of reducing transmission beyond 8 months in discordant couples has not been established.

*HIV-infected patients:* In HIV-infected patients with CD4 cell count at least 100 cells/mm$^3$, the recommended dosage of valacyclovir for chronic suppressive therapy of recurrent genital herpes is 500 mg twice daily. The safety and efficacy of therapy with valacyclovir beyond 6 months in patients with HIV infection have not been established.

*Herpes labialis:* The recommended dosage of valacyclovir for the treatment of cold sores is 2 g twice daily for 1 day taken approximately 12 hours apart. Initiate therapy at the earliest symptom of a cold sore (eg, tingling, itching, burning). There are no data on the effectiveness of treatment initiated after the development of clinical signs of a cold sore (eg, papule, vesicle, ulcer). Therapy beyond 1 day does not appear to provide additional clinical benefit.

*Acute or chronic renal impairment:*

| Valacyclovir Dosage Adjustments for Renal Impairment | | | | |
|---|---|---|---|---|
| | Normal dosage (Ccr ≥ 50) | Ccr (mL/min) | | |
| Indication | | 30 to 49 | 10 to 29 | < 10 |
| Herpes zoster | 1 g q 8 h | 1 g q 12 h | 1 g q 24 h | 500 mg q 24 h |
| Genital herpes | | | | |
| Initial treatment | 1 g q 12 h | No reduction | 1 g q 24 h | 500 mg q 24 h |
| Recurrent episodes | 500 mg q 12 h | No reduction | 500 mg q 24 h | 500 mg q 24 h |
| Suppressive therapy | 1 g q 24 h | No reduction | 500 mg q 24 h | 500 mg q 24 h |
| Suppressive therapy (≤ 9 recurrences/yr) | 500 mg q 24 h | No reduction | 500 mg q 48 h | 500 mg q 48 h |
| Suppressive therapy in HIV-infected patients | 500 mg q 12 h | No reduction | 500 mg q 24 h | 500 mg q 24 h |
| Herpes labialis (cold sores) (do not exceed 1 day of treatment) | Two 2 g doses taken ≈ 12 h apart | Two 1 g doses taken ≈ 12 h apart | Two 500 mg doses taken ≈ 12 h apart | 500 mg single dose |

*Hemodialysis:* Following valacyclovir administration to volunteers with end-stage renal disease, the average acyclovir half-life is approximately 14 hours. During hemodialysis, the half-life of acyclovir after administration of valacyclovir is approximately 4 hours. About 33% of acyclovir in the body is removed by dialysis during a 4-hour hemodialysis session. Patients requiring hemodialysis should receive the recommended dose of valacyclovir after hemodialysis.

*Peritoneal dialysis:* Supplemental doses of valacyclovir should not be required following chronic ambulatory peritoneal dialysis (CAPD) or continuous arteriovenous hemofiltration/hemodialysis (CAVHD).

*Peritoneal dialysis:* Supplemental doses of valacyclovir should not be required following chronic ambulatory peritoneal dialysis (CAPD) or continuous arteriovenous hemofiltration/hemodialysis (CAVHD).

**Actions**

*Pharmacology:* Valacyclovir is the hydrochloride salt of L-valyl ester of the antiviral drug acyclovir. Valacyclovir is rapidly converted to acyclovir, which has in vitro and in vivo inhibitory activity against herpes simplex virus types I (HSV-1) and II (HSV-2), and varicella-zoster virus (VZV). In cell culture, acyclovir has the highest antiviral activity against HSV-1, followed by (in decreasing order of potency) HSV-2 and VZV.

In vitro, acyclovir triphosphate stops replication of herpes viral DNA in 3 ways: 1) Competitive inhibition of viral DNA polymerase; 2) incorporation and termination of the growing viral DNA chain; and 3) inactivation of the viral DNA polymerase.

*Pharmacokinetics:*

*Absorption/Distribution* – Valacyclovir is rapidly absorbed and is rapidly and nearly completely converted to acyclovir and L-valine by first-pass metabolism. The absolute bioavailability of acyclovir after administration of valacyclovir is 54.5%.

*Metabolism* – Neither valacyclovir nor acyclovir metabolism is metabolized by cytochrome P450 enzymes.

*Excretion* – Acyclovir accounted for 88.6% excreted in the urine. Renal clearance of acyclovir following the administration of a single 1 g valacyclovir dose to 12 healthy volunteers was approximately 255 mL/min, which represents 41.9% of total acyclovir apparent plasma clearance.

The plasma elimination half-life of acyclovir typically averaged 2.5 to 3.3 hours in volunteers with normal renal function.

### Contraindications

Hypersensitivity or intolerance to valacyclovir, acyclovir, or any component of the formulation.

### Warnings

*Thrombotic thrombocytopenic purpura/hemolytic uremic syndrome (TTP/HUS):* TTP/HUS, in some cases resulting in death, has been reported in patients with advanced HIV disease and in bone marrow and renal transplant recipients.

*Renal function impairment:* Dosage reduction is recommended with renal impairment (see Administration and Dosage). Acute renal failure and CNS symptoms have been reported in patients with underlying renal disease who have received inappropriately high doses for their level of renal function. Exercise similar caution when administering valacyclovir to elderly patients and patients receiving potentially nephrotoxic agents.

*Hepatic function impairment:* Administration of valacyclovir to patients with moderate (biopsy-proven cirrhosis) or severe (with and without ascites and biopsy-proven cirrhosis) liver disease indicated that the rate but not the extent of conversion of valacyclovir to acyclovir was reduced, and the acyclovir half-life was not affected. Dosage modification is not recommended for patients with cirrhosis.

*Elderly:* Dosage reduction may be required in geriatric patients, depending on the underlying renal status of the patient.

*Pregnancy: Category B.*

*Lactation:* Consider temporary discontinuation of nursing, as the safety of valacyclovir has not been established in infants.

*Children:* Safety and efficacy have not been established.

### Drug Interactions

Drugs that may affect valacyclovir include cimetidine/probenecid.

### Adverse Reactions

Adverse reactions occurring in 3% or more of patients include nausea, headache, vomiting, dizziness, abdominal pain, depression, AST abnormalities, dysmenorrhea, and arthralgia.

## AMANTADINE HCl

| | |
|---|---|
| **Tablets:** 100 mg (*Rx*) | *Symmetrel* (Endo) |
| **Capsules:** 100 mg (*Rx*) | Various |
| **Syrup:** 50 mg/5 mL (*Rx*) | Various, *Symmetrel* (Endo) |

### Indications

*Influenza A viral infection:* Amantadine is indicated for the prophylaxis and treatment of signs and symptoms of infection caused by various strains of influenza A virus.

*Prophylaxis* – Chemoprophylaxis against influenza A virus infection when early vaccination is not feasible or when the vaccine is contraindicated or not available. Following vaccination during an influenza A outbreak, consider amantadine prophylaxis for the 2- to 4-week time period required to develop an antibody response.

*Treatment* – Treatment of uncomplicated respiratory tract illness caused by influenza A virus, especially when administered early in the course of illness.

*Prophylaxis recommendations:*

1.) High-risk patients vaccinated after influenza outbreak has begun: Consider prophylaxis until immunity from the influenza vaccine has developed (up to 2 weeks).

2.) Caretakers of those at high risk: Consider prophylaxis for unvaccinated caretakers of high-risk patients during peak influenza activity.

3.) Patients with immune deficiency: Consider prophylaxis for high-risk patients who are expected to have inadequate antibody response to influenza vaccine (eg, HIV).

4.) Other: Consider prophylaxis in high-risk patients who should not be vaccinated. Prophylaxis also may be offered to those patients who desire to avoid influenza illness.

*Parkinsonism and drug-induced extrapyramidal reactions:* See amantadine in the Antiparkinson Agents section.

### Administration and Dosage

*Influenza A virus illness:*

*Prophylaxis* – Start in anticipation of contact or as soon as possible after exposure. Use daily for at least 10 days following a known exposure. The infectious period extends from shortly before onset of symptoms to up to 1 week after. Because amantadine does not appear to suppress antibody response, it can be used in conjunction with inactivated influenza A virus vaccine until protective antibody responses develop; administer for 2 to 4 weeks after vaccine has been given. When the vaccine is unavailable or contraindicated, give amantadine for the duration of known influenza A in the community because of repeated and unknown exposure.

*Symptomatic management* – Start as soon as possible after onset of symptoms and continue for 24 to 48 hours after symptoms disappear.

*Dosage:*

| Amantadine Dosage by Patient Age and Renal Function ||
| --- | --- |
| Renal function | Dosage |
| *No recognized renal disease* ||
| 1 to 9 yrs[1] | 4.4 to 8.8 mg/kg/day given once daily or divided twice daily, not to exceed 150 mg/day |
| 9 to 12 yrs | 100 mg twice daily |
| 13 to 64 yrs | 200 mg once daily or divided twice daily |
| ≥ 65 yrs | 100 mg once daily |
| *Renal function impairment – Ccr (mL/min/1.73 m$^2$)* ||
| 30 to 50 | 200 mg 1st day; 100 mg daily thereafter |
| 15 to 29 | 200 mg 1st day; then 100 mg on alternate days |
| < 15 | 200 mg every 7 days |
| Hemodialysis patients | 200 mg every 7 days |

[1] Use in children younger than 1 year of age has not been evaluated adequately.

*Dosage adjustments:* For adults younger than 65 years of age, if CNS effects develop in a once-daily dosage, a split dosage schedule may reduce such complaints.

*Special risk patients:* Dose may need reduction in patients with CHF, peripheral edema, orthostatic hypotension, or impaired renal function.

### Actions

*Pharmacology:* Inhibits the replication of influenza A virus isolates from each of the subtypes. Amantadine's antiviral activity is not completely understood. Its mode of action appears to be the prevention of the release of infectious viral nucleic acid into the host cell. Amantadine does not appear to interfere with the immunogenicity of inactivated influenza A virus vaccine.

Amantadine is 70% to 90% effective in preventing illnesses caused by type A influenza viruses.

*Pharmacokinetics:*

*Absorption/Distribution* – After administration of a single dose of 100 mg, maximum blood levels are reached in approximately 4 hours, based on the mean time of the peak urinary excretion rate; the peak excretion rate is approximately 5 mg/h; the mean half-life of the excretion rate is approximately 15 hours.

Clearance of amantadine is significantly reduced in adults with renal insufficiency. Elimination half-life increases 2- to 3-fold when Ccr is less than 40 mL/min/1.73 m$^2$ and averages 8 days in patients on chronic maintenance hemodialysis.

*Metabolism/Excretion* – Amantadine is readily absorbed, is not metabolized, and is excreted in the urine. The renal clearance of amantadine is reduced and plasma levels are increased in otherwise healthy elderly patients 65 years of age and older. The drug plasma levels in elderly patients receiving 100 mg daily have been reported to approximate those determined in younger adults taking 200 mg daily.

## Contraindications
Hypersensitivity to amantadine.

## Warnings
*Deaths:* Deaths have been reported from overdose with amantadine (see Overdosage).

*Suicide attempts:* Suicide attempts, some of which have been fatal, have been reported in patients treated with amantadine, many of whom received short courses for influenza treatment or prophylaxis. Suicide attempts and suicidal ideation have been reported in patients with and without prior history of psychiatric illness. Amantadine can exacerbate mental problems in patients with a history of psychiatric disorders or substance abuse. Patients who attempt suicide may exhibit abnormal mental states, which include disorientation, confusion, depression, personality changes, agitation, aggressive behavior, hallucinations, paranoia, other psychotic reactions, and somnolence or insomnia. Because of the possibility of serious adverse effects, observe caution when prescribing amantadine to patients being treated with drugs having CNS effects, or for whom the potential risks outweigh the benefit of treatment.

*Seizures and other CNS effects:* Closely observe patients with a history of seizures for increased seizure activity. Caution patients who note CNS effects or blurring of vision against driving or working in situations where alertness and adequate motor coordination are important.

*CHF or peripheral edema:* Closely follow patients with a history of CHF or peripheral edema as there are patients who developed CHF while receiving amantadine.

*Glaucoma:* Because amantadine has anticholinergic effects and may cause mydriasis, do not give to patients with untreated angle closure glaucoma.

*Other:* Exercise care when administering to patients with a history of recurrent eczematoid rash, or to patients with psychosis or severe psychoneurosis not controlled by chemotherapeutic agents.

*Renal function impairment:* Reduce the dose in renal impairment.

*Elderly:* Reduce dose in individuals 65 years of age and older.

*Pregnancy:* Category C.

*Lactation:* Amantadine is excreted in breast milk. Use is not recommended in nursing mothers.

*Children:* Safety and efficacy for use in neonates and infants younger than 1 year of age have not been established.

## Precautions
*Abrupt withdrawal:* Do not discontinue amantadine abruptly in patients with Parkinson's disease. A few patients have experienced a parkinsonian crisis (a sudden marked clinical deterioration) when this medication was suddenly stopped. Abrupt

discontinuation also may precipitate delirium, agitation, delusions, hallucinations, paranoid reaction, stupor, anxiety, depression, and slurred speech.

*Neuroleptic malignant syndrome (NMS):* Sporadic cases of possible NMS have been reported in association with dose reduction or withdrawal of amantadine therapy. Observe patients carefully when the dosage of amantadine is reduced abruptly or discontinued, especially if the patient is receiving neuroleptics.

### Drug Interactions

Drugs that may affect amantadine include anticholinergic drugs, triamterene and thiazide diuretics, quinidine, quinine, and trimethoprim/sulfamethoxazole.

Drugs that may be affected by amantadine include CNS stimulants.

### Adverse Reactions

Adverse reactions occurring in ≥ 3% of patients include nausea; dizziness; lightheadedness; insomnia; depression; anxiety; irritability; hallucinations; confusion; anorexia; dry mouth; constipation; ataxia; livedo reticularis; peripheral edema; orthostatic hypotension; headache.

# RIBAVIRIN

| | |
|---|---|
| **Tablets**: 200 mg (*Rx*) | *Copegus* (Roche) |
| **Capsules**: 200 mg (*Rx*) | *Rebetol* (Schering), *Ribaspheres*(Three Rivers) |
| **Lyophilized powder for aerosol reconstitution**: 6 g ribavirin/100 mL vial. Contains 20 mg/mL when reconstituted with 300 mL sterile water (*Rx*) | *Virazole* (ICN) |
| **Oral solution**: 40 mg/mL (*Rx*) | *Rebetol* (Schering) |

**Warning:**

*Capsules/Tablets/Oral solution:* Ribavirin monotherapy poop is not effective for the treatment of chronic hepatitis C virus (HCV) infection and should not be used alone for this indication.

The primary toxicity of ribavirin is hemolytic anemia that may result in worsening of cardiac disease and lead to fatal and nonfatal myocardial infarctions (MIs). Do not treat patients with a history of significant or unstable cardiac disease with ribavirin.

Significant teratogenic or embryocidal effects have been demonstrated in all animal species exposed to ribavirin. In addition, ribavirin has a multiple-dose half-life of 12 days, and it may persist in nonplasma compartments for as long as 6 months. Therefore, ribavirin therapy is contraindicated in women who are pregnant and in the male partners of women who are pregnant. Extreme care must be taken to avoid pregnancy during therapy and for 6 months after completion of treatment in these individuals. At least 2 reliable forms of effective contraception must be used during treatment and during the 6-month posttreatment follow-up period.

*Aerosol:* Use of aerosolized ribavirin in patients requiring mechanical ventilator assistance should be undertaken only by health care providers and support staff familiar with the specific ventilator being used and this mode of administration of the drug. Pay strict attention to procedures that have been shown to minimize the accumulation of drug precipitate that can result in mechanical ventilator dysfunction and associated increased pulmonary pressures.

**Warning: (cont.)**

Sudden deterioration of respiratory function has been associated with initiation of aerosolized ribavirin use in infants. Carefully monitor respiratory function during treatment. If initiation of aerosolized ribavirin treatment appears to produce sudden deterioration of respiratory function, stop treatment and reinstitute only with extreme caution, continuous monitoring, and consideration of concomitant administration of bronchodilators (see Warnings).

Ribavirin aerosol is not indicated for use in adults. Health care providers and patients should be aware that ribavirin has been shown to produce testicular lesions in rodents and to be teratogenic in all animal species in which adequate studies have been conducted (rodents and rabbits).

## Indications

*Tablets:*

*Chronic HCV* – In combination with peginterferon alfa-2a for the treatment of adults with chronic HCV infection who have compensated liver disease and have not been previously treated with interferon alpha. Patients in whom efficacy was demonstrated included patients with compensated liver disease and histological evidence of cirrhosis (Child-Pugh class A).

*Capsules/Oral solution:*

*Chronic HCV* – In combination with interferon alfa-2b injection for the treatment of chronic HCV in patients 3 years of age (oral solution) or 5 years of age (capsules) and older with compensated liver disease previously untreated with alpha interferon or in patients who have relapsed following alpha interferon therapy. Note: *Ribaspheres* is only indicated in combination with interferon alfa-2b in patients 18 years of age and older.

In combination with peginterferon alfa-2b injection for the treatment of chronic HCV in patients with compensated liver disease who have not been previously treated with interferon alpha and are at least 18 years of age.

The safety and efficacy of ribavirin capsules or oral solution with interferons other than interferon alfa-2b or peginterferon alfa-2b products have not been established.

*Pediatric use* – Consider evidence of disease progression, such as hepatic inflammation and fibrosis, as well as prognostic factors for response, HCV genotype, and viral load, when deciding to treat a pediatric patient. Weigh the benefits of treatment against the safety findings observed for pediatric patients in clinical trials.

*Aerosol:*

*Severe lower respiratory tract infections* – Treatment of hospitalized infants and young children with severe lower respiratory tract infections caused by respiratory syncytial virus (RSV).

## Administration and Dosage

*Tablets:* The daily dose of ribavirin tablets is 800 to 1200 mg administered orally in 2 divided doses with food.

The recommended duration of treatment for patients previously untreated with ribavirin and interferon is 24 to 48 weeks.

| Peginterferon alfa-2a and Ribavirin Tablet Dosing Recommendations | | | |
|---|---|---|---|
| Genotype[1] | Peginterferon alfa-2a dose | Ribavirin tablet dose | Duration |
| Genotype 1, 4 | 180 mcg | < 75 kg = 1000 mg | 48 wk |
| | | ≥ 75 kg = 1200 mg | 48 wk |
| Genotype 2, 3 | 180 mcg | 800 mg | 24 wk |

[1] Genotypes non-1 showed no increased response to treatment beyond 24 weeks. Data on genotypes 5 and 6 are insufficient for dosing recommendations.

*Dose modifications –*

| Ribavirin Tablet Dosage Modification Guidelines | | |
|---|---|---|
| Laboratory values | Reduce only ribavirin tablet dose to 600 mg/day[1] if: | Discontinue ribavirin tablets if: |
| Hemoglobin in patients with no cardiac disease | < 10 g/dL | < 8.5 g/dL |
| Hemoglobin in patients with history of stable cardiac disease | ≥ 2 g/dL decrease in hemoglobin during any 4-wk treatment period | < 12 g/dL despite 4 wk at reduced dose |

[1] One 200 mg tablet in the morning and two 200 mg tablets in the evening.

Once ribavirin tablets have been withheld because of a laboratory abnormality or clinical manifestation, an attempt may be made to restart ribavirin tablets at 600 mg/day and further increase the dose to 800 mg/day depending upon the physician's judgement. However, it is not recommended that ribavirin tablets be increased to the original assigned dose (1000 to 1200 mg).

*Renal impairment* – Do not use ribavirin tablets in patients with creatinine clearance (Ccr) less than 50 mL/min.

*Capsules/Oral solution:* When given in combination with peginterferon alfa-2b, it is recommended that ribavirin be administered in the evening with food.

Do not open, crush, or break capsules.

| Recommended Dosing | |
|---|---|
| Body weight | Ribavirin capsules |
| ≤ 75 kg | 2 × 200 mg capsules AM, 3 × 200 mg capsules PM daily PO |
| > 75 kg | 3 × 200 mg capsules AM, 3 × 200 mg capsules PM daily PO |

Ribavirin may be administered without regard to food but should be administered in a consistent manner with respect to food intake.

*Treatment duration* – The recommended duration of treatment for patients previously untreated with interferon is 24 to 48 weeks. Assess virologic response after 24 weeks of treatment. Consider treatment discontinuation in any patient who has not achieved an HCV-RNA below the limit of detection by 24 weeks.

The recommended duration of treatment is 48 weeks for pediatric patients with genotype 1 and 24 weeks for genotype 2/3.

*Therapy relapse* – In patients who relapse following interferon therapy, the recommended duration of treatment is 24 weeks. There are no safety and efficacy data on treatment for more than 24 weeks in the relapse patient population.

*Pediatric* – The recommended dose is 15 mg/kg/day orally (divided dose AM and PM). For children weighing 25 kg or less or who cannot swallow capsules, ribavirin oral solution is supplied in a concentration of 40 mg/mL. For children weighing more than 25 kg, administer either the oral solution or 200 mg capsule.

| Pediatric Dosing for Interferon Alfa-2b and Ribavirin | | |
|---|---|---|
| Body weight | Ribavirin capsules | Interferon alfa-2b injection |
| 25 to 36 kg | 1 × 200 mg capsules AM, 1 × 200 mg capsules PM daily by mouth | 3 million units/m² 3 times weekly subcutaneously |
| 37 to 49 kg | 1 × 200 mg capsules AM, 2 × 200 mg capsules PM daily by mouth | 3 million units/m² 3 times weekly subcutaneously |
| 50 to 61 kg | 2 × 200 mg capsules AM, 2 × 200 mg capsules PM daily by mouth | 3 million units/m² 3 times weekly subcutaneously |
| > 61 kg | Refer to adult dosing table | Refer to adult dosing table |

*Ribavirin capsules/Peginterferon alfa-2b combination therapy (adults)* – The recommended dose of ribavirin capsules is 800 mg/day in 2 divided doses: 2 capsules (400 mg) in the morning with food and 2 capsules (400 mg) in the evening with food.

*Dose modifications* – If severe adverse reactions or laboratory abnormalities develop during combination therapy, modify or discontinue the dose, if appropriate, until the adverse reactions abate. If intolerance persists after dose adjustment, discontinue combination therapy.

A permanent dose reduction is required for patients with a history of stable cardiovascular disease if the hemoglobin decreases by 2 g/dL or more during any 4-week period. In addition, discontinue combination therapy in cardiac history patients if the hemoglobin remains less than 12 g/dL after 4 weeks on a reduced dose.

It is recommended that a patient whose hemoglobin level falls below 10 g/dL have his/her ribavirin dose reduced to 600 mg daily (1 × 200 mg capsule AM, 2 × 200 mg capsules PM) for adults and 7.5 mg/kg/day (divided dose AM and PM) for pediatric patients. Permanently discontinue ribavirin therapy in patients whose hemoglobin level falls below 8.5 g/dL.

| Guidelines for Dose Modifications and Discontinuation for Anemia Based on Hemoglobin Levels | | |
|---|---|---|
| | Dose reduction ribavirin capsules 600 mg daily | Permanent discontinuation of ribavirin treatment |
| Hemoglobin in patients with no cardiac history | < 10 g/dL | < 8.5 g/dL |
| Hemoglobin in patients with a cardiac history | ≥ 2 g/dL decrease during any 4-wk period during treatment | < 12 g/dL after 4 wks of dose reduction |

*Aerosol:* For aerosol administration only. Do not administer with any other aerosol-generating device or together with other aerosolized medications.

The recommended treatment regimen is 20 mg/mL as the starting solution in the drug reservoir of the Small Particle Aerosol Generator (SPAG-2) unit. Treatment is carried out for 12 to 18 hours/day for 3 to 7 days.

*Mechanically ventilated infants* – The recommended dose and administration schedule for infants who require mechanical ventilation is the same as for those who do not.

*Nonmechanically ventilated infants* – The aerosol is delivered to an infant oxygen hood from the SPAG-2 aerosol generator. Administration by face mask or oxygen tent may be necessary if a hood cannot be used. However, the volume and condensation area are larger in a tent, and this may alter the drug's delivery dynamics.

*Reconstitution* – Reconstitute drug with a minimum of 75 mL sterile water for injection or inhalation in the original 100 mL vial. Shake well. Transfer to the clean, sterilized 500 mL SPAG-2 reservoir and further dilute to a final volume of 300 mL with sterile water for injection or inhalation. The final concentration should be 20 mg/mL.

*Important:* This water should not have any antimicrobial agent or other substance added. Discard solutions placed in the SPAG-2 unit at least every 24 hours and when the liquid level is low before adding newly reconstituted solution. Using the recommended drug concentration of 20 mg/mL ribavirin as the starting solution in the SPAG-2 unit's drug reservoir, the average aerosol concentration for a 12-hour period is 190 mcg/L of air.

### Actions

*Pharmacology:* Ribavirin is a synthetic nucleoside analog. It has antiviral activity in vitro against RSV, influenza A and B viruses, and herpes simplex virus.

*Pharmacokinetics:*

*Absorption* –

*Tablets:* The average time to reach $C_{max}$ was 2 hours.

*Capsules:* Ribavirin was rapidly and extensively absorbed following oral administration. However, because of first-pass metabolism, the absolute bioavailability averaged 64%.

*Aerosol:* Ribavirin administered by aerosol is absorbed systemically. The plasma half-life was 9.5 hours.

*Distribution –*

*Capsules:* Following oral dosing with 600 mg twice daily, steady-state was reached by about 4 weeks.

*Aerosol:* Bioavailability of the aerosol is unknown and may depend on mode of delivery.

Accumulation of drug or metabolites in red blood cells occurs, with plateauing in red cells in about 4 days. Accumulation gradually declines with an apparent half-life of 40 days.

*Metabolism –*

*Capsules:* Ribavirin is hepatically metabolized.

*Excretion –*

*Tablets:* The terminal half-life following a single dose administration is approximately 120 to 170 hours. The total apparent clearance is about 26 L/h.

*Capsules:* Ribavirin and its metabolites are excreted renally. Upon discontinuation of dosing, the mean half-life was 298 hours.

## Contraindications

*Tablets/Capsules/Oral solution:* Ribavirin may cause birth defects or death of the exposed fetus. Ribavirin is contraindicated in women who are pregnant or in men whose female partners are pregnant (see Warnings), in patients with a history of hypersensitivity to ribavirin or any component of the drug, and in patients with hemoglobinopathies (eg, thalassemia major, sickle-cell anemia).

*Aerosol:* Hypersensitivity to the drug or its components; pregnancy or the potential for pregnancy during exposure to the drug (see Warnings).

*Ribavirin tablets/Peginterferon alfa-2a:* Ribavirin tablets/peginterferon alfa-2a combination therapy is contraindicated in patients with autoimmune hepatitis and hepatic decompensation (Child-Pugh class B and C) before or during treatment.

*Ribavirin capsules/oral solution/interferon alfa-2b:* Patients with autoimmune hepatitis must not be treated with combination ribavirin capsules/interferon alfa-2b therapy because using these medicines can make the hepatitis worse.

## Warnings

*Monotherapy:*

*Capsules/Tablets/Oral solution –* Ribavirin monotherapy is not effective for the treatment of chronic HCV infection. The safety and efficacy of ribavirin capsules and oral solution have only been established when used together with interferon alfa-2b, recombinant as interferon alfa-2b/ribavirin capsule combination therapy or with peginterferon alfa-2b injection.

*Combination therapy adverse events:*

*Capsules/Tablets/Oral solution –* There are significant adverse events caused by ribavirin capsules/interferon alfa-2b or peginterferon alfa-2b therapy, and ribavirin tablets/peginterferon alfa-2a therapy, including severe depression and suicidal ideation, hemolytic anemia, suppression of bone marrow function, autoimmune and infectious disorders, pulmonary dysfunction, pancreatitis, and diabetes.

*Cardiovascular effects:*

*Capsules/Tablets/Oral solution –* Fatal and nonfatal MIs have been reported in patients with anemia caused by ribavirin.

*Aerosol –* Events associated with aerosolized ribavirin have included cardiac arrest, hypotension, bradycardia, and digitalis toxicity. Bigeminy, bradycardia, and tachycardia have been described in patients with underlying congenital heart disease.

*Coadministration with nucleoside analogs (eg, didanosine):*

*Tablets –* Coadministration of ribavirin and didanosine is not recommended. Reports of fatal hepatic failure, as well as peripheral neuropathy, pancreatitis, and symptomatic hyperlactatemia/lactic acidosis have been reported in clinical trials.

*Underlying conditions:*

*Aerosol* – The presence of underlying conditions such as prematurity, immuno-suppression, or cardiopulmonary disease may increase the severity of the infection and its risk to the patient.

*Assisted ventilation:*

*Aerosol* – Some subjects requiring assisted ventilation have experienced serious difficulties because of inadequate ventilation and gas exchange. Drug precipitation within the ventilatory apparatus, including the endotracheal tube, has resulted in increased positive and expiratory pressure and increased positive inspiratory pressure. Accumulation of fluid in tubing ("rain out") also has been noted.

*Pancreatitis:* Suspend ribavirin, interferon alfa-2b, peginterferon alfa-2b, or peginterferon alfa-2a therapy in patients with signs and symptoms of pancreatitis and discontinue in patients with confirmed pancreatitis.

*Suicidal ideation (capsules/oral solution):* Severe psychiatric adverse events including depression, psychoses, aggressive behavior, hallucinations, violent behavior (suicidal ideation, suicidal attempts, suicides) and rare instances of homicidal ideation have occurred during combination ribavirin capsules/*Intron A* therapy, both in patients with and without a previous psychiatric disorder.

*Pulmonary effects:*

*Aerosol* – Several serious adverse events occurred in severely ill infants with life-threatening underlying diseases, many of whom required assisted ventilation. Additional reports of worsening of respiratory status, bronchospasm, pulmonary edema, hypoventilation, cyanosis, dyspnea, bacterial pneumonia, pneumothorax, apnea, atelectasis, and ventilator dependence have occurred. Sudden deterioration of respiratory function has been associated with initiation of aerosolized ribavirin use in infants. If ribavirin aerosol treatment produces sudden deterioration of respiratory function, stop treatment and reinstitute only with extreme caution, continuous monitoring, and consideration of coadministration of bronchodilators.

*Capsules/Tablets/Oral solution* – Pulmonary symptoms, including dyspnea, pulmonary infiltrates, pneumonitis, and pneumonia have been reported during therapy with ribavirin and interferon. Occasional cases of fatal pneumonia have occurred. In addition, sarcoidosis or the exacerbation of sarcoidosis has been reported.

*Hemolytic anemia:*

*Capsules/Tablets/Oral solution* – The primary toxicity of ribavirin is hemolytic anemia, which occurs within 1 to 2 weeks of initiation of therapy.

*Aerosol* – Although anemia has not been reported with aerosol use, it occurs frequently with experimental oral and IV ribavirin. Cases of anemia, reticulocytosis, and hemolytic anemia associated with aerosolized ribavirin use have been reported in postmarketing reporting systems.

*Renal function impairment:*

*Capsules/Tablets/Oral solution* – Do not treat patients with Ccr less than 50 mL/min with ribavirin.

*Carcinogenesis:*

*Capsules/Oral solution* – Ribavirin has produced positive findings in multiple in vitro and animal in vivo genotoxicity assays, and should be considered a potential carcinogen.

*Aerosol* – Chronic feeding of ribavirin to rats at doses of 16 to 100 mg/kg/day (estimated human equivalent of 2.3 to 14.3 mg/kg/day, based on body surface area adjustment for adults) suggest that ribavirin may induce benign mammary, pancreatic, pituitary, and adrenal tumors.

*Mutagenesis:*

*Tablets* – The in vitro mouse lymphoma assay demonstrated mutagenic activity.

*Aerosol* – An increased incidence of cell transformations and mutations was shown.

*Fertility impairment:*

*Capsules/Tablets/Oral solution* – Use ribavirin with caution in fertile men. Upon cessation of treatment, essentially total recovery from ribavirin-induced testicular toxicity was apparent within 1 or 2 spermatogenesis cycles.

*Aerosol* – Doses administered to mice between 35 and 150 mg/kg/day resulted in significant seminiferous tubule atrophy, decreased sperm concentrations, and increased numbers of sperm with abnormal morphology. Partial recovery of sperm production was apparent 3 to 6 months following dose cessation. Testicular lesions (tubular atrophy) in adult rats at oral dose levels as low as 16 mg/kg/day was shown.

*Elderly:*

*Capsules/Oral solution* – In clinical trials, elderly subjects had a higher frequency of anemia than did younger patients (see Warnings).

In general, cautiously administer ribavirin capsules to elderly patients, starting at the lower end of the dosing range, reflecting the greater frequency of decreased hepatic, renal, or cardiac function, and of concomitant disease or other drug therapy. Do not use ribavirin in elderly patients with Ccr less than 50 mL/min.

*Pregnancy: Category X.*

*Lactation:*

*Aerosol* – Ribavirin is toxic to lactating animals and their offspring.

*Capsules/Tablets/Oral solution* – It is not known whether ribavirin is excreted in human milk. Because of the potential for serious adverse reactions from the drug in nursing infants, a decision should be made whether to discontinue nursing or to delay or discontinue ribavirin.

*Children:*

*Tablets* – Safety and efficacy of ribavirin tablets have not been established in pediatric patients younger than 18 years of age.

*Capsules/Oral solution* – Suicidal ideation or attempts occurred more frequently among pediatric patients, primarily adolescents, compared with adult patients during treatment and off-therapy follow-up. Safety and efficacy of ribavirin in combination with peginterferon alfa-2b has not been established in pediatric patients.

During a 48-week course of therapy there was a decrease in the rate of linear growth (mean percentile assignment decrease of 9%) and a decrease in the rate of weight gain (mean percentile assignment decrease of 13%). A general reversal of these trends was noted during the 24-week posttreatment period.

## Precautions

*Monitoring:*

*Capsules/Tablets/Oral solution* – Assess patients for underlying cardiac disease before initiation of ribavirin therapy and appropriately monitor them during therapy. The recommended monitoring for all patients treated with ribavirin prior to beginning treatment and then periodically thereafter:

- Standard hematologic tests: Including hemoglobin (pretreatment, week 2 and week 4 of therapy, and as clinically appropriate) (see Warnings), complete and differential white blood cell counts, and platelet count.
- Blood chemistries: Liver function tests and TSH.
- Pregnancy: Including monthly monitoring for women of childbearing potential and for 6 months after discontinuing therapy.
- ECG

*Aerosol* – Monitor respiratory function and fluid status during treatment.

*HIV or HBV coinfection:*

*Capsules/Tablets/Oral solution* – The safety and efficacy of ribavirin and interferon alfa-2b or peginterferon alfa-2a combination therapy for the treatment of HCV have not been established in patients coinfected with HIV or HBV.

*Hepatitis C:*

*Capsules/Tablets/Oral solution* – The safety and efficacy of ribavirin and interferon alfa-2b or peginterferon alfa-2a combination therapy for the treatment of HCV in patients who have received liver or other organ transplants have not been established.

*Other infections:*

*Capsules/Tablets/Oral solution* – The safety and efficacy of ribavirin and peginterferon alfa-2a, interferon alfa-2b, and peginterferon alfa-2b combination therapy for the treatment of HIV infection, adenovirus RSV, parainfluenza, or influenza infections have not been established. Do not use ribavirin for these indications.

*Health care personnel:*

*Aerosol* – Health care workers directly providing care to patients receiving aerosolized ribavirin should be aware that ribavirin is teratogenic in all animal species in which adequate studies have been conducted.

Health care workers who are pregnant should consider avoiding direct care of patients receiving aerosolized ribavirin. If close patient contact cannot be avoided, take precautions to limit exposure.

## Drug Interactions

Drugs that may interact with ribavirin capsules/oral solution include antacids. Drugs that may interact with ribavirin tablets include nucleoside analogs (eg, didanosine, zidovudine, stavudine).

## Adverse Reactions

*Aerosol:* Adverse reactions may include anemia and hemolytic anemia; apnea; atelectasis; bacterial pneumonia; bigeminy; bradycardia; bronchospasm; cardiac arrest; conjunctivitis; cyanosis; digitalis toxicity; dyspnea; hypotension; hypoventilation; pneumothorax; pulmonary edema; rash; reticulocytosis; tachycardia; ventilator dependence; worsening of respiratory status.

*Healthcare workers:* Headache (51%); conjunctivitis (32%); rhinitis, nausea, rash, dizziness, pharyngitis, lacrimation (10% to 20%).

*Capsule combination therapy:* Adverse reactions occurring in at least 3% of patients include abdominal pain; agitation; alopecia; anemia; anorexia; anxiety/emotional lability/ irritability; arthralgia; asthenia; blurred vision; chest pain; concentration impaired; conjunctivitis; constipation; coughing; depression; diarrhea; dizziness; dry mouth; dry skin; dyspnea; dyspepsia; fatigue; fever; flushing; fungal/viral infection; headache; hepatomegaly; hypothyroidism; increased sweating; influenza-like symptoms; injection site inflammation; injection site reaction; insomnia; irritability; leukopenia; malaise; menstrual disorder; musculoskeletal pain; myalgia; nausea; nervousness; neutropenia; pharyngitis; pruritus; rash; rhinitis; right upper quadrant pain; rigors; sinusitis; taste perversion; thrombocytopenia; vomiting; weight decrease.

*Tablet combination therapy:* Adverse reactions occurring in at least 3% of patients include the following: Abdominal pain; alopecia; anemia; anorexia; anxiety; arthralgia; back pain; bacterial infection; blurred vision; concentration impairment; cough; depression; dermatitis; diarrhea; dizziness; dry mouth/skin; dyspepsia; dyspnea; eczema; fatigue/ asthenia; headache; hypothyroidism; increased sweating; injection site reaction; insomnia; irritability/anxiety/nervousness; lymphopenia; memory impairment; mood alteration; myalgia; nausea; neutropenia; pain; pruritus; pyrexia; rash; resistance mechanism disorders; rigors; thrombocytopenia; vomiting; weight decrease.

# RIMANTADINE HCl

| | |
|---|---|
| **Tablets**: 100 mg *(Rx)* | *Flumadine* (Forest) |
| **Syrup**: 50 mg/5 mL *(Rx)* | |

## Indications

*Adults:* Prophylaxis/treatment of illness caused by various strains of influenza A virus.

*Children:* Prophylaxis against influenza A virus.

*Prophylaxis recommendations:*

1.) High-risk patients vaccinated after influenza outbreak has begun: Consider prophylaxis until immunity from the influenza vaccine has developed (up to 2 weeks).

2.) Caretakers of those at high risk: Consider prophylaxis for unvaccinated caretakers of high-risk patients during peak influenza activity.

3.) Patients with immune deficiency: Consider prophylaxis for high-risk patients who are expected to have inadequate antibody response to influenza vaccine (eg, patients with HIV).

4.) Other: Consider prophylaxis in high-risk patients who should not be vaccinated. Prophylaxis also may be offered to those patients who desire to avoid influenza illness.

## Administration and Dosage

*Prophylaxis:*

*Adults* – The recommended dose of rimantadine is 100 mg twice daily. In patients with severe hepatic dysfunction or renal failure (Ccr less than or equal to 10 mL/min) and in elderly nursing home patients, a dose reduction to 100 mg daily is recommended.

*Children (younger than 10 years of age)* – Administer once daily at a dose of 5 mg/kg, not exceeding 150 mg. For children 10 years of age and older, use the adult dose.

*Treatment:*

*Adults* – The recommended dose is 100 mg twice daily. In patients with severe hepatic dysfunction or renal failure (Ccr less than or equal to 10 mL/min) and in elderly nursing home patients, a dose reduction to 100 mg daily is recommended. Initiate therapy as soon as possible, preferably within 48 hours after onset of signs and symptoms of influenza A infection. Continue therapy for approximately 7 days from the initial onset of symptoms.

## Actions

*Pharmacology:* Rimantadine is a synthetic antiviral agent that appears to exert its inhibitory effect early in the viral replicative cycle, possibly inhibiting the uncoating of the virus.

*Pharmacokinetics:* The tablet and syrup formulations of rimantadine are equally absorbed after oral administration. The time to peak concentration was 6 hours in healthy adults. The single dose elimination half-life in this population was 25.4 hours. The single-dose elimination half-life in a group of healthy 71- to 79-year-old subjects was 32 hours.

In a group (n = 10) of children 4 to 8 years of age who were given a single dose (6.6 mg/kg) of syrup, plasma concentrations ranged from 446 to 988 ng/mL at 5 to 6 hours and from 170 to 424 ng/mL at 24 hours. In some children, the drug was detected in plasma 72 hours after the last dose. Following oral administration, rimantadine is extensively metabolized in the liver with less than 25% of the dose excreted in the urine as unchanged drug. Three hydroxylated metabolites have been found in plasma. These metabolites, an additional conjugated metabolite and parent drug account for 74% of a single 200 mg dose excreted in urine over 72 hours.

## Contraindications

Hypersensitivity to drugs of the adamantine class, including rimantadine and amantadine.

## Warnings

*Renal/Hepatic function impairment:* The safety and pharmacokinetics of rimantadine in renal and hepatic insufficiency only have been evaluated after single dose administration. In a single dose study of patients with anuric renal failure, the apparent clearance was approximately 40% lower and the elimination half-life was 1.6-fold greater than that in healthy controls. In a study of 14 people with chronic liver disease (mostly stabilized cirrhotics), no alterations in the pharmacokinetics were observed after a single dose of rimantadine. However, the apparent clearance of rimantadine following a single dose to 10 patients with severe liver dysfunction was 50% lower than that reported for healthy subjects. Because of the potential for accumulation of rimantadine and its metabolites in plasma, exercise caution when patients with renal or hepatic insufficiency are treated with rimantadine.

*Pregnancy:* Category C.

*Lactation:* Rimantadine should not be administered to nursing mothers because of the adverse affects noted in offspring of rats treated with rimantadine during the nursing period.

*Children:* In children, rimantadine is recommended for the prophylaxis of influenza A. Safety and efficacy of rimantadine in the treatment of symptomatic influenza infection in children have not been established. Prophylaxis studies with rimantadine have not been performed in children younger than 1 year of age.

**Precautions**

*Seizures:* An increased incidence of seizures has been reported in patients with a history of epilepsy who received the related drug amantadine. In clinical trials, the occurrence of seizure-like activity was observed in a small number of patients with a history of seizures who were not receiving anticonvulsant medication while taking rimantadine. If seizures develop, discontinue the drug.

*Resistance:* Consider transmission of rimantadine-resistant virus when treating patients whose contacts are at high risk for influenza A illness. Influenza A virus strains resistant to rimantadine can emerge during treatment and may be transmissible and cause typical influenza illness. Of patients with initially sensitive virus upon treatment with rimantadine, 10% to 30% shed rimantadine-resistant virus. Clinical response, although slower in those patients, was not significantly different from those who did not shed resistant virus.

**Drug Interactions**

Drugs that may affect rimantadine include acetaminophen, aspirin, and cimetidine.

**Adverse Reactions**

Adverse reactions occurring in at least 3% of patients included insomnia.

Geriatric subjects who received 200 or 400 mg of rimantadine daily experienced considerably more CNS and GI adverse events than comparable geriatric subjects receiving placebo. CNS events, including dizziness, headache, anxiety, asthenia, and fatigue occurred up to 2 times more often with rimantadine than with placebo. GI symptoms, particularly nausea, vomiting, and abdominal pain occurred at least twice as frequently with rimantadine than with receiving placebo. The GI symptoms appeared to be dose-related.

# ZANAMIVIR

**Blisters of powder for inhalation:** 5 mg (*Rx*)          *Relenza* (GlaxoSmithKline)

**Indications**

*Influenza treatment:* Treatment of uncomplicated acute illness caused by influenza A and B virus in adults and children 7 years of age and older who have been symptomatic for no more than 2 days.

Zanamivir is not recommended for treatment of patients with underlying airways disease such as asthma or chronic obstructive pulmonary disease (COPD) (see Warnings).

**Administration and Dosage**

Zanamivir is for administration to the respiratory tract by oral inhalation only, using the *Diskhaler* device provided. Instruct patients in the use of the delivery system. Include a demonstration whenever possible. If zanamivir is prescribed for children, it should be used only under adult supervision and instruction, and the supervising adult should first be instructed by a health care professional.

The recommended dose of zanamivir for the treatment of influenza in patients 7 years of age and older is 2 inhalations (one 5 mg blister per inhalation for a total dose of 10 mg) twice daily (about 12 hours apart) for 5 days. Two doses should be taken on the first day of treatment whenever possible, provided there is at least 2 hours between doses. On subsequent days, doses should be approximately 12 hours apart (eg, morning and evening) at approximately the same time each day. There are no data on the effectiveness of treatment with zanamivir when initiated more than 2 days after the onset of signs or symptoms.

Patients scheduled to use an inhaled bronchodilator at the same time as zanamivir should use their bronchodilator before taking zanamivir.

### Actions

*Pharmacology:* The proposed mechanism of action of zanamivir is via inhibition of influenza virus neuraminidase with the possibility of alteration of virus particle aggregation and release.

*Drug resistance* – Influenza viruses with reduced susceptibility to zanamivir have been recovered in vitro by passage of the virus in the presence of increasing concentrations of the drug. Genetic analysis of these viruses showed that the reduced susceptibility in vitro to zanamivir is associated with mutations that result in amino acid changes in the viral neuraminidase or viral hemagglutinin or both.

*Cross-resistance* – Cross-resistance has been observed between zanamivir-resistant and oseltamivir-resistant influenza virus mutants generated in vitro.

*Pharmacokinetics:*

*Absorption* – Approximately 4% to 17% of the inhaled dose is systemically absorbed. Peak serum concentrations ranged from 17 to 142 ng/mL within 1 to 2 hours after a 10 mg dose.

*Distribution* – Zanamivir has limited plasma protein binding (less than 10%).

*Metabolism* – Zanamivir is renally excreted as unchanged drug. No metabolites have been detected.

*Excretion* – The serum half-life of zanamivir following oral inhalation ranges from 2.5 to 5.1 hours. It is excreted unchanged in the urine with excretion of a single dose completed within 24 hours. Total clearance ranges from 2.5 to 10.9 L/h. Unabsorbed drug is excreted in the feces.

### Contraindications

Hypersensitivity to any component of the formulation.

### Warnings

*Underlying respiratory disease:* Zanamivir has not been shown to be effective and may carry risk in patients with severe or decompensated COPD or asthma, and serious adverse events have been reported in such patients. Therefore, zanamivir is not generally recommended for treatment of patients with underlying airways disease such as asthma or COPD.

*Pregnancy: Category C.*

There are no adequate and well-controlled studies in pregnant women. Use during pregnancy only if the potential benefit justifies the potential risk to the fetus.

*Lactation:* It is not known whether zanamivir is excreted in human breast milk. Exercise caution when zanamivir is administered to a nursing mother.

*Children:* Safety and efficacy of zanamivir have not been established in pediatric patients younger than 7 years of age.

### Precautions

*Start of treatment:* No data are available to support safety or efficacy in patients who begin treatment after 48 hours of symptoms.

*Repeated courses:* Safety and efficacy of repeated treatment courses have not been studied.

*Allergic reactions:* Allergic-like reactions, including oropharyngeal edema and serious skin rashes, have been reported in postmarketing experience with zanamivir. Stop zanamivir and institute appropriate treatment if an allergic reaction occurs or is suspected.

*Bacterial infections:* Serious bacterial infections may begin with influenza-like symptoms or may coexist with or occur as complications during the course of influenza. Zanamivir has not been shown to prevent such complications.

*Other illness:* There is no evidence for efficacy of zanamivir in any illness caused by agents other than influenza virus A and B.

*Prevention of influenza:* Safety and efficacy of zanamivir have not been established for pro-phylactic use to prevent influenza. Use of zanamivir should not affect the evaluation of individuals for annual influenza vaccination in accordance with guidelines of the Centers for Disease Control and Prevention Advisory Committee on Immunization Practices.

*High-risk patients:* Safety and efficacy have not been demonstrated in patients with high-risk underlying medical conditions. No information is available regarding treatment of influenza in patients with any medical condition sufficiently severe or unstable to be considered at imminent risk of requiring inpatient management.

### Drug Interactions

Zanamivir is not a substrate nor does it affect cytochrome P450 (CYP) isoenzymes (CYP1A1/2, 2A6, 2C9, 2C18, 2D6, 2E1, and 3A4) in human liver microsomes.

### Adverse Reactions

Adverse reactions occurring in at least 3% of patients include diarrhea, nasal signs and symptoms, nausea, sinusitis, and ear, nose, and throat infections.

*Lab test abnormalities:* Elevations of liver enzymes and CPK, lymphopenia, and neutropenia occurred. These were reported in similar proportions of zanamivir and lactose-vehicle placebo recipients with acute influenza-like illness.

# OSELTAMIVIR PHOSPHATE

**Capsules**: 75 mg (75 mg free base equivalent of the phos-phate salt) (*Rx*)  *Tamiflu* (Roche)

**Powder for oral suspension**: 12 mg/mL after reconstitution  *Tamiflu* (Roche)
(*Rx*)

### Indications

*Influenza infection:*

*Treatment* – Treatment of uncomplicated acute illness caused by influenza infection in patients older than 1 year of age who have been symptomatic for no more than 2 days.

*Prophylaxis* – For prophylaxis of influenza in adults and adolescents 13 years of age and older.

Oseltamivir is not a substitute for early vaccination on an annual basis as recommended by the CDC Immunization Practices Advisory Committee.

### Administration and Dosage

Oseltamivir may be taken without regard to food. However, when taken with food, tolerability may be enhanced.

*Treatment of influenza:*

*Adults and adolescents 13 years of age and older* – The recommended oral dose of oseltamivir is 75 mg twice daily for 5 days. Begin treatment within 2 days of onset of symptoms of influenza.

*Children* – The recommended oral dose of oseltamivir oral suspension for children 1 year of age and older or adults who cannot swallow a capsule is in the following table.

| Oseltamivir Oral Suspension Dosing | | | |
|---|---|---|---|
| Body weight (kg) | Body weight (lbs) | Recommended dose for 5 days | Volume |
| ≤ 15 | ≤ 33 | 30 mg twice daily | 2.5 mL (½ tsp) |
| > 15 to 23 | > 33 to 51 | 45 mg twice daily | 3.8 mL (¾ tsp) |
| > 23 to 40 | > 51 to 88 | 60 mg twice daily | 5 mL (1 tsp) |
| > 40 | > 88 | 75 mg twice daily | 6.2 mL (1¼ tsp) |

An oral dosing dispenser with 30, 45, and 60 mg graduations is provided with the oral suspension; the 75 mg dose can be measured using a combination of 30 and 45 mg. It is recommended that patients use this dispenser.

*Influenza prophylaxis:* The recommended oral dose of oseltamivir for influenza prophylaxis in adults and adolescents 13 years of age and older following close contact with an infected individual is 75 mg once daily for at least 7 days. Therapy should begin within 2 days of exposure. The recommended dose for prophylaxis during a community outbreak of influenza is 75 mg once daily. Safety and efficacy have been demonstrated for up to 6 weeks. The duration of protection lasts for as long as dosing is continued.

*Renal function impairment:*
  *Influenza treatment* – Dose adjustment is recommended for patients with Ccr between 10 and 30 mL/min receiving oseltamivir for treatment of influenza. In these patients, it is recommended that the dose be reduced to 75 mg oseltamivir once daily for 5 days.

  *Influenza prophylaxis* – For prophylaxis of influenza, dose adjustment is recommended for patients with Ccr between 10 and 30 mL/min receiving oseltamivir. In these patients, it is recommended that the dose be reduced to 75 mg every other day.

**Actions**

*Pharmacology:* Oseltamivir is an ethyl ester prodrug requiring ester hydrolysis for conversion to the active form, oseltamivir carboxylate. The proposed mechanism of action of oseltamivir is via inhibition of influenza virus neuraminidase with the possibility of alteration of virus particle aggregation and release.

  *Drug resistance* – In clinical studies of naturally acquired infection with influenza virus, 1.3% of posttreatment isolates in adults and adolescents, and 8.6% in children from 1 to 12 years of age showed emergence of influenza variants with decreased neuraminidase susceptibility to oseltamivir carboxylate.

  The contribution of resistance because of alterations in the viral hemagglutinin has not been fully evaluated.

*Pharmacokinetics:*
  *Absorption* – Oseltamivir phosphate is readily absorbed from the GI tract after oral administration.

  The mean $C_{max}$ of oseltamivir and oseltamivir carboxylate were 65.2 ng/mL and 348 ng/mL, respectively, after multiple doses of 75 mg twice daily. The mean $AUC_{(0 \text{ to } 12 \text{ h})}$ for oseltamivir was 112 ng•h/mL and 2719 ng•h/mL for oseltamivir carboxylate.

  Coadministration with food has no significant effect on the peak plasma concentration and the area under the plasma concentration time curve of oseltamivir carboxylate.

  *Distribution* – The binding of oseltamivir carboxylate to human plasma protein is low (3%). The binding of oseltamivir to human plasma protein is 42%, which is insufficient to cause significant displacement-based drug interactions.

  *Metabolism* – Oseltamivir is extensively converted to oseltamivir carboxylate by esterases located predominantly in the liver. Neither oseltamivir nor oseltamivir carboxylate is a substrate for, or inhibitor of, cytochrome P450 isoforms.

  *Excretion* – Absorbed oseltamivir is primarily (more than 90%) eliminated by conversion to oseltamivir carboxylate. Plasma concentrations of oseltamivir declined with a half-life of 1 to 3 hours in most subjects after oral administration. Oseltamivir carboxylate is not further metabolized and is eliminated in the urine. Plasma concentrations of oseltamivir carboxylate declined with a half-life of 6 to 10 hours in most subjects. Oseltamivir carboxylate is eliminated entirely (more than 99%) by renal excretion. Renal clearance (18.8 L/h) exceeds glomerular filtration rate (7.5 L/h) indicating that tubular secretion occurs, in addition to glomerular filtration. Less than 20% of an oral dose is eliminated in feces.

**Contraindications**

Hypersensitivity to any of the components of the product.

**Warnings**

*Renal function impairment:* Dose adjustment is recommended for patients with a serum Ccr less than 30 mL/min (see Administration and Dosage).

*Pregnancy:* Category C.

*Lactation:* It is not known whether oseltamivir or oseltamivir carboxylate is excreted in human breast milk. Therefore, use oseltamivir only if the potential benefit for the lactating mother justifies the potential risk to the breast-fed infant.

*Children:* The safety and efficacy in children less than 1 year of age have not been established.

### Precautions

*Bacterial infections:* Serious bacterial infections may begin with influenza-like symptoms or may coexist with or occur as complications during the course of influenza.

*Other illnesses:* There is no evidence for efficacy of oseltamivir in any illness caused by agents other than influenza viruses Types A and B.

*Start of treatment:* Efficacy of oseltamivir in patients who begin treatment after 40 hours of symptoms has not been established.

*High-risk patients:* Efficacy of oseltamivir in subjects with chronic cardiac disease or respiratory disease has not been established.

*Prevention of influenza:* Use of oseltamivir should not affect the evaluation of individuals for annual influenza vaccination in accordance with guidelines of the Center for Disease Controls and Prevention Advisory Committee on Immunization Practices. Efficacy of oseltamivir has not been established for prophylactic use to prevent influenza.

*Repeated courses:* Safety and efficacy of repeated treatment courses have not been established.

### Drug Interactions

*Probenecid:* Coadministration of probenecid results in an approximate 2-fold increase in exposure to oseltamivir carboxylate because of a decrease in active anionic tubular secretion in the kidney.

### Adverse Reactions

Adverse reactions occurring in at least 3% of patients include abdominal pain, cough, diarrhea, fatigue, headache, nausea, and vomiting.

## ADEFOVIR DIPIVOXIL

**Tablets:** 10 mg (*Rx*)                    *Hepsera* (Gilead Sciences)

**Warning:**

Severe acute exacerbations of hepatitis have been reported in patients who have discontinued anti-hepatitis B therapy, including adefovir. Closely monitor hepatic function in patients who discontinue anti-hepatitis B therapy.

In patients at risk of or having renal dysfunction, chronic administration of adefovir may result in nephrotoxicity. Closely monitor for renal function and adjust dose as required.

Human immunodeficiency virus (HIV) resistance may emerge in chronic hepatitis B patients with unrecognized or untreated HIV infection treated with anti-hepatitis B therapies, such as adefovir.

Lactic acidosis and severe hepatomegaly with steatosis, including fatal cases, have been reported with the use of nucleoside analogs alone or in combination with other antiretrovirals.

### Indications

*Chronic hepatitis B:* Treatment of chronic hepatitis B in adults with active viral replication and persistent elevations in serum aminotransferases (ALT or AST) or histologically active disease.

### Administration and Dosage

The recommended dose is 10 mg once daily without regard to food.

*Dosage adjustment in renal impairment:*

| **Adefovir Dosage Adjustment in Renal Impairment** | | | | |
|---|---|---|---|---|
| | Ccr (mL/min) | | | |
| | ≥ 50 | 20 to 49 | 10 to 19 | Hemodialysis patients |
| Recommended dose and dosing interval | 10 mg q 24 h | 10 mg q 48 h | 10 mg q 72 h | 10 mg q 7 days following dialysis |

The pharmacokinetics of adefovir have not been evaluated in nonhemodialysis patients with Ccr below 10 mL/min; therefore, no dosing recommendation is available for these patients.

### Actions

*Pharmacology:* Adefovir is an acyclic nucleotide analog of adenosine monophosphate.

*Pharmacokinetics:*

> *Absorption* – The oral bioavailability of adefovir is 59%. Adefovir may be taken without regard to food.

> *Distribution* – Binding of adefovir to plasma or proteins is less than or equal to 4%.

> *Metabolism/Excretion* – Elimination half-life is approximately 7.48 hours. Adefovir is renally excreted.

> *Special populations* –

>> *Renal impairment:* In subjects with impaired renal function or with end-stage renal disease requiring hemodialysis, $C_{max}$, AUC, and $T_{1/2}$ were increased. It is recommended that the dosing interval of adefovir be modified in these patients.

### Contraindications

Previously demonstrated hypersensitivity to any of the components of the product.

### Warnings

*Exacerbations of hepatitis after discontinuation of treatment:* Severe acute exacerbation of hepatitis has been reported in patients who have discontinued anti-hepatitis B therapy, including adefovir. Monitor patients who discontinue adefovir for hepatic function.

*Nephrotoxicity:* Nephrotoxicity characterized by a delayed onset of gradual increases in serum creatinine and decreases in serum phosphorus was shown to be the treatment-limiting toxicity of adefovir therapy at higher doses in HIV-infected patients (60 and 120 mg/day) and in chronic hepatitis B patients (30 mg/day). Chronic administration of adefovir (10 mg once daily) may result in nephrotoxicity. The overall risk of nephrotoxicity in patients with normal renal function is low. This is of special importance in patients at risk of or having renal dysfunction and patients taking concomitant nephrotoxic agents (eg, cyclosporine, tacrolimus, aminoglycosides, vancomycin, nonsteroidal anti-inflammatory drugs).

*Lactic acidosis/severe hepatomegaly with steatosis:* Lactic acidosis and severe hepatomegaly with steatosis, including fatal cases, have been reported with nucleoside analogs alone or in combination with antiretrovirals. A majority of these cases have been in women. Obesity and prolonged nucleoside exposure may be risk factors. Suspend treatment with adefovir in any patient who develops clinical or laboratory findings of lactic acidosis or hepatotoxicity (which may include hepatomegaly and steatosis even in the absence of marked transaminase elevations).

*Elderly:* Exercise caution in elderly patients who may have a greater frequency of decreased renal or cardiac function caused by concomitant disease or other drug therapy.

*Pregnancy: Category* C. To monitor fetal outcomes of pregnant women exposed to adefovir, a pregnancy registry has been established. Health care providers are encouraged to register patients by calling (800) 258-4263.

*Lactation:* It is not known whether adefovir is excreted in human milk. Instruct mothers not to breastfeed if they are taking adefovir.

## Precautions

*Monitoring:*

Renal function – Monitor renal function in all patients during treatment with adefovir, particularly for those with pre-existing or other risks for renal impairment. Patients with renal insufficiency at baseline or during treatment may require dose adjustment. Evaluate the risks and benefits of adefovir treatment prior to discontinuing adefovir in a patient with treatment-emergent nephrotoxicity.

*HIV resistance* – Prior to initiating adefovir, offer HIV antibody testing to all patients. Treatment with anti-hepatitis B therapies, such as adefovir, that have activity against HIV in a chronic hepatitis B patient with unrecognized or untreated HIV infection may result in emergence of HIV resistance.

*Drug coadministration* – Closely monitor patients when adefovir is coadministered with drugs that are excreted renally or with other drugs known to affect renal function.

## Drug Interactions

Drugs that may interact with adefovir include ibuprofen.

Coadministration of adefovir with drugs that reduce renal function or compete for active tubular secretion may increase serum concentrations of adefovir or these coadministered drugs.

## Adverse Reactions

Adverse reactions may include the following: Asthenia, headache, abdominal pain, nausea, flatulence, diarrhea, dyspepsia. Laboratory abnormalities may include the following: Increased ALT or AST, hematuria, increased creatine kinase, increased amylase, glycosuria, increased serum creatinine greater than or equal to 0.3 mg/dL from baseline 4% (compared with 2% placebo).

# SAQUINAVIR MESYLATE

| | |
|---|---|
| **Capsules**: 200 mg (as mesylate) (*Rx*) | *Invirase* (Roche) |
| **Capsules, soft gelatin**: 200 mg (*Rx*) | *Fortovase* (Roche) |

**Warning:**
> Saquinivir mesylate capsules (*Invirase*) and saquinavir soft gelatin capsules (*Fortovase*) are not bioequivalent and cannot be used interchangeably. When using saquinavir as part of an antiviral regimen, *Fortovase* is the recommended formulation. In rare circumstances, *Invirase* may be considered if it is to be combined with antiretrovirals that significantly inhibit saquinavir's metabolism.

## Indications

*HIV infection:* In combination with nucleoside analogs for the treatment of advanced HIV infection in selected patients.

## Administration and Dosage

Saquinavir soft gelatin capsules (*Fortovase*) and saquinavir mesylate capsules (*Invirase*) are not bioequivalent and cannot be used interchangeably.

*Invirase:* Three 200 mg capsules 3 times daily taken within 2 hours after a full meal in combination with a nucleoside analog.

Use saquinavir mesylate only in combination with an active antiretroviral nucleoside analog regimen. Base concomitant therapy on a patient's prior drug exposure.

*Fortovase:* Six 200 mg capsules 3 times daily taken with a meal or up to 2 hours after a meal. When used in combination with nucleoside analogs, do not reduce the dosage of saquinavir, as this will lead to greater than dose-proportional decreases in saquinavir plasma levels.

*Dose adjustment for combination therapy with saquinavir:* For toxicities that may be associated with saquinavir, interrupt the drug. Saquinavir at doses less than 600 mg 3 times daily are not recommended because lower doses have not shown antiviral activity. For recipients of combination therapy with saquinavir and nucleoside analogs, dose adjustment of the nucleoside analog should be based on the known toxicity profile of the individual drug.

## Actions

*Pharmacology:* Saquinavir is an inhibitor of HIV protease which cleaves viral polyprotein precursors to generate functional proteins in HIV-infected cells. The cleavage of viral polyprotein precursors is essential for maturation of infectious virus. Saquinavir is a synthetic peptide-like substrate analog that inhibits the activity of HIV protease and prevents the cleavage of viral polyproteins.

*Pharmacokinetics:*

*Absorption/Distribution* – Saquinavir exhibits a low absolute bioavailability of 4% following a single dose of *Invirase* after a high-fat breakfast (48 g protein, 60 g carbohydrate, 57 g fat, 1006 kcal). This is considered to be the result of incomplete absorption and extensive first-pass metabolism. However, the relative bioavailability is approximately 331% when saquinavir is administered as *Fortovase* compared with *Invirase*.

In HIV-infected patients, multiple dosing yields steady-state AUC values approximately 2.5 times higher than a single *Invirase* dose and 80% higher than a single *Fortovase* dose. AUCs and peak levels in these patients are about twice those observed in healthy volunteers. Greater than dose-proportional increases in plasma levels occur following single and multiple doses when saquinavir is administered as *Fortovase*.

The mean steady-state Vd following 12 mg IV is 700 L, suggesting saquinavir partitions into tissues. Saquinavir is approximately 98% bound to plasma proteins over a concentration range of 15 to 700 ng/mL. CSF levels are negligible.

*Metabolism/Excretion* – In vitro, the metabolism of saquinavir is cytochrome P450 mediated with specific isoenzyme, CYP3A4, responsible for greater than 90% of the hepatic metabolism. In vitro, saquinavir is rapidly metabolized to a range of mono- and di-hydroxylated inactive compounds; 88% and 1% of the oral dose was recovered in feces and urine, respectively, within 48 hours of dosing; 81% and 3% of an IV dose was recovered in feces and urine, respectively, within 48 hours of dosing. In mass balance studies, 13% of circulating radioactivity in plasma was attributed to unchanged drug after oral administration and the remainder attributed to saquinavir metabolites. Following IV administration, 66% of circulating radioactivity was attributed to unchanged drug and the remainder attributed to saquinavir metabolites, suggesting that saquinavir undergoes extensive first-pass metabolism.

Systemic clearance of saquinavir was rapid, 1.14 L/h/kg after IV doses of 6, 36, and 72 mg. The mean residence time of saquinavir was 7 hours.

### Contraindications
Clinically significant hypersensitivity to saquinavir or any components in the capsules; coadministration with terfenadine, cisapride, astemizole, triazolam, midazolam, or ergot derivatives.

### Warnings
*Diabetes mellitus, new onset:* Exacerbation of pre-existing diabetes mellitus and hyperglycemia have been reported in HIV-infected patients receiving protease inhibitors.

*Hepatic function impairment:* Exercise caution when administering saquinavir to patients with hepatic insufficiency. Exacerbation of chronic liver dysfunction, including portal hypertension, in patients with underlying hepatitis B or C, cirrhosis or other underlying liver abnormalities have been reported.

*Elderly:* In general, take caution when dosing *Fortovase* in elderly patients because of the greater frequency of decreased hepatic, renal, or cardiac function, and of concomitant disease or other drug therapy.

*Pregnancy: Category B.*

*Lactation:* It is not known whether saquinavir is excreted in breast milk. Because of the potential for serious adverse reactions in nursing infants from saquinavir, decide whether to discontinue nursing or discontinue the drug, taking into account the importance of saquinavir to the mother.

The Centers for Disease Control and Prevention advises HIV-infected women not to breastfeed to avoid postnatal transmission of HIV to a child who may not be infected.

*Children:* Safety and efficacy in HIV-infected children or adolescents < 16 years of age have not been established.

### Precautions
*Monitoring:* Perform clinical chemistry tests prior to initiating saquinavir therapy and at appropriate intervals thereafter. Periodically monitor triglyceride levels during therapy.

*General:* Saquinavir soft gelatin capsules (*Fortovase*) and saquinavir mesylate capsules (*Invirase*) are not bioequivalent and cannot be used interchangeably. Only *Fortovase* should be used for the initiation of saquinavir therapy (see Administration and Dosage) because *Fortovase* capsules provide greater bioavailability and efficacy than *Invirase*. For patients taking *Invirase* capsules with a viral load below the limit of quantification, a switch to *Fortovase* is recommended to maintain a virologic response. For patients taking *Invirase* capsules who have not had an adequate response or are failing therapy, if saquinavir resistance is clinically suspected, then do not use *Fortovase*. If resistance to saquinavir is not clinically suspected, consider a switch to *Fortovase*.

*Hemophilia:* There have been reports of spontaneous bleeding in patients with hemophilia A and B treated with protease inhibitors. In some patients, additional Factor VIII was required.

*Fat redistribution:* Redistribution/Accumulation of body fat, including central obesity, dorsocervical fat enlargement (buffalo hump), peripheral wasting, breast enlargement, and "cushingoid appearance" have been observed in patients receiving protease inhibitors.

*Use with HMG-CoA reductase inhibitors:* Concomitant use of saquinavir with lovastatin or simvastatin is not recommended. Exercise caution if HIV protease inhibitors, including saquinavir, are used concurrently with other HMG-CoA reductase inhibitors that are also metabolized by the CYP3A4 pathway (eg, atorvastatin, cerivastatin).

*Toxicity:* If a serious or severe toxicity occurs during treatment with saquinavir, interrupt therapy until the etiology of the event is identified or the toxicity resolves. At the time, resumption of treatment with full-dose saquinavir may be considered.

*Photosensitivity:* Photosensitization (photoallergy or phototoxicity) may occur.

### Drug Interactions

Drugs that may interact with saquinavir include ketoconazole, delavirdine, nevirapine, ritonavir, clarithromycin, indinavir, nelfinavir, and rifamycins.

Other drugs that induce CYP3A4 (eg, phenobarbital, phenytoin, dexamethasone, carbamazepine) may reduce saquinavir plasma concentrations.

Saquinavir may affect clarithromycin, nelfinavir, and sildenafil.

Competition for CYP3A by saquinavir could result in inhibition of the metabolism of astemizole, cisapride, ergot derivatives, midazolam, and triazolam and create the potential for serious or life-threatening reactions such as cardiac arrhythmias or prolonged sedation.

*Drug/Food interactions:* The mean 24-hour AUC after a single 600 mg oral dose in healthy volunteers was increased from 24 (under fasting conditions) to 161 ng•h/mL when saquinavir was given following a high-fat breakfast. Saquinavir 24-hour AUC and $C_{max}$ following the administration of a higher calorie meal (943 kcal, 54 g fat) were on average 2 times higher than after a lower calorie, lower fat meal. The effect of food persists for up to 2 hours.

### Adverse Reactions

Adverse reactions occurring in at least 3% of patients include diarrhea, abdominal discomfort; nausea; buccal mucosa ulceration; paresthesia; peripheral neuropathy; asthenia; rash; headache; fatigue; pain; taste alteration; insomnia; dyspepsia; flatulence; vomiting; constipation; lab test abnormalities of creatine phosphokinase, glucose (low), AST, ALT, and neutrophils (low).

# RITONAVIR

**Capsules:** 100 mg (*Rx*)                                *Norvir* (Abbott)
**Oral solution:** 80 mg/mL (*Rx*)

---

**Warning:**
Coadministration of ritonavir with certain sedative hypnotics, antiarrhythmics, or ergot alkaloid preparations may result in potentially serious or life-threatening adverse events because of possible effects of ritonavir on the hepatic metabolism of certain drugs (see Contraindications and Drug Interactions).

---

### Indications

*HIV infection:* In combination with other antiretroviral agents for the treatment of HIV infection.

### Administration and Dosage

*Adults:* The recommended dosage is 600 mg twice daily. Use of a dose titration schedule may help to reduce treatment-emergent adverse events while maintaining appropriate ritonavir plasma levels. Start ritonavir at no less than 300 mg twice daily and increase at 2 to 3 days intervals by 100 mg twice daily. If saquinavir and riton-avir are used in combination, reduce the dosage of saquinavir by 400 mg twice daily. The optimum dosage of ritonavir (400 or 600 mg twice daily) in combina-tion with saquinavir has not been determined; however, the combination regimen was better tolerated in patients who received ritonavir 400 mg twice daily.

*Children:* Use ritonavir in combination with other antiretroviral agents. The recom-mended dosage of ritonavir is 400 mg/m² twice daily by mouth and should not exceed 600 mg twice daily. Start ritonavir at 250 mg/m² and increase at 2- to 3-day intervals by 50 mg/m² twice daily. If patients do not tolerate 400 mg/m² twice daily because of adverse events, the highest tolerated dose may be used for mainte-nance therapy in combination with other antiretroviral agents; however, consider alternative therapy. When possible, administer dose using a calibrated dosing syringe.

| Pediatric Dosage Guidelines | | | | |
|---|---|---|---|---|
| Body surface area¹ (m²) | Twice-daily dose 250 mg/m² | Twice-daily dose 300 mg/m² | Twice-daily dose 350 mg/m² | Twice-daily dose 400 mg/m² |
| 0.25 | 0.8 mL (62.5 mg) | 0.9 mL (75 mg) | 1.1 mL (87.5 mg) | 1.25 mL (100 mg) |
| 0.5 | 1.6 mL (125 mg) | 1.9 mL (150 mg) | 2.2 mL (175 mg) | 2.5 mL (200 mg) |
| 1 | 3.1 mL (250 mg) | 3.75 mL (300 mg) | 4.4 mL (350 mg) | 5 mL (400 mg) |
| 1.25 | 3.9 mL (312.5 mg) | 4.7 mL (375 mg) | 5.5 mL (437.5 mg) | 6.25 mL (500 mg) |
| 1.5 | 4.7 mL (375 mg) | 5.6 mL (450 mg) | 6.6 mL (525 mg) | 7.5 mL (600 mg) |

¹ Body surface area can be calculated with the following equation:

$$\text{BSA (m}^2) = \sqrt{\frac{\text{ht (cm)} \times \text{wt (kg)}}{3600}}$$

*Dosing guidelines:* Alert patients that frequently observed adverse events, such as mild to moderate GI disturbances and paresthesias, may diminish as therapy is contin-ued. In addition, patients initiating combination regimens with ritonavir and nucleosides may improve GI tolerance by initiating ritonavir alone and subsequently adding nucleosides before completing 2 weeks of ritonavir monotherapy.

If possible, take with food. Patients may improve the taste of ritonavir oral solu-tion by mixing with chocolate milk, *Ensure*, or *Advera* within 1 hour of dosing. The effects of antacids on the absorption of ritonavir have not been studied.

**Actions**

*Pharmacology:* Ritonavir is a petidomimetic inhibitor of the HIV-1 and HIV-2 prote-ases. Inhibition of HIV protease renders the enzyme incapable of processing the *gag-pol* polyprotein precursor which leads to production of noninfectious immature HIV particles. Cross-resistance between ritonavir and reverse transcriptase inhibi-tors is unlikely because of the different enzyme targets involved.

*Pharmacokinetics:* After a 600 mg dose of oral solution, peak concentrations of ritonavir were achieved approximately 2 and 4 hours after dosing under fasting and nonfast-ing conditions, respectively. Relative to fasting conditions, the extent of absorp-tion of ritonavir from the capsule formulation was 15% higher when administered with a meal.

Cytochrome P450 3A (CYP3A) is a major isoform involved in ritonavir metabo-lism, although CYP2D6 also contributes to the formation of M-2.

| Ritonavir Pharmacokinetic Characteristics | | | |
|---|---|---|---|
| Parameter | Values (mean) | Parameter | Values (mean) |
| $C_{max}$ $SS^1$ | 11.2 mcg/mL | $CL/F^2$ | 4.6 L/h |
| $C_{trough}$ $SS^1$ | 3.7 mcg/mL | $CL_R$ | < 0.1 L/h |
| $V_\beta/F^2$ | 0.41 L/kg | RBC/Plasma ratio | 0.14 |
| $CL/F^2$ | 8.8 L/h | Percent bound[3] | 98% to 99% |

[1] SS = Steady state; ritonavir doses of 600 mg q 12 h.
[2] Single ritonavir 600 mg dose.
[3] Primarily bound to human serum albumin and alpha-1 acid glycoprotein over the ritonavir concentration range of 0.01 to 30 μg/mL.

## Contraindications

Hypersensitivity to the drug or any of its ingredients.

Do not administer ritonavir concurrently with any of the following listed drugs because competition for primarily CYP3A by ritonavir could result in inhibition of the metabolism of these drugs and create the potential for serious or life-threatening reactions such as cardiac arrhythmias, prolonged or increased sedation, and respiratory depression:

Postmarketing reports indicate that coadministration of ritonavir with ergotamine or dihydroergotamine has been associated with acute ergot toxicity characterized by peripheral vasospasm and ischemia of the extremities.

Drugs contraindicated with ritonavir include the following: Amiodarone, bepridil, flecainide, propafenone, quinidine, dihydroergotamine, ergotamine, midazolam, triazolam, cisapride, pimozide (see Drug Interactions for more information).

## Warnings

*Allergic reactions:* Allergic reactions including urticaria, mild skin eruptions, bronchospasm, and angioedema have been reported. Rare cases of anaphylaxis and Stevens-Johnson syndrome also have been reported.

*Pancreatitis:* Pancreatitis has been observed in patients receiving ritonavir therapy, including those who developed hypertriglyceridemia. Patients with advanced HIV disease may be at increased risk of elevated triglycerides and pancreatitis.

*Diabetes mellitus/Hyperglycemia:* New-onset diabetes mellitus, exacerbation of pre-existing diabetes mellitus, diabetic ketoacidosis, and hyperglycemia have been reported in HIV-infected patients receiving protease inhibitors.

*Hepatic function impairment:* Ritonavir is principally metabolized by the liver. Exercise caution when administering this drug to patients with pre-existing liver diseases, liver enzyme abnormalities, or hepatitis.

*Pregnancy: Category B.*

*Lactation:* It is not known whether this drug is excreted in breast milk. The CDC advises HIV-infected women not to breastfeed to avoid postnatal transmission of HIV to a child who may not be infected.

*Children:* Safety and efficacy in children under 2 years of age have not been established.

## Precautions

*Resistance/Cross-resistance:* Varying degrees of cross-resistance among protease inhibitors have been observed. Continued administration of ritonavir therapy following loss of viral suppression may increase the likelihood of cross-resistance to other protease inhibitors.

*Hemophilia:* There have been reports of increased bleeding, including spontaneous skin hematomas and hemarthrosis, in patients with hemophilia type A and B treated with protease inhibitors. In some patients, additional factor VIII was given.

*Fat redistribution:* Redistribution/accumulation of body fat including central obesity, dorsocervical fat enlargement (buffalo hump), peripheral wasting, breast enlargement, and "cushingoid appearance" have been observed in patients receiving protease inhibitors.

*Lipid disorders:* Treatment with ritonavir alone or in combination with saquinavir has resulted in substantial increases in the concentration of total triglycerides and cholesterol.

*Lab test abnormalities:* Ritonavir has been associated with alterations in triglycerides, AST, ALT, GGT, CPK, and uric acid. It also has been associated with decreases in hemoglobin, hematocrit, neutrophils, RBC, and WBC.

### Drug Interactions

*CYP450:* Ritonavir has been found to be an inhibitor of cytochrome P450 3A (CYP3A) and also inhibits CYP2D6 to a lesser extent. It appears to induce CYP3A, as well as other enzymes, including glycuronosyl transferase, CYP1A2, possibly CYP2C9.

Drugs that may affect ritonavir include clarithromycin, didanosine, azole antifungals, St. John's wort, interleukins, and rifampin.

Drugs that may be affected by ritonavir include clarithromycin, didanosine, desipramine, disulfiram, metronidazole, ethinyl estradiol, narcotic analgesics, rifabutin, saquinavir, theophylline, antiarrhythmic agents (eg, amiodarone, bepridil, flecainide, encainide, propafenone), benzodiazepines (eg, alprazolam, flurazepam, triazolam), bupropion, clozapine, ergot alkaloids, indinavir, piroxicam, quinidine, sildenafil, and zolpidem.

Drugs contraindicated with ritonavir include the following: Amiodarone, bepridil, flecainide, propafenone, quinidine, dihydroergotamine, ergotamine, midazolam, triazolam, cisapride, pimozide.

Drugs whose AUCs may be increased by administration with ritonavir include the following: Narcotic analgesics, antiarrhythmic agents, anticonvulsants (eg, carbamazepine, clonazepam, ethosuximide), antidepressants, antiemetics, antiparasitics (eg, quinine), beta blockers, calcium channel blockers, HMG-CoA reductase inhibitors, immunosuppressants, neuroleptics, sedative/hypnotics, steroids, stimulants.

Drugs whose AUCs may be decreased by ritonavir include the following: Anticoagulants, anticonvulsants (eg, phenytoin, divalproex, lamotrigine), antiparasitics (eg, atovaquone).

*Drug/Food interactions:* When the oral solution was given under nonfasting conditions, peak ritonavir concentrations decreased 23% and extent of absorption decreased 7% relative to fasting conditions. Extent of absorption of ritonavir from the capsule was 15% higher when given with a meal relative to fasting conditions. If possible, take ritonavir with meals.

### Adverse Reactions

The most frequent clinical adverse events, other than asthenia, among patients receiving ritonavir were GI and neurological disturbances including nausea, diarrhea, vomiting, anorexia, abdominal pain, taste perversion, and circumoral and peripheral paresthesias.

Adverse reactions occurring in at least 2% of treatment-naïve patients include the following: Paresthesias, dizziness, headache, insomnia, somnolence, sweating, diarrhea, nausea, vomiting, abdominal pain, asthenia, pharyngitis, taste perversion.

# INDINAVIR SULFATE

**Capsules:** 200, 333, and 400 mg (Rx)          *Crixivan* (Merck)

### Indications

*HIV infection:* Treatment of HIV infection in combination with other antiretroviral agents.

### Administration and Dosage

*Adults:* The recommended dosage is 800 mg (two 400 mg capsules) orally every 8 hours.

Administer at intervals of 8 hours. For optimal absorption, administer without food, but with water, 1 hour before or 2 hours after a meal or administer with other liquids such as skim milk, juice, coffee or tea, or with a light meal (eg, dry toast with jelly, juice, and coffee with skim milk and sugar; or corn flakes, skim milk, and sugar).

To ensure adequate hydration, it is recommended that adults drink at least 1.5 L (about 48 oz) of liquids during the course of 24 hours.

*Delavirdine:* Consider dose reduction of indinavir to 600 mg every 8 hours when administering delavirdine 400 mg 3 times/day.

*Didanosine:* If indinavir and didanosine are administered concomitantly, administer them at least 1 hour apart on an empty stomach.

*Efavirenz:* Dose increase of indinavir to 1000 mg every 8 hours is recommended when concurrently administering efavirenz.

*Itraconazole:* Dose reduction of indinavir to 600 mg every 8 hours is recommended when concurrently administering itraconazole 200 mg twice daily.

*Ketoconazole:* Dose reduction of indinavir to 600 mg every 8 hours is recommended when concurrently administering ketoconazole.

*Rifabutin:* Dose reduction of rifabutin to half the standard dose and a dose increase of indinavir to 1000 mg (three 333 mg capsules) every 8 hours are recommended when rifabutin and indinavir are coadministered.

*Cirrhosis:* Reduce the dosage of indinavir to 600 mg every 8 hours in patients with mild to moderate hepatic insufficiency caused by cirrhosis.

*Nephrolithiasis/Urolithiasis:* In addition to adequate hydration, medical management in patients who experience nephrolithiasis may include temporary interruption of therapy (eg, 1 to 3 days) or discontinuation of therapy.

### Actions

*Pharmacology:* Indinavir is an inhibitor of the HIV protease. HIV protease is an enzyme required for the proteolytic cleavage of the viral polyprotein precursors into the individual functional proteins found in infectious HIV. Indinavir binds to the protease active site and inhibits the activity of the enzyme. This inhibition prevents cleavage of the viral polyproteins resulting in the formation of immature noninfectious viral particles. The relationship between in vitro susceptibility of HIV to indinavir and inhibition of HIV replication in humans has not been established.

*Drug resistance* – Isolates of HIV with reduced susceptibility to the drug have been recovered from some patients treated with indinavir.

Cross-resistance between indinavir and HIV reverse transcriptase inhibitors is unlikely because the enzyme targets involved are different. Cross-resistance was noted between indinavir and the protease inhibitor ritonavir. Varying degrees of cross-resistance have been observed between indinavir and other HIV-protease inhibitors.

*Pharmacokinetics:*

*Absorption* – Indinavir was rapidly absorbed in the fasted state with a time to peak plasma concentration ($T_{max}$) of 0.8 hours. A greater than dose-proportional increase in indinavir plasma concentrations was observed over the 200 to 1000 mg dose range. At a dosing regimen of 800 mg every 8 hours, steady-state AUC was 30,691 nM•h, $C_{max}$ was 12,617 nM, and plasma concentration 8 hours post-dose (trough) was 251 nM.

*Distribution* – Indinavir was approximately 60% bound to human plasma proteins over a concentration range of 81 to 16,300 nM.

*Metabolism* – Following a 400 mg dose of $^{14}$C-indinavir, 83% and 19% of the total radioactivity was recovered in feces and urine, respectively; radioactivity caused by parent drug in feces and urine was 19.1% and 9.4%, respectively. Seven metabolites have been identified: 1 glucuronide conjugate and 6 oxidative metabolites. In vitro studies indicate that cytochrome P450 3A4 (CYP3A4) is the major enzyme responsible for formation of the oxidative metabolites.

*Excretion* – Indinavir is excreted (less than 20%) unchanged in the urine. Mean urinary excretion of unchanged drug was 10.4% and 12% following a single 700 and 1000 mg dose, respectively. Indinavir was rapidly eliminated with a half-life of 1.8 hours. Significant accumulation was not observed after multiple dosing at 800 mg every 8 hours.

## Contraindications

Hypersensitivity to any component of the product.

*Concomitant agents:* Do not administer indinavir concurrently with terfenadine, cisapride, triazolam, and midazolam because competition for CYP3A4 by indinavir could result in inhibition of the metabolism of these drugs and create the potential for serious or life-threatening events.

## Warnings

*Nephrolithiasis/Urolithiasis:* Nephrolithiasis/Urolithiasis has occurred with indinavir. The frequency of nephrolithiasis is substantially higher in pediatric patients (29%) than in adult patients (9.3%).

*Hemolytic anemia:* Acute hemolytic anemia, including cases resulting in death, has been reported in patients treated with indinavir.

*Hyperglycemia:* New-onset diabetes mellitus, exacerbation of pre-existing diabetes mellitus, and hyperglycemia have been reported during postmarketing surveillance in HIV-infected patients receiving protease inhibitor therapy.

*Hepatic function impairment:* Hepatitis including cases resulting in hepatic failure and death has been reported in patients treated with indinavir. Patients with hepatic insufficiency because of cirrhosis should have the dosage of indinavir lowered because of decreased metabolism.

*Pregnancy: Category C.*

*Lactation:* Although it is not known whether indinavir is excreted in breast milk, there exists the potential for adverse effects from indinavir in nursing infants. Instruct mothers to discontinue nursing if they are receiving indinavir.

*Children:* Safety and efficacy have not been established.

## Precautions

*Hyperbilirubinemia:* Asymptomatic hyperbilirubinemia (total bilirubin at least 2.5 mg/dL), reported predominantly as elevated indirect bilirubin, has occurred in about 10% of patients. In less than 1%, this was associated with elevations in ALT or AST.

*Hemophilia:* There have been reports of spontaneous bleeding in patients with hemophilia A and B treated with protease inhibitors.

*Fat redistribution:* Redistribution/Accumulation of body fat including central obesity, dorsocervical fat enlargement (buffalo hump), peripheral wasting, breast enlargement, and "cushingoid appearance" have been observed in patients receiving protease inhibitors.

## Drug Interactions

Drugs that may affect indinavir include didanosine, azole antifungals, rifamycins, delavirdine, efavirenz, interleukins, St. John's wort.

Drugs that may be affected by indinavir include cisapride, amiodarone, benzodiazepines, ergot alkaloids, fentanyl, rifamycins, ritonavir, sildenafil.

*Drug/Food interactions:* Administration of indinavir with a meal high in calories, fat, and protein (784 kcal, 48.6 g fat, 31.3 g protein) resulted in a 77% reduction in AUC and an

84% reduction in $C_{max}$. Administration with lighter meals resulted in little or no change in AUC, $C_{max}$, or trough concentration. A single 400 mg dose of indinavir with 8 oz of grapefruit juice resulted in a decrease in indinavir AUC (26%).

### Adverse Reactions

Adverse reactions occurring in at least 3% of patients include abdominal pain; nausea; diarrhea; vomiting; headache; dizziness; pruritus; nephrolithiasis/urolithiasis; back pain; fever; increased ALT, AST, and total serum bilirubin; decreased neutrophils.

# NELFINAVIR MESYLATE

**Tablets**: 250 and 625 mg (as base) (*Rx*)
**Powder**: 50 mg/g (as base) (*Rx*)

*Viracept* (Agouron)

**Warning:**
Nelfinavir is indicated for the treatment of human immunodeficiency virus (HIV) infection when antiretroviral therapy is warranted. At present, there are no results from controlled trials evaluating the effect of therapy with nelfinavir on clinical progression of HIV infection, such as survival or the incidence of opportunistic infections.

### Indications

*HIV*: For the treatment of HIV infection when antiretroviral therapy is warranted.

### Administration and Dosage

Take with a meal.

*Adults*: The recommended dose is 1250 mg (five 250 mg tablets or two 625 mg tablets) twice daily or 750 mg (three 250 mg tablets) 3 times/day.

*Pediatric patients (2 to 13 years of age)*: 20 to 30 mg/kg/dose 3 times/day. Doses as high as 45 mg/kg every 8 hours have been used.

| Pediatric Dose of Nelfinavir (administered 3 times/day) | | | | |
|---|---|---|---|---|
| Body weight | | Number of level 1 g scoops | Number of level teaspoons | Number of 250 mg tablets |
| kg | lbs | | | |
| 7 to < 8.5 | 15.5 to < 18.5 | 4 | 1 | - |
| 8.5 to < 10.5 | 18.5 to < 23 | 5 | 1¼ | - |
| 10.5 to < 12 | 23 to < 26.5 | 6 | 1½ | - |
| 12 to < 14 | 26.5 to < 31 | 7 | 1¾ | - |
| 14 to < 16 | 31 to < 35 | 8 | 2 | - |
| 16 to < 18 | 35 to < 39.5 | 9 | 2¼ | - |
| 18 to < 23 | 39.5 to < 50.5 | 10 | 2½ | 2 |
| ≥ 23 | ≥ 50.5 | 15 | 3¾ | 3 |

*Oral powder* – The oral powder may be mixed with a small amount of water, milk, formula, soy formula, soy milk, or dietary supplement; once mixed, the entire contents must be consumed in order to obtain the full dose. Acidic food or juice (eg, orange juice, apple juice, or apple sauce) are not recommended because of bitter taste. Do not reconstitute with water in its original container. Once mixed, store the oral powder for no more than 6 hours. May be refrigerated for up to 6 hours.

### Actions

*Pharmacology*: Nelfinavir is an inhibitor of the HIV-1 protease. Inhibition of the viral protease prevents cleavage of the gagpol polyprotein resulting in the production of immature, noninfectious virus.

*Pharmacokinetics*:

*Absorption* – After multiple oral doses of 750 mg 3 times/day or 1250 mg 2 times/day for 28 days (steady-state), peak plasma concentrations averaged 3 to 4 mg/mL, plasma concentrations prior to the morning dose were 1.4 to 2.2 mg/L, and prior to afternoon or evening dose were 0.7 to 1 mg/L.

*Effect of food:* Maximum plasma concentrations and area under the plasma concentration-time curve (AUC) were 2- to 3-fold higher under fed conditions compared with fasting.

*Distribution* – The apparent volume of distribution following oral administration of nelfinavir was 2 to 7 L/kg. Nelfinavir in serum is extensively protein-bound (greater than 98%).

*Metabolism* – Unchanged nelfinavir comprised 82% to 86% of the total plasma. In vitro multiple cytochrome P450 isoforms including CYP3A and CYP2C19 are responsible for metabolism of nelfinavir. One major and several minor oxidative metabolites were found in plasma. The major oxidative metabolite has in vitro antiviral activity comparable with the parent drug.

*Excretion* – The terminal half-life in plasma was typically 3.5 to 5 hours. The majority (87%) of an oral 750 mg dose was recovered in the feces, which consisted of numerous oxidative metabolites (78%) and unchanged nelfinavir (22%). Only 1% to 2% of the dose was recovered in the urine, of which unchanged nelfinavir was the major component.

## Contraindications

Hypersensitivity to any component of the product. Coadministration of nelfinavir is contraindicated with drugs that are highly dependent on CYP3A for clearance and for which elevated plasma concentrations are associated with serious and/or life-threatening events (eg, amiodarone, quinidine, ergot derivatives, pimozide, midazolam, triazolam, lovastatin, simvastatin; see Drug Interactions).

## Warnings

*Diabetes mellitus/hyperglycemia:* New-onset diabetes mellitus, exacerbation of pre-existing diabetes mellitus and hyperglycemia have been reported during postmarketing surveillance in HIV-infected patients receiving protease inhibitor therapy. Some patients required either initiation or dose adjustments of insulin or oral hypoglycemic agents for treatment of these events. In some cases, diabetic ketoacidosis has occurred.

*Phenylketonurics:* Nelfinavir oral powder contains 11.2 mg phenylalanine per g of powder.

*Hepatic function impairment:* Nelfinavir is principally metabolized by the liver. Exercise caution when administering this drug to patients with hepatic impairment.

*Pregnancy: Category B.*

*Lactation:* The US Public Health Service Centers for Disease Control and Prevention advises HIV-infected women not to breastfeed to avoid postnatal transmission of HIV to a child who may not yet be infected. It is not known whether nelfinavir is excreted in breast milk.

*Children:* A similar adverse event profile was seen during the pediatric clinical trial as in adult patients. The evaluation of the antiviral activity of nelfinavir in pediatric patients is ongoing.

The safety, efficacy, and pharmacokinetics of nelfinavir have not been evaluated in pediatric patients younger than 2 years of age.

## Precautions

*Fat redistribution:* Redistribution/accumulation of body fat including central obesity, dorsocervical fat enlargement (buffalo hump), peripheral wasting, facial wasting, breast enlargement, and "cushingoid appearance" have been observed in patients receiving antiretroviral therapy.

*Hemophilia:* There have been reports of increased bleeding, including spontaneous skin hematomas and hemarthrosis, in patients with hemophilia type A and B treated with protease inhibitors.

## Drug Interactions

*CYP450:* Nelfinavir is an inhibitor of CYP3A (cytochrome P450 3A). Coadministration of nelfinavir and drugs primarily metabolized by CYP3A may result in increased plasma concentrations of the other drug, which could increase or prolong its therapeutic and adverse effects.

Drugs that may affect nelfinavir include anticonvulsants, azithromycin, azole antifungals, efavirenz, delavirdine, HMG-CoA reductase inhibitors, indinavir, interleukins, nevirapine, rifabutin, rifampin, ritonavir, saquinavir, St. John's wort.

Drugs that may be affected by nelfinavir include amiodarone, antiarrhythmics (amiodarone, quinidine), azithromycin, benzodiazepines, efavirenz, ergot alkaloids, delavirdine, didanosine, fentanyl, indinavir, lamivudine; methadone, nonsedating antihistamines, oral contraceptives, phenytoin, pimozide, quinidine, rifabutin, saquinavir, sildenafil, sirolimus, tacrolimus, zidovudine.

*Drug/Food interactions:* Maximum plasma concentrations and AUC were 2- to 3-fold higher under fed conditions compared with fasting.

### Adverse Reactions

Adverse effects occurring in at least 3% of patients include diarrhea, nausea, flatulence, hematologic abnormalities, rash, and increases in ALT, AST, and creatine kinase.

# AMPRENAVIR

**Capsules:** 50 mg (*Rx*)                           *Agenerase* (GlaxoSmithKline)
**Oral solution:** 15 mg/mL (*Rx*)

---

**Warning:**
Because of the potential risk of toxicity from the large amount of the excipient propylene glycol, amprenavir oral solution is contraindicated in infants and children below 4 years of age, pregnant women, patients with hepatic or renal failure, and patients treated with disulfiram or metronidazole (see Contraindications and Warnings).

Use amprenavir oral solution only when amprenavir capsules or other protease inhibitor formulations are not therapeutic options.

---

### Indications

*HIV infection:* In combination with other antiretroviral agents for the treatment of HIV-1 infection.

### Administration and Dosage

Amprenavir may be taken with or without food; however, a high-fat meal decreases the absorption of amprenavir and should be avoided. Advise adult and pediatric patients not to take supplemental vitamin E since the vitamin E content of amprenavir capsules and oral solution exceeds the Reference Daily Intake (adults, 30 units; pediatrics, about 10 units).

Amprenavir capsules and oral solution are not interchangeable on a mg per mg basis.

*Adults:* The recommended oral dose of amprenavir capsules for adults is 1200 mg (eight 150 mg capsules) twice daily in combination with other antiretroviral agents.

    *Concomitant therapy* – If amprenavir and ritonavir are used in combination, the recommended dosage regimens are the following: Amprenavir 1200 mg with ritonavir 200 mg once daily or amprenavir 600 mg with ritonavir 100 mg twice daily.

*Pediatric patients:*
    *Capsules* – For adolescents (13 to 16 years of age), the recommended dose is 1200 mg (eight 150 mg capsules) twice daily in combination with other antiretroviral agents. For patients between 4 and 12 years of age or for patients 13 to 16 years of age with weight of less than 50 kg, the recommended dose is 20 mg/kg twice daily or 15 mg/kg 3 times daily (to a maximum daily dose of 2400 mg) in combination with other antiretroviral agents.

*Oral solution* – The recommended dose for patients between 4 and 12 years of age or for patients 13 to 16 years of age with weight less than 50 kg is 22.5 mg/kg (1.5 mL/kg) twice daily or 17 mg/kg (1.1 mL/kg) 3 times daily (to a maximum daily dose of 2800 mg) in combination with other antiretroviral agents. The recommended dose for patients between 13 and 16 years of age and weighing 50 kg or more or for patients older than 16 years of age is 1400 mg twice daily.

*Concomitant therapy* – Concomitant use of amprenavir oral solution and ritonavir oral solution is not recommended because the large amount of propylene glycol in amprenavir oral solution and ethanol in ritonavir oral solution may compete for the same metabolic pathway for elimination.

*Hepatic function impairment:*

*Capsules* – Use with caution in patients with moderate or severe hepatic impairment. Patients with Child-Pugh scores ranging from 5 to 8 should receive a reduced dose of amprenavir capsules of 450 mg twice daily, and patients with a Child-Pugh score ranging from 9 to 12 should receive a reduced dose of amprenavir capsules of 300 mg twice daily.

*Oral solution* – Amprenavir oral solution is contraindicated in patients with hepatic failure

*Renal function impairment:* Amprenavir oral solution is contraindicated in patients with renal failure.

### Actions

*Pharmacology:* Amprenavir is an inhibitor of human immunodeficiency virus (HIV)-1 protease. Amprenavir binds to the active site of HIV-1 protease and thereby prevents the processing of viral gag and gag-pol polyprotein precursors, resulting in the formation of immature noninfectious viral particles.

*Pharmacokinetics:*

*Absorption* – Amprenavir was rapidly absorbed after oral administration in HIV-1 infected patients with a time to peak concentration ($t_{max}$) typically between 1 and 2 hours after a single oral dose.

Amprenavir oral solution was 14% less bioavailable compared to the capsules.

*Distribution* – The apparent volume of distribution is about 430 L in healthy adult subjects. In vitro binding is about 90% to plasma proteins.

*Metabolism* – Amprenavir is metabolized in the liver by the cytochrome CYP3A4 enzyme system.

*Excretion* – Excretion of unchanged amprenavir in urine and feces is minimal. The plasma elimination half-life of amprenavir ranged from 7.1 to 10.6 hours.

### Contraindications

Concurrent use with cisapride, dihydroergotamine, ergotamine, ergonovine, methylergonovine, pimozide, midazolam, and triazolam. Coadministration of amprenavir is contraindicated with drugs that are highly dependent on CYP3A4 for clearance and for which elevated plasma concentrations are associated with serious and/or life-threatening events.

If amprenavir is coadministered with ritonavir, the antiarrhythmic agents flecainide and propafenone also are contraindicated.

Hypersensitivity to any of the components of this product.

*Oral solution:* Because of the potential risk of toxicity from the large amount of the excipient propylene glycol, amprenavir oral solution is contraindicated in infants and children below 4 years of age, pregnant women, patients with renal or hepatic failure, and patients treated with disulfiram or metronidazole.

### Warnings

*Drug interactions:* Serious and/or life-threatening drug interactions could occur between amprenavir and amiodarone, lidocaine (systemic), tricyclic antidepressants, and quinidine. Concentration monitoring of these agents is recommended if these agents are used concomitantly with amprenavir.

*Oral solution:* Because of the possible toxicity associated with the large amount of propylene glycol and the lack of information on chronic exposure to large amounts of propylene glycol, use amprenavir oral solution only when amprenavir capsules or other protease inhibitor formulations are not therapeutic options. Certain ethnic populations (Asians, Eskimos, Native Americans) and women may be at increased risk of propylene glycol-associated adverse events because of diminished ability to metabolize propylene glycol; no data are available on propylene glycol metabolism in these groups.

Closely monitor patients who require treatment with amprenavir oral solution for propylene glycol-associated adverse events, including seizures, stupor, tachycardia, hyperosmolality, lactic acidosis, renal toxicity, and hemolysis. Switch patients from amprenavir oral solution to amprenavir capsules as soon as they are able to take the capsule formulation.

Concurrent use of amprenavir oral solution and ritonavir oral solution is not recommended because the large amount of propylene glycol in amprenavir oral solution and ethanol in ritonavir oral solution may compete for the same metabolic pathway for elimination.

Use of alcoholic beverages is not recommended in patients treated with amprenavir oral solution.

*Skin reactions:* Severe and life-threatening skin reactions, including Stevens-Johnson syndrome, have occurred in patients treated with amprenavir (see Adverse Reactions).

*Anemia:* Acute hemolytic anemia has occurred in a patient treated with amprenavir.

*Diabetes mellitus/hyperglycemia:* New-onset diabetes mellitus, exacerbation of pre-existing diabetes mellitus, and hyperglycemia have been reported during postmarketing surveillance in HIV-infected patients receiving protease inhibitor therapy.

*Renal function impairment:* Amprenavir oral solution is contraindicated in patients with renal failure. Patients with renal impairment are at increased risk of propylene glycol-associated adverse events.

*Hepatic function impairment:* Amprenavir is principally metabolized by the liver; exercise caution when administering this drug to patients with hepatic impairment.

*Elderly:* In general, dose selection for an elderly patient should be cautious, reflecting the greater frequency of decreased hepatic, renal, or cardiac function and of concomitant disease or other drug therapy.

*Pregnancy:* Category C.

*Antiretroviral pregnancy registry* – To monitor maternal-fetal outcomes of pregnant women exposed to amprenavir, an Antiretroviral Pregnancy Registry has been established. Physicians are encouraged to register patients by calling (800) 258-4263.

*Lactation:* The Centers for Disease Control and Prevention recommend that HIV-infected mothers not breastfeed their infants to avoid risking postnatal transmission of HIV. Because of both the potential for HIV transmission and any possible adverse effects of amprenavir, instruct mothers not to breastfeed if they are receiving amprenavir.

*Children:* Two hundred fifty-one patients 4 years of age and above have received amprenavir as single or multiple doses in studies. An adverse event profile similar to that seen in adults was seen in pediatric patients. The safety, efficacy, and pharmacokinetics of amprenavir capsules have not been evaluated in pediatric patients below 4 years of age.

**Precautions**

*Doseform interchangeability:* Amprenavir capsules and oral solution are not interchangeable on a mg per mg basis.

*Sulfonamide cross-sensitivity:* Amprenavir is a sulfonamide. The potential for cross-sensitivity between drugs in the sulfonamide class and amprenavir is unknown. Treat patients with a known sulfonamide allergy with caution.

*Vitamin E:* Formulations of amprenavir provide high daily doses of vitamin E.

*Hemophilia:* There have been reports of spontaneous bleeding in patients with hemophilia A and B treated with protease inhibitors.

*Fat redistribution:* Redistribution/accumulation of body fat including central obesity, dorsocervical fat enlargement (buffalo hump), peripheral wasting, breast enlargement, and "cushingoid appearance" have been observed in patients receiving protease inhibitors.

*Lipid elevations:* Treatment with amprenavir alone or in combination with ritonavir has resulted in increases in the concentration of total cholesterol and triglycerides.

*Resistance/Cross-resistance:* Because the potential for HIV cross-resistance among protease inhibitors has not been fully explored, it is unknown what effect amprenavir therapy will have on the activity of subsequently administered protease inhibitors.

## Drug Interactions

Amprenavir is metabolized by the cytochrome P450 enzyme system and inhibits CYP3A4. Use caution when coadministering medications that are substrates, inhibitors, or inducers of CYP3A4, or potentially toxic medications that are metabolized by CYP3A4.

Drugs that might affect amprenavir include abacavir, aldesleukin, antacids, anticonvulsants, azole antifungals, clarithromycin, cyclosporine, dexamethasone, buffered didanosine, disulfiram, ethanol, indinavir, methadone, metronidazole, nelfinavir, nonnucleoside reverse transcriptase inhibitors, oral contraceptives, rifamycins, ritonavir, saquinavir, St. John's wort, and zidovudine.

Drugs that might be affected by amprenavir include antiarrhythmics, anticonvulsants, azole antifungals, benzodiazepines, calcium channel blockers, cisapride, clarithromycin, cyclosporine, ergot alkaloids, fentanyl, HMG-CoA reductase inhibitors, indinavir, methadone, nelfinavir, oral contraceptives, pimozide, rifabutin, ritonavir, saquinavir, sildenafil, tacrolimus, tricyclic antidepressants, warfarin, and zidovudine.

## Adverse Reactions

Adverse reactions occurring in at least 3% of patients include paresthesia, nausea, vomiting, diarrhea, depression, taste disorder, and rash.

# ATAZANAVIR SULFATE

| Capsules: 100, 150, and 200 mg (as base) (*Rx*) | *Reyataz* (Bristol-Myers Squibb Virology) |
|---|---|

## Indications

*HIV infection:* In combination with other antiretroviral agents for the treatment of HIV-1 infection.

## Administration and Dosage

*Dosage:* The recommended dose is 400 mg (two 200 mg capsules) once daily taken with food.

*Concomitant therapy:* When coadministered with efavirenz, it is recommended that 300 mg atazanavir and 100 mg ritonavir be given with 600 mg efavirenz (all as a single daily dose with food). Do not coadminister atazanavir without ritonavir with efavirenz.

When coadministered with didanosine buffered formulations, give atazanavir (with food) 2 hours before or 1 hour after didanosine.

*Hepatic function impairment:* Give with extreme caution in patients with mild to moderate hepatic insufficiency. Consider a dose reduction to 300 mg once daily for patients with moderate hepatic insufficiency (Child-Pugh class B). Do not use atazanavir in patients with severe hepatic insufficiency (Child-Pugh class C).

## Actions

*Pharmacology:* Atazanavir is an azapeptide HIV-1 protease inhibitor. The compound selectively inhibits the virus-specific processing of viral Gag and Gag-Pol polyproteins in HIV-1 infected cells, thus preventing formation of mature virions.

*Pharmacokinetics:*
  *Absorption –*

| Atazanavir Steady-State Pharmacokinetics in the Fed State After 400 mg Once Daily | | |
|---|---|---|
| Parameter | Healthy subjects (n = 14) | HIV-infected patients (n = 13) |
| $C_{max}$ (ng/mL) Mean | 5358 | 3152 |
| $T_{max}$ (h) Median | 2.5 | 2 |
| AUC (ng•h/mL) Mean | 29,303 | 22,262 |
| $t_{-\frac{1}{2}}$ (h) Mean | 7.9 | 6.5 |
| $C_{min}$ (ng/mL) Mean | 218 | 273 |

Atazanavir is rapidly absorbed with a $T_{max}$ of approximately 2.5 hours.

*Distribution* – Atazanavir is 86% bound to human serum proteins, and protein binding is independent of concentration. Atazanavir binds to both alpha-1-acid glycoprotein (AAG) and albumin to a similar extent (89% and 86%, respectively).

*Metabolism* – Atazanavir is extensively metabolized. The major biotransformation pathways of atazanavir in humans consisted of mono-oxygenation and dioxygenation. Other minor biotransformation pathways for atazanavir or its metabolites consisted of glucuronidation, N-dealkylation, hydrolysis, and oxygenation with dehydrogenation.

*Excretion* – Following a single 400 mg dose of atazanavir, 79% and 13% was recovered in the feces and urine, respectively. Unchanged drug accounted for approximately 20% and 7% of the administered dose in the feces and urine, respectively. The mean elimination half-life of atazanavir was approximately 7 hours at steady-state.

*Effect of food* – Administration of atazanavir with food enhances bioavailability and reduces pharmacokinetic variability.

**Contraindications**

Known hypersensitivity to atazanavir or any of its ingredients.

Coadministration of atazanavir is contraindicated with drugs (eg, midazolam, triazolam, ergot derivatives, cisapride, pimozide) that are highly dependent on CYP3A for clearance and for which elevated plasma concentrations are associated with serious and/or life-threatening events.

**Warnings**

*PR interval prolongation:* Concentration- and dose-dependent prolongation of the PR interval in the electrocardiogram has been observed in healthy volunteers receiving atazanavir.

In healthy volunteers and in patients, abnormalities in atrioventricular (AV) conduction were asymptomatic and limited to first-degree AV block with rare exceptions. There has been no second- or third-degree AV block. Because of limited clinical experience, use atazanavir with caution in patients with pre-existing conduction system disease (eg, marked first-degree AV block or second- or third-degree AV block).

*Diabetes mellitus/hyperglycemia:* New-onset diabetes mellitus, exacerbation of pre-existing diabetes mellitus, and hyperglycemia have been reported during postmarketing surveillance in HIV-infected patients receiving protease inhibitor therapy. Some patients required either initiation or dose adjustments of insulin or oral hypoglycemia agents for treatment of these events. In some cases, diabetic ketoacidosis has occurred.

*Hepatic function impairment:* Atazanavir is principally metabolized by the liver; exercise caution when administering this drug to patients with hepatic impairment because atazanavir concentrations may be increased.

*Elderly:* In general, exercise appropriate caution in the administration and monitoring of atazanavir in elderly patients.

*Pregnancy: Category B.*

*Antiretroviral pregnancy registry* – To monitor maternal-fetal outcomes of pregnant women exposed to atazanavir, an antiretroviral pregnancy registry has been established. Physicians are encouraged to register patients by calling (800) 258-4263.

*Lactation:* It is not known whether atazanavir is secreted in human breast milk. Because of the potential for HIV transmission and the potential for serious adverse reactions in breastfeeding infants, instruct mothers not to breastfeed if they are receiving atazanavir.

*Children:* Do not administer atazanavir to pediatric patients below 3 months of age because of the risk of kernicterus.

## Precautions

*Monitoring:* Monitor LFTs in patients with a history of hepatitis B or C.

*Hyperbilirubinemia:* Most patients taking atazanavir experience asymptomatic elevations in indirect (unconjugated) bilirubin related to inhibition of UDP-glucuronosyl transferase (UGT). This hyperbilirubinemia is reversible upon discontinuation of atazanavir.

*Resistance/Cross-resistance:* Various degrees of cross-resistance among protease inhibitors have been observed. Resistance to atazanavir may not preclude the subsequent use of other protease inhibitors.

*Hemophilia:* There have been reports of increased bleeding, including spontaneous skin hematomas and hemarthrosis in patients with hemophilia type A and B treated with protease inhibitors.

*Lactic acidosis syndrome:* Cases of lactic acidosis syndrome (LAS), sometimes fatal, and symptomatic hyperlactatemia have been reported in patients receiving atazanavir in combination with nucleoside analogs, which are known to be associated with increased risk of LAS.

*Fat redistribution:* Redistribution/accumulation of body fat including central obesity, dorsocervical fat enlargement (buffalo hump), peripheral wasting, facial wasting, breast enlargement, and cushingoid appearance have been observed in patients receiving antiretroviral therapy.

*Photosensitivity:* Photosensitization may occur; therefore, caution patients to take protective measures (ie, sunscreens, protective clothing) against exposure to ultraviolet light or sunlight until tolerance is determined.

## Drug Interactions

*CYP450:* Atazanavir is an inhibitor of CYP3A, CYP1A2, CYP2C9, and UGT1A1. Coadmistration of atazanavir and drugs primarily metabolized by CYP3A (eg, calcium channel blockers, HMG-CoA reductase inhibitors, immunosuppressants, and sildenafil) or UGT1A1 (eg, irinotecan) may result in increased plasma concentrations of the other drug that could increase or prolong its therapeutic and adverse effects.

Drugs that may be affected by atazanavir include the following: Antiarrhythmics, benzodiazepines, calcium channel blockers, cisapride, clarithromycin, ergot derivatives, HMG-CoA reductase inhibitors, immunosuppressants, indinavir, irinotecan, oral contraceptives, pimozide, rifabutin, saquinavir, sildenafil, tricyclic antidepressants, warfarin.

Drugs that may affect atazanavir include the following: Antacids and buffered medications, clarithromycin, didanosine (buffered formulation only), efavirenz, $H_2$-receptor antagonists, indinavir, proton pump inhibitors, rifampin, ritonavir, St. John's wort.

## Adverse Reactions

Moderate to severe adverse events associated with atazanavir administration in at least 3% of patients include the following: Abdominal pain, amylase/lipase (at least 2.1 x ULN), arthralgia, AST/ALT at least 5.1 x ULN, back pain, Depression, diarrhea, dizziness, fatigue, fever, headache, hemoglobin (less than 8 g/dL), increased cough, insomnia, jaundice/scleral icterus, lipodystrophy, nausea, neutrophils (less than 750 cells/mm$^3$, pain, peripheral neurologic symptoms, platelets (less than 50,000/mm$^3$rash, total bilirubin (at least 2.6 x ULN), vomiting.

# LOPINAVIR/RITONAVIR

**Capsules**: 133.3 mg lopinavir/33.3 mg ritonavir (*Rx*)     *Kaletra* (Abbott)
**Solution, oral**: 80 mg lopinavir/20 mg ritonavir per mL (*Rx*)

## Indications

*HIV treatment:* In combination with other antiretroviral agents for the treatment of HIV infection. This indication is based on analyses of plasma HIV RNA levels and CD4 cell counts in a controlled study of lopinavir/ritonavir combination of 24 weeks duration and in smaller uncontrolled dose-ranging studies of 72 weeks duration. At present, there are no results from controlled trials evaluating the effect on clinical progression of HIV.

## Administration and Dosage

*Adults:* The recommended dosage is 400/100 mg of lopinavir/ritonavir (3 capsules or 5 mL) twice daily taken with food.

*Concomitant therapy with efavirenz or nevirapine –* Consider a dose increase to 533/133 mg lopinavir/ritonavir (4 capsules or 6.5 mL) twice daily taken with food when used in combination with efavirenz or nevirapine in treatment-experienced patients where reduced susceptibility to lopinavir is clinically suspected (by treatment history or laboratory evidence).

*Children (6 months to 12 years of age):*

| Lopinavir/Ritonavir Pediatric Dosage Without Efavirenz or Nevirapine | | |
|---|---|---|
| Weight (kg)[1] | Dose (mg/kg)[2] | Volume of oral solution BID (80 mg lopinavir/20 mg ritonavir per mL) |
| *7 to < 15* | 12 mg/kg BID | |
| 7 to 10 | | 1.25 mL |
| > 10 to < 15 | | 1.75 mL |
| *15 to 40* | 10 mg/kg BID | |
| 15 to 20 | | 2.25 mL |
| > 20 to 25 | | 2.75 mL |
| > 25 to 30 | | 3.5 mL |
| > 30 to 35 | | 4 mL |
| > 35 to 40 | | 4.75 mL |
| > 40 | Adult dose | 5 mL (or 3 capsules) |

[1] Note: Use adult dosage recommendation for children above 12 years of age.
[2] Dosing based on the lopinavir component of lopinavir/ritonavir solution (80 mg/20 mg per mL).

*Concomitant therapy with efavirenz or nevirapine –*

| Lopinavir/Ritonavir Pediatric Dosage With Efavirenz or Nevirapine | | |
|---|---|---|
| Weight (kg)[1] | Dose (mg/kg)[2] | Volume of oral solution BID (80 mg lopinavir/20 mg ritonavir per mL) |
| *7 to < 15* | 13 mg/kg BID | |
| 7 to 10 | | 1.5 mL |
| > 10 to < 15 | | 2 mL |
| *15 to 45* | 11 mg/kg BID | |
| 15 to 20 | | 2.5 mL |
| > 20 to 25 | | 3.25 mL |

| Lopinavir/Ritonavir Pediatric Dosage With Efavirenz or Nevirapine | | |
|---|---|---|
| Weight (kg)[1] | Dose (mg/kg)[2] | Volume of oral solution BID (80 mg lopinavir/20 mg ritonavir per mL) |
| > 25 to 30 | | 4 mL |
| > 30 to 35 | | 4.5 mL |
| > 35 to 40 | | 5 mL (or 3 capsules) |
| > 40 to 45 | | 5.75 mL |
| > 45 | Adult dose | 6.5 mL (or 4 capsules) |

[1] Note: Use adult dosage recommendation for children over 12 years of age.
[2] Dosing based on the lopinavir component of lopinavir/ritonavir solution (80 mg/ 20 mg per mL).

**Actions**

*Pharmacology:* Lopinavir, an HIV protease inhibitor, prevents cleavage of the Gag-Pol polyprotein, resulting in the production of immature, noninfectious viral particles. As coformulated in the lopinavir/ritonavir combination, ritonavir inhibits the CYP3A-mediated metabolism of lopinavir, providing increased lopinavir plasma levels.

*Pharmacokinetics:*

*Absorption* – Administration of a single 400/100 mg dose of lopinavir/ritonavir with a moderate-fat meal was associated with a mean increase of 48% and 23% in lopinavir AUC and $C_{max}$, respectively, relative to fasting. To enhance bioavailability and minimize pharmacokinetic variability, take lopinavir/ritonavir with food.

*Distribution* – At steady state, lopinavir is approximately 98% to 99% bound to plasma proteins.

*Metabolism* – Lopinavir is extensively metabolized by the hepatic cytochrome P450 system, almost exclusively by the CYP3A isozyme. Ritonavir is a potent CYP3A inhibitor that inhibits the metabolism of lopinavir and, therefore, increases plasma levels of lopinavir. Ritonavir has been shown to induce metabolic enzymes, resulting in the induction of its own metabolism.

*Excretion* – Less than 3% of the lopinavir dose is excreted unchanged in the urine. The half-life of lopinavir over a 12-hour dosing interval averaged 5 to 6 hours; the apparent oral clearance (CL/F) of lopinavir is 6 to 7 L/h.

**Contraindications**

Hypersensitivity to any of its ingredients, including ritonavir.

Coadministration of lopinavir/ritonavir is contraindicated with drugs that are highly dependent on CYP3A or CYP2D6 for clearance and for which elevated plasma concentrations are associated with serious or life-threatening events. These drugs include the following: Flecainide, propafenone, dihydroergotamine, ergonovine, ergotamine, methylergonovine, pimozide, midazolam, cisapride, triazolam.

**Warnings**

*Hepatic function impairment:* Lopinavir/ritonavir is principally metabolized by the liver; therefore, exercise caution when administering this drug to patients with hepatic impairment because lopinavir concentrations may be increased. Consider increased AST/ALT monitoring in these patients, especially during the first several months of lopinavir/ritonavir treatment.

*Elderly:* Exercise appropriate caution in the administration and monitoring of lopinavir/ ritonavir in elderly patients, reflecting the greater frequency of decreased hepatic, renal, or cardiac function and of concomitant disease or other drug therapy.

*Pregnancy:* Category C. To monitor maternal-fetal outcomes of pregnant women exposed to lopinavir/ritonavir, an antiretroviral pregnancy registry has been established. Physicians are encouraged to register patients by calling (800) 258-4263.

*Lactation:* The Centers for Disease Control and Prevention recommend that HIV-infected mothers not breastfeed their infants to avoid risking postnatal transmission of HIV.

*Children:* The safety and pharmacokinetic profiles of lopinavir/ritonavir in children under 6 months of age have not been established. In HIV-infected patients

6 months to 12 years of age, the adverse event profile seen during a clinical trial was similar to that for adult patients. The evaluation of the antiviral activity of lopinavir/ritonavir in pediatric patients in clinical trials is ongoing.

## Precautions

*Pancreatitis:* Pancreatitis has been observed in patients receiving lopinavir/ritonavir therapy, including those who developed marked triglyceride elevations. Fatalities have been observed. Although a causal relationship to lopinavir/ritonavir has not been established, marked triglyceride elevation is a risk factor for development of pancreatitis.

Evaluate patients who exhibit signs or symptoms of pancreatitis and suspend lopinavir/ritonavir or other antiretroviral therapy as clinically appropriate.

*Diabetes mellitus/hyperglycemia:* New-onset diabetes mellitus, exacerbation of pre-existing diabetes mellitus, and hyperglycemia have been reported during postmarketing surveillance in HIV-infected patients receiving protease inhibitor therapy. Some patients required initiation or dose adjustments of insulin or oral hypoglycemic agent for treatment of these events.

*Resistance/Cross-resistance:* Various degrees of cross-resistance among protease inhibitors have been observed.

*Hemophilia:* There have been reports of increased bleeding, including spontaneous skin hematomas and hemarthrosis, in patients with hemophilia types A and B treated with protease inhibitors.

*Fat redistribution:* Redistribution/accumulation of body fat, including central obesity, dorsocervical fat enlargement (buffalo hump), peripheral wasting, breast enlargement, and "cushingoid appearance" have been observed in patients receiving antiretroviral therapy.

*Lipid elevations:* Treatment with lopinavir/ritonavir has resulted in large increases in the concentration of total cholesterol and triglycerides. Perform triglyceride and cholesterol testing prior to initiating therapy and at periodic intervals during therapy. Manage lipid disorders as clinically appropriate.

## Drug Interactions

*CYP 450:* Lopinavir/ritonavir is metabolized by CYP3A. Drugs that induce CYP3A activity would be expected to increase the clearance of lopinavir, resulting in lowered plasma concentrations of lopinavir. Although not noted with concurrent ketoconazole, coadministration of lopinavir/ritonavir and other drugs that inhibit CYP3A may increase lopinavir plasma concentrations.

Drugs that might decrease plasma concentrations of lopinavir/ritonavir include rifampin, phenobarbital, carbamazepine, phenytoin, azole antifungals, delavirdine, rifabutin, St. John's wort, efavirenz, nevirapine, and corticosteroids.

Drugs that might be affected by lopinavir/ritonavir include ergot derivatives, oral contraceptives, antiarrhythmics, HMG-CoA reductase inhibitors, HIV protease inhibitors, atovaquone, calcium channel blockers, ketoconazole, itraconazole, pimozide, cisapride, clarithromycin, disulfiram, metronidazole, immunosuppressants, midazolam, triazolam, narcotic analgesics, rifabutin and rifabutin metabolite, sildenafil, warfarin, bupropion, clozapine, desipramine, piroxicam, quinidine, theophylline, and zolpidem.

*Drug/Food interactions:*

*Didanosine* – It is recommended that didanosine be administered on an empty stomach. Give didanosine 1 hour before or 2 hours after lopinavir/ritonavir (give with food).

## Adverse Reactions

Adverse reactions occurring in at least 3% of patients include the following: Abdominal pain, nausea, diarrhea, headache, abnormal stools, vomiting, rash, and asthenia. Lab abnormalities include the following: Elevations of AST, ALT, GGT, total cholesterol, triglycerides, glucose, uric acid, and amylase.

*Children* – Lab abnormalities occurring in at least 3% of patients include the following: Total bilirubin, AST, ALT, amylase, sodium, total cholesterol, and platelet count.

# TENOFOVIR DISOPROXIL FUMARATE (PMPA)

**Tablets**: 300 mg (equivalent to 245 mg tenofovir disoproxil)    *Viread* (Gilead Sciences)
(*Rx*)

> **Warning:**
> Lactic acidosis and severe hepatomegaly with steatosis, including fatal cases, have been reported with the use of nucleoside analogs alone or in combination with other antiretrovirals (see Warnings).

## Indications

*HIV infection:* In combination with other antiretroviral agents for the treatment of HIV-1 infection.

## Administration and Dosage

300 mg once daily taken orally without regard to food.

*Renal function impairment:* Adjust the dosing interval of tenofovir in patients with baseline creatinine clearance (Ccr) less than 50 mL/min using the recommendations in the following table. The safety and effectiveness of these dosing interval recommendations have not been clinically evaluated; closely monitor clinical response to treatment and renal function in these patients.

| Tenofovir Dosage Adjustment for Patients with Altered Ccr | | | | |
| --- | --- | --- | --- | --- |
| | Ccr (mL/min)[a] | | | Hemodialysis patients |
| | ≥ 50 | 30 to 49 | 10 to 29 | |
| Recommended 300 mg dosing interval | Every 24 hours | Every 48 hours | Twice a week | Every 7 days or after a total of ≈ 12 hours of dialysis[b] |

[a] Calculated using ideal (lean) body weight.
[b] Generally once weekly assuming 3 hemodialysis sessions/week of approximately 4-hours duration. Administer tenofovir following completion of dialysis.

The pharmacokinetics of tenofovir have not been evaluated in nonhemodialysis patients with Ccr less than 10 mL/min; therefore, no dosing recommendation is available for these patients.

## Actions

*Pharmacology:* Tenofovir disoproxil, an acyclic nucleoside phosphonate diester analog of adenosine monophosphate, inhibits the activity of HIV reverse transcriptase.

*Pharmacokinetics:*

*Absorption* – The oral bioavailability of tenofovir in fasted patients is about 25%. Maximum serum concentrations ($C_{max}$) are achieved in about 1 hour.

Administration of tenofovir disoproxil following a high-fat meal increases the oral bioavailability with an increase in tenofovir $AUC_{0-\infty}$ of about 40% and an increase in $C_{max}$ of about 14%. Food delays the time to $C_{max}$ by approximately 1 hour.

*Distribution* – Binding of tenofovir to serum proteins is 7.2%. The volume of distribution at steady state is about 1.3 L/kg.

*Metabolism/Excretion* – Following a single oral dose of tenofovir, the terminal elimination half-life is approximately 17 hours. Tenofovir is eliminated by a combination of glomerular filtration and active tubular secretion.

## Warnings

*Coinfection:* It is recommended that all patients with HIV be tested for the presence of hepatitis B virus (HBV) before initiating antiretroviral therapy. The safety and efficacy of tenofovir have not been established in patients coinfected with HBV and HIV. Exacerbations of HBV have been reported in patients after the discontinuation of tenofovir. Closely monitor patients coinfected with HBV and HIV for at least several months after stopping tenofovir treatment.

*Lactic acidosis/severe hepatomegaly with steatosis:* Lactic acidosis and severe hepatomegaly with steatosis, including fatal cases, have been reported with the use of nucleoside analogs alone or in combination with other antiretrovirals. Exercise particular caution when administering nucleoside analogs to any patient with known risk factors for liver disease.

*Virologic failure:* A high rate of early virologic failure and emergence of nucleoside reverse transcriptase inhibitor (NRTI) resistance mutations have been observed in studies of HIV-infected treatment-naive patients receiving once-daily 3-drug combination therapies with either lamivudine, abacavir, and tenofovir or didanosine, lamivudine and tenofovir. It is recommended not to use abacavir and lamivudine or didanosine and lamivudine in combination with tenofovir as a triple antiretroviral therapy when considering a new treatment regimen for therapy-naive or pretreated patients with HIV infection.

*Renal function impairment:* Renal impairment, including cases of acute renal failure and Fanconi syndrome, has been reported in association with the use of tenofovir.

Avoid tenofovir with concurrent or recent use of a nephrotoxic agent. Carefully monitor patients at risk for, or with a history of, renal dysfunction and patients receiving concomitant nephrotoxic agents for changes in serum creatinine and phosphorus.

*Hepatic function impairment:* Tenofovir pharmacokinetics may be altered in patients with hepatic insufficiency.

*Elderly:* In general, dose selection for the elderly patient should be cautious, keeping in mind the greater frequency of decreased hepatic, renal, or cardiac function, and of concomitant disease or other drug therapy.

*Pregnancy: Category B.*

*Antiretroviral Pregnancy Registry* – To monitor fetal outcomes of pregnant women exposed to tenofovir, an Antiretroviral Pregnancy Registry has been established. Health care providers are encouraged to register patients by calling (800) 258-4263.

*Lactation:* The Centers for Disease Control and Prevention recommend that HIV-infected mothers not breastfeed their infants to avoid risking postnatal transmission of HIV.

*Children:* Safety and efficacy in pediatric patients have not been established.

**Precautions**

*Monitoring:* Bone monitoring should be considered for HIV infected patients who have a history of pathologic bone fracture or are at substantial risk for osteopenia. Supplementation with calcium and vitamin D may be considered for HIV-associated osteopenia or osteoporosis

*Bone toxicity:* It is not known if long-term administration of tenofovir (more than 1 year) will cause bone abnormalities. If bone abnormalities are suspected, obtain appropriate consultation.

*Fat redistribution:* Redistribution and accumulation of body fat have been observed in patients receiving antiretroviral therapy.

**Drug Interactions**

*Drugs eliminated by the kidneys:* Coadministration of tenofovir with drugs that are eliminated by active tubular secretion may increase serum concentrations of tenofovir and/or the coadministered drug. Some examples include, but are not limited to, acyclovir, adefovir dipivoxil, cidofovir, ganciclovir, valacyclovir, and valganciclovir. Drugs that decrease renal function also may increase serum concentrations of tenofovir.

Drugs that may affect tenofovir include indinavir and lopinavir/ritonavir.

Drugs that may be affected by tenofovir include abacavir, atazanavir, didanosine (buffered formulation or enteric coated), indinavir, and lamivudine.

**Adverse Reactions**

Adverse reactions occurring in at least 3% of treatment-experienced and treatment-naive patients include the following: abdominal pain, abnormal dreams, anorexia, arthralgia, asthenia, back pain, chest pain, depression, diarrhea, dizziness, dyspepsia, fever, flatulence, headache, insomnia, myalgia, nausea, pain, paresthesia, peripheral neuropathy, pneumonia, rash event, sweating, vomiting, weight loss.

Lab test abnormalities include the following: triglycerides, creatine kinase, serum amylase, urine glucose, AST, ALT, serum glucose, hematuria, neutrophils.

# DIDANOSINE (ddI; dideoxyinosine)

| | |
|---|---|
| **Tablets, buffered, chewable/dispersible:** 25, 50, 100, and 200 mg (*Rx*) | *Videx* (Bristol-Myers Squibb) |
| **Capsules, delayed release (with enteric-coated beadlets):** 125, 200, 250, and 400 mg (*Rx*) | *Videx EC* (Bristol-Myers Squibb) |
| **Powder for oral solution, buffered:** 100 and 250 mg (*Rx*) | *Videx* (Bristol-Myers Squibb) |
| **Powder for oral solution, pediatric:** 2 and 4 g (*Rx*) | *Videx* (Bristol-Myers Squibb) |

---

**Warning:**

Fatal and nonfatal pancreatitis has occurred during therapy with didanosine alone or in combination regimens in treatment-naive and treatment-experienced patients, regardless of degree of immunosuppression. Suspend didanosine in patients with suspected pancreatitis, and discontinue therapy in patients with confirmed pancreatitis (see Warnings).

Lactic acidosis and severe hepatomegaly with steatosis, including fatal cases, have been reported with the use of nucleoside analogs alone or in combination, including didanosine and other antiretrovirals. Fatal lactic acidosis has been reported in pregnant women who received the combination of didanosine and stavudine with other antiretroviral agents. The combination of didanosine and stavudine should be used with caution during pregnancy and is recommended only if the potential benefit clearly outweighs the potential risk (see Warnings).

---

**Indications**

*Didanosine (Videx):* In combination with other antiretroviral agents for treatment of HIV-1 infection.

*Didanosine EC (Videx EC):* In combination with other antiretroviral agents for treatment of HIV-1 infection in adults whose management requires once-daily administration of didanosine or an alternative didanosine formulation. There are limited data to date to support the long-term durability of response with a once-daily regimen of didanosine.

**Administration and Dosage**

*Dosage:*

*Didanosine (Videx)* – Administer all didanosine formulations on an empty stomach, at least 30 minutes before or 2 hours after eating. For either a once-daily or twice-daily regimen, patients must take at least 2 of the appropriate strength tablets at each dose to provide adequate buffering and prevent gastric acid degradation of didanosine. Because of the need for adequate buffering, use the 200 mg strength buffered tablet only as a component of the once-daily regimen. To reduce the risk of GI side effects, patients should take no more than 4 tablets at each dose.

*Adults:*

*Didanosine (Videx)* – The preferred dosing frequency of didanosine buffered is twice daily because there is more evidence to support the effectiveness of this dosing regimen. Once-daily dosing should be considered only for adult patients whose management requires once-daily dosing of didanosine.

*Didanosine EC (Videx EC)* – Didanosine EC should be administered on an empty stomach and should be swallowed intact.

| Adult Didanosine Dosing | | | |
|---|---|---|---|
| Patient weight (kg) | Tablets[1] | Buffered powder[2] | Enteric-coated capsules |
| ≥ 60 | 400 mg qd or 200 mg bid | 250 mg bid | 400 mg qd |
| < 60 | 250 mg qd or 125 mg bid | 167 mg bid | 250 mg qd |

[1] Use the 200 mg strength tablet only as a component of the once-daily regimen.
[2] Not suitable for once-daily dosing except for patients with renal impairment.

*Children:*
    *Didanosine (Videx)* – The recommended dose of didanosine in pediatric patients is 120 mg/m$^2$ twice daily. There are no data on once-daily dosing of didanosine in pediatric patients.
    *Didanosine EC (Videx EC)* – Didanosine EC has not been studied in pediatric patients. Please consult the complete prescribing information for didanosine buffered formulation and pediatric powder for oral solution for dosage and administration of didanosine to pediatric patients.

*Dose adjustment:* If clinical and laboratory signs suggest pancreatitis, promptly suspend dose and carefully evaluate the possibility of pancreatitis. Discontinue in patients with confirmed pancreatitis.
    Based on data with buffered didanosine formulations, patients with symptoms of peripheral neuropathy may tolerate a reduced dose after resolution of these symptoms following drug discontinuation. If neuropathy recurs after resumption of didanosine, consider permanent discontinuation.
    *Renal function impairment* – In adult patients with impaired renal function, adjust the dose of didanosine to compensate for the slower rate of elimination.

| | ≥ 60 kg | | | < 60 kg | | |
|---|---|---|---|---|---|---|
| Ccr (mL/min) | Tablet (mg)[1] | Buffered powder (mg)[2] | Enteric-coated capsules | Tablet (mg)[1] | Buffered powder (mg)[2] | Enteric-coated capsules |
| ≥ 60 | 400 qd or 200 bid | 250 bid | 400 mg qd | 250 qd or 125 bid | 167 bid | 250 mg qd |
| 30 to 59 | 200 qd or 100 bid | 100 bid | 200 mg qd | 150 qd or 75 bid | 100 bid | 125 mg qd |
| 10 to 29 | 150 qd | 167 qd | 125 mg qd | 100 qd | 100 qd | 125 mg qd |
| < 10 | 100 qd | 100 qd | 125 mg qd | 75 qd | 100 qd | —[3] |

*Table title: Recommended Dose (mg) of Didanosine by Body Weight in Renal Function Impairment*

[1] Didanosine chewable/dispersible buffered tablets. Two didanosine tablets must be taken with each dose; different strengths of tablets may be combined to yield the recommended dose.
[2] Didanosine buffered powder for oral solution.
[3] Didanosine EC capsules are not suitable for patients less than 60 kg with Ccr less than 10 mL/min. An alternate didanosine formulation should be used.

    *Didanosine (Videx):* Urinary excretion is also a major route of didanosine elimination in pediatric patients; therefore, the clearance of didanosine may be altered in children with renal impairment. Although there are insufficient data to recommend a specific dose adjustment in this patient population, consider a reduction in the dose or an increase in the interval between doses.
    *Patients requiring continuous ambulatory peritoneal dialysis (CAPD) or hemodialysis* –
    *Didanosine (Videx):* It is recommended that ¼ of the total daily dose of didanosine be administered once daily. For patients with Ccr less than 10 mL/min, it is not necessary to administer a supplemental dose of didanosine following hemodialysis.
    *Didanosine EC (Videx EC):* For patients 60 kg or more, administer 125 mg once daily. Didanosine EC is not suitable for use in patients less than 60 kg with Ccr less than 10 mL/min. It is not necessary to administer a supplemental dose of didanosine EC following hemodialysis.

*Method of preparation:*
  *Adults –*
    *Chewable/Dispersible buffered tablets:* To provide adequate buffering, thoroughly chew at least 2 of the appropriate strength tablets, but no more than 4 tablets, or disperse in at least 1 ounce of water prior to consumption. To disperse tablets, add 2 tablets to at least 1 ounce of water. Stir until a uniform dispersion forms, and drink entire dispersion immediately. If additional flavoring is desired, the dispersion may be diluted with 1 ounce of clear apple juice. Stir the further diluted dispersion just prior to consumption. The dispersion with clear apple juice is stable at room temperature for up to 1 hour.
    *Buffered powder for oral solution:*
1.) Open packet carefully and pour contents into approximately 4 ounces of water. Do not mix with fruit juice or other acid-containing liquid.
2.) Stir until the powder completely dissolves (approximately 2 to 3 minutes).
3.) Drink the entire solution immediately.
  *Children –*
    *Chewable/Dispersible buffered tablets:* Chew tablets or manually crush or disperse 1 or 2 tablets in water prior to consumption, as described for adults.
    *Pediatric powder for oral solution:* Prior to dispensing, the pharmacist must constitute dry powder with Purified Water, USP, to an initial concentration of 20 mg/mL and immediately mix the resulting solution with antacid to a final concentration of 10 mg/mL as follows:
      *20 mg/mL initial solution –* Reconstitute the product to 20 mg/mL by adding 100 or 200 mL Purified Water, USP, to the 2 or 4 g of powder, respectively, in the product bottle. Prepare final admixture as described below.
      *10 mg/mL final admixture –*
1.) Immediately mix 1 part of the 20 mg/mL initial solution with 1 part of either *Mylanta Double Strength Liquid, Extra Strength Maalox Plus Suspension,* or *Maalox TC Suspension* for a final dispensing concentration of 10 mg/mL. For patient home use, dispense the admixture in flint-glass or plastic bottles with child-resistant closures. This admixture is stable for 30 days under refrigeration at 2° to 8°C (36° to 46°F).
2.) Instruct the patient or caregiver to shake the admixture thoroughly prior to use and to store the tightly closed container in the refrigerator at 2° to 8°C (36° to 46°F) up to 30 days.

## Actions

*Pharmacology:* Didanosine is a synthetic purine nucleoside analog of deoxyadenosine, in which the 3′-hydroxyl group is replaced by hydrogen. Intracellularly, it is converted by cellular enzymes to the active metabolite, dideoxyadenosine 5′-triphosphate. It inhibits the activity of HIV-1 reverse transcriptase by competing with the natural substrate, deoxyadenosine 5′-triphosphate, and by incorporating in viral DNA causing termination of viral DNA chain elongation.

*Pharmacokinetics:*
  *Effect of food on oral absorption –* Didanosine $C_{max}$ and AUC were decreased by approximately 55% when didanosine tablets were administered up to 2 hours after a meal. Administration of didanosine tablets up to 30 minutes before a meal did not result in any significant changes in bioavailability.
  *Enteric-coated capsules:* In the presence of food, $C_{max}$ and AUC for didanosine capsules were reduced by approximately 46% and 19%, respectively, compared with the fasting state. Take didanosine capsules on an empty stomach.

| Pharmacokinetic Parameters of Didanosine in Adult and Pediatric Patients | | |
|---|---|---|
| Parameter | Adult patients[1] | Pediatric patients |
| Oral bioavailability | ≈ 42% | ≈ 25% |
| Apparent volume of distribution[2] | ≈ 1.08 L/kg | ≈ 28 L/m² |
| CSF[3]-plasma ratio[4] | ≈ 21% | 46% (range, 12% to 85%) |
| Systemic clearance[2] | ≈ 13 mL/min/kg | ≈ 516 mL/min/m² |

| Pharmacokinetic Parameters of Didanosine in Adult and Pediatric Patients | | |
| --- | --- | --- |
| Parameter | Adult patients[1] | Pediatric patients |
| Renal clearance[5] | $\approx$ 5.5 mL/min/kg | $\approx$ 240 mL/min/m$^2$ |
| Elimination half-life[5] | $\approx$ 1.5 h | $\approx$ 0.8 h |
| Urine recovery of didanosine[5] | $\approx$ 18% | $\approx$ 18% |

[1] Administered as buffered formulation.
[2] Following IV administration.
[3] CSF = cerebrospinal fluid.
[4] Following IV administration in adults and IV or oral administration in pediatric patients.
[5] Following oral administration.

*Children* – The pharmacokinetics of didanosine administered as *Videx EC* has not been studied in pediatric patients.

*Comparison of didanosine formulations* – In didanosine EC (*Videx EC*), the active ingredient, didanosine, is protected against degradation by stomach acid by the use of an enteric coating on the beadlets in the capsule. The enteric coating dissolves when the beadlets empty into the small intestine, the site of drug absorption. With buffered formulations of didanosine, administration with antacid provides protection from degradation by stomach acid.

## Contraindications

Hypersensitivity to any of the components of the formulations.

## Warnings

*Pancreatitis:* Fatal and nonfatal pancreatitis has occurred during didanosine therapy used alone or in combination regimens in treatment-naive and treatment-experienced patients regardless of degree of immunosuppression (see Warning Box).

*Lactic acidosis/Severe hepatomegaly with steatosis:* Lactic acidosis and severe hepatomegaly with steatosis, including fatal cases, have been reported with the use of nucleoside analogs alone or in combination, including didanosine and other antiretrovirals. A majority of these cases have been in women. Obesity and prolonged nucleoside exposure may be risk factors (see Warning Box).

*Retinal changes and optic neuritis:* Retinal changes and optic neuritis have been reported in adult and pediatric patients. Consider periodic retinal examinations for patients receiving didanosine.

*Peripheral neuropathy:* Peripheral neuropathy, manifested by numbness, tingling, or pain in the hands or feet, has been reported in patients receiving didanosine therapy.

*Myopathy:* Human myopathy has been associated with administration of other nucleoside analogs.

*Renal function impairment:* Patients with renal impairment (serum creatinine greater than 1.5 mg/dL or Ccr less than 60 mL/min) may be at greater risk of toxicity from didanosine because of decreased drug clearance; consider a dose reduction. The magnesium hydroxide content of each buffered tablet (8.6 mEq) may present an excessive magnesium load to patients with significant renal impairment, particularly after prolonged dosing.

*Hepatic function impairment:* It is unknown if hepatic impairment significantly affects didanosine pharmacokinetics. Therefore, monitor these patients closely for evidence of didanosine toxicity.

*Elderly:* In an expanded access program using a buffered formulation of didanosine for the treatment of advanced HIV infection, patients 65 years of age and older had a higher frequency of pancreatitis (10%) than younger patients (5%).

*Pregnancy: Category B.*

To monitor maternal-fetal outcomes of pregnant women exposed to didanosine and other antiretroviral agents, an Antiretroviral Pregnancy Registry has been established. Physicians are encouraged to register patients by calling (800) 258-4263.

*Lactation:* It is not known whether didanosine is excreted in breast milk. Because of the potential for serious adverse reactions from didanosine in nursing infants, instruct mothers to discontinue nursing when taking didanosine; this is consistent with the CDC's recommendation that HIV-infected mothers not breastfeed their infants to avoid risking postnatal transmission of HIV infection.

*Children:* Safety and efficacy of didanosine EC have not been established in pediatric patients (see Administration and Dosage).

**Precautions**

*Frequency of dosing:* The preferred dosing frequency of didanosine is twice daily because there is more evidence to support the effectiveness of this dosing frequency. Once daily dosing should be considered only for adult patients whose management requires once daily dosing of didanosine.

*Phenylketonuria:* Didanosine chewable/dispersible buffered tablets contain the following quantities of phenylalanine: 73 mg phenylalanine per 2-tablet dose (36.5 mg phenylalanine per tablet).

*Sodium-restricted diets:* Each buffered tablet contains 264.5 mg sodium. Each single-dose packet of buffered powder for oral solution contains 1380 mg sodium.

*Hyperuricemia:* Didanosine has been associated with asymptomatic hyperuricemia; consider suspending treatment if clinical measures aimed at reducing uric acid levels fail.

**Drug Interactions**

Drugs that may affect didanosine include allopurinol, methadone, and ganciclovir.

Drugs that may be affected by didanosine include ganciclovir, antacids, antifungal agents, antiretroviral drugs, fluoroquinolones, and stavudine.

Coadministration of didanosine buffered tablets, buffered powder for oral solution, and pediatric powder for oral solution with drugs that are known to cause peripheral neuropathy or pancreatitis or patients who have a history of neuropathy or neurotoxic drug therapy may have increased risk of toxicities. Closely observe patients who receive these drugs or have a history of neuropathy or neurotoxic drug therapy.

*Drug/Food interactions:* Ingestion of didanosine with food reduces the absorption of didanosine by as much as 50%. Therefore, administer on an empty stomach, at least 30 minutes before or 2 hours after eating.

**Adverse Reactions**

A serious toxicity of didanosine is pancreatitis, which may be fatal (see Warnings). Other important toxicities include lactic acidosis/severe hepatomegaly with steatosis; retinal changes and optic neuritis; and peripheral neuropathy (see Warnings and Precautions).

When didanosine is used in combination with other agents with similar toxicities, the incidence of these toxicities may be higher than when didanosine is used alone. Thus, patients treated with didanosine in combination with stavudine, with or without hydroxyurea, may be at increased risk for pancreatitis and liver function abnormalities (see Warnings). Patients treated with didanosine in combination with stavudine may also be at increased risk for peripheral neuropathy (see Precautions).

Adverse reactions occurring in at least 3% of patients include diarrhea, neuropathy (all grades), rash/pruritus, abdominal pain, headache, pain, nausea/vomiting, pancreatitis, and laboratory abnormalities including amylase, ALT, AST, and uric acid.

# LAMIVUDINE (3TC)

| | |
|---|---|
| **Tablets:** 100 mg (*Rx*) | *Epivir-HBV* (GlaxoSmithKline) |
| 150 and 300 mg (*Rx*) | *Epivir* (GlaxoSmithKline) |
| **Oral solution:** 5 mg/mL (*Rx*) | *Epivir-HBV* (GlaxoSmithKline) |
| 10 mg/mL (*Rx*) | *Epivir* (GlaxoSmithKline) |

**Warning:**
> Lactic acidosis and severe hepatomegaly with steatosis, including fatal cases, have been reported with the use of antiretroviral nucleoside analogs alone or in combination, including lamivudine and other antiretroviral agents (see Warnings).
>
> Offer human immunodeficiency virus (HIV) counseling and testing to patients before beginning *Epivir-HBV* and periodically during treatment. *Epivir-HBV* tablets and oral solution contain a lower dose of the same active ingredient (lamivudine) as the *Epivir* tablets and oral solution used to treat HIV infection. If treatment with *Epivir-HBV* is prescribed for chronic hepatitis B for a patient with unrecognized or untreated HIV infection, rapid emergence of HIV resistance is likely because of subtherapeutic dose and inappropriate monotherapy.
>
> *Epivir* tablets and oral solution (used to treat HIV infection) contain a higher dose of the active ingredient (lamivudine) than *Epivir-HBV* tablets and oral solution (used to treat chronic hepatitis B). Patients with HIV infection should receive only dosing forms appropriate for the treatment of HIV (see Warnings and Precautions).

### Indications
*HIV infection (Epivir):* Lamivudine in combination with other antiretroviral agents is indicated for the treatment of HIV infection.

*Chronic hepatitis B (Epivir-HBV):* Treatment of chronic hepatitis B associated with evidence of hepatitis B viral replication and active liver inflammation.

### Administration and Dosage
*HIV infection:*
> *Adults* – 300 mg/day, administered as either 150 mg twice daily or 300 mg once daily, in combination with other antiretroviral agents.
>
> *Children (3 months up to 16 years of age)* – 4 mg/kg twice daily (up to a maximum of 150 mg twice a day) administered with other antiretroviral agents.
>
> *Renal function impairment* – Adjust lamivudine dose in accordance with renal function. Insufficient data are available to recommend a dosage of lamivudine in dialysis.

| Adjustment of Lamivudine Dosage in HIV-Infected Adult and Adolescent Patients with Renal Function Impairment | |
|---|---|
| Ccr (mL/min) | Recommended lamivudine dosage |
| ≥ 50 | 150 mg twice daily or 300 mg once daily |
| 30 to 49 | 150 mg once daily |
| 15 to 29 | 150 mg first dose, then 100 mg once daily |
| 5 to 14 | 150 mg first dose, then 50 mg once daily |
| < 5 | 50 mg first dose, then 25 mg once daily |

*Chronic hepatitis B:*
> *Adults* – 100 mg once daily. Safety and efficacy of treatment beyond 1 year have not been established, and the optimum duration of treatment is not known.
>
> *Children (2 to 17 years of age)* – 3 mg/kg once daily up to a maximum daily dose of 100 mg. Safety and effectiveness of treatment beyond 1 year have not been established, and the optimum duration of treatment is not known.
>
> *HIV co-infection* – The formulation and dosage of lamivudine in *Epivir-HBV* are not appropriate for patients dually infected with HBV and HIV. If lamivudine is administered to such patients, use the higher dosage indicated for HIV therapy as part of an appropriate combination regimen.

*Renal function impairment* – Adjust the dose of lamivudine in accordance with renal function. No additional dosing of lamivudine is required after routine (4-hour) hemodialysis. Insufficient data are available to recommend a dosage of lamivudine in patients undergoing peritoneal dialysis.

| Adjustment of Lamivudine Dosage in Chronic Hepatitis B Adult Patients with Renal Function Impairment | |
| --- | --- |
| Ccr (mL/min) | Recommended lamivudine dosage |
| ≥ 50 | 100 mg once daily |
| 30 to 49 | 100 mg first dose, then 50 mg once daily |
| 15 to 29 | 100 mg first dose, then 25 mg once daily |
| 5 to 14 | 35 mg first dose, then 15 mg once daily |
| < 5 | 35 mg first dose, then 10 mg once daily |

## Actions

*Pharmacology:* Lamivudine is a synthetic nucleoside analog with activity against HIV and hepatitis B virus (HBV). Lamivudine is phosphorylated intracellularly to lamivudine 5'-triphosphate (L-TP). Incorporation of the monophosphate form into viral DNA by HBV polymerase results in DNA chain termination. L-TP also inhibits the RNA- and DNA-dependent DNA polymerase activities of HIV-1 reverse transcriptase.

*Pharmacokinetics:*

*Absorption/Distribution* – Lamivudine is rapidly absorbed after oral administration. Absolute bioavailability as demonstrated in HIV-infected patients is 86% for the tablet and 87% for the oral solution. The solution and tablet may be used interchangeably. The apparent volume of distribution ($V_d$) is 1.3 L/kg. Binding of lamivudine to plasma proteins is less than 36% and independent of dose.

*Metabolism/Excretion* – Metabolism is a minor route of elimination. The mean elimination half-life of lamivudine ranges from 5 to 7 hours. The majority of the dose is eliminated in the urine as unchanged drug, with about 5% excreted as the metabolite within 12 hours of dose administration.

*Special populations:*

*Children* – In HIV-infected pediatric patients approximately 4 months to 16 years of age and chronic hepatitis B pediatric patients 2 to 12 years of age, lamivudine was rapidly absorbed with a $T_{max}$ of 0.5 to 1 hour and an absolute bioavailability of 66%. After 8 mg/kg/day, $C_{max}$ was 1.1 mcg/mL and half-life was 2 hours (vs 3.7 hours in adults). Weight-corrected oral clearances were higher, resulting in lower AUCs compared with adults. Total exposure to lamivudine, as reflected by mean AUC values, was comparable between pediatric patients receiving 8 mg/kg/day and adults receiving 4 mg/kg/day. Age-stratified oral clearance was highest at 2 years of age and declined from 2 to 12 years of age, where values were then similar to those seen in adults.

## Contraindications

Hypersensitivity to any of the components of the products.

## Warnings

*Lactic acidosis/severe hepatomegaly with steatosis:* Lactic acidosis and severe hepatomegaly with steatosis, including fatal cases, have occurred with the use of antiretroviral nucleoside analogs alone or in combination. A majority of these cases have been in women. Obesity and prolonged nucleoside exposure may be risk factors. Exercise caution when administering lamivudine to any patient, particularly to those with known risk factors for liver disease. Suspend treatment with lamivudine in any patient who develops clinical or laboratory findings suggestive of lactic acidosis or pronounced hepatotoxicity, which may include hepatomegaly and steatosis even in the absence of marked transaminase elevations.

*Differences between lamivudine-containing products/risk of emergence of resistant HIV: Epivir-HBV* tablets and oral solution contain a lower dose of the same active ingredient (lamivudine) as *Epivir* tablets and oral solution, lamivudine/zidovudine tablets (*Combivir*), and abacavir/lamivudine/zidovudine tablets (*Trizivir*) used to treat HIV infection. The formulation and dosage of lamivudine in *Epivir-HBV* are not appropriate for patients infected with both HBV and HIV. If treatment with *Epivir-HBV* is prescribed for chronic hepatitis B for a patient with unrecognized or untreated HIV infection, rapid emergence of HIV resistance is likely to result because of the subtherapeutic dose and the inappropriateness of monotherapy HIV treatment. If a decision is made to administer lamivudine to patients dually infected with HIV and HBV, use *Epivir* tablets or oral solution or *Combivir* tablets as a part of an appropriate combination regimen. Do not administer *Combivir* concomitantly with *Epivir*, *Epivir-HBV*, *Retrovir*, or *Trizivir*.

*Posttreatment exacerbations of hepatitis:* Clinical and laboratory evidence of exacerbations of hepatitis have occurred after discontinuation of lamivudine (these have been primarily detected by serum ALT elevations in addition to the re-emergence of HBV DNA commonly observed after stopping treatment). Although most events appear to have been self-limited, fatalities have been reported in some cases. Closely monitor patients with clinical and laboratory follow-up for at least several months after stopping treatment.

*Elderly:* Because elderly patients are more likely to have decreased renal function, monitor renal function and make dose adjustments accordingly.

*Pregnancy: Category C.*
   Lamivudine has not affected the transmission of HBV from mother to infant; immunize infants appropriately to prevent neonatal acquisition of HBV.
   *Antiretroviral pregnancy registry* – To monitor maternal-fetal outcomes of women exposed to lamivudine, an Antiretroviral Pregnancy Registry has been established. Physicians are encouraged to register patients by calling (800) 258-4263.

*Lactation:* Lamivudine is excreted in human breast milk. Instruct mothers to discontinue nursing if they are receiving lamivudine, which is consistent with the CDC recommendation that HIV-infected mothers not breastfeed their infants to avoid risking postnatal transmission of HIV infection.

*Children:*
   *Hepatitis B* – Safety and efficacy in pediatric patients under 2 years of age have not been established.
   *HIV infection* – The safety and effectiveness of twice-daily lamivudine in combination with other antiretroviral agents have been established in pediatric patients 3 months of age and older.
   *Pancreatitis* – Pancreatitis has been observed in antiretroviral nucleoside-experienced pediatric patients receiving lamivudine. Use lamivudine with caution in pediatric patients with a history of prior antiretroviral nucleoside exposure, a history of pancreatitis, or other significant risk factors for the development of pancreatitis. Stop lamivudine treatment immediately if clinical signs, symptoms, or lab abnormalities suggestive of pancreatitis occur (see Adverse Reactions).

**Precautions**
   *Monitoring:*
      *Epivir-HBV* – Monitor patients regularly during treatment. The safety and efficacy of treatment with *Epivir-HBV* beyond 1 year have not been established. During treatment, combinations of events such as return of persistently elevated ALT, increasing levels of HBV DNA over time after an initial decline below assay limit, progression of clinical signs or symptoms of hepatic disease, and/or worsening of hepatic necroinflammatory findings may be considered as potentially reflecting loss of therapeutic response. Consider such observations when determining the advisability of continuing therapy.
      *Emergence of resistance-associated HBV mutations:* Progression of hepatitis B, including death, has been reported in some patients with YMDD-mutant HBV, including patients from the liver transplant setting and from other clinical trials. The long-term clinical significance of YMDD-mutant HBV is not known. Increased clinical and laboratory monitoring may aid in treatment decisions if emergence of viral mutants is suspected.

*Fat redistribution:* Redistribution/Accumulation of body fat, including central obesity, dorsocervical fat enlargement (buffalo hump), peripheral wasting, facial wasting, breast enlargement, and "cushingoid appearance," have been observed in patients receiving antiretroviral therapy. The mechanism and long-term consequences of these events are currently unknown. A causal relationship has not been established.

*Special risk:* Safety and efficacy of *Epivir-HBV* have not been established in patients with decompensated liver disease or organ transplants; pediatric patients under 2 years of age (use appropriate infant immunizations to prevent HBV); patients dually infected with HBV and HCV, hepatitis delta, or HIV; or other populations not included in the principal Phase III controlled studies.

### Drug Interactions
Drugs that may interact with lamivudine include zalcitabine and trimethoprim/sulfamethoxazole.

### Adverse Reactions
*HIV* – Adverse reactions occurring in at least 5% of patients include abdominal pain/cramps, anorexia, arthralgia, chills, cough, depression, diarrhea, dizziness, dyspepsia, fatigue, fever, headache, insomnia, malaise, musculoskeletal pain, myalgia, nasal symptoms, nausea, neuropathy, rash, and vomiting. Lab abnormalities may include anemia, neutropenia, thrombocytopenia, and elevations in amylase, AST, ALT, and bilirubin.

*Chronic hepatitis B* – Adverse reactions occurring in at least 3% of patients include abdominal discomfort/pain; arthralgia; diarrhea; ear, nose, and throat infections; fever or chills; headache; malaise/fatigue; myalgia; nausea/vomiting; rash; sore throat. Lab abnormalities may include decreased platelets and elevations in ALT, CPK, and serum lipase.

*Children* – Adverse reactions in children are similar to adults and include abnormal breath sounds/wheezing, cough, diarrhea, ear signs or symptoms, fever, hepatomegaly, lymphadenopathy, nasal discharge or congestion, nausea and vomiting, pancreatitis, skin rashes, splenomegaly, and stomatitis. Lab abnormalities may include elevated lipase and amylase, neutropenia, and thrombocytopenia.

# STAVUDINE (d4T)

| | |
|---|---|
| **Capsules**: 15, 20, 30, and 40 mg (*Rx*) | *Zerit* (BMS Virology) |
| **Powder for oral solution**: 1 mg/mL when reconstituted (*Rx*) | |
| **Capsules, extended-release**: 37.5, 50, 75, and 100 mg (*Rx*) | *Zerit XR* (BMS Virology) |

---

**Warning:**
Lactic acidosis and severe hepatomegaly with steatosis, including fatal cases, have been reported with the use of nucleoside analogs alone or in combination, including stavudine and other antiretrovirals (see Warnings). Fatal lactic acidosis has been reported in pregnant women who received the combination of stavudine and didanosine with other antiretroviral agents. Use the combination of stavudine and didanosine with caution during pregnancy; it is recommended only if the potential benefit clearly outweighs the potential risk (see Warnings).

Fatal and nonfatal pancreatitis have occurred during therapy when stavudine was part of a combination regimen that included didanosine, with or without hydroxyurea, in both treatment-naive and treatment-experienced patients, regardless of degree of immunosuppression (see Warnings).

---

### Indications
*Human immunodeficiency virus (HIV) infection:* For the treatment of HIV-1 infection in combination with other antiretroviral agents.

## Administration and Dosage

*Stavudine immediate-release:*

*Adults –* The recommended starting dose based on body weight is as follows:

*Patients weighing 60 kg or greater:* 40 mg every 12 hours.

*Patients weighing less than 60 kg:* 30 mg every 12 hours.

Stavudine may be taken without regard to meals.

*Children –* The recommended dose for newborns from birth to 13 days of age is 0.5 mg/kg/dose given every 12 hours. The recommended dose for pediatric patients at least 14 days of age and weighing less than 30 kg is 1 mg/kg/dose, given every 12 hours without regard to meals. Pediatric patients weighing 30 kg or greater should receive the recommended adult dosage.

*Dosage adjustment in renal function impairment –* Stavudine may be administered to adult patients with impaired renal function. The following schedule is recommended:

| Stavudine Dosage in Renal Function Impairment | | |
|---|---|---|
| Creatinine clearance (mL/min) | Recommended stavudine dose by patient weight | |
| | ≥ 60 kg | < 60 kg |
| > 50 | 40 mg every 12 hours | 30 mg every 12 hours |
| 26 to 50 | 20 mg every 12 hours | 15 mg every 12 hours |
| 10 to 25 | 20 mg every 24 hours | 15 mg every 24 hours |

Because urinary excretion is a major route of elimination of stavudine in pediatric patients, the clearance also may be altered in children with renal impairment. Although there are insufficient data to recommend a specific dose adjustment in this patient population, consider a reduction in the dose or an increase in the interval between doses.

*Hemodialysis patients:* The recommended dose is 20 mg every 24 hours (60 kg or more) or 15 mg every 24 hours (less than 60 kg) administered after the completion of hemodialysis and at the same time of day on nondialysis days.

*Stavudine, extended-release:*

*Adults –* The recommended daily dose is based on body weight and is administered in a once-daily schedule as follows:

*Patients weighing 60 kg or more:* 100 mg once daily.

*Patients weighing less than 60 kg:* 75 mg once daily

For patients who have difficulty swallowing intact capsules, the capsule can be carefully opened and the contents mixed with 30 mL of yogurt or applesauce. Patients should be cautioned not to chew or crush the beads while swallowing.

*Children –* Extended-release stavudine has not been studied in pediatric patients.

*Renal impairment –* Extended-release stavudine has not been studied in patients with renal impairment.

*Dosage adjustment in peripheral neuropathy:* Monitor patients for the development of peripheral neuropathy, which is usually characterized by numbness, tingling, or pain in the feet or hands. These symptoms may be difficult to detect in young children. If these symptoms develop, interrupt stavudine therapy. Symptoms may resolve if therapy is withdrawn promptly. In some cases, symptoms may worsen temporarily following discontinuation of therapy. Switching the patient to an alternate treatment regimen should be considered. If switching to an alternate regimen is not suitable and if symptoms resolve satisfactorily, resumption of treatment may be considered at 50% of the recommended dose using the following dosage schedule:

*Patients weighing 60 kg or greater –*

*Immediate-release:* 20 mg every 12 hours.

*Extended-release:* 50 mg once daily.

*Patients weighing less than 60 kg –*

*Immediate-release:* 15 mg every 12 hours.

*Extended-release:* 37.5 mg once daily.

If peripheral neuropathy recurs after resumption of stavudine, consider permanent discontinuation.

## Actions

*Pharmacology:* Stavudine is a synthetic thymidine nucleoside analog active against HIV. It inhibits the replication of HIV in human cells in vitro.

*Pharmacokinetics:*

*Absorption/Distribution –* Following oral administration, stavudine is rapidly absorbed with peak plasma concentrations occurring within 1 hour after dosing. The systemic exposure to stavudine is the same following administration as capsules or solution. Binding to serum proteins was negligible. Oral bioavailability in adults is approximately 86%. The apparent oral volume of distribution is about 66 L.

*Excretion –* Renal elimination accounted for about 40% of the overall clearance regardless of the route of administration. The elimination half-life is about 1.4 hours.

*Special populations –*

*Renal function impairment:* Adjust dosage in patients with reduced Ccr and in patients receiving maintenance hemodialysis (see Administration and Dosage).

## Contraindications

Hypersensitivity to stavudine or to any components of the formulation.

## Warnings

*Lactic acidosis/severe hepatomegaly with steatosis/hepatic failure:* Lactic acidosis and severe hepatomegaly with steatosis, including fatal cases, have been reported with the use of nucleoside analogs alone or in combination, including stavudine and other antiretrovirals. Female gender, obesity, and prolonged nucleoside exposure may be risk factors. Fatal lactic acidosis has been reported in pregnant women who received the combination of stavudine and didanosine with other antiretroviral agents. Use the combination of stavudine and didanosine with caution during pregnancy; it is recommended only if the potential benefit clearly outweighs the potential risk (see Pregnancy). Deaths attributed to hepatotoxicity have occurred in patients receiving the combination of stavudine, didanosine, and hydroxyurea. Exercise caution when administering stavudine to any patient with known risk factors for liver disease; however, cases also have been reported in patients with no known risk factors. Suspend treatment with stavudine in any patient who develops clinical or laboratory findings suggestive of lactic acidosis or pronounced hepatotoxicity (which may include hepatomegaly and steatosis even in the absence of marked transaminase elevations). An increased risk of hepatotoxicity, which may be fatal, may occur in patients treated with stavudine in combination with didanosine and hydroxyurea compared with when stavudine is used alone. Closely monitor patients treated with this combination for signs of liver toxicity.

*Neurologic symptoms:* Motor weakness has been reported rarely. Most of these cases occurred in the setting of lactic acidosis. The evolution of motor weakness may mimic the clinical presentation of Guillain-Barré syndrome (including respiratory failure). Symptoms may continue or worsen following discontinuation of therapy.

Stavudine therapy has been associated with peripheral neuropathy, which can be severe and is dose-related. Peripheral neuropathy has occurred more frequently in patients with advanced HIV disease, a history of neuropathy, or concurrent neurotoxic drug therapy, including didanosine (see Adverse Reactions).

Monitor patients for development of neuropathy. Stavudine-related peripheral neuropathy may resolve if therapy is withdrawn promptly. Symptoms may worsen temporarily following therapy discontinuation. If symptoms resolve completely, resumption of treatment may be considered at 50% of the dose (see Administration and Dosage). If stavudine must be given in this clinical setting, careful monitoring is essential. If neuropathy recurs after resumption of stavudine, consider permanent discontinuation.

*Pancreatitis:* Fatal and nonfatal pancreatitis have occurred during therapy when stavudine was part of a combination regimen that included didanosine, with or without hydroxyurea, in treatment-naive and treatment-experienced patients, regardless of degree of immunosuppression. In patients with suspected pancreatitis, suspend the combination of stavudine and didanosine (with or without hydroxyurea) and any other agents that are toxic to the pancreas. Reinstitution of stavudine after a confirmed diagnosis of pancreatitis should be undertaken with particular caution and close patient monitoring. The new regimen should not contain either didanosine or hydroxyurea.

*Fat redistribution:* Redistribution/accumulation of body fat including central obesity, dorsocervical fat enlargement (buffalo hump), peripheral wasting, facial wasting, breast enlargement, and "cushingoid appearance" have been observed in patients receiving antiretroviral therapy. The mechanism and long-term consequences of these events are currently unknown. A causal relationship has not been established.

*Elderly:* Clinical studies of stavudine did not include sufficient numbers of patients 65 years of age or older to determine whether they respond differently than younger patients. Closely monitor elderly patients for signs and symptoms of peripheral neuropathy. Because elderly patients are more likely to have decreased renal function, it may be useful to monitor renal function.

*Pregnancy: Category* C.

To monitor maternal-fetal outcomes of pregnant women exposed to stavudine and other antiretroviral agents, an Antiretroviral Pregnancy Registry has been established. Physicians are encouraged to register patients by calling (800) 258-4263.

Fatal lactic acidosis has been reported in pregnant women who received the combination of stavudine and didanosine with other antiretroviral agents (see Warning Box).

*Lactation:* Because of the potential for adverse reactions in nursing infants, instruct mothers to discontinue nursing if they are receiving stavudine. To avoid risking postnatal transmission of HIV infection, instruct HIV-infected mothers not to breastfeed their infants; this is consistent with the CDC's recommendation.

*Children:* Use of stavudine in pediatric patients is supported by evidence from adequate and well-controlled studies of stavudine in adults with additional pharmacokinetic and safety data in pediatric patients.

**Drug Interactions**

Drugs that may interact with stavudine include didanosine, doxorubicin, hydroxyurea, methadone, ribavirin, and zidovudine.

**Adverse Reactions**

When stavudine is used in combination with other agents with similar toxicities, the incidence of adverse events may be higher than when stavudine is used alone. Pancreatitis, peripheral neuropathy, and liver function abnormalities occur more frequently in patients treated with the combination of stavudine and didanosine, with or without hydroxyurea. Fatal pancreatitis and hepatotoxicity may occur more frequently in patients treated with stavudine in combination with didanosine and hydroxyurea (see Warnings).

Adverse reactions occurring in at least 3% of patients include headache, diarrhea, peripheral neurologic symptoms/neuropathy, rash, nausea, and vomiting. Lab abnormalities include elevations in AST, ALT, and amylase.

# ZALCITABINE (Dideoxycytidine; ddC)

**Tablets:** 0.375 and 0.75 mg (Rx)          Hivid (Roche)

**Warning:**
> The use of zalcitabine has been associated with significant clinical adverse reactions, some of which are potentially fatal. Zalcitabine can cause severe peripheral neuropathy; therefore, use with extreme caution in patients with pre-existing neuropathy. Zalcitabine may also rarely cause pancreatitis, and patients who develop any symptoms suggestive of pancreatitis while using zalcitabine should have therapy suspended immediately until this diagnosis is excluded.
>
> Lactic acidosis and severe hepatomegaly with steatosis, including fatal cases, have been reported with the use of antiretroviral nucleoside analogs alone or in combination, including zalcitabine. In addition, rare cases of hepatic failure and death, considered possibly related to underlying hepatitis B and zalcitabine have been reported (see Warnings).

## Indications
*Combination therapy with antiretrovirals:* For the treatment of human immunodeficiency virus (HIV) infection.

## Administration and Dosage
*Combination therapy with antiretrovirals:* The recommended regimen is one 0.75 mg tablet of zalcitabine orally every 8 hours (2.25 mg zalcitabine total daily dose) in combination with other antiretroviral agents.

*Renal function impairment:* Dosage reduction is recommended: Ccr 10 to 40 mL/min, 0.75 mg every 12 hours; Ccr less than 10 mL/min, 0.75 mg every 24 hours.

*Dose adjustment:*

*Combination therapy* – For toxicities likely to be associated with zalcitabine (eg, peripheral neuropathy, severe oral ulcers, pancreatitis, elevated liver function tests, especially in patients with chronic hepatitis B; see Warnings and Precautions), interrupt or reduce dose. For severe toxicities or those persisting after dose reduction, interrupt zalcitabine therapy. For recipients of combination therapy with zalcitabine and other antiretrovirals, base dose adjustments or interruption for either drug on the known toxicity profile of the individual drugs.

*Peripheral neuropathy* – Patients developing moderate discomfort with signs or symptoms of peripheral neuropathy should stop zalcitabine. Zalcitabine-associated peripheral neuropathy may continue to worsen despite interruption of therapy. Reintroduce the drug at 50% dose (0.375 mg every 8 hours) only if all findings related to peripheral neuropathy have improved to mild symptoms. Permanently discontinue the drug when patients experience severe discomfort related to peripheral neuropathy or moderate discomfort progresses. If other moderate to severe clinical adverse reactions or lab abnormalities (eg, increased liver function tests) occur, interrupt zalcitabine (or both zalcitabine and the other potential causative agent(s) in combination therapy) until the adverse reaction abates. Carefully reintroduce zalcitabine or the other agent at lower doses if appropriate. If adverse reactions recur, discontinue therapy. The minimum effective dose of zalcitabine in combination with zidovudine for the treatment of adults with advanced HIV infection has not been established.

*Hematologic toxicities* – Significant toxicities, such as anemia (hemoglobin less than 7.5 g/dL or reduction of greater than 25% of baseline) or granulocytopenia (granulocyte count of less than 750/mm$^3$ or reduction of greater than 50% from baseline), may require a treatment interruption of zalcitabine and zidovudine until evidence of marrow recovery is observed (see Warnings). For less severe anemia or granulocytopenia, a reduction in the daily dose of zidovudine in those patients receiving combination therapy may be adequate. In patients who develop significant anemia, dose modification does not necessarily eliminate the need for transfusion. If marrow recovery occurs following dose modification, gradual increases in dose may be appropriate, depending on hematologic indices and patient intolerance.

### Actions

*Pharmacology:* Zalcitabine, active against HIV, is a synthetic pyrimidine nucleoside analog of the naturally occurring nucleoside deoxycytidine in which the 3'-hydroxyl group is replaced by hydrogen. Within cells, zalcitabine is converted to the active metabolite, dideoxycytidine 5'-triphosphate (ddCTP), by cellular enzymes. ddCTP inhibits the activity of the HIV-reverse transcriptase both by competing for utilization of the natural substrate, deoxycytidine 5'-triphosphate (dCTP), and by its incorporation into viral DNA.

*Pharmacokinetics:*

   *Adults –*

   *Absorption/Distribution:* Following oral administration to HIV-infected patients, the mean absolute bioavailability of zalcitabine was greater than 80%. The absorption rate of a 1.5 mg oral dose was reduced when administered with food. This resulted in a 39% decrease in mean maximum plasma concentrations ($C_{max}$) from 25.2 to 15.5 ng/mL, and a 2-fold increase in time to achieve $C_{max}$ from a mean of 0.8 hours under fasting conditions to 1.6 hours when the drug was given with food. The extent of absorption was decreased by 14% (from 72 to 62 ng•h/mL).

   The steady-state volume of distribution following IV administration of a 1.5 mg dose averaged 0.534 L/kg. Cerebrospinal fluid obtained from 9 patients at 2 to 3.5 hours following 0.06 or 0.09 mg/kg IV infusion showed measurable concentrations of zalcitabine. The CSF:plasma concentration ratio ranged from 9% to 37% (mean, 20%), demonstrating drug penetration through the blood-brain barrier.

   *Metabolism/Excretion:* Zalcitabine is phosphorylated intracellularly to zalcitabine triphosphate, the active substrate for HIV-reverse transcriptase. Concentrations of zalcitabine triphosphate are too low for quantitation. Metabolism has not been fully evaluated. Zalcitabine does not appear to undergo a significant degree of metabolism by the liver. Renal excretion appears to be the primary route of elimination, and accounted for approximately 70% of an orally administered dose within 24 hours after dosing. The mean elimination half-life is 2 hours. Total body clearance following an IV dose averages 285 mL/min. Less than 10% of a dose appears in the feces.

   *Children –* Limited pharmacokinetic data have been reported for 5 HIV-positive children using doses of 0.03 and 0.04 mg/kg administered orally every 6 hours. The mean bioavailability of zalcitabine in this study was 54% and mean apparent systemic clearance was 150 mL/min/m².

### Contraindications

Hypersensitivity to zalcitabine or any components of the product.

### Warnings

Significant clinical adverse reactions, some of which are potentially fatal, have been reported with zalcitabine. Patients with decreased $CD_4$ cell counts appear to have an increased incidence of adverse events.

*Peripheral neuropathy:* The major clinical toxicity is peripheral neuropathy (22% to 35%) of subjects.

   In some patients, symptoms of neuropathy may initially progress despite discontinuation of zalcitabine. With prompt discontinuation, the neuropathy is usually slowly reversible.

   Use with extreme caution in patients with pre-existing peripheral neuropathy. Avoid zalcitabine in individuals with moderate or severe peripheral neuropathy, as evidenced by symptoms accompanied by objective findings.

   Zalcitabine should be used with caution in the following patients with a risk of developing peripheral neuropathy: Patients with low CD4 cell counts (CD4 less than 50 cells/mm³), diabetes, weight loss, or patients receiving zalcitabine concomitantly with drugs that have the potential to cause peripheral neuropathy. Careful monitoring is strongly recommended for these individuals.

Stop zalcitabine promptly if signs or symptoms of peripheral neuropathy occurs, such as when moderate discomfort from numbness, tingling, burning, or pain of the extremities progresses, or any related symptoms occur that are accompanied by an objective finding (see Administration and Dosage).

*Pancreatitis:* Pancreatitis, fatal in some cases, has been observed with zalcitabine administration. Pancreatitis is an uncommon complication of zalcitabine therapy, occurring in up to 1.1% of patients.

*Lactic acidosis/severe hepatomegaly with steatosis/hepatic toxicity:* Lactic acidosis and severe hepatomegaly with steatosis, including fatal cases, have been reported with the use of nucleoside analogs alone or in combination, including zalcitabine and other antiretrovirals. A majority of these cases have been in women. Obesity and prolonged nucleoside exposure may be risk factors. Exercise particular caution when administering zalcitabine to any patient with known risk factors for liver disease; however, cases also have been reported in patients with no known risk factors. Suspend treatment with zalcitabine in any patient who develops clinical or laboratory findings suggestive of lactic acidosis or pronounced hepatotoxicity (which may include hepatomegaly and steatosis even in the absence of marked transaminase elevations).

Suspend treatment with zalcitabine in any patient who develops clinical or laboratory findings suggestive of pronounced hepatotoxicity. In clinical trials, drug interruption was recommended if liver function tests exceeded 5 times the upper limit of normal.

*Hematologic toxicities:* In patients with poor bone marrow reserve, particularly those patients with advanced symptomatic HIV disease, frequent monitoring of hematologic indices is recommended to detect serious anemia or granulocytopenia. In patients who experience hematologic toxicity, reduction in hemoglobin may occur as early as 2 to 4 weeks after initiation of therapy and granulocytopenia usually occurs after 6 to 8 weeks of therapy.

*Oral ulcers:* Severe oral ulcers occurred in approximately 3% of patients in 2 trials. Less severe oral ulcerations occurred at higher frequencies in other clinical trials.

*Esophageal ulcers:* Infrequent cases of esophageal ulcers have been attributed to zalcitabine therapy. Consider interruption of therapy in patients who develop esophageal ulcers that do not respond to specific treatment for opportunistic pathogens in order to assess a possible relationship to zalcitabine.

*Cardiomyopathy/CHF:* Cardiomyopathy and CHF have occurred with the use of nucleoside antiretroviral agents in AIDS patients; infrequent cases have occurred in patients receiving zalcitabine. Approach treatment with caution in patients with baseline cardiomyopathy or history of CHF.

*Anaphylactoid reaction:* There has been 1 report of an anaphylactoid reaction occurring in a patient receiving zalcitabine and zidovudine. In addition, there have been several reports of urticaria without other signs of anaphylaxis.

*Carcinogenesis:* No increase in tumor incidence was observed in rats or male mice treated with zalcitabine.

*Mutagenesis:* Human peripheral blood lymphocytes were exposed to zalcitabine, and at 1.5 mcg/mL or more, dose-related increases in chromosomal aberrations were seen. Oral doses of zalcitabine at 2500 and 4500 mg/kg were clastogenic in the mouse micronucleus assay.

*Elderly:* Clinical studies of zalcitabine did not include sufficient numbers of subjects 65 years of age and older to determine whether they respond differently than younger subjects. In general, dose selection for an elderly patient should be cautious, reflecting the greater frequency of decreased hepatic, renal, or cardiac function, and of concomitant disease or other drug therapy.

*Pregnancy:* Category C.

*Lactation:* It is not known whether zalcitabine is excreted in breast milk. Decide whether to discontinue nursing or the drug, taking into account the importance of the drug to the mother. In the US, it currently is recommended that HIV-infected women do not breastfeed infants regardless of the use of antiretroviral agents.

*Children:* Safety and efficacy of zalcitabine in combination with zidovudine or as monotherapy in HIV-infected children younger than 13 years of age have not been established.

### Precautions

*Monitoring:* Perform periodic complete blood counts and clinical chemistry tests. Monitor serum amylase levels in those individuals who have a history of elevated amylase, pancreatitis, ethanol abuse, who are on parenteral nutrition, or who are otherwise at high risk of pancreatitis.

### Drug Interactions

Drugs that may interact with zalcitabine include antacids, chloramphenicol, cisplatin, dapsone, didanosine, disulfiram, ethionamide, glutethimide, gold, hydralazine, iodoquinol, isoniazid, metronidazole, nitrofurantoin, phenytoin, ribavirin, vincristine, cimetidine, metoclopramide, amphotericin, aminoglycosides, foscarnet, antiretroviral nucleoside analogs, pentamidine, and probenecid.

*Drug/Food interactions:* The absorption rate of a 1.5 mg dose is reduced when administered with food resulting in a 39% decrease in mean $C_{max}$ and a 2-fold increase in time to achieve $C_{max}$. The extent of absorption is decreased by 14%.

### Adverse Reactions

Adverse reactions occurring in ≥ 3% of patients include malaise/fatigue; abdominal pain; oral lesions/stomatitis; vomiting/nausea; peripheral neuropathy; elevated amylase; rash/pruritus/urticaria; diarrhea; oral ulcers; dysphagia; hypoglycemia; hyponatremia; bilirubin increased; loss of appetite; abnormal weight loss; abnormal hepatic function; hyperglycemia; myalgia; headache; nasal discharge; cough; pruritic disorder; fever; thrombocytopenia; neutropenia; leukopenia; eosinophilia; anemia.

# ZIDOVUDINE (Azidothymidine; AZT; Compound S)

**Tablets:** 300 mg (*Rx*)  
**Capsules:** 100 mg (*Rx*)  
**Syrup:** 50 mg/5 mL (*Rx*)  
**Injection:** 10 mg/mL (*Rx*)

*Retrovir* (GlaxoSmithKline)

---

**Warning:**

Zidovudine has been associated with hematologic toxicity, including neutropenia and severe anemia, particularly in patients with advanced human immunodeficiency (HIV) disease (see Warnings). Prolonged use of zidovudine has been associated with symptomatic myopathy.

Lactic acidosis and severe hepatomegaly with steatosis, including fatal cases, have been reported with the use of nucleoside analogs alone or in combination, including zidovudine and other antiretrovirals (see Warnings).

---

### Indications

*HIV infection:* In combination with other antiretroviral agents for the treatment of HIV infection.

*Maternal-fetal HIV transmission –* Prevention of maternal-fetal HIV transmission as part of a regimen that includes oral zidovudine beginning between 14 and 34 weeks of gestation, IV zidovudine during labor, and administration of zidovudine syrup to the neonate after birth. The efficacy of this regimen for preventing HIV transmission in women who have received zidovudine for a prolonged period before pregnancy has not been evaluated. The safety of zidovudine for the mother or fetus during the first trimester of pregnancy has not been assessed.

## Administration and Dosage

*HIV infection:*

*Adults (oral)* – Recommended dose is 600 mg/day in divided doses in combination with other antiretroviral agents.

*Adults (IV)* – Recommended IV dose is 1 mg/kg infused over 1 hour. Administer this dose 5 to 6 times daily (5 to 6 mg/kg/day). Patients should receive zidovudine IV infusion only until oral therapy can be administered. The IV dosing regimen equivalent to the oral administration of 100 mg every 4 hours is approximately 1 mg/kg IV every 4 hours. Avoid rapid infusion or bolus injection. Do not give IM.

*Children (oral)* – Recommended dose in children 6 weeks to 12 years of age is 160 mg/m$^2$ every 8 hours (480 mg/m$^2$/day up to a maximum of 200 mg every 8 hours) in combination with other antiretroviral agents.

*Maternal-fetal HIV transmission:* Recommended dosing regimen to pregnant women (greater than 14 weeks of pregnancy) and their neonates is as follows:

*Maternal dosing (oral)* – 100 mg orally 5 times per day until the start of labor.

*Maternal dosing (IV)* – During labor and delivery, administer IV zidovudine at 2 mg/kg (total body weight) over 1 hour followed by a continuous IV infusion of 1 mg/kg/h (total body weight) until clamping of the umbilical cord.

*Neonatal dosing (oral)* – 2 mg/kg orally every 6 hours starting within 12 hours after birth and continuing through 6 weeks of age.

*Neonatal dosing (IV)* – Neonates unable to receive oral dosing may be given zidovudine IV at 1.5 mg/kg, infused over 30 minutes, every 6 hours.

*Dose adjustment:* Significant anemia (hemoglobin of less than 7.5 g/dL or reduction of greater than 25% from baseline) and/or significant neutropenia (granulocyte count of less than 750 cells/mm$^3$ or reduction of greater than 50% from baseline) may require a dose interruption until evidence of marrow recovery is observed. In patients who develop significant anemia, dose interruption does not necessarily eliminate the need for transfusion. If marrow recovery occurs following dose interruption, resumption in dose may be appropriate using adjunctive measures such as epoetin alfa at recommended doses, depending on hematologic indices such as serum erythropoietin level and patient tolerance.

*Renal function impairment* – In end-stage renal disease patients maintained on hemodialysis or peritoneal dialysis, the recommended dosing is 100 mg every 6 to 8 hours.

*Hepatic function impairment* – Because zidovudine is primarily eliminated by hepatic metabolism, a reduction in the daily dose may be necessary in these patients. Frequent monitoring for hematologic toxicities is advised.

## Actions

*Pharmacology:* Zidovudine is a synthetic nucleoside analog of the naturally occurring nucleoside thymidine. The active metabolite, zidovudine 5′-triphosphate (AztTP), inhibits the activity of the HIV reverse transcriptase by competing for utilization with the natural substrate deoxythymidine 5′-triphosphate (dTTP) and by its incorporation into viral DNA.

*Pharmacokinetics:*

*Adults* – Following oral administration, zidovudine is rapidly absorbed and extensively distributed, with peak serum concentrations occurring within 0.5 to 1.5 hours. Zidovudine is primarily eliminated by hepatic metabolism.

| Zidovudine Pharmacokinetic Parameters in Fasting Adult Patients | |
| --- | --- |
| Parameter | Mean value |
| Oral bioavailability (%) | ≈ 64 |
| Apparent volume of distribution (L/kg) | ≈ 1.6 |
| Plasma protein binding (%) | < 38 |
| CSF:plasma ratio[1] | 0.6 (0.04 to 2.62) |
| Systemic clearance (L/h/kg) | ≈ 1.6 |
| Renal clearance (L/h/kg) | ≈ 0.34 |
| Elimination half-life (h)[2] | 0.5 to 3 (oral); 1.1 (IV) |

[1] Median (range).
[2] Approximate range.

*Adults with impaired renal function* – A dose adjustment should not be necessary for patients with creatinine clearance (Ccr) greater than or equal to 15 mL/min.

| Zidovudine Pharmacokinetics Parameters in Patients with Severe Renal Impairment | | |
|---|---|---|
| Parameter | Control subjects (normal renal function) (n = 6) | Patients with renal impairment (n = 14) |
| Ccr (mL/min) | ≈ 120 | ≈ 18 |
| Zidovudine AUC (ng•h/mL) | ≈ 1400 | ≈ 3100 |
| Zidovudine half-life (h) | ≈ 1 | ≈ 1.4 |

A dosage adjustment is recommended for patients undergoing hemodialysis or peritoneal dialysis.

*Patients younger than 3 months of age* – The half-life was about 13 hours. In neonates 14 days of age or less, bioavailability was greater, total body clearance was slower, and half-life was longer than in pediatric patients more than 14 days old.

| Zidovudine Pharmacokinetic Parameters in Pediatric Patients | | | |
|---|---|---|---|
| Parameter | Birth to 14 days of age | 14 days to 3 months of age | 3 months to 12 years of age |
| Oral bioavailability (%) | ≈ 89 | ≈ 61 | ≈ 65 |
| CSF:Plasma ratio | no data | no data | ≈ 0.68 (0.03 to 3.25)[1] (oral); ≈ 0.26[1] (IV) |
| CL (L/h/kg) | ≈ 0.65 | ≈ 1.14 | ≈ 1.85 |
| Elimination half-life (h) | ≈ 3.1 | ≈ 1.9 | ≈ 1.5 |

[1] Median (range).

## Contraindications

Potentially life-threatening allergic reactions to any of the components of the product.

## Warnings

*Hematologic effects:* Use with extreme caution in patients who have bone marrow compromise evidenced by granulocyte count less than 1000/mm$^3$ or hemoglobin less than 9.5 g/dL. Anemia and granulocytopenia are the most significant adverse events observed. Reversible pancytopenia has been reported.

*Myopathy:* Myopathy and myositis with pathological changes, similar to that produced by HIV disease, have been associated with prolonged use of zidovudine.

*Lactic acidosis/severe hepatomegaly with steatosis:* Rare occurrences of lactic acidosis in the absence of hypoxemia, and severe hepatomegaly with steatosis have been reported with the use of antiretroviral nucleoside analogs, including zidovudine and zalcitabine, and are potentially fatal.

*Combination therapy:* Lamivudine/zidovudine and abacavir/lamivudine/zidovudine are combination product tablets that contain zidovudine as one of their components. Do not administer zidovudine concomitantly with lamivudine/zidovudine or abacavir/lamivudine/zidovudine.

*Renal/Hepatic function impairment:* Zidovudine is eliminated from the body primarily by renal excretion following metabolism in the liver (glucuronidation). In patients with severely impaired renal function (Ccr less than 15 mL/min), dosage reduction is recommended. Although very little data are available, patients with severely impaired hepatic function may be at greater risk of toxicity.

*Pregnancy: Category C.*

*Antiretroviral pregnancy registry* – Physicians are encouraged to register patients by calling (800) 258-4263.

*Lactation:* The Centers for Disease Control and Prevention recommend that HIV-infected women not breastfeed to avoid postnatal transmission of HIV.

Zidovudine is excreted in breast milk. Because of the potential for HIV transmission and for serious adverse reactions in nursing infants, instruct mothers not to breastfeed if they are receiving zidovudine.

*Children:* Zidovudine has been studied in HIV-infected pediatric patients over 3 months of age who had HIV-related symptoms or who were asymptomatic with abnormal laboratory values indicating significant HIV-related immunosuppression. Zidovudine also has been studied in neonates perinatally exposed to HIV.

### Drug Interactions

Drugs that may affect zidovudine include acetaminophen, atovaquone, bone marrow suppressive/cytotoxic agents (eg, adriamycin, dapsone), clarithromycin, doxorubicin, fluconazole, ganciclovir, methadone, nelfinavir/ritonavir, phenytoin, probenecid, ribavirin, rifamycins, stavudine, trimethoprim, and valproic acid.

Drugs that may be affected by zidovudine include phenytoin.

### Adverse Reactions

The frequency and severity of adverse events associated with the use of zidovudine are greater in patients with more advanced infection at the time of initiation of therapy.

The most frequent adverse events and abnormal laboratory values reported in the placebo-controlled clinical trial of oral zidovudine were granulocytopenia and anemia.

Adverse reactions occurring in at least 5% of patients with asymptomatic HIV infection include nausea, anorexia, vomiting, constipation, headache, malaise, and asthenia.

Other adverse events observed in clinical studies were abdominal cramps, abdominal pain, arthralgia, chills, dyspepsia, fatigue, hyperbilirubinemia, insomnia, musculoskeletal pain, myalgia, and neuropathy.

# ABACAVIR SULFATE

**Tablets:** 300 mg *(Rx)*                              *Ziagen* (GlaxoSmithKline)
**Oral solution:** 20 mg/mL *(Rx)*

---

**Warning:**
Fatal hypersensitivity reactions have been associated with abacavir sulfate therapy. Discontinue abacavir in patients developing signs or symptoms of hypersensitivity (eg, fever, rash, fatigue; GI symptoms such as nausea, vomiting, diarrhea, abdominal pain; respiratory symptoms such as pharyngitis, dyspnea, cough) as soon as a hypersensitivity reaction is suspected. To avoid a delay in diagnosis and minimize the risk of a life-threatening hypersensitivity reaction, permanently discontinue abacavir therapy if hypersensitivity cannot be ruled out, even when other diagnoses are possible (eg, acute onset respiratory diseases, gastroenteritis, reactions to other medications). Do not restart abacavir following a hypersensitivity reaction because more severe symptoms will recur within hours and may include life-threatening hypotension and death. Severe or fatal hypersensitivity reactions can occur within hours after reintroduction of abacavir in patients who have no identified history or unrecognized symptoms of hypersensitivity to abacavir therapy.

Lactic acidosis and severe hepatomegaly with steatosis, including fatal cases, have been reported with the use of nucleoside analogs alone or in combination, including abacavir and other antiretrovirals.

---

### Indications

*HIV infection:* In combination with other antiretroviral agents for the treatment of HIV-1 infection.

## Administration and Dosage

Dispense Medication Guide and Warning Card that provide information about recognition of hypersensitivity reactions with each new prescription and refill.

Always use abacavir in combination with other antiretroviral agents. Do not add abacavir as a single agent when antiretroviral regimens are changed because of loss of virologic response.

Abacavir may be taken with or without food.

*Adults:* The recommended dose is 300 mg twice daily in combination with other antiretroviral agents.

*Children (3 months to up to 16 years of age):* 8 mg/kg twice daily (up to a maximum of 300 mg twice daily) in combination with other antiretroviral agents.

*Dose adjustment in hepatic impairment:* The recommended dose of abacavir in patients with mild hepatic impairment (Child-Pugh score 5 to 6) is 200 mg twice daily. To enable dose reduction, abacavir oral solution (10 mL twice daily) should be used for the treatment of these patients. The safety, efficacy, and pharmacokinetic properties of abacavir have not been established in patients with moderate to severe hepatic impairment; therefore, abacavir is contraindicated in these patients.

## Actions

*Pharmacology:* Abacavir is a synthetic carbocyclic synthetic nucleoside analog with inhibitory activity against HIV. Intracellularly, abacavir is converted by cellular enzymes to the active metabolite carbovir triphosphate, an analog of deoxyguanosine-5'-triphosphate (dGTP). Carbovir triphosphate inhibits the activity of HIV-1 reverse transcriptase both by competing with the natural substrate dGTP and by its incorporation into viral DNA. Abacavir has synergistic activity in combination with amprenavir, nevirapine, and zidovudine and additive activity in combination with didanosine, lamivudine, stavudine, and zalcitabine in vitro.

*Cross-resistance* – In vitro, recombinant laboratory strains of HIV-1 (HXB2) containing multiple reverse transcriptase mutations conferring abacavir resistance exhibited cross-resistance to lamivudine, didanosine, and zalcitabine.

*Pharmacokinetics:*

*Absorption* – Abacavir was rapidly and extensively absorbed after oral administration with bioavailability at 83%. Systemic exposure to abacavir was comparable after administration of oral solution and tablets. Therefore, these products may be used interchangeably.

*Distribution* – The apparent volume of distribution after IV administration of abacavir was approximately 0.86 L/kg, suggesting that abacavir distributes into extravascular space. Binding to human plasma proteins is approximately 50% and was independent of concentration.

*Metabolism* – Abacavir is not significantly metabolized by cytochrome P450 enzymes.

*Excretion* – Of the 99% of the total abacavir dose recovered, 1.2% was excreted in the urine as abacavir. Fecal elimination accounted for 16% of the dose. In single-dose studies, the observed elimination half-life was approximately 1.54 hours.

## Contraindications

Hypersensitivity to any of the components of the product.

Moderate or severe hepatic impairment (Child-Pugh score greater than 6).

## Warnings

*Lactic acidosis/severe hepatomegaly with steatosis:* Lactic acidosis and severe hepatomegaly with steatosis, including fatal cases, have been reported with the use of nucleoside analogs alone or in combination, including abacavir and other antiretrovirals. A majority of these cases have been in women. Obesity and prolonged nucleoside exposure may be risk factors. Suspend treatment with abacavir in any patient who develops clinical or laboratory findings suggestive of lactic acidosis or pronounced hepatotoxicity (which may include hepatomegaly and steatosis even in the absence of marked transaminase elevations).

*Hypersensitivity reactions:* Fatal hypersensitivity reactions have been associated with abacavir therapy. Discontinue abacavir in patients developing signs or symptoms of hypersensitivity as soon as a hypersensitivity reaction is first suspected; seek medical attention immediately. Do not restart abacavir following a hypersensitivity reaction because more severe symptoms will recur within hours and may include life-threatening hypotension and death.

*Abacavir hypersensitivity reaction registry* – Physicians should register patients by calling (800) 270-0425.

*Pregnancy:* Category C.

*Antiretroviral pregnancy registry* – Physicians are encouraged to register patients by calling (800) 258-4263.

*Lactation:* The Centers for Disease Control and Prevention recommend that HIV-infected mothers not breastfeed their infants to avoid risking postnatal transmission of HIV infection. Because of the potential for HIV transmission and any possible adverse effects of abacavir, instruct mothers not to breastfeed if they are receiving abacavir.

*Children:* Use of abacavir in pediatric patients 3 months to 13 years of age is safe and effective and is supported by pharmacokinetic studies and evidence from adequate and well-controlled studies of abacavir in adults and pediatric patients.

## Precautions

*Cross-resistance:* In clinical trials, patients with prolonged prior nucleoside reverse transcriptase inhibitor (NRTI) exposure or who had HIV-1 isolates that contained multiple mutations conferring resistance to NRTIs had limited response to abacavir. Consider the potential for cross-resistance between abacavir and other NRTIs when choosing new therapeutic regimens in therapy-experienced patients.

*Fat redistribution* – Redistribution/accumulation of body fat, including central obesity, dorsocervical fat enlargement (buffalo hump), peripheral wasting, facial wasting, breast enlargement, and "cushingoid appearance" have been observed in patients receiving antiretroviral therapy.

## Drug Interactions

*Ethanol:* Ethanol decreases the elimination of abacavir, causing an increase in overall exposure.

*Methadone:* Coadministration increased oral methadone clearance by 22% (90% CI 6% to 42%). This alteration will not result in a methadone dose modification in the majority of patients; however, an increased methadone dose may be required in a small number of patients.

## Adverse Reactions

*Adults:* Adverse effects occurring in at least 5% of adults include the following: Diarrhea; fever and/or chills; headache; insomnia and other sleep disorders; loss of appetite/anorexia; malaise; nausea and vomiting.

*Children:* Adverse effects occurring in at least 5% of children include the following: Diarrhea; fever; headache; loss of appetite/anorexia; nausea and vomiting; rash.

*Hypersensitivity:* Fatal hypersensitivity reactions have been associated with abacavir therapy (see Warnings and Warning Box).

*Lab test abnormalities:* Mild elevations of blood glucose; anemia; neutropenia; liver function test abnormalities; CPK or creatinine elevations; lymphopenia; triglyceride elevations.

# LAMIVUDINE/ZIDOVUDINE (3TC/ZDV, 3TC/AZT)

**Tablets:** 150 mg lamivudine/300 mg zidovudine (*Rx*)        *Combivir* (GlaxoSmithKline)

Consult the complete prescribing information for each agent, lamivudine and zidovudine, prior to administration of lamivudine/zidovudine combination tablets.

**Warning:**
Zidovudine may result in hematologic toxicity (eg, neutropenia, severe anemia), especially in patients with advanced human immunodeficiency virus (HIV). Prolonged use has been associated with symptomatic myopathy (see Warnings section in zidovudine monograph).

Lactic acidosis and severe hepatomegaly with steatosis, including fatal cases, have been reported with use of nucleoside analogs alone or in combination.

## Indications
*HIV infection:* In combination with other antiretrovirals for the treatment of HIV infection.

## Administration and Dosage
*Adults and children at least 12 years of age:* One lamivudine/zidovudine combination tablet (150 mg/300 mg) orally twice daily without regard to food.

*Renal function impairment:* Because it is a fixed-dose combination, do not prescribe lamivudine/zidovudine for patients requiring dosage adjustment, such as those with reduced renal function (Ccr less than 50 mL/min) or those experiencing dose-limiting adverse events.

*Hepatic function impairment:* A reduction in the daily dose of zidovudine may be necessary in patients with mild to moderate hepatic function impairment or liver cirrhosis. Because lamivudine/zidovudine is a fixed-dose combination that cannot be adjusted for this patient population, it is not recommended for patients with impaired hepatic function.

## Actions
*Pharmacology:* Lamivudine/zidovudine combination tablets contain 2 synthetic nucleoside analog reverse transcriptase inhibitors with activity against HIV. Lamivudine in combination with zidovudine has exhibited synergistic antiretroviral activity. Refer to lamivudine and zidovudine individual monographs.

*Pharmacokinetics:* One combination lamivudine/zidovudine (150/300 mg) tablet is bioequivalent to a 150 mg lamivudine tablet plus a 300 mg zidovudine tablet.

| Select Pharmacokinetic Parameters for Lamivudine and Zidovudine[1] | | | | | | |
|---|---|---|---|---|---|---|
| | Bioavailability (%) | $V_d$ (L/kg) | CSF:Plasma ratio | Clearance (L/h/kg) | Renal clearance (L/h/kg) | $t_{1/2}$ (h) |
| Lamivudine | ≈ 86 | ≈ 1.3 | ≈ 0.12 | ≈ 0.33 | ≈ 0.22 | 5 to 7 |
| Zidovudine | ≈ 64 | ≈ 1.6 | ≈ 0.6 | ≈ 1.6 | ≈ 0.34 | 0.5 to 3 |

[1] In adults.

## Contraindications
Hypersensitivity to any of the components of this product.

Because this product is a fixed-dose combination doseform, avoid use in patients requiring dosage reduction.

## Warnings
*Fixed-dose combination:* Lamivudine/zidovudine tablets are a fixed-dose combination doseform that does not allow for dose reduction. Avoid use in patients requiring lamivudine or zidovudine dosage reduction including children under 12 years of age, renally impaired patients with Ccr less than 50 mL/min, or those experiencing dose-limiting adverse effects.

*Hematologic:* Use lamivudine/zidovudine with caution in patients who have bone marrow compromise evidenced by granulocyte count less than 1000 cells/mm³ or hemoglobin less than 9.5 g/dL.

*Lactic acidosis/severe hepatomegaly with steatosis:* Lactic acidosis and severe hepatomegaly with steatosis, including fatal cases, have been reported with the use of nucleoside analogs alone or in combination, including lamivudine, zidovudine, and other antiretrovirals. Suspend treatment with lamivudine/zidovudine in any patient who develops clinical or laboratory findings suggestive of lactic acidosis or pronounced hepatotoxicity (which may include hepatomegaly and steatosis even in the absence of marked transaminase elevations).

*Pregnancy:* Category C.

**Precautions**

*Monitoring:* Blood counts are recommended frequently for patients with advanced HIV disease and periodically for patients with asymptomatic or early HIV disease.

# ABACAVIR SULFATE/LAMIVUDINE/ZIDOVUDINE

| | |
|---|---|
| **Tablets**: 300 mg abacavir sulfate/150 mg lamivudine/ 300 mg zidovudine (*Rx*) | *Trizivir* (GlaxoSmithKline) |

Consult the complete prescribing information for each agent, abacavir, lamivudine, and zidovudine, prior to administration of abacavir/lamivudine/zidovudine combination tablets.

**Warning:**
This product contains 3 nucleoside analogs (abacavir sulfate, lamivudine, and zidovudine) and is intended only for patients whose regimen would otherwise include these 3 components.

Abacavir sulfate has been associated with fatal hypersensitivity reactions (see Warnings). Patients developing signs or symptoms of hypersensitivity (eg, fever; skin rash; fatigue; GI symptoms such as nausea, vomiting, diarrhea, or abdominal pain; respiratory symptoms such as pharyngitis, dyspnea, or cough) should discontinue abacavir/lamivudine/zidovudine as soon as a hypersensitivity reaction is suspected. To avoid a delay in diagnosis and minimize the risk of a life-threatening hypersensitivity reaction, permanently discontinue abacavir/lamivudine/zidovudine if hypersensitivity cannot be ruled out, even when other diagnoses are possible (eg, acute onset respiratory diseases, gastroenteritis, reactions to other medications).

Do not restart abacavir following a hypersensitivity reaction because more severe symptoms will recur within hours and may include life-threatening hypotension and death.

Severe or fatal hypersensitivity reactions can occur within hours after reintroduction of abacavir in patients who have no identified history or unrecognized symptoms of hypersensitivity to abacavir therapy (see Warnings and Adverse Reactions).

Zidovudine has been associated with hematologic toxicity, including neutropenia and severe anemia, particularly in patients with advanced HIV disease (see Warnings). Prolonged use of zidovudine has been associated with symptomatic myopathy.

---

**Warning: (cont.)**

Lactic acidosis and severe hepatomegaly with steatosis, including fatal cases, have been reported with the use of nucleoside analogs alone or in combination, including abacavir, lamivudine, zidovudine, and other antiretrovirals (see Warnings).

There are limited data on the use of this triple-combination regimen in patients with higher viral load levels (more than 100,000 copies/mL) at baseline.

---

### Indications

HIV infection: Alone or in combination with other antiretroviral agents for the treatment of HIV-1 infection.

### Administration and Dosage

Dispense a Medication Guide and Warning Card that provide information about recognition of hypersensitivity reactions with each new prescription or refill. To facilitate reporting hypersensitivity reactions and collection of information on each case, an Abacavir Hypersensitivity Registry has been established. Physicians should register patients by calling (800) 270-0425.

Adults and adolescents (40 kg or greater): 1 tablet twice daily. Not recommended in adults or adolescents who weigh less than 40 kg because it is a fixed-dose tablet.

Dose adjustment: Because it is a fixed-dose tablet, do not prescribe for patients requiring dosage adjustments such as those with Ccr less than 50 mL/min or those experiencing dose-limiting adverse events.

### Actions

Pharmacology: The combination tablets contain the following 3 synthetic nucleoside analogs: Abacavir sulfate, lamivudine, and zidovudine. Abacavir is a carbocyclic synthetic nucleoside analog. Lamivudine and zidovudine are synthetic nucleoside analogs.

Pharmacokinetics: Following oral administration, abacavir, lamivudine, and zidovudine are rapidly absorbed and extensively distributed. Binding of abacavir to human plasma proteins is about 50%; binding of lamivudine and zidovudine to plasma proteins is low.

The pharmacokinetic properties of abacavir, lamivudine, and zidovudine in fasting patients are summarized below.

| Pharmacokinetic Parameters for Abacavir, Lamivudine, and Zidovudine in Adults | | | |
|---|---|---|---|
| Parameter | Abacavir | Lamivudine | Zidovudine |
| Oral bioavailability (%) | ≈ 86 | ≈ 86 | ≈ 64 |
| Apparent volume of distribution (L/kg) | ≈ 0.86 | ≈ 1.3 | ≈ 1.6 |
| Systemic clearance (L/h/kg) | ≈ 0.8 | ≈ 0.33 | ≈ 1.6 |
| Renal clearance (L/h/kg) | ≈ 0.007 | ≈ 0.22 | ≈ 0.34 |
| Elimination half-life (h)[1] | ≈ 1.45 | 5 to 7 | 0.5 to 3 |

[1] Approximate range.

### Contraindications

Abacavir sulfate has been associated with fatal hypersensitivity reactions. Do not restart abacavir following a hypersensitivity reaction (see Warnings and Adverse Reactions).

Abacavir/lamivudine/zidovudine tablets are contraindicated in patients with previously demonstrated hypersensitivity to any of the components of the product (see Warnings).

### Warnings

Lactic acidosis/severe hepatomegaly with steatosis: Lactic acidosis and severe hepatomegaly with steatosis, including fatal cases, have been reported with the use of nucleoside analogs alone or in combination, including abacavir, lamivudine, zidovudine, and other antiretrovirals. A majority of these cases have been in women. Obesity and prolonged nucleoside exposure may be risk factors. Exercise particular caution when administering abacavir/lamivudine/zidovudine to any patient with known risk factors for liver disease; however, cases also have been reported in patients with no known risk factors. Suspend treatment in any patient who develops clinical or laboratory findings suggestive of lactic acidosis or pronounced hepatotoxicity (which may include hepatomegaly and steatosis even in the absence of marked transaminase elevations).

*Hematologic effects:* Because the combination contains zidovudine, use with caution in patients who have bone marrow compromise evidenced by granulocyte count less than 1000 cells/mm$^3$ or hemoglobin less than 9.5 g/dL.

*Hypersensitivity reactions:* Abacavir sulfate has been associated with fatal hypersensitivity reactions. Patients developing signs or symptoms of hypersensitivity (eg, fever; skin rash; fatigue; GI symptoms such as nausea, vomiting, diarrhea, or abdominal pain; and respiratory symptoms such as pharyngitis, dyspnea, or cough) should discontinue abacavir/lamivudine/zidovudine combination tablets as soon as a hypersensitivity reaction is first suspected and should seek medical evaluation immediately. To avoid a delay in diagnosis and minimize the risk of a life-threatening hypersensitivity reaction, permanently discontinue the combination tablets if hypersensitivity cannot be ruled out, even when other diagnoses are possible (eg, acute onset respiratory diseases, gastroenteritis, reactions to other medications). Do not restart abacavir following a hypersensitivity reaction because more severe symptoms will recur within hours and may include life-threatening hypotension and death.

*Pregnancy:* Category C.

*Antiretroviral pregnancy registry* – Physicians are encouraged to register patients by calling (800) 258-4263.

# EMTRICITABINE/TENOFOVIR DISOPROXIL FUMARATE

| | |
|---|---|
| **Tablets**: 200 mg emtricitabine/300 mg tenofovir disoproxil fumarate (equivalent to 245 mg tenofovir disoproxil) (*Rx*) | *Truvada* (Gilead) |

Consult the complete prescribing information for each agent prior to administration of emtricitabine/tenofovir disoproxil fumarate combination tablets.

---

**Warning:**

Lactic acidosis and severe hepatomegaly with steatosis, including fatal cases, have been reported with the use of nucleoside analogs alone or in combination with other antiretrovirals (see Warnings).

Emtricitabine/tenofovir disoproxil fumarate is not indicated for the treatment of chronic hepatitis B virus (HBV) infection; safety and efficacy have not been established in patients coinfected with HBV and HIV. Severe acute exacerbations of hepatitis B have been reported in patients who have discontinued emtricitabine or tenofovir disoproxil fumarate. Closely monitor hepatic function with clinical and laboratory follow-up for at least several months in patients who discontinue emtricitabine/tenofovir disoproxil fumarate and are coinfected with HIV and HBV. If appropriate, initiation of antihepatitis B therapy may be warranted (see Warnings).

---

**Indications**

*HIV infection:* In combination with other antiretroviral agents (such as nonnucleoside reverse transcriptase inhibitors or protease inhibitors) for the treatment of HIV-1 infection in adults.

In treatment-naïve patients, consider emtricitabine/tenofovir disoproxil fumarate as an alternative to the combination of tenofovir disoproxil fumarate plus lamivudine (3TC) for those patients who might benefit from a once-daily regimen. In treatment-experienced patients, guide the use of emtricitabine/tenofovir disoproxil fumarate by laboratory testing and treatment history.

## Administration and Dosage

The dose of emtricitabine/tenofovir disoproxil fumarate is 1 tablet taken orally once daily with or without food.

*Renal function impairment:* Significantly increased drug exposures occurred when emtricitabine or tenofovir disoproxil fumarate were administered to patients with moderate to severe renal impairment. Because the safety and efficacy of the dosing interval adjustment recommendations below have not been clinically evaluated, closely monitor clinical response to treatment and renal function in these patients.

| Dosage Adjustment for Patients with Altered Ccr | | | |
|---|---|---|---|
| Ccr (mL/min)[a] | ≥ 50 | 30 to 49 | < 30 (including patients requiring hemodialysis) |
| Recommended dosing interval | Every 24 hours | Every 48 hours | Not to be administered |

[a] Calculated using ideal (lean) body weight.

## Actions

*Pharmacology:* Refer to individual monographs for a complete explanation of mechanisms of action.

*Pharmacokinetics:* One emtricitabine/tenofovir disoproxil fumarate tablet was bioequivalent to 1 emtricitabine capsule (200 mg) plus 1 tenofovir disoproxil fumarate tablet (300 mg) following single-dose administration to fasting healthy subjects.

| Single Dose Pharmacokinetic Parameters for Emtricitabine and Tenofovir in Adults | | |
|---|---|---|
| | Emtricitabine | Tenofovir |
| Fasted oral bioavailability[a] (%) | ≈ 92 | ≈ 25 |
| Plasma terminal elimination half-life[a] (h) | ≈ 10 | ≈ 17 |
| $C_{max}$[b] (mcg/mL) | ≈ 1.8[c] | ≈ 0.30 |
| $AUC$[b] (mcg•h/mL) | ≈ 10[c] | ≈ 2.29 |
| $CL/F$[b] (mL/min) | ≈ 302 | ≈ 1,043 |
| $CL_{renal}$[b] (mL/min) | ≈ 213 | ≈ 243 |

[a] Median (range).
[b] Mean (approximately SD).
[c] Data presented as steady-state values.

## Contraindications

Previously demonstrated hypersensitivity to any of the components of the product.

## Warnings

*Fixed dose combination:* This combination contains fixed doses of 2 nucleoside analogs: emtricitabine and tenofovir disoproxil fumarate. Do not administer concomitantly with emtricitabine or tenofovir disoproxil fumarate.

*Lactic acidosis/severe hepatomegaly with steatosis:* Lactic acidosis and severe hepatomegaly with steatosis, including fatal cases, have been reported with the use of nucleoside analogs alone or in combination with other antiretrovirals. A majority of these cases have been in women. Obesity and prolonged nucleoside exposure may be risk factors. Exercise particular caution when administering nucleoside analogs to any patient with known risk factors for liver disease. Suspend treatment in any patient who develops clinical or laboratory findings suggestive of lactic acidosis or pronounced hepatotoxicity (which may include hepatomegaly and steatosis even in the absence of marked transaminase elevations).

*Patients with HIV and hepatitis B coinfection:* It is recommended that all patients with HIV be tested for the presence of HBV before initiating antiretroviral therapy. Emtricitabine/tenofovir disoproxil fumarate is not indicated for the treatment of chronic HBV infection; safety and efficacy have not been established in patients coinfected with HBV and HIV. Severe acute exacerbations of hepatitis B have been reported in patients after the discontinuation of emtricitabine/tenofovir disoproxil fumarate. Closely monitor hepatic function with clinical and laboratory follow-up for at least several months in patients who discontinue emtricitabine/tenofovir diso-proxil fumarate and are coinfected with HIV and HBV. If appropriate, initia-tion of antihepatitis B therapy may be warranted.

*Renal function impairment:* Emtricitabine and tenofovir disoproxil fumarate are princi-pally eliminated by the kidney. Dosing interval adjustment is recommended in all patients with Ccr 30 to 49 mL/min; do not administer the combination to patients with Ccr less than 30 mL/min or patients requiring hemodialysis.

Renal impairment, including cases of acute renal failure and Fanconi syndrome (renal tubular injury with severe hypophosphatemia), has been reported in associa-tion with the use of tenofovir disoproxil fumarate.

Avoid emtricitabine/tenofovir disoproxil fumarate with concurrent or recent use of a nephrotoxic agent. Carefully monitor patients at risk for or with a history of renal dysfunction and those receiving concomitant nephrotoxic agents for changes in serum creatinine and phosphorus.

*Pregnancy:* Category B.

*Antiretroviral pregnancy registry* – To monitor fetal outcomes of pregnant women exposed to emtricitabine/tenofovir disoproxil fumarate, an Antiretroviral Preg-nancy Registry has been established. Health care providers are encouraged to regis-ter patients by calling 1-800-258-4263.

*Lactation:* The Centers for Disease Control and Prevention recommend that HIV-infected mothers not breastfeed their infants to avoid risking postnatal transmis-sion of HIV.

# ABACAVIR/LAMIVUDINE

**Tablets:** 600 mg abacavir (as sulfate)/300 mg lamivudine **(Rx)** *Epzicom* (GlaxoSmithKline)

---

**Warning:**
This product contains 2 nucleoside analogs (abacavir sulfate and lamivudine) and is intended only for patients whose regimen would otherwise include these 2 com-ponents.

*Hypersensitivity reactions:* Serious and sometimes fatal hypersensitivity reactions have been associated with abacavir, a component of *Epzicom*. Discontinue abacavir/lamivudine as soon as a hypersensitivity reaction is suspected. Permanently discontinue abacavir/lamivudine if hypersensitivity cannot be ruled out, even when other diagnoses are possible.

Following a hypersensitivity reaction to abacavir, never restart abacavir/lamivu-dine or any other abacavir-containing product because more severe symptoms can occur within hours and may include life-threatening hypotension and death.

Reintroduction of abacavir/lamivudine or any other abacavir-containing product, even in patients who have no identified history or unrecognized symp-toms of hypersensitivity to abacavir therapy, can result in serious or fatal hyper-sensitivity reactions. Such reactions can occur within hours.

*Lactic acidosis and severe hepatomegaly:* Lactic acidosis and severe hepatomegaly with ste-atosis, including fatal cases, has been reported with the use of nucleoside ana-logs alone or in combination, including abacavir, lamivudine, and other antiretrovirals.

**Warning: (cont.)**

*Exacerbations of hepatitis B:* Severe acute exacerbations of hepatitis B have been reported in patients who are co-infected with hepatitis B virus (HBV) and human immunodeficiency virus (HIV) and have discontinued lamivudine, which is one component of abacavir/lamivudine. Closely monitor hepatic function with clinical and laboratory follow-up for at least several months in patients who discontinued abacavir/lamivudine and are co-infected with HIV and HBV. If appropriate, initiation of anti-hepatitis B therapy may be warranted.

### Indications

*HIV infection:* For use in combination with other antiretroviral agents for the treatment of HIV-1 infection.

### Administration and Dosage

*Adults:* 1 tablet daily, in combination with other antiretroviral agents. May be taken without regard to food.

*Dose adjustment:* Do not prescribe abacavir/lamivudine to patients requiring dosage adjustment such as those with Ccr less than 50 mL/min, those with hepatic impairment, or those experiencing dose-limiting adverse events.

### Actions

*Pharmacology:* The combination tablets contain 2 synthetic nucleoside analogs, abacavir sulfate and lamivudine, with inhibitory activity against HIV.

*Pharmacokinetics:* Following oral administration, abacavir and lamivudine are absorbed rapidly and distributed extensively. Binding of abacavir to human plasma proteins is about 50%; binding of lamivudine to plasma proteins is low.

The pharmacokinetic properties of abacavir and lamivudine in fasting patients are summarized below.

| Pharmacokinetic Parameters for Abacavir and Lamivudine in Adults | | |
| --- | --- | --- |
| Parameter | Abacavir | Lamivudine |
| Oral bioavailability (%) | ≈ 86 | ≈ 86 |
| Apparent volume of distribution (L/kg) | ≈ 0.86 | ≈ 1.3 |
| Systemic clearance (L/h/kg) | ≈ 0.8 | ≈ 0.33 |
| Renal clearance (L/h/kg) | ≈ 0.007 | ≈ 0.22 |
| Elimination half-life (h) | ≈ 1.45 | 5 to 7[1] |

[1] Approximate range.

*Special populations –*

*Renal function impairment:* Lamivudine requires dose adjustment in the presence of renal insufficiency; abacavir/lamivudine is not recommended for use in patients with Ccr less than 50mL/min.

*Liver function impairment:* Abacavir is contraindicated in patients with moderate to severe hepatic impairment, and dose reduction is required in patients with mild hepatic impairment. Because abacavir/lamivudine is a fixed-dose combination and cannot be dose adjusted, abacavir/lamivudine is contraindicated for patients with hepatic impairment.

### Contraindications

Abacavir sulfate has been associated with fatal hypersensitivity reactions. Do not restart abacavir following a hypersensitivity reaction to any abacavir containing product (see Warning box); hepatic impairment; previously demonstrated hypersensitivity to any of the components of the product.

### Warnings

*Lactic acidosis/severe hepatomegaly with steatosis:* Lactic acidosis and severe hepatomegaly with steatosis, including fatal cases, have been reported with the use of nucleoside analogs alone or in combination, including abacavir and lamivudine and other antiretrovirals.

*Posttreatment exacerbations of hepatitis:* In clinical trials in non-HIV-infected patients treated with lamivudine for chronic HBV, clinical and laboratory evidence of exacerbations of hepatitis have occurred after discontinuation of lamivudine. These exacerbations have been detected primarily by serum ALT elevations in addition to re-emergence of HBV DNA. Although most events appear to have been self-limited, fatalities have been reported in some cases.

*Fixed-dose combination:* This combination contains fixed doses of 2 nucleoside analogs, abacavir and lamivudine, and should not be administered concomitantly with other abacavir-containing and/or lamivudine-containing products.

*Hypersensitivity reactions:* Serious and sometimes fatal hypersensitivity reactions have been associated with abacavir/lamivudine and other abacavir-containing products.

*Pregnancy:* Category C.

*Lactation:* Because of the potential for HIV transmission and the potential for serious adverse reactions in nursing infants, instruct mothers not to breastfeed if they are receiving abacavir/lamivudine. Lamivudine is excreted in human breast milk.

# NEVIRAPINE

**Tablets:** 200 mg (*Rx*)  Viramune (Boehringer Ingelheim)
**Oral suspension:** 50 mg/5 mL (as hemihydrate) (*Rx*)

**Warning:**
Severe, life-threatening, and, in some cases, fatal hepatotoxicity, including fulminant and cholestatic hepatitis, hepatic necrosis, and hepatic failure, has been reported in patients treated with nevirapine (see Warnings).

Nevirapine has been associated with severe, life-threatening rash (Stevens-Johnson syndrome, toxic epidermal necrolysis), which in some cases, has been fatal. When severe rash occurs, discontinue nevirapine.

It is essential that patients be monitored intensively during the first 18 weeks of nevirapine therapy to detect potentially life-threatening hepatotoxicity or skin reactions. The greatest risk of severe rash or hepatic events (often associated with rash) occurs in the first 6 weeks of therapy. However, the risk of any hepatic event, with or without rash, continues past this period and monitoring should continue at frequent intervals. In some cases, hepatic injury has progressed despite discontinuation of treatment. Do not restart nevirapine following severe hepatic, skin, or hypersensitivity reactions. In addition, strictly follow the 14-day lead-in period with 200 mg/day nevirapine dosing (see Warnings).

## Indications
*Human immunodeficiency virus type 1 (HIV-1) infection:* In combination with other antiretroviral agents for the treatment of HIV-1 infection.

## Administration and Dosage
*Adults:*
    *Initial therapy* – 200 mg tablet daily for 14 days. Use this lead-in period because it has been found to lessen the frequency of rash. May administer with or without food.
    *Maintenance* – 200 mg tablet twice daily in combination with other antiretroviral agents.
*Children:*
    *2 months to 8 years of age* – 4 mg/kg once daily for 14 days followed by 7 mg/kg twice daily.
    *8 years of age and older* – 4 mg/kg once daily for 14 days followed by 4 mg/kg twice daily.
    The total daily dose should not exceed 400 mg for any patient.
    *Suspension* – Shake nevirapine suspension gently prior to administration. Administer the entire measured dose of suspension by using an oral dosing syringe or dosing cup. If a dosing cup is used, thoroughly rinse with water and administer the rinse to the patient.

*Dosage adjustment:* Discontinue nevirapine if patients experience severe rash or a rash accompanied by constitutional findings (see Warnings). Patients experiencing rash during the 14-day lead-in period of 200 mg/day (4 mg/kg/day in children) should not have their nevirapine dose increased until the rash has resolved.

If clinical hepatitis occurs, permanently discontinue nevirapine and do not restart after recovery.

*Missed doses:* Patients who interrupt nevirapine dosing for more than 7 days should restart the recommended dosing, using one 200 mg tablet daily (4 mg/kg/day in children) for the first 14 days (lead-in), followed by one 200 mg tablet twice daily (4 or 7 mg/kg twice daily, according to age, for children).

## Actions

*Pharmacology:* Nevirapine is a nonnucleoside reverse transcriptase inhibitor (NNRTI) with activity against HIV-1.

Nevirapine binds directly to reverse transcriptase (RT) and blocks the RNA-dependent and DNA-dependent DNA polymerase activities by causing a disruption of the enzyme's catalytic site. The activity of nevirapine does not compete with template or nucleoside triphosphates. HIV-2 RT and eukaryotic DNA polymerases are not inhibited by nevirapine.

*Pharmacokinetics:*

*Absorption* – Nevirapine is readily absorbed (more than 90%) after oral administration. Peak plasma nevirapine concentrations of 2 mcg/mL (7.5 micromolar) were attained within 4 hours following a single 200 mg dose. Following multiple doses, nevirapine peak concentrations appear to increase linearly in the dose range of 200 to 400 mg/day. Steady-state trough nevirapine concentrations of 4.5 mcg/mL were attained at 400 mg/day. Nevirapine tablets and suspension have been shown to be comparably bioavailable and interchangeable at doses 200 mg or less.

*Distribution* – Nevirapine is highly lipophilic and is essentially nonionized at physiologic pH. Following IV administration to healthy adults, the volume of distribution of nevirapine was 1.21 L/kg, suggesting that nevirapine is widely distributed in humans. Nevirapine is approximately 60% bound to plasma proteins in the plasma concentration range of 1 to 10 mcg/mL.

*Metabolism/Excretion* – Nevirapine is extensively biotransformed via cytochrome P450 (oxidative) metabolism to several hydroxylated metabolites.

Nevirapine has been shown to be an inducer of hepatic cytochrome P450 metabolic enzymes 3A4 and 2B6. The pharmacokinetics of autoinduction are characterized by an approximately 1.5- to 2-fold increase in the apparent oral clearance of nevirapine as treatment continues from a single dose to 2 to 4 weeks of dosing with 200 to 400 mg/day. Auto-induction also results in a corresponding decrease in the terminal phase half-life of nevirapine in plasma from approximately 45 hours (single dose) to approximately 25 to 30 hours following multiple dosing with 200 to 400 mg/day.

## Contraindications

Hypersensitivity to any of the components contained in the product.

## Warnings

*Skin reactions:* Severe and life-threatening skin reactions, including fatal cases, have occurred in patients treated with nevirapine, including Stevens-Johnson syndrome and toxic epidermal necrolysis. Discontinue nevirapine in patients developing a severe rash accompanied by constitutional symptoms such as fever, blistering, oral lesions, conjunctivitis, swelling muscle or joint aches, or general malaise. Do not restart nevirapine following severe skin rash or hypersensitivity reaction.

The majority of rashes associated with nevirapine occur within the first 6 weeks of initiation of therapy. Instruct patients not to increase the 200 mg/day (4 mg/kg/day in children) dosage if any rash occurs during the 2-week lead-in dosing period until the rash resolves.

Rashes are usually mild to moderate, maculopapular, erythematous cutaneous eruptions with or without pruritus, located on the trunk, face, and extremities. Closely monitor patients if isolated rash of any severity occurs.

*Resistant virus:* Resistant virus emerges rapidly and uniformly when nevirapine is administered as monotherapy. Therefore, always administer nevirapine in combination with other antiretroviral agents.

*Renal function impairment:* An additional 200 mg dose of nevirapine following each dialysis treatment is indicated in patients requiring dialysis. Patients with Ccr 20 mL/min or greater do not require an adjustment in nevirapine dosing.

*Hepatic function impairment:* Exercise caution when nevirapine is administered to patients with moderate hepatic impairment. Do not administer nevirapine to patients with severe hepatic impairment.

*Hepatotoxicity* – Severe, life-threatening, and in some cases fatal hepatotoxicity, including fulminant and cholestatic hepatitis, hepatic necrosis, and hepatic failure, have been reported in patients treated with nevirapine. The risk of hepatic events regardless of severity was greatest in the first 6 weeks of therapy; however, hepatic events may occur at any time during treatment. Discontinue nevirapine in patients with signs or symptoms of hepatitis.

Increased AST or ALT levels and/or coinfection with hepatitis B or C at the start of antiretroviral therapy are associated with a greater risk of hepatic adverse events. The patients at greatest risk of hepatic events, including potentially fatal events, are women with high CD4 counts.

Physicians and patients should be vigilant for the appearance of signs or symptoms of hepatitis, such as fatigue, malaise, anorexia, nausea, jaundice, bilirubinuria, acholic stools, liver tenderness, or hepatomegaly. Consider the diagnosis of hepatotoxicity in this setting, even if liver function tests are initially normal or alternative diagnoses are possible.

*Carcinogenesis:* Hepatocellular adenomas and carcinomas were increased at all doses in rats and mice.

*Fertility impairment:* Evidence of impaired fertility was seen in female rats.

*Elderly:* Make dose selection with caution, reflecting the greater frequency of decreased hepatic, renal, or cardiac function, and of concomitant disease or other drug therapy.

*Pregnancy:* Category C.

*Lactation:* Nevirapine readily crosses the placenta and is found in breast milk. Instruct patients receiving nevirapine to discontinue nursing, consistent with the recommendation by the US Public Health Service Centers for Disease Control and Prevention that HIV-infected mothers not breastfeed their infants to avoid risking postnatal transmission of HIV.

*Children:* Nevirapine apparent clearance adjusted for body weight was at least 2-fold greater in children younger than 8 years of age compared with adults.

**Precautions**

*Monitoring:* The first 18 weeks of therapy with nevirapine are a critical period during which intensive patient monitoring is required to detect potentially life-threatening hepatic events and skin reactions. The optimal frequency of monitoring during this time period has not been established. After the initial 18-week period, continue frequent clinical and laboratory monitoring throughout treatment. Immediately perform liver function tests if a patient experiences signs or symptoms suggestive of hepatitis, hypersensitivity reaction, and/or rash.

*Fat redistribution:* Redistribution/accumulation of body fat, including central obesity, dorsocervical fat enlargement (buffalo hump), peripheral wasting, facial wasting, breast enlargement, and "cushingoid appearance," has been observed in patients receiving antiretroviral therapy.

**Drug Interactions**

Nevirapine induces hepatic CYP3A4 and 2B6. Coadministration of nevirapine and drugs primarily metabolized by CYP3A4 or CYP2B6 may result in decreased plasma concentrations of these drugs and attenuate their therapeutic effects.

Drugs that may affect nevirapine include rifamycins (eg, rifampin, rifabutin), fluconazole, St. John's wort.

Drugs that may be affected by nevirapine include rifamycins, clarithromycin, oral contraceptives, efavirenz, ketoconazole, methadone, protease inhibitors, warfarin, zidovudine.

The following drug classes may have a potential drug interaction with nevirapine: Antiarrhythmics, anticonvulsants, antifungals, calcium channel blockers, cancer chemotherapy (cyclophosphamide), ergot alkaloids, immunosuppressants, motility agents, opiate agonists.

### Adverse Reactions

The most frequent adverse events related to nevirapine therapy are abnormal liver function tests, fatigue, headache, nausea, and rash.

*Lab test abnormalities:* Decreased hemoglobin and neutrophils. Increased ALT and AST.

*Children* – The most frequently reported adverse events related to nevirapine in children were similar to those observed in adults, with the exception of granulocytopenia, which was more commonly observed in children.

# DELAVIRDINE MESYLATE

**Tablets:** 100 and 200 mg (*Rx*)                    *Rescriptor* (Agouron)

> **Warning:**
> Delavirdine tablets are indicated for the treatment of HIV-1 infection in combination with appropriate antiretroviral agents when therapy is warranted. This indication is based on surrogate marker changes in clinical studies. Clinical benefit was not demonstrated for delavirdine based on survival or incidence of AIDS-defining clinical events in a completed trial comparing delavirdine plus didanosine with didanosine monotherapy.
>
> Resistant virus emerges rapidly when delavirdine is administered as monotherapy. Therefore, always administer delavirdine in combination with appropriate antiretroviral therapy.

### Indications

*Human immunodeficiency virus-1 (HIV-1):* For the treatment of HIV-1 infection in combination with appropriate antiretroviral agents when therapy is warranted.

### Administration and Dosage

The recommended dosage for delavirdine is 400 mg (four 100 mg or two 200 mg tablets) 3 times daily. Use delavirdine in combination with appropriate other antiretroviral therapy. Consult the complete prescribing information for other antiretroviral agents for information on dosage and administration.

The 100 mg delavirdine tablets may be dispersed in water prior to consumption. To prepare a dispersion, add four 100 mg tablets to at least 3 ounces of water, allow to stand for a few minutes, and then stir until a uniform dispersion occurs. Consume the dispersion promptly. Rinse the glass and swallow the rinse to ensure the entire dose is consumed. Take the 200 mg tablets intact because they are not readily dispersed in water.

Administer delavirdine with or without food. Patients with achlorhydria should take delavirdine with an acidic beverage (eg, orange or cranberry juice). However, the effect of an acidic beverage on the absorption of delavirdine in patients with achlorhydria has not been investigated.

### Actions

*Pharmacology:* Delavirdine is a nonnucleoside reverse transcriptase inhibitor (NNRTI) of HIV-1. Delavirdine binds directly to reverse transcriptase (RT) and blocks RNA-dependent and DNA-dependent DNA polymerase activities.

*Cross-resistance* – Rapid emergence of HIV strains that are cross-resistant to certain NNRTIs has been observed in vitro. Delavirdine may confer cross-resistance to other non-nucleoside reverse transcriptase inhibitors when used alone or in combination. The potential for cross-resistance between delavirdine and protease inhibitors and between NNRTIs and nucleoside analog RT inhibitors is low.

*Pharmacokinetics:*

*Absorption* – Delavirdine is rapidly absorbed following oral administration with peak plasma concentrations occurring at approximately 1 hour. The single-dose bioavailability of delavirdine tablets was increased by approximately 20% when a slurry of drug was prepared by allowing the tablets to disintegrate in water before administration.

*Distribution* – Delavirdine is extensively bound (approximately 98%) to plasma proteins, primarily albumin. CSF concentrations of delavirdine averaged 0.4% of the corresponding plasma delavirdine concentrations.

*Metabolism/Excretion* – Delavirdine is extensively converted to several inactive metabolites. Delavirdine is primarily metabolized by cytochrome P450 3A (CYP3A), but in vitro data suggest that delavirdine may also be metabolized by CYP2D6. The apparent plasma half-life of delavirdine increases with dose; mean half-life following 400 mg 3 times daily is 5.8 hours (range, 2 to 11 hours).

Delavirdine reduces CYP3A activity and inhibits its own metabolism. In vitro studies have also shown that delavirdine reduces CYP2C9 and CYP2C19 activity. Inhibition of CYP3A by delavirdine is reversible within 1 week after discontinuation of the drug.

*Gender* – Following administration of delavirdine (400 mg every 8 hours), median delavirdine AUC was 31% higher in female patients than in male patients.

### Contraindications

Hypersensitivity to any of the components of the formulation.

### Warnings

*Cytochrome P450 inhibition:* Coadministration of delavirdine tablets with certain nonsedating antihistamines, sedative hypnotics, antiarrhythmics, calcium channel blockers, ergot alkaloid preparations, amphetamines, and cisapride may result in potentially serious or life-threatening adverse events caused by possible effects of delavirdine on the hepatic metabolism of certain drugs metabolized by CYP3A and CYP2C9.

*Hepatic function impairment:* Delavirdine is metabolized primarily by the liver. Therefore, exercise caution when administering to patients with impaired hepatic function.

*Pregnancy: Category C.*

*Lactation:* The US Public Health Services Centers for Disease Control and Prevention advises HIV-infected women not to breastfeed to avoid postnatal transmission of HIV to a child who may not yet be infected.

*Children:* Safety and efficacy of delavirdine in combination with other antiretroviral agents has not been established in HIV-1-infected individuals < 16 years of age.

### Precautions

*Monitoring:* Monitor hepatocellular enzymes (ALT/AST) frequently if delavirdine is prescribed with saquinavir.

*Resistance/Cross-resistance:* NNRTIs, when used alone or in combination, may confer cross-resistance to other NNRTIs.

*Skin rash:* Skin rash attributable to delavirdine has occurred in 18% of patients in combination regimens in clinical trials who received delavirdine 400 mg 3 times daily.

### Drug Interactions

Drugs that may affect delavirdine include the following: Anticonvulsants, antacids, clarithromycin, didanosine, fluoxetine, histamine $H_2$ antagonists, ketoconazole, rifabutin, rifampin, and saquinavir.

Drugs that may be affected by delavirdine include the following: Clarithromycin, indinavir, amprenavir, benzodiazepines, cisapride, dihydropyridine calcium channel blockers, ergot derivatives, quinidine, sildenafil, warfarin, saquinavir, and didanosine.

## Adverse Reactions

Adverse reactions occurring in at least 3% of patients include the following: Headache; fatigue; nausea; diarrhea; increased ALT and AST; rash; maculopapular rash; neutropenia; increased amylase; pruritus.

# EFAVIRENZ

**Tablets:** 600 mg (*Rx*)
**Capsules:** 50, 100, and 200 mg (*Rx*)

*Sustiva* (Bristol-Myers Squibb Oncology/Immunology)

## Indications

*Human immunodeficiency virus (HIV) infection:* In combination with other antiretroviral agents for the treatment of HIV-1 infection.

## Administration and Dosage

*Adults:* The recommended dosage is 600 mg once daily in combination with a protease inhibitor or nucleoside analog reverse transcriptase inhibitors (NRTIs). It is recommended that efavirenz be taken on an empty stomach, preferably at bedtime. The increased efavirenz concentration following administration of efavirenz with food may lead to an increase in adverse events.

To improve the tolerability of nervous system side effects, bedtime dosing is recommended during the first 2 to 4 weeks of therapy and in patients who continue to experience these symptoms.

*Concomitant antiretroviral therapy:* Efavirenz must be given in combination with other antiretroviral medications.

*Children:* It is recommended that efavirenz be taken on an empty stomach, preferably at bedtime. The following table describes the recommended dose for pediatric patients 3 years of age and older and weighing between 10 and 40 kg (22 and 88 lbs). The recommended dosage for pediatric patients weighing more than 40 kg (88 lbs) is 600 mg once daily.

| Pediatric Dose of Efavirenz to be Administered Once Daily | | |
|---|---|---|
| Body weight | | Efavirenz dose (mg) |
| kg | lbs | |
| 10 to < 15 | 22 to < 33 | 200 |
| 15 to < 20 | 33 to < 44 | 250 |
| 20 to < 25 | 44 to < 55 | 300 |
| 25 to < 32.5 | 55 to < 71.5 | 350 |
| 32.5 to < 40 | 71.5 to < 88 | 400 |
| ≥ 40 | ≥ 88 | 600 |

## Actions

*Pharmacology:* Efavirenz is a nonnucleoside reverse transcriptase inhibitor (NNRTI) of HIV-1. Its activity is mediated predominantly by noncompetitive inhibition of HIV-1 reverse transcriptase (RT). It does not inhibit HIV-2 RT and human cellular DNA polymerases alpha, beta, gamma, and delta.

*Pharmacokinetics:* Time-to-peak plasma concentrations were approximately 3 to 5 hours and steady-state plasma concentrations were reached in 6 to 10 days. Efavirenz is highly protein-bound (approximately 99.5% to 99.75%), predominantly to albumin. It is principally metabolized by the cytochrome P450 system (CYP3A4 and CYP2B6) to hydroxylated metabolites with subsequent glucuronidation of these hydroxylated metabolites. Efavirenz induces P450 enzymes, resulting in the induction of its own metabolism. It has a terminal half-life of 52 to 76 hours after single doses and 40 to 55 hours after multiple doses.

## Contraindications

Do not administer concurrently with cisapride, midazolam, triazolam, or ergot derivatives. Competition for CYP3A4 by efavirenz could result in inhibition of metabolism of these drugs and create the potential for serious or life-threatening adverse events (eg, cardiac arrhythmias, prolonged sedation, respiratory depression; see Drug Interactions).

Clinically significant hypersensitivity to any components of the product.

**Warnings**

*Monotherapy:* Resistant virus emerges rapidly when NNRTIs are administered as monotherapy. Therefore, efavirenz must not be used as a single agent to treat HIV or added on as a sole agent to a failing regimen. The choice of new antiretroviral agents to be used in combination with efavirenz should take into consideration the potential for viral cross-resistance.

*Psychiatric symptoms:* Serious psychiatric adverse experiences have been reported in patients treated with efavirenz. Patients with a history of psychiatric disorders appear to be at greater risk for serious psychiatric adverse experiences.

*CNS symptoms:* Inform patients that common symptoms were likely to improve with continued therapy and were not predictive of subsequent onset of the less frequent psychiatric symptoms. Dosing at bedtime improves the tolerability of these CNS symptoms. Alert patients to the potential for additive CNS effects when efavirenz is used concomitantly with alcohol or psychoactive drugs.

*Pregnancy: Category* C.

*Lactation:* Instruct mothers not to breastfeed during treatment.

*Children:* Efavirenz has not been studied in pediatric patients under 3 years of age or who weigh less than 13 kg (29 lbs).

**Precautions**

*Skin rash:* In controlled clinical trials, 26% of patients treated with 600 mg efavirenz experienced new onset skin rash compared with 17% of patients treated in control groups. Rash associated with blistering, moist desquamation, or ulceration occurred in 0.9% of patients treated with efavirenz. The incidence of Grade 4 rash in patients treated with efavirenz in all studies and expanded access was 0.1%. The median time to onset of rash in adults was 11 days and the median duration, 16 days. Appropriate antihistamines or corticosteroids may improve the tolerability and hasten the resolution of rash.

Rash was reported in 46% of children treated with efavirenz capsules. The median time to onset of rash in children was 8 days. Consider prophylaxis with appropriate antihistamines prior to initiating therapy in children.

*Hepatic enzymes:* Monitor liver enzymes in patients with known or suspected history of hepatitis B or C infection and in patients treated with other medications associated with liver toxicity.

*Cholesterol:* Consider monitoring of cholesterol and triglycerides in patients treated with efavirenz.

*Fat redistribution:* Redistribution/accumulation of body fat including central obesity, dorsocervical fat enlargement (buffalo hump), peripheral wasting, facial wasting, breast enlargement, and "cushingoid appearance" have been observed in patients receiving antiretroviral therapy.

**Drug Interactions**

*P450 system:* Efavirenz induces CYP3A4 in vitro. Compounds that are substrates of CYP3A4 may have decreased plasma concentrations when coadministered with efavirenz. Drugs that induce CYP3A4 activity would be expected to increase the clearance of efavirenz, resulting in lowered plasma concentrations.

In vitro, efavirenz inhibits 2C9, 2C19, and 3A4 isozymes. Coadministration with drugs metabolized by these isozymes may result in altered plasma concentrations of the coadministered drug. Dose adjustments may be necessary for these drugs.

Drugs that may affect efavirenz include phenytoin, phenobarbital, carbamazepine, St. John's wort, rifamycins, and ritonavir. Drugs that may be affected by efavirenz include phenytoin, phenobarbital, carbamazepine, itraconazole, ketoconazole, methadone, ritonavir, amprenavir, benzodiazepines, clarithromycin, ethinyl estradiol, indinavir, nelfinavir, saquinavir, and warfarin.

*Drug/Lab test interactions:*

*Cannabinoid test interaction* – False-positive urine cannabinoid test results have been reported in uninfected volunteers who received efavirenz. False-positive test results have been observed only with the CEDIA DAU Multi-Level THC assay used for screening and have not been observed with tests used for confirmation of positive results. Efavirenz does not bind to cannabinoid receptors.

*Drug/Food interactions:* Food increases efavirenz concentrations and may increase the frequency of adverse events (see Administration and Dosage).

### Adverse Reactions

The most significant adverse events with efavirenz are nervous system symptoms and rash. Of patients receiving efavirenz, 52% reported CNS and psychiatric symptoms.

Adverse events occurring in at least 3% of patients include dizziness, fatigue, headache, concentration impaired, insomnia, abnormal dreams, somnolence, depression, anxiety, pruritus, nervousness, rash, nausea, vomiting, diarrhea, dyspepsia, abdominal pain.

*Skin rash* – Rashes are usually mild to moderate maculopapular skin eruptions that occur within the first 2 weeks of initiating therapy. Rash is more common in children and more often of higher grade (ie, more severe). In most patients, rash resolves with continuing therapy within 1 month. Efavirenz can be reinitiated in patients interrupting therapy because of rash.

*Lab test abnormalities:* Increased hepatic enzymes, lipids, and serum amylase.

*Miscellaneous:*

*Children* – Clinical adverse experiences observed in 10% or more of pediatric patients 3 to 16 years of age who received efavirenz capsules were the following: Rash, diarrhea/loose stools, fever, cough, dizziness/lightheadedness/fainting; ache/pain/discomfort, nausea/vomiting, headache.

# ENFUVIRTIDE

**Powder for injection, lyophilized:** 108 mg (≈ 90 mg/mL when reconstituted) (*Rx*)    *Fuzeon* (Hoffman-La Roche)

### Indications

*HIV-1 infection:* In combination with other antiretroviral agents for the treatment of HIV-1 infection in treatment-experienced patients with evidence of HIV-1 replication despite ongoing antiretroviral therapy.

### Administration and Dosage

*Adults:* 90 mg (1 mL) twice daily injected subcutaneously into the upper arm, anterior thigh, or abdomen.

*Children:* In pediatric patients 6 through 16 years of age, the recommended dosage is 2 mg/kg twice daily up to a maximum dose of 90 mg twice daily injected subcutaneously into the upper arm, anterior thigh, or abdomen. Monitor weight periodically and adjust the enfuvirtide dose accordingly.

| Enfuvirtide Pediatric Dosing Guidelines | | | |
|---|---|---|---|
| Weight | | Dose per bid injection (mg/dose) | Injection volume (90 mg enfuvirtide per mL) |
| Kilograms (kg) | Pounds (lb) | | |
| 11 to 15.5 | 24 to 34 | 27 | 0.3 mL |
| 15.6 to 20 | > 34 to 44 | 36 | 0.4 mL |
| 20.1 to 24.5 | > 44 to 54 | 45 | 0.5 mL |
| 24.6 to 29 | > 54 to 64 | 54 | 0.6 mL |
| 29.1 to 33.5 | > 64 to 74 | 63 | 0.7 mL |
| 33.6 to 38 | > 74 to 84 | 72 | 0.8 mL |

| Enfuvirtide Pediatric Dosing Guidelines | | | |
|---|---|---|---|
| Weight | | Dose per bid injection (mg/dose) | Injection volume (90 mg enfuvirtide per mL) |
| Kilograms (kg) | Pounds (lb) | | |
| 38.1 to 42.5 | > 84 to 94 | 81 | 0.9 mL |
| ≥ 42.6 | > 94 | 90 | 1 mL |

*Administration:* Give each injection at a site different from the preceding injection site, and only where there is no current injection site reaction from an earlier dose. Do not inject enfuvirtide into moles, scar tissue, bruises, or the navel.

*Preparation for administration:* Enfuvirtide must only be reconstituted with 1.1 mL of sterile water for injection.

Enfuvirtide contains no preservatives. Once reconstituted, inject enfuvirtide immediately or keep refrigerated in the original vial; use within 24 hours. The subsequent dose can be reconstituted in advance, stored in the refrigerator in the original vial, and used within 24 hours.

## Actions

*Pharmacology:* Enfuvirtide is an inhibitor of the fusion of HIV-1 with CD4+ cells. Enfuvirtide interferes with the entry of HIV-1 into cells by inhibiting fusion of viral and cellular membranes.

*Pharmacokinetics:*

*Absorption* – The absolute bioavailability (using a 90 mg IV dose as a reference) was 84.3% ± 15.5%.

*Distribution* – The volume of distribution after IV administration of enfuvirtide is 5.5 ± 1.1 L.

Enfuvirtide is approximately 92% bound to plasma proteins in HIV-infected plasma over a concentration range of 2 to 10 mcg/mL.

*Metabolism/Excretion* – As a peptide, enfuvirtide is expected to undergo catabolism to its constituent amino acids, with subsequent recycling of the amino acids in the body pool.

Following a single 90 mg subcutaneous dose of enfuvirtide the mean ± SD elimination half-life of enfuvirtide is 3.8 ± 0.6 hours and the mean ± SD apparent clearance was 24.8 ± 4.1 mL/h/kg.

## Contraindications

Enfuvirtide is contraindicated in patients with known hypersensitivity to enfuvirtide or any of its components (see Warnings).

## Warnings

*Local injection site reactions:* The most common adverse events associated with enfuvirtide use are local injection site reactions. Manifestations may include pain and discomfort, induration, erythema, nodules and cysts, pruritus, and ecchymosis.

*Pneumonia:* An increased rate of bacterial pneumonia was observed in subjects treated with enfuvirtide in the phase 3 clinical trials compared with the control arm.

*Hypersensitivity reactions:* Hypersensitivity reactions have been associated with enfuvirtide therapy and may recur on rechallenge. Hypersensitivity reactions have included individually and in combination: Rash, fever, nausea and vomiting, chills, rigors, hypotension, and elevated serum liver transaminases. Other adverse events that may be immune mediated and have been reported in subjects receiving enfuvirtide include primary immune complex reaction, respiratory distress, glomerulonephritis, and Guillain-Barre syndrome.

*Pregnancy: Category B.*

*Antiretroviral pregnancy registry* – To monitor maternal-fetal outcomes of pregnant women exposed to enfuvirtide and other antiretroviral drugs, an antiretroviral pregnancy registry has been established. Physicians are encouraged to register patients by calling 1-800-258-4263.

*Lactation:* It is not known whether enfuvirtide is excreted in human milk. Because of the potential for HIV transmission and the potential for serious adverse reactions in nursing infants, mothers should be instructed not to breastfeed if they are receiving enfuvirtide.

*Children:* The safety and pharmacokinetics of enfuvirtide have not been established in pediatric subjects below 6 years of age.

**Precautions**

*Non-HIV infected individuals:* There is a theoretical risk that enfuvirtide use may lead to the production of antienfuvirtide antibodies that cross react with HIV gp41. This could result in a false positive HIV test with an ELISA assay; a confirmatory western blot test would be expected to be negative. Enfuvirtide has not been studied in non-HIV infected individuals.

**Adverse Reactions**

Local injection site reactions including pain/discomfort, induration, erythema, nodules and cysts, pruritus, and ecchymosis were the most frequent adverse events associated with the use of enfuvirtide.

Other frequently reported events in subjects receiving enfuvirtide plus background regimen were diarrhea, nausea, and fatigue.

Adverse reactions occurring in at least 3% of patients included the following: Upper abdominal pain, anxiety, appetite decrease, asthenia, constipation, cough, depression, herpes simplex, influenza, insomnia, myalgia, peripheral neuropathy, pruritus (not otherwise specified), sinusitis, skin papilloma, weight decreased.

# EMTRICITABINE

**Capsules:** 200 mg *(Rx)*                              *Emtriva* (Gilead Sciences)

---

**Warning:**

Lactic acidosis and severe hepatomegaly with steatosis, including fatal cases, have been reported with the use of nucleoside analogs alone or in combination with other antiretrovirals (see Warnings).

---

**Indications**

*HIV infection:* In combination with other antiretroviral agents for the treatment of HIV-1 infection in adults.

**Administration and Dosage**

*Adults:* 200 mg once daily taken orally with or without food.

*Renal function impairment:* Adjust the dosing interval of emtricitabine in patients with baseline creatinine clearance less than 50 mL/min (see table). Clinical response to treatment and renal function should be closely monitored in these patients.

| Emtricitabine Dosing Interval Adjustment in Patients with Renal Impairment | | | | |
|---|---|---|---|---|
| | Creatinine clearance (mL/min) | | | |
| | ≥ 50 | 30 to 49 | 15 to 29 | < 15 (including patients requiring hemodialysis)[1] |
| Recommended dose and dosing interval | 200 mg q 24 h | 200 mg q 48 h | 200 mg q 72 h | 200 mg q 96 h |

[1] Hemodialysis patients: If dosing on day of dialysis, give dose after dialysis.

## Actions

*Pharmacology:* Emtricitabine is a synthetic nucleoside analog of cytosine. Emtricitabine inhibits the activity of the HIV-1 reverse transcriptase, which results in chain termination.

*Pharmacokinetics:*

*Absorption* – Emtricitabine is rapidly and extensively absorbed following oral administration with peak plasma concentrations occurring at 1 to 2 hours postdose. The mean steady-state plasma trough concentration at 24 hours postdose was 0.09 mcg/mL. The mean absolute bioavailability of emtricitabine was 93%.

The multiple dose pharmacokinetics of emtricitabine are dose-proportional over a dose range of 25 to 200 mg.

*Distribution* – Binding of emtricitabine to human plasma proteins was less than 4%. At peak plasma concentration, the mean plasma to blood drug concentration ratio was approximately 1 and the mean semen to plasma drug concentration ratio was approximately 4.

*Metabolism/Excretion* – Emtricitabine is not an inhibitor of human CYP450 enzymes. Following administration of emtricitabine, complete recovery of the dose was achieved in urine (approximately 86%) and feces (approximately 14%). The plasma emtricitabine half-life is approximately 10 hours. The renal clearance of emtricitabine is greater than the estimated creatinine clearance, suggesting elimination by both glomerular filtration and active tubular secretion.

## Contraindications

Previously demonstrated hypersensitivity to any of the components of the products.

## Warnings

*Lactic acidosis/Severe hepatomegaly with steatosis:* Lactic acidosis and severe hepatomegaly with steatosis, including fatal cases, have been reported with the use of nucleoside analogs alone or in combination, including emtricitabine and other antiretrovirals. A majority of these cases have been in women. Obesity and prolonged nucleoside exposure may be risk factors. Treatment with emtricitabine should be suspended in any patient who develops clinical or laboratory findings suggestive of lactic acidosis or pronounced hepatotoxicity.

*Posttreatment exacerbation of hepatitis:* Patients with HIV should be tested for the presence of chronic hepatitis B virus (HBV) before initiating antiretroviral therapy. Patients coinfected with HIV and HBV should be closely monitored for at least several months after stopping treatment.

*Renal function impairment:* Emtricitabine is principally eliminated by the kidney. Reduction of the dosage of emtricitabine is recommended for patients with impaired renal function (see Administration and Dosage).

*Elderly:* Dose selection for elderly patients should be cautious, keeping in mind the greater frequency of decreased hepatic, renal, or cardiac function, and of concomitant disease or other drug therapy.

*Pregnancy:* Category B.

*Antiretroviral pregnancy registry* – To monitor fetal outcomes of pregnant women exposed to emtricitabine, an antiretroviral pregnancy registry has been established. Health care providers are encouraged to register patients by calling (800) 258-4263.

*Lactation:* The Centers for Disease Control and Prevention recommend that HIV-infected mothers not breastfeed their infants to avoid risking postnatal transmission of HIV.

*Children:* Safety and effectiveness in pediatric patients have not been established.

## Precautions

*Fat redistribution:* Redistribution/accumulation of body fat including central obesity, dorsocervical fat enlargement (buffalo hump), peripheral wasting, facial wasting, breast enlargement, and "cushingoid appearance" have been observed in patients receiving antiretroviral therapy.

### Adverse Reactions

The most common adverse events that occurred in patients receiving emtricitabine were headache, diarrhea, nausea, and rash.

Skin discoloration, manifested by hyperpigmentation on the palms and/or soles was generally mild and asymptomatic.

Adverse events that occurred in at least 3% of patients included the following: Abdominal pain; abnormal dreams; ALT (greater than 5 times the ULN); arthralgia; asthenia; AST (greater than 5 times the ULN); cough increased; creatine kinase (greater than 4 times the ULN); depressive disorders; diarrhea; dizziness; dyspepsia; headache; insomnia; myalgia; nausea; neuropathy/peripheral neuritis; neutrophils (less than 750 mm$^3$); rash event; rhinitis; paresthesia; serum amylase (greater than 2 times the ULN); serum glucose (less than 40 or greater than 250 mg/dL); triglycerides (greater than 750 mg/dL); vomiting.

# FOSAMPRENAVIR CALCIUM

**Tablets:** 700 mg (equivalent to 600 mg amprenavir) (Rx)          *Lexiva* (GlaxoSmithKline)

### Indications

*HIV infection:* In combination with other antiretroviral agents for the treatment of human immunodeficiency virus (HIV) infection in adults.

### Administration and Dosage

Fosamprenavir may be taken with or without food.

*Therapy-naive patients:* Fosamprenavir 1400 mg twice daily (without ritonavir); fosamprenavir 1400 mg once daily plus ritonavir 200 mg once daily; fosamprenavir 700 mg twice daily plus ritonavir 100 mg twice daily.

*Protease inhibitor (PI)-experienced patients:* Fosamprenavir 700 mg twice daily plus ritonavir 100 mg twice daily. Once-daily administration of fosamprenavir plus ritonavir is not recommended in PI-experienced patients.

*Ritonavir dose adjustment when fosamprenavir plus ritonavir are administered with efavirenz:* An additional 100 mg/day (300 mg total) of ritonavir is recommended when efavirenz is administered with fosamprenavir plus ritonavir once daily.

*Hepatic function impairment:* Reduce fosamprenavir dose to 700 mg twice daily, in patients with mild or moderate hepatic impairment (Child-Pugh score ranging from 5 to 8) receiving fosamprenavir without concurrent ritonavir. Do not use fosamprenavir in patients with severe hepatic impairment (Child-Pugh score ranging from 9 to 12).

### Actions

*Pharmacology:* Fosamprenavir is a prodrug of amprenavir, an inhibitor of HIV protease.

*Pharmacokinetics:*

*Absorption/Distribution* – Fosamprenavir is a prodrug that is rapidly hydrolyzed to amprenavir by enzymes in the gut epithelium as it is absorbed. After administration of a single dose of fosamprenavir to HIV-1-infected patients, the time to peak amprenavir concentration ($T_{max}$) occurred between 1.5 and 4 hours (median 2.5 hours).

| Mean Steady-State Plasma Amprenavir Pharmacokinetic Parameters | | | | |
|---|---|---|---|---|
| Regimen | $C_{max}$ (mcg/mL) | $T_{max}$ (hours)[1] | $AUC_{24}$ (mcg•h/mL) | $C_{min}$ (mcg/mL) |
| Fosamprenavir 1400 mg bid | 4.82 | 1.3 | 33 | 0.35 |
| Fosamprenavir 1400 mg qd plus ritonavir 200 mg qd | 7.24 | 2.1 | 69.4 | 1.45 |
| Fosamprenavir 700 mg bid plus ritonavir 100 mg bid | 6.08 | 1.5 | 79.2 | 2.12 |

[1] Data shown are median (range).

Amprenavir is approximately 90% bound to plasma proteins, primarily to alpha$_1$-acid glycoprotein.

*Metabolism/Excretion* – Fosamprenavir is rapidly and almost completely hydrolyzed to amprenavir. Amprenavir is metabolized in the liver by the cytochrome P450 3A4 (CYP3A4) enzyme system.

The plasma elimination half-life of amprenavir is approximately 7.7 hours.

### Contraindications

Hypersensitivity to any of the components of this product or to amprenavir; coadministration with dihydroergotamine, ergonovine, ergotamine, methylergonovine, cisapride, pimozide, midazolam, or triazolam.

If fosamprenavir is coadministered with ritonavir, the antiarrhythmic agents flecainide and propafenone also are contraindicated.

### Warnings

*Drug interactions:* Serious and/or life-threatening drug interactions could occur between fosamprenavir and amiodarone, lidocaine (systemic), tricyclic antidepressants, and quinidine.

*Skin reactions:* Severe or life-threatening skin reactions, including Stevens-Johnson syndrome, were reported in less than 1% of patients treated with fosamprenavir in the clinical studies. Discontinue treatment with fosamprenavir for severe or life-threatening rashes and moderate rashes accompanied by systemic symptoms.

*Hemolytic anemia:* Acute hemolytic anemia has been reported.

*Diabetes mellitus/hyperglycemia:* New-onset diabetes mellitus, exacerbation of preexisting diabetes mellitus, and hyperglycemia have been reported during postmarketing surveillance in HIV-infected patients receiving PI therapy.

*Hepatic function impairment:* Exercise caution when administering fosamprenavir to patients with hepatic impairment. Patients with impaired hepatic function receiving fosamprenavir without concurrent ritonavir may require dose reduction.

*Elderly:* In general, dose selection for an elderly patient should be cautious, reflecting the greater frequency of decreased hepatic, renal, or cardiac function, and of concomitant disease or other drug therapy.

*Pregnancy:* Category C.

*Antiretroviral pregnancy registry* – To monitor maternal-fetal outcomes of pregnant women exposed to fosamprenavir, an Antiretroviral Pregnancy Registry has been established. Physicians are encouraged to register patients by calling 1-800-258-4263.

*Lactation:* The Centers for Disease Control and Prevention recommend that HIV-infected mothers not breastfeed their infants to avoid risking postnatal transmission of HIV.

*Children:* The safety and efficacy of fosamprenavir have not been established in pediatric patients.

### Precautions

*Sulfa sensitivity:* Use fosamprenavir with caution in patients with a known sulfonamide allergy. Fosamprenavir contains a sulfonamide moiety.

*Hemophilia:* There have been reports of spontaneous bleeding in patients with hemophilia A and B treated with PI.

*Opportunistic infections:* During the initial phase of treatment, patients responding to antiretroviral therapy may develop an inflammatory response to indolent or residual opportunistic infections.

*Fat redistribution:* Redistribution/accumulation of body fat has been observed in patients receiving antiretroviral therapy, including fosamprenavir.

*Lipid elevations:* Treatment with fosamprenavir plus ritonavir has resulted in increases in the concentration of triglycerides.

*Resistance/Cross-resistance:* Because the potential for HIV cross-resistance among PI has not been fully explored, it is unknown what effect therapy with fosamprenavir will have on the activity of subsequently administered PI.

### Drug Interactions

*CYP3A4:* Amprenavir is metabolized by CYP3A4 and is an inhibitor (and possibly an inducer) of CYP3A4. Coadministration of fosamprenavir and drugs that induce CYP3A4, such as rifampin, may decrease amprenavir concentrations and reduce its therapeutic effect. Coadministration of fosamprenavir and drugs that inhibit CYP3A4 may increase amprenavir concentrations and increase the incidence of adverse effects.

The potential for drug interactions with fosamprenavir changes when fosamprenavir is coadministered with the potent CYP3A4 inhibitor ritonavir. Because ritonavir is a CYP2D6 inhibitor, clinically significant interactions with drugs metabolized by CYP2D6 are possible when coadministered with fosamprenavir plus ritonavir.

Drugs that may be affected by fosamprenavir include the following: Amiodarone, amitriptyline, benzodiazepines, calcium channel blockers, cisapride, contraceptives (oral), cyclosporine, ergot derivatives, HMG-CoA reductase inhibitors, imipramine, itraconazole, ketoconazole, lidocaine (systemic), methadone, pimozide, quinidine, rifabutin, sildenafil, tacrolimus, vardenafil, warfarin.

Drugs that may affect fosamprenavir include antacids, carbamazepine, delavirdine, dexamethasone, histamine $H_2$-receptor antagonists, HMG-CoA reductase inhibitors, indinavir, nelfinavir, nevirapine, phenobarbital, phenytoin, proton pump inhibitors, ranitidine, rifampin, saquinavir, St. John's wort.

Fosamprenavir plus ritonavir may interact with flecainide, propafenone, efavirenz plus ritonavir, and lopinavir plus ritonavir. Efavirenz may affect fosamprenavir with or without ritonavir.

### Adverse Reactions

Adverse reactions occurring in at least 3% of patients include the following: Abdominal pain, ALT greater than 5 times the ULN, AST greater than 5 times the ULN, depressive mood disorders, diarrhea, fatigue, headache, hypertriglyceridemia (greater than 750 mg/dL), nausea, neutropenia (less than 750 cells/mm$^3$), paresthesia (oral), pruritus, rash, serum lipase greater than 2 times the ULN, vomiting.

# TRIMETHOPRIM AND SULFAMETHOXAZOLE (Co-Trimoxazole; TMP-SMZ)

| | |
|---|---|
| **Tablets:** 80 mg trimethoprim and 400 mg sulfamethoxazole (*Rx*) | Various, *Bactrim* (Roche), *Septra* (GlaxoSmithKline) |
| **Tablets, double strength:** 160 mg trimethoprim and 800 mg sulfamethoxazole (*Rx*) | Various, *Bactrim DS* (Roche), *Septra DS* (GlaxoSmithKline) |
| **Oral suspension:** 40 mg trimethoprim and 200 mg sulfamethoxazole/5 mL (*Rx*) | Various, *Bactrim Pediatric* (Roche), *Septra* (GlaxoSmithKline) |
| **Injection:** 80 mg trimethoprim and 400 mg sulfamethoxazol/5 mL (*Rx*) | Various, *Bactrim IV* (Roche), *Septra IV* (GlaxoSmithKline) |

## Indications

*Oral and parenteral:*

*Urinary tract infections (UTIs)* – Urinary tract infections (UTIs) caused by susceptible strains of *Escherichia coli*, *Klebsiella* and *Enterobacter* sp., *Morganella morganii*, *Proteus mirabilis*, and *Proteus vulgaris*.

*Shigellosis* – Shigellosis enteritis caused by susceptible strains of *Shigella flexneri* and *Shigella sonnei* in children and adults.

*Pneumocystis carinii pneumonia (PCP)* – Treatment in children and adults.

*Oral:*

*Pneumocystis carinii pneumonia* – Prophylaxis in individuals who are immunosuppressed and considered to be at increased risk.

*Acute otitis media in children* – Acute otitis media in children due to susceptible strains of *Haemophilus influenzae* or *Streptococcus pneumoniae*. There are limited data on the safety of repeated use in children younger than 2 years of age. Not indicated for prophylactic use or prolonged administration.

*Acute exacerbations of chronic bronchitis in adults* – Acute exacerbations of chronic bronchitis in adults caused by susceptible strains of *H. influenzae* and *S. pneumoniae*.

*Travelers' diarrhea in adults* – Travelers' diarrhea in adults caused by susceptible strains of enterotoxigenic *E. coli*.

*Unlabeled uses:* TMP 40 mg and SMZ 200 mg daily at bedtime, a minimum of 3 times weekly or postcoitally has been used to prevent recurrent UTIs in females.

*Treatment of acute and chronic prostatitis* – 160 mg TMP/800 mg SMZ twice daily has been used for chronic bacterial prostatitis for up to 12 weeks.

## Administration and Dosage

| Administration and Dosage of TMP-SMZ | |
|---|---|
| Organisms/Infections | Dosage |
| *Urinary tract infections, shigellosis and acute otitis media:* | |
| Adults: | 160 mg TMP/800 mg SMZ every 12 hours for 10 to 14 days (5 days for shigellosis). |
| Children (≥ 2 months of age): | 8 mg/kg TMP/40 mg/kg SMZ per day given in 2 divided doses every 12 hours for 10 days (5 days for shigellosis). |

| Guideline for proper dosage: | Dose every 12 hours: | |
|---|---|---|
| Weight (kg) | Teaspoonfuls | Tablets |
| 10 | 1 (5 mL) | - |
| 20 | 2 (10 mL) | 1 |
| 30 | 3 (15 mL) | 1½ |
| 40 | 4 (20 mL) | 2 (or 1 double strength tablet) |

| | |
|---|---|
| Patients with impaired renal function Ccr (mL/min): | Recommended dosage regimen: |
| > 30 | Usual regimen |
| 15 to 30 | ½ usual regimen |
| < 15 | Not recommended |
| IV: Adults and children > 2 months with normal renal function for severe UTIs and shigellosis. | 8 to 10 mg/kg/day (based on TMP) in 2 to 4 divided doses every 6, 8 or 12 hours for up to 14 days for severe UTIs and 5 days for shigellosis. |

| Administration and Dosage of TMP-SMZ | |
|---|---|
| Organisms/Infections | Dosage |
| *Travelers' diarrhea in adults:* | 160 mg TMP/800 mg SMZ every 12 h for 5 days. |
| *Acute exacerbations of chronic bronchitis in adults:* | 160 mg TMP/800 mg SMZ every 12 h for 14 days. |
| *Pneumocystis carinii pneumonia:* | |
| Treatment: | 15 to 20 mg/kg TMP/100 mg/kg SMZ per day in divided doses every 6 hours for 14 to 21 days. |

| Guideline for proper dosage in children | Dose every 6 hours: | |
|---|---|---|
| Weight (kg) | Teaspoonfuls | Tablets |
| 8 | 1 (5 mL) | - |
| 16 | 2 (10 mL) | 1 |
| 24 | 3 (15 mL) | 1½ |
| 32 | 4 (20 mL) | 2 (or 1 double strength tablet) |

| | |
|---|---|
| IV for adults and children > 2 months: | 15 to 20 mg/kg/day (based on TMP) in 3 or 4 divided doses every 6 to 8 hours for up to 14 days. |
| *Prophylaxis:* | |
| Adults: | 160 mg TMP/800 mg SMZ given orally every 24 hours. |
| Children: | 150 mg/m$^2$ TMP/ 750 mg/m$^2$ SMZ per day given orally in equally divided doses twice a day, on 3 consecutive days per week. The total daily dose should not exceed 320 mg TMP/1600 mg SMZ. |

| Guideline for proper dosage in children | Dose every 12 hours | |
|---|---|---|
| Body surface area (m$^2$) | Teaspoonfuls | Tablets |
| 0.26 | ½ (2.5 mL) | - |
| 0.53 | 1 (5 mL) | ½ |
| 1.06 | 2 (10 mL) | 1 |

*Parenteral:*
   *IV* – Administer over 60 to 90 minutes. Avoid rapid infusion or bolus injection. Do not give IM.

### Actions

*Pharmacology:* SMZ inhibits bacterial synthesis of dihydrofolic acid by competing with para-aminobenzoic acid. TMP blocks the production of tetrahydrofolic acid by inhibiting the enzyme dihydrofolate reductase.

*Pharmacokinetics:*
   *Absorption/Distribution* – TMP-SMZ is rapidly and completely absorbed following oral administration. Approximately 44% of TMP and 70% of SMZ are protein bound. Following oral administration, the half-lives of TMP (8 to 11 hours) and SMZ (10 to 12 hours) are similar. Following IV administration, the mean plasma half-life was 11.3 hours for TMP and 12.8 hours for SMZ.

   *Metabolism/Excretion* – TMP is metabolized to a small extent; SMZ undergoes bio-transformation to inactive compounds.

   Urine concentrations are considerably higher than serum concentrations.

### Contraindications

Hypersensitivity to TMP or SMZ; megaloblastic anemia caused by folate deficiency; pregnancy at term and lactation; infants younger than 2 months of age.

The sulfonamides are chemically similar to some goitrogens, diuretics (acetazolamide and the thiazides) and oral hypoglycemic agents. Goiter production, diuresis, and hypoglycemia occur rarely in patients receiving sulfonamides. Cross-sensitivity may exist with these agents.

### Warnings

*Streptococcal pharyngitis:* Do not use to treat streptococcal pharyngitis.

*Hematologic effects:* Sulfonamide-associated deaths, although rare, have occurred from hypersensitivity of the respiratory tract, Stevens-Johnson syndrome, toxic epidermal necrolysis, fulminant hepatic necrosis, agranulocytosis, aplastic anemia, and other blood dyscrasias.

IV use at high doses or for extended periods of time may cause bone marrow depression manifested as thrombocytopenia, leukopenia, or megaloblastic anemia.

*PCP in patients with Acquired Immunodeficiency Syndrome (AIDS):* AIDS patients may not tolerate or respond to TMP-SMZ.

*Renal/Hepatic function impairment:* Use with caution. Maintain adequate fluid intake to prevent crystalluria and stone formation. Patients with severely impaired renal function exhibit an increase in the half-lives of both TMP and SMZ, requiring dosage regimen adjustment.

*Elderly:* There may be an increased risk of severe adverse reactions, particularly when complicating conditions exist.

*Pregnancy:* Category C.

*Lactation:* TMP-SMZ is not recommended in the nursing period because sulfonamides are excreted in breast milk and may cause kernicterus. Premature infants and infants with hyperbilirubinemia or G-6-PD deficiency are also at risk for adverse effects.

*Children:* Not recommended for infants younger than 2 months of age. See Indications.

## Precautions

*Extravascular infiltration:* If local irritation and inflammation caused by extravascular infiltration of the infusion occurs, discontinue the infusion and restart at another site.

*Benzyl alcohol:* Benzyl alcohol, contained in some of these products as a preservative, has been associated with a fatal "gasping syndrome" in premature infants.

*Special risk:* Use with caution in patients with possible folate deficiency, severe allergy or bronchial asthma. In G-6-PD deficient individuals, hemolysis may occur; it is frequently dose-related.

## Drug Interactions

Drugs that may be affected by TMP-SMZ include anticoagulants, cyclosporine, dapsone, diuretics, hydantoins, methotrexate, sulfonylureas, and zidovudine. Drugs that may affect TMP-SMZ include dapsone.

## Adverse Reactions

Adverse reactions may include GI disturbances; allergic skin reactions; agranulocytosis; aplastic, hemolytic or megaloblastic anemia; thrombocytopenia; leukopenia; neutropenia; hypoprothrombinemia; eosinophilia; methemoglobinemia; hyperkalemia; hyponatremia; erythema multiforme; Stevens-Johnson syndrome; generalized skin eruptions; rash; toxic epidermal necrolysis; urticaria; pruritus; exfoliative dermatitis; anaphylactoid reactions; photosensitization; allergic myocarditis; angioedema; drug fever; chills; systemic lupus erythematosus; generalized allergic reactions; glossitis; anorexia; stomatitis; pancreatitis; elevation of serum transaminase and bilirubin; headache; mental depression; convulsions; ataxia; hallucinations; tinnitus; vertigo; insomnia; apathy; fatigue; weakness; nervousness; peripheral neuritis; renal failure; interstitial nephritis; BUN and serum creatinine elevation; toxic nephrosis with oliguria and anuria; crystalluria; arthralgia; myalgia.

# ERYTHROMYCIN ETHYLSUCCINATE AND SULFISOXAZOLE

**Granules for oral suspension**: Erythromycin ethylsuccinate (equivalent to 200 mg erythromycin activity) and sulfisoxazole acetyl (equivalent to 600 mg sulfisoxazole)/5 mL when reconstituted (*Rx*)

Various, *Eryzole* (Alra), *Pediazole* (Ross)

### Indications

*Children:* Acute otitis media caused by susceptible strains of *Haemophilus influenzae*.

### Administration and Dosage

Do not administer to infants younger than 2 months of age; systemic sulfonamides are contraindicated in this age group.

*Acute otitis media:* 50 mg/kg/day erythromycin and 150 mg/kg/day (to a maximum of 6 g/day) sulfisoxazole. Give in equally divided doses 4 times daily for 10 days. Administer without regard to meals.

| Erythromycin/Sulfisoxazole Dosage Based on Weight | | |
|---|---|---|
| Weight | | |
| kg | lb | Dose (every 6 hours) |
| < 8 | < 18 | Adjust dosage by body weight |
| 8 | 18 | 2.5 mL |
| 16 | 35 | 5 mL |
| 24 | 53 | 7.5 mL |
| > 45 | > 100 | 10 mL |

# PENTAMIDINE ISETHIONATE

**Injection**: 300 mg (*Rx*)
**Powder for injection, lyophilized**: 300 mg (*Rx*)
**Aerosol**: 300 mg (*Rx*)

*Pentam 300* (Lyphomed), *Pentacarinat* (Armour)
*Pentamidine Isethionate* (Abbott)
*NebuPent* (Lyphomed)

### Indications

*Injection:* Treatment of *Pneumocystis carinii* pneumonia (PCP).

*Inhalation:* Prevention of PCP in high-risk, HIV-infected patients defined by one or both of the following criteria: History of 1 or more episodes of PCP; a peripheral CD4+ (T4 helper/inducer) lymphocyte count less than or equal to 200 mm$^3$.

### Administration and Dosage

*Injection:*

*Adults and children* – 4 mg/kg once a day for 14 days administered deep IM or IV only. The benefits and risks of therapy for longer than 14 days are not well defined. Dosage in renal failure should be patient-specific. If necessary, reduce dosage, use a longer infusion time or extend the dosing interval.

*Preparation of solution:*

IM – Dissolve the contents of 1 vial in 3 mL of Sterile Water for Injection.

IV – Dissolve the contents of 1 vial in 3 to 5 mL of Sterile Water for Injection or 5% Dextrose Injection. Further dilute the calculated dose in 50 to 250 mL of 5% Dextrose solution.

Infuse the diluted IV solution over 60 minutes.

*Aerosol:*

*Prevention of PCP* – 300 mg once every 4 weeks administered via the *Respirgard* II nebulizer by Marquest.

Deliver the dose until the nebulizer chamber is empty (approximately 30 to 45 minutes). The flow rate should be 5 to 7 L/min from a 40 to 50 lbs/in$^2$ (PSI) air or oxygen source. Alternatively, a 40 to 50 PSI air compressor can be used with flow limited by setting the flowmeter at 5 to 7 L/min or by setting the pressure at 22 to 25 PSI. Do not use low pressure (less than 20 PSI) compressors.

*Reconstitution* – The contents of 1 vial must be dissolved in 6 mL Sterile Water for Injection, USP. It is important to use *only* sterile water; saline solution will cause the drug to precipitate. Place the entire reconstituted contents of the vial into the

*Respirgard II* nebulizer reservoir for administration. Do not mix the pentamidine solution with any other drugs.

### Actions
*Pharmacology:* Pentamidine isethionate, an aromatic diamidine antiprotozoal agent, has activity against *P. carinii*. In vitro studies indicate that the drug interferes with nuclear metabolism and inhibits the synthesis of DNA, RNA, phospholipids, and protein synthesis.

*Pharmacokinetics:*

*Absorption/Distribution* – Pentamidine is well absorbed after IM administration.

*Metabolism/Excretion* – Pentamidine may accumulate in renal failure.

Plasma concentrations after aerosol administration are substantially lower than those observed after a comparable IV dose. The extent of pentamidine accumulation and distribution following chronic inhalation therapy are not known.

### Contraindications
*Injection:* Once the diagnosis of PCP has been established, there are no absolute contraindications to the use of pentamidine.

*Inhalation:* Patients with a history of an anaphylactic reaction to inhaled or parenteral pentamidine isethionate.

### Warnings
*Development of acute PCP:* Development of acute PCP still exists in patients receiving pentamidine prophylaxis. The use of pentamidine may alter the clinical and radiographic features of PCP and could result in an atypical presentation, including but not limited to mild diseases or focal infection.

Prior to initiating pentamidine prophylaxis, evaluate symptomatic patients to exclude the presence of PCP. The recommended dose for the prevention of PCP is insufficient to treat acute PCP.

*Fatalities:* Fatalities caused by severe hypotension, hypoglycemia, and cardiac arrhythmias have been reported, both by the IM and IV routes. Severe hypotension may result after a single dose. Limit administration of the drug to patients in whom *P. carinii* has been demonstrated.

*Pregnancy: Category* C.

*Lactation:* It is not known whether pentamidine is excreted in breast milk. Because of the potential for serious adverse reactions in nursing infants, decide whether to discontinue nursing or to discontinue the drug, taking into account the importance of the drug to the mother.

*Children:* Safety and efficacy of inhalation solution have not been established.

### Precautions
*Use with caution:* Use with caution in patients with hypertension, hypotension, hypoglycemia, hyperglycemia, hypocalcemia, leukopenia, thrombocytopenia, anemia, hepatic or renal dysfunction, ventricular tachycardia, pancreatitis, and Stevens-Johnson syndrome.

*Hypotension:* Patients may develop sudden, severe hypotension after a single dose, whether given IV or IM. Therefore, patients receiving the drug should be supine; monitor blood pressure closely during drug administration and several times thereafter until the blood pressure is stable. Have equipment for emergency resuscitation readily available. If pentamidine is administered IV, infuse over 60 minutes.

*Hypoglycemia:* Pentamidine-induced hypoglycemia has been associated with pancreatic islet cell necrosis and inappropriately high plasma insulin concentrations. Hyperglycemia and diabetes mellitus, with or without preceding hypoglycemia, also have occurred, sometimes several months after therapy. Therefore, monitor blood glucose levels daily during therapy and several times thereafter.

*Pulmonary:* Inhalation of pentamidine isethionate may induce bronchospasm or cough, particularly in patients who have a history of smoking or asthma. In patients who experience bronchospasm or cough, administration of an inhaled bronchodilator prior to giving each pentamidine dose may minimize recurrence of the symptoms.

Extrapulmonary infection with *P. carinii* has been reported infrequently with inhalation use.

*Laboratory tests* – Laboratory tests to perform before, during, and after therapy:

1.) Daily BUN, serum creatinine and blood glucose.
2.) Complete blood count and platelet counts.
3.) Liver function test, including bilirubin, alkaline phosphatase, AST, and ALT.
4.) Serum calcium.
5.) ECG at regular intervals.

**Adverse Reactions**

*Injection* – 244 of 424 (57.5%) patients treated with pentamidine injection developed some adverse reaction. Most of the patients had acquired immunodeficiency syndrome (AIDS). In the following, "severe" refers to life-threatening reactions or reactions that required immediate corrective measures and led to discontinuation of pentamidine.

*Severe* – Leukopenia (less than 1000/mm³) 2.8%; hypoglycemia (less than 25 mg/dL) 2.4%; thrombocytopenia (less than 20,000/mm³) 1.7%; hypotension (less than 60 mm Hg systolic) 0.9%; acute renal failure (serum creatinine greater than 6 mg/dL) 0.5%; hypocalcemia (0.2%); Stevens-Johnson syndrome and ventricular tachycardia (0.2%); fatalities caused by severe hypotension, hypoglycemia, and cardiac arrhythmias.

Adverse reactions occurring in at least 3 % of patients include elevated serum creatinine; sterile abscess, pain, or induration at the IM injection site; elevated liver function tests; leukopenia; nausea; anorexia; hypotension; fever; hypoglycemia; rash; bad taste in mouth; shortness of breath; dizziness; cough; pharyngitis; chest pain/congestion; night sweats; chills; vomiting; bronchospasm; pneumothorax; diarrhea; headache; anemia (generally associated with zidovudine use), myalgia; abdominal pain; edema.

Adverse reactions may also include tachycardia; hypertension; palpitations; syncope; cerebrovascular accident; vasodilation; vasculitis; gingivitis; dyspepsia; oral ulcer/abscess; gastritis; gastric ulcer; hypersalivation; dry mouth; splenomegaly; melena; hematochezia; esophagitis; colitis; pancreatitis; pancytopenia; neutropenia; eosinophilia; thrombocytopenia; hepatitis; hepatomegaly; hepatic dysfunction; renal failure; flank pain; nephritis; tremors; confusion; anxiety; memory loss; seizure; neuropathy; paresthesia; insomnia; hypesthesia; drowsiness; emotional lability; vertigo; paranoia; neuralgia; hallucination; depression; unsteady gait; rhinitis; laryngitis; pneumonitis; pleuritis; cyanosis; tachypnea; rales; pruritus; erythema; dry skin; desquamation; urticaria; eye discomfort; conjunctivitis; blurred vision; blepharitis; loss of taste and smell; incontinence; miscarriage; arthralgia; allergic reactions; extrapulmonary pneumocystosis.

# TINIDAZOLE

**Tablets:** 250 and 500 mg (*Rx*)                    *Tindamax* (Presutti)

---

**Warning:**
Carcinogenicity has been seen in mice and rats treated chronically with another agent in the nitroimidazole class (metronidazole) (see Warnings). Although such data have not been reported for tinidazole, avoid unnecessary use. Reserve tinidazole use for the conditions described in Indications.

**Indications**

*Amebiasis:* For the treatment of intestinal amebiasis and amebic liver abscess caused by *Entamoeba histolytica* in adults and pediatric patients older than 3 years of age.

*Giardiasis:* For the treatment of giardiasis caused by *Giardia duodenalis* (also termed *Giardia lamblia*) in adults and pediatric patients older than 3 years of age.

*Trichomoniasis:* For the treatment of trichomoniasis caused by *Trichomonas vaginalis* in female and male patients. Because trichomoniasis is a sexually transmitted disease with potentially serious sequelae, partners of infected patients should be treated simultaneously in order to prevent reinfection.

## Administration and Dosage

*Approved by the FDA:* May 17, 2004.

Take tinidazole with food to minimize the incidence of epigastric discomfort and other GI side effects.

| Tinidazole Dosing Regimens | | | |
|---|---|---|---|
| Indication | Adult dose | Pediatric dose (≥ 3 years of age) | Duration of therapy |
| Amebiasis | | | |
|   Amebic liver abscess | 2 g/day | 50 mg/kg/day (up to 2 g) | 3 to 5 days |
|   Intestinal | 2 g/day | 50 mg/kg/day (up to 2 g) | 3 days |
| Giardiasis | 2 g | 50 mg/kg (up to 2 g) | Single dose |
| Trichomoniasis | 2 g | — | Single dose |

*Dosing in hemodialysis patients:* If tinidazole is administered on a day when dialysis is performed, administer an additional dose of tinidazole equivalent to one half the recommended dose after the end of the hemodialysis.

*Extemporaneous oral suspension:* Grind four 500 mg oral tablets to a fine powder with a mortar and pestle. Add approximately 10 mL of cherry syrup to the powder and mix until smooth. Transfer the suspension to a graduated amber container. Use several small rinses of cherry syrup to transfer any remaining drug in the mortar to the final suspension for a final volume of 30 mL. The suspension of crushed tablets in artificial cherry syrup (*Humco*) is stable for 7 days at room temperature. When this suspension is used, shake well before each administration.

## Actions

*Pharmacology:*

   *Mechanism of action* – Tinidazole is an antiprotozoal agent.

*Pharmacokinetics:*

   *Absorption* – After oral administration, tinidazole is rapidly and completely absorbed. Steady-state conditions are reached in 2½ to 3 days of multi-day dosing. Administration of tinidazole tablets with food resulted in a delay in $T_{max}$ of approximately 2 hours and a decline in $C_{max}$ of approximately 10% compared with fasted conditions. Administration of tinidazole with food did not affect AUC or half-life in this study.

   *Distribution* – Tinidazole is distributed into virtually all tissues and body fluids and crosses the blood-brain barrier. The apparent volume of distribution is approximately 50 L. Plasma protein binding of tinidazole is 12%. Tinidazole crosses the placental barrier and is secreted in breast milk.

   *Metabolism* – Tinidazole is partly metabolized by oxidation, hydroxylation, and conjugation. Tinidazole is biotransformed mainly by CYP3A4.

   *Excretion* – The plasma half-life of tinidazole is approximately 12 to 14 hours. Tinidazole is excreted by the liver and the kidneys.

   During hemodialysis, clearance of tinidazole is significantly increased; the half-life is reduced from 12 to 4.9 hours.

## Contraindications

Hypersensitivity to tinidazole, any component of the tablet, or other nitroimidazole derivatives; during the first trimester of pregnancy (see Warnings).

## Warnings

*Neurologic effects:* Convulsive seizures and peripheral neuropathy, the latter characterized mainly by numbness or paresthesia of an extremity, have been reported in patients treated with nitroimidazole drugs including tinidazole and metronidazole. The appearance of abnormal neurologic signs demands the prompt discontinuation of tinidazole therapy. Administer tinidazole with caution to patients with central nervous system diseases.

*Hepatic function impairment:* Patients with severe hepatic disease metabolize nitroimid-azoles slowly, with resultant accumulation of parent drug in the plasma. For patients with hepatic dysfunction, cautiously administer the usual recommended doses of tinidazole.

*Elderly:* In general, dose selection for an elderly patient should be cautious, reflecting the greater frequency of decreased hepatic, renal, or cardiac function, and of concomitant disease or other drug therapy.

*Pregnancy: Category* C.

*Lactation:* Tinidazole is excreted in breast milk in concentrations similar to those seen in serum. Tinidazole can be detected in breast milk for up to 72 hours following administration. Interruption of breastfeeding is recommended during tinidazole therapy and for 3 days following the last dose.

*Children:* Other than for use in the treatment of giardiasis and amebiasis in pediatric patients older than 3 years of age, safety and efficacy of tinidazole in pediatric patients have not been established.

## Precautions

*Candidiasis:* Known or previously unrecognized candidiasis may present more prominent symptoms during therapy with tinidazole and requires treatment with an antifungal agent.

*Hematologic effects:* Use with caution in patients with evidence of or history of blood dyscrasia. Tinidazole may produce transient leukopenia and neutropenia. Total and differential leukocyte counts are recommended if retreatment is necessary.

## Drug Interactions

The following drug interactions were reported for metronidazole, a chemically related nitroimidazole. Therefore, these drug interactions may occur with tinidazole. Drugs that may affect tinidazole include cholestyramine, CYP3A4 inducers and inhibitors and oxytetracycline. Drugs that may be affected by tinidazole include alcohols, anticoagulants, cyclosporine, tacrolimus, disulfiram, fluorouracil, hydantoins, and lithium.

*Drug/Lab test interactions:* Tinidazole may interfere with certain serum chemistry values, such as aspartate aminotransferase (AST), alanine aminotransferase (ALT), lactate dehydrogenase (LDH), triglycerides, and hexokinase glucose.

## Adverse Reactions

Adverse reactions occurring in at least 3% of patients include the following: metallic/bitter taste and nausea.

# ATOVAQUONE

| **Suspension:** 750 mg/5 mL *(Rx)* | *Mepron* (GlaxoSmithKline) |
|---|---|

## Indications

*Pneumocystitis carinii pneumonia (PCP):* Prevention of PCP in patients who are intolerant to trimethoprim-sulfamethoxazole (TMP-SMZ).

Acute oral treatment of mild to moderate PCP in patients who are intolerant to TMP-SMZ.

## Administration and Dosage

*Prevention of PCP:*

*Adults and adolescents 13 to 16 years of age –* 1500 mg once daily with a meal.

*Treatment of mild to moderate PCP:*

*Adults and adolescents 13 to 16 years of age –* 750 mg administered with food twice daily for 21 days (total daily dose 1500 mg).

Failure to administer with food may result in lower atovaquone plasma concentrations and may limit response to therapy.

## Actions

*Pharmacology:* Atovaquone, an analog of ubiquinone, is an antiprotozoal with antipneumocystis activity.

*Pharmacokinetics:* Absorption is enhanced approximately 2-fold when given with food. Atovaquone is extensively bound to plasma proteins (greater than 99.9%). CSF concentratons are less than 1% of plasma concentrations. Half-life ranged from 67 to 77.6 hours following the suspension. The long half-life is caused by presumed enterohepatic cycling and eventual fecal elimination. There is indirect evidence that atovaquone may undergo limited metabolism; however, a specific metabolite has not been identified.

## Contraindications

Development or history of potentially life-threatening allergic reactions to any of the components of the formulation.

## Warnings

*Severe PCP:* Clinical experience has been limited to patients with mild to moderate PCP. Treatment of more severe episodes of PCP has not been systematically studied. Atovaquone efficacy in patients who are failing therapy with TMP-SMZ has not been systematically studied.

*Hepatic function impairment:* Use caution in patients with severe hepatic impairment, and closely monitor administration.

*Elderly:* Dose selection for an elderly patient should be cautious. Exercise caution when treating elderly patients reflecting the greater frequency of decreased hepatic, renal, and cardiac function.

*Pregnancy:* Category C.

*Lactation:* It is not known whether atovaquone is excreted into breast milk.

*Children:* Safety and efficacy have not been established. Preliminary analysis suggests that the pharmacokinetics are age-dependent.

## Precautions

*Absorption:* Absorption of atovaquone is limited but can be significantly increased when the drug is taken with food. Plasma concentrations correlate with the likelihood of successful treatment and survival. GI disorders may limit absorption of orally administered drugs. Patients with these disorders also may not achieve plasma concentrations of atovaquone associated with response to therapy in controlled trials.

*Concurrent pulmonary conditions:* Atovaquone is not effective therapy for concurrent pulmonary conditions such as bacterial, viral, or fungal pneumonia or mycobacterial diseases. Clinical deterioration in patients may be due to infections with other pathogens, as well as progressive PCP.

## Drug Interactions

Use caution when administering atovaquone concurrently with other highly plasma protein bound drugs with narrow therapeutic indices as competition for binding sites may occur.

Drugs that may interact include rifamycins, TMP-SMZ, and zidovudine.

*Drug/Food interactions:* Administering atovaquone with food enhances its absorption by approximately 2-fold.

## Adverse Reactions

Adverse reactions occurring in at least 3% of patients include rash (including maculopapular), nausea, diarrhea, headache, vomiting, fever, cough, insomnia, asthenia, pruritus, monilia (oral), abdominal pain, constipation, dizziness, anemia, neutropenia, elevated ALT and AST, elevated alkaline phosphatase, elevated amylase, hyponatremia, pain, sweating, anxiety, anorexia, sinusitis, dyspepsia, rhinitis, and taste perversion.

# TRIMETREXATE GLUCURONATE

**Powder for injection, lyophilized:** 25 mg trimetrexate *(Rx)*   *Neutrexin* (US Bioscience)

---

**Warning:**
   Trimetrexate must be used with concurrent leucovorin (leucovorin protection) to
   avoid potentially serious or life-threatening toxicities.

---

### Indications
   As an alternative therapy with concurrent leucovorin administration (leucovorin protection) for the treatment of moderate to severe *Pneumocystis carinii* pneumonia
   (PCP) in immunocompromised patients, including patients with acquired immunodeficiency syndrome (AIDS), who are intolerant of or refractory to TMP-SMZ
   therapy, or for whom TMP-SMZ is contraindicated.

### Administration and Dosage
   Trimetrexate must be given with concurrent leucovorin (leucovorin protection) to
   avoid potentially serious or life-threatening toxicities. Leucovorin must be given
   daily during trimetrexate treatment and for 72 hours past the last trimetrexate dose.

   Trimetrexate is administered at a dose of 45 mg/m$^2$ once daily by IV infusion over 60
   to 90 minutes. Leucovorin may be administered IV at a dose of 20 mg/m$^2$ over 5
   to 10 minutes every 6 hours for a total daily dose of 80 mg/m$^2$, or orally as 4 doses
   of 20 mg/m$^2$ spaced equally throughout the day. Round up the oral dose to the
   next higher 25 mg increment. The recommended course of therapy is 21 days of trimetrexate and 24 days of leucovorin.

   *Dosage modifications:*
      *Hematologic toxicity* – Modify trimetrexate and leucovorin doses based on the worst
      hematologic toxicity according to the following table. If leucovorin is given orally,
      round up doses to the next higher 25 mg increment.

| Dose Modifications for Hematologic Toxicity | | | | |
|---|---|---|---|---|
| Toxicity grade | Neutrophils/ mm$^3$ | Platelets/ mm$^3$ | Trimetrexate | Leucovorin |
| 1 | > 1000 | > 75,000 | 45 mg/m$^2$ once daily | 20 mg/m$^2$ every 6 hours |
| 2 | 750 to 1000 | 50,000 to 75,000 | 45 mg/m$^2$ once daily | 40 mg/m$^2$ every 6 hours |
| 3 | 500 to 749 | 25,000 to 49,999 | 22 mg/m$^2$ once daily | 40 mg/m$^2$ every 6 hours |
| 4 | < 500 | < 25,000 | Day 1 to 9 discontinue Day 10 to 21 interrupt up to 96 hours[1] | 40 mg/m$^2$ every 6 hours |

[1] If Grade 4 hematologic toxicity occurs prior to day 10, discontinue trimetrexate. Administer leucovorin
(40 mg/m$^2$ every 6 hours) for an additional 72 hours. If Grade 4 hematologic toxicity occurs at day 10 or
later, trimetrexate may be held up to 96 hours to allow counts to recover. If counts recover to Grade 3
within 96 hours, administer trimetrexate at a dose of 22 mg/m$^2$ and maintain leucovorin at 40 mg/m$^2$
every 6 hours. When counts recover to Grade 2 toxicity, trimetrexate dose may be increased to 45 mg/
m$^2$, but the leucovorin dose should be maintained at 40 mg/m$^2$ for the duration of treatment. If counts do
not improve to Grade 3 toxicity or lower within 96 hours, discontinue trimetrexate. Administer leucovorin at a dose of 40 mg/m$^2$ every 6 hours for 72 hours following the last dose of trimetrexate.

### Actions
   *Pharmacology:* Trimetrexate, a 2.4-diaminoquinazoline, nonclassical folate antagonist, is
   a synthetic inhibitor of the enzyme dihydrofolate reductase. The end result is disruption of DNA, RNA, and protein synthesis, with consequent cell death.

   *Pharmacokinetics:* Clearance was 38 ± 15 mL/min/m$^2$ and volume of distribution at
   steady state (Vd$_{ss}$) was 20 ± 8 L/m$^2$. The plasma concentration time profile
   declined in a biphasic manner over 24 hours with a terminal half-life of 11 ±
   4 hours.

      Renal clearance in cancer patients has varied from about 4 ± 2 to 10 ± 6 mL/
   min/m$^2$ and 10% and 30% is excreted unchanged in the urine. Considering the free
   fraction of trimetrexate, active tubular secretion may possibly contribute to the
   renal clearance.

**Contraindications**
Clinically significant sensitivity to trimetrexate, leucovorin, or methotrexate.

**Warnings**
*Concurrent leucovorin:* Trimetrexate must be used with concurrent leucovorin to avoid
potentially serious or life-threatening complications, including bone marrow suppression, oral and GI mucosal ulceration, and renal and hepatic dysfunction. Leucovorin therapy must extend for 72 hours past the last dose of trimetrexate. Inform
patients that failure to take the recommended dose and duration of leucovorin can
lead to fatal toxicity. Closely monitor patients for the development of serious
hematologic adverse reactions.

*Pregnancy: Category D.*

*Lactation:* It is not known if trimetrexate is excreted in breast milk.

*Children:* Safety and efficacy of trimetrexate for the treatment of histologically confirmed PCP has not been established for patients younger than 18 years of age.

**Precautions**
*Monitoring:* Perform blood tests at least twice a week during therapy to assess the following parameters: Hematology (absolute neutrophil counts [ANC], platelets);
renal function (serum creatinine, BUN); hepatic function (AST, ALT, alkaline
phosphatase).

*Pulmonary conditions:* Trimetrexate has not been evaluated clinically for the treatment
of concurrent pulmonary conditions such as bacterial, viral, or fungal pneumonia
or mycobacterial diseases.

*Special risk:* Patients receiving trimetrexate may experience hematologic, hepatic, renal,
and GI toxicities. Use caution in treating patients with impaired hematologic, renal,
or hepatic function.

**Drug Interactions**
Because trimetrexate is metabolized by a P450 enzyme system, drugs that induce or
inhibit this drug metabolizing enzyme system may elicit important drug interactions that may alter trimetrexate plasma concentrations, which include erythromycin, rifampin, rifabutin, ketoconazole, fluconazole, cimetidine, nitrogen
substituted imidazole drugs (eg, clotrimazole, ketoconazole, miconazole).

**Adverse Reactions**
Adverse reactions occurring in at least 3% of patients include fever, rash/pruritus, nau-
sea/vomiting, neutropenia, thrombocytopenia, anemia, increased AST and ALT,
increased alkaline phosphatase, hyponatremia.

# ANTHELMINTICS

The following table lists the major parasitic infections, causative organisms, and drugs of choice for treatment.

| Major Parasite Infections | | |
|---|---|---|
| Infection (common name) | Organism | Drug(s) of Choice |
| **Intestinal Nematodes** | | |
| Ascariasis[1] (Roundworm) | *Ascaris lumbricoides* | Mebendazole, Pyrantel pamoate, or Diethylcarbamazine |
| Uncinariasis (Hookworm) | *Ancylostoma duodenale Necator americanus* | Mebendazole or Pyrantel pamoate[2] |
| Strongyloidiasis (Threadworm) | *Strongyloides stercoralis* | Thiabendazole |
| Trichuriasis (Whipworm) | *Trichuris trichiura* | Mebendazole |
| Enterobiasis[3] (Pinworm) | *Enterobius vermicularis* | Mebendazole, Pyrantel pamoate, or Albendazole |
| Capillariasis | *Capillaria philippinensis* | Mebendazole or Thiabendazole |
| **Tissue Nematodes** | | |
| Trichinosis | *Trichinella spiralis* | Steroids for severe symptoms plus Thiabendazole, Albendazole, Flubendazole[4], or Mebendazole[2] |
| Cutaneous larva migrans (creeping eruption) | *Ancylostoma braziliense* and others | Thiabendazole, Albendazole, or Ivermectin[5] |
| Onchocerciasis (River blindness) | *Onchocerca volvulus* | Suramin,[6] Diethylcarbamazine, or Ivermectin[5] |
| Dracontiasis (guinea worm) | *Dracunculus medinensis* | Thiabendazole or Mebendazole |
| Angiostrongyliasis (rat lungworm) | *Angiostrongylus cantonensis* | Thiabendazole or Mebendazole |
| Loiasis | *Loa loa* | Diethylcarbamazine |
| **Cestodes** | | |
| Taeniasis (Beef tapeworm) | *Taenia saginata* | Praziquantel[2] or Niclosamide |
| (Pork tapeworm) | *Taenia solium* | Praziquantel,[2] Niclosamide, or Albendazole |
| Diphyllobothriasis (Fish tapeworm) | *Diphyllobothrium latum* | Praziquantel[2] or Niclosamide |
| Dog tapeworm | *Dipylidium caninum* | Praziquantel[2] |
| Hymenolepiasis (Dwarf tapeworm) | *Hymenolepis nana* | Praziquantel[2] or Niclosamide[4] |
| Hydatid cysts | *Echinococcus granulosus* | Albendazole or Praziquantel |
| **Trematodes** | | |
| Schistosomiasis | *Schistosoma mansoni* | Praziquantel or Oxamniquine |
| | *Schistosoma japonicum* | Praziquantel |
| | *Schistosoma haematobium* | Praziquantel |
| | *Schistosoma mekongi* | Praziquantel |
| Hermaphroditic Flukes Fasciolopsiasis (Intestinal fluke) | *Fasciolopsis buski* | Praziquantel |
| | *Heterophyes heterophyes Metagonimus yokogawai* | Praziquantel |
| Clonorchiasis (Chinese liver fluke) | *Clonorchis sinensis* | Praziquantel |
| Fascioliasis (Sheep liver fluke) | *Fasciola hepatica* | Praziquantel or Bithionol[5] |
| Opisthorchiasis (Liver fluke) | *Opisthorchis viverrini* | Praziquantel |
| Paragonimiasis (Lung fluke) | *Paragonimus westermani* | Praziquantel or Bithionol[5] (alternate) |

[1] The following drugs also are indicated in *Ascariasis*: Piperazine citrate (if intestinal or biliary obstruction); thiabendazole.
[2] Unlabeled use.
[3] The following drugs also are indicated in *Enterobiasis*: Piperazine and thiabendazole.
[4] Not available in the US.
[5] Available from the CDC.
[6] Available from the CDC, although generally not recommended.

# Chapter 10

# BIOLOGIC AND IMMUNOLOGIC AGENTS

# AZATHIOPRINE

**Tablets:** 50 mg (*Rx*)                 *Imuran* (GlaxoSmithKline)
**Injection:** 100 mg (as sodium)/vial (*Rx*)     Various, *Imuran* (GlaxoSmithKline)

---

**Warning:**
Chronic immunosuppression with azathioprine increases the risk of neoplasia. Physicians using this drug should be familiar with this risk as well as with the mutagenic potential to men and women and with possible hematologic toxicities.

---

### Indications
*Renal homotransplantation:* As an adjunct for the prevention of rejection in renal homotransplantation.

*Rheumatoid arthritis:* Indicated only in adult patients meeting criteria for classic or definite rheumatoid arthritis as specified by the American Rheumatism Association. Restrict use to patients with severe, active, and erosive disease not responsive to conventional management.

### Administration and Dosage
*Renal homotransplantation:* Initial dose is usually 3 to 5 mg/kg/day, given as a single daily dose on the day of transplantation, and in a minority of cases, 1 to 3 days before transplantation. It is often initiated IV, with subsequent use of tablets (at the same dose level) after the postoperative period. Reserve IV administration for patients unable to tolerate oral medications. Maintenance levels are 1 to 3 mg/kg/day.

    *Children* – An initial dose of 3 to 5 mg/kg/day IV or orally followed by a maintenance dose of 1 to 3 mg/kg/day has been recommended.

*Rheumatoid arthritis:* Initial dose is approximately 1 mg/kg (50 to 100 mg) given as a single dose or twice daily. The dose may be increased, beginning at 6 to 8 weeks and thereafter by steps at 4-week intervals, if there are no serious toxicities and if initial response is unsatisfactory. Use dose increments of 0.5 mg/kg/day, up to a maximum dose of 2.5 mg/kg/day.

    Use the lowest effective dose for maintenance therapy; lower decrementally with changes of 0.5 mg/kg or approximately 25 mg/day every 4 weeks while other therapy is kept constant.

*Renal function impairment:* Relatively oliguric patients, especially those with tubular necrosis in the immediate postcadaveric transplant period, may have delayed clearance of azathioprine or its metabolites.

*Use with allopurinol:* Reduce dose of azathioprine to approximately 25% to 33% of the usual dose.

### Actions
*Pharmacology:* Azathioprine, an imidazoyl derivative of 6-mercaptopurine (6-MP), has many biological effects similar to those of the parent compound.

    *Homograft survival* – Although the use of azathioprine for inhibition of renal homograft rejection is well established, the mechanism(s) for this action are obscure.

    *Immuno-inflammatory response* – The severity of adjuvant arthritis is reduced by azathioprine. The mechanisms whereby it affects autoimmune diseases are not known.

*Pharmacokinetics:* Azathioprine is well absorbed following oral administration. Blood levels are of little value for therapy because the magnitude and duration of clinical effects correlate with thiopurine nucleotide levels in tissues rather than with plasma drug levels.

### Contraindications
Hypersensitivity to azathioprine; pregnancy in rheumatoid arthritis patients.

### Warnings
*Hematologic effects:* Severe leukopenia or thrombocytopenia, macrocytic anemia, severe bone marrow depression, and selective erythrocyte aplasia may occur in patients on azathioprine. Hematologic toxicities are dose-related, may occur late in the

course of therapy, and may be more severe in renal transplant patients whose homograft is undergoing rejection. Perform complete blood counts, including platelet counts, weekly during the first month, twice monthly for the second and third months of treatment, then monthly or more frequently if dosage alterations or other therapy changes are necessary.

*Infections:* Serious infections are a constant hazard for patients on chronic immunosuppression, especially for homograft recipients. The incidence of infection in renal homotransplantation is 30 to 60 times that in rheumatoid arthritis. Fungal, viral, bacterial, and protozoal infections may be fatal and should be treated vigorously.

*GI toxicity:* A GI hypersensitivity reaction characterized by severe nausea and vomiting has been reported. These symptoms also may be accompanied by diarrhea, rash, fever, malaise, myalgias, elevations in liver enzymes, and, occasionally, hypotension.

*Hepatotoxicity:* Hepatotoxicity with elevated serum alkaline phosphatase and bilirubin may occur primarily in allograft recipients. Periodically measure serum transaminases, alkaline phosphatase and bilirubin for early detection of hepatotoxicity.

*Carcinogenesis:* Azathioprine is carcinogenic in animals and may increase the patient's risk of neoplasia.

*Mutagenesis:* Azathioprine is mutagenic in animals and humans.

*Pregnancy:* Category D.

*Lactation:* Use of azathioprine in nursing mothers is not recommended.

*Children:* Safety and efficacy in children have not been established. However, azathioprine has been used in children.

## Drug Interactions

Drugs that may affect azathioprine include ACE inhibitors, allopurinol, and methotrexate.

Drugs that may be affected by azathioprine include anticoagulants, cyclosporine, and nondepolarizing neuromuscular blockers.

## Adverse Reactions

The principal and potentially serious toxic effects are hematologic and GI. Adverse reactions may include leukopenia, infections, and neoplasia.

# TACROLIMUS (FK506)

**Capsules**: 0.5, 1, and 5 mg (*Rx*)  
**Injection**: 5 mg/mL (*Rx*)  

*Prograf* (Fujisawa)

Tacrolimus also is available as a cream for moderate to severe atopic dermatitis; refer to the Dermatologics chapter.

**Warning:**
> Increased susceptibility to infection and the possible development of lymphoma may result from immunosuppression. Manage patients receiving the drug in facilities equipped and staffed with adequate laboratory and supportive medical resources.

## Indications

*Organ rejection prophylaxis:* Prophylaxis of organ rejection in patients receiving allogeneic liver or kidney transplants. It is recommended that tacrolimus be used concomitantly with adrenal corticosteroids. Because of the risk of anaphylaxis, reserve the injection for patients unable to take the capsules orally.

## Administration and Dosage

*Injection:* For IV infusion only.

In patients unable to take the capsules, therapy may be initiated with the injection. Administer the initial dose no sooner than 6 hours after transplantation. The recommended starting dose is 0.03 to 0.05 mg/kg/day as a continuous IV infusion. Give adult patients doses at the lower end of the dosing range. Concomitant adrenal corticosteroid therapy is recommended early posttransplantation. Proceed with continuous IV infusion only until the patient can tolerate oral administration.

*Oral:*

Liver transplantation –

| Summary of Initial Oral Dosage Recommendations and Typical Whole Blood Trough Concentrations | | |
|---|---|---|
| Patient population | Recommended initial oral dose[1] | Typical whole blood trough concentrations |
| Adult kidney transplant patients | 0.2 mg/kg/day | Months 1 through 3: 7 to 20 ng/mL Months 4 through 12: 5 to 15 ng/mL |
| Adult liver transplant patients | 0.1 to 0.15 mg/kg/day | Months 1 through 12: 5 to 20 ng/mL |
| Pediatric liver transplant patients | 0.15 to 0.2 mg/kg/day | Months 1 through 12: 5 to 20 ng/mL |

[1] 2 divided doses, every 12 hours.

It is recommended that patients be converted from IV to oral therapy as soon as oral therapy can be tolerated. This usually occurs within 2 to 3 days. Give the first dose of oral therapy 8 to 12 hours after discontinuing the IV infusion. The recommended starting oral dose is 0.1 to 0.15 mg/kg/day administered in 2 divided daily doses every 12 hours. Administer the initial dose no sooner than 6 hours after transplantation. Give adult patients doses at the lower end of the dosing range.

*Children (under 12 years of age):* It is recommended that therapy be initiated in pediatric patients at the high end of the recommended adult IV and oral dosing ranges (0.0.3 to 0.05 mg/kg/day IV and 0.15 to 0.2 mg/kg/day oral).

*Kidney transplantation:* The recommended starting oral dose is 0.2 mg/kg/day administered every 12 hours in 2 divided doses. The initial dose of tacrolimus may be administered within 24 hours of transplantation, but should be delayed until renal function has recovered (as indicated, for example, by a serum creatinine of 4 mg/dL or less). Black patients may require higher doses to achieve comparable blood concentrations.

The data in kidney transplant patients indicate that the black patients required a higher dose to attain comparable trough concentrations compared with Caucasian patients.

*Hepatic/Renal function impairment:* Because of the potential for nephrotoxicity, give patients with renal or hepatic impairment doses at the lowest value of the recommended IV and oral dosing ranges. Therapy may need to be delayed by up to 48 hours or longer in patients with postoperative oliguria.

*Conversion from one immunosuppressive regimen to another:* Do not use tacrolimus simultaneously with cyclosporine. Discontinue either agent at least 24 hours before initiating the other.

**Actions**

*Pharmacology:* Tacrolimus is a macrolide immunosuppressant that prolongs the survival of the host and transplanted graft and inhibits T-lymphocyte activation, although the exact mechanism of action is not known.

*Pharmacokinetics:*

| Pharmacokinetic Parameters of Tacrolimus | | | | | | | | |
|---|---|---|---|---|---|---|---|---|
| Population | N | Route (dose) | $C_{max}$ (ng/mL) | $T_{max}$ (h) | AUC (ng•h/mL) | $t\frac{1}{2}$ (h) | Clearance (L/h/kg) | Vd (L/kg) |
| Healthy volunteers | 8 | IV (0.025 mg/kg/4 h) | — | — | ≈ 598[1] | ≈ 34.2 | ≈ 0.04 | ≈ 1.91 |
| | 16 | PO (5 mg) | ≈ 29.7 | ≈ 1.6 | ≈ 243[2] | ≈ 34.8 | ≈ 0.041[3] | ≈ 1.94[3] |
| Kidney transplant patients | 26 | IV (0.02 mg/kg/12 h) | — | — | ≈ 294[4] | ≈ 18.8 | ≈ 0.083 | 1.41 |
| | | PO (0.2 mg/kg/day) | ≈ 19.2 | 3 | ≈ 203[4] | NA[5] | NA | NA |
| | | PO (0.3 mg/kg/day) | ≈ 24.2 | 1.5 | ≈ 288[4] | NA | NA | NA |
| Liver transplant patients | 17 | IV (0.05 mg/kg/12 h) | — | — | ≈ 3300[4] | ≈ 11.7 | ≈ 0.053 | ≈ 0.85 |
| | | PO (0.3 mg/kg/day) | ≈ 68.5 | ≈ 2.3 | ≈ 519[4] | NA | NA | NA |

[1] $AUC_{0-120}$
[2] $AUC_{0-72}$
[3] Corrected for individual bioavailability.
[4] $AUC_{0-\infty}$
[5] NA = Not available
– = Not applicable

The plasma protein binding of tacrolimus is approximately 99%. Tacrolimus is bound mainly to albumin and alpha-1-acid glycoprotein and has a high level of association with erythrocytes. It is extensively metabolized by the mixed-function oxidase system, primarily the cytochrome P450 system (CYP3A). The disposition of tacrolimus from whole blood was biphasic with a terminal elimination half-life of 11.7 hours in liver transplant patients.

### Contraindications

Hypersensitivity to tacrolimus; hypersensitivity to HCO-60 polyoxyl 60 hydrogenated castor oil (used in vehicle for injection).

### Warnings

*Insulin-dependent posttransplant diabetes mellitus (PTDM):* Insulin-dependent PTDM was reported in 20% of tacrolimus-treated kidney patients without pretransplant history of diabetes mellitus in the Phase 3 study. The median time to onset of PTDM was 68 days. Insulin dependence was reversible in 15% of these PTDM patients at 1 year and in 50% at 2 years posttransplant. Black and Hispanic kidney transplant patients were at an increased risk of development of PTDM.

*Nephrotoxicity:* Tacrolimus can cause nephrotoxicity, particularly when used in high doses. Nephrotoxicity has been noted in approximately 52% of kidney transplantation patients and in 33% to 40% of liver transplantation patients receiving the drug.

*Hyperkalemia:* Mild to severe hyperkalemia has been noted with tacrolimus and may require treatment.

*Neurotoxicity:* Neurotoxicity, including tremor, headache, and other changes in motor function, mental status, and sensory function occurred in approximately 55% of liver transplant recipients. Tremor occurred more often in tacrolimus-treated kidney transplant patients (54%) compared with cyclosporine-treated patients. Tremor and headache have been associated with high whole-blood concentrations of tacrolimus and may respond to dosage adjustment. Seizures have occurred in adult and pediatric patients. Coma and delirium also have been associated with high plasma concentrations of tacrolimus.

*Lymphomas:* As with other immunosuppressants, patients receiving tacrolimus are at increased risk of developing lymphomas and other malignancies, particularly of the skin.

*Myocardial hypertrophy:* Myocardial hypertrophy has been reported in association with the administration of tacrolimus and generally is manifested by echocardiographically demonstrated concentric increases in left ventricular posterior wall and interventricular septum thickness. Hypertrophy has been observed in infants, children, and adults. This condition appears reversible in most cases following dose reduction or discontinuance of therapy.

*Hypersensitivity reactions:* A few patients receiving the injection have experienced anaphylactic reactions. Although the exact cause of these reactions is not known, other drugs with castor oil derivatives in the formulation have been associated with anaphylaxis in a small percentage of patients.

Continuously observe patients receiving the injection for at least the first 30 minutes following the start of the infusion and at frequent intervals thereafter.

*Renal/Hepatic function impairment:* The use of tacrolimus in liver transplant recipients experiencing posttransplant hepatic impairment may be associated with increased risk of developing renal insufficiency related to high whole-blood levels of tacrolimus.

*Carcinogenesis:* An increased incidence of malignancy is a recognized complication of immunosuppression in recipients of organ transplants.

*Pregnancy: Category* C. The use of tacrolimus during pregnancy has been associated with neonatal hyperkalemia and renal dysfunction.

*Lactation:* Tacrolimus is excreted in breast milk; avoid nursing.

## Precautions

*Monitoring:* Regularly assess serum creatinine and potassium. Perform routine monitoring of metabolic and hematologic systems as clinically warranted.

*Hypertension:* Hypertension is a common adverse effect of tacrolimus therapy. Mild or moderate hypertension is reported more frequently than severe hypertension.

*Hyperglycemia:* Hyperglycemia was associated with the use of tacrolimus in 29% to 47% of liver transplant recipients and may require treatment.

## Drug Interactions

Drugs that may affect tacrolimus include nephrotoxic agents (aminoglycosides, amphotericin B, cisplatin, cyclosporine), antifungals, bromocriptine, calcium channel blockers, cimetidine, clarithromycin, danazol, diltiazem, erythromycin, methylprednisolone, metoclopramide, carbamazepine, phenobarbital, phenytoin, rifamycins, cisapride, chloramphenicol, metronidazole, nefazodone, omeprazole, protease inhibitors, macrolide antibiotics, fosphenytoin, and St. John's wort.

Drugs that may be affected by tacrolimus include vaccines and mycophenolate mofetil.

Because tacrolimus is metabolized mainly by the cytochrome P450 3A enzyme systems, substances known to inhibit or induce these enzymes may affect the metabolism of tacrolimus with resultant increases or decreases in whole blood or plasma levels.

*Drug/Food interactions:* The presence of food reduced the absorption of tacrolimus (decrease in AUC and $C_{max}$ and increase in $T_{max}$). The relative oral bioavailability (whole blood) was reduced by 27% compared with the fasting state.

Coadministered grapefruit juice has been reported to increase tacrolimus blood trough concentrations in liver transplant patients.

## Adverse Reactions

The principal adverse reactions of tacrolimus are tremor, headache, diarrhea, hypertension, nausea, and renal dysfunction. Other reactions may include insomnia, paresthesia, constipation, anorexia, vomiting, anemia, leukocytosis, thrombocytopenia, hyperglycemia, dyspnea, pruritus, rash, abdominal pain, fever, asthenia, back pain, ascites and peripheral edema, abnormal dreams, agitation, anxiety, confusion, convulsion, depression, dizziness, hallucinations, incoordination, nervousness, somnolence, abnormal thinking, abnormal vision, tinnitus, dyspepsia, flatulence, GI hemorrhage, GI perforation, hepatitis, increased appetite, jaundice, liver damage, oral moniliasis, chest pain, hypotension, tachycardia, hematuria, hyperlipemia, hyperphosphatemia, hyperuricemia, hypocalcemia, hypophosphatemia, hyponatremia, diabetes mellitus, coagulation disorder, ecchymosis, leukopenia, prothrombin decreased, abdomen enlarged, chills, peritonitis, photosensitivity reaction, arthralgia, generalized spasm, leg cramps, myalgia, asthma, bronchitis, cough increased, pulmonary edema, pharyngitis, rhinitis, sinusitis, voice alteration, alopecia, hirsutism, sweating.

# SIROLIMUS

**Tablets**: 1 and 2 mg (Rx)                    *Rapamune* (Wyeth Labs.)
**Solution, oral**: 1 mg/mL (Rx)                *Rapamune* (Wyeth Labs.)

---

**Warning:**
Increased susceptibility to infection and the possible development of lymphoma may result from immunosuppression. Only physicians experienced in immunosuppressive therapy and management of renal transplant patients should use sirolimus. Manage patients receiving the drug in facilities equipped and staffed with adequate laboratory and supportive medical resources. The physician responsible for maintenance therapy should have complete information needed for the follow-up of the patient.

*Liver transplantation-excess mortality, graft loss, and hepatic artery thrombosis (HAT):* The use of sirolimus in combination with tacrolimus was associated with excess mortality and graft loss in a study in de novo liver transplant recipients. Many of these patients had evidence of infection at or near the time of death.

In this and another study in de novo liver transplant recipients, the use of sirolimus in combination with cyclosporine or tacrolimus was associated with an increase in HAT; most cases of HAT occurred within 30 days post-transplantation and most led to graft loss or death.

*Lung transplantation-bronchial anastomotic dehiscence:* Cases of bronchial anastomotic dehiscence, most fatal, have been reported in de novo lung transplant patients when sirolimus has been used as part of an immunosuppressive regimen.

The safety and efficacy of sirolimus as immunosuppressive therapy have not been established in liver or lung transplant patients, and therefore, such use is not recommended.

---

## Indications
*Organ rejection:* Prophylaxis of organ rejection in patients receiving renal transplants. It is recommended that sirolimus be used in a regimen with cyclosporine and corticosteroids. In patients at low to moderate immunological risk, cyclosporine should be withdrawn 2 to 4 months after transplantation and sirolimus dose should be increased to reach recommended blood concentrations.

*Unlabeled uses:* Treatment of psoriasis.

## Administration and Dosage
*Concomitant use with cyclosporine and corticosteroids:* It is recommended that sirolimus be used initially in a regimen with cyclosporine and corticosteroids. It is recommended that sirolimus be taken 4 hours after cyclosporine. Cyclosporine withdrawal is recommended 2 to 4 months after transplantation in patients at low to moderate immunological risk.

*Sirolimus and cyclosporine combination therapy:* Administer the initial dose as soon as possible after transplantation. For de novo transplant recipients, give a loading dose of sirolimus 3 times the maintenance dose. A daily maintenance dose of 2 mg is recommended for use in renal transplant patients, with a 6 mg loading dose. Although a 5 mg/day maintenance dose with a 15 mg loading dose was found to be safe and effective, no efficacy advantage over the 2 mg dose could be established for renal transplant patients.

*Sirolimus following cyclosporine withdrawal:* Initially, patients considered for cyclosporine withdrawal should be receiving sirolimus and cyclosporine combination therapy. At 2 to 4 months following transplantation, progressively discontinue cyclosporine over 4 to 8 weeks and adjust the sirolimus dose to obtain whole blood trough concentrations within the range of 12 to 24 ng/mL. Therapeutic drug monitoring should not be the sole basis for adjusting sirolimus therapy. Careful attention should be made to clinical signs/symptoms, tissue biopsy, and laboratory parameters. The sirolimus dose will need to be approximately 4-fold higher to account for both the absence of the pharmacokinetic interaction (approximately 2-fold increase) and the augmented immunosuppressive requirement in the absence of cyclosporine (approximately 2-fold increase).

*Dosage adjustment:* Frequent sirolimus dose adjustments based on non-steady-state sirolimus concentrations can lead to overdosing or underdosing because sirolimus has a long half-life. Once sirolimus maintenance dose is adjusted, retain patients on the new maintenance dose for at least 7 to 14 days before further dosage adjustment with concentration monitoring. In most patients dose adjustments can be based on simple proportion: new sirolimus dose = current dose × (target concentration/current concentration). Consider a loading dose in addition to a new maintenance dose when it is necessary to considerably increase sirolimus trough concentration: sirolimus loading dose = 3 × (new maintenance dose - current maintenance dose). The maximum sirolimus dose administered on any day should not exceed 40 mg. If an estimated daily dose exceeds 40 mg because of the addition of a loading dose, administer the loading dose over 2 days. Monitor sirolimus trough concentrations for at least 3 to 4 days after a loading dose(s).

To minimize the variability of exposure to sirolimus, this drug should be taken consistently with or without food. Grapefruit juice reduces CYP3A4-mediated metabolism of sirolimus and must not be administered with sirolimus or used for dilution.

*Oral solution:* 2 mg of oral solution has been demonstrated to be clinically equivalent to 2 mg oral tablets, making them interchangeable on a milligram-to-milligram basis. However, it is not known if higher doses of oral solution are clinically equivalent to higher doses of tablets on a milligram-to-milligram basis. Patients receiving 2 mg/day oral solution demonstrated an overall better safety profile than did patients receiving 5 mg/day oral solution.

*Patients 13 years of age or older weighing less than 40 kg (88 lb):* Adjust the initial dosage based on body surface area to 1 mg/m$^2$/day. The loading dose should be 3 mg/m$^2$ in this population.

*Hepatic function impairment:* Reduce the maintenance dose of sirolimus by approximately 33% in patients with hepatic function impairment. It is not necessary to modify the sirolimus loading dose.

*Blood concentration monitoring:* Whole blood trough concentrations of sirolimus should be monitored in patients receiving concentration-controlled sirolimus. Monitor blood sirolimus levels in pediatric patients, in patients with hepatic function impairment, during coadministration of strong CYP3A4 and/or P-glyco-protein inducers and inhibitors, and/or if cyclosporine dosing is markedly reduced or discontinued. In controlled clinical trials with concomitant cylcosporine, mean sirolimus whole blood trough levels, as measured by immunoassay, were 9 ng/mL for the 2 mg/day treatment group, and 17 ng/mL for the 5 mg/day dose. Results from other assays may differ from those with an immunoassay.

*Instructions for dilution and administration of oral solution:*
Bottles – Use the amber oral dose syringe to withdraw the prescribed amount of sirolimus oral solution from the bottle. Empty the correct amount of sirolimus from

the syringe into a glass or plastic container holding 2 ounces or more (¼ cup, 60 mL) of water or orange juice. No other liquids, including grapefruit juice, should be used for dilution. Stir vigorously and drink at once. Refill the container with an additional volume (minimum of 4 ounces [½ cup, 120 mL]) of water or orange juice, stir vigorously, and drink at once.

*Pouches* – When using the pouch, squeeze the entire contents of the pouch into a glass or plastic container holding 2 or more ounces (¼ cup, 60 mL) of water or orange juice. No other liquids, including grapefruit juice, should be used for dilution. Stir vigorously and drink at once. Refill the container with an additional volume (minimum of 4 ounces [½ cup, 120 mL]) of water or orange juice, stir vigorously, and drink at once.

## Actions

*Pharmacology:* Sirolimus, a macrolide immunosuppressive agent, inhibits both T-lymphocyte activation and proliferation that occurs in response to antigenic and cytokine (interleukin-2, -4, and -15) stimulation and also inhibits antibody production. In cells, sirolimus binds to the immunophilin, FK binding protein-12 (FKBP-12), to generate an immunosuppressive complex.

*Pharmacokinetics:*

*Absorption* – Sirolimus is rapidly absorbed following oral administration, with a mean time-to-peak concentration of approximately 1 hour after a single dose in healthy subjects and approximately 2 hours after multiple oral doses in renal transplant recipients. The systemic bioavailability of sirolimus was estimated to be approximately 14%.

*Distribution* – The mean volume of distribution is 12 L/kg. Sirolimus is extensively bound (approximately 92%) to human plasma proteins. The binding of sirolimus was shown mainly to be associated with serum albumin (97%), $\alpha_1$-acid glycoprotein, and lipoproteins. The majority of sirolimus is sequestered in erythrocytes, resulting in considerably higher whole blood concentrations vs plasma concentrations. Sirolimus also is distributed in high concentrations to the heart, intestines, kidneys, liver, lungs, muscle, spleen, and testes.

*Metabolism* – Sirolimus is a substrate for both cytochrome P450 IIIA4 (CYP3A4) and P-glycoprotein. Sirolimus is extensively metabolized by O-demethylation and hydroxylation. Seven major metabolites, including hydroxy, demethyl, and hydroxydemethyl, are identifiable in whole blood. Some of these metabolites are also detectable in plasma, fecal, and urine samples. Glucuronide and sulfate conjugates are not present in any of the biologic matrices. Sirolimus is the major component in human whole blood and contributes to more than 90% of the immunosuppressive activity.

*Excretion* – After a single dose of sirolimus in healthy volunteers, 91% was recovered from the feces and 2.2% was excreted in urine.

## Contraindications

Hypersensitivity to sirolimus, its derivatives, or any component of the drug product.

## Warnings

*Interstitial lung disease:* Cases of interstitial lung disease (including pneumonitis, and infrequently bronchiolitis obliterans organizing pneumonia [BOOP] and pulmonary fibrosis), some fatal, have occurred in patients receiving immunosuppressive regiments including sirolimus. In some cases, the interstitial lung disease has resolved upon discontinuation of sirolimus.

*High-risk patients:* The safety and efficacy of cyclosporine withdrawal in high-risk patients have not been adequately studied and it is therefore not recommended. This includes patients with Banff grade II acute rejection or vascular rejection prior to cyclosporine withdrawal, those who are dialysis-dependent, or with serum creatinine greater than 4.5 mg/dL, black patients, retransplants, multi-organ transplants, or patients with high panel of reactive antibodies.

*Hepatic artery thrombosis:* In de novo liver transplant recipients, the use of sirolimus in combination with cyclosporine or tacrolimus was associated with an increase in hepatic artery thrombosis. Most cases occurred within 30 days post-transplantation and most led to graft loss or death.

*Infection/Lymphoma/Other malignancies:* Increased susceptibility to infection and the possible development of lymphoma may result from immunosuppression.

*Lipids:* Increased serum cholesterol and triglycerides that may require treatment occurred more frequently in patients treated with sirolimus compared to azathioprine or placebo controls.

Renal transplant patients have a higher prevalence of clinically significant hyperlipidemia. Accordingly, carefully consider the risk/benefit in patients with established hyperlipidemia before initiating an immunosuppressive regimen including sirolimus.

Monitor patients who are administered sirolimus for hyperlipidemia using laboratory tests. If hyperlipidemia is detected, initiate subsequent interventions such as diet, exercise, and lipid-lowering agents, as outlined by the National Cholesterol Education Program guidelines.

*Concurrent immunosuppressants:* Sirolimus has been administered concurrently with cyclosporine and corticosteroids. The efficacy and safety of the use of sirolimus in combination with other immunosuppressive agents have not been determined.

*Renal function impairment:* Mean serum creatinine was increased and mean glomerular filtration rate was decreased in patients treated with sirolimus and cyclosporine compared with those treated with cyclosporine and placebo or azathioprine controls. Monitor renal function during the administration of maintenance immunosuppression regimens including sirolimus in combination with cyclosporine, and consider appropriate adjustment of the immunosuppression regimen in patients with elevated serum creatinine levels. Exercise caution when using agents that are known to impair renal function (eg, aminoglycosides, amphotericin B).

*Carcinogenesis:* Animal studies have shown that sirolimus caused an increase in malignant lymphoma and testicular adenoma.

*Fertility impairment:* Animal studies have shown that sirolimus caused a reduction of testicular weight and histological lesions and reduced sperm counts.

*Pregnancy: Category C.*

*Lactation:* It is not known whether sirolimus is excreted in human breast milk. The pharmacokinetic and safety profiles of sirolimus in infants are not known. Because of the potential for adverse reactions in nursing infants from sirolimus, decide whether to discontinue nursing or to discontinue the drug, taking into account the importance of the drug to the mother.

*Children:* The safety and efficacy of sirolimus in pediatric patients younger than 13 years of age have not been established.

### Precautions

*Monitoring:* Monitor whole blood sirolimus concentrations in patients receiving concentration-controlled sirolimus. Monitoring is also necessary in patients likely to have altered drug metabolism, in patients at least 13 years of age who weigh less than 40 kg, in patients with hepatic impairment, and during coadministration of potent CYP3A4 inducers and inhibitors.

*Lymphocele:* Lymphocele, a known surgical complication of renal transplantation, occurred significantly more often in a dose-related fashion in sirolimus-treated patients. Consider appropriate postoperative measures to minimize this complication.

*Antimicrobial prophylaxis:* Cases of *Pneumocystis carinii* pneumonia (PCP) have been reported in patients not receiving antimicrobial prophylaxis. Therefore, administer antimicrobial prophylaxis for PCP for 1 year following transplantation. Cytomegalovirus (CMV) prophylaxis is recommended for 3 months after transplantation, particularly for patients at increased risk for CMV disease.

### Drug Interactions

*P450 system:* Sirolimus is extensively metabolized by the CYP3A4 isoenzyme in the gut wall and liver. Therefore, absorption and the subsequent elimination of systemically absorbed sirolimus may be influenced by drugs that affect this isoenzyme. Exercise care when concomitantly administering drugs metabolized by CYP3A4 with sirolimus.

Drugs that may increase sirolimus blood concentrations include the following: Nicardipine, verapamil, clotrimazole, fluconazole, itraconazole, clarithromycin, erythromycin, troleandomycin, cisapride, metoclopramide, bromocriptine, cimetidine, danazol, HIV-protease inhibitors, cyclosporine, diltiazem, azole antifungals.

Drugs that may decrease sirolimus levels include the following: Carbamazepine, phenobarbital, phenytoin, rifabutin, rifapentine, rifampin, St. John's wort.

Drugs that may be affected by sirolimus include vaccines.

*Drug/Food interactions:* To minimize variability, sirolimus should be taken consistently with or without food (see Administration and Dosage).

Grapefruit juice reduced CYP3A4-mediated metabolism of sirolimus and must not be used for dilution.

### Adverse Reactions

Adverse reactions occurring in 3% or more of patients include tremor, acne, constipation, diarrhea, nausea, increased serum creatinine, edema, hypercholesterolemia, hyperkalemia, hypokalemia, hyperlipemia, hypophosphatemia, peripheral edema, weight gain, rash, dyspepsia, vomiting, anemia, thrombocytopenia, leukopenia, dyspnea, pharyngitis, upper respiratory tract infection, abdominal pain, asthenia, back/chest pain, fever, headache, pain, arthralgia, urinary tract infection, hypertension.

Among the adverse events that were reported at a rate of 3% or more and less than 20%, the following were more prominent in patients maintained on sirolimus 5 mg/day vs 2 mg/day: Epistaxis, lymphocele, insomnia, thrombotic thrombocytopenic purpura (hemolytic-uremic syndrome), skin ulcer, increased LDH, hypotension, facial edema.

# MYCOPHENOLATE MOFETIL

| | |
|---|---|
| **Tablets:** 500 mg (*Rx*) | *CellCept* (Roche) |
| **Tablets, extended-release:** 180 and 360 mg (*Rx*) | *Myfortic* (Novartis) |
| **Capsules:** 250 mg (*Rx*) | *CellCept* (Roche) |
| **Powder for Oral Suspension:** 200 mg/mL (constituted) (*Rx*) | *CellCept* (Roche) |
| **Powder for Injection, lyophilized:** 500 mg (as HCl) | *CellCept* (Roche) |

---

**Warning:**

Increased susceptibility to infection and the possible development of lymphoma may result from immunosuppression. Only physicians experienced in immunosuppressive therapy and management of renal, hepatic, or cardiac transplant patients should use mycophenolate. Manage patients receiving the drug in facilities equipped and staffed with adequate laboratory and supportive medical resources. The physician responsible for maintenance therapy should have complete information requisite for the follow-up of the patient.

---

### Indications

*Allogeneic transplants:* For the prophylaxis of organ rejection in patients receiving allogeneic renal, hepatic, or cardiac transplants. Use mycophenolate concomitantly with cyclosporine and corticosteroids.

*Unlabeled uses:* Refractory uveitis (2 g/day alone or in combination with previous corticosteroid, cyclosporine, or tacrolimus therapy); second-line therapy for Churg-Strauss syndrome; in combination with prednisolone for the treatment of diffuse proliferative lupus nephritis.

### Administration and Dosage

*Renal transplantation:* 1 g administered orally or IV (over 2 hours or more) twice a day (daily dose of 2 g). Although a dose of 1.5 g twice daily (daily dose of 3 g) was used in clinical trials and was shown to be safe and effective, no efficacy advantage could be established for renal transplant patients. Patients receiving 2 g/day demonstrate an overall better safety profile than patients receiving 3 g/day.

*Tablets, ER:*

> *Adults* – 720 mg administered twice daily (1440 mg total daily dose) on an empty stomach, 1 hour before or 2 hours after food intake.
>
> The mycophenolate mofetil ER tablets and mycophenolate mofetil tablets and capsules should not be used interchangeably without physician supervision because the rate of absorption following the administration of these two products is not equivalent.
>
> *Children* – The recommended dose of mycophenolate mofetil ER in stable pediatric patients is 400 mg/m² body surface area (BSA) administered twice daily (up to a maximum dose of 720 mg administered twice daily). Patients with a BSA of 1.19 to 1.58 m² may be dosed either with three 180 mg ER tablets or one 180 mg ER tablet plus one 360 mg ER tablet twice daily (1080 mg daily dose). Patients with a BSA of more than 1.58 m² may be dosed either with four 180 mg ER tablets or two 360 mg ER tablets twice daily (1440 mg daily dose). Pediatric doses for patients with BSA more than 1.19 m² cannot be accurately administered using currently available formulations of ER tablets.
>
> *Elderly* – The maximum recommended dose is 720 mg administered twice daily.

*Cardiac transplantation:* 1.5 g administered orally or IV (over 2 hours or more) twice daily (daily dose of 3 g) is recommended.

*Hepatic transplantation:* 1 g twice daily administered IV (over 2 hours or more) or 1.5 g twice daily orally (daily dose of 3 g) is recommended.

*Capsules, oral suspension, and tablets:* Give the initial oral dose as soon as possible following transplantation. It is recommended that mycophenolate be administered on an empty stomach. However, in stable renal transplant patients, it may be administered with food if necessary.

> If required, the oral suspension can be administered via a nasogastric tube with a minimum size of 8 French (minimum 1.7 mm interior diameter).

*IV administration:* Do not administer IV solution by rapid or bolus IV injection. Mycophenolate IV is recommended for patients unable to take capsules or tablets. Administer no more than 24 hours following transplantation and for no longer than 14 days; switch patients to oral mycophenolate as soon as they can tolerate oral medication. Following reconstitution, administer by slow IV infusion over a period of at least 2 hours by peripheral or central vein.

*Preparation of oral suspension:* Tap the closed bottle several times to loosen the powder. Measure 94 mL of water in a graduated cylinder. Add approximately ½ the total amount of water for constitution to the bottle and shake the closed bottle well for approximately 1 minute. Add the remainder of water and shake the closed bottle well for approximately 1 minute. Remove the child-resistant cap and push bottle adapter into neck of bottle. Close bottle with child-resistant cap tightly. This will assure the proper seating of the bottle adapter in the bottle and child-resistant status of the cap.

*Preparation of infusion solution (6 mg/mL):* Mycophenolate IV must be reconstituted and diluted to a concentration of 6 mg/mL using 5% Dextrose Injection. Mycophenolate IV is incompatible with other IV infusion solutions.

> Mycophenolate IV does not contain an antibacterial preservative; use within 4 hours of reconstitution and dilution.
>
> Reconstitute the contents of each vial with 14 mL of 5% Dextrose Injection. Gently shake the vial to dissolve the drug. The resulting solution is slightly yellow. Discard the vial if particulate matter or discoloration is observed.

Further dilute the contents of 2 reconstituted vials (for a 1 g dose) into 140 mL of 5% Dextrose Injection or 3 reconstituted vials (for a 1.5 g dose) into 210 mL of 5% Dextrose Injection. The final concentration of both solutions is 6 mg/mL. Discard the infusion solution if particulate matter or discoloration is observed.

*Dosage adjustments:* In patients with severe chronic renal impairment (GFR less than 25 mL/min/1.73 m$^2$) outside of the immediate post-transplant period, avoid doses greater than 1 g administered twice a day; carefully observe these patients. No dose adjustments are needed in patients experiencing delayed graft function post-operatively. If neutropenia develops (ANC less than 1.3 x 10$^3$/mcL), interrupt dosing or reduce the dose, perform appropriate diagnostic tests, and appropriately manage the patient.

*Handling/Disposal:* Because mycophenolate has demonstrated teratogenic effects in rats and rabbits, do not crush tablets, and do not open or crush the capsules. Avoid inhalation or direct contact with skin or mucous membranes of the powder contained in mycophenolate capsules, oral suspension, and injection (before or after constitution). If such contact occurs, wash thoroughly with soap and water; rinse eyes with plain water. Should a spill occur, wipe up using paper towels wetted with water to remove spilled powder or suspension.

*Admixture incompatibility:* Do not mix or administer mycophenolate IV concurrently via the same infusion catheter with other IV drugs or infusion admixtures.

## Actions

*Pharmacology:* Mycophenolate is rapidly absorbed following oral administration and hydrolyzed to form MPA, which is the active metabolite. MPA is a potent, selective, uncompetitive and reversible inhibitor of inosine monophosphate dehydrogenase (IMPDH), and therefore inhibits the de novo pathway of guanosine nucleotide synthesis without incorporation into DNA.

*Pharmacokinetics:*

*Absorption/Distribution* – Following oral and IV administration, mycophenolate undergoes rapid and extensive absorption and complete presystemic metabolism to MPA, the active metabolite.

In 12 healthy volunteers, the mean absolute bioavailability of oral mycophenolate relative to IV mycophenolate (based on MPA AUC) was 94%. The AUC for MPA appears to increase in a dose-proportional fashion in renal transplant patients receiving multiple doses of mycophenolate up to a daily dose of 3 g.

Immediately post-transplant (less than 40 days), mean AUC and $C_{max}$ are approximately 45% to 50% and 20% to 30% lower, respectively, as compared with healthy volunteers or with stable renal and cardiac transplant patients.

*Metabolism* – In addition to MPA, other metabolites of the 2-hydroxyethyl-morpholino moiety are also recovered in the urine.

*Excretion* – Negligible amount of drug is excreted as MPA (less than 1% of dose) in the urine. Oral administration resulted in complete recovery of the administered dose; 93% was recovered in the urine and 6% recovered in feces. Most (about 87%) of the administered dose is excreted in the urine as MPAG (phenolic glucuronide of MPA).

| Mean Pharmacokinetic Parameters for MPA Following Mycophenolate Administration | | | | |
|---|---|---|---|---|
| Parameter | Dose/ Route | $T_{max}$ (h) | $C_{max}$ (mcg/mL) | AUC (mcg•h/mL) |
| Healthy volunteers (n = 129) (single dose) | 1 g/oral | ≈ 0.8 | ≈ 24.5 | ≈ 63.9 (n = 117) |
| Renal transplant patients Time after renal transplantation | | | | |
| 5 days (n = 31) | 1 g bid/IV | ≈ 1.58 | ≈ 12 | ≈ 40.8[1] |
| 6 days (n = 31) | 1 g bid/oral | ≈ 1.33 | ≈ 10.7 | ≈ 32.9[1] |
| Early (< 40 days; n = 25) | 1 g bid/oral | ≈ 1.31 | ≈ 8.16 | ≈ 27.3[1] |
| Early (< 40 days; n = 27) | 1.5 g bid/oral | ≈ 1.21 | ≈ 13.5 | ≈ 38.4[1] |
| Late (> 3 months; n = 23) | 1.5 g bid/oral | ≈ 0.9 | ≈ 24.1 | ≈ 65.3[1] |

| Mean Pharmacokinetic Parameters for MPA Following Mycophenolate Administration | | | | |
|---|---|---|---|---|
| Parameter | Dose/ Route | $T_{max}$ (h) | $C_{max}$ (mcg/mL) | AUC (mcg•h/mL) |
| *Cardiac transplant patients* | | | | |
| Time after cardiac transplantation | | | | |
| Early (day before discharge) | 1.5 g bid/oral | $\approx 1.8$ (n = 11) | $\approx 11.5$ (n = 11) | $\approx 43.3$ (n = 9)[1] |
| Late (> 6 months) | 1.5 g bid/oral | $\approx 1.1$ (n = 52) | $\approx 20$ (n = 52) | $\approx 54.1$ (n = 49)[2] |
| *Hepatic transplant patients* | | | | |
| Time after hepatic transplantation | | | | |
| 4 to 9 days (n = 22) | 1 g bid/IV | $\approx 1.5$ | $\approx 17$ | $\approx 34$[1] |
| Early (5 to 8 days) (n = 20) | 1.5 g bid/oral | $\approx 1.15$ | $\approx 13.1$ | $\approx 29.2$[1] |
| Late (> 6 months) (n = 6) | 1.5 g bid/oral | $\approx 1.54$ | $\approx 19.3$ | $\approx 49.3$[1] |
| *Renal impairment (single dose)* (GFR, mL/min/1.73 $m^2$) | | | | |
| Healthy volunteers (GFR> 80; n = 6) | 1 g/oral | $\approx 0.75$ | $\approx 25.3$ | $\approx 45$[3] |
| Mild renal impairment (GFR 50 to 80; n = 6) | 1 g/oral | $\approx 0.75$ | $\approx 26$ | $\approx 59.9$[3] |
| Moderate renal impairment (GFR 25 to 49; n = 6) | 1 g/oral | $\approx 0.75$ | $\approx 19$ | $\approx 52.9$[3] |
| Severe renal impairment (GFR < 25; n = 7) | 1 g/oral | $\approx 1$ | $\approx 16.3$ | $\approx 78.6$[3] |
| *Hepatic impairment (single dose)* | | | | |
| Healthy volunteers (n = 6) | 1 g/oral | $\approx 0.63$ | $\approx 24.3$ | $\approx 29$[4] |
| Alcoholic cirrhosis (n = 18) | 1 g/oral | $\approx 0.85$ | $\approx 22.4$ | $\approx 29.8$[4] |

[1] Interdosing interval $AUC_{0-12}$.
[2] $AUC_{0-12}$ values quoted are extrapolated from data from samples collected over 4 hours.
[3] Interdosing interval $AUC_{0-96}$.
[4] Interdosing interval $AUC_{0-48}$.

## Contraindications

Hypersensitivity to the drug, mycophenolic acid, or any component of the drug product; people with a sensitivity to polysorbate 80 (*Tween*) (IV only).

## Warnings

*Lymphomas/Malignancies:* Patients receiving immunosuppressive regimens involving combinations of drugs, including mycophenolate, as part of an immunosuppressive regimen are at increased risk of developing lymphomas and other malignancies, particularly of the skin. Lymphoproliferative disease or lymphoma developed in 0.4% to 1% of patients in the controlled studies of prevention of rejection.

Instruct patients to limit exposure to sunlight and UV light by wearing protective clothing and using a strong sunscreen.

*Neutropenia:* Up to 2% of renal transplant patients, up to 3.6% of hepatic transplant patients, and up to 2.8% of cardiac transplant patients receiving mycophenolate developed severe neutropenia. Neutropenia has been observed most frequently in the period from 31 to 180 days posttransplant in patients treated for prevention of rejection.

*Renal function impairment:* Avoid mycophenolate doses greater than 1 g administered twice a day and carefully observe patients.

No data are available for cardiac or hepatic transplant patients with severe chronic renal impairment. Mycophenolate may be used for cardiac or hepatic transplant patients with severe chronic renal impairment if the potential benefits outweigh the potential risks.

*Elderly:* Elderly patients, particularly those who are receiving mycophenolate as part of a combination immunosuppressive regimen, may be at increased risk of certain infections (including CMV tissue invasive disease) and possibly GI hemorrhage and pulmonary edema, compared with younger individuals.

*Pregnancy:* Category C.

*Lactation:* It is not known whether this drug is excreted in human milk. Because of the potential for serious adverse reactions in nursing infants from mycophenolate, decide whether to discontinue nursing or discontinue the drug, taking into account the importance of the drug to the mother.

*Children:* Safety and efficacy have not been established.

**Precautions**

*Monitoring:* Perform CBCs weekly during the first month of treatment, twice monthly for the second and third months, then monthly through the first year.

*GI hemorrhage:* GI tract hemorrhage has been observed in approximately 3% of renal transplants, 5.4% of hepatic transplants, and 1.7% of cardiac transplants treated with mycophenolate 3 g/day. GI tract perforations rarely have been observed.

*Delayed graft function:* In patients with delayed graft function posttransplant, mean MPA AUC was comparable, but MPAG AUC was 2- to 3-fold higher, compared to that seen in posttransplant patients without delayed graft function. No dose adjustment is recommended for these patients; however, they should be carefully observed.

*Rare hereditary deficiency:* On theoretical grounds, because mycophenolate is an inosine monophosphate dehydrogenase (IMPDH) inhibitor, avoid in patients with rare hereditary deficiency of hypoxanthine-guanine phosphoribosyl-transferase (HGPRT), such as Lesch-Nyhan and Kelley-Seegmiller syndromes.

*Phenylketonuria:* Mycophenolate oral suspension contains aspartame, a source of phenylalanine (0.56 mg phenylalanine/mL suspension). Therefore, take care if the oral suspension is administered to patients with phenylketonuria.

**Drug Interactions**

*Drugs that alter the GI flora:* Drugs that alter the GI flora may interact with mycophenolate by disrupting enterohepatic recirculation. Interference of MPAG hydrolysis may lead to less MPA available for absorption.

Drugs that may be affected by mycophenolate include acyclovir, ganciclovir, live attenuated vaccines, oral contraceptives, phenytoin, and theophylline.

Drugs that may affect mycophenolate include acyclovir, antacids, azathioprine, cholestyramine, ganciclovir, iron, probenecid, and salicylates.

*Drug/Food interactions:* Food (27 g fat, 650 calories) had no effect on the extent of absorption (MPA AUC) of mycophenolate when administered at doses of 1.5 g twice daily to renal transplant patients. However, MPA $C_{max}$ was decreased by 40% in the presence of food.

**Adverse Reactions**

The principal adverse reactions associated with mycophenolate include diarrhea, leukopenia, sepsis, and vomiting, and there is evidence of a higher frequency of certain types of infections.

Adverse reactions occurring in at least 10% of patients include pain; abdominal pain; fever; headache; infection; pain; accidental injury; chills; ascites; hernia; amblyopia; peritonitis; sepsis; asthenia; chest pain; back pain; hypertension; hypotension; cardiovascular disorder; tachycardia; arrhythmia; bradycardia; pericardial effusion; heart failure; anemia; leukopenia; ecchymosis; thrombocytopenia; hypochromic anemia; leukocytosis; urinary tract infection; oliguria; kidney tubular necrosis; hematuria; kidney tubular necrosis; peripheral edema; hypercholesterolemia; hypophosphatemia; edema; hyperglycemia; liver function tests, abnormal; creatinine increased; BUN increased; LDH increased; bilirubinemia; hypervolemia; hyperuricemia; AST increased; hypomagnesemia; acidosis; weight gain; ALT increased; hyponatremia; hyperlipemia; hypocalcemia; hypoproteinemia; hypoglycemia; healing abnormal; hypokalemia; hyperkalemia; diarrhea; constipation; nausea; dyspepsia; vomiting; flatulence; abdomen enlarged; anorexia; cholangitis; hepatitis; cholestatic jaundice; oral moniliasis; dyspnea; cough increased; lung disorder; sinusitis; rhinitis; pleural effusion; asthma; atelectasis; pharyngitis; pneumonia; acne; rash; skin disorder; pruritus; sweating; tremor; insomnia; anxiety; paresthesia; hypertonia; depression; agitation; somnolence; confusion; nervousness; dizziness; leg cramps; myasthenia; myalgia.

Patients receiving mycophenolate 2 g/day had an overall better safety profile than did patients receiving 3 g/day. Sepsis, which was generally CMV viremia, was slightly more common in renal transplant patients treated with mycophenolate, compared with patients receiving azathioprine. The incidence of sepsis was comparable to mycophenolate and in azathioprine-treated patients in cardiac and hepatic studies. In the digestive system, diarrhea was increased in renal and cardiac transplant patients receiving mycophenolate compared with patients receiving azathioprine, but was comparable in hepatic transplant patients treated with mycophenolate or azathioprine. Severe neutropenia developed in less than or equal to 2% of renal transplant patients, less than or equal to 2.8% of cardiac transplant patients, and less than or equal to 3.6% of hepatic transplant patients receiving mycophenolate 3 g daily (see Warnings).

| Viral and Fungal Infections in Prevention of Renal, Cardiac, or Hepatic Transplant Rejection with Mycophenolate (%)[1] | | | | | | |
|---|---|---|---|---|---|---|
| | Renal studies | | | Cardiac study | | Hepatic study | |
| Infection | Mycophenolate 2 g/day (n = 336) | Mycophenolate 3 g/day (n = 330) | Azathioprine 1 to 2 mg/ kg/day or 100 to 150 mg/day (n = 326) | Mycophenolate 3 g/day (n = 289) | Azathioprine 1.5 to 3 mg/ kg/day (n = 289) | Mycophenolate 3 g/day (n = 277) | Azathioprine 1 to 2 mg/ kg/day (n = 287) |
| Herpes simplex | 16.7 | 20 | 19 | 20.8 | 14.5 | 10.1 | 5.9 |
| CMV | | | | | | | |
| Viremia/ Syndrome | 13.4 | 12.4 | 13.8 | 12.1 | 10 | 14.1 | 12.2 |
| Tissue invasive disease | 8.3 | 11.5 | 6.1 | 11.4 | 8.7 | 5.8 | 8 |
| Herpes zoster | 6 | 7.6 | 5.8 | 10.7 | 5.9 | 4.3 | 4.9 |
| Cutaneous disease | 6 | 7.3 | 5.5 | 10 | 5.5 | 4.3 | 4.9 |
| Candida | 17 | 17.3 | 18.1 | 18.7 | 17.6 | 22.4 | 24.4 |
| Muco-cutaneous | 15.5 | 16.4 | 15.3 | 18 | 17.3 | 18.4 | 17.4 |

[1] Data pooled from 3 separate studies and are not necessarily comparable.

# DACLIZUMAB

**Injection**: 25 mg per 5 mL (*Rx*)        *Zenapax* (Roche)

**Warning:**
  Only physicians experienced in immunosuppressive therapy and management of organ transplant patients should prescribe daclizumab. The physician responsible for daclizumab administration should have complete information requisite for the follow-up of the patient. Daclizumab should only be administered by health care personnel trained in the administration of the drug who have available adequate laboratory and supportive medical resources.

### Indications
  *Organ rejection, prophylaxis:* Prophylaxis of acute organ rejection in patients receiving renal transplants. It is used as part of an immunosuppressive regimen that includes cyclosporine and corticosteroids.

### Administration and Dosage
  The recommended dose for daclizumab in adults and children is 1 mg/kg IV used as part of an immunosuppressive regimen that includes cyclosporine and corticosteroids. Mix the calculated volume of daclizumab with 50 mL of sterile 0.9% sodium chloride solution, and administer via a peripheral or central vein over a 15-minute period. Not for direct injection.

  The standard course of daclizumab therapy is 5 doses. Give the first dose no more than 24 hours before transplantation. Give the 4 remaining doses at intervals of 14 days.

## Actions

*Pharmacology:* Daclizumab is an immunosuppressive, humanized IgG1 monoclonal antibody produced by recombinant DNA technology that binds specifically to the alpha subunit (Tac subunit) of the human high-affinity interleukin-2 (IL-2) receptor that is expressed on the surface of activated lymphocytes. Daclizumab is a composite of human (90%) and murine (10%) antibody sequences.

*Pharmacokinetics:* Population pharmacokinetic analysis gave the following values for a reference patient (white male, 45 years of age, with a body weight of 80 kg and no proteinuria): Systemic clearance is 15 mL/h, volume of central compartment is 2.5 L, volume of peripheral compartment is 3.4 L. The estimated terminal elimination half-life for the reference patient was 20 days (480 hours), which is similar to the terminal elimination half-life for human IgG (18 to 23 days). Bayesian estimates of terminal elimination half-life ranged from 11 to 38 days for the 123 patients included in the population analysis.

The influence of body weight on systemic clearance supports the dosing of daclizumab on a mg/kg basis. For patients studied, this dosing maintained drug exposure within 30% of the reference exposure.

## Contraindications

Hypersensitivity to daclizumab or to any components of this product.

## Warnings

*Mortality:* The use of daclizumab as part of an immunosuppressive regimen including cyclosporine, mycophenolate mofetil, and corticosteroids may be associated with an increase in mortality.

*Benefit/Risk:* Inform patients of the potential benefits of therapy and the risks associated with administration of immunosuppressive therapy.

*Lymphoproliferative disorders:* While the incidence of lymphoproliferative disorders and opportunistic infections in the limited clinical trial experience was no higher in daclizumab-treated patients compared with placebo-treated patients, patients on immunosuppressive therapy are at increased risk for developing lymphoproliferative disorders and opportunistic infections and should be monitored accordingly.

*Hypersensitivity reactions:* Severe, acute (onset within 24 hours) hypersensitivity reactions including anaphylaxis have been observed both on initial exposure to daclizumab and following re-exposure. These reactions may include hypotension, bronchospasm, wheezing, laryngeal edema, pulmonary edema, cyanosis hypoxia, respiratory arrest, cardiac arrhythmia, cardiac arrest, peripheral edema, loss of consciousness, fever, rash, urticaria, diaphoresis, pruritus, and/or injection site reactions. If a severe hypersensitivity reaction occurs, permanently discontinue therapy with daclizumab.

*Elderly:* Use caution in giving immunosuppressive drugs to elderly patients.

*Pregnancy: Category C.*

*Lactation:* It is not known whether daclizumab is excreted in human milk. Because of the potential for adverse reactions, decide whether to discontinue nursing or discontinue the drug, taking into account the importance of the drug to the mother.

*Children:* The safety and efficacy of daclizumab have been established in pediatric patients from 11 months to 17 years of age.

## Precautions

*Immune system effects:* It is not known whether daclizumab use will have a long-term effect on the ability of the immune system to respond to antigens first encountered during daclizumab-induced immunosuppression.

*Readministration:* Readministration of daclizumab after an initial course of therapy has not been studied in humans. The potential risks of such readministration, specifically those associated with immunosuppression and/or the occurrence of anaphylaxis/anaphylactoid reactions, are not known.

*Immunogenicity:* Low titers of anti-idiotype antibodies to daclizumab were detected in the adult patients treated with daclizumab with an overall incidence of 14%. The incidence of anti-daclizumab antibodies observed in the pediatric patients was 34%. No antibodies that affected efficacy, safety, serum daclizumab levels or any other clinically related parameter were detected.

**Adverse Reactions**

*Cardiovascular:* Aggravated hypertension, bleeding, hypertension, hypotension, tachycardia, thrombosis (5% or more).

*CNS:* Dizziness, headache, insomnia, tremor, (5% or more); anxiety, depression, prickly sensation (2% to less than 5%).

*Dermatologic:* Acne , impaired wound healing without infection (5% or more); hirsutism, increased sweating, night sweats, pruritus, rash (2% to less than 5%).

*GI:* Abdominal distension, abdominal pain, constipation, diarrhea, dyspepsia, epigastric pain (not food-related), nausea, pyrosis, vomiting (5% or more); flatulence, gastritis, hemorrhoids (2% to less than 5%).

*GU:* Dysuria, oliguria, renal tubular necrosis (5% or more); hydronephrosis, renal damage, renal insufficiency, urinary retention, urinary tract bleeding, urinary tract disorder (2% to less than 5%).

*Metabolic/Nutritional:* Edema, peripheral edema (5% or more); dehydration, diabetes mellitus, fluid overload (2% to less than 5%).

*Hyperglycemia* – A total of 32% of daclizumab-treated patients (16% for placebo) had high fasting blood-glucose values. Most of these high values occurred either on the first day post-transplant when patients received high doses of corticosteroids or in patients with diabetes.

*Musculoskeletal:* Back pain, musculoskeletal pain (5% or more); arthralgia, leg cramps, myalgia (2% to less than 5%).

*Respiratory:* Coughing, dyspnea, pulmonary edema (5% or more); abnormal breath sounds, atelectasis, congestion, hypoxia, pharyngitis, pleural effusion, rales, rhinitis (2% to less than 5%).

*Miscellaneous:* Chest pain, fatigue, fever, lymphocele, pain, post-traumatic pain (5% or more); blurred vision, generalized weakness, injection site reaction, shivering (2% to less than 5%).

# CYCLOSPORINE (Cyclosporin A)

| | |
|---|---|
| **Capsules**: 25 and 100 mg (*Rx*) | *Gengraf* (Abbott) |
| **Capsules, soft gelatin**: 25 and 50 mg (*Rx*) | *Sandimmune* (Novartis, Various) |
| **Capsules, soft gelatin for microemulsion**: 25 and 100 mg (*Rx*) | *Neoral* (Novartis) |
| **Oral solution**: 100 mg/mL (*Rx*) | *Gengraf* (Abbott), *Sandimmune* (Novartis) |
| **Oral solution for microemulsion**: 100 mg/mL (*Rx*) | *Neoral* (Novartis) |
| **IV solution**: 50 mg/mL (*Rx*) | *Sandimmune* (Novartis, Bedford) |

> **Warning:**
> Only physicians experienced in the management of systemic immunosuppressive therapy for the indicated disease should prescribe cyclosporine. Patients receiving the drug should be managed in facilities equipped and staffed with adequate laboratory and supportive medical resources. The physician responsible for maintenance therapy should have complete information requisite for the follow-up of the patient.
>
> Administer *Sandimmune* with adrenal corticosteroids but not with other immunosuppressive agents. Increased susceptibility to infection and other possible development of lymphoma may result from immunosuppression.

**Warning: (cont.)**

*Neoral* and *Gengraf* may increase the susceptibility to infection and the development of neoplasia. In kidney, liver, and heart transplant patients, *Gengraf* and *Neoral* may be administered with other immunosuppressive agents. Increased susceptibility to infection and the possible development of lymphoma and other neoplasms may result from the increase in the degree of immunosuppression in transplant patients.

The absorption of *Sandimmune* during chronic administration was found to be erratic. It is recommended that patients taking *Sandimmune* over a period of time be monitored at repeated intervals to avoid toxicity from high levels and possible organ rejection from low absorption. This is of special importance in liver transplants.

*Sandimmune* capsules and oral solution have decreased bioavailability in comparison with *Neoral* capsules, *Neoral* oral solution, *Gengraf* capsules, and *Gengraf* oral solution. *Gengraf* and *Neoral* are not bioequivalent to *Sandimmune* and cannot be used interchangeably without physician supervision. For given trough concentrations, cyclosporine exposure will be greater with *Neoral* and *Gengraf* than with *Sandimmune*. If a patient receiving exceptionally high doses of *Sandimmune* is converted to *Neoral* or *Gengraf*, exercise particular caution. Monitor cyclosporine blood levels in transplant and rheumatoid arthritis (RA) patients taking *Gengraf* and *Neoral* to minimize possible organ rejection due to high concentrations. Make dose adjustments in transplant patients to minimize possible organ rejection due to low concentrations. Comparison of blood concentrations in the published literature with blood concentrations obtained using current assays must be done with detailed knowledge of the assay methods employed.

Psoriasis patients previously treated with PUVA and to a lesser extent, methotrexate or other immunosuppressive agents, UVB, coal tar, or radiation therapy, are at an increased risk of developing skin malignancies when taking *Neoral* or *Gengraf*.

Cyclosporine, in recommended doses, can cause systemic hypertension and nephrotoxicity. The risk increases with increasing dose and duration of cyclosporine therapy. Renal dysfunction, including structural kidney damage, is a potential consequence of cyclosporine, and therefore, renal function must be monitored during therapy.

## Indications

*Allogeneic transplants:* For prophylaxis of organ rejection in kidney, liver, and heart allogeneic transplants. *Gengraf* and *Neoral* have been used in combination with azathioprine and corticosteroids. *Sandimmune* always is to be used with adrenal corticosteroids. *Sandimmune* also may be used in the treatment of chronic rejection in patients previously treated with other immunosuppressive agents. Because of the risk of anaphylaxis, reserve *Sandimmune* injection for patients who are unable to take the soft gelatin capsule or oral solution.

*Psoriasis:* *Neoral* and *Gengraf* are indicated for the treatment of adult, nonimmunocompromised patients with severe (ie, extensive and/or disabling), recalcitrant, plaque psoriasis who have failed to respond to at least 1 systemic therapy (eg, PUVA, retinoids, methotrexate) or in patients for whom other systemic therapies are contraindicated or cannot be tolerated. While rebound rarely occurs, most patients will experience relapse with *Neoral* or *Gengraf* as with other therapies upon cessation of treatment.

*RA:* *Neoral* and *Gengraf* are indicated for the treatment of patients with severe, active, RA where the disease has not adequately responded to methotrexate. *Neoral* and *Gengraf* can be used in combination with methotrexate in RA patients who do not respond adequately to methotrexate alone.

### Administration and Dosage

*Bioequivalency:* Sandimmune capsules and oral solution have decreased bioavailability in comparison with Neoral capsules, Neoral oral solution, Gengraf capsules, and Gengraf oral solution. Gengraf and Neoral are not bioequivalent to Sandimmune and cannot be used interchangeably without physician supervision.

*Adjunct therapy:* Adjunct therapy with adrenal corticosteroids is recommended.

*Sandimmune:*

*Initial* – 15 mg/kg/day 4 to 12 hours prior to transplantation. There is a trend toward use of even lower initial doses for renal transplantation in the ranges of 10 to 14 mg/kg/day. Continue dose postoperatively for 1 to 2 weeks, then taper by 5% per week to a maintenance level of 5 to 10 mg/kg/day. Some centers successfully tapered the dose to as low as 3 mg/kg/day in selected renal transplant patients without an apparent rise in rejection rate.

*Parenteral* – For infusion only. Patients unable to take the oral solution or capsules preoperatively or postoperatively may be given the IV concentrate. Use the IV form at ⅓ the oral dose.

*Initial dose:* 5 to 6 mg/kg/day given 4 to 12 hours prior to transplantation as a single IV dose. Continue this daily single dose postoperatively until the patient can tolerate the oral doseforms. Switch patients to oral therapy as soon as possible.

*Children* – May use same dose and dosing regimen, but higher doses may be required.

*Neoral and Gengraf:* Always give the daily dosage of Neoral and Gengraf in 2 divided doses (bid) on a consistent schedule with regard to time of day and relation to meals.

*Initial dose* – The initial dose of Neoral and Gengraf can be given 4 to 12 hours prior to transplantation or postoperatively. In newly transplanted patients, the initial dose of Neoral and Gengraf are the same as the initial oral dose of Sandimmune. The mean doses were 9 mg/kg/day for heart transplant patients, 8 mg/kg/day for liver transplant patients and 7 mg/kg/day for heart transplant patients. Divide total daily dose into 2 equal daily doses. The Neoral or Gengraf dose is subsequently adjusted to achieve a predefined cyclosporine blood concentration. If cyclosporine trough blood concentrations are used, the target range is the same for Neoral or Gengraf as for Sandimmune. Using the same trough concentration target range as for Sandimmune results in greater cyclosporine exposure when Neoral is administered. Titrate dosing based on clinical assessments of rejection and tolerability. Lower Neoral or Gengraf doses may be sufficient as maintenance therapy.

*Conversion from Sandimmune* – In transplanted patients who are considered for conversion to Neoral or Gengraf from Sandimmune, start Neoral or Gengraf with the same daily dose as was previously used with Sandimmune (1:1 dose conversion). Subsequently adjust Neoral or Gengraf to attain the preconversion cyclosporine blood trough concentration. Using the same trough concentration target range for Neoral or Gengraf as for Sandimmune results in greater cyclosporine exposure when Neoral or Gengraf is administered. Monitor blood trough concentration every 4 to 7 days until preconversion value is obtained.

*Poor Sandimmune absorption* – Patients with lower than expected cyclosporine blood trough concentrations in relation to the oral dose of Sandimmune may have poor or inconsistent absorption. After conversion to Neoral or Gengraf, patients tend to have higher cyclosporine concentrations. Because of the increase in bioavailability following conversion to Neoral or Gengraf, the cyclosporine blood trough concentration may exceed the target range. Exercise particular caution when converting patients to Neoral at doses more than 10 mg/kg/day. Individually titrate Neoral or Gengraf dose based on cyclosporine trough concentrations, tolerability, and clinical response. Measure cyclosporine blood trough concentration more frequently, at least twice a week (daily, if initial dose exceeds 10 mg/kg/day) until concentration stabilizes within desired range.

*Rheumatoid arthritis (Neoral or Gengraf only)* – Initial dose of Neoral or Gengraf is 2.5 mg/kg/day, taken twice daily as a divided oral dose. Salicylates, NSAIDs and oral corticosteroids may be continued. Onset of action generally occurs between 4 and 8 weeks. If insufficient benefit is seen and tolerability is good (including serum creatinine less than 30% above baseline), the dose may be increased by 0.5 to 0.75 mg/kg/day after 8 weeks and again after 12 weeks to a maximum of 4 mg/kg/day. If no benefit is seen by 16 weeks of therapy, discontinue. There is limited long-term treatment data. Recurrence of disease activity is generally apparent within 4 weeks after stopping cyclosporine.

With methotrexate: Use the same initial dose and dosage range if Neoral is combined with the recommended dose of methotrexate. Most patients can be treated with Neoral doses of 3 mg/kg/day or less when combined with methotrexate doses of 15 mg/week or less.

Psoriasis (Neoral or Gengraf only) – The initial dose of Neoral or Gengraf is 2.5 mg/kg/day. Take Neoral or Gengraf twice daily, as a 1.25 mg/kg oral dose. Keep patients at that dose for 4 weeks or more, barring adverse events. If significant clinical improvement has not occurred in patients by that time, increase the patient's dosage at 2-week intervals. Based on patient response, make dose increases of approximately 0.5 mg/kg/day to a maximum of 4 mg/kg/day.

Patients generally show some improvement in the clinical manifestations of psoriasis in 2 weeks. Satisfactory control and stabilization of the disease may take 12 to 16 weeks to achieve. Discontinue treatment if satisfactory response cannot be achieved after 6 weeks at 4 mg/kg/day or the patient's maximum tolerated dose. Once a patient is adequately controlled and appears stable, lower the dose.

Upon stopping treatment with cyclosporine, relapse will occur in approximately 6 weeks (50% of patients) to 16 weeks (75% of patients). In the majority of patients, rebound does not occur after cessation of treatment with cyclosporine. Continuous treatment for extended periods longer than 1 year is not recommended. Consider alternation with other forms of treatment in the long-term management of patients with this disease.

Admixture compatibility/incompatibility:
Magnesium sulfate – Magnesium sulfate and cyclosporine in 5% dextrose stored in glass bottles at room temperature is stable for 6 hours.

**Actions**

Pharmacology: Cyclosporine is a potent immunosuppressive agent that in animals prolongs survival of allogenic transplants involving skin, kidney, liver, heart, pancreas, bone marrow, small intestine, and lung. Cyclosporine has been demonstrated to suppress some humoral immunity and to a greater extent, cell-mediated immune reactions such as allograft rejection, delayed hypersensitivity, experimental allergic encephalomyelitis, Freund's adjuvant arthritis, and graft vs host disease in many animal species for a variety of organs.

The effectiveness of cyclosporine results from specific and reversible inhibition of immunocompetent lymphocytes in the $G_0$ and $G_1$-phase of the cell cycle. T-lymphocytes are preferentially inhibited. The T-helper cell is the main target, although the T-suppressor cell also may be suppressed. Cyclosporine also inhibits lymphokine production and release including interleukin-2.

Pharmacokinetics:
Absorption –

| Select Pharmacokinetic Parameters of Cyclosporine Formulations | | | | |
|---|---|---|---|---|
| | Absolute bioavailability (%) | $T_{max}$ (hours) | $C_{max}$ (ng/mL/mg of dose) | $t_{1/2}$ (hours) |
| Conventional: Sandimmune | 30[1] | 3.5 | ≈ 1 (2.7 to 1.4)[2] | 19 (10 to 27) |
| Lipid microemulsion: Neoral | ND | 1.5 to 2 | ↑ (40% to 106%)[3] | 8.4 (5 to 18) |
| Gengraf | ND | 1.5 to 2 | ↑ (40% to 106%)[3] | 8.4 (5 to 18) |

[1] < 10% in liver transplant and approximately 89% in renal transplant patients.
[2] Blood levels for low to high doses, respectively.
[3] In renal transplant patients treated with Neoral or Gengraf, peak levels were 40% to 106% greater than those following Sandimmune administration.

Absorption from the GI tract is incomplete and variable. There is very little difference in absorption between *Gengraf* and *Neoral*.

*Distribution* – Largely outside the blood volume; approximately 33% to 47% is in plasma, 4% to 9% in lymphocytes, 5% to 12% in granulocytes and 41% to 58% in erythrocytes. In plasma, approximately 90% is bound to proteins, primarily lipoproteins. Blood level monitoring is useful in patient management.

*Metabolism* – Cyclosporine is metabolized by the cytochrome P-450 3A4 hepatic enzyme system.

*Excretion* – Primarily biliary. Only 6% of the dose is excreted in urine.

### Contraindications

Hypersensitivity to polyoxyethylated castor oil (injection only; see Warnings and Administration and Dosage), cyclosporine, or any component of the products; *Gengraf* and *Neoral* in psoriasis or RA patients with abnormal renal function, uncontrolled hypertension, or malignancies; *Gengraf* and *Neoral* concomitantly with PUVA or UVB, methotrexate or other immunosuppressive agents, coal tar or radiation therapy in psoriasis patients.

### Warnings

*Nephrotoxicity:* Nephrotoxicity has been noted in 25% of cases of renal transplantation, 38% of cases of cardiac transplantation, and 37% of cases of liver transplantation. Mild nephrotoxicity was generally noted 2 to 3 months after transplant and consisted of an arrest in the fall of the preoperative elevations of BUN and creatinine at a range of 35 to 45 mg/dL and 2 to 2.5 mg/dL, respectively. These elevations are often responsive to dosage reductions. More overt nephrotoxicity was seen early after transplantation and was characterized by a rapidly rising BUN and creatinine. Because these events are similar to rejection episodes, care must be taken to differentiate between them. This form of toxicity is usually responsive to cyclosporine dosage reduction.

*Hepatotoxicity:* Hepatotoxicity has been noted in 4%, 7%, and 4% of renal, cardiac, and liver transplantation cases, respectively. This usually occurred during the first month of therapy when high doses were used, and consisted of elevated hepatic enzymes and bilirubin.

*Glomerular capillary thrombosis:* Glomerular capillary thrombosis, which may result in graft failure, occasionally develops.

*Convulsions:* Convulsions have occurred in adult and pediatric patients receiving cyclosporine, particularly in combination with high-dose methylprednisolone.

*Bioequivalency: Sandimmune* is not bioequivalent to *Neoral* or *Gengraf.*

*Thrombocytopenia and microangiopathic hemolytic anemia:* Occasionally patients have developed a syndrome of thrombocytopenia and microangiopathic hemolytic anemia that may result in graft failure.

*Hyperkalemia:* Significant hyperkalemia (sometimes associated with hyperchloremic metabolic acidosis) and hyperuricemia have been seen occasionally in individual patients.

*Encephalopathy:* Encephalopathy has been described in postmarketing reports and in the literature. Manifestations include impaired consciousness, convulsions, visual disturbances (including blindness), loss of motor function, movement disorders, and psychiatric disturbances.

*Hypomagnesemia:* Hypomagnesemia has been reported in some, but not all, patients exhibiting convulsions while on cyclosporine therapy.

*Vaccination:* During treatment with cyclosporine, vaccination may be less effective; avoid the use of live attenuated vaccines.

*Nephrotoxic drugs:* Care should be taken in using cyclosporine with nephrotoxic drugs.

*Elderly:* Patients at least 65 years of age are more likely to develop systolic hypertension on therapy, and more likely to show serum creatinine rises greater than or equal to 50% above the baseline after 3 to 4 months of therapy. Monitor elderly patients with particular care, because decreases in renal function also occur with age. If patients are not properly monitored and dosages are not properly adjusted, cyclosporine therapy can cause structural kidney damage and persistent renal dysfunction.

*Elevated BUN and serum creatinine:* It is not unusual for serum creatinine and BUN levels to be elevated during cyclosporine therapy. These elevations in renal transplant patients do not necessarily indicate rejection, and each patient must be fully evaluated before dosage adjustment is indicated. These increases reflect a reduction in the glomerular filtration rate. Impaired renal function at any time requires close monitoring, and frequent dosage adjustments may be indicated. The frequency and severity of serum creatinine elevations increase with dose and duration of cyclosporine therapy. These elevations are likely to become more pronounced without dose reduction or discontinuation.

*Hypersensitivity reactions:* Anaphylactic reactions are rare (approximately 1 in 1000) in patients on cyclosporine injection. Continuously observe patients on IV cyclosporine for at least the first 30 minutes after start of infusion and frequently thereafter. If anaphylaxis occurs, stop infusion.

*Renal function impairment:* Requires close monitoring and possibly frequent dosage adjustment. In patients with persistent high elevations of BUN and creatinine who are unresponsive to dosage adjustments, consider switching to other immunosuppressive therapy.

*Carcinogenesis:* The risk of malignancies in cyclosporine recipients is higher than in the healthy population but similar to that in patients receiving other immunosuppressive therapies.

   With cyclosporine, some patients have developed a lymphoproliferative disorder, which regresses when the drug is discontinued. Patients receiving cyclosporine are at increased risk for development of lymphomas and other malignancies, particularly those of the skin. The increased risk appears related to the intensity and duration of immunosuppression rather than to the use of specific agents. Because of the danger of oversuppression of the immune system, which can also increase susceptibility to infection, do not give *Sandimmune* with other immunosuppressive agents except adrenal corticosteroids. Because of the danger of oversuppression of the immune system resulting in increased risk of infection or malignancy caused by *Neoral*, use a treatment regimen containing multiple immunosuppressants with caution.

*Pregnancy: Category C.*

*Lactation:* Avoid nursing; cyclosporine is excreted in breast milk.

*Children:* Patients as young as 6 months of age have received *Sandimmune* with no unusual adverse effects. Transplant recipients as young as 1 year of age have received *Neoral* or *Gengraf* with no unusual adverse effects. The safety and efficacy of *Neoral* or *Gengraf* treatment in children younger than 18 years of age with juvenile rheumatoid arthritis or psoriasis have not been established.

## Precautions
*Monitoring:*
   Blood levels – Blood level monitoring of cyclosporine is a useful and essential component in patient management. While no fixed relationships have been established, blood concentration monitoring may assist in the clinical evaluation of rejection and toxicity, dose adjustments, and the assessment of compliance.
   Of major importance to blood level analysis are the type of assay used, the transplanted organ, and the other immunosuppressant agents being administered.
   While several assays and assay matrices are available, there is a consensus that parent-compound-specific assays correlate best with clinical events. Of these, HPLC

is the standard reference, but the monoclonal antibody RIAs and the monoclonal antibody FPIA offer sensitivity, reproducibility, and convenience.

Repeatedly assess renal and liver functions by measurement of BUN, serum creatinine, serum bilirubin, and liver enzymes.

*Malabsorption:* Patients with malabsorption may have difficulty achieving therapeutic levels with oral *Sandimmune* use.

*Hypertension:* Hypertension is a fairly common side effect. Mild or moderate hypertension, which may occur in approximately 50% of patients following renal transplantation and in most cardiac transplant patients, is more frequently encountered than severe hypertension and the incidence decreases over time. Control of blood pressure can be accomplished with any of the common antihypertensive agents. Because cyclosporine may cause hyperkalemia, do not use potassium-sparing diuretics. While calcium antagonists can be effective agents in treating cyclosporine-associated hypertension, use care because interference with cyclosporine metabolism may require a dosage adjustment.

### Drug Interactions

*P-450 system:* Monitoring of circulating cyclosporine levels and appropriate dosage adjustment are essential when drugs that affect hepatic microsomal enzymes, particularly the cytochrome P-450 3A enzymes, are used concomitantly (eg, HIV protease inhibitors, anticonvulsants, azole antifungals).

*Nephrotoxic drugs:* Use with caution in patients receiving cyclosporine. The following drugs may potentiate renal dysfunction: *antibiotics:* gentamicin, tobramycin, vancomycin, TMP-SMZ; *antineoplastics:* melphalan; *antifungals:* amphotericin B, ketoconazole; *anti-inflammatory drugs:* diclofenac, naproxen, sulindac; *GI agents:* cimetidine, ranitidine; *immunosuppressives:* tacrolimus.

Drugs that may affect cyclosporine include: allopurinol, amiodarone, androgens (eg, danazol, methyltestosterone), anticonvulsants (eg, carbamazepine, phenobarbital, phenytoin), azole antifungals (eg, fluconazole, ketoconazole), beta-blockers, bosentan, bromocriptine, calcium channel blockers, colchicine, oral contraceptives, corticosteroids, fluoroquinolones (eg, ciprofloxacin), foscarnet, HMG-CoA reductase inhibitors, imipenem-cilastatin, macrolide antibiotics, methotrexate, metoclopramide, nafcillin, nefazodone, orlistat, potassium-sparing diuretics, probucol, rifamycins (rifampin, rifabutin), serotonin reuptake inhibitors (SSRIs; eg, fluoxetine, sertraline), sirolimus, St. John's wort, sulfamethoxazole/trimethoprim, terbinafine, and ticlopidine.

Drugs that may be affected by cyclosporine include bosentan, digoxin, etopisode, and HMG-CoA reductase inhibitors, methotrexate, potassium-sparing diuretics, and sirolimus.

*Drug/Food interactions:* Administration of food with *Neoral* decreases the AUC and $C_{max}$ of cyclosporine. A high-fat meal consumed within 30 minutes of *Neoral* administration decreased the AUC by 13% and $C_{max}$ by 33%. The effects of a low-fat meal were similar. In addition, do not take cyclosporine simultaneously with grapefruit juice unless specifically instructed to do so; trough cyclosporine concentrations may be increased.

### Adverse Reactions

Adverse reactions may include renal dysfunction; tremor; infectious complications; hirsutism; hypertension; gum hyperplasia; cramps; acne; convulsions; paresthesia.

# METHOTREXATE

| | |
|---|---|
| **Tablets:** 2.5 mg (Rx) | Various, *Rheumatrex Dose Pack* (STADA) |
| 5, 7.5, 10, and 15 mg (Rx) | *Trexall* (Barr) |
| **Injection:** 25 mg/mL (as base) (Rx) | Various, *Methotrexate LPF Sodium* (Xanodyne) |
| **Powder for injection, lyophilized:** 20 mg and 1 g (as base) (Rx) | Various |

**Warning:**

Methotrexate should be used only by physicians whose knowledge and experience include the use of antimetabolite therapy.

*Severe reactions:* Because of the possibility of severe toxic reactions (which can be fatal), fully inform patients of the risks involved and assure constant supervision.

*Deaths:* Use methotrexate only in life-threatening neoplastic diseases, or in patients with psoriasis or rheumatoid arthritis (RA) with severe, recalcitrant, disabling disease that is not adequately responsive to other forms of therapy. Deaths have occurred with the use of methotrexate in malignancy, psoriasis, and RA. Closely monitor patients for bone marrow, liver, lung, and kidney toxicities.

Marked bone marrow depression may occur with resultant anemia, leukopenia, or thrombocytopenia.

Unexpectedly severe (sometimes fatal) bone marrow suppression, aplastic anemia, and GI toxicity have occurred with coadministration of methotrexate (usually in high dosage) along with some NSAIDs (see Precautions, Drug Interactions).

*Monitoring:* Periodic monitoring for toxicity, including CBC with differential and platelet counts, and liver and renal function testing is mandatory. Periodic liver biopsies may be indicated in some situations. Monitor patients at increased risk for impaired methotrexate elimination (eg, renal dysfunction, pleural effusions, ascites) more frequently (see Precautions).

*Liver:* Methotrexate causes hepatotoxicity, fibrosis, and cirrhosis, but generally only after prolonged use. Acutely, liver enzyme elevations are frequent, usually transient and asymptomatic, and also do not appear predictive of subsequent hepatic disease. Liver biopsy after sustained use often shows histologic changes, and fibrosis and cirrhosis have occurred; these latter lesions often are not preceded by symptoms or abnormal liver function tests (see Precautions). For this reason, periodic liver biopsies are usually recommended for psoriatic patients who are under long-term treatment. Persistent abnormalities in liver function tests may precede appearance of fibrosis or cirrhosis in the RA population.

*Methotrexate-induced lung disease:* Methotrexate-induced lung disease is a potentially dangerous lesion that may occur acutely at any time during therapy and has occurred at doses as low as 7.5 mg/week. It is not always fully reversible. Pulmonary symptoms (especially a dry, nonproductive cough) may require interruption of treatment and careful investigation.

*Pregnancy:* Fetal death and/or congenital anomalies have occurred; do not use in women of childbearing potential unless benefits outweigh possible risks. Pregnant women with psoriasis or RA should not receive methotrexate (see Contraindications).

*Renal use:* Use methotrexate in patients with impaired renal function with extreme caution, and at reduced dosages, because renal dysfunction will prolong elimination.

*GI:* Diarrhea and ulcerative stomatitis require interruption of therapy; hemorrhagic enteritis and death from intestinal perforation may occur.

**Warning: (cont.)**

*Diluents:* Do not use methotrexate formulations and diluents containing preservatives for intrathecal or high-dose methotrexate therapy.

*Malignant lymphomas:* Malignant lymphomas, which may regress following withdrawal of methotrexate, may occur in patients receiving low-dose methotrexate and, thus, may not require cytotoxic treatment. Discontinue methotrexate first and, if the lymphoma does not regress, institute appropriate treatment.

*Tumor lysis syndrome:* Like other cytotoxic drugs, methotrexate may induce tumor lysis syndrome in patients with rapidly growing tumors.

*Skin reactions:* Severe, occasionally fatal skin reactions have been reported following single or multiple doses of methotrexate. Reactions have occurred within days of oral, IM, IV, or intrathecal methotrexate administration. Recovery has been reported with discontinuation of therapy.

*Potentially fatal opportunistic infections:* Potentially fatal opportunistic infections, especially *Pneumocystis carinii* pneumonia, may occur with methotrexate therapy.

*Radiotherapy:* Methotrexate given concomitantly with radiotherapy may increase the risk of soft tissue necrosis and osteonecrosis.

## Indications

*Severe, active, classical or definite adult RA:* (ACR criteria) in selected adults who have had an insufficient therapeutic response to, or are intolerant of, an adequate trial of first-line therapy including full-dose NSAIDs.

*Polyarticular-course juvenile rheumatoid arthritis (JRA):* Management of children with active polyarticular-course JRA who have had an insufficient therapeutic response to, or are intolerant of, an adequate trial of first-line therapy including full-dose NSAIDs.

*Psoriasis:* Symptomatic control of severe, recalcitrant, disabling psoriasis that is not adequately responsive to other forms of therapy.

*Other:* Methotrexate also is indicated as an antineoplastic chemotherapy in various types of cancers and acute lymphocytic leukemia.

## Administration and Dosage

*Arthritis:* Therapeutic response for adult RA and polyarticular-course JRA usually begins within 3 to 6 weeks and the patient may continue to improve for another 12 weeks or more.

Adult RA –

Starting dose: Single oral doses of 7.5 mg/week or divided oral dosages of 2.5 mg at 12-hour intervals for 3 doses given as a course once weekly.

Polyarticular-course JRA –

Starting dose: 10 mg/m$^2$ given once weekly.

Dose adjustment – Dosages may be adjusted gradually to achieve an optimal response. Limited experience shows a significant increase in the incidence and severity of serious toxic reactions, especially bone marrow suppression, at doses greater than 20 mg/week in adults. Although there is experience with doses up to 30 mg/m$^2$/week in children, there are too few published data to assess how doses over 20 mg/m$^2$/week might affect the risk of serious toxicity in children. Experience suggests that children receiving 20 to 30 mg/m$^2$/week (0.65 to 1 mg/kg/week) may have better absorption and fewer GI side effects if methotrexate is administered either IM or subcutaneously.

Duration of therapy – Optimal duration of therapy is unknown. Limited data from long-term studies in adults indicate that initial clinical improvement is maintained at least 2 years with continued therapy. When methotrexate is discontinued, the arthritis usually worsens within 3 to 6 weeks.

Weekly therapy may be instituted with the *Rheumatrex Dose Packs*, which are designed to provide doses over a range of 5 to 15 mg administered as a single weekly dose. The dose packs are not recommended for weekly doses greater than 15 mg. Tailor schedules to the individual patient. An initial test dose may be given prior to the regular dosing schedule to detect any extreme sensitivity to adverse effects. Maximal myelosuppression usually occurs in 7 to 10 days.

*Concomitant therapy* – Aspirin, NSAIDs, and/or low-dose steroids may be continued, although the possibility of increased toxicity with concomitant use of NSAIDs, including salicylates, has not been fully explored. Steroids may be reduced gradually in patients who respond to methotrexate. Combined use of methotrexate with gold, penicillamine, hydroxychloroquine, sulfasalazine, or cytotoxic agents has not been studied and may increase the incidence of adverse effects. Note that the doses used in RA (7.5 to 15 mg/week) are somewhat lower than those used in psoriasis and that larger doses could lead to toxicity. Rest and physiotherapy as indicated should be continued.

*Psoriasis:*

> *Weekly single oral, IM, or IV dose schedule* – 10 to 25 mg/week until adequate response is achieved. Do not exceed 30 mg/week.

> *Divided oral dose schedule* – 2.5 mg at 12-hour intervals for 3 doses.

> Dosages in each schedule may be gradually adjusted to achieve optimal clinical response; do not exceed 30 mg/week.

> Once optimal clinical response has been achieved, reduce each schedule to the lowest possible amount of drug and to the longest possible rest period. The use of methotrexate may permit the return to conventional topical therapy, which should be encouraged.

> Assess hematologic, hepatic, renal, and pulmonary function before beginning, periodically during, and before reinstituting therapy.

## Actions

*Pharmacology:* The mechanism of action in RA is unknown; it may affect immune function. Methotrexate inhibits dihydrofolic acid reductase and interferes with DNA synthesis, repair, and cellular replication.

*Pharmacokinetics:*

> *Absorption* – Peak serum levels are reached within 1 to 2 hours. The mean bioavailability is approximately 60%. Food delayed absorption and reduced peak concentration.

> *Distribution* – Methotrexate is approximately 50% protein bound.

> *Metabolism* – Methotrexate undergoes hepatic and intracellular metabolism. The terminal half-life reported is approximately 3 to 10 for patients receiving treatment for psoriasis, RA, or low-dose antineoplastic therapy (less than 30 mg/m$^2$).

> *Excretion* – Renal excretion is the primary route of elimination and is dependent upon dosage and route of administration.

## Contraindications

Hypersensitivity to the drug.

Patients with psoriasis or RA who have any of the following: alcoholism, alcoholic liver disease, or other chronic liver disease; overt or laboratory evidence of immunodeficiency syndromes; preexisting blood dyscrasias (eg, bone marrow hypoplasia, leukopenia, thrombocytopenia, significant anemia).

*Pregnancy:* Methotrexate can cause fetal death or teratogenic effects when administered to a pregnant woman. Methotrexate is contraindicated in pregnant women with psoriasis or RA and should be used in the treatment of neoplastic diseases only when the potential benefit outweighs the risk to the fetus. Women of childbearing potential should not be started on methotrexate until pregnancy is excluded and should be fully counseled on the serious risk to the fetus should they become pregnant while undergoing treatment. Pregnancy should be avoided if either partner is receiving methotrexate; during and for a minimum of 3 months after therapy for male patients, and during and for at least 1 ovulatory cycle after therapy for female patients.

*Lactation* – Because of the potential for serious adverse reactions from methotrexate in breastfed infants, it is contraindicated in nursing mothers.

**Warnings**

*Toxic effects:* Toxic effects, potentially serious, may be related in frequency and severity to dose or frequency of administration, but have been seen at all doses. These effects can occur at any time during therapy; follow patients closely. Most adverse reactions are reversible if detected early. When reactions occur, reduce dosage or discontinue drug and take appropriate corrective measures; this could include use of leucovorin calcium. Use caution if therapy is reinstituted.

*Renal function impairment:* See Precautions.

*Fertility impairment:* Impairment of fertility, oligospermia, and menstrual dysfunction in humans has been reported during and for a short period after cessation of therapy.

*Pregnancy: Category X.* Avoid pregnancy if either partner is receiving methotrexate: During and for a minimum of 3 months after therapy for male patients, and during and for at least one ovulatory cycle after therapy for female patients.

*Lactation:* Methotrexate has been detected in human breast milk. Methotrexate is contraindicated in nursing mothers.

*Children:* Safety and efficacy in children have been established only in cancer chemotherapy and in polyarticular-course JRA.

**Precautions**

*Monitoring:* Monitor hematology at least monthly, and liver and renal function every 1 to 2 months during therapy. During initial or changing doses, or periods of increased risk of elevated methotrexate blood levels (eg, dehydration), more frequent monitoring may be indicated. Stop methotrexate immediately if there is a significant drop in blood counts.

Transient liver function test abnormalities are observed frequently after methotrexate administration and are usually not cause for modification of therapy. Persistent liver function test abnormalities and/or depression of serum albumin may be indicators of serious liver toxicity and require evaluation.

*Weekly dose:* Physicians and pharmacists should emphasize that the dose is taken weekly. Mistaken daily use has led to fatal toxicity. Encourage patients to read the Patient Instructions in the Dose Pack. Do not write or refill prescriptions on a PRN basis.

*Organ system toxicity:*

GI – If vomiting, diarrhea, or stomatitis occur, which may result in dehydration, discontinue methotrexate until recovery occurs. Use with extreme caution in the presence of peptic ulcer disease or ulcerative colitis.

Hematologic – Methotrexate can suppress hematopoiesis and cause anemia, aplastic anemia, pancytopenia, leukopenia, neutropenia, and/or thrombocytopenia. Use with caution, if at all, in patients with malignancy and preexisting hematopoietic impairment.

In psoriasis and RA, stop methotrexate immediately if there is a significant drop in blood counts.

Hepatic – Methotrexate has the potential for acute (elevated transaminases) and chronic (fibrosis and cirrhosis) hepatotoxicity. Chronic toxicity is potentially fatal; it generally occurs after prolonged use (generally 2 years or more) and after a total dose of at least 1.5 g.

Periodically perform liver function tests, including serum albumin, prior to dosing.

Psoriasis: The usual recommendation is to obtain a liver biopsy at 1) pretherapy or shortly after initiation of therapy (2 to 4 months), 2) a total cumulative dose of 1.5 g, and 3) after each additional 1 to 1.5 g. Moderate fibrosis or any cirrhosis normally leads to discontinuation of the drug; mild fibrosis normally suggests a repeat biopsy in 6 months.

RA: In RA, first use of methotrexate and duration of therapy have been reported as risk factors for hepatotoxicity. Persistent abnormalities in liver function tests may precede appearance of fibrosis or cirrhosis in this population.

Infection or immunologic states – Use with extreme caution in the presence of active infection.

Potentially fatal opportunistic infections, especially *P. carinii* pneumonia may occur with methotrexate therapy.

*Neurologic* – A transient acute neurologic syndrome has been observed in patients treated with high-dosage regimens. Manifestations of this stroke-like encephalopathy may include confusion, hemiparesis, transient blindness, seizures, and coma.

*Pulmonary* – Pulmonary symptoms (especially a dry, nonproductive cough) or a nonspecific pneumonitis indicate a potentially dangerous lesion and require interruption of treatment and careful investigation. The typical patient presents with fever, cough, dyspnea, hypoxemia, and an infiltrate on chest x-ray.

*Renal* – Methotrexate may cause renal damage that may lead to acute renal failure. Close attention to renal function including adequate hydration, urine alkalinization and measurement of serum methotrexate and creatinine levels are essential for safe administration.

*Skin* – Severe, occasionally fatal dermatologic reactions, including toxic epidermal necrolysis, Stevens-Johnson syndrome, exfoliative dermatitis, skin necrosis, and erythema multiforme, have been reported within days of methotrexate administration.

*Vaccines:* Immunization may be ineffective when given during methotrexate therapy. Immunization with live virus vaccines is generally not recommended. Disseminated vaccinia infections after smallpox immunization have occurred in patients receiving methotrexate.

*Debility:* Use with extreme caution in the presence of debility.

*Pleural effusions or ascites:* In patients with significant third space accumulations, evacuate the fluid before treatment and monitor plasma methotrexate levels.

*Psoriasis lesions:* Lesions of psoriasis may be aggravated by concomitant exposure to ultraviolet radiation. Radiation dermatitis and sunburn may be "recalled" by the use of methotrexate.

*Folate deficiency:* Folate deficiency states may increase methotrexate toxicity.

*Benzyl alcohol:* Methotrexate sodium for injection contains the preservative benzyl alcohol and is not recommended for use in neonates.

## Drug Interactions

Drugs that may affect methotrexate include oral aminoglycosides, charcoal, chloramphenicol, folic acid, NSAIDs, PCNs, probenecid, salicylates, sulfonamides, TCN, trimethoprim.

Drugs that may be affected by methotrexate include sulfonamides, digoxin, phenytoin, theophylline, and thiopurines (eg, azathioprine).

*Drug/Food interactions:* Food may delay the absorption and reduce the peak concentration of methotrexate.

## Adverse Reactions

The most common adverse reactions include the following: Abdominal distress, chills, decreased resistance to infection, dizziness, fatigue, fever, leukopenia, malaise, nausea, ulcerative stomatitis.

*Adult RA:* Alopecia, diarrhea, dizziness, elevated liver function tests, leukopenia (WBC below 3,000/mm$^3$), nausea/vomiting, pancytopenia, rash/pruritus/dermatitis, stomatitis, thrombocytopenia (platelet count below 100,000/mm$^3$).

*Polyarticular-course JRA:* Virtually all patients were receiving concomitant NSAIDs, and some also were taking low doses of corticosteroids. Elevated liver function tests, GI reactions (eg, diarrhea, nausea, vomiting).

*Psoriasis:* Alopecia, photosensitivity, "burning of skin" lesions.

# MUROMONAB-CD3

| | |
|---|---|
| Injection: 5 mg/5 mL (Rx) | *Orthoclone OKT3* (Ortho Biotech) |

> **Warning:**
> Only physicians experienced in immunosuppressive therapy and management of renal transplant patients should use muromonab-CD3.
>
> Anaphylactic or anaphylactoid reactions may occur following administration of any dose or course of muromonab-CD3. Serious and occasionally life-threatening systemic, cardiovascular, and CNS reactions have been reported. These have included the following: Pulmonary edema, especially in patients with volume overload; shock; cardiovascular collapse; cardiac or respiratory arrest; seizures; coma. Hence, a patient being treated with muromonab-CD3 must be managed in a facility equipped and staffed for cardiopulmonary resuscitation.

### Indications

*Renal allograft rejection:* Treatment of acute allograft rejection in renal transplant patients.

*Cardiac/Hepatic allograft rejection:* Treatment of steroid-resistant acute allograft rejection in cardiac and hepatic transplant patients.

### Administration and Dosage

Muromonab-CD3 is for IV use only.

Administer as an IV bolus in less than 1 minute. Do not give by IV infusion or in conjunction with other drug solutions.

*Renal allograft rejection, acute:* 5 mg/day for 10 to 14 days. Begin treatment once acute renal rejection is diagnosed.

*Cardiac/hepatic allograft rejection, steroid resistant:* 5 mg/day for 10 to 14 days. Begin treatment when it is determined that a rejection has not been reversed by an adequate course of corticosteroid therapy.

*Monitor:* Monitor patients closely for the first few doses. Methylprednisolone sodium succinate 8 mg/kg IV given 1 to 4 hours prior to muromonab-CD3 administration is strongly recommended to decrease the incidence of reactions to the first dose. Acetaminophen and antihistamines, given concomitantly, may reduce early reactions. Patient temperature should not exceed 37.8°C (100°F) prior to first administration.

### Actions

*Pharmacology:* Muromonab-CD3 is a murine monoclonal antibody to the T3 (CD3) antigen of human T cells which functions as an immunosuppressant. The antibody is a biochemically purified $IgG_{2a}$ immunoglobulin. It reverses graft rejection, probably by blocking the T-cell function, which plays a major role in acute renal rejection.

*Pharmacokinetics:* Serum levels are measured with an enzyme-linked immunosorbent assay (ELISA). During treatment with 5 mg/day for 14 days, mean serum trough levels rose over the first 3 days and then averaged 0.9 mcg/mL on days 3 to 14. Circulating serum levels greater than 0.8 mcg/mL block the function of cytotoxic T cells in vitro and in vivo.

### Contraindications

Hypersensitivity to this or any product of murine origin; anti–mouse antibody titers greater than or equal to 1:1000; patients in fluid overload or uncompensated heart failure, as evidenced by chest x-ray or greater than 3% weight gain within the week prior to treatment; history of seizures or predisposition to seizures; pregnancy; breastfeeding.

### Warnings

*Cytokine release syndrome (CRS):* Temporally associated with the administration of the first few doses of muromonab-CD3 (particularly, the first 2 to 3 doses), most patients have developed CRS that has been attributed to the release of cytokines by activated lymphocytes or monocytes. This clinical syndrome has ranged from a more frequently reported mild, self-limited, "flu-like" illness to a less frequently reported severe, life-threatening shock-like reaction, which may include serious cardiovascular and CNS manifestations. The syndrome typically begins approximately 30 to 60 minutes after administration of a dose (but may occur later) and may persist for several hours. The frequency and severity of this symptom complex usually are greatest with the first dose.

*Pulmonary edema* – Severe pulmonary edema has occurred in patients who appeared to be euvolemic. The pathogenesis of pulmonary edema may involve some or all of the following: Volume overload; increased pulmonary vascular permeability; reduced left ventricular compliance/contractility.

*Serum creatinine* – During the first 1 to 3 days of therapy, some patients have experienced an acute and transient decline in the glomerular filtration rate (GFR) and diminished urine output with a resulting increase in the level of serum creatinine.

*Common clinical manifestations* – High fever (often spiking, up to 107°F); chills/rigors; headache; tremor; nausea/vomiting; diarrhea; abdominal pain; malaise; muscle/joint aches and pains; generalized weakness. Less frequently reported adverse experiences include minor dermatologic reactions (eg, rash, pruritus) and a spectrum of often serious, occasionally fatal, cardiorespiratory and neuro-psychiatric adverse experiences.

*Fluid status* – Prior to administration, assess the patient's volume (fluid) status carefully. It is imperative, especially prior to the first few doses, that there be no clinical evidence of volume overload or uncompensated heart failure, including a clear chest X-ray and weight restriction of less than or equal to 3% above the patient's minimum weight during the week prior to injection.

*Prevention/Minimization* – Manifestations of the CRS may be prevented or minimized by pretreatment with 8 mg/kg methylprednisolone, given 1 to 4 hours prior to administration of the first dose of muromonab-CD3 and by closely following recommendations for dosage and treatment duration.

*Neuropsychiatric events:* Seizures, encephalopathy, cerebral edema, aseptic meningitis, and headaches have occurred during therapy with muromonab-CD3, even following the first dose, resulting in part from T-cell activation and subsequent systemic release of cytokines.

*Aseptic meningitis syndrome* – The incidence of this syndrome was 6%. Fever, headache, meningismus, and photophobia were the most commonly reported symptoms; a combination of these 4 symptoms occurred in 5% of patients.

*Headache* – Headache is frequently seen after any of the first few doses and may occur in any of the aforementioned neurologic syndromes or by itself.

*Seizures* – Seizures, some accompanied by loss of consciousness or cardiorespiratory arrest, or death, have occurred independently or in conjunction with any of the neurologic syndromes described below. Patients predisposed to seizures may include those with the following conditions: Acute tubular necrosis/uremia; fever; infection; a precipitous fall in serum calcium; fluid overload; hypertension; hypoglycemia, history of seizures and electrolyte imbalances; those who are taking a medication concomitantly that may, by itself, cause seizures.

*Encephalopathy* – Impaired cognition; confusion; obtundation; altered mental status; auditory/visual hallucinations; psychosis (delirium, paranoia); mood changes (eg, mania, agitation, combativeness); diffuse hypotonus; hyperreflexia; myoclonus; tremor; asterixis; involuntary movements; major motor seizures; lethargy/stupor/coma; diffuse weakness. Approximately one-third of patients with a diagnosis of encephalopathy may have had coexisting aseptic meningitis syndrome.

*Cerebral edema* – Cerebral edema and other signs of increased vascular permeability (eg, otitis media, nasal and ear stuffiness) have been seen in patients treated with muromonab-CD3 and may accompany some of the other neurologic manifestations.

*Patients who may be at greater risk for CNS adverse experiences* – Patients who may be at greater risk for CNS adverse experiences include the following: Known or suspected CNS disorders; cerebrovascular disease (small or large vessel); conditions having associated neurologic problems; underlying vascular diseases; concomitant medication that may, by itself, affect the CNS.

*Infections:* Muromonab-CD3 is usually added to immunosuppressive therapeutic regimens, thereby augmenting the degree of immunosuppression. This increase in the total burden of immunosuppression may alter the spectrum of infections observed and increase the risk, the severity and the potential gravity (morbidity) of infectious complications.

*Carcinogenesis:* As a result of depressed cell-mediated immunity, organ transplant patients have an increased risk of developing malignancies.

*Hypersensitivity reactions:* Serious and occasionally fatal, immediate (usually within 10 minutes) hypersensitivity reactions have occurred. Manifestations of anaphylaxis may appear similar to manifestations of the CRS.

*Pregnancy:* Category C.

*Lactation:* It is not known whether muromonab-CD3 is excreted in breast milk.

*Children:* Safety and efficacy in children have not been established. Muromonab-CD3 has been used in infants/children, beginning with a dose of 5 mg or less.

## Precautions
*Monitoring:* Monitor the following tests prior to and during therapy:
- *Renal:* BUN, serum creatinine, etc.;
- *Hepatic:* Transaminases, alkaline phosphatase, bilirubin;
- *Hematopoietic:* WBCs and differential, platelet count, etc.;
- *Chest X-ray:* within 24 hours before initiating treatment, which should be free of any evidence of heart failure or fluid overload.

Monitor one of the following immunologic tests during therapy:
- Plasma levels determined by an ELISA; (target levels should be at least 800 ng/mL); or
- Quantitative T lymphocyte surface phenotyping (CD3, CD4, CD8); target CD3 positive T cells less than 25 cells/mm$^3$.

Testing for human-mouse antibody titers is strongly recommended; a titer greater than or equal to 1:1000 is a contraindication for use.

*Intravascular thrombosis:* As with other immunosuppressive therapies, arterial or venous thromboses of allografts and other vascular beds have been reported.

## Drug Interactions
Drugs that may affect muromonab include indomethacin.

## Adverse Reactions
Adverse reactions associated with CRS may include high (often spiking, up to 107°F) fever, chills/rigors, abdominal pain, malaise, muscle/joint aches and pains, dyspnea, shortness of breath, tachypnea, respiratory arrest/failure/distress, cardiovascular collapse, cardiac arrest, angina/MI, nausea, vomiting, chest pain/tightness, hemodynamic instability, heart failure, pulmonary edema, adult respiratory distress syndrome, hypoxemia, apnea, arrhythmias, diarrhea, tremor, bronchospasm/wheezing, headache, tachycardia, rigor, and hypertension.

Other adverse events may include pancytopenia, aplastic anemia, neutropenia, leukopenia, thrombocytopenia, lymphopenia, leukocytosis, lymphadenopathy, coagulation disturbances, hypotension/shock, heart failure, angina/MI, tachycardia, bradycardia, tachypnea/hyperventilation, abnormal chest sounds, pneumonia/pneumonitis, rash, urticaria, pruritus, erythema, flushing, diaphoresis, diarrhea, bowel infarction, arthralgia, arthritis, blindness, blurred vision, diplopia, hearing loss, otitis media, tinnitus, vertigo, photophobia, conjunctivitis, nasal/ear stuffiness, and anuria/oliguria.

# PEGINTERFERON ALFA-2a

| Injection: 180 mcg/mL (Rx) | Pegasys (Roche) |
|---|---|

**Warning:**
> Alpha interferons, including peginterferon alfa-2a, may cause or aggravate fatal or life-threatening neuropsychiatric, autoimmune, ischemic, and infectious disorders. Closely monitor patients with periodic clinical and laboratory evaluations. Patients with persistently severe or worsening signs or symptoms of these conditions should be withdrawn from therapy. In many, but not all cases, these disorders resolve after stopping peginterferon alfa-2a (see Warnings and Adverse Reactions).
>
> *Use with ribavirin:* Ribavirin may cause birth defects and/or death of the fetus. Extreme care must be taken to avoid pregnancy in female patients and in female partners of male patients. Ribavirin causes hemolytic anemia. The anemia associated with ribavirin therapy may result in a worsening of cardiac disease. Ribavirin is genotoxic and mutagenic and should be considered a potential carcinogen.

## Indications
*Chronic hepatitis C:* Alone or in combination with ribavirin tablets for the treatment of adults with chronic hepatitis C who have compensated liver disease and have not been treated previously with interferon alfa.

## Administration and Dosage
The recommended dose of peginterferon alfa-2a is 180 mcg (1 mL) once weekly for 48 weeks by subcutaneous administration in the abdomen or thigh.

There are no safety and efficacy data on treatment for longer than 48 weeks. Consider discontinuing therapy after 12 to 24 weeks of therapy if the patient has failed to demonstrate an early virologic response.

A patient should self-inject peginterferon alfa-2a only if the physician determines that it is appropriate, the patient agrees to medical follow-up as necessary, and training in proper injection technique has been provided.

*Peginterferon alfa-2a/Ribavirin tablet combination:* The recommended dose of ribavirin and duration for the peginterferon alfa-2a/ribavirin tablet combination therapy is based on viral genotype.

The daily dose of ribavirin tablets is 800 to 1200 mg administered orally in 2 divided doses. Individualize the dose depending on baseline disease characteristics (eg, genotype), response to therapy, and tolerability of the regimen.

Because ribavirin tablet absorption increases when administered with a meal, advise patients to take the tablet with food.

| Peginterferon Alfa-2a/Ribavirin Tablet Combination Dosing Recommendations | | | |
|---|---|---|---|
| Genotype | Peginterferon alfa-2a dose | Ribavirin tablet dose | Duration |
| Genotype 1, 4 | 180 mcg | < 75 kg = 1000 mg | 48 weeks |
| | | ≥ 75 kg = 1200 mg | 48 weeks |
| Genotype 2, 3 | 180 mcg | 800 mg | 24 weeks |

*Dose reduction:* When dose modification is required for moderate to severe adverse reactions (clinical or laboratory), initial dose reduction to 135 mcg (0.75 mL) is generally adequate. However, in some cases, dose reduction to 90 mcg (0.5 mL) may be needed. Following improvement of the adverse reaction, re-escalation of the dose may be considered. If intolerance persists after dose adjustment, discontinue therapy.
> *Hematologic toxicity* –
> *Peginterferon alfa-2a:* Dose reduction to 135 mcg peginterferon alfa-2a is recommended if the neutrophil count is less than 750 cells/mm$^3$. For patients with absc-

lute neutrophil count (ANC) values below 500 cells/mm$^3$, suspend treatment until ANC values return to more than 1000 cells/mm$^3$. Initially reinstitute therapy at 90 mcg peginterferon alfa-2a, and monitor the neutrophil count.

Dose reduction to 90 mcg peginterferon alfa-2a is recommended if the platelet count is less than 50,000 cells/mm$^3$. Cessation of therapy is recommended when platelet count is below 25,000 cells/mm$^3$.

*Ribavirin tablets:*

| **Ribavirin Tablet Dosage Modification Guidelines** | | |
|---|---|---|
| Laboratory values | Reduce only ribavirin tablet dose to 600 mg/day[1] if: | Discontinue ribavirin tablet if: |
| Hemoglobin in patients with no cardiac disease | < 10 g/dL | < 8.5 g/dL |
| Hemoglobin in patients with history of stable cardiac disease | ≥ 2 g/dL decrease in hemoglobin during any 4-week period treatment | < 12 g/dL despite 4 weeks at reduced dose. |

[1] One 200 mg tablet in the morning and two 200 mg tablets in the evening.

Once the ribavirin tablet has been withheld because of a laboratory abnormality or clinical manifestation, an attempt may be made to restart the ribavirin tablet at 600 mg/day and further increase the dose to 800 mg/day depending upon the physician's judgment. However, it is not recommended that the ribavirin tablet be increased to the original dose (1000 or 1200 mg).

*Psychiatric depression –*

| **Guidelines for Modification or Discontinuation of Peginterferon alfa-2a and for Scheduling Visits for Patients with Depression** | | | | | |
|---|---|---|---|---|---|
| | Initial management (4 to 8 weeks) | | Depression | | |
| Depression severity | Dose modification | Visit schedule | Remains stable | Improves | Worsens |
| Mild | No change | Evaluate once weekly by visit and/or phone | Continue weekly visit schedule | Resume normal visit schedule | (see moderate or severe depression) |
| Moderate | Decrease peginterferon alfa-2a dose to 135 mcg (in some cases dose reduction to 90 mcg may be needed) | Evaluate once weekly (office visit at least every other week) | Consider psychiatric consultation. Continue reduced dosing | If symptoms improve and are stable for 4 weeks, may resume normal visit schedule. Continue reduced dosing or return to normal dose. | (see severe depression) |
| Severe | Discontinue peginterferon alfa-2a permanently | Obtain immediate psychiatric consultation | Psychiatric therapy necessary. | | |

*Renal function impairment* – In patients with end-stage renal disease requiring hemodialysis, dose reduction to 135 mcg peginterferon alfa-2a is recommended. Closely monitor for signs and symptoms of interferon toxicity. Do not use ribavirin in patients with creatinine clearance less than 50 mL/min.

*Liver function impairment* – In patients with progressive ALT increases above baseline values, reduce the dose of peginterferon alfa-2a to 135 mcg. Immediately discontinue therapy if ALT increases are progressive despite dose reduction or are accompanied by increased bilirubin or evidence of hepatic decompensation.

**Actions**

*Pharmacology:* Interferons bind to specific receptors on the cell surface, initiating intracellular signaling via a complex cascade of protein-protein interactions and leading to rapid activation of gene transcription. Interferon-stimulated genes modulate many biological effects, including the inhibition of viral replication in infected cells, inhibition of cell proliferation, and immunomodulation. Peginterferon alfa-2a stimulates the production of effector proteins such as serum neopterin and 2′,5′-oligoadenylate synthetase.

*Pharmacokinetics:*

*Absorption/Distribution* – Maximal serum concentrations ($C_{max}$) occur between 72 to 96 hours postdose. Steady-state serum levels are reached within 5 to 8 weeks of once-weekly dosing. The peak-to-trough ratio at week 48 is approximately 2.

*Metabolism/Excretion* – The mean systemic clearance in healthy subjects given peginterferon alfa-2a was 94 mL/h. The mean terminal half-life after subcutaneous dosing in patients with chronic hepatitis C was 80 hours (range, 50 to 140 hours).

*Special populations* –

*Elderly:* The AUC was increased from 1295 to 1663 ng•h/mL in subjects older than 62 years of age taking 180 mcg peginterferon alfa-2a, but peak concentrations were similar (9 vs 10 ng/mL) in those older and younger than 62 years of age.

*Renal impairment:* In patients with end-stage renal disease undergoing hemodialysis, there is a 25% to 45% reduction in clearance (see Warnings).

## Contraindications

*Peginterferon alfa-2a:* Contraindicated for use in neonates and infants because it contains benzyl alcohol (see Warnings).

Contraindicated in patients with the following:

- Hypersensitivity to peginterferon alfa-2a or any of its components,
- Autoimmune hepatitis, or
- Decompensated hepatic disease (Child-Pugh class B and C) prior to or during treatment with peginterferon alfa-2a.

*Peginterferon alfa-2a/Ribavirin tablets combination:*

- Patients with known hypersensitivity to ribavirin tablets or to any component of the tablet.
- Women who are pregnant.
- Men whose female partners are pregnant.
- Patients with hemoglobinopathies (eg, thalassemia major, sickle-cell anemia).

## Warnings

*Autoimmune disorders:* Development or exacerbation of autoimmune disorders, including myositis, hepatitis, idiopathic thrombocytopenic purpura, psoriasis, rheumatoid arthritis, interstitial nephritis, thyroiditis, and systemic lupus erythematosus have been reported in patients receiving alpha interferon.

*Hemolytic anemia:* The primary toxicity of ribavirin is hemolytic anemia. The anemia associated with ribavirin tablets occurs within 1 to 2 weeks of initiation of therapy with maximum drop in hemoglobin observed during the first 8 weeks.

*Benzyl alcohol:* Peginterferon alfa-2a is contraindicated in neonates and infants because it contains benzyl alcohol.

*Bone marrow toxicity:* Peginterferon alfa-2a suppresses bone marrow function and may result in severe cytopenias. Ribavirin may potentiate the neutropenia and lymphopenia induced by alpha interferons including peginterferon alfa-2a. Alpha interferons may be associated with aplastic anemia very rarely.

*Cardiovascular events:* Hypertension, supraventricular arrhythmias, chest pain, and MI have been observed in patients treated with peginterferon alfa-2a.

Fatal and nonfatal MIs have been reported in patients with anemia caused by ribavirin.

*Colitis:* Ulcerative and hemorrhagic/ischemic colitis, sometimes fatal, has been observed within 12 weeks of starting alpha interferon treatment. Abdominal pain, bloody diarrhea, and fever are the typical manifestations of colitis.

*Endocrine disorders:* Peginterferon alfa-2a causes or aggravates hypothyroidism and hyperthyroidism. Hyperglycemia, hypoglycemia, and diabetes mellitus have developed in patients treated with peginterferon alfa-2a.

*Hypersensitivity reactions:* Severe acute hypersensitivity reactions (eg, urticaria, angio-edema, bronchoconstriction, anaphylaxis) have been rarely observed during alpha interferon and ribavirin therapy.

*Neuropsychiatric events:* Life-threatening or fatal neuropsychiatric reactions may manifest in patients receiving therapy with peginterferon alfa-2a. Depression, suicidal ide-ation, suicide, relapse of drug addiction, and drug overdose may occur in patients with and without previous psychiatric illness.

*Infections:* Serious and severe bacterial infections, some fatal, have been observed in patients treated with alfa interferons including peginterferon alfa-2a.

*Ophthalmologic disorders:* Decrease or loss of vision, retinopathy (including macular edema, retinal artery or vein thrombosis), retinal hemorrhages and cotton wool spots, optic neuritis, and papilledema are induced or aggravated by treatment with peginter-feron alfa-2a or other alpha interferons. All patients should receive an eye exami-nation at baseline.

*Pancreatitis:* Pancreatitis, sometimes fatal, has occurred during alpha interferon and riba-virin treatment.

*Pulmonary disorders:* Dyspnea, pulmonary infiltrates, pneumonia, bronchiolitis obliter-ans, interstitial pneumonitis, and sarcoidosis, some resulting in respiratory failure and/or patient deaths, may be induced or aggravated by peginterferon alfa-2a or alpha interferon therapy.

*Renal function impairment:* A 25% to 45% higher exposure to peginterferon alfa-2a is seen in subjects undergoing hemodialysis. In patients with impaired renal function, closely monitor for signs and symptoms of interferon toxicity. Use peginterferon alfa-2a with caution in patients with creatinine clearance less than 50 mL/min.

*Fertility impairment:* Peginterferon alfa-2a may impair fertility in women.

*Pregnancy:* Category C.

   *Use with ribavirin – Category X.*

      If pregnancy occurs in a patient or partner of a patient during treatment or dur-ing the 6 months after treatment cessation, such cases should be reported to the ribavirin tablet Pregnancy Registry at (800) 526-6367.

*Lactation:* It is not known whether peginterferon alfa-2a or ribavirin or its compo-nents are excreted in breast milk.

*Children:* The safety and efficacy in children below 18 years of age have not been estab-lished.

**Precautions**

*Monitoring:* Before beginning peginterferon alfa-2a or peginterferon/ribavirin tablet com-bination therapy, standard hematological and biochemical laboratory tests are rec-ommended for all patients. Pregnancy screening for women of childbearing potential must be performed. After initiation of therapy, perform hematological tests at 2 and 4 weeks and biochemical tests at 4 weeks. Periodically perform additional test-ing during therapy.

*Immunogenicity:* Nine percent of patients treated with peginterferon alfa-2a with or with-out ribavirin tablets developed binding antibodies to interferon alfa-2a, as assessed by an ELISA assay. The clinical and pathological significance of the appearance of serum neutralizing antibodies is unknown.

*HIV or HBV coinfections:* The safety and efficacy of peginterferon alfa-2a alone or in com-bination with ribavirin tablets for the treatment of hepatitis C have not been estab-lished in patients co-infected with HIV or HBV.

*Hepatitis C:* The safety and efficacy of peginterferon alfa-2a alone or in combination with ribavirin tablets for the treatment of hepatitis C in patients who have received liver or other organ transplants have not been established.

*Lab test abnormalities:* Peginterferon alfa-2a treatment was associated with decreases in WBC, ANC, lymphocytes, and platelet counts, often starting within the first 2 weeks of treatment.

Transient elevations in ALT (2- to 5-fold above baseline) were observed in some patients receiving peginterferon alfa-2a and were not associated with deterioration of other liver function tests.

**Drug Interactions**

Drugs that may be affected by peginterferon alfa-2a include theophylline.

**Adverse Reactions**

The most common life-threatening or fatal events induced or aggravated by peginterferon alfa-2a and ribavirin tablets were depression, suicide, relapse of drug abuse/ overdose, and bacterial infections; each occurred at a frequency of less than 1%. The most commonly reported adverse reactions were psychiatric reactions, including anxiety, depression, irritability, and flu-like symptoms such as fatigue, headache, myalgia, pyrexia, and rigors.

Peginterferon alfa-2a dose was reduced in 12% of patients receiving 1000 to 1200 mg ribavirin tablets for 48 weeks and in 7% of patients receiving 800 mg ribavirin tablets for 24 weeks. Ribavirin tablet dose was reduced in 21% of patients receiving 1000 to 1200 mg ribavirin tablets for 48 weeks and 12% in patients receiving 800 mg ribavirin tablets for 24 weeks.

Adverse reactions occurring in at least 3% of patients include the following: Abdominal pain, alopecia, anorexia, arthralgia, back pain, concentration impairment, cough, depression, dermatitis, diarrhea, dizziness, dry mouth, dry skin, dyspnea, fatigue/asthenia, headache, hypothyroidism, injection-site reaction, insomnia, irritability/anxiety/nervousness, lymphopenia, memory impairment, mood alteration, myalgia, nausea/vomiting, neutropenia, pain, pruritus, pyrexia, rash, overall resistance mechanism disorders, rigors, sweating increased, thrombocytopenia, vision blurred, weight decrease.

# PEGINTERFERON ALFA-2B

**Powder for injection, lyophilized:** 50, 80, 120, 150 mcg/ 0.5 mL (*Rx*)    *PEG-Intron*[1] (Schering)

[1] Effective October 22, 2001, *PEG-Intron* only will be made available through the *PEG-Intron* Access Assurance program. Pharmacists must obtain an order authorization number prior to placing an order with their wholesaler. To obtain this number, call (888) 437-2608 to provide the patient's Access Assurance ID# and the quantity to be dispensed (maximum 4 units). Patients without an Access Assurance ID# also may call this number to enroll. Next, contact the wholesaler and provide the authorization number and order information.

---

**Warning:**

Alpha interferons, including peginterferon alfa-2b, cause or aggravate fatal or life-threatening neuropsychiatric, autoimmune, ischemic, and infectious disorders. Closely monitor patients with periodic clinical and laboratory evaluations. Withdraw from therapy patients with persistently severe or worsening signs or symptoms of these conditions. In many but not all cases, these disorders resolve after stopping peginterferon alfa-2b therapy.

*Ribavirin use:* Ribavirin may cause birth defects and/or death of the unborn child. Take extreme care to avoid pregnancy in female patients and in female partners of male patients. Ribavirin causes hemolytic anemia. The anemia associated with ribavirin therapy may result in a worsening of cardiac disease. Ribavirin is genotoxic and mutagenic; consider it a potential carcinogen (see Ribavirin monograph for additional information and warnings).

---

**Indications**

*Chronic hepatitis C:* For use alone or in combination with ribavirin capsules for the treatment of chronic hepatitis C in patients with compensated liver disease who have not been previously treated with interferon alpha and are at least 18 years of age.

When used in combination with ribavirin, refer to ribavirin monograph for additional prescribing information.

**Administration and Dosage**

Patients should self-inject only if the physician determines that it is appropriate and patients agree to medical follow-up as necessary and receive training in proper injection technique.

*Monotherapy:* 1 mcg/kg/week subcutaneously for 1 year. Administer the dose on the same day of the week. Base initial dosing on the patient's weight as described in the following table.

| Recommended Dosing of Peginterferon Alfa-2b | | | |
|---|---|---|---|
| *Redipen* or vial strength to use (mcg/0.5 mL) | Body weight (kg) | Amount of peginterferon alfa-2b to administer (mcg) | Volume[1] of peginterferon alfa-2b to administer (mL) |
| 50 | ≤ 45 | 40 | 0.4 |
| | 46 to 56 | 50 | 0.5 |
| 80 | 57 to 72 | 64 | 0.4 |
| | 73 to 88 | 80 | 0.5 |
| 120 | 89 to 106 | 96 | 0.4 |
| | 107 to 136 | 120 | 0.5 |
| 150 | 137 to 160 | 150 | 0.5 |

[1] When reconstituted as directed.

*Peginterferon alfa-2b/Ribavirin capsules combination therapy:* When administered in combination with ribavirin capsules, the recommended dose of peginterferon alfa-2b is 1.5 mcg/kg/week. The volume of peginterferon alfa-2b to be injected depends on the strength of peginterferon alfa-2b and the patient's body weight.

| Recommended Peginterferon Alfa-2b Combination Therapy Dosing | | | |
|---|---|---|---|
| *Redipen* or vial strength to use (mcg/0.5 mL) | Body weight (kg) | Amount of peginterferon alfa-2b to administer (mcg) | Volume[1] of peginterferon alfa-2b to administer (mL) |
| 50 | < 40 | 50 | 0.5 |
| 80 | 40 to 50 | 64 | 0.4 |
| | 51 to 60 | 80 | 0.5 |
| 120 | 61 to 75 | 96 | 0.4 |
| | 76 to 85 | 120 | 0.5 |
| 150 | > 85 | 150 | 0.5 |

[1] When reconstituted as directed.

The recommended dose of ribavirin capsules is 800 mg/day in 2 divided doses; 2 capsules (400 mg) with breakfast and 2 capsules (400 mg) with dinner. Do not use ribavirin capsules in patients with Ccr less than 50 mL/min.

*Discontinuation:* It is recommended that patients receiving peginterferon alfa-2b alone or in combination with ribavirin be discontinued from therapy if hepatitis C virus (HCV) viral levels remain high after 6 months of therapy.

*Dose reduction:* If a serious adverse reaction develops during the course of treatment (see Warnings, Precautions), discontinue or modify the dosage of peginterferon alfa-2b and/or ribavirin capsules until the adverse reaction abates or decreases in severity. If persistent or recurrent serious adverse reactions develop despite adequate dosage adjustment, discontinue treatment. Decreases in hemoglobin, neutrophils, and platelets may require dose reduction or permanent discontinuation from therapy. For guidelines for dose modifications and discontinuation based on laboratory parameters, see the tables below.

| Guidelines for Modification or Discontinuation of Peginterferon Alfa-2b or Peginterferon Alfa-2b/Ribavirin Capsules and for Scheduling Visits for Patients with Depression | | | | | |
|---|---|---|---|---|---|
| | Initial management (4 to 8 weeks) | | Depression | | |
| Depression severity[1] | Dose modification | Visit schedule | Remains stable | Improves | Worsens |
| Mild | No change. | Evaluate once/week by visit or phone. | Continue weekly visit schedule. | Resume normal visit schedule. | (See moderate or severe depression.) |
| Moderate | Decrease IFN dose 50%. | Evaluate once/week (office visit at least every other week). | Consider psychiatric consultation. Continue reduced dosing. | If symptoms improve and are stable for 4 weeks, may resume normal visit schedule. Continue reduced dosing or return to normal dose. | (See severe depression.) |
| Severe | Discontinue IFN/R permanently. | Obtain immediate psychiatric consultation. | Psychiatric therapy necessary. | | |

[1] See DSM-IV for definitions.

| Guidelines for Dose Modification and Discontinuation of Peginterferon Alfa-2b or Peginterferon Alfa-2b/Ribavirin Capsules for Hematologic Toxicity | | | |
|---|---|---|---|
| Laboratory values | | Peginterferon alfa-2b | Ribavirin capsules |
| Hemoglobin[1] | < 10 g/dL | — | Decrease by 200 mg/day |
| | < 8.5 g/dL | Permanently discontinue | Permanently discontinue |
| WBC | $< 1.5 \times 10^9$/L | Reduce dose by 50% | — |
| | $< 1 \times 10^9$/L | Permanently discontinue | Permanently discontinue |
| Neutrophils | $< 0.75 \times 10^9$/L | Reduce dose by 50% | — |
| | $< 0.5 \times 10^9$/L | Permanently discontinue | Permanently discontinue |
| Platelets | $< 80 \times 10^9$/L | Reduce dose by 50% | — |
| | $< 50 \times 10^9$/L | Permanently discontinue | Permanently discontinue |

[1] For patients with a history of stable cardiac disease receiving peginterferon alfa-2b in combination with ribavirin capsules, reduce the peginterferon alfa-2b dose by half and the ribavirin capsule dose by 200 mg/day if a more than 2 g/dL decrease in hemoglobin is observed during any 4-week period. Permanently discontinue peginterferon alfa-2b and ribavirin capsules if patient has hemoglobin levels less than 12 g/dL after this ribavirin dose reduction.

*Reconstitution:*

   *Redipen* – To reconstitute the lyophilized peginterferon alfa-2b in the *Redipen*, hold the *Redipen* upright (dose button down) and press the two halves of the pen together until there is an audible click. Gently invert the pen to mix the solution. Do not shake. Keeping the pen upright, attach the supplied needle and select the appropriate peginterferon alfa-2b dose by pulling back on the dosing button until the dark bands are visible and turning the button until the dark band is aligned with the correct dose. The *Redipen* is for single use only.

*Vials* – Reconstitute the peginterferon alfa-2b lyophilized product with only 0.7 mL of supplied diluent (sterile water for injection). The diluent vial is for single use only. Discard the remaining diluent. Do not add any other medication to solutions containing peginterferon alfa-2b, and do not reconstitute peginterferon alfa-2b with other diluents. Swirl gently to hasten complete dissolution of the powder.

## Actions

*Pharmacology:* The biological activity of peginterferon alfa-2b is derived from its interferon alfa-2b moiety. Interferons exert their cellular activities by binding to specific membrane receptors on the cell surface and initiate a complex sequence of intracellular events.

*Pharmacokinetics:*

*Absorption/Distribution* – Maximal serum concentrations ($C_{max}$) occur between 15 and 44 hours postdose and are sustained for up to 48 to 72 hours.

*Metabolism/Excretion* – The mean peginterferon alfa-2b elimination half-life is approximately 40 hours (range, 22 to 60 hours) in patients with HCV infection. The apparent clearance of peginterferon alfa-2b is estimated to be approximately 22 mL/h•kg. Renal elimination accounts for 30% of the clearance.

Pegylation of interferon alfa-2b produces a product (peginterferon alfa-2b) whose clearance is lower than that of nonpegylated interferon alfa-2b. When compared to interferon alfa-2b, peginterferon alfa-2b (1 mcg/kg) has an approximately 7-fold lower mean apparent clearance and a 5-fold greater mean half life permitting a reduced dosing frequency.

## Contraindications

*Peginterferon alfa-2b:* Hypersensitivity to peginterferon alfa-2b or any component of the product; autoimmune hepatitis; decompensated liver disease.

*Peginterferon alfa-2b/Ribavirin capsules combination:* Hypersensitivity to ribavirin capsules or any other component of the product; pregnant women; men whose female partners are pregnant; patients with hemoglobinopathies (eg, thalassemia major, sickle-cell anemia).

## Warnings

*Neuropsychiatric events:* Life-threatening or fatal neuropsychiatric events, including suicide, suicidal and homicidal ideation, depression, relapse of drug addiction/overdose, and aggressive behavior have occurred in patients with and without a previous psychiatric disorder during peginterferon alfa-2b treatment and follow-up. Psychoses, hallucinations, bipolar disorders, and mania have been observed in patients treated with alpha interferons.

*Bone marrow toxicity:* Peginterferon alfa-2b suppresses bone marrow function, sometimes resulting in severe cytopenias. Ribavirin may potentiate the neutropenia induced by interferon alpha. Very rarely, alpha interferons may be associated with aplastic anemia.

*Colitis:* Fatal and nonfatal ulcerative or hemorrhagic/ischemic colitis have been observed within 12 weeks of the start of alpha interferon treatment. Abdominal pain, bloody diarrhea, and fever are the typical manifestations.

*Pancreatitis:* Fatal and nonfatal pancreatitis have been observed in patients treated with alpha interferons.

*Pulmonary disorders:* Dyspnea, pulmonary infiltrates, pneumonia, bronchiolitis obliterans, interstitial pneumonitis, and sarcoidosis, some resulting in respiratory failure and/or patient deaths, may be induced or aggravated by peginterferon alfa-2b or alpha-interferon therapy.

*Endocrine disorders:* Peginterferon alfa-2b causes or aggravates hypothyroidism and hyperthyroidism. Hyperglycemia has been observed in patients treated with peginterferon alfa-2b. Diabetes mellitus has been observed in patients treated with alpha interferons.

*Cardiovascular events:* Cardiovascular events, including hypotension, arrhythmia, tachycardia, cardiomyopathy, angina pectoris, and MI have been observed in patients treated with peginterferon alfa-2b.

*Autoimmune disorders:* Development or exacerbation of autoimmune disorders (eg, thyroiditis, thrombocytopenia, rheumatoid arthritis, interstitial nephritis, systemic lupus erythematosus, psoriasis) has been observed in patients receiving peginterferon alfa-2b.

*Ophthalmologic disorders:* Decrease or loss of vision, retinopathy (including macular edema), retinal artery or vein thrombosis, retinal hemorrhages and cotton wool spots, optic neuritis, and papilledema may be induced or aggravated by treatment with peginterferon alfa-2b or other alpha interferons. All patients should receive an eye examination at baseline.

*Anemia:* Ribavirin caused hemolytic anemia in 10% of peginterferon alfa-2b/ribavirin capsule-treated patients within 1 to 4 weeks of initiation of therapy. Obtain complete blood counts pretreatment and at weeks 2 and 4 of therapy or more frequently if clinically indicated.

*Hypersensitivity reactions:* Serious, acute hypersensitivity reactions (eg, urticaria, angioedema, bronchoconstriction, anaphylaxis) have been rarely observed during alpha interferon therapy.

*Renal function impairment:* Closely monitor patients with impairment of renal function for signs and symptoms of interferon toxicity and adjust doses of peginterferon alfa-2b accordingly. Use peginterferon alfa-2b with caution in patients with Ccr less than 50 mL/min.

*Elderly:* Treatment with alpha interferons, including peginterferon alfa-2b, is associated with CNS, cardiac, and systemic (flu-like) adverse effects. Because these adverse reactions may be more severe in the elderly, exercise caution in the use of interferon alfa-2b in this population.

*Pregnancy: Category* C (*Category* X if used with ribavirin). Peginterferon alfa-2b should be assumed to have abortifacient potential. Use during pregnancy only if the potential benefit justifies the potential risk to the fetus. Therefore, peginterferon alfa-2b is recommended for use in fertile women only when they are using effective contraception during the treatment period.

*Lactation:* It is not known whether the components of interferon alfa-2b are excreted in human milk.

*Children:* Safety and efficacy in pediatric patients younger than 18 years of age have not been established.

## Precautions

*Monitoring:* Patients on peginterferon alfa-2b or peginterferon alfa-2b/ribavirin capsules combination therapy should have hematology and blood chemistry testing before the start of treatment and then periodically thereafter. Measure HCV RNA at 6 months of treatment. Discontinue peginterferon alfa-2b or peginterferon alfa-2b/ribavirin capsules combination therapy in patients with persistent high viral levels. Administer an ECG to patients who have preexisting cardiac abnormalities before treatment with peginterferon alfa-2b/ribavirin capsules.

*Immunogenicity:* Approximately 2% of patients receiving peginterferon alfa-2b or interferon alfa-2b with or without ribavirin capsules developed low-titer (160 or less) neutralizing antibodies to peginterferon alfa-2b or interferon alfa-2b.

*HIV or HBV coinfections:* The safety and efficacy of peginterferon alfa-2b/ribavirin capsules for the treatment of patients with HCV coinfected with HIV or HBV have not been established.

*Organ transplants:* The safety and efficacy of peginterferon alfa-2b alone or in combination with ribavirin capsules for the treatment of hepatitis C in patients who have received liver or other organ transplants have not been studied. Preliminary data indicate that interferon alpha therapy may be associated with an increased rate of kidney graft rejection. Liver graft rejection also has been reported, but a causal association to interferon alpha therapy has not been established.

*Triglycerides:* Elevated triglyceride levels have been observed in patients treated with interferons, including peginterferon alfa-2b therapy. Manage elevated triglyceride levels as clinically appropriate. Hypertriglyceridemia may result in pancreatitis. Consider discontinuation of peginterferon alfa-2b therapy for patients with persistently elevated triglycerides (ie, triglycerides greater than 1000 mg/dL) associated with symptoms of potential pancreatitis, such as abdominal pain, nausea, or vomiting.

*Lab test abnormalities:* Peginterferon alfa-2b alone or in combination with ribavirin capsules may cause severe decreases in neutrophil and platelet counts and abnormality of TSH. In 10% of patients treated with peginterferon alfa-2b, ALT levels rose 2- to 5-fold above baseline. The elevations were transient and were not associated with deterioration of other liver functions.

## Adverse Reactions

Adverse reactions occurring in at least 3% of patients include the following: Abdominal pain; agitation; alopecia; anemia; anorexia; anxiety/emotional lability/irritability; arthralgia; asthenia; blurred vision; chest pain; concentration impaired; conjunctivitis; constipation; coughing; depression; diarrhea; dizziness; dry mouth; dry skin; dyspepsia; dyspnea; fatigue; fever; flushing; headache; hepatomegaly; hypothyroidism; injection site inflammation/reaction; insomnia; leukopenia; malaise; menstrual disorder; musculoskeletal pain; myalgia; nausea; nervousness; neutropenia; pharyngitis; pruritus; rash; rhinitis; right upper quadrant pain; rigors; sinusitis; sweating increased; taste perversion; thrombocytopenia; viral/fungal infection; vomiting; weight decrease.

# INTERFERON GAMMA-1B

**Injection:** 100 mcg (2 million units/0.5 mL) *(Rx)*       *Actimmune* (InterMune Pharm.)

## Indications

*Chronic granulomatous disease (GCD):* For reducing the frequency and severity of serious infections associated with chronic granulomatous disease.

*Osteopetrosis:* For delaying time to disease progression in patients with severe, malignant osteopetrosis.

## Administration and Dosage

*Chronic granulomatous disease:* 50 mcg/m$^2$ (1 million units/m$^2$) for patients whose body surface area is greater than 0.5 m$^2$ and 1.5 mcg/kg/dose for patients whose body surface area is less than or equal to 0.5 m$^2$. Administer subcutaneously 3 times/week (eg, Monday, Wednesday, Friday). The optimum sites of injection are the right and left deltoid and anterior thigh.

Higher doses are not recommended. Safety and efficacy have not been established for interferon gamma given in doses greater or less than the recommended dose of 50 mcg/m$^2$. The minimum effective dose has not been established.

If severe reactions occur, modify the dosage (50% reduction) or discontinue therapy until the adverse reaction abates.

The formulation does not contain a preservative. Discard the unused portion of any vial.

## Actions

*Pharmacology:* Interferon gamma-1b, a biologic response modifier, is a single-chain polypeptide containing 140 amino acids. Interferon gamma has potent phagocyte-activating effects not seen with other interferon preparations, including generation of toxic oxygen metabolites within phagocytes, which are capable of mediating the killing of microorganisms such as *Staphylococcus aureus*, *Toxoplasma gondii*, *Leishmania donovani*, *Listeria monocytogenes*, and *Mycobacterium avium intracellulare*. Interferon gamma-1b was found to enhance osteoclast function in vitro.

*Pharmacokinetics:* After IM or subcutaneous injection, the apparent fraction of dose absorbed was greater than 89%. The mean elimination half-life after IV administration was 38 minutes. The mean elimination half-lives for IM and subcutaneous dosing were 2.9 and 5.9 hours, respectively. Peak plasma concentrations occurred approximately 4 hours after IM dosing and 7 hours after subcutaneous dosing.

## Contraindications

Hypersensitivity to interferon gamma, *Escherichia coli* derived products, or any component of the product.

## Warnings

*CNS disorders:* CNS adverse reactions including decreased mental status, gait disturbance, and dizziness have been observed, particularly in patients receiving doses greater than 250 mcg/m$^2$/day. Most of these abnormalities were mild and reversible within a few days upon dose reduction or discontinuation of therapy. Exercise caution in patients with seizure disorders and compromised CNS function.

*Cardiac disease:* Use with caution in patients with pre-existing cardiac disease, including symptoms of ischemia, CHF, or arrhythmia.

*Myelosuppression:* Exercise caution in patients with myelosuppression. Reversible neutropenia and elevation of hepatic enzymes can be dose-limiting at doses greater than 250 mcg/m$^2$/day.

*Hypersensitivity reactions:* Acute serious hypersensitivity reactions have not been observed in patients receiving interferon gamma; however, if such an acute reaction develops, discontinue the drug immediately and institute appropriate medical therapy. Refer to Management of Acute Hypersensitivity Reactions.

*Pregnancy:* Category C.

*Lactation:* It is not known whether interferon gamma is excreted in breast milk.

*Children:* Safety and efficacy in children younger than 1 year of age has not been established.

## Precautions

*Monitoring:* In addition to tests normally required for monitoring patients with chronic granulomatous disease, the following laboratory tests are recommended for all patients prior to beginning therapy and at 3-month intervals during treatment: Hematologic tests including complete blood counts, differential and platelet counts; blood chemistries including renal and liver function tests; urinalysis.

## Drug Interactions

Exercise caution when administering interferon gamma in combination with other potentially myelosuppressive agents. Possible depression of CYP450 hepatic metabolism of drugs.

## Adverse Reactions

Adverse reactions may include fever, headache, rash, chills, injection site erythema or tenderness, fatigue, diarrhea, vomiting, nausea, abdominal pain, myalgia, and depression.

# INTERFERON BETA

**INTERFERON BETA-1a**
**Powder for injection, lyophilized:** 22 and 44 mcg *(Rx)*    *Rebif* (Serono)
**Powder for injection, lyophilized:** 33 mcg (6.6 mIU) *(Rx)*    *Avonex* (Biogen)
**Prefilled syringe:** 30 mcg/0.5 mL *(Rx)*

**INTERFERON BETA-1b**
**Powder for injection, lyophilized:** 0.3 mg (9.6 mIU) *(Rx)*    *Betaseron* (Berlex)

## Indications

*Interferon beta-1a:*

*Multiple sclerosis (MS)* – For the treatment of relapsing forms of MS to slow the accumulation of physical disability and decrease the frequency of clinical exacerbations.

*Interferon beta-1b:*

*MS* – For use in ambulatory patients with relapsing-remitting MS to reduce the frequency of clinical exacerbations. Relapsing-remitting MS is characterized by recurrent attacks of neurologic dysfunction followed by complete or incomplete recovery.

## Administration and Dosage

*Interferon beta-1a:*

*Avonex* – 30 mcg IM once/week.

*Rebif* – 44 mcg subcutaneously 3 times/week. Administer, if possible, at the same time on the same 3 days at least 48 hours apart each week. Generally, start patients at 8.8 mcg subcutaneously 3 times/week and increase over a 4-week period to 44 mcg 3 times/week. A starter kit containing 22 mcg syringes is available for use in titrating the dose during the first 4 weeks of treatment.

| *Rebif* Schedule for Patient Titration | | | | |
|---|---|---|---|---|
| | Recommended titration (%) | Dose (mcg) | Volume (mL) | Syringe strength (per 0.5 mL) (mcg) |
| Weeks 1 to 2 | 20 | 8.8 | 0.2 | 22 |
| Weeks 3 to 4 | 50 | 22 | 0.5 | 22 |
| Weeks 5+ | 100 | 44 | 0.5 | 44 |

Leukopenia or elevated liver function tests may necessitate dose reductions of 20% to 50% until toxicity is resolved.

*Interferon beta-1b:*

*Relapsing/Remitting MS* – 0.25 mg subcutaneously every other day.

| Interferon Beta-1b Schedule for Dose Titration | | | |
|---|---|---|---|
| | Recommended titration (%) | Interferon beta-1b dose (mg) | Volume (mL) |
| Weeks 1 to 2 | 25 | 0.0625 | 0.25 |
| Weeks 3 to 4 | 50 | 0.125 | 0.50 |
| Weeks 5 to 6 | 75 | 0.1875 | 0.75 |
| Weeks 7+ | 100 | 0.25 | 1 |

*Administration:* Sites for self-injection include arms, abdomen, hips, and thighs.

## Actions

*Pharmacology:* Interferon beta-1a and beta-1b have antiviral, antiproliferative, and immunoregulatory activities. The mechanisms by which they exert their actions in MS are not clearly understood.

*Pharmacokinetics:*

*Interferon beta-1a* – Biological response marker levels increase within 12 hours of dosing and remain elevated for at least 4 days. Peak biological response marker levels typically are observed 48 hours after dosing.

| Interferon Beta-1a Pharmacokinetic Parameters[a] | | | | |
|---|---|---|---|---|
| Route | Mean $C_{max}$ (IU/mL) | $T_{max}$ (h) | Mean AUC (IU•h/mL) | $t_{1/2}$ (h) |
| IM | 4.9 | 3 to 15 | 65 | 10 |
| Subcutaneous[b] | 5.1 | 16 (median) | 294 | 69 |

[a] Data are pooled from different studies and are not necessarily comparable.
[b] Based on a single dose of 60 mcg.

*Interferon beta-1b* – Peak serum concentrations occurred between 1 and 8 hours. Bioavailability, based on a total dose of 0.5 mg given as 2 subcutaneous injections at different sites, was approximately 50%.

Mean serum clearance values ranged from 9.4 to 28.9 mL/min/kg and were independent of dose. Mean terminal elimination half-life values ranged from 8 minutes to 4.3 hours and mean steady-state volume of distribution values ranged from 0.25 to 2.88 L/kg. IV dosing 3 times/week for 2 weeks resulted in no accumulation of interferon beta-1a or beta-1b in the serum of patients.

## Contraindications

Hypersensitivity to natural or recombinant interferon beta, albumin human, or any other component of the formulation.

## Warnings

*Chronic progressive MS:* The safety and efficacy of interferon beta in chronic progressive MS have not been evaluated.

*Depression:* Use interferon beta with caution in patients with depression or other mood disorders, conditions that are common with MS. Depression and suicide have been reported in patients receiving interferon compounds. Advise patients treated with interferon beta to immediately report any symptoms of depression or suicidal ideation.

*Injection-site necrosis (ISN):* ISN has been reported. Typically, ISN occurs within the first 4 months of therapy. Periodically re-evaluate patient understanding and use of aseptic self-injection techniques, particularly if ISN has occurred.

*Anaphylaxis:* Anaphylaxis has been reported as a rare complication of interferon beta use.

*Decreased peripheral blood counts:* Decreased peripheral blood counts in all cell lines, including rare pancytopenia and thrombocytopenia, have been reported from postmarketing experience.

*Albumin (human):* Some of these products contain albumin, a derivative of human blood. Based on effective donor screening and product manufacturing processes, it carries an extremely remote risk for transmission of viral diseases.

*Special risk patients:* Exercise caution when administering **interferon beta-1a** to patients with pre-existing seizure disorders. Seizures have been associated with the use of beta interferons.

*Cardiac disease:* Closely monitor patients with cardiac disease, such as angina, CHF, or arrhythmia, for worsening of their clinical condition during initiation and continued treatment.

*Hepatic function impairment:* Severe liver dysfunction, leading to hepatic failure requiring liver transplantation, has been reported very rarely in patients taking interferon beta.

*Fertility impairment:* Menstrual irregularities were observed in monkeys administered **interferon beta-1a** at a dose 100 times the recommended weekly human dose.

*Pregnancy:* Category C.

*Lactation:* It is not known whether interferon beta is excreted in breast milk.

*Children:* Safety and efficacy in children under 18 years of age have not been established.

## Precautions

*Monitoring:* In addition to the laboratory tests normally required for monitoring patients with MS, blood cell counts and liver function tests are recommended at baseline and regular intervals (1, 3, and 6 months) following introduction of interferon beta therapy and then periodically thereafter in the absence of clinical symptoms. Thyroid function tests are recommended every 6 months in patients with a history of thyroid dysfunction or as clinically indicated. Patients with myelosuppression may require more intensive monitoring of complete blood cell counts, with differential and platelet counts.

*Self-administration:* Instruct patients in injection techniques to ensure the safe self-administration of interferon beta.

*Flu-like symptoms complex:* Flu-like symptoms, including headache, fever, fatigue, rigors, chest pain, back pain, and myalgia, have been commonly reported with interferon beta therapy. Symptoms usually occur 4 hours after injection and subside within 24 hours. Acetaminophen or NSAIDs prior to and/or following injection may help to prevent or treat these symptoms.

*Autoimmune disorders:* Autoimmune disorders of multiple target organs have been reported postmarketing, including idiopathic thrombocytopenia, hyper- and hypothyroidism, and rare cases of autoimmune hepatitis.

*Hepatic injury:* Hepatic injury, including elevated serum hepatic enzyme levels and hepatitis, some of which have been severe, has been reported postmarketing. Monitor patients for signs of hepatic injury and exercise caution when interferons are used concomitantly with other drugs associated with hepatic injury.

*Immunogenicity:* As with all therapeutic proteins, there is a potential for immunogenicity.

*Latex sensitivity:* Administer with caution to patients with a possible history of latex sensitivity; packaging may contain dry natural rubber.

*Photosensitivity:* Photosensitization (photoallergy or phototoxicity) may occur.

## Adverse Reactions

Adverse reactions occurring in at least 3% of patients may include injection site reaction, headache, fever, flu-like symptoms, pain, asthenia, chills, infection, abdominal pain, chest pain, malaise, generalized edema, pelvic pain, injection site necrosis/inflammation, cyst/ovarian cyst, suicide attempt, hypersensitivity reaction, migraine, palpitation, hypertension, tachycardia, peripheral vascular disorder, hemorrhage, syncope, vasodilation, lymphocytes less than 1500/mm$^3$, ANC less than 3000/mm$^3$, lymphadenopathy, anemia, eosinophils at least 10%, HCT (%) up to 37, sinusitis, upper respiratory tract infection, dyspnea, laryngitis, myalgia, myasthenia, arthralgia, nausea, diarrhea, constipation, vomiting, dyspepsia, anorexia, GI disorder, ALT more than 5 times baseline, glucose less than 55 mg/dL, total bilirubin more than 2.5 times baseline, urine protein more than 1 +, AST more than 5 times baseline, weight gain/loss, AST at least 3 times the upper limit of normal, mental symptoms, hypertonia, sleep difficulty, dizziness, muscle spasm, somnolence, speech disorder, convulsion, sweating, urticaria, alopecia, nevus, herpes zoster, conjunctivitis, abnormal vision, otitis media, hearing decreased, dysmenorrhea, menstrual disorder, metrorrhagia, cystitis, breast pain, menorrhagia, urinary urgency, vaginitis, fibrocystic breast.

# ETANERCEPT

**Powder for Injection, lyophilized:** 25 mg *(Rx)*        *Enbrel*[1] (Immunex)

---

[1] Because of a probable temporary limited supply of etanercept, beginning January 1, 2001, patients must register for an *Enbrel Enrollment Card*. The enrollment cards will be needed by the pharmacy to order etanercept to fill prescriptions. Without prior enrollment, patients will be unable to receive the drug as of January 1, 2001. To register, patients need to call 1-888-4ENBREL (1-888-436-2735) 24 hours/day, 7 days/week.

## Indications

*Ankylosing spondylitis:* For reducing signs and symptoms in patients with active ankylosing spondylitis.

*Polyarticular-course juvenile rheumatoid arthritis (JRA):* For reducing signs and symptoms of moderately to severely active polyarticular-course JRA in patients who have had an inadequate response to at least 1 disease-modifying antirheumatic drug (DMARD).

*Psoriatic arthritis:* For reducing signs and symptoms of active arthritis in patients with psoriatic arthritis. It can be used in combination with MTX in patients who do not respond adequately to MTX alone.

*Rheumatoid arthritis (RA):* For reduction in signs and symptoms and inhibiting the progression of structural damage and improving physical function in moderately to severely active RA. It can be used in combination with methotrexate (MTX) in patients who do not respond adequately to MTX alone.

### Administration and Dosage

*Adults (RA, psoriatic arthritis, or ankylosing spondylitis):* 50 mg/week given as two 25 mg subcutaneous injections at separate sites. Administer dose as two 25 mg injections given either on the same day or 3 or 4 days apart. MTX, glucocorticoids, salicylates, nonsteroidal anti-inflammatory drugs (NSAIDs), or analgesics may be continued during treatment. Doses higher than 50 mg/week are not recommended.

*Children (4 to 17 years of age):* 0.8 mg/kg/week (up to a maximum of 50 mg/week). The maximum dose that should be administered at a single injection site is 25 mg (1 mL). Therefore, for pediatric patients weighing more than 31 kg (68 lb), administer the total weekly dose as 2 subcutaneous injections either on the same day or 3 or 4 days apart. Administer the dose for pediatric patients weighing 31 kg (68 lb) or less as a single subcutaneous injection once weekly. Glucocorticoids, NSAIDs, or analgesics may be continued during treatment with etanercept. Concurrent use with methotrexate and higher doses of etanercept have not been studied in pediatric patients.

*Admixture incompatibilities:* Do not add other medications to solutions containing etanercept, and do not reconstitute with other diluents.

*Self-administration:* Etanercept is intended for use under the guidance and supervision of a physician. Patients may self-inject only if the physician determines that it is appropriate and medical follow-up is provided, as necessary, after proper training in injection technique and how to measure the correct dose.

Rotate injection sites (thigh, abdomen, or upper arm). Give new injections at least 1 inch from an old site and never into areas where the skin is tender, bruised, red, or hard.

### Actions

*Pharmacology:* Etanercept is a dimeric fusion protein consisting of the extracellular ligand-binding portion of the human 75 kd (p75) tumor necrosis factor receptor (TNFR) linked to the Fc portion of human IgG1. Etanercept binds specifically to tumor necrosis factor (TNF) and blocks its interaction with cell surface TNFRs. TNF is a naturally occurring cytokine that is involved in normal inflammatory and immune responses. It plays an important role in the inflammatory processes of RA, polyarticular-course JRA, and the resulting joint pathology.

*Pharmacokinetics:*

*Absorption/Distribution* – After administration of 25 mg of etanercept by a single subcutaneous injection to 25 patients with RA, a mean half-life of approximately 102 hours was observed with a clearance of approximately 160 mL/h. A maximum serum concentration ($C_{max}$) of approximately 1.1 mcg/mL and time to $C_{max}$ of approximately 69 hours was observed in these patients. Patients exhibited a 2- to 7-fold increase in peak serum concentrations and an approximately 4-fold increase in $AUC_{0-72\ h}$ (range, 1- to 17-fold) with repeated dosing.

Pediatric patients 4 to 17 years of age with JRA were administered 0.4 mg/kg of etanercept twice weekly for up to 18 weeks. The mean serum concentration after repeated subcutaneous dosing was 2.1 mcg/mL (range, 0.7 to 4.3 mcg/mL).

### Contraindications

Sepsis; hypersensitivity to etanercept or any of its components.

### Warnings

*Infections:* In postmarketing reports, serious infections and sepsis, including fatalities, have been reported with the use of etanercept. Many of these serious infections have occurred in patients on concomitant immunosuppressive therapy that, in addition to their underlying disease, could predispose them to infections. Rare cases of tuberculosis have been observed in patients treated with TNF antagonists, including etanercept.

*Neurologic events:* Treatment with etanercept and other agents that inhibit TNF have been associated with rare cases of new onset or exacerbation of CNS demyelinating disorders, some presenting with mental status changes and some associated with permanent disability. Cases of transverse myelitis, optic neuritis, multiple sclerosis (MS), and new onset or exacerbation of seizure disorders have been observed in association with etanercept therapy. Other TNF antagonists administered to patients with multiple sclerosis have been associated with increases in disease activity. Exercise caution in considering the use of etanercept in patients with pre-existing or recent-onset CNS demyelinating disorders.

*Hematologic events:* Rare reports of pancytopenia including aplastic anemia, some fatal, have been reported in patients with RA treated with etanercept. Advise all patients to seek immediate medical attention if they develop signs and symptoms suggestive of blood dyscrasias or infection (eg, persistent fever, bruising, bleeding, pallor) while on etanercept.

*Malignancies:* In the controlled portions of clinical trials of all the TNF-blocking agents, more cases of lymphoma have been observed among patients receiving the TNF blocker compared with control patients.

Fifty-five malignancies other than lymphoma were observed. Of these, the most common malignancies were colon, breast, lung, and prostate, which were similar in type and number to what would be expected in the general population.

*Heart failure:* There have been postmarketing reports of worsening of CHF, with and without identifiable precipitating factors, in patients taking etanercept. There also have been rare reports of new onset CHF, including CHF in patients without known preexisting cardiovascular disease. Some of these patients have been younger than 50 years of age.

*Hypersensitivity reactions:* Allergic reactions associated with etanercept during clinical trials have been reported in less than 2% of patients.

*Elderly:* No overall differences in safety or effectiveness were observed in clinical trials between elderly and younger patients. However, because there is a higher incidence of infections in the elderly population in general, use caution in treating the elderly.

*Pregnancy:* Category B.

*Lactation:* It is not known whether etanercept is excreted in breast milk or absorbed systemically after ingestion. Because many drugs and immunoglobulins are excreted in breast milk and because of the potential for serious adverse reactions in nursing infants from etanercept, decide whether to discontinue nursing or to discontinue the drug.

*Children:* Etanercept has not been studied in children under 4 years of age. Preliminary data suggest the clearance of etanercept is reduced slightly in children 4 to 8 years of age.

### Precautions

*Immunogenicity:* Antibodies, all non-neutralizing, were detected at least once in sera of 5% of adult RA, psoriatic arthritis, or ankylosing spondylitis patients. No apparent correlation of antibody development to clinical response or adverse events was observed. Results from the JRA patients were similar to those seen in adult RA patients treated with etanercept.

*Injection site reactions:* In controlled trials, 37% of patients developed injection site reactions. Reactions were mild to moderate (erythema or itching, pain, or swelling) and generally did not necessitate drug discontinuation.

*Malignancies/Infections:* Anti-TNF therapies, including etanercept, affect host defenses against infections and malignancies because TNF mediates inflammation and modulates cellular immune responses.

*Vaccinations:* Do not give live vaccines concurrently with etanercept.

It is recommended that JRA patients, if possible, be brought up to date with all immunizations in agreement with current immunization guidelines prior to initiating therapy.

*Autoantibodies:* Treatment with etanercept may result in the formation of autoimmune antibodies.

*Benzyl alcohol:* Benzyl alcohol, a preservative contained in the diluent supplied, has been associated with a fatal "gasping syndrome" in premature infants.

**Adverse Reactions**

The following adverse events were reported in at least 3% of all patients: Infection; headache; rhinitis; nausea; dizziness; pharyngitis; cough; asthenia; abdominal pain; rash; respiratory disorder; dyspepsia; sinusitis; vomiting; peripheral edema; mouth ulcer; alopecia; injection site reaction.

*Children:*

*Miscellaneous* – Adverse events in children were similar in frequency and type as those in adults. Differences from adults and other special considerations are discussed below.

Severe adverse reactions reported in 69 JRA patients from 4 to 17 years of age included the following: Varicella, gastroenteritis, depression/personality disorder, cutaneous ulcer, esophagitis/gastritis, group A streptococcal septic shock, type I diabetes mellitus, soft tissue and postoperative wound infection.

The following adverse reactions were reported more commonly in 69 JRA patients receiving 3 months of etanercept compared with the 349 adult RA patients in placebo-controlled trials. These included headache (19%; 1.7 events per patient year), nausea (9%; 1 event per patient year), abdominal pain (19%; 0.74 events per patient year), and vomiting (13%; 0.74 events per patient year).

# ANAKINRA

| Injection: 100 mg/0.67 mL (*Rx*) | *Kineret* (Amgen) |
|---|---|

**Indications**

*Rheumatoid arthritis (RA):* For the reduction in signs and symptoms and slowing the progression of structural damage in moderately to severely active RA in patients 18 years of age and older who have failed 1 or more disease-modifying antirheumatic drugs (DMARDs). Anakinra can be used alone or in combination with DMARDs other than tumor necrosis factor (TNF)-blocking agents.

**Administration and Dosage**

The recommended dose of anakinra is 100 mg/day administered at approximately the same time daily by subcutaneous injection. Higher doses did not result in a higher response. Administer the dose at approximately the same time every day.

**Actions**

*Pharmacology:* Anakinra is a recombinant, nonglycosylated form of the human interleukin-1 receptor antagonist (IL-1Ra). Anakinra differs from native human IL-1Ra in that it has a single methionine residue at its amino terminus. It is produced by recombinant DNA technology using an *Escherichia coli* bacterial expression system.

Anakinra blocks the biologic activity of IL-1 by competitively inhibiting IL-1 binding to the interleukin-1 type I receptor (IL-1RI), which is expressed in a wide variety of tissues and organs.

*Pharmacokinetics:* The absolute bioavailability after a 70 mg subcutaneous bolus injection in healthy subjects (n = 11) is 95%. In subjects with RA, maximum plasma concentrations occurred 3 to 7 hours after subcutaneous administration of anakinra at clinically relevant doses (1 to 2 mg/kg; n = 18); the terminal half-life ranged from 4 to 6 hours. In RA patients, no unexpected accumulation was observed after daily subcutaneous doses for up to 24 weeks. The estimated clearance increased with increasing Ccr and body weight.

Special populations –

Renal function impairment: The mean plasma clearance decreased 70% to 75% in normal subjects with severe or end-stage renal disease (Ccr less than 30 mL/min).

## Contraindications

Patients with known hypersensitivity to *E. coli*-derived proteins, anakinra, or any component of the product.

## Warnings

*Infections:* Anakinra has been associated with an increased incidence of serious infections (2%) vs placebo (less than 1%). Discontinue administration if a patient develops a serious infection. Do not initiate treatment with anakinra in patients with active infections. The safety and efficacy of anakinra in immunocompromised patients or in patients with chronic infections have not been evaluated. Coadministration of anakinra and etanercept has not demonstrated increased clinical benefit. Carefully monitor patients when considering initiation of anakinra therapy concurrently with etanercept therapy.

*Immunosuppression:* The impact of treatment with anakinra on active and/or chronic infections and the development of malignancies is not known.

*Vaccinations:* Do not give live vaccines concurrently with anakinra. No data are available on the secondary transmission of infections by live vaccines in patients receiving anakinra. Because anakinra interferes with normal immune response mechanisms to new antigens such as vaccines, vaccination may not be effective in patients receiving anakinra.

*Hematologic events:* Patients may experience a decrease in neutrophil counts.

*Hypersensitivity reactions:* Hypersensitivity reactions associated with anakinra administration are rare. If a severe hypersensitivity reaction occurs, discontinue anakinra administration and initiate appropriate therapy.

*Renal function impairment:* This drug is known to be substantially excreted by the kidney, and the risk of toxic reactions to this drug may be greater in patients with impaired renal function.

*Elderly:* Because there is a higher incidence of infections in the elderly population in general, use caution in treating the elderly.

*Pregnancy:* Category B.

*Lactation:* It is not known whether anakinra is secreted in human milk. Because many drugs are secreted in human milk, exercise caution if anakinra is administered to nursing women.

*Children:* Safety and efficacy in patients with juvenile RA have not been established.

## Precautions

*Monitoring:* Assess neutrophil counts prior to initiating anakinra treatment, and while receiving anakinra, monthly for 3 months, and thereafter quarterly for a period up to 1 year.

*Immunogenicity:* In 2 studies, 26% of patients tested positive for anti-anakinra antibodies at month 12 in a highly sensitive, anakinra-binding biosensor assay. Of the 1318 subjects with available data at week 12 or later, 1% were seropositive in a cell-based bioassay for antibodies capable of neutralizing the biologic effects of anakinra. Two of the 15 of these subjects were positive for neutralizing antibodies at more than 1 time point up to the week 52 visit and 4 were positive at week 52. No correlation between antibody development and clinical response or adverse events was observed. The long-term immunogenicity of anakinra is unknown.

**Adverse Reactions**

The most serious adverse reactions were serious infection and neutropenia, particularly when used in combination with TNF-blocking agents. The most common adverse reaction with anakinra is injection site reactions, the majority of which were reported as mild. These typically lasted for 14 to 28 days and were characterized by 1 or more of the following reactions: Erythema, ecchymosis, inflammation, and pain.

Adverse reactions occurring in at least 5% of RA patients include injection site reaction, worsening of RA, infection (eg, upper respiratory infection, sinusitis, influenza-like symptoms, other infections), headache, nausea, diarrhea, sinusitis, arthralgia, and abdominal pain.

# MITOXANTRONE

**Injection:** 2 mg/mL (*Rx*)                              *Novantrone* (Serono)

---

**Warning:**

Administer mitoxantrone for injection concentrate under the supervision of a physician experienced in the use of cytotoxic chemotherapy agents.

Give mitoxantrone slowly into a freely flowing IV infusion. Never give subcutaneously, IM, or intra-arterially. Severe local tissue damage may occur if there is extravasation during administration (see Adverse Reactions).

Not for intrathecal use. Severe injury with permanent sequelae can result from intrathecal administration (see Warnings).

Except for the treatment of acute nonlymphocytic leukemia, mitoxantrone therapy generally should not be given to patients with baseline neutrophil counts less than 1500 cells/mm$^3$. In order to monitor the occurrence of bone marrow suppression, primarily neutropenia, which may be severe and result in infection, it is recommended that frequent peripheral blood cell counts be performed on all patients receiving mitoxantrone.

Myocardial toxicity, manifested in its most severe form by potentially fatal CHF, may occur either during therapy with mitoxantrone or months to years after termination of therapy. Mitoxantrone use has been associated with cardiotoxicity; this risk increases with cumulative dose. In cancer patients, the risk of symptomatic CHF was estimated to be 2.6% for patients receiving up to a cumulative dose of 140 mg/m$^2$. For this reason, monitor patients for evidence of cardiac toxicity and question them about symptoms of heart failure prior to initiation of treatment. Monitor patients with multiple sclerosis (MS) who reach a cumulative dose of 100 mg/m$^2$ for evidence of cardiac toxicity prior to each subsequent dose. Ordinarily, patients with MS should not receive a cumulative dose greater than 140 mg/m$^2$. Active or dormant cardiovascular disease, prior or concomitant radiotherapy to the mediastinal/pericardial area, previous therapy with other anthracyclines or anthracenediones, or concomitant use of other cardiotoxic drugs may increase the risk of cardiac toxicity. Cardiac toxicity with mitoxantrone may occur at lower cumulative doses whether or not cardiac risk factors are present (see Warnings and Administration and Dosage).

> **Warning: (cont.)**
> Secondary acute myelogenous leukemia (AML) has been reported in cancer patients
> treated with anthracyclines. Mitoxantrone is an anthracenedione, a related drug.
> Secondary AML has also been reported in cancer patients and MS patients who
> have been treated with mitoxantrone. The occurrence of refractory second-
> ary leukemia is more common when anthracyclines are given in combination with
> DNA-damaging antineoplastic agents, when patients have been heavily pre-
> treated with cytotoxic drugs, or when doses of anthracyclines have been esca-
> lated. The cumulative risk of developing treatment-related AML, in 1774 patients
> with breast cancer who received mitoxantrone concomitantly with other cyto-
> toxic agents and radiotherapy, was estimated as 1.1% and 1.6% at 5 and 10 years,
> respectively (see Warnings).

### Indications
MS: For reducing neurologic disability and/or the frequency of clinical relapses in
patients with secondary (chronic) progressive, progressive relapsing, or worsening relapsing-remitting MS (ie, patients whose neurologic status is significantly
abnormal between relapses). Mitoxantrone is not indicated in the treatment of
patients with primary progressive MS.

Mitoxantrone also is used in combination with other medications for prostate cancer
and acute nonlymphocytic leukemia in adults.

### Administration and Dosage
MS: 12 mg/m$^2$ given as a short (approximately 5 to 15 minutes) IV infusion every
3 months.

Evaluation of left ventricular ejection fraction (LVEF) is recommended prior to
administration of the initial dose of mitoxantrone. Subsequent LVEF evaluations are
recommended if signs or symptoms of CHF develop, and prior to all doses administered to patients who have received a cumulative dose of 100 mg/m$^2$ or more.
Do not administer mitoxantrone to MS patients who have received a cumulative
lifetime dose of 140 mg/m$^2$ or more, or those with either LVEF of less than 50% or
a clinically significant reduction in LVEF.

Monitor complete blood counts, including platelets, prior to each course of mitoxantrone and in the event that signs or symptoms of infection develop. Mitoxantrone
generally should not be administered to MS patients with neutrophil counts less
than 1500 cells/mm$^3$. Monitor liver function tests prior to each course. Mitoxantrone therapy in MS patients with abnormal liver function tests is not recommended because mitoxantrone clearance is reduced by hepatic impairment.

*Preparation and administration:* Dilute to at least 50 mL with either 0.9% Sodium Chloride Injection or 5% Dextrose Injection. Mitoxantrone may be further diluted into
Dextrose 5% in Water, Normal Saline, or 5% Dextrose with Normal Saline, and
used immediately. Introduce this solution slowly into the tubing as a freely running IV infusion over a period of not less than 3 minutes. The tubing should be
attached to a butterfly needle or other suitable device and inserted preferably into
a large vein. If possible, avoid veins over joints or in extremities with compromised venous or lymphatic drainage.

If extravasation occurs, stop administration immediately and restart in another
vein. Carefully monitor the extravasation site for signs of necrosis or phlebitis.

*IV incompatibility:* Do not mix in the same infusion as heparin. Mitoxantrone not be
mixed in the same infusion with other drugs.

Women with MS who are biologically capable of becoming pregnant, even if they
are using birth control, should have a pregnancy test, and the results must be
known before receiving each dose of mitoxantrone.

### Actions
*Pharmacology:* Mitoxantrone is a synthetic antineoplastic anthracenedione.

It has a cytocidal effect on both proliferating and nonproliferating cultured human cells, suggesting lack of cell cycle phase specificity.

*Pharmacokinetics:*

*Absorption/Distribution* – The mean alpha half-life of mitoxantrone is 6 to 12 minutes, the mean beta half-life is 1.1 to 3.1 hours, and the mean gamma (terminal or elimination) half-life is 23 to 215 hours. Distribution to tissues is extensive: Steady-state volume of distribution exceeds 1000 L/m$^2$. Mitoxantrone is 78% bound to plasma proteins.

*Metabolism/Excretion* – Mitoxantrone is excreted in urine and feces as either unchanged drug or as inactive metabolites.

## Contraindications

Hypersensitivity to mitoxantrone.

## Warnings

*Myelosuppression:* When mitoxantrone is used in high doses (more than 14 mg/m$^2$/day for 3 days), severe myelosuppression will occur. Assure full hematologic recovery before undertaking consolidation therapy and monitor patients closely during this phase.

Patients with preexisting myelosuppression as the result of prior drug therapy should not receive mitoxantrone unless the possible benefit warrants the risk of further suppression.

*Cardiac:*

MS – Functional cardiac changes may occur in patients with MS treated with mitoxantrone.

Functional cardiac changes including irreversible CHF and decreases in LVEF can occur. Cardiac toxicity may be more common in patients with prior treatment with anthracyclines, prior mediastinal radiotherapy, or with preexisting cardiovascular disease. Such patients should have regular cardiac monitoring of LVEF from the initiation of therapy.

*Secondary leukemia:* Secondary leukemia has been reported in cancer patients and multiple sclerosis patients treated with mitoxantrone.

*Acute leukemia/myelodysplasia:* Topoisomerase II inhibitors, including mitoxantrone, have been associated with the development of acute leukemia and myelodysplasia.

*Hepatic function impairment:* Patients with severe hepatic dysfunction have an AUC more than 3 times greater than that of patients with normal hepatic function receiving the same dose. Administer mitoxantrone with caution to other patients with hepatic impairment; a dosage adjustment may be required.

*Pregnancy: Category D.*

*Lactation:* Mitoxantrone is excreted in breast milk. Because of the potential for serious adverse reactions in infants, discontinue breastfeeding before starting treatment.

*Children:* Safety and efficacy for use in children have not been established.

## Precautions

*Monitoring:* Frequently observe the patient and monitor hematologic and chemical laboratory parameters. Obtain a complete blood count, including platelets, prior to each course of mitoxantrone and in the event that signs and symptoms of infection develop. Liver function tests should also be performed prior to each course of therapy.

Women with MS who are biologically capable of becoming pregnant, even if they are using birth control, should have a pregnancy test and the results should be known before receiving each dose of mitoxantrone (see Warnings).

*Hyperuricemia* – Monitor serum uric acid levels and institute hypouricemic therapy prior to the initiation of antileukemic therapy.

*For IV use only:* Mitoxantrone is not indicated for subcutaneous, IM, or intra-arterial injection.

Mitoxantrone must not be given by intrathecal injection. Neuropathy and neurotoxicity have been reported. These reports have included seizures leading to coma and severe neurologic sequelae, and paralysis with bowel and bladder dysfunction.

*Systemic infections:* Treat concomitantly with or just before starting mitoxantrone.

### Adverse Reactions
*Use in MS:* Adverse drug reactions occurring in at least 3% of patients include the following: Alopecia; amenorrhea; anemia; arrhythmia; ALT high; ANC low (less than 1500 cells/mm$^3$); aphthosis; AST high; asthenia; back pain; constipation; cutaneous mycosis; diarrhea; ECG abnormal; gamma-GT increased; gastralgia/stomach burn/epigastric pain; glucose high; granulocytopenia (less than 2000 cells/mm$^3$); headache; hemoglobin low; infection; leukopenia (less than 4000 cells/mm$^3$); lymphocytes low; menorrhagia (female patients); menstrual disorder; nausea; pharyngitis/throat infection; platelets low (less than 100,000 cells/mm$^3$); potassium low; rhinitis; sinusitis; stomatitis; UTI; urine abnormal; upper respiratory tract infection; WBC low (less than 4000 cells/mm$^3$).

## HYDROXYCHLOROQUINE SULFATE

| **Tablets**: 200 mg (equiv. to 155 mg base) | Various, *Plaquenil* (Sanofi Synthelabo) |
| --- | --- |

> **Warning:**
> Physicians should completely familiarize themselves with the complete contents of the package insert before prescribing hydroxychloroquine.

### Indications
*Lupus erythematosus:* For the treatment of chronic discoid and systemic lupus erythematosus (SLE) in patients who have not responded satisfactorily to drugs with less potential for serious side effects.

*Malaria:* For the suppressive treatment and treatment of acute attacks of malaria caused by *Plasmodium vivax, P. malariae, P. ovale,* and susceptible strains of *P. falciparum.*

*Rheumatoid arthritis (RA):* For the treatment of acute or chronic RA in patients who have not responded satisfactorily to drugs with less potential for serious side effects.

### Administration and Dosage
*Lupus erythematosus:* Initially, 400 mg once or twice daily in adults, continued for several weeks or months depending on response. For prolonged maintenance therapy, 200 to 400 mg daily frequently will suffice.

*RA:* Initially, 400 to 600 mg daily, taken with a meal or a glass of milk. Side effects may require temporary reduction. Later (usually from 5 to 10 days), dose may be increased gradually to optimum response level. For maintenance therapy, when a good response is obtained (usually in 4 to 12 weeks), reduce dosage by 50% and continue at a level of 200 to 400 mg daily.

Maximum effects may not be obtained for several months. If objective improvement (reduced joint swelling, increased mobility) does not occur within 6 months, discontinue the drug.

If relapse occurs after drug withdrawal, resume therapy or continue on an intermittent schedule if there are no ocular contraindications.

Corticosteroids and salicylates may be used with this compound; generally they can be decreased gradually or eliminated after hydroxychloroquine has been used for several weeks.

### Actions
*Pharmacology:* The precise mechanism of action is not known.

*Pharmacokinetics:*

*Absorption/Distribution* – Hydroxychloroquine is absorbed very rapidly and almost completely after oral administration. Hydroxychloroquine is distributed widely into body tissues and concentrates in the spleen, liver, kidney, melanin-containing tissues, and lungs. It has a large apparent volume of distribution (more than 100 L/kg). It is bound approximately 60% to plasma proteins.

## Contraindications

Retinal or visual field changes attributable to any 4-aminoquinoline compound; hypersensitivity to 4-aminoquinoline compounds; long-term therapy in children.

## Warnings

*Psoriasis:* Use in patients with psoriasis may precipitate a severe attack. Porphyria may be exacerbated. Do not use unless the benefit to the patient outweighs possible risks.

*Ophthalmic effects:* Irreversible retinal damage has been observed in some patients who had received long-term or high-dosage 4-aminoquinoline therapy for discoid and SLE or RA. When prolonged therapy is contemplated, perform initial (baseline) and periodic (every 3 months) ophthalmologic examinations (including visual acuity, expert slit-lamp, funduscopic, and visual field tests).

*Retinal changes* – Retinal changes and visual disturbances may progress even after cessation of therapy.

*Muscular weakness:* Examine patients on long-term therapy periodically, and test knee and ankle reflexes to detect evidence of muscular weakness. If weakness occurs, discontinue drug.

*RA:* In RA, discontinue if objective improvement does not occur within 6 months.

*Renal/Hepatic function impairment:* Use with caution.

*Pregnancy:* According to *Drugs in Pregnancy and Lactation* by Briggs, the pregnancy risk factor is a *Category* C. The Centers for Disease Control and Prevention recommends use for prophylaxis in pregnant women who are traveling to areas with chloroquine-sensitive *P. falciparum* malaria.

Avoid use during pregnancy, except in the suppression of malaria when the benefit outweighs the possible hazard.

*Lactation:* The drug has been detected in breast milk from 2 mothers receiving 400 mg daily doses for SLE or RA.

*Children:* Children are especially sensitive to 4-aminoquinolines. Safe use of the drug in the treatment of JRA and SLE has not been established.

## Precautions

*Monitoring:* Perform periodic blood cell counts during prolonged therapy. If a severe blood disorder appears, consider discontinuation. Use caution in glucose-6-phosphate dehydrogenase (G-6-PD) deficiency.

*Hepatic disease:* Use with caution in patients with hepatic disease or in conjunction with hepatotoxic drugs.

*Alcoholism:* Use with caution in patients with alcoholism.

*Dermatologic reactions:* Dermatologic reactions may occur; exercise care when given to any patient receiving a drug with significant tendency to produce dermatitis.

*Toxic symptoms:* If serious toxic symptoms occur, administer ammonium chloride (8 g daily in divided doses for adults) 3 or 4 days a week for several months after therapy has been stopped; acidification of the urine increases renal excretion by 20% to 90%. Exercise caution in renal function impairment and/or metabolic acidosis.

## Drug Interactions

Drugs that may affect hydroxychloroquine include cimetidine. Drugs that may be affected by hydroxychloroquine include beta blockers, cyclosporine, digoxin, magnesium salts, and mefloquine.

**Adverse Reactions**

The following have occurred with 1 or more of the 4-aminoquinoline compounds.

*CNS:* Ataxia; convulsions; dizziness; emotional changes; headache; irritability; nerve deafness; nervousness; nightmares; nystagmus; psychosis; tinnitus; vertigo.

*Dermatologic:* Alopecia; bleaching of hair; photosensitivity; precipitation of nonlight-sensitive psoriasis; pruritus; skin and mucosal pigmentation; skin eruptions (urticarial, morbilliform, lichenoid, maculopapular, purpuric, erythema annulare centrifugum, Stevens-Johnson syndrome, acute generalized exanthematous pustulosis, and exfoliative dermatitis).

*GI:* Abdominal cramps; anorexia; diarrhea; nausea; vomiting.

*Hematologic:* Agranulocytosis; aplastic anemia; hemolysis in individuals with G-6-PD deficiency; leukopenia; thrombocytopenia.

*Musculoskeletal:* Skeletal muscle palsies, myopathy, or neuromyopathy leading to progressive weakness and atrophy of proximal muscle groups, depression of tendon reflexes, and abnormal nerve conduction.

*Ophthalmic:*

   *Ciliary body* – See Warnings. Disturbance of accommodation with blurred vision. This reaction is dose-related and reversible with cessation of therapy.

   *Cornea* – Decreased corneal sensitivity; punctate to lineal opacities; transient edema.

   *Retina* – Abnormal pigmentation (mild pigment stippling to a "bull's eye" appearance); atrophy; edema; elevated retinal threshold to red light in macular, paramacular, and peripheral retinal areas; increased macular recovery time following exposure to a bright light (photo-stress test); loss of foveal reflex.

   *Retinopathy* – Reading and seeing difficulties (ie, words, letters, or parts of objects missing); photophobia; blurred distance vision; missing or blacked out areas in the central or peripheral visual field; light flashes and streaks.

   *Other fundus changes* – Attenuation of retinal arterioles; fine granular pigmentary disturbances in the peripheral retina; optic disc pallor and atrophy; prominent choroidal patterns in advanced stage.

   *Visual field defects* – Central scotoma with decreased visual acuity; field constriction (rare); pericentral or paracentral scotoma.

*Miscellaneous:* Weight loss; lassitude; exacerbation or precipitation of porphyria.

# Chapter 11

# DERMATOLOGICAL AGENTS

# ISOTRETINOIN (13-cis-Retinoic Acid)

**Capsules:**[1] 10, 20, and 40 mg         *Accutane* (Roche), *Claravis* (Barr Laboratories)

[1] Capsule contains suspension of drug in soybean oil; also contains parabens and EDTA.

**Warning:**

Isotretinoin must not be used by females who are pregnant. Although not every fetus exposed to isotretinoin has resulted in a deformed child, there is an extremely high risk that a deformed infant can result if pregnancy occurs while taking isotretinoin in any amount even for short periods of time. Potentially any fetus exposed during pregnancy can be affected. Presently, there are no accurate means of determining, after isotretinoin exposure, which fetus has been affected and which fetus has not been affected.

Major human fetal abnormalities related to isotretinoin administration in females have been documented. There is an increased risk of spontaneous abortion. In addition, premature births have been reported.

Documented external abnormalities include the following: Skull abnormality; ear abnormalities (including anotia, micropinna, small or absent external auditory canals); eye abnormalities (including microphthalmia); facial dysmorphia; cleft palate. Documented internal abnormalities include the following: CNS abnormalities (including cerebral abnormalities, cerebellar malformation, hydrocephalus, microcephaly, cranial nerve deficit); cardiovascular abnormalities; thymus gland abnormality; parathyroid hormone deficiency. In some cases death has occurred with certain of the abnormalities previously noted.

Cases of IQ scores less than 85 with or without obvious CNS abnormalities also have been reported.

Isotretinoin is contraindicated in females of childbearing potential unless the patient meets all of the following conditions:

- Must not be pregnant or breastfeeding,
- Must be capable of complying with mandatory contraceptive measures required for isotretinoin therapy and understand behaviors associated with an increased risk of pregnancy, and
- Must be reliable in understanding and carrying out instructions.

*Accutane* must be prescribed under the System to Manage Accutane-Related Teratogenicity (SMART). The prescriber must obtain a supply of yellow self-adhesive *Accutane* qualification stickers. To obtain these stickers: 1) Read the booklet entitled *SMART Guide to Best Practices*; 2) sign and return the completed SMART letter of understanding containing the prescriber checklist; and 3) use the yellow self-adhesive *Accutane* qualification sticker. *Accutane* should not be prescribed or dispensed to any patient (male or female) without a yellow self-adhesive *Accutane* qualification sticker.

**Warning: (cont.)**

*Female patients:* For female patients, the yellow self-adhesive *Accutane* qualification sticker signifies that she understands the following:

- Must have had 2 negative urine or serum pregnancy tests with a sensitivity of at least 25 milliunits/mL before receiving the initial isotretinoin prescription. The first test (a screening test) is obtained by the prescriber when the decision is made to pursue qualification of the patient for isotretinoin. The second pregnancy test (a confirmation test) should be done during the first 5 days of the menstrual period immediately preceding the beginning of isotretinoin therapy. For patients with amenorrhea, the second test should be done at least 11 days after the last act of unprotected sexual intercourse (without using 2 effective forms of contraception). Each month of therapy, the patient must have a negative result from a urine or serum pregnancy test. A pregnancy test must be repeated every month prior to the female patient receiving each prescription. The manufacturer will make available urine pregnancy test kits for female isotretinoin patients for the initial, second, and monthly testing during therapy.

- Must have selected and has committed to using 2 forms of effective contraception simultaneously, at least 1 of which must be a primary form, unless absolute abstinence is the chosen method, or the patient has undergone a hysterectomy. Patients must use 2 forms of effective contraception for at least 1 month prior to initiation of isotretinoin therapy, during isotretinoin therapy, and for 1 month after discontinuing isotretinoin therapy. Counseling about contraception and behaviors associated with an increased risk of pregnancy must be repeated on a monthly basis.

Effective forms of contraception include both primary and secondary forms of contraception. Primary forms of contraception include: Tubal ligation, partner's vasectomy, intrauterine devices, birth control pills, and injectable/implantable/insertable hormonal birth control products. Secondary forms of contraception include diaphragms, latex condoms, and cervical caps; each must be used with a spermicide.

Any birth control method can fail. Therefore, it is critically important that women of childbearing potential use 2 effective forms of contraception simultaneously. A drug interaction that decreases effectiveness of hormonal contraceptives has not been entirely ruled out for isotretinoin. Although hormonal contraceptives are highly effective, there have been reports of pregnancy from women who have used oral contraceptives, as well as injectable/implantable contraceptive products. These reports occurred while these patients were taking isotretinoin. These reports are more frequent for women who use only a single method of contraception. Patients must receive written warnings about the rates of possible contraception failure (included in patient education kits).

Prescribers are advised to consult the package insert of any medication administered concomitantly with hormonal contraceptives, because some medications may decrease the effectiveness of these birth control products. Patients should be prospectively cautioned not to self-medicate with the herbal supplement St. John's wort because a possible interaction has been suggested with hormonal contraceptives based on reports of breakthrough bleeding while on oral contraceptives shortly after starting St. John's wort. Pregnancies have been reported by users of combined hormonal contraceptives who also used some form of St. John's wort.

- Must have signed a patient information/consent form that contains warnings about the risk of potential birth defects if the fetus is exposed to isotretinoin.

- Must have been informed of the purpose and importance of participating in the *Accutane* survey and have been given the opportunity to enroll.

**Warning: (cont.)**
The yellow self-adhesive *Accutane* qualification sticker documents that the female patient is qualified and includes the date of qualification, patient gender, cut-off date for filling the prescription, and up to a 30-day supply limit with no refills.

If a pregnancy does occur during treatment with isotretinoin, the prescriber and patient should discuss the desirability of continuing the pregnancy. Prescribers are strongly encouraged to report all cases of pregnancy to Roche at (800) 526-6367 where a Roche pregnancy prevention program specialist will be available to discuss Roche pregnancy information, or prescribers may contact the FDA MedWatch program at (800) FDA-1088.

Isotretinoin should be prescribed only by prescribers who have demonstrated special competence in the diagnosis and treatment of severe recalcitrant nodular acne, are experienced in the use of systemic retinoids, have read the *SMART Guide to Best Practices*, signed and returned the completed SMART letter of understanding, and obtained yellow self-adhesive *Accutane* qualification stickers. Do not prescribe or dispense *Accutane* without a yellow self-adhesive *Accutane* qualification sticker.

*Male patients:* These yellow self-adhesive *Accutane* qualification stickers also should be used for male patients.

*Information for pharmacists:* Isotretinoin must only be dispensed as follows:
- In no more than 30-day supply.
- Only on presentation of an *Accutane* prescription with a yellow self-adhesive *Accutane* qualification sticker.
- Prescription written within the previous 7 days.
- Refills require a new prescription with a yellow self-adhesive *Accutane* qualification sticker.
- No telephone or computerized prescriptions are permitted.

An *Accutane* medication guide must be given to the patient each time isotretinoin is dispensed, as required by law. This guide is an important part of the risk management program for the patient.

### Indications

*Severe recalcitrant nodular acne:* Nodules are inflammatory lesions with a diameter of 5 mm or greater. The nodules may become suppurative or hemorrhagic. "Severe," by definition, means "many" as opposed to "few or several" nodules.

Adverse effects are significant; reserve treatment for patients unresponsive to conventional therapy, including systemic antibiotics. In addition, isotretinoin is indicated only for those females who are not pregnant, because isotretinoin can cause severe birth defects. A single course of therapy for 15 to 20 weeks has resulted in complete, prolonged remission in many patients. If a second course is needed, do not initiate therapy until at least 8 weeks after completion of the first course. Patients may continue to improve while not receiving the drug. The optimal interval before retreatment has not been defined for patients who have not completed skeletal growth.

### Administration and Dosage

Individualize dosage. Adjust the dose according to side effects and disease response.

*Recommended course of therapy:* The recommended dose is 0.5 to 1 mg/kg/day divided into 2 doses for 15 to 20 weeks. Administer isotretinoin with food. Adult patients whose disease is very severe with scarring or is primarily manifested on the trunk may require up to the maximum recommended dose, 2 mg/kg/day, as tolerated. Failure to take isotretinoin with food will significantly decrease absorption. Before upward dose adjustments are made, question patients about their compliance with food instructions. The safety of once-daily dosing with isotretinoin has not been established. Once-daily dosing is not recommended. If the total nodule count decreases by more than 70% prior to completing 15 to 20 weeks of treatment, the drug may be discontinued. After 2 months or more off therapy, and if warranted by persistent or recurring severe nodular acne, a second course of therapy may be initiated.

In studies comparing 0.1, 0.5, and 1 mg/kg/day, all doses provided initial clearing of disease, but there was a greater need for retreatment with the lower doses.

| Isotretinoin Dosing by Body Weight | | | | |
|---|---|---|---|---|
| Body weight | | Total mg/day | | |
| kg | lbs | 0.5 mg/kg | 1 mg/kg | 2 mg/kg[1] |
| 40 | 88 | 20 | 40 | 80 |
| 50 | 110 | 25 | 50 | 100 |
| 60 | 132 | 30 | 60 | 120 |
| 70 | 154 | 35 | 70 | 140 |
| 80 | 176 | 40 | 80 | 160 |
| 90 | 198 | 45 | 90 | 180 |
| 100 | 220 | 50 | 100 | 200 |

[1] The recommended dosage range is 0.5 to 1 mg/kg/day.

## Actions

*Pharmacology:* Isotretinoin is a retinoid that, when administered in pharmacologic dosages of 0.5 to 1 mg/kg/day, inhibits sebaceous gland function and keratinization. The exact mechanism of action of isotretinoin is unknown.

Clinical improvement in nodular acne occurs in association with a reduction in sebum secretion. The decrease in sebum secretion is temporary, is related to the dose and duration of treatment with isotretinoin, and reflects a reduction in sebaceous gland size and an inhibition of sebaceous gland differentiation.

*Pharmacokinetics:*

*Absorption* – Because of its high lipophilicity, oral absorption of isotretinoin is enhanced when given with a high-fat meal. In a crossover study, 74 healthy adult subjects received a single 80 mg oral dose (two 40 mg capsules) of isotretinoin under fasted and fed conditions. Peak plasma concentration ($C_{max}$) and the total exposure (AUC) of isotretinoin were more than doubled following a standardized high-fat meal when compared with isotretinoin given under fasted conditions. The observed elimination half-life was unchanged. This lack of change in half-life suggests that food increases the bioavailability of isotretinoin without altering its disposition. The time to peak concentration ($T_{max}$) also was increased with food and may be related to a longer absorption phase. Therefore, isotretinoin always should be taken with food.

| Pharmacokinetic Parameters of Isotretinoin Mean (%CV), N = 74 | | | | |
|---|---|---|---|---|
| Isotretinoin 2 × 40 mg capsules | $AUC_{(0-\infty)}$ (ng•h/mL) | $C_{max}$ (ng/mL) | $T_{max}$ (h) | $t_{1/2}$ (h) |
| Fed[1] | 10,004 (22%) | 862 (22%) | 5.3 (77%) | 21 (39%) |
| Fasted | 3703 (46%) | 301 (63%) | 3.2 (56%) | 21 (30%) |

[1] Eating a standardized high-fat meal.

*Distribution* – Isotretinoin is more than 99.9% bound to plasma proteins, primarily albumin.

*Metabolism* – Following oral administration of isotretinoin, at least 3 metabolites have been identified in human plasma: 4-*oxo*-isotretinoin, retinoic acid (tretinoin), and 4-*oxo*-retinoic acid (4-*oxo*-tretinoin). Retinoic acid and 13-*cis*-retinoic acid are geometric isomers and show reversible interconversion. The administration of one isomer will give rise to the other. Isotretinoin also is irreversibly oxidized to 4-*oxo*-isotretinoin, which forms its geometric isomer 4-*oxo*-tretinoin.

After a single 80 mg oral dose of isotretinoin to 74 healthy adult subjects, concurrent administration of food increased the extent of formation of all metabolites in plasma when compared with the extent of formation under fasted conditions.

All of these metabolites possess retinoid activity that is in some in vitro models more than that of the parent isotretinoin. However, the clinical significance of these models is unknown. After multiple oral dose administration of isotretinoin to adult cystic acne patients (18 years of age and older), the exposure of patients to 4-oxo-isotretinoin at steady state under fasted and fed conditions was approximately 3.4 times higher than that of isotretinoin. In vitro studies indicated that the primary P450 isoforms involved in isotretinoin metabolism are 2C8, 2C9, 3A4, and 2B6. Isotretinoin and its metabolites are further metabolized into conjugates, which are then excreted in urine and feces.

*Excretion* – Following oral administration of an 80 mg dose of $^{14}$C-isotretinoin as a liquid suspension, $^{14}$C-activity in blood declined with a half-life of 90 hours. The metabolites of isotretinoin and any conjugates are ultimately excreted in the feces and urine in relatively equal amounts (total of 65% to 83%). After a single 80 mg oral dose of isotretinoin to 74 healthy adult subjects under fed conditions, the mean elimination half-lives of isotretinoin and 4-oxo-isotretinoin were approximately 21 and 24 hours, respectively. After single and multiple doses, the observed accumulation ratios of isotretinoin ranged from 0.9 to 5.43 in patients with cystic acne.

## Contraindications

Pregnancy (see Warning Box); hypersensitivity to this medication or any of its components; hypersensitivity to parabens (used as a preservative in the formulation).

## Warnings

*Psychiatric disorders:* Isotretinoin may cause depression, psychosis, and rarely, suicidal ideation, suicide attempts, suicide, and aggressive or violent behavior. Discontinuation of isotretinoin therapy may be insufficient; further evaluation may be necessary. No mechanism of action has been established for these events.

*Pseudotumor cerebri (benign intracranial hypertension):* Isotretinoin use has been associated with a number of cases of pseudotumor cerebri, some of which involved concomitant use of tetracyclines. Therefore, avoid concomitant treatment with tetracyclines. Early signs and symptoms include papilledema, headache, nausea, vomiting, and visual disturbances. Screen patients with these symptoms for papilledema; if present, discontinue drug immediately and consult a neurologist.

*Pancreatitis:* Acute pancreatitis has been reported in patients with elevated or normal serum triglyceride levels. In rare instances, fatal hemorrhagic pancreatitis has been reported. Stop isotretinoin if hypertriglyceridemia cannot be controlled at an acceptable level or if symptoms of pancreatitis occur.

*Visual impairment:* Carefully monitor visual problems. If visual difficulties occur, discontinue the drug and have an ophthalmological examination.

*Corneal opacities* – These have appeared in patients receiving isotretinoin for acne and more frequently in patients on higher dosages for keratinization disorders. Corneal opacities have either completely resolved or were resolving at followup 6 to 7 weeks after discontinuation.

*Decreased night vision* – Decreased night vision has occurred during therapy and in some cases persisted after therapy was discontinued. Because the onset in some patients was sudden, advise patients of this potential problem and warn them to be cautious when driving or operating any vehicle at night.

*Inflammatory bowel disease:* Inflammatory bowel disease, including regional ileitis, has been associated with isotretinoin in patients without a history of intestinal disorders. In some instances, symptoms have been reported to persist after isotretinoin therapy has been stopped. Discontinue treatment immediately if abdominal pain, rectal bleeding, or severe diarrhea occurs.

*Hypertriglyceridemia:* Hypertriglyceridemia in excess of 800 mg/dL occurred in approximately 25% of patients; approximately 15% developed a decrease in high density lipoproteins (HDL) and approximately 7% showed an increase in cholesterol levels. Perform blood lipid determinations before isotretinoin is given and then at intervals until the lipid response to isotretinoin is established, which usually occurs within 4 weeks.

These effects are reversible after cessation of therapy. Patients who are at high risk of developing hypertriglyceridemia include those with diabetes, obesity, increased alcohol intake, a lipid metabolism disorder, and a familial history.

Reduction of weight, dietary fat intake, alcohol intake, and dose may reverse the effects on serum triglycerides, allowing patients to continue therapy.

*Musculoskeletal effects:* In a clinical trial (N = 217) of a single course of therapy for isotretinoin, 7.9% of patients had decreases in lumbar spine bone mineral density greater than 4%, and 10.6% of patients had decreases in total hip bone mineral density greater than 5%.

Spontaneous reports of osteoporosis, osteopenia, bone fractures, and delayed healing of bone fractures have been seen in the isotretinoin population. While causality to isotretinoin has not been established, an effect cannot be ruled out. Physicians should use caution when prescribing isotretinoin to patients with a genetic predisposition for age-related osteoporosis, a history of childhood osteoporosis conditions, osteomalacia, or other disorders of bone metabolism. This would include patients diagnosed with anorexia nervosa and those who are on chronic drug therapy that causes drug-induced osteoporosis/osteomalacia and/or affects vitamin D metabolism, such as systemic corticosteroids and any anticonvulsants.

There are spontaneous reports of premature epiphyseal closure in acne patients receiving recommended doses of isotretinoin.

In clinical trials for disorders of keratinization, a high prevalence of skeletal hyperostosis was noted with a mean dose of 2.24 mg/kg/day.

Minimal skeletal hyperostosis and calcification of ligaments and tendons has been observed by x-ray in prospective studies of nodular acne patients treated with a single course of therapy at recommended doses. The skeletal effects of multiple isotretinoin treatment courses for acne are unknown.

*Hepatotoxicity:* Clinical hepatitis possibly or probably related to isotretinoin therapy has been reported. Additionally, mild to moderate elevations of liver enzymes have been seen in approximately 15% of patients, some of whom normalized with dosage reduction or continued administration of the drug. If normalization does not readily occur, or if hepatitis is suspected, stop the drug and further investigate etiology.

*Hearing impairment:* Impaired hearing has been reported in patients taking isotretinoin; in some cases, the hearing impairment has been reported to persist after therapy has been discontinued. Mechanisms and causality for this event have not been established. Patients who experience tinnitus or hearing impairment should discontinue isotretinoin treatment and be referred to specialized care for further evaluation.

*Hormonal contraceptives:* Microdosed progesterone preparations (minipills) may be an inadequate method of contraception during isotretinoin therapy. Although other hormonal contraceptives are highly effective, there have been reports of pregnancy from women who have used combined oral contraceptives, as well as injectable/implantable contraceptive products. These reports are more frequent for women who use only a single method of contraception. It is not known if hormonal contraceptives differ in their effectiveness when used with isotretinoin. Therefore, it is critically important that women of childbearing potential use 2 effective forms of contraception simultaneously, at least 1 of which must be a primary form, unless absolute abstinence is the chosen method, or the patient has undergone a hysterectomy (see Warning Box).

*Hypersensitivity reactions:* Anaphylactic reactions and other allergic reactions have been reported. Cutaneous allergic reactions and serious cases of allergic vasculitis, often with purpura (bruises and red patches), of the extremities and extracutaneous involvement (including renal) have been reported. Severe allergic reaction necessitates discontinuation of therapy and appropriate medical management.

*Carcinogenesis:* In male and female Fischer 344 rats given oral isotretinoin at dosages of 8 or 32 mg/kg/day (1.3 to 5.3 times the recommended clinical dose of 1 mg/kg/day, respectively, after normalization for total body surface area) for more than 18 months, there was a dose-related increased incidence of pheochromocytoma relative to controls. The incidence of adrenal medullary hyperplasia also was increased at the higher dosage in both sexes.

*Pregnancy: Category* X (see Warning Box).

*Lactation:* It is not known whether this drug is excreted in breast milk. Because of the potential for adverse effects, do not give to a nursing mother.

*Children:* The use of isotretinoin in pediatric patients less than 12 years of age has not been studied. Carefully consider isotretinoin use in pediatric patients 12 to 17 years of age, especially for those patients in whom a known metabolic or structural bone disease exists.

## Precautions

*Monitoring:*

*Pregnancy test* – Female patients of childbearing potential must have negative results from 2 urine or serum pregnancy tests with a sensitivity of at least 25 milliunits/mL before receiving the initial isotretinoin prescription. The first test is obtained by the prescriber when the decision is made to pursue qualification of the patient for isotretinoin (a screening test). Perform the second pregnancy test (a confirmation test) during the first 5 days of the menstrual period immediately preceding the beginning of isotretinoin therapy. For patients with amenorrhea, the second test should be done at least 11 days after the last act of unprotected sexual intercourse (without using 2 effective forms of contraception).

Each month of therapy, the patient must have a negative result from a urine or serum pregnancy test. Repeat the pregnancy test each month prior to the female patient receiving each prescription.

*Lipids* – Obtain pretreatment and followup blood lipids under fasting conditions. After consumption of alcohol, at least 36 hours should elapse before these determinations are made. It is recommended that these tests be performed at weekly or biweekly intervals until the lipid response to isotretinoin is established. The incidence of hypertriglyceridemia is 1 patient in 4 on isotretinoin therapy.

*Liver function tests* – Because elevations of liver enzymes have been observed during clinical trials and hepatitis has been reported, perform pretreatment and followup liver function tests at weekly or biweekly intervals until the response to isotretinoin has been established.

*Exacerbation of acne (transient):* Transient exacerbation of acne has occurred, generally during the initial therapy period.

*Contact lens:* Tolerance may decrease.

*Diabetes:* Certain patients have experienced problems in the control of their blood sugar. In addition, new cases of diabetes have been diagnosed during therapy, although no causal relationship has been established.

*Blood donation:* Because of isotretinoin's teratogenic potential, patients receiving the drug should not donate blood for transfusion during treatment and for 1 month after discontinuing therapy.

*Neutropenia/Agranulocytosis:* Neutropenia and rare cases of agranulocytosis have been reported. Discontinue isotretinoin if clinically significant decreases in white cell counts occur.

*Photosensitivity:* Photosensitization (photoallergy or phototoxicity) may occur; caution patients to take protective measures (eg, sunscreens, protective clothing) against exposure to ultraviolet light or sunlight until tolerance is determined.

## Drug Interactions

Isotretinoin may interact with vitamin A and tetracyclines.

**Adverse Reactions**

Most adverse reactions are reversible upon discontinuation; however, some have persisted after cessation of therapy. Many are similar to those described in patients taking high doses of vitamin A (dryness of the skin and mucous membranes, eg, of the lips, nasal passage, eyes).

*Cardiovascular:* Palpitation; tachycardia; vascular thrombotic disease.

*CNS:* Fatigue; headache; pseudotumor cerebri, including headache, visual disturbances, and papilledema; dizziness; drowsiness; insomnia; lethargy; malaise; nervousness; paresthesias; seizures; stroke; syncope; weakness; suicidal ideation; suicide attempts; suicide; psychosis; emotional instability; aggression; violent behaviors. Depression has occurred and has subsided with discontinuation of therapy and recurred upon reinstitution.

*Dermatologic:* Acne fulminans; alopecia (which persists in some cases); bruising; cheilitis (dry lips); dry skin; eruptive xanthomas; flushing; fragility of skin; hair abnormalities; hirsutism; hyperpigmentation and hypopigmentation; infections (including disseminated herpes simplex); nail dystrophy; paronychia; peeling of palms and soles; photoallergic/photosensitizing reactions; pruritus; pyogenic granuloma; rash (including facial erythema, seborrhea, and eczema); sunburn susceptibility increased; sweating; urticaria; abnormal wound healing (delayed healing or exuberant granulation tissue with crusting).

*GI:* Dry mouth; nausea; nonspecific GI symptoms; inflammatory bowel disease; bleeding and inflammation of the gums; hepatitis; pancreatitis; colitis; ileitis; esophagitis/esophageal ulceration.

*GU:* White cells in urine; proteinuria; microscopic or gross hematuria; nonspecific urogenital findings; abnormal menses; glomerulonephritis.

*Hypersensitivity:* Allergic reactions; systemic hypersensitivity.

*Musculoskeletal:* Mild to moderate musculoskeletal symptoms, including arthralgia, that occasionally require drug discontinuation and rarely persist after discontinuation (16%); skeletal hyperostosis (see Warnings); calcification of tendons and ligaments; premature epiphyseal closure; arthritis; tendonitis; other bone abnormalities; decreases in bone mineral density; back pain; rhabdomyolysis (rare postmarketing reports).

*Ophthalmic:* Conjunctivitis; optic neuritis; photophobia; eyelid inflammation; corneal opacities (see Warnings); cataracts; visual disturbances; color vision disorder; keratitis; dry eyes; decreased night vision that may persist.

*Respiratory:* Bronchospasms, with or without a history of asthma; respiratory infections; voice alterations.

*Miscellaneous:* Epistaxis; dry nose or mouth; transient chest pain (rarely persists after discontinuation); vasculitis (including Wegener's granulomatosis); anemia; lymphadenopathy; edema; tinnitus; hearing impairment; weight loss.

*Lab test abnormalities:* Hypertriglyceridemia; elevated sedimentation rate; decreased red blood cell parameters and white blood cell counts, including severe neutropenia and rare reports of agranulocytosis; elevated platelet counts; decrease in serum HDL levels; elevations of serum cholesterol; increased alkaline phosphatase, AST, ALT, GGTP, and LDH; increased fasting blood sugar; hyperuricemia; thrombocytopenia; elevated CPK levels in patients who undergo vigorous physical activity.

# CORTICOSTEROIDS, TOPICAL

**ACLOMETASONE DIPROPIONATE**
**Ointment**: 0.05% (*Rx*)                                  *Aclovate* (GlaxoSmithKline)
**Cream**: 0.05% (*Rx*)

**AMCINONIDE**
**Ointment**: 0.1% (*Rx*)                                   *Cyclocort* (Fujisawa)
**Cream**: 0.1% (*Rx*)
**Lotion**: 0.1% (*Rx*)

**AUGMENTED BETAMETHASONE DIPROPIONATE**
**Ointment**: 0.05% (*Rx*)                                  *Diprolene* (Schering)
**Cream**: 0.05% (*Rx*)                                     *Diprolene AF* (Schering)
**Lotion**: 0.05% (*Rx*)                                    *Diprolene* (Schering)
**Gel**: 0.05% (*Rx*)                                       *Diprolene* (Schering)

**BETAMETHASONE BENZOATE**
**Cream**: 0.025% (*Rx*)                                    *Uticort* (Parke-Davis)
**Lotion**: 0.025% (*Rx*)
**Gel**: 0.025% (*Rx*)

**BETAMETHASONE DIPROPIONATE**
**Ointment**: 0.05% (*Rx*)                                  Various, *Maxivate* (Westwood-Squibb)
**Cream**: 0.05% (*Rx*)
**Lotion**: 0.05% (*Rx*)
**Aerosol**: 0.1% (*Rx*)

**BETAMETHASONE VALERATE**
**Ointment**: 0.1% (*Rx*)                                   Various, *Valisone* (Schering)
**Cream**: 0.01%, 0.05%, 0.1% (*Rx*)                        Various, *Valisone* (Schering)
**Lotion**: 0.1% (*Rx*)                                     Various, *Valisone* (Schering)
**Powder for compounding** (*Rx*)                           *Betamethasone Valerate* (Paddock)

**CLOBETASOL PROPIONATE**
**Ointment**: 0.05% (*Rx*)                                  Various, *Temovate* (GlaxoSmithKline)
**Cream**: 0.05% (*Rx*)
**Scalp application**: 0.05% (*Rx*)                         *Temovate* (GlaxoSmithKline)
**Gel**: 0.05% (*Rx*)                                       Various, *Temovate* (GlaxoSmithKline), *Clobevate* (Stiefel)

**CLOCORTOLONE PIVALATE**
**Cream**: 0.1% (*Rx*)                                      *Cloderm* (Hermal)

**DESONIDE**
**Ointment**: 0.05% (*Rx*)                                  Various, *DesOwen* (Owen/Galderma), *Tridesilon* (Miles Inc)
**Cream**: 0.05%, 0.25% (*Rx*)                              *DesOwen* (Owen/Galderma), *Tridesilon* (Miles Inc)
**Lotion**: 0.05% (*Rx*)                                    *DesOwen* (Owen/Galderma)

**DESOXIMETASONE**
**Ointment**: 0.25% (*Rx*)                                  *Topicort* (Taro)
**Cream**: 0.05%, 0.25% (*Rx*)                              Various, *Topicort* (Taro)
**Gel**: 0.05% (*Rx*)                                       *Topicort* (Taro)

**DEXAMETHASONE SODIUM PHOSPHATE**
**Aerosol**: 0.01%, 0.04% (*Rx*)                            *Aeroseb-Dex* (Herbert)

**DIFLORASONE DIACETATE**
**Ointment**: 0.05% (*Rx*)                                  *Maxiflor* (Herbert)
**Cream**: 0.05% (*Rx*)                                     *Psorcon* (Dermik)

**FLUOCINOLONE ACETONIDE**
**Ointment**: 0.025% (*Rx*)                                 Various, *Synalar* (Syntex)
**Cream**: 0.01%, 0.025%, 0.2% (*Rx*)
**Solution**: 0.01% (*Rx*)                                  Various, *Synalar* (Syntex)
**Shampoo**: 0.01% (*Rx*)                                   *FS Shampoo* (Hill), *Capex* (Galderma)
**Oil**: 0.01% (*Rx*)                                       *Derma-Smoothe/FS* (Hill)

**FLUOCINONIDE**
**Cream**: 0.05% (*Rx*) — Various, *Lidex* (Syntex)
**Ointment**: 0.05% (*Rx*) — Various, *Lidex* (Syntex)
**Solution**: 0.05% (*Rx*)
**Gel**: 0.05% (*Rx*)

**FLURANDRENOLIDE**
**Ointment**: 0.05% (*Rx*) — *Cordran* (Oclassen)
**Cream**: 0.05% (*Rx*) — *Cordran SP* (Oclassen)
**Lotion**: 0.05% (*Rx*) — Various, *Cordran* (Oclassen)
**Tape**: 4 mcg/cm$^2$ (*Rx*) — *Cordran* (Oclassen)

**FLUTICASONE PROPIONATE**
**Cream**: 0.05% (*Rx*) — *Cutivate* (GlaxoSmithKline)
**Ointment**: 0.005% (*Rx*)

**HALCINONIDE**
**Ointment**: 0.1% (*Rx*) — *Halog* (Westwood Squibb)
**Cream**: 0.025%, 0.1% (*Rx*) — *Halog* (Westwood Squibb), *Halog-E* (Westwood Squibb)
**Solution**: 0.1% (*Rx*) — *Halog* (Westwood Squibb)

**HALOBETASOL PROPIONATE**
**Ointment**: 0.05% (*Rx*) — *Ultravate* (Westwood-Squibb)
**Cream**: 0.05% (*Rx*)

**HYDROCORTISONE**
**Ointment**: 0.5%, 1%, 2.5% (*Rx/OTC*) — Various, *Cortizone•10* (Thompson)
**Cream**: 0.5%, 1%, 2.5% (*Rx/OTC*) — Various, *Hytone* (Dermik), *Dermacort* (Solvay), *LactiCare-HC* (Stiefel)
**Lotion**: 0.25%, 0.5%, 1%, 2%, 2.5% (*Rx*) — Various, *Ala-Scalp* (Del-Ray), *Cetacort* (Healthpoint), *Hytone* (Dermik), *SARNOL-HC* (Stiefel)
**Liquid**: 1% (*OTC*) — *Scalpicin* (Combe), *T/Scalp* (Neutrogena)
**Gel**: 0.5%, 1% (*OTC*) — *Extra Strength CortaGel* (Norstar)
**Solution**: 1% (*Rx*) — *Texacort* (GenDerm)
**Aerosol/Pump spray**: 0.5% (*Rx/OTC*) — *Aeroseb-HC* (Herbert), *Cortaid* (Pharmacia)

**HYDROCORTISONE ACETATE**
**Ointment**: 0.5%, 1% (*OTC*) — *Lanacort-5* (Combe), *Maximum Strength Lanacort 10* (Combe), *Anusol HC-1* (Parke-Davis)
**Cream**: 0.5%, 1% (*Rx*) — *Cortaid with Aloe* (Pharmacia), *U-Cort* (Thames)

**HYDROCORTISONE BUTEPRATE**
**Cream**: 1% (*Rx*) — *Pandel* (Collagenex)

**HYDROCORTISONE BUTYRATE**
**Solution**: (*Rx*) — *Locoid* (Ferndale)

**HYDROCORTISONE VALERATE**
**Ointment**: 0.2% (*Rx*) — *Westcort* (Westwood-Squibb)
**Cream**: 0.2% (*Rx*)

**MOMETASONE FUROATE**
**Ointment**: 0.1% (*Rx*) — *Elocon* (Schering)
**Cream**: 0.1% (*Rx*)
**Lotion**: 0.1% (*Rx*)

**PREDNICARBATE**
**Cream**: 0.1% (*Rx*) — *Dermatop* (Aventis)

**TRIAMCINOLONE ACETONIDE**
**Ointment**: 0.025%, 0.1%, 0.5% (*Rx*) — Various, *Kenalog* (Westwood-Squibb), *Aristocort* (Fujisawa)
**Cream**: 0.025%, 0.1%, 0.5% (*Rx*)
**Lotion**: 0.025% and 0.1% (*Rx*) — Various, *Kenalog* (Westwood-Squibb)
**Aerosol**: (2 sec. spray) (*Rx*) — *Kenalog* (Westwood-Squibb)

## Indications

*Pruritus*:
Relief of inflammatory and pruritic manifestations of corticosteroid-responsive dermatoses – Contact dermatitis, atopic dermatitis, nummular eczema, stasis eczema, asteatotic eczema, lichen planus, lichen simplex chronicus, insect and arthropod bite reactions, first- and second-degree localized burns, and sunburns.

*Alternative/Adjunctive treatment:* Psoriasis, seborrheic dermatitis, severe diaper rash, dishidrosis, nodular prurigo, chronic discoid lupus erythematosus, alopecia areata, lymphocytic infiltration of the skin, mycosis fungoides, and familial benign pemphigus of Hailey-Hailey.

*Possibly effective:* Possibly effective in the following conditions: Bullous pemphigoid, cutaneous mastocytosis, lichen sclerosus et atrophicus, and vitiligo.

*Nonprescription hydrocortisone preparations:* Temporary relief of itching associated with minor skin irritations, inflammation, and rashes caused by eczema, insect bites, poison ivy, poison oak, poison sumac, soaps, detergents, cosmetics, jewelry, seborrheic dermatitis, psoriasis, and external genital and anal itching.

## Administration and Dosage
*Usual dose:* Apply sparingly to affected areas 1 to 4 times/day.

## Actions
*Pharmacology:* The primary therapeutic effects of the topical corticosteroids are caused by their antiinflammatory activity, which is nonspecific (ie, they act against most causes of inflammation including mechanical, chemical, microbiological, and immunological).

*Pharmacokinetics:* The amount of corticosteroid absorbed from the skin depends on the intrinsic properties of the drug itself, the vehicle used, the duration of exposure, and the surface area and condition of the skin to which it is applied.

*Vehicles* – Ointments are more occlusive and are preferred for dry scaly lesions. Use creams on oozing lesions or in intertriginous areas where the occlusive effects of ointments may cause maceration and folliculitis.

*Relative potency* – The relative potency of a product depends on several factors including the characteristics and concentration of the drug and the vehicle used.

Topical corticosteroids are ranked into several classes according to their potency based on vasoconstrictor activity; Group I has the highest potency and highest potential for localized as well as systemic side effects. The percent of the corticosteroid agent is NOT an indication of potency. Use high potency agents for very short periods of time for acute exacerbations and only on areas that are lichenified; avoid use of these agents on facial areas, skin folds, and on infants. Intermediate and lower potency agents can be used for longer durations and to treat chronic symptoms on areas of the torso and extremities.

| Relative Potency of Selected Topical Corticosteroid Products | | |
|---|---|---|
| Drug | Dosage Form | Strength |
| **I. Very high potency** | | |
| Augmented betamethasone dipropionate | Ointment | 0.05% |
| Clobetasol propionate | Cream, Ointment | 0.05% |
| Diflorasone diacetate | Ointment | 0.05% |
| Halobetasol propionate | Cream, Ointment | 0.05% |
| **II. High potency** | | |
| Amcinonide | Cream, Lotion, Ointment | 0.1% |
| Augmented betamethasone dipropionate | Cream | 0.05% |
| Betamethasone dipropionate | Cream, Ointment | 0.05% |
| Betamethasone valerate | Ointment | 0.1% |
| Desoximetasone | Cream, Ointment | 0.25% |
| | Gel | 0.05% |
| Diflorasone diacetate | Cream, Ointment (emollient base) | 0.05% |
| Fluocinolone acetonide | Cream | 0.2% |
| Fluocinonide | Cream, Ointment, Gel | 0.05% |
| Halcinonide | Cream, Ointment | 0.1% |
| Triamcinolone acetonide | Cream, Ointment | 0.5% |

| Relative Potency of Selected Topical Corticosteroid Products | | |
|---|---|---|
| Drug | Dosage Form | Strength |
| **III. Medium potency** | | |
| Betamethasone benzoate | Cream, Gel, Lotion | 0.025% |
| Betamethasone dipropionate | Lotion | 0.05% |
| Betamethasone valerate | Cream | 0.1% |
| Clocortolone pivalate | Cream | 0.1% |
| Desoximetasone | Cream | 0.05% |
| Fluocinolone acetonide | Cream, Ointment | 0.025% |
| Flurandrenolide | Cream, Ointment | 0.025% |
| | Cream, Ointment, Lotion | 0.05% |
| | Tape | 4 mcg/cm$^2$ |
| Fluticasone propionate | Cream | 0.05% |
| | Ointment | 0.005% |
| Hydrocortisone butyrate | Ointment, Solution | 0.1% |
| Hydrocortisone valerate | Cream, Ointment | 0.2% |
| Mometasone furoate | Cream, Ointment, Lotion | 0.1% |
| Triamcinolone acetonide | Cream, Ointment, Lotion | 0.025% |
| | Cream, Ointment, Lotion | 0.1% |
| **IV. Low potency** | | |
| Aclometasone dipropionate | Cream, Ointment | 0.05% |
| Desonide | Cream | 0.05% |
| Dexamethasone | Aerosol | 0.01% |
| | Aerosol | 0.04% |
| Dexamethasone sodium phosphate | Cream | 0.1% |
| Fluocinolone acetonide | Cream, Solution | 0.01% |
| Hydrocortisone | Lotion | 0.25% |
| | Cream, Ointment, Lotion, Aerosol | 0.5% |
| | Cream, Ointment, Lotion, Solution | 1% |
| | Cream, Ointment, Lotion | 2.5% |
| Hydrocortisone acetate | Cream, Ointment | 0.5% |
| | Cream, Ointment | 1% |

**Contraindications**

Hypersensitivity to any component; monotherapy in primary bacterial infections such as impetigo, paronychia, erysipelas, cellulitis, angular cheilitis, erythrasma (clobetasol), treatment of rosacea, perioral dermatitis, or acne; use on the face, groin, or axilla (very high or high potency agents); ophthalmic use.

**Warnings**

*Pregnancy: Category C.*

*Lactation:* It is not known whether topical corticosteroids could result in sufficient systemic absorption to produce detectable quantities in breast milk.

*Children:* Children may be more susceptible to topical corticosteroid-induced hypothalamic-pituitary-adrenal (HPA) axis suppression and Cushing syndrome than adults because of a larger skin surface area to body weight ratio.

**Precautions**

*Systemic effects:* Systemic absorption of topical corticosteroids has produced reversible HPA axis suppression, Cushing syndrome, hyperglycemia, and glycosuria.

As a general rule, little effect on the HPA axis will occur with a potent topical corticosteroid in amounts of less than 50 g weekly for an adult and 15 g weekly for a small child, without occlusion. To cover the adult body 1 time requires 12 to 26 g.

*Local irritation:* If local irritation develops, discontinue use and institute appropriate therapy.

*Psoriasis:* Do not use topical corticosteroids as sole therapy in widespread plaque psoriasis.

*Atrophic changes:* Skin atrophy is common and may be clinically significant in 3 to 4 weeks with potent preparations. Certain areas of the body, such as the face, groin, and axillae, are more prone to atrophic changes than other areas of the body following treatment with corticosteroids.

*Infections:* Treating skin infections with topical corticosteroids can extensively worsen the infection.

*Occlusive therapy:* Occlusive dressings such as a plastic wrap increase skin penetration by 10-fold. Discontinue the use of occlusive dressings if infection develops and institute appropriate antimicrobial therapy.

Do not use occlusive dressings in augmented betamethasone dipropionate, betamethasone dipropionate, clobetasol, halobetasol propionate, and mometasone treatment regimens.

**Adverse Reactions**

Adverse reactions may include burning; itching; irritation; erythema; dryness; folliculitis; hypertrichosis; pruritus; acneiform eruptions; hypopigmentation; perioral dermatitis; allergic contact dermatitis; numbness of fingers; stinging and cracking/tightening of skin; maceration of the skin; secondary infection; skin atrophy; striae; miliaria; telangiectasia. These may occur more frequently with occlusive dressings.

# TRETINOIN (trans-Retinoic Acid; Vitamin A Acid)

| | |
|---|---|
| **Cream**: 0.02% (*Rx*) | *Renova* (Ortho Dermatological) |
| 0.025% (*Rx*) | Tretinoin (Various), *Avita* (Bertek), *Retin-A* (Ortho) |
| 0.05% (*Rx*) | Tretinoin (Spear Dermatology), *Renova* (Ortho Dermatological), *Retin-A* (Ortho) |
| 0.1% (*Rx*) | Tretinoin (Spear Dermatology), *Retin-A* (Ortho) |
| **Gel**: 0.01% (*Rx*) | Tretinoin (Spear Dermatology), *Retin-A* (Ortho) |
| 0.025% (*Rx*) | Tretinoin (Spear Dermatology), *Avita* (Bertek), *Retin-A* (Ortho) |
| 0.04% and 0.1% (*Rx*) | *Retin-A Micro* (Ortho) |
| **Liquid**: 0.05% (*Rx*) | *Retin-A* (Ortho) |

### Indications

*Acne (except Renova):* Topical treatment of acne vulgaris.

*Renova:*
   Dermatologic conditions –
      *0.02% cream:* Adjunctive agent for use in the mitigation (palliation) of fine wrinkles in patients who use comprehensive skin care and sun avoidance programs.
      *0.05% cream:* Adjunctive agent for use in the mitigation (palliation) of fine wrinkles, mottled hyperpigmentation, and tactile roughness of facial skin in patients who do not achieve such palliation using comprehensive skin care and sun avoidance programs alone.

### Administration and Dosage

*Acne treatment:* Apply once a day before bedtime or in the evening. Cover the entire affected area lightly.

Closely monitor alterations of vehicle, drug concentration, or dose frequency. During the early weeks of therapy, an apparent exacerbation of inflammatory lesions may occur due to the action of the medication on deep, previously undetected lesions; this is not a reason to discontinue therapy.

Therapeutic results should be seen after 2 to 3 weeks, but may not be optimal until after 6 weeks. Once lesions have responded satisfactorily, maintain therapy with less frequent applications or other dosage forms.

Patients may use cosmetics, but thoroughly cleanse area to be treated before applying medication.

*Liquid:* Apply with fingertip, gauze pad, or cotton swab. Do not oversaturate gauze or cotton to the extent that liquid will run into unaffected areas.

*Gel:* Excessive application results in "piling" of the gel, which minimizes the likelihood of overapplication by the patient.

*Renova:* Gently wash face with a mild soap, pat the skin dry, and wait 20 to 30 minutes before applying. Apply tretinoin to the face once a day in the evening, using only enough to cover the entire affected area lightly. Apply a pea-sized amount of cream to cover the entire face. Take caution to avoid contact with eyes, ears, nostrils, and mouth.

For best results, do not apply another skin care product or cosmetic for at least 1 hour after applying tretinoin.

Do not wash face for at least 1 hour after applying tretinoin.

Application of tretinoin may cause a transitory feeling of warmth or slight stinging.

Mitigation (palliation) of fine facial wrinkling, mottled hyperpigmentation, and tactile roughness may occur gradually over the course of therapy. Up to 6 months of therapy may be required before the effects are seen. Most of the improvement noted with tretinoin is seen during the first 24 weeks of therapy. Thereafter, therapy primarily maintains the improvement noticed during the first 24 weeks.

Patients treated with tretinoin may use cosmetics, but the areas to be treated should be cleansed thoroughly before the medication is applied.

### Actions

*Pharmacology:* Tretinoin is a retinoid metabolite of vitamin A. Although the exact mode of action of tretinoin is unknown, current evidence suggests that topical tretinoin decreases cohesiveness of follicular epithelial cells with decreased microcomedo formation. Additionally, tretinoin stimulates mitotic activity and increases turnover of follicular epithelial cells, causing extrusion of the comedones.

*Pharmacokinetics:* The transdermal absorption of tretinoin from various topical formulations ranged from 1% to 31% of applied dose, depending on whether it was applied to healthy skin or dermatitic skin.

In vitro and in vivo pharmacokinetic studies with tretinoin cream and gel indicated that less than 0.3% of the topically applied dose is bioavailable. Circulating plasma levels of tretinoin are only slightly elevated above those found in healthy normal controls. Estimates of in vivo bioavailability of *Retin-A Micro* following single and multiple daily applications, for a period of 28 days with the 0.1% gel, were approximately 0.82% and 1.41%, respectively. When percutaneous absorption of *Renova* was assessed in healthy male subjects (n = 14) after a single application, as well as after repeated daily applications for 28 days, the absorption of tretinoin was less than 2% and endogenous concentrations of tretinoin and its major metabolites were unaltered.

## Contraindications

Hypersensitivity to any component of the product (discontinue if hypersensitivity to any ingredient is noted).

## Warnings

*For external use only:* Keep tretinoin away from the eyes, mouth, angles of the nose, and mucous membranes.

*Renova:*

Mitigating effects – Tretinoin has shown no mitigating effects on significant signs of chronic sun exposure (eg, coarse or deep wrinkling, skin yellowing, lentigines, telangiectasia, skin laxity, keratinocytic atypia, melanocytic atypia, dermal elastosis).

Tretinoin 0.02% cream has shown no mitigating effects on tactile roughness or mottled hyperpigmentation.

Tretinoin does not eliminate wrinkles, repair sun damaged skin, reverse photoaging, or restore a more youthful or younger dermal histologic pattern.

Many patients achieve desired palliative effect on fine wrinkling, mottled hyperpigmentation, and tactile roughness of facial skin with the use of comprehensive skin care and sun avoidance programs including sunscreens, protective clothing, and nonprescription emollient creams.

Long-term use – Tretinoin is a dermal irritant, and the results of continued irritation of the skin for greater than 48 weeks are not known. There is evidence of atypical changes in melanocytes and keratinocytes and of increased dermal elastosis in some patients treated with tretinoin 0.05% for longer than 52 weeks.

*Pregnancy: Category* C.

*Lactation:* It is not known whether this drug is excreted in breast milk. Exercise caution when tretinoin is administered to a nursing mother.

*Children:*

Renova – Safety and efficacy in patients less than 18 years of age have not been established.

## Precautions

*Irritation:* Tretinoin may induce severe local erythema, pruritus, burning, stinging, and peeling at the application site. If the degree of local irritation warrants, use medication less frequently or discontinue use temporarily or completely. Tretinoin may cause severe irritation to eczematous skin; use with caution in patients with this condition.

*Photosensitivity:* It is advisable to "rest" a patient's skin until effects of keratolytic agents subside before beginning tretinoin. Minimize exposure to sunlight and sunlamps, and advise patients with sunburn not to use tretinoin until fully recovered because of heightened susceptibility to sunlight as a result of tretinoin use. Patients who undergo considerable sun exposure due to occupation and those with inherent sun sensitivity should exercise particular caution. Use sunscreen products and wear protective clothing over treated areas. Weather extremes, such as wind and cold, also may irritate treated areas.

### Drug Interactions

*Sulfur, resorcinol, benzoyl peroxide, or salicylic acid:* Cautiously use concomitant topical medications because of possible interactions with tretinoin. Significant skin irritation may result. It also is advisable to "rest" a patient's skin until the effects of such preparations subside before use of tretinoin is begun.

*Topical preparations:* Cautiously use medicated or abrasive soaps and cleansers, soaps, and cosmetics that have a strong drying effect, and products with high concentrations of alcohol, astringents, spices, or lime, permanent wave solutions, electrolysis, hair depilatories or waxes, and products that may irritate the skin in patients being treated with tretinoin because they may increase irritation.

*Photosensitizers:* Do not use tretinoin if the patient also is taking drugs known to be photosensitizers (eg, thiazides, tetracyclines, fluoroquinolones, phenothiazines, sulfonamides) because of the possibility of augmented phototoxicity.

### Adverse Reactions

Almost all patients reported 1 or more local reactions such as peeling, dry skin, burning, stinging, erythema, and pruritus during therapy with tretinoin.

Sensitive skin may become excessively red, edematous, blistered, or crusted. If these effects occur, discontinue medication until skin integrity is restored or adjust to a tolerable level. True contact allergy is rare.

Temporary hyperpigmentation or hypopigmentation has been reported with repeated application. Some individuals have a heightened susceptibility to sunlight while under treatment.

All adverse effects have been reversible upon discontinuation.

# CAPSAICIN

| | |
|---|---|
| **Cream:** 0.025% and 0.075% in an emollient base (*otc*) | *Zostrix* (GenDerm), *Zostrix-HP* (GenDerm) |
| 0.025% (*otc*) | *Capzasin•P* (Thompson Medical) |
| **Gel:** 0.025% (*otc*) | *R-Gel* (Healthline Labs) |
| **Lotion:** 0.025% and 0.075% (*otc*) | *Capsin* (Fleming) |
| **Roll-on:** 0.075% (*otc*) | *No pain-HP* (Young Again Products) |

### Indications

Temporary relief of pain from rheumatoid arthritis, osteoarthritis, and relief of neuralgias such as the pain following shingles (herpes zoster) or painful diabetic neuropathy.

### Administration and Dosage

*Adults and children 2 years of age and older:* Apply to affected area not more than 3 or 4 times daily. May cause transient burning on application. This is observed more frequently when application schedules of less than 3 or 4 times daily are used. If applied with the fingers, wash hands immediately after application.

### Actions

*Pharmacology:* Capsaicin is a natural chemical derived from plants. Although the precise mechanism of action is not fully understood, evidence suggests that the drug renders skin and joints insensitive to pain by depleting and preventing reaccumulation of substance P in peripheral sensory neurons.

### Warnings

*For external use only:* Avoid contact with eyes or broken or irritated skin. Use care when handling contact lenses following application of capsaicin.

*Bandage use:* Do not bandage tightly.

*Worsened condition:* If condition worsens or if symptoms persist 14 to 28 days, discontinue use and consult physician.

### Adverse Reactions

Adverse reactions include burning; stinging; erythema; cough; respiratory irritation.

# ACYCLOVIR (Acycloguanosine)

**Ointment:** 5% (50 mg/g) (*Rx*)
**Cream:** 5% (50 mg/g) (*Rx*)

*Zovirax* (Biovail)

### Indications
*Ointment:* Management of initial episodes of herpes genitalis and in limited non-life-threatening mucocutaneous herpes simplex virus infections in immunocompromised patients.

*Cream:* Treatment of recurrent herpes labialis (cold sores) in adults and adolescents (12 years of age and older).

### Administration and Dosage
Initiate therapy as early as possible following onset of signs and symptoms.

*Ointment:* Apply sufficient quantity to adequately cover all lesions every 3 hours 6 times daily for 7 days. Use approximately a one-half inch ribbon of ointment per 4 square inches of surface area. Use a finger cot or rubber glove when applying acyclovir to prevent autoinoculation of other body sites and transmission of infection to other people.

*Cream:* Apply 5 times/day for 4 days. For adolescents 12 years of age and older the dosage is the same as in adults.

### Actions
*Pharmacokinetics:*
   *Ointment* – Systemic absorption of acyclovir after topical application is minimal.
   *Cream* – Systemic absorption of acyclovir from the cream is minimal in adults.

### Warnings
*For cutaneous use only:* Do not use in eyes, nose, or mouth.

*Pregnancy:* Category B.

*Lactation:* Systemic exposure following topical administration is minimal.

### Adverse Reactions
Mild pain with transient burning/stinging; pruritus.

*Post-marketing events:* Edema and/or pain at application site; rash (ointment). Angioedema, anaphylaxis, contact dermatitis, eczema, and application site reactions including inflammation (cream).

# PENCICLOVIR

**Cream:** 10 mg/kg (*Rx*)

*Denavir* (GlaxoSmithKline)

### Indications
*Herpes labialis:* For the treatment of recurrent herpes labialis (cold sores) in adults.

### Administration and Dosage
Apply penciclovir every 2 hours while awake for 4 days. Start treatment as early as possible (eg, during the prodrome or when lesions appear).

### Actions
*Pharmacology:* Penciclovir is an antiviral agent active against herpes viruses. It has in vitro inhibitory activity against herpes simplex virus types 1 (HSV-1) and 2 (HSV-2).

*Pharmacokinetics:* Measurable penciclovir concentrations were not detected in plasma or urine of healthy male volunteers following single or repeat application of the 1% cream at a dose of 180 mg penciclovir daily (about 67 times the estimated usual clinical dose).

### Contraindications
Hypersensitivity to the product or any of its components.

### Warnings
*Pregnancy:* Category B.

*Lactation:* There is no information on whether penciclovir is excreted in breast milk after topical administration.

*Children:* Safety and efficacy in pediatric patients have not been established.

**Precautions**

*Mucous membranes:* Use penciclovir on herpes labialis on the lips and face only. Application to human mucous membranes is not recommended. Avoid application in or near the eyes because it may cause irritation.

*Immunocompromised patients:* Penciclovir's effect in immunocompromised patients has not been established.

**Adverse Reactions**

Adverse reactions occurring in at least 3% of patients include headache.

# ALUMINUM CHLORIDE (HEXAHYDRATE)

**Solution**: 20% in 88.5% SD alcohol 40-2 (*Rx*)      *Aluminum Chloride Hexahydrate* (Glades)
20% in 93% SD alcohol 40 (*Rx*)                        *Drysol* (Person & Covey)

**Indications**
An astringent used as an aid in the management of hyperhidrosis.

**Administration and Dosage**
Apply to the affected area once daily, only at bedtime. To help prevent irritation, completely dry area prior to application. Do not apply to broken, irritated, or recently shaved skin.

For maximum effect, cover the treated area with plastic wrap, held in place by a snug fitting T-shirt or body shirt, mitten, or sock (never hold plastic wrap in place with tape). Wash the treated area the following morning. Excessive sweating may stop after 2 or more treatments. Thereafter, apply once or twice weekly or as needed.

**Warnings**
*For external use only:* Avoid contact with the eyes.

*Discontinue use:* If irritation or sensitization occurs, discontinue use.

*Metals/Fabrics:* Aluminum chloride (hexahydrate) may be harmful to certain metals and fabrics.

**Adverse Reactions**
Burning or prickling sensation may occur.

# FORMALDEHYDE

**Spray**: 10% (*Rx*)                                  *Formaldehyde-10* (Pedinol)
**Solution**: 10% (*Rx*)                               *Lazer Formaldehyde* (Pedinol)

**Indications**
Drying agent for presurgical and postsurgical removal of warts or for *Histofreezer* treatment of warts where dryness is required. Safeguards against offensive odor and dries excessive moisture of feet.

**Administration and Dosage**
Apply once daily to affected areas as directed.

**Contraindications**
Hypersensitivity to any ingredients of the product.

**Precautions**
*For external use only:* Avoid contact with and keep away from face, eyes, nose, and mucous membranes.

*Irritation/Sensitivity:* May be irritating and sensitizing to the skin of some patients; check skin for sensitivity prior to application. If redness or irritation persists, consult physician.

# COLLAGENASE

**Ointment:** 250 units collagenase enzyme/g (*Rx*)    *Collagenase Santyl* (Ross)

### Indications
For debriding chronic dermal ulcers and severely burned areas.

### Administration and Dosage
Apply once daily (or more frequently if the dressing becomes soiled, as from incontinence). When clinically indicated, crosshatching thick eschar with a No. 10 blade allows collagenase more surface contact with necrotic debris. It also is more desirable to remove, with forceps and scissors, as much loosened detritus as can be done readily.

*Instructions for use:*
1.) Prior to application, cleanse the wound of debris and digested material by gently rubbing with a gauze pad saturated with normal saline solution, or with the desired cleansing agent compatible with collagenase, followed by a normal saline solution rinse.
2.) Whenever infection is present, it is desirable to use an appropriate topical antibiotic powder. Apply the antibiotic to the wound prior to the application of collagenase ointment. If the infection does not respond, discontinue therapy with collagenase until remission of the infection.
3.) Collagenase may be applied directly to the wound or to a sterile gauze pad, which is applied to the wound and secured.
4.) Terminate use of collagenase when debridement of necrotic tissue is completed and granulation tissue is well established.

### Actions
*Pharmacology:* Because collagen accounts for 75% of the dry weight of skin tissue, the ability of collagenase to digest collagen in the physiological pH and temperature range makes it particularly effective in the removal of detritus. Collagenase thus contributes toward the formation of granulation tissue and subsequent epithelization of dermal ulcers and severely burned areas. Collagen in healthy tissue or in newly formed granulation tissue is not attacked.

### Contraindications
Local or systemic hypersensitivity to collagenase.

### Warnings
*Children:* Safety and efficacy in children are not established.

### Precautions
*For external use only:* Avoid contact with the eyes.

*Optimal pH range:* The optimal pH range of collagenase is 6 to 8. Higher or lower pH conditions will decrease the enzyme's activity; take appropriate precautions. The enzymatic activity also is adversely affected by certain detergents and heavy metal ions, such as mercury and silver, which are used in some antiseptics. When it is suspected that such materials have been used, carefully cleanse the site by repeatedly washing with normal saline before collagenase is applied. Avoid soaks containing metal ions or acidic solutions because of the metal ion and low pH. Cleansing materials such as hydrogen peroxide, Dakin's solution, and normal saline are compatible with the collagenase ointment.

*Systemic bacterial infections:* Closely monitor debilitated patients for systemic bacterial infections because of the theoretical possibility that debriding enzymes may increase the risk of bacteremia.

*Erythema:* Slight transient erythema has been noted in the surrounding tissue, particularly when collagenase was not confined to the wound. Therefore, apply carefully within the wound area.

### Adverse Reactions
*Hypersensitivity:* One case of systemic manifestations of hypersensitivity to collagenase occurred with treatment of more than 1 year with both collagenase and cortisone.

# ENZYME COMBINATIONS, TOPICAL

| | |
|---|---|
| **Aerosol:** 0.1 mg trypsin, 72.5 mg balsam peru, and 650 mg castor oil per 0.82 mL *(Rx)* | *Granul-Derm* (Qualitest) |
| 0.12 mg trypsin, 87 mg balsam peru, and 788 mg castor oil per g *(Rx)* | *Granulex* (Bertek) |
| **Ointment:** $1.1 \times 10^6$ units papain and 100 mg urea per g *(Rx)* | *Ethezyme* (Ethex) |
| $8.3 \times 10^5$ units papain and 100 mg urea per g *(Rx)* | *Accuzyme* (Healthpoint), *Ethezyme 830* (Ethex), *Gladase* (Smith & Nephew) |
| $\geq$ 521,700 units papain, 10% urea, 0.5% chlorophyllin copper complex sodium per g *(Rx)* | *Papain-Urea-Chlorophyllin* (Cypress), *Panafil* (Healthpoint) |
| **Spray:** $\geq$ 521,700 units papain, 10% urea, 0.5% chlorophyllin copper complex sodium per g *(Rx)* | *Panafil* (Healthpoint) |
| $8.3 \times 10^5$ units papain and 10% urea per g *(Rx)* | *Accuzyme* (Healthpoint) |

## Indications
For debridement of necrotic tissue and liquefication of slough in acute and chronic lesions such as pressure ulcers, varicose, diabetic, and decubitus ulcers, burns, postoperative wounds, pilonidal cyst wounds, carbuncles, and miscellaneous traumatic or infected wounds. Also stimulates vascular bed activity to improve epithelization.

## Administration and Dosage
Cleanse the wound prior to application with wound cleanser or saline. For papain-containing products, avoid cleansing with hydrogen peroxide solution.

*Aerosol:* Shake well. Hold upright and approximately 12 inches from the area to be treated. Press valve and coat wound rapidly. Wound may be left unbandaged or a wet dressing may be applied. Apply 2 to 3 times daily, or as often as necessary. To remove, wash gently with water.

*Ointment:* Apply ointment directly to the wound, cover with appropriate dressing, and secure into place. Daily or twice daily applications are preferred. Irrigate the wound at each redressing to remove any accumulation of liquefied necrotic material.

Longer intervals between redressings (2 or 3 days) have proved satisfactory, and ointment may be applied under pressure dressings.

*Spray:* Shake well. Begin initial use by holding spray upright directly over the wound, and prime the pump 6 to 8 times.

Hold the spray bottle approximately 2 to 3 inches from the wound and use even, firm, and consistent pressure to dispense product. When sprayed from the appropriate distance, the spray should appear in a nickel-sized diameter.

Completely cover the wound site with spray. Cover wound with appropriate dressing of choice (eg, saline-moistened gauze, semi-occlusive dressings), and secure into place.

## Contraindications
Sensitivity to papain or any other components of these preparations.

## Warnings
*Arterial clots:* Do not spray aerosol products on fresh arterial clots.

*For external use only:* Avoid contact with the eyes.

*Transient burning:* Transient burning may occur upon application.

*Papain:* Papain may be inactivated by the salts of heavy metals such as lead, silver, and mercury. Avoid contact with medications containing these metals.

## Adverse Reactions
Generally well-tolerated and nonirritating. A transient burning sensation may be experienced by a small percentage of patients upon application. Occasionally, the profuse exudate from enzymatic digestion may irritate the skin. In such cases, more frequent dressing changes will alleviate discomfort until exudate decreases.

# IMIQUIMOD

| Cream: 5% (*Rx*) | *Aldara* (3M Pharm) |

### Indications

*Genital and perianal warts:* Treatment of external genital and perianal warts/condyloma acuminata in patients 12 years of age and older.

### Administration and Dosage

Apply imiquimod 3 times/week, prior to normal sleeping hours, and leave on the skin for 6 to 10 hours. Following the treatment period, remove cream by washing the treated area with mild soap and water. Continue imiquimod treatment until there is total clearance of the genital/perianal warts or for at least 16 weeks. A rest period of several days may be taken if required by the patient's discomfort or severity of the local skin reaction. Treatment may resume once the reaction subsides. Nonocclusive dressings such as cotton gauze or cotton underwear may be used in the management of skin reactions.

Hand-washing before and after cream application is recommended. Avoid use of excessive amounts of cream. Apply a thin layer to the wart area and rub in until the cream is no longer visible. Do not occlude the application site.

### Actions

*Pharmacology:* Imiquimod is an immune response modifier. The mechanism of action of imiquimod in treating genital/perianal warts is unknown.

*Pharmacokinetics:* Less than 0.9% of the dose was excreted in the urine and feces following topical application.

### Contraindications

None known.

### Warnings

*Other conditions:* Imiquimod has not been evaluated for the treatment of urethral, intravaginal, cervical, rectal, or intra-anal human papilloma viral disease and is not recommended for these conditions.

*Pregnancy:* Category B.

*Lactation:* It is not known whether imiquimod is excreted in breast milk.

*Children:* Safety and efficacy in patients younger than 12 years of age have not been established.

### Precautions

*Skin reactions:* The most frequently reported adverse reactions were local skin and application-site reactions. These reactions were usually mild to moderate in intensity. These reactions were more frequent and more intense with daily application than with 3 times/week application.

Local skin reactions such as erythema, erosion, excoriation/flaking, and edema are common. Should severe local skin reaction occur, remove the cream by washing the treatment area with mild soap and water. Resume treatment with imiquimod cream after the skin reaction has subsided. Imiquimod cream administration is not recommended until genital/perianal tissue is healed from any previous drug or surgical treatment. Imiquimod has the potential to exacerbate inflammatory conditions of the skin.

### Adverse Reactions

The adverse reactions with an incidence of at least 3% include burning, edema, erosion, erythema, excoriation, flaking, fungal infection, headache, induration, influenza-like symptoms, itching, local pain, scabbing, soreness, ulceration, and vesicles.

# TACROLIMUS

| **Ointment:** 0.03%, 0.1% (*Rx*) | *Protopic* (Fujisawa) |
| --- | --- |

### Indications
*Moderate to severe atopic dermatitis:* Tacrolimus ointment, both 0.03% and 0.1% for adults, and only 0.03% for children 2 to 15 years of age, is indicated for short-term and intermittent long-term therapy in the treatment of patients with moderate to severe atopic dermatitis.

### Administration and Dosage
*Adults:*
> *0.03% and 0.1%* – Apply a thin layer to the affected skin areas twice daily and rub in gently and completely. Continue treatment for 1 week after clearing of signs and symptoms of atopic dermatitis.

*Children:*
> *0.03%* – Apply a thin layer to the affected skin areas twice daily and rub in gently and completely. Continue treatment for 1 week after clearing of signs and symptoms of atopic dermatitis.

The safety of tacrolimus ointment under occlusion, which may promote systemic exposure, has not been evaluated. Do not use tacrolimus ointment with occlusive dressings.

### Actions
*Pharmacology:* Tacrolimus is a macrolide immunosuppressant produced by *Streptomyces tsukubaensis*. The mechanism of action of tacrolimus in atopic dermatitis is not known. It has been demonstrated that tacrolimus inhibits T-lymphocyte activation by first binding to an intracellular protein, FKBP-12.

*Pharmacokinetics:*
> *Absorption/Distribution* – In atopic dermatitis patients, tacrolimus is absorbed after topical application of 0.1% tacrolimus ointment.
>
> There was no evidence based on blood concentrations that tacrolimus accumulates systemically upon intermittent topical application for periods of up to 1 year. The absolute bioavailability of topical tacrolimus is unknown.

### Contraindications
A history of hypersensitivity to tacrolimus or any other component of the preparation.

### Warnings
*Pregnancy:* Category C.

*Lactation:* Tacrolimus is excreted in human milk. Decide whether to discontinue nursing or to discontinue the drug, taking into account the importance of the drug to the mother.

*Children:* Tacrolimus 0.03% ointment may be used in children 2 years of age and older.

### Precautions
*Infected atopic dermatitis:* Before commencing treatment with tacrolimus ointment, clear clinical infections at treatment sites.

*Viral infection:* Treatment with tacrolimus ointment may be associated with an increased risk of varicella zoster virus infection (chicken pox or shingles), herpes simplex virus infection, or eczema herpeticum.

*Lymphadenopathy:* Patients who receive tacrolimus ointment and who develop lymphadenopathy should have the etiology of their lymphadenopathy investigated. In the absence of a clear etiology for the lymphadenopathy, or in the presence of acute infectious mononucleosis, consider discontinuation of tacrolimus ointment. Monitor patients who develop lymphadenopathy to ensure that the lymphadenopathy resolves.

*Phototoxicity:* It is prudent for patients to minimize or avoid natural or artificial sunlight exposure.

*Other skin disorders:* The use of tacrolimus ointment in patients with Netherton syndrome is not recommended because of the potential for increased systemic absorption of tacrolimus. The safety of tacrolimus ointment has not been established in patients with generalized erythroderma.

### Drug Interactions

Coadminister known CYP3A4 inhibitors (eg, erythromycin, itraconazole, ketoconazole, fluconazole, calcium channel blockers, cimetidine) with caution in patients with widespread or erythrodermic disease.

### Adverse Reactions

Adverse events that occurred in at least 3% of patients include the following: Skin burning, pruritus, skin erythema, skin infection, herpes simplex, pustular rash, folliculitis, urticaria, maculopapular rash, rash, fungal dermatitis, acne, sunburn, skin disorder, vesiculobullous rash, skin tingling, dry skin, benign skin neoplasm, contact dermatitis, eczema, exfoliative dermatitis, diarrhea, vomiting, abdominal pain, gastroenteritis, nausea, cough increased, asthma, pharyngitis, rhinitis, sinusitis, bronchitis, flu-like symptoms, allergic reaction, headache, fever, infection, accidental injury, otitis media, lack of drug effect, alcohol intolerance, conjunctivitis, pain, lymphadenopathy, face edema, hyperesthesia, back pain, peripheral edema, varicella zoster/herpes zoster, asthenia, insomnia, dysmenorrhea, periodontal abscess, myalgia, cyst.

# Chapter 12

# OPHTHALMIC AND OTIC AGENTS

# TOPICAL OPHTHALMICS

*General considerations in topical ophthalmic drug therapy:* Proper administration is essential to optimal therapeutic response. In many instances, health professionals may be too casual when instructing patients on proper use of ophthalmics. The administration technique used often determines drug safety and efficacy.

- The normal eye retains approximately 10 mcL of fluid (adjusted for blinking). The average dropper delivers 25 to 50 mcL/drop. The value of more than 1 drop is questionable.
- Minimize systemic absorption of ophthalmic drops by compressing lacrimal sac for 3 to 5 minutes after instillation. This retards passage of drops via nasolacrimal duct into areas of potential absorption such as nasal and pharyngeal mucosa.
- Because of rapid lacrimal drainage and limited eye capacity, if multiple drop therapy is indicated, the best interval between drops is 5 minutes. This ensures the first drop is not flushed away by the second or the second is not diluted by the first.
- Topical anesthesia will increase the bioavailability of ophthalmic agents by decreasing the blink reflex and the production and turnover of tears.
- Factors that may increase absorption from ophthalmic dosage forms include lax eyelids of some patients, usually the elderly, which creates a greater reservoir for retention of drops, and hyperemic or diseased eyes.
- Eyecup use is discouraged because of the risk of contamination and spreading disease.
- Ophthalmic suspensions mix with tears less rapidly and remain in the cul-de-sac longer than solutions.
- Ophthalmic ointments maintain contact between the drug and ocular tissues by slowing the clearance rate to as little as 0.5%/min. Ophthalmic ointments provide maximum contact between drug and external ocular tissues.
- Ophthalmic ointments may impede delivery of other ophthalmic drugs to the affected side by serving as a barrier to contact.
- Ointments may blur vision during waking hours. Use with caution in conditions where visual clarity is critical (eg, operating motor equipment, reading).
- Monitor expiration dates closely. Do not use outdated medication.
- Solutions and ointments are frequently misused. Do not assume that patients know how to maximize safe and effective use of these agents. Combine appropriate patient education and counseling with prescribing and dispensing of ophthalmics.

Topical application is the most common route of administration for ophthalmic drugs. Advantages include convenience, simplicity, noninvasive nature, and the ability of the patient to self-administer. Because of blood and aqueous losses of drug, topical medications typically do not penetrate in useful concentrations to posterior ocular structures and therefore are of no therapeutic benefit for diseases of the retina, optic nerve, and other posterior segment structures.

*Medications:*

*Solutions and suspensions* – Most topical ocular preparations are commercially available as solutions or suspensions that are applied directly to the eye from the bottle, which serves as the eye dropper. Avoid touching the dropper tip to the eye because this can lead to contamination of the medication and also may cause ocular injury. Resuspend suspensions (notably, many ocular steroids) by shaking to provide an accurate dosage of drug.

*Recommended procedures for administration of solutions or suspensions* –

- Wash hands thoroughly before administration.
- Tilt head backward or lie down and gaze upward.
- Gently grasp lower eyelid below eyelashes and pull the eyelid away from the eye to form a pouch.
- Place dropper directly over eye. Avoid contact of the dropper with the eye, finger or any surface.

- Look upward just before applying a drop.
- After instilling the drop, look downward for several seconds.
- Release the lid slowly.
- With eyes closed, apply gentle pressure with fingers to the inside corner of eye for 3 to 5 minutes. This retards drainage of solution from intended solution.
- Do not rub the eye. Minimize blinking.
- Do not rinse the dropper.
- Do not use eye drops that have changed color.
- If more than 1 type of ophthalmic drop is used, wait at least 5 minutes before administering the second agent.
- When the instillation of eye drops is difficult (eg, pediatric patients, adults with particularly strong blink reflex), the close-eye method may be used. This involves lying down, placing the prescribed number of drops on the eyelid in the inner corner of the eye, then opening eye so that drops will fall into the eye by gravity.

*Ointments* – The primary purpose for an ophthalmic ointment vehicle is to prolong drug contact time with the external ocular surface. This is particularly useful for treating children, who may "cry out" topically applied solutions, and for medicating ocular injuries, such as corneal abrasions, when the eye is to be patched. Administer solutions before ointments. Ointments preclude entry of subsequent drops.

*Recommended procedures for administration of ointments* –
- Wash hands thoroughly before administration.
- Holding the ointment tube in the hand for a few minutes will warm the ointment and facilitate flow.
- When opening the ointment tube for the first time, squeeze out and discard the first 0.25 inch of ointment as it may be too dry.
- Tilt head backward or lie down and gaze upward.
- Gently pull down the lower lid to form a pouch.
- Place 0.25 to 0.5 inch of ointment with a sweeping motion inside the lower lid by squeezing the tube gently.
- Close the eye for 1 to 2 minutes and roll the eyeball in all directions.
- Temporary blurring of vision may occur. Avoid activities requiring visual acuity until blurring clears.
- Remove excessive ointment around the eye or ointment tube tip with a tissue.
- If using more than 1 kind of ointment, wait about 10 minutes before applying the second drug.

# AGENTS FOR GLAUCOMA

Glaucoma is a condition of the eye in which an elevation of the intraocular pressure (IOP) leads to progressive cupping and atrophy of the optic nerve head, deterioration of the visual fields, and, ultimately, to blindness. Primary open-angle glaucoma is the most common type of glaucoma. Angle-closure glaucoma and congenital glaucoma are treated primarily by surgical methods, although short-term drug therapy is used to decrease IOP prior to surgery.

Drugs used in the therapy of primary open-angle glaucoma include a variety of agents with different mechanisms of action. The therapeutic goal in treating glaucoma is reducing the elevated IOP, a major risk factor in the pathogenesis of glaucomatous visual field loss. The higher the level of IOP, the greater the likelihood of glaucomatous visual field loss and optic nerve damage. Reduction of IOP may be accomplished by: 1) Decreasing the rate of production of aqueous humor or 2) increasing the rate of outflow (drainage) of aqueous humor from the anterior chamber of the eye.

The 5 groups of agents used in therapy of primary open-angle glaucoma are listed in the table, which summarizes their mechanism of decreasing IOP, effects on pupil size and ciliary muscle and duration of action.

| Agents for Glaucoma | | | | | | |
|---|---|---|---|---|---|---|
| Drug | Strength | Duration (h) | Decrease aqueous production | Increase aqueous outflow | Effect on pupil | Effect on ciliary muscle |
| *Sympathomimetics* | | | | | | |
| Apraclonidine[1] | 0.5 to 1% | 7 to 12 | +++ | NR | NR | NR |
| Brimonidine | 0.2% | 12 | ++ | ++ | NR | NR |
| Dipivefrin | 0.1% | 12 | + | ++ | mydriasis | NR |
| Epinephrine | 0.1% to 2% | 12 to 24 | + | ++ | mydriasis | NR |
| *Beta blockers* | | | | | | |
| Betaxolol | 0.25% to 0.5% | 12 | +++ | NR | NR | NR |
| Carteolol | 1% | 12 | +++ | nd | NR | NR |
| Levobunolol | 0.25% to 0.5% | 12 to 24 | +++ | NR | NR | NR |
| Metipranolol | 0.3% | 12 to 24 | +++ | + | NR | NR |
| Timolol | 0.25% to 0.5% | 12 to 24 | +++ | + | NR | NR |
| *Miotics, direct-acting* | | | | | | |
| Acetylcholine[2] | 1% | 10 to 20 min | NR | +++ | miosis | accommodation |
| Carbachol[2] | 0.75% to 3% | 6 to 8 | NR | +++ | miosis | accommodation |
| Pilocarpine[3] | 0.25% to 10% | 4 to 8 | NR | +++ | miosis | accommodation |
| *Miotics, cholinesterase inhibitors* | | | | | | |
| Echothiophate | 0.03% to 0.25% | days/wks | NR | +++ | miosis | accommodation |
| Physostigmine | 0.25% to 0.5% | 12 to 36 | NR | +++ | miosis | accommodation |
| *Carbonic anhydrase inhibitors* | | | | | | |
| Acetazolamide[4] | 125 to 500 mg | 8 to 12 | +++ | NR | NR | NR |
| Brinzolamide[5] | 1% | ≈ 8 | +++ | NR | NR | NR |
| Dichlorphenamide[4] | 50 mg | 6 to 12 | +++ | NR | NR | NR |
| Dorzolamide[5] | 2% | ≈ 8 | +++ | NR | NR | NR |
| Methazolamide[4] | 25 to 50 mg | 10 to 18 | +++ | NR | NR | NR |

| Agents for Glaucoma | | | | | | |
|---|---|---|---|---|---|---|
| Drug | Strength | Duration (h) | Decrease aqueous production | Increase aqueous outflow | Effect on pupil | Effect on ciliary muscle |
| *Prostaglandin analog* | | | | | | |
| Bimatoprost | 0.03% | ≈ 24 | NR | +++ | NR | NR |
| Latanoprost | 0.0005% | 24 | NR | +++ | NR | NR |
| Travoprost | 0.004% | ≈ 24 | NR | +++ | NR | NR |

+++ = significant activity    ++ = moderate activity    + = some activity    NR = no activity reported
nd = No data available
[1] 1% used only to decrease IOP in surgery.
[2] Intraocular administration only for miosis during surgery; carbachol also available as a topical agent.
[3] Also available as a gel and an insert; the duration of these doseforms is longer (18 to 24 hours and 1 week, respectively) than the solution.
[4] Systemic agents; for detailed information, see group monograph in Cardiovascular section.
[5] Topical ophthalmic agent.

*Prostaglandin analogs:* Prostaglandin analogs increase uveoscleral outflow through a new mechanism of action; selective prostanoid receptor agonism. Latanoprost, currently the only agent available in this class, can be used concurrently with other topical ophthalmic drug products to reduce IOP.

# BRIMONIDINE TARTRATE

**Solution: 0.15% (Rx)**            *Alphagan, Alphagan-P* (Allergan)

## Indications
*Intraocular pressure (IOP):* To lower IOP in patients with open-angle glaucoma or ocular hypertension.

## Administration and Dosage
The recommended dose is 1 drop of brimonidine tartrate in the affected eye(s) 3 times daily, approximately 8 hours apart.

## Actions
*Pharmacology:* Brimonidine is an alpha-2 adrenergic receptor agonist. It has a peak ocular hypotensive effect occurring at 2 hours postdose. Brimonidine has a dual mechanism of action; it reduces aqueous humor production and increases uveoscleral outflow.

*Pharmacokinetics:* After ocular administration of a 0.1% or 0.2% solution, plasma concentrations peaked within 0.5 to 2.5 hours and declined with a systemic half-life of approximately 2 hours.

Brimonidine is metabolized primarily by the liver. Urinary excretion is the major route of elimination of the drug and its metabolites. Approximately 87% of an orally administered radioactive dose was eliminated within 120 hours, with 74% found in the urine.

## Contraindications
Hypersensitivity to brimonidine tartrate or any component of this medication; patients receiving monoamine oxidase inhibitor (MAOI) therapy.

## Warnings
*Soft contact lenses:* The preservative in brimonidine, benzalkonium chloride, may be absorbed by soft contact lenses. Instruct patients wearing soft contact lenses to wait at least 15 minutes after instilling brimonidine to insert soft contact lenses.

*Renal/Hepatic function impairment:* Use caution when treating patients with hepatic or renal impairment.

*Pregnancy:* Category B.

*Lactation:* It is not known whether brimonidine is excreted in breast milk.

*Children:* Safety and efficacy in pediatric patients have not been established.

#### Precautions

*Cardiovascular disease:* Exercise caution in treating patients with severe cardiovascular disease.

*Use with caution:* Use with caution in patients with depression, cerebral or coronary insufficiency, Raynaud phenomenon, orthostatic hypotension, or thromboangitis obliterans.

*Loss of effect:* Loss of effect in some patients may occur. The IOP-lowering efficacy observed with brimonidine during the first month of therapy may not always reflect the long-term level of IOP reduction. Therefore, routinely monitor IOP.

#### Drug Interactions

Drugs that may be affected by brimonidine include CNS depressants, beta-blockers, antihypertensives, MAOIs, and cardiac glycosides.

Drugs that may affect brimonidine include tricyclic antidepressants.

#### Adverse Reactions

Adverse events occurring in 10% to 30% of patients in descending order include oral dryness, ocular hyperemia, burning and stinging, headache, blurring, foreign body sensation, fatigue/drowsiness, conjunctival follicles, ocular allergic reactions, and ocular pruritus.

Adverse events occurring in 3% to 9% in descending order include corneal staining/erosion, photophobia, eyelid erythema, ocular ache/pain, ocular dryness, tearing, upper respiratory symptoms, eyelid edema, conjunctival edema, dizziness, blepharitis, ocular irritation, GI symptoms, asthenia, conjunctival blanching, abnormal vision, and muscular pain.

## EPINEPHRINE

**EPINEPHRINE (as Borate)**
**Solution: 0.5%, 1%, and 2% (Rx)**                    *Epinal* (Alcon)

#### Indications

*Glaucoma:* Management of open-angle (chronic simple) glaucoma; may be used in combination with miotics, beta blockers, hyperosmotic agents, or carbonic anhydrase inhibitors.

#### Administration and Dosage

Instill 1 drop into affected eye(s) once or twice daily. Determine frequency of instillation by tonometry.

More frequent instillation than 1 drop twice daily does not usually elicit any further improvement in therapeutic response.

When used in conjunction with miotics, instill the miotic first.

#### Actions

*Pharmacology:* Epinephrine, a direct-acting sympathomimetic agent, acts on $\alpha$ and $\beta$ receptors. Topical application, therefore, causes conjunctival decongestion (vasoconstriction), transient mydriasis (pupillary dilation), and reduction in intraocular pressure (IOP). It is believed IOP reduction primarily is caused by reduced aqueous production and increased aqueous outflow. The duration of decrease in IOP is 12 to 24 hours.

#### Contraindications

Hypersensitivity to epinephrine or any component of the formulation; narrow- or shallow-angle (angle Y closure) glaucoma; aphakia; patients with a narrow angle but no glaucoma; if the nature of the glaucoma is not clearly established. Do not use while wearing soft contact lenses; discoloration of lenses may occur.

#### Warnings

*For ophthalmic use only:* Not for injection or intraocular use.

*Gonioscopy:* Because pupil dilation may precipitate an acute attack of narrow-angle glaucoma, evaluate anterior chamber angle by gonioscopy prior to beginning therapy.

*Anesthesia:* Discontinue use prior to general anesthesia with anesthetics that sensitize the myocardium to sympathomimetics (eg, cyclopropane, halothane).

*Aphakic patients:* Maculopathy with associated decrease in visual acuity may occur in the aphakic eye; if this occurs, promptly discontinue use.

*Elderly:* Use with caution.

*Pregnancy: Category C.*

*Lactation:* It is not known whether this drug is excreted in breast milk.

*Children:* Safety and efficacy for use in children have not been established.

### Precautions

*Installation discomfort:* Epinephrine is relatively uncomfortable upon instillation. Discomfort lessens as concentration of epinephrine decreases.

*Special risk:* Use with caution in the presence or history of the following: Hypertension; diabetes; hyperthyroidism; heart disease; cerebral arteriosclerosis; bronchial asthma.

*Hazardous tasks:* Epinephrine may cause temporarily blurred or unstable vision after instillation; observe caution while driving, operating machinery, or performing other tasks requiring physical dexterity.

### Drug Interactions

Consider interactions that occur with systemic use of epinephrine, including beta blockers and chymotrypsin.

### Adverse Reactions

Adverse reactions may include transient stinging and burning; eye pain/ache; browache; headache; allergic lid reaction; conjunctival hyperemia; conjunctival or corneal pigmentation; ocular irritation (hypersensitivity); localized adrenochrome deposits in conjunctiva and cornea (prolonged use); reversible cystoid macular edema (may result from use in aphakic patients); palpitations; tachycardia; extrasystoles; cardiac arrhythmia; hypertension; faintness.

## DIPIVEFRIN HCl (Dipivalyl epinephrine)

| Solution: 0.1% (*Rx*) | Various, *Propine* (Allergan), *AKPro* (Akorn) |
| --- | --- |

### Indications

*Glaucoma:* Initial therapy or as an adjunct with other antiglaucoma agents for the control of intraocular pressure (IOP) in chronic open-angle glaucoma.

### Administration and Dosage

*Initial glaucoma therapy:* Instill 1 drop into the eye(s) every 12 hours.

### Actions

*Pharmacology:* Dipivefrin is a prodrug of epinephrine. Dipivefrin, converted to epinephrine in the eye by enzymatic hydrolysis, appears to act by decreasing aqueous production and enhancing outflow facility. It has the same therapeutic effects as epinephrine with fewer local and systemic side effects.

*Pharmacokinetics:* The onset of action with 1 drop occurs approximately 30 minutes after treatment, with maximum effect seen at about 1 hour.

### Contraindications

Hypersensitivity to dipivefrin or any formulation component; narrow-angle glaucoma.

### Warnings

*Pregnancy: Category B.*

*Lactation:* It is not known whether this drug is excreted in breast milk.

*Children:* Safety and efficacy for use in children have not been established.

## Precautions

*Aphakic patients:* Macular edema occurs in up to 30% of aphakic patients treated with epinephrine. Discontinuation generally results in reversal of the maculopathy.

## Adverse Reactions

Adverse reactions may include tachycardia; arrhythmias; hypertension; burning and stinging; conjunctival injection.

# APRACLONIDINE HYDROCHLORIDE

**Solution**: 0.5% and 0.01% *(Rx)*                         *Iopidine* (Alcon)

## Indications

*1%:* To control or prevent postsurgical elevations in IOP that occur in patients after argon laser trabeculoplasty or iridotomy.

*0.5%:* Short-term adjunctive therapy in patients on maximally tolerated medical therapy who require additional IOP reduction.

## Administration and Dosage

*0.5%:* Instill 1 to 2 drops in the affected eye(s) 3 times daily. Because apraclonidine 0.5% will be used with other ocular glaucoma therapies, use an approximate 5-minute interval between instillation of each medication to prevent washout of the previous dose. Not for injection into the eye.

*1%:* Instill 1 drop in scheduled operative eye 1 hour before initiating anterior segment laser surgery. Instill second drop into same eye immediately upon completion of surgery.

## Actions

*Pharmacology:* Apraclonidine HCl is a relatively selective α-adrenergic agonist. When instilled into the eyes, apraclonidine reduces intraocular pressure (IOP) and has minimal effect on cardiovascular parameters.

*Pharmacokinetics:* Topical use of apraclonidine 0.5% leads to systemic absorption. The onset of action is usually within 1 hour and the maximum IOP reduction occurs 3 to 5 hours after application of a single dose.

## Contraindications

Hypersensitivity to any component of this medication or to clonidine; concurrent monamine oxidase inhibitor therapy.

## Warnings

*Concomitant therapy:* The addition of 0.5% apraclonidine to patients already using 2 aqueous suppressing drugs (eg, beta blocker plus carbonic anhydrase inhibitor) as part of their maximally tolerated medical therapy may not provide additional benefit.

*Tachyphylaxis:* The IOP-lowering efficacy of 0.5% apraclonidine diminishes over time in some patients. The benefit for most patients is less than 1 month.

*Hypersensitivity reactions:* Apraclonidine can lead to an allergic-like reaction characterized wholly or in part by the symptoms of hyperemia, pruritus, discomfort, tearing, foreign body sensation, and edema of the lids and conjunctiva. If ocular allergic-like symptoms occur, discontinue therapy.

*Renal/Hepatic function impairment:* Although the topical use of apraclonidine has not been studied in renal failure patients, structurally related clonidine undergoes a significant increase in half-life in patients with severe renal impairment. Close monitoring of cardiovascular parameters in patients with impaired renal function is advised if they are candidates for topical apraclonidine therapy. Close monitoring of cardiovascular parameters in patients with impaired liver function is also advised as the systemic dosage form of clonidine is partly metabolized in the liver.

*Pregnancy: Category C.*

*Lactation:* Consider discontinuing nursing for the day on which apraclonidine is used.

*Children:* Safety and efficacy for use in children have not been established.

**Precautions**

*Monitoring:* Glaucoma patients on maximally tolerated medical therapy who are treated with 0.5% apraclonidine to delay surgery should have their visual fields monitored periodically. Discontinue treatment if IOP rises significantly.

*IOP reduction:* Because apraclonidine is a potent depressor of IOP, closely monitor patients who develop exaggerated reductions in IOP.

*Cardiovascular disease:* Acute administration of 2 drops of apraclonidine has had minimal effect on heart rate or blood pressure; however, observe caution in treating patients with severe cardiovascular disease, including hypertension.

Use 0.5% apraclonidine with caution in patients with coronary insufficiency, recent MI, cerebrovascular disease, chronic renal failure, Raynaud disease, or thromboangiitis obliterans.

*Depression:* Use caution and monitor depressed patients because apraclonidine has been infrequently associated with depression.

**Drug Interactions**

Drugs that may interact include cardiovascular agents and MAOIs.

**Adverse Reactions**

Adverse reactions from 1% solution may include upper lid elevation; conjunctival blanching; mydriasis; burning; discomfort; foreign body sensation; dryness; itching; hypotony; blurred or dimmed vision; allergic response; conjunctival microhemorrhage; dry mouth; bradycardia; vasovagal attack; palpitations; orthostatic episode; headache; taste abnormalities; nasal burning or head-cold sensation; shortness of breath.

Adverse reactions from 0.5% solution may include hyperemia; pruritus; discomfort; tearing; taste perversion; use can lead to an allergic-type reaction.

# BETA-ADRENERGIC BLOCKING AGENTS

| | |
|---|---|
| **BETAXOLOL HCl** | |
| **Solution:** 5.6 mg (equiv. to 5 mg base) per mL (0.5%) (*Rx*) | Various, *Betoptic* (Alcon) |
| **Suspension:** 2.8 mg (equiv. to 2.5 mg base) per mL (0.25%) (*Rx*) | *Betoptic S* (Alcon) |
| **CARTEOLOL HCl** | |
| **Solution:** 1% (*Rx*) | Various |
| **LEVOBETAXOLOL HCl** | |
| **Suspension:** 0.5% as base (5.6 mg/mL) (*Rx*) | *Betaxon* (Alcon) |
| **LEVOBUNOLOL HCl** | |
| **Solution:** 0.25% and 0.5% (*Rx*) | Various, *AKBeta* (Akorn), *Betagan Liquifilm* (Allergan) |
| **METIPRANOLOL HCl** | |
| **Solution:** 0.3% (*Rx*) | *OptiPranolol* (Bausch & Lomb) |
| **TIMOLOL MALEATE** | |
| **Solution:** 0.25% and 0.5% (*Rx*) | Various, *Timoptic* (Merck) |
| **Gel:** 0.25% and 0.5% (*Rx*) | Various, *Timoptic-XE* (Merck) |

**Indications**

*Glaucoma:* Lowering intraocular pressure (IOP) in patients with chronic open-angle glaucoma and intraocular hypertension.

**Administration and Dosage**

*BETAXOLOL HCl:* Instill 1 to 2 drops twice daily.

*CARTEOLOL HCl:* One drop in the affected eye(s) twice daily.

*LEVOBETAXOLOL HCl:* Instill 1 drop in the affected eye(s) twice daily. In some patients, the IOP-lowering responses may require a few weeks to stabilize.

*LEVOBUNOLOL HCl:*

    0.5% – 1 to 2 drops in the affected eye(s) once daily.

    0.25% – 1 to 2 drops in the affected eye(s) twice daily.

In patients with more severe or uncontrolled glaucoma, the 0.5% solution can be administered twice daily.

METIPRANOLOL HCl: One drop in the affected eye(s) twice a day. If the patient's IOP is not at a satisfactory level on this regimen, more frequent administration or a larger dose is not known to be of benefit.

TIMOLOL MALEATE:
> Solution –
>> Initial therapy: 1 drop of 0.25% or 0.5% twice daily. If clinical response is not adequate, change the dosage to 1 drop of 0.5% solution twice a day. If the IOP is maintained at satisfactory levels, change the dosage to 1 drop once a day.
>
> Gel – Administer other ophthalmics at least 10 minutes before the gel. Dose is 1 drop (0.25% or 0.5%) once daily. Dosages more than 1 drop of 0.5% have not been studied. Consider concomitant therapy if IOP is not at a satisfactory level.

## Actions

Pharmacology: The exact mechanism of ocular antihypertensive action is not established, but it appears to be a reduction of aqueous production. However, some studies show a slight increase in outflow facility with **timolol** and **metipranolol**.

Pharmacokinetics:

| Pharmacokinetics of Ophthalmic β-Adrenergic Blocking Agents | | | | |
|---|---|---|---|---|
| Drug | β-receptor selectivity | Onset (min) | Maximum effect (h) | Duration (h) |
| Carteolol | $\beta_1$ and $\beta_2$ | nd[1] | 2 | 12 |
| Betaxolol | $\beta_1$ | ≤ 30 | 2 | 12 |
| Levobunolol | $\beta_1$ and $\beta_2$ | < 60 | 2 to 6 | ≤ 24 |
| Metipranolol | $\beta_1$ and $\beta_2$ | ≤ 30 | ≈ 2 | 24 |
| Timolol | $\beta_1$ and $\beta_2$ | ≤ 30 | 1 to 2 | ≤ 24 |
| Levobetaxolol | $\beta_1$ | ≤ 30 | 2 | ≈ 12 |

[1] nd = No data

## Contraindications

Bronchial asthma, a history of bronchial asthma, or severe chronic obstructive pulmonary disease; sinus bradycardia; second- and third-degree AV block; overt cardiac failure; cardiogenic shock; hypersensitivity to any component of the products.

## Warnings

Systemic absorption: These agents may be absorbed systemically. The same adverse reactions found with systemic β-blockers may occur with topical use.

Cardiovascular: These agents can decrease resting and maximal exercise heart rate, even in healthy subjects.

Cardiac failure: Sympathetic stimulation may be essential for circulation support in diminished myocardial contractility; its inhibition by β-receptor blockade may precipitate more severe failure.

Bronchospasm: Nonallergic bronchospasm patients or patients with a history of chronic bronchitis, emphysema, etc., should receive β-blockers with caution; they may block bronchodilation produced by catecholamine stimulation of $\beta_2$-receptors.

Diabetes mellitus: Administer with caution to patients subject to spontaneous hypoglycemia or to diabetic patients (especially labile diabetics). Beta-blocking agents may mask signs and symptoms of acute hypoglycemia.

Thyroid: Beta-adrenergic blocking agents may mask clinical signs of hyperthyroidism (eg, tachycardia).

Cerebrovascular insufficiency: Because of potential effects of β-blockers on blood pressure and pulse, use with caution in patients with cerebrovascular insufficiency.

Pregnancy: Category C.

Lactation: It is not known whether these agents are excreted in human breast milk.

Children: Safety and efficacy for use in children have not been established.

## Precautions

*Angle-closure glaucoma:* The immediate objective is to reopen the angle, requiring constriction of the pupil with a miotic. These agents have little or no effect on the pupil.

*Muscle weakness:* Beta-blockade may potentiate muscle weakness consistent with certain myasthenic symptoms (eg, diplopia, ptosis, generalized weakness).

*Long-term therapy:* In long-term studies (2 and 3 years), no significant differences in mean IOP were observed after initial stabilization.

## Drug Interactions

Ophthalmic beta blockers may affect oral beta blockers, catecholamine-depleting drugs, calcium antagonists, digitalis, and phenothiazines.

Drugs that may affect ophthalmic beta blockers include catecholamine-depleting drugs, digitalis, and quinidine.

Other drugs that may interact with systemic β-adrenergic blocking agents also may interact with ophthalmic agents.

## Adverse Reactions

Adverse reactions may include headache; depression; arrhythmia; syncope; heart block; cerebral vascular accident; cerebral ischemia; CHF; palpitation; nausea; hypersensitivity, including localized and generalized rash; bronchospasm; respiratory failure; eratitis; blepharoptosis; visual disturbances including refractive changes; diplopia; ptosis.

*Systemic β-adrenergic blocker-associated reactions* – Consider potential effects with ophthalmic use. The following adverse reactions have occurred with each individual agent:

*Carteolol –*

*Ophthalmic:* Transient irritation, burning, tearing, conjunctival hyperemia, edema (approximately 25%).

*Betaxolol –*

*Ophthalmic:* Brief discomfort (more than 25%); occasional tearing (5%).

*Metipranolol –*

*Ophthalmic:* Transient local discomfort; conjunctivitis; eyelid dermatitis; blepharitis; blurred vision; tearing; browache; abnormal vision; photophobia; edema; uveitis.

*Levobetaxolol –*

*Ophthalmic:* Transient ocular discomfort upon installation (11%).

*Levobunolol –*

*Ophthalmic:* Transient burning/stinging (up to 33%); blepharoconjunctivitis (up to 5%).

*Timolol –*

*Ophthalmic:* Ocular irritation including conjunctivitis; blepharitis; keratitis; blepharoptosis; decreased corneal sensitivity; visual disturbances including refractive changes; diplopia; ptosis.

# MIOTICS, DIRECT-ACTING

| | |
|---|---|
| **ACETYLCHOLINE CHLORIDE, INTRAOCULAR** | |
| **Solution:** 1:100 acetylcholine chloride when reconstituted (*Rx*) | *Miochol-E* (Novartis Ophthalmic) |
| **CARBACHOL, INTRAOCULAR** | |
| **Solution:** 0.01% (*Rx*) | *Miostat* (Alcon), *Carbastat* (Novartis Ophthalmic) |
| **CARBACHOL, TOPICAL** | |
| **Solution:** 0.75%, 1.5%, 2.25%, and 3% (*Rx*) | *Isopto Carbachol* (Alcon), *Carboptic* (Optopics) |
| **PILOCARPINE HCl** | |
| **Solution:** 0.25%, 0.5%, 1%, 2%, 3%, 4%, 5%, 6%, 8%, and 10% (*Rx*) | Various, *Pilocar* (Novartis Ophthalmic), *Isopto Carpine* (Alcon) |
| **Gel:** 4% (*Rx*) | *Pilopine HS* (Alcon) |
| **PILOCARPINE NITRATE** | |
| **Solution:** 1%, 2%, and 4% (*Rx*) | *Pilagan* (Allergan) |
| **PILOCARPINE OCULAR THERAPEUTIC SYSTEM** | |
| **Ocular Therapeutic System:** Releases 20 or 40 mcg pilocarpine/hour for 1 week (*Rx*) | *Ocusert Pilo-20*, *Ocusert Pilo-40* (Alza) |

**Indications**
> *Carbachol, topical; pilocarpine:*
>> *Glaucoma* – To decrease elevated intraocular pressure (IOP) in glaucoma.
>
> *Acetylcholine; carbachol, intraocular:*
>> *Miosis* – To induce miosis during surgery.

**Administration and Dosage**
> ACETYLCHOLINE CHLORIDE, INTRAOCULAR:
>> *Solution* – 0.5 to 2 mL produces satisfactory miosis. Solution need not be flushed from the chamber after miosis occurs.
>
> CARBACHOL, INTRAOCULAR: Gently instill no more than 0.5 mL into the anterior chamber before or after securing sutures. Miosis is usually maximal 2 to 5 minutes after application.
>
> CARBACHOL, TOPICAL: Instill 2 drops into eye(s) up to 3 times daily.
>
> PILOCARPINE:
>> *Solution* –
>>> *Initial:* 1 or 2 drops 3 to 4 times daily. Individuals with heavily pigmented irides may require higher strengths.
>>
>> *Gel* – Apply a 0.5 inch ribbon in the lower conjunctival sac of affected eye(s) once daily at bedtime.
>
> PILOCARPINE NITRATE:
>> *Glaucoma* – 1 to 2 drops 2 to 4 times daily.
>>
>> *Emergency miosis* – 1 to 2 drops of higher concentrations.
>>
>> *Reversal of mydriasis* – Dosage and strength required are dependent on the cycloplegic used.
>
> PILOCARPINE OCULAR THERAPEUTIC SYSTEM:
>> *Initiation of therapy* – It has been estimated that 20 mcg *Ocusert* is roughly equal to 0.5% or 1% drops and 40 mcg is roughly equal to 2% or 3% drops. Therapy may be started with the 20 mcg system, regardless of the strength of pilocarpine solution the patient previously required. Because of the patient's age, family history, and disease status or progression, however, therapy may be started with the 40 mcg system.
>>
>> If pressure is satisfactorily reduced with the 30 mcg system, the patient should continue its use, replacing each unit every 7 days. If IOP reduction greater than that achieved by 20 mcg is needed, transfer the patient to the 40 mcg system.

**Actions**
> *Pharmacology:* Direct-acting miotics are parasympathomimetic (cholinergic) drugs which duplicate the muscarinic effects of **acetylcholine**. When applied topically, these drugs produce pupillary constriction, stimulate ciliary muscles, and increase aqueous humor outflow facility. With the increase in outflow facility, there is a decrease in IOP. Topical ophthalmic instillation of acetylcholine causes no discernible

response, as cholinesterase destroys the molecule more rapidly than it can penetrate the cornea; therefore, acetylcholine only is used intraocularly.

*Pharmacokinetics:*

| Miosis Induction of Direct-Acting Miotics | | | |
|---|---|---|---|
| Miotic | Onset | Peak | Duration |
| Acetylcholine, intraocular | seconds | — | 10 min |
| Carbachol<br>Intraocular<br>Topical | seconds<br>10 to 20 min | 2 to 5 min<br>— | 1 to 2 days<br>4 to 8 hours |
| Pilocarpine, topical | 10 to 30 min | — | 4 to 8 hours |

## Contraindications

Hypersensitivity to any component of the formulation; where constriction is undesirable (eg, acute iritis, acute or anterior uveitis, some forms of secondary glaucoma, pupillary block glaucoma, acute inflammatory disease of the anterior chamber).

## Warnings

*Corneal abrasion:* Use carbachol with caution in the presence of corneal abrasion to avoid excessive penetration.

*Pregnancy:* Category C (carbachol, pilocarpine).

*Lactation:* It is not known whether these drugs are excreted in breast milk.

*Children:* Safety and efficacy for use in children have not been established.

## Precautions

*Systemic reactions:* Caution is advised in patients with acute cardiac failure, bronchial asthma, peptic ulcer, hyperthyroidism, GI spasm, urinary tract obstruction, Parkinson's disease, recent MI, hypertension, or hypotension.

*Retinal detachment:* Retinal detachment has been caused by miotics in susceptible individuals, in individuals with pre-existing retinal disease, or in those who are predisposed to retinal tears.

*Miosis:* Miosis usually causes difficulty in dark adaptation. Advise patients to use caution while night driving or performing hazardous tasks in poor light.

*Angle-closure:* Although withdrawal of the peripheral iris from the anterior chamber angle by miosis may reduce the tendency for narrow-angle closure, miotics occasionally can precipitate angle closure by increasing resistance to aqueous flow from posterior to anterior chamber.

*Pilocarpine ocular therapeutic system (Ocusert):* Carefully consider and evaluate patients with acute infectious conjunctivitis or keratitis prior to use.

## Adverse Reactions

*Acetylcholine:*

   Ophthalmic – Corneal edema; corneal clouding; corneal decompensation.

   Systemic – Bradycardia; hypotension; flushing; breathing difficulties; sweating.

*Carbachol:*

   Ophthalmic – Transient stinging and burning; corneal clouding; persistent bullous keratopathy; retinal detachment; transient ciliary and conjunctival injection; ciliary spasm with resultant temporary decrease of visual acuity.

   Systemic – Headache; salivation; GI cramps; vomiting; diarrhea; asthma; syncope; cardiac arrhythmia; flushing; sweating; epigastric distress; tightness in bladder; hypotension; frequent urge to urinate.

*Pilocarpine:*

   Ophthalmic – Transient stinging and burning; tearing; ciliary spasm; conjunctival vascular congestion; temporal, peri-, or supra-orbital headache; superficial keratitis-induced myopia; blurred vision; poor dark adaptation; reduced visual acuity in poor illumination in older individuals and in individuals with lens opacity.

# MIOTICS, CHOLINESTERASE INHIBITORS

**ECHOTHIOPHATE IODIDE**

**Powder for Reconstitution:** 1.5 mg to make 0.03%, 3 mg to make 0.06%, 6.25 mg to make 0.125%, 12.5 mg to make 0.25% *(Rx)*

*Phospholine Iodide* (Wyeth-Ayerst)

**PHYSOSTIGMINE (Eserine)**

**Ointment:** 0.25% (as sulfate) *(Rx)*

*Eserine Sulfate* (Novartis Ophthalmic)

### Indications

*Glaucoma:* Therapy of open-angle glaucoma.

### Administration and Dosage

ECHOTHIOPHATE IODIDE:

*Glaucoma* – Two doses per day are preferred to maintain as smooth a diurnal tension curve as possible, although 1 dose/day or every other day has been used with satisfactory results. Instill the daily dose or 1 of the 2 daily doses just before bedtime to avoid inconvenience due to miosis.

*Early chronic simple glaucoma:* Instill a 0.03% solution just before retiring and in the morning in cases not controlled with pilocarpine.

*Advanced chronic simple glaucoma and glaucoma secondary to cataract surgery:* Instill 0.03% solution twice daily, as above.

*Accommodative esotropia –*

*Diagnosis:* Instill 1 drop of 0.125% solution once a day into both eyes at bedtime for 2 or 3 weeks. If the esotropia is accommodative, a favorable response may begin within a few hours.

*Treatment:* After initial period of treatment for diagnostic purposes, reduce schedule to 0.125% every other day or 0.06% every day. The 0.03% strength has proven effective in some cases. The maximum recommended dose is 0.125% once a day, although more intensive therapy has been used for short periods.

PHYSOSTIGMINE (ESERINE):

*Ointment* – Apply small quantity to lower fornix, up to 3 times daily.

### Actions

*Pharmacology:* Topical application to the eye produces intense miosis and muscle contraction. IOP is reduced by a decreased resistance to aqueous outflow.

| Cholinesterase-Inhibiting Miotics | | | | | |
|---|---|---|---|---|---|
| | Miosis | | IOP reduction | | |
| Miotics | Onset (minutes) | Duration | Onset (h) | Peak (h) | Duration |
| Reversible Physostigmine | 20 to 30 | 12 to 36 h | — | 2 to 6 | 12 to 36 h |
| Irreversible Echothiophate | 10 to 30 | 1 to 4 weeks | 4 to 8 | 24 | 7 to 28 days |

### Contraindications

Hypersensitivity to cholinesterase inhibitors or any component of the formulation; active uveal inflammation or any inflammatory disease of the iris or ciliary body; glaucoma associated with iridocyclitis.

*Echothiophate:* Most cases of angle-closure glaucoma (because of the possibility of increasing angle-block).

### Warnings

*Myasthenia gravis:* Because of possible additive adverse effects, administer **echothiophate** only with extreme caution to patients with myasthenia gravis who are receiving systemic anticholinesterase therapy.

*Surgery:* In patients receiving cholinesterase inhibitors, administer succinylcholine with extreme caution before and during general anesthesia. Use prior to ophthalmic surgery only as a considered risk because of the possible occurrence of hyphema.

*Pregnancy: Category C.*

*Lactation:* It is not known whether these drugs are excreted in breast milk.

*Children:* The occurrence of iris cysts is more frequent in children. Safety and efficacy for use of **physostigmine** have not been established.

**Precautions**

*Concomitant therapy:* Cholinesterase inhibitors may be used in combination with adrenergic agents, β-blockers, carbonic anhydrase inhibitors, or hyperosmotic agents.

*Narrow-angle glaucoma:* Use with caution in patients with chronic angle-closure (narrow-angle) glaucoma or in patients with narrow angles, because of the possibility of producing pupillary block and increasing angle blockage. Temporarily discontinue if cardiac irregularities occur.

*Ophthalmic ointments:* Ophthalmic ointments may retard corneal healing.

*Miosis:* Miosis usually causes difficulty in dark adaptation. Use caution while driving at night or performing hazardous tasks in poor light.

*Gonioscopy:* Use only when shorter-acting miotics have proven inadequate. Gonioscopy is recommended prior to use of medication.

*Concomitant ocular conditions:* When an intraocular inflammatory process is present, breakdown of the blood-aqueous barrier from anticholinesterase therapy requires abstention from, or cautious use of, these drugs. Use with great caution where there is a history of quiescent uveitis.

*Systemic effects:* Repeated administration may cause depression of the concentration of cholinesterase in the serum and erythrocytes, with resultant systemic effects.

*Iris cysts:* Iris cysts may form, enlarge, and obscure vision (more frequent in children).

*Special risk:* Use caution in patients with marked vagotonia, bronchial asthma, spastic GI disturbances, peptic ulcer, pronounced bradycardia/hypotension, recent MI, epilepsy, parkinsonism, and other disorders that may respond adversely to vagotonic effects.

**Drug Interactions**

Drugs that may interact with cholinesterase inhibitors include carbamate/organophosphate insecticides and pesticides, succinylcholine, and systemic anticholinesterases.

**Adverse Reactions**

*Ophthalmic:* Iris cysts; burning; lacrimation; lid muscle twitching; conjunctival and ciliary redness; browache; headache; activation of latent iritis or uveitis; induced myopia with visual blurring.

*Systemic:* Nausea; vomiting; abdominal cramps; diarrhea; urinary incontinence; fainting; sweating; salivation; difficulty in breathing; cardiac irregularities.

# CARBONIC ANHYDRASE INHIBITORS

| **BRINZOLAMIDE** | |
|---|---|
| **Suspension:** 1% *(Rx)* | *Azopt* (Alcon) |
| **DORZOLAMIDE** | |
| **Solution:** 2% *(Rx)* | *Trusopt* (Merck) |

**Indications**

*Elevated intraocular pressure (IOP):* Treatment of elevated IOP in patients with ocular hypertension or open-angle glaucoma.

**Administration and Dosage**

*Dosage:* One drop in the affected eye(s) 3 times daily.

*Concomitant therapy:* If more than one ophthalmic drug is being used, administer the drugs at least 10 minutes apart.

**Actions**

*Pharmacology:* **Brinzolamide** and **dorzolamide** are carbonic anhydrase inhibitors formulated for topical ophthalmic use.

*Pharmacokinetics:* When topically applied, **brinzolamide** and **dorzolamide** reach the systemic circulation and accumulate in RBCs during chronic dosing. Extensive distribution into RBCs yields a long half-life, approximately 3.5 to 4 months. The drugs primarily are excreted unchanged in the urine and the metabolite also is excreted in urine.

### Contraindications
Hypersensitivity to any component of this product.

### Warnings
*Systemic effects:* These agents are sulfonamides and, although administered topically, are absorbed systemically. Therefore, the same types of adverse reactions attributable to sulfonamides may occur with topical administration of **brinzolamide** and **dorzolamide**.

*Renal function impairment:* These agents have not been studied in patients with severe renal impairment (Ccr less than 30 mL/min). However, because the drugs and their metabolites are excreted predominantly by the kidney, these agents are not recommended in such patients.

*Elderly:* No overall differences in efficacy or safety were observed between these patients and younger patients.

*Pregnancy:* Category C.

*Lactation:* It is not known whether these drugs are excreted in breast milk.

*Children:* Safety and efficacy in children have not been established.

### Precautions
*Corneal endothelium effects:* The effect of continued administration of **brinzolamide** and **dorzolamide** on the corneal endothelium has not been fully evaluated.

*Acute angle-closure glaucoma:* The management of patients with acute angle-closure glaucoma requires therapeutic interventions in addition to ocular hypotensive agents. These agents have not been studied in patients with acute angle-closure glaucoma.

*Ocular effects:* Local ocular adverse effects, primarily conjunctivitis and lid reactions, were reported with chronic administration.

*Concomitant oral carbonic anhydrase inhibitors:* There is a potential for an additive effect of the known systemic effects of carbonic anhydrase (CA) inhibition in patients receiving an oral and ophthalmic CA inhibitor. The concomitant administration of ocular and oral CA inhibitors is not recommended.

*Contact lenses:* The preservative in these products, benzalkonium chloride, may be absorbed by soft contact lenses. Do not administer these agents while wearing soft contact lenses; reinsert lenses 15 minutes or more after drug administration.

### Drug Interactions
Although acid-base and electrolyte disturbances were not reported in the clinical trials, these disturbances have been reported with oral CA inhibitors and have, in some instances, resulted in drug interactions (eg, toxicity associated with high-dose salicylate therapy).

### Adverse Reactions
Adverse reactions occurring in at least 3% of patients include ocular burning, stinging, or discomfort immediately following administration; bitter taste following administration; superficial punctate keratitis; signs and symptoms of ocular allergic reaction; blurred vision; tearing; dryness; photophobia; blepharitis; dermatitis, foreign body sensation, hyperemia, ocular discharge/keratitis/pain/pruritus; rhinitis.

# PROSTAGLANDIN AGONISTS

| **BIMATOPROST** | |
|---|---|
| **Solution:** 0.03% (*Rx*) | *Lumigan* (Allergan) |
| **LATANOPROST** | |
| **Solution:** 0.005% (50 mcg/mL) (*Rx*) | *Xalatan* (Pharmacia) |
| **TRAVOPROST** | |
| **Solution:** 0.004% (*Rx*) | *Travatan* (Alcon) |

### Indications
Elevated intraocular pressure (IOP): For reduction of elevated IOP in patients with open-angle glaucoma and ocular hypertension who are intolerant of other IOP-lowering medications or insufficiently responsive to another IOP-lowering medication.

### Administration and Dosage
BIMATOPROST, LATANOPROST, TRAVOPROST: The recommended dosage is 1 drop in the affected eye(s) once daily in the evening. Do not exceed once-daily dosage because it has been shown that more frequent administration may decrease the IOP-lowering effect. Reduction of IOP starts about 2 to 4 hours after administration and the maximum effect is reached after 8 to 12 hours.

Bimatoprost, latanoprost, and travoprost may be used concomitantly with other topical ophthalmic drug products to lower IOP. If more than 1 topical ophthalmic drug is being used, administer the drugs at least 5 minutes apart.

### Actions
Pharmacology: Prostaglandin agonists lower IOP by increasing outflow of aqueous humor, although the exact mechanism is unknown at this time.

### Contraindications
Hypersensitivity to any component of these products, including benzalkonium chloride. Travoprost may interfere with the maintenance of pregnancy and should not be used by women during pregnancy or by women attempting to become pregnant.

### Warnings
Eye pigment changes: Prostaglandin agonists may gradually change eye color, increasing the amount of brown pigment in the iris by increasing the number of melanosomas (pigment granules) in melanocytes.

Pregnancy: Category C. Because prostaglandins are biologically active and may be absorbed through the skin, women who are pregnant or attempting to become pregnant should exercise appropriate precautions to avoid direct exposure to the contents of the bottle.

Lactation: It is not known whether these drugs or their metabolites are excreted in breast milk.

Children: Safety and efficacy in children have not been established.

### Precautions
Bacterial keratitis: There have been reports of bacterial keratitis associated with the use of multiple-dose containers of topical ophthalmic products. These containers had been inadvertently contaminated by patients who, in most cases, had a concurrent corneal disease or a disruption of the ocular epithelial surface.

Contact lenses: Do not administer prostaglandin agonists while wearing contact lenses.

Macular edema: Macular edema, including cystoid edema, has been reported during treatment with prostaglandin agonists. These reports mainly have occurred in aphakic patients, pseudoaphakic patients with torn posterior lens capsule, or patients with known risk factors for macular edema.

Cornea: Latanoprost is hydrolyzed in the cornea. The effect of continued administration of latanoprost on the corneal endothelium has not been fully evaluated.

Active intraocular inflammation: Use bimatoprost with caution in patients with active intraocular inflammation (eg, uveitis).

### Drug Interactions

In vitro studies have shown that precipitation occurs when eye drops containing thimerosal are mixed with **latanoprost**. If such drugs are used, administer with an interval of at least 5 minutes between applications.

### Adverse Reactions

*Prostaglandin agonists:*
  *Systemic* – The most common systemic adverse events seen with prostaglandin agonists were upper respiratory tract infection/cold/flu (4% to 10%).

*Bimatoprost:*
  *Ophthalmic* – Bimatoprost-associated ocular adverse events that occurred in 3% to 10% of patients, in descending order of incidence, included the following: Ocular dryness, visual disturbances, ocular burning, foreign body sensation, eye pain, pigmentation of the periocular skin, blepharitis, cataract, superficial punctate keratitis, eyelid erythema, ocular irritation, eyelash darkening.

*Latanoprost:*
  *Ophthalmic* – Latanoprost-associated ocular adverse events reported at an incidence of 5% to 15% included the following: Blurred vision, burning and stinging, conjunctival hyperemia, foreign body sensation, itching, increased pigmentation of the iris, punctate epithelial keratopathy.

*Travoprost:*
  *Ophthalmic* – Travoprost-associated ocular adverse events reported at an incidence of 5% to 15% included the following: Decreased visual acuity, eye discomfort, foreign body sensation, pain, pruritus.

# CORTICOSTEROIDS

**DEXAMETHASONE**

**Solution:** 0.1% dexamethasone phosphate (Rx) | Various, *AK-Dex* (Akorn), *Decadron Phosphate* (Merck)

**Suspension:** 0.1% (Rx) | *Maxidex* (Alcon)

**Ointment:** 0.05% dexamethasone phosphate (Rx) | Various, *Decadron Phosphate* (Merck)

**FLUOROMETHOLONE**

**Suspension:** 0.1% and 0.25% (Rx) | Various, *Fluor-Op* (Novartis Ophthalmic), *FML* (Allergan), *FML Forte* (Allergan)

**Suspension:** 0.1% fluorometholone acetate (Rx) | *Flarex* (Alcon)

**Ointment:** 0.1% (Rx) | *FML S.O.P.* (Allergan)

**LOTEPREDNOL ETABONATE**

**Suspension:** 0.5% (Rx) | *Lotemax* (Bausch & Lomb)

**Suspension:** 0.2% (Rx) | *Alrex* (Bausch & Lomb)

**MEDRYSONE**

**Suspension:** 1% (Rx) | *HMS* (Allergan)

**PREDNISOLONE**

**Suspension:** 0.12%, 0.125%, 1% prednisolone acetate (Rx) | *Econopred* (Alcon), *Econopred Plus* (Alcon), *Pred Mild* (Allergan), *Pred Forte* (Allergan), *Prednisolone Acetate Ophthalmic* (Falcon)

**Solution:** 0.125% and 1% prednisolone sodium phosphate (Rx) | Various, *AK-Pred* (Akorn), *Inflamase Mild* (Novartis Ophthalmic), *Inflamase Forte* (Novartis Ophthalmic)

**RIMEXOLONE**

**Suspension:** 1% (Rx) | *Vexol* (Alcon)

## Indications

*Inflammatory conditions:* Treatment of steroid-responsive inflammatory conditions of the palpebral and bulbar conjunctiva, lid, sclera, cornea, and anterior segment of the globe, such as: Allergic conjunctivitis; acne rosacea; superficial punctate keratitis; herpes zoster keratitis; iritis; cyclitis; and selected infective conjunctivitis (when the inherent hazard of steroid use is accepted to obtain an advisable diminution in edema and inflammation [prednisolone]); vernal conjunctivitis; episcleritis; epinephrine sensitivity; and anterior uveitis.

*Mild to moderate* – For the treatment of mild to moderate noninfectious allergic and inflammatory disorders of the lid, conjunctiva, cornea, and sclera (including chemical and thermal burns) (**prednisolone**).

*Moderate to severe* – Use higher strengths for moderate to severe inflammations. In difficult cases of anterior segment eye disease, systemic therapy may be required. When deeper ocular structures are involved, use systemic therapy (**prednisolone**).

*Ocular surgery:* For treatment of postoperative inflammation following ocular surgery.

*Corneal injury:* For corneal injury from chemical, radiation, or thermal burns, or from penetration of foreign bodies.

## Administration and Dosage

Treatment duration varies with type of lesion and may extend from a few days to several weeks, depending on therapeutic response. If signs and symptoms fail to improve after 2 days, reevaluate the patient. Relapse may occur if therapy is reduced too rapidly; taper over several days. Relapses, more common in chronic active lesions than in self-limited conditions, usually respond to retreatment.

*DEXAMETHASONE:*

*Solutions* – Instill 1 to 2 drops into the conjunctival sac every hour during the day and every 2 hours during the night as initial therapy. When a favorable response is observed, reduce dosage to 1 drop every 4 hours. Further reduction in dosage to 1 drop 3 or 4 times daily may suffice to control symptoms.

*Suspension* – Shake well before using. Instill 1 or 2 drops in the conjunctival sac(s). In severe disease, drops may be used hourly, being tapered to discontinuation as inflammation subsides. In mild disease, drops may be used up to 4 to 6 times daily.

*Ointment* – Apply a thin coating of ointment 3 to 4 times a day. When a favorable response is observed, reduce the number of daily applications to twice daily and later to once daily as a maintenance dose if this is sufficient to control symptoms.

The ointment is particularly convenient when an eye pad is used. It also may be the preparation of choice for patients in whom therapeutic benefit depends on prolonged contact of the active ingredients with ocular tissues.

FLUOROMETHALONE: Consult a physician if there is no improvement after 2 days. Do not discontinue therapy prematurely. In chronic conditions, withdraw treatment by gradually decreasing the frequency of applications.

*Suspension* – Shake well before using. Instill 1 to 2 drops into the conjunctival sac(s) 2 to 4 times daily. During the initial 24 to 48 hours, the dosage may be increased to 2 drops every 2 hours.

*Ointment* – Apply a small amount (about a ½ inch ribbon) of ointment to the conjunctival sac 1 to 3 times daily. During the first 24 to 48 hours, the dosing frequency may be increased to one application every 4 hours.

LOTEPREDNOL ETABONATE: Shake well before using.

*0.2% suspension* – Instill 1 drop into the affected eye(s) 4 times daily.

*0.5% suspension* –

*Steroid responsive disease:* Apply 1 to 2 drops into the conjunctival sac of the affected eye(s) 4 times daily. During the initial treatment within the first week, the dosing may be increased up to 1 drop every hour. Advise patients not to discontinue therapy prematurely. If signs and symptoms fail to improve after 2 days, reevaluate the patient.

*Postoperative inflammation:* Apply 1 to 2 drops into the conjunctival sac of the operated eye(s) 4 times daily beginning 24 hours after surgery and continuing throughout the first 2 weeks of the postoperative period.

MEDRYSONE: Shake well before using. Instill 1 drop into the conjunctival sac up to every 4 hours.

PREDNISOLONE:

*Solutions* – Depending on the severity of inflammation, instill 1 or 2 drops of solution into the conjunctival sac up to every hour during the day and every 2 hours during the night as necessary as initial therapy.

When a favorable response is observed, reduce dosage to 1 drop every 4 hours. Further reduction in dosage to 1 drop 3 to 4 times daily may suffice to control symptoms.

*Suspensions* – Shake well before using. Instill 1 to 2 drops into the conjunctival sac 2 to 4 times daily. During the initial 24 to 48 hours, the dosing frequency may be increased if necessary.

In cases of bacterial infections, concomitant use of anti-infective agents is mandatory.

If signs and symptoms do not improve after 2 days, reevaluate the patient.

Dosing may be reduced, but advise patients not to discontinue therapy prematurely. In chronic conditions, withdraw treatment by gradually decreasing the frequency of applications.

RIMEXOLONE: Shake well before using.

*Postoperative inflammation* – Apply 1 to 2 drops into the conjunctival sac of the affected eye(s) 4 times daily beginning 24 hours after surgery and continuing throughout the first 2 weeks of the postoperative period.

*Anterior uveitis* – Apply 1 to 2 drops into the conjunctival sac of the affected eye every hour during waking hours for the first week, 1 drop every 2 hours during waking hours of the second week, and then taper until uveitis is resolved.

## Actions

*Pharmacology:* Topical corticosteroids exert an antiinflammatory action. Steroids inhibit inflammatory response to inciting agents of mechanical, chemical, or immunological nature.

## Contraindications

Acute epithelial herpes simplex keratitis (dendritic keratitis); fungal diseases of ocular structures; vaccinia, varicella and most other viral diseases of the cornea and conjunctiva; ocular tuberculosis; hypersensitivity; after uncomplicated removal of a superficial corneal foreign body; mycobacterial eye infection; acute, purulent, untreated eye infections that may be masked or enhanced by the presence of steroids.

*Medrysone:* Medrysone is not for use in iritis and uveitis; its efficacy has not been demonstrated.

## Warnings

*Moderate to severe inflammation:* Use higher strengths for moderate to severe inflammations. In difficult cases of anterior segment eye disease, systemic therapy may be required. When deeper ocular structures are involved, use systemic therapy.

*Ocular damage:* Prolonged use may result in glaucoma, elevated IOP, optic nerve damage, defects in visual acuity and fields of vision, posterior subcapsular cataract formation or secondary ocular infections from pathogens liberated from ocular tissues.

*Cataract surgery:* The use of steroids after cataract surgery may delay healing and increase the incidence of bleb formation.

*Mustard gas keratitis or Sjogren's keratoconjunctivitis:* Topical steroids are not effective.

*Infections:* Prolonged use may result in secondary ocular infections caused by suppression of host response. Acute, purulent, untreated eye infections may be masked or activity enhanced by steroids. Fungal infections of the cornea have been reported with long-term local steroid applications.

*Pregnancy:* Category C.

*Lactation:* It is not known whether topical steroids are excreted in breast milk.

*Children:* Safety and efficacy have not been established in children.

## Precautions

*Bacterial keratitis:* Bacterial keratitis associated with the use of multiple-dose containers of topical ophthalmic products has been reported. Serious damage to the eye and subsequent loss of vision may result from using contaminated preparations.

*Benzalkonium chloride:* Benzalkonium chloride is a preservative used in some of these products that may be absorbed by soft contact lenses. Patients wearing soft contact lenses should wait at least 15 minutes after instilling products containing this preservative before inserting their lenses.

## Adverse Reactions

Glaucoma (elevated IOP) with optic nerve damage, loss of visual acuity and field defects; posterior subcapsular cataract formation; delayed wound healing; secondary ocular infection from pathogens, including herpes simplex and fungi liberated from ocular tissues; acute uveitis; perforation of globe where there is corneal or scleral thinning; exacerbation of viral, bacterial, and fungal corneal infections; transient stinging or burning; chemosis; dry eyes; epiphora; photophobia; keratitis; conjunctivitis; corneal ulcers; mydriasis; ptosis; blurred vision, discharge, discomfort, ocular pain, foreign body sensation, hyperemia, pruritus (**rimexolone**).

*Systemic:* Systemic side effects may occur with extensive use.

# LODOXAMIDE TROMETHAMINE

**Solution:** 0.1% (*Rx*)                                    *Alomide* (Alcon)

## Indications
Treatment of the ocular disorders referred to by the terms vernal keratoconjunctivitis, vernal conjunctivitis, and vernal keratitis.

## Administration and Dosage
*Adults and children older than 2 years of age:* 1 to 2 drops in each affected eye 4 times daily for up to 3 months.

## Actions
*Pharmacology:* Lodoxamide is a mast cell stabilizer that inhibits the in vivo Type I immediate hypersensitivity reaction. Although lodoxamide's precise mechanism of action is unknown, the drug may prevent calcium influx into mast cells upon antigen stimulation.

*Pharmacokinetics:* The disposition of lodoxamide was studied in 6 healthy adult volunteers receiving a 3 mg oral dose. Urinary excretion was the major route of elimination. The elimination half-life was 8.5 hours in urine. In a study in 12 healthy adult volunteers, topical administration of 1 drop in each eye 4 times/day for 10 days did not result in any measurable lodoxamide plasma levels at a detection limit of 2.5 ng/mL.

## Contraindications
Hypersensitivity to any component of this product.

## Warnings
*For ophthalmic use only.* Not for injection.

*Contact lenses:* As with all ophthalmic preparations containing benzalkonium chloride, instruct patients not to wear soft contact lenses during treatment with lodoxamide.

*Pregnancy: Category B.*

*Lactation:* It is not known whether lodoxamide is excreted in breast milk.

*Children:* Safety and efficacy in children younger than 2 years of age have not been established.

## Precautions
*Burning/Stinging:* Patients may experience a transient burning or stinging upon instillation of lodoxamide. Should these symptoms persist, advise patients to contact their physicians.

## Adverse Reactions
Adverse reactions occurring in at least 3% of patients include transient burning, stinging or discomfort upon instillation; ocular itching/pruritus; blurred vision; dry eye; tearing/discharge; hyperemia; crystalline deposits; and foreign body sensation.

# ANTIBIOTICS

| | |
|---|---|
| **BACITRACIN** | |
| **Ointment:** 500 units/g (Rx) | Various, *AK-Tracin* (Akorn) |
| **CHLORAMPHENICOL** | |
| **Ointment:** 10 mg/g (Rx) | Various, *Chloroptic S.O.P.* (Allergan) |
| **Solution:** 5 mg/mL (Rx) | Various, *Chloroptic* (Allergan), *AK-Chlor* (Akorn) |
| **CIPROFLOXACIN** | |
| **Solution:** 3.5 mg/mL (equivalent to 3 mg base) (Rx) | *Ciloxan* (Alcon) |
| **ERYTHROMYCIN** | |
| **Ointment:** 5 mg/g (Rx) | Various, *Ilotycin* (Dista) |
| **GATIFLOXACIN** | |
| **Solution:** 0.3% (3 mg/mL) | *Zymar* (Allergan) |
| **GENTAMICIN SULFATE** | |
| **Ointment:** 3 mg/g (Rx) | Various, *Genoptic S.O.P.* (Allergan) |
| **Solution:** 3 mg/mL (Rx) | Various, *Garamycin* (Schering), *Genoptic* (Allergan) |
| **LEVOFLOXACIN** | |
| **Solution:** 5 mg/mL (Rx) | *Quixin* (Santen) |
| **MOXIFLOXACIN HCl** | |
| **Solution:** 0.5% (5 mg/mL) | *Vigamox* (Alcon) |
| **NORFLOXACIN** | |
| **Solution:** 3 mg/mL (Rx) | *Chibroxin* (Merck) |
| **OFLOXACIN** | |
| **Solution:** 3 mg/mL (Rx) | *Ocuflox* (Allergan) |
| **POLYMYXIN B SULFATE** | |
| **Powder for solution:** 500,000 units (Rx) | *Polymyxin B Sulfate Sterile* (Roerig) |
| **TOBRAMYCIN** | |
| **Ointment:** 3 mg/g (Rx) | Various, *Tobrex* (Alcon) |
| **Solution:** 0.3% (Rx) | Various, *AKTob* (Akorn), *Tobrex* (Alcon) |

**Indications**

*Infections:* Treatment of superficial ocular infections involving the conjunctiva or cornea (eg, conjunctivitis, keratitis, keratoconjunctivitis, corneal ulcers, blepharitis, blepharoconjunctivitis, acute meibomianitis, dacryocystitis) caused by strains of microorganisms susceptible to antibiotics.

*Tetracycline and erythromycin:* Tetracycline and erythromycin also are indicated for the prophylaxis of ophthalmia neonatorum caused by *Neisseria gonorrhoeae* or *Chlamydia trachomatis.*

*Chloramphenicol:* Use chloramphenicol only in those serious infections for which less potentially dangerous drugs are ineffective or contraindicated (see Warnings).

## Topical Ophthalmic Antibiotic Preparations

| Organism/Infection | Bacitracin | Chloramphenicol | Erythromycin | Gramicidin | Polymyxin B | Trimethoprim | Ciprofloxacin | Gatifloxacin | Levofloxacin | Moxifloxacin | Norfloxacin | Ofloxacin | Gentamicin | Neomycin | Tobramycin | Chlortetracycline | Oxytetracycline | Tetracycline | Sodium sulfacetamide | Sulfisoxazole |
|---|---|---|---|---|---|---|---|---|---|---|---|---|---|---|---|---|---|---|---|---|
| | | | Miscellaneous | | | | | | Quinolones | | | | | Aminoglycosides | | | Tetracyclines | | | Sulfonamides |
| **Gram-Positive** | | | | | | | | | | | | | | | | | | | | |
| Staphylococcus sp. | ✓ | | | ✓ | | | ✓ | | ✓ | | ✓ | ✓ | ✓ | | ✓ | | | | | |
| S. aureus | ✓ | ✓ | ✓ | ✓ | | ✓ | ✓ | ✓ | ✓ | ✓ | ✓ | ✓ | ✓ | ✓ | ✓ | ✓ | | ✓ | ✓ | |
| S. epidermidis | | | | | | | | ✓ | | ✓ | | | | | | | | | | |
| S. hominis | | | | | | | | | | ✓ | | | | | | | | | | |
| S. warneri | | | | | | | | | | ✓[1] | | | | | | | | | | |
| Streptococcus sp. | ✓ | ✓ | | ✓ | | | ✓ | | ✓ | | | ✓ | | | ✓ | | | ✓ | ✓ | |
| S. mitis | | | | | | | ✓[1] | | | | | | | | | | | | | |
| S. pneumoniae | ✓ | ✓ | ✓ | ✓ | | ✓ | ✓ | ✓ | ✓ | ✓ | ✓ | ✓ | ✓[2] | | ✓ | | | ✓ | | |
| α-hemolytic streptococci (viridans group) | | | ✓ | | | | | | ✓ | ✓ | | | | | | | | | | |
| β-hemolytic streptococci | ✓ | | | | | | | | | | | | ✓[2] | ✓ | | | | | | |
| S. pyogenes | ✓ | | ✓ | | ✓ | ✓ | | | | | | ✓ | ✓ | | | | ✓ | | | |
| Corynebacterium sp. | ✓ | | ✓ | ✓ | | | | ✓ | | ✓[1] | | | ✓ | ✓ | ✓ | | | | | |
| Micrococcus luteus | | | | | | | | | | ✓[1] | | | | | | | | | | |
| **Gram-Negative** | | | | | | | | | | | | | | | | | | | | |
| Escherichia coli | | ✓ | | | ✓ | ✓ | ✓ | | | | ✓ | ✓ | ✓ | ✓ | ✓ | ✓ | ✓ | ✓ | ✓ | ✓ |
| Haemophilus aegyptius | | ✓ | | | | ✓ | | | | | ✓ | | | | ✓ | | | | ✓ | ✓ |
| H. ducreyi | | ✓ | | | | | | | | | ✓ | | | | | ✓ | ✓ | ✓ | | |
| H. influenzae | | ✓ | ✓ | | ✓ | ✓ | ✓ | ✓ | ✓ | ✓ | ✓ | ✓ | ✓ | ✓ | ✓ | ✓ | ✓ | ✓ | | |
| H. parainfluenzae | | | | | | | | | | ✓[1] | | | | | | | | | | |
| Klebsiella sp. | | ✓ | | | | | ✓ | | | | ✓ | ✓ | | | ✓ | | | ✓ | | |
| K. pneumoniae | | | | | ✓ | ✓ | ✓ | | | | ✓ | ✓ | ✓ | ✓ | | ✓ | | | | |
| Neisseria sp. | ✓ | ✓ | | | | | ✓ | | | | | | ✓ | ✓ | ✓ | | | ✓ | | |
| N. gonorrhoeae | ✓ | | ✓[3] | | | | ✓ | | | | | | ✓ | ✓ | ✓ | | | ✓ | ✓[3] | ✓ |
| Proteus sp. | | | | | ✓ | ✓ | | | | | | | ✓ | ✓ | ✓ | ✓ | ✓ | | | |
| Acinetobacter calcoaceticus | | | | | | | ✓ | | | | | | ✓ | ✓ | ✓ | ✓ | | | | |
| A. lwoffi | | | | | | | | | | | ✓ | ✓[1] | | | | | | | | |
| Enterobacter aerogenes | | | | | ✓ | ✓ | ✓ | | | | | | ✓ | ✓ | ✓ | ✓ | | ✓ | | |
| Enterobacter sp. | | ✓ | | | | | ✓ | | | | | | ✓ | ✓ | ✓ | ✓ | ✓ | | | |
| Serratia marcescens | | | | | | | ✓ | | ✓ | | | | ✓ | ✓ | ✓ | ✓ | | | | |
| Moraxella sp. | | ✓ | | | | | | | | | | | ✓ | ✓ | | ✓ | | | | |
| Chlamydia trachomatis | | | ✓[3] | | | | ✓ | | | ✓ | | | ✓ | | | ✓[4] | | ✓[4] | ✓[5] | ✓ |
| Pasteurella tularensis | | | | | | | | | | | | | | | | ✓ | ✓ | | | |
| Pseudomonas aeruginosa | | ✓ | | ✓ | | | ✓ | | | | | | ✓ | ✓ | ✓[5] | ✓ | | | | |
| Bartonella bacilliformis | | | | | | | | | | | | | | | | | ✓ | | | |
| Bacteroides sp. | | | ✓ | | | | | | | | | | | | | ✓ | ✓ | ✓ | | |
| Vibrio sp. | | ✓ | | | | | ✓ | | | | ✓ | | ✓ | | ✓ | | ✓ | | | |
| Yersinia pestis | | | | | | | | | | | | | | | | ✓ | ✓ | | | |

[1] Efficacy for this organism was studied in fewer than 10 infections.
[2] Increasing resistance has been seen.
[3] For prophylaxis.
[4] In conjunction with oral therapy
[5] Adjunct in systemic sulfonamide therapy.

### Administration and Dosage

Administration and dosage varies for the individual products. Refer to individual manufacturer inserts.

#### Contraindications

Hypersensitivity to any component of these products; epithelial herpes simplex keratitis (dendritic keratitis); vaccinia; varicella; mycobacterial infections of the eye;
fungal diseases of the ocular structure; use of steroid combinations after uncomplicated removal of a corneal foreign body.

#### Warnings

*Sensitization:* Sensitization from the topical use of an antibiotic may contraindicate the
drug's later systemic use in serious infections.

*Cross-sensitivity:* Allergic cross-reactions may occur that could prevent future use of any
or all of these antibiotics – Kanamycin, neomycin, paromomycin, streptomycin,
and possibly, gentamicin.

*Chloramphenicol* – Hematopoietic toxicity has occurred occasionally with the systemic use of chloramphenicol and rarely with topical administration.

*Pregnancy: Category B* (tobramycin); *Category C* (gentamicin, ciprofloxacin, norfloxacin, ofloxacin).

*Lactation:* It is not known whether **ciprofloxacin, norfloxacin,** or **ofloxacin** appears in
breast milk following ophthalmic use. Exercise caution when administering ciprofloxacin to a nursing mother.

*Children:* **Tobramycin** is safe and effective in children. Safety and efficacy of **ciprofloxacin** in children younger than 12 years of age and **norfloxacin** and **ofloxacin** in
infants younger than 1 year of age have not been established.

#### Precautions

*Superinfection:* Do not use topical antibiotics in deep-seated ocular infections or in those
that are likely to become systemic.

*Systemic antibiotics* – In all except very superficial infections, supplement the topical use of antibiotics with appropriate systemic medication.

*Crystalline precipitate* – A white crystalline precipitate located in the superficial portion of the corneal defect was observed in about 17% of patients on **ciprofloxacin.**

#### Adverse Reactions

Sensitivity reactions such as transient irritation, burning, stinging, itching, inflammation, angioneurotic edema, urticaria, and vesicular and maculopapular dermatitis
have occurred in some patients.

*Chloramphenicol:* Hematological events (including aplastic anemia) have been reported.

*Ciprofloxacin:* White crystalline precipitates; lid margin crusting; crystals/scales; foreign body sensation; itching; conjunctival hyperemia; bad taste in mouth; corneal
staining; keratopathy/keratitis; allergic reactions; lid edema; tearing; photophobia; corneal infiltrates; nausea; decreased vision.

*Norfloxacin:* Conjunctival hyperemia; chemosis; photophobia; bitter taste in mouth.

# NATAMYCIN

**Suspension: 5% (Rx)**                     *Natacyn* (Alcon)

#### Indications

*Fungal infections:* Fungal blepharitis, conjunctivitis, and keratitis caused by susceptible
organisms. Natamycin is the initial drug of choice in Fusarium solani keratitis.

#### Administration and Dosage

*Fungal keratitis:* Instill 1 drop into the conjunctival sac at 1 or 2 hour intervals. The frequency of application can usually be reduced to 1 drop 6 to 8 times daily after the
first 3 to 4 days. Generally, continue therapy for 14 to 21 days, or until there is
resolution of active fungal keratitis. In many cases, it may help to reduce the dosage gradually at 4 to 7 day intervals to ensure that the organism has been eliminated.

*Fungal blepharitis and conjunctivitis:* 4 to 6 daily applications may be sufficient.

### Actions

*Pharmacology:* Natamycin, a tetraene polyene antibiotic, is derived from *Streptomyces natalensis.*

It possesses in vitro activity against a variety of yeast and filamentous fungi, including *Candida, Aspergillus, Cephalosporium, Fusarium,* and *Penicillium.* The mechanism of action appears to be through binding of the molecule to the fungal cell membrane. The polyenesterol complex alters membrane permeability, depleting essential cellular constituents. Although activity against fungi is dose-related, natamycin is predominantly fungicidal.

*Pharmacokinetics:* Topical administration appears to produce effective concentrations within the corneal stroma, but not in intraocular fluid. Absorption from the GI tract is very poor. Systemic absorption should not occur after topical administration.

### Contraindications

Hypersensitivity to any component of the formulation.

### Warnings

*Pregnancy:* Safety for use during pregnancy has not been established.

### Precautions

*For topical use only:* Not for injection.

*Fungal endophthalmitis:* The effectiveness of topical natamycin as a single agent in fungal endophthalmitis has not been established.

*Resistance:* Failure of keratitis to improve following 7 to 10 days of administration suggests that the infection may be caused by a microorganism not susceptible to natamycin. Base continuation of therapy on clinical reevaluation and additional laboratory studies.

*Toxicity:* Adherence of the suspension to areas of epithelial ulceration or retention in the fornices occurs regularly. Should suspicion of drug toxicity occur, discontinue the drug.

*Diagnosis/Monitoring:* Determine initial and sustained therapy of fungal keratitis by the clinical diagnosis (laboratory diagnosis by smear and culture of corneal scrapings) and by response to the drug. Whenever possible, determine the in vitro activity of natamycin against the responsible fungus. Monitor tolerance to natamycin at least twice weekly.

### Adverse Reactions

One case of conjunctival chemosis and hyperemia, thought to be allergic in nature, was reported.

# TOPICAL OPHTHALMIC ANTIVIRAL PREPARATIONS

The topical ophthalmic antiviral preparations appear to interfere with viral reproduction by altering DNA synthesis. Trifluridine is effective treatment for herpes simplex infections of the conjunctiva and cornea. Ganciclovir is indicated for use in immunocompromised patients with cytomegalovirus (CMV) retinitis and for prevention of CMV retinitis in transplant patients. Foscarnet is indicated for use only in AIDS patients with CMV retinitis.

The trifluridine monograph follows this introduction. Prescribing information for foscarnet and ganciclovir appear in the Antivirals section of the Anti-Infectives chapter.

Viral infection, especially epidemic keratoconjunctivitis (EKC), more often is associated with a follicular conjunctivitis, a serous conjunctival discharge, and preauricular lymphadenopathy. The exceptionally contagious organism causing EKC is not susceptible to antiviral therapy at this time.

# TRIFLURIDINE (Trifluorothymidine)

| **Ophthalmic solution:** 1% (Rx) | *Viroptic* (Burroughs Wellcome) |
| --- | --- |

**Indications**

Primary keratoconjunctivitis and recurrent epithelial keratitis caused by herpes simplex virus types 1 and 2.

Epithelial keratitis that has not responded clinically to topical idoxuridine, or when ocular toxicity or hypersensitivity to idoxuridine has occurred. In a smaller number of patients resistant to topical vidarabine, trifluridine was also effective.

**Administration and Dosage**

Instill 1 drop onto the cornea of the affected eye(s) every 2 hours while awake for a maximum daily dosage of 9 drops until the corneal ulcer has completely re-epithelialized. Following re-epithelialization, treat for an additional 7 days with 1 drop every 4 hours while awake for a minimum daily dosage of 5 drops.

If there are no signs of improvement after 7 days, or if complete re-epithelialization has not occurred after 14 days, consider other forms of therapy. Avoid continuous administration for periods exceeding 21 days because of potential ocular toxicity.

**Actions**

*Pharmacology:* A fluorinated pyrimidine nucleoside with in vitro and in vivo activity against herpes simplex virus types 1 and 2, and vaccinia virus. Some strains of adenovirus are also inhibited in vitro. Its antiviral mechanism of action is not completely known.

*Pharmacokinetics:*

   *Absorption* – Intraocular penetration occurs after topical instillation. Decreased corneal integrity or stromal or uveal inflammation may enhance the penetration into the aqueous humor. Systemic absorption following therapeutic dosing appears negligible.

**Contraindications**

Hypersensitivity reactions or chemical intolerance to trifluridine.

**Warnings**

*Efficacy in other conditions:* The clinical efficacy in the treatment of stromal keratitis and uveitis caused by herpes simplex or ophthalmic infections caused by vaccinia virus and adenovirus, or in the prophylaxis of herpes simplex virus keratoconjunctivitis and epithelial keratitis has not been established by well-controlled clinical trials. Not effective against bacterial, fungal, or chlamydial infections of the cornea or trophic lesions.

*Dosage/Frequency:* Do not exceed the recommended dosage or frequency of administration.

*Pregnancy:* Safety for use during pregnancy has not been established.

*Lactation:* Safety and efficacy have not been established.

**Precautions**

*Viral resistance:* Viral resistance, although documented in vitro, has not been reported following multiple exposure to trifluridine; this possibility may exist.

**Adverse Reactions**

Adverse reactions may include mild, transient burning or stinging upon instillation; palpebral edema; superficial punctate keratopathy; epithelial keratopathy; hypersensitivity reaction; stromal edema; irritation; keratitis sicca; hyperemia and increased intraocular pressure.

# Chapter 13
# ANTINEOPLASTIC AGENTS

# ANTINEOPLASTICS INTRODUCTION

The chemotherapeutic agents include a wide range of compounds that work by various mechanisms. Although development has been directed toward agents capable of selective actions on neoplastic tissues, those presently available manifest significant toxicity on normal tissues as a major complication of therapy. Thoroughly consider the risks vs benefits of therapy when using these agents.

Because of the complexities and dangers in cancer chemotherapy, use should be restricted to, or under the direct supervision of, physicians experienced in its use. In addition to drug therapy, surgical excision and radiation therapy also are employed when appropriate.

*Handling of cytotoxic agents:* Most antineoplastics are toxic compounds known to be carcinogenic, mutagenic, or teratogenic. Direct contact may cause irritation of the skin, eyes, and mucous membranes. Safe and aseptic handling of parenteral chemotherapeutic drugs by medical personnel involved in preparation and administration of these agents is mandatory. Potential risks from repeated contact with parenteral antineoplastics can be controlled by a combination of specific containment equipment and proper work techniques. The NIH Division of Safety brochure outlines recommendations for safe handling of these agents.

*Mechanisms of action:* The mechanism of action by which these agents suppress proliferation of neoplasms is not fully understood. Generally, they affect at least 1 stage of cell growth or replication. Those more active at one specific phase of cellular growth are referred to as *cell cycle specific* agents; those that are active on both proliferating and resting cells are *cell cycle nonspecific* agents. The selectivity of cytotoxic agents inversely follows cell cycle specificity. Rapidly dividing normal tissues including bone marrow, blood components, hair follicles, and mucous membranes of the GI tract also may experience major adverse effects.

*Alkylating agents:* Alkylating agents form highly reactive carbonium ions that react with essential cellular components, thereby altering normal biological function. Alkylating agents replace hydrogen atoms with an alkyl radical, causing cross-linking and abnormal base pairing in deoxyribonucleic acid (DNA) molecules. They also react with sulfhydryl, phosphate, and amine groups, resulting in multiple lesions in dividing and nondividing cells. The resultant defective DNA molecules are unable to carry out normal cellular reproductive functions. Examples of alkylating agents include the following:

| | |
|---|---|
| busulfan | lomustine |
| carboplatin | mechlorethamine |
| carmustine | melphalan |
| chlorambucil | oxaliplatin |
| cisplatin | pipobroman |
| cyclophosphamide | streptozocin |
| dacarbazine | thiotepa |
| estramustine | uracil mustard |
| ifosfamide | |

*Antimetabolites:* Antimetabolites include a diverse group of compounds that interfere with various metabolic processes, thereby disrupting normal cellular functions. These agents may act by the following 2 general mechanisms: Incorporating the drug, rather than a normal cellular constituent, into an essential chemical compound; or inhibiting a key enzyme from functioning normally. Their primary benefit is the ability to disrupt nucleic acid synthesis. These agents work only on dividing cells during the S phase of nucleic acid synthesis and are most effective on rapidly proliferating neoplasms. Examples of antimetabolites include the following:

| | |
|---|---|
| cytarabine | hydroxyurea |
| floxuridine | mercaptopurine |
| fludarabine | methotrexate |
| 5-fluorouracil | thioguanine |
| gemcitabine | |

*Hormones:* Hormones have been used to treat several types of neoplasms. Hormonal therapy interferes at the cellular membrane level with growth stimulatory receptor proteins. The mechanism of action, however, is still unclear. Adrenocortical steroids are used primarily for their suppressant effect on lymphocytes in leukemias and lymphomas and as a component in many combination regimens. The counterbalancing effect of androgens, estrogens, and progestins has been used to advantage in the therapy of malignancies of tissues dependent upon these sex-related hormones (eg, tumors of the breast, endometrium, prostate). These agents have the advantage of greater specificity for tissues responsive to their effects, thus inhibiting proliferation without a direct cytotoxic action.

Examples of hormone agents include the following:

| | |
|---|---|
| aminoglutethimide | leuprolide |
| anastrozole | medroxyprogesterone |
| bicalutamide | megestrol |
| diethylstilbestrol | mitotane |
| estramustine | polyestradiol |
| flutamide | tamoxifen |
| goserelin | testolactone |

*Antibiotic:* Antibiotic-type agents, unlike their anti-infective relatives, are capable of disrupting cellular functions of host (mammalian) tissues. Their primary mechanisms of action are to inhibit DNA-dependent RNA synthesis and to delay or inhibit mitosis. The antibiotics are cell cycle nonspecific. Examples of antineoplastic antibiotics include the following:

| | |
|---|---|
| bleomycin | mitomycin |
| dactinomycin | mitoxantrone |
| daunorubicin | pentostatin |
| doxorubicin | plicamycin |
| idarubicin | |

*Mitotic inhibitors:* Mitotic inhibitor mechanisms are not fully understood. Podophyllotoxin derivatives inhibit DNA synthesis at specific phases of the cell cycle. Vinca alkaloids bind to tubulin, the subunits of the microtubules that form the mitotic spindle. This complex inhibits microtubule assembly, causing metaphase arrest. In contrast, paclitaxel enhances the polymerization of tubulin and induces the production of stable, nonfunctional microtubules, thus inhibiting cell replication. Podophyllotoxin derivatives include etoposide and teniposide. Vinca alkaloids include vinblastine, vincristine, and vincrelbine. A new class of agents called taxanes includes paclitaxel and docetaxel.

*Radiopharmaceuticals:* Radiopharmaceuticals exert direct toxic effects on exposed tissue via radiation emission. Primary activity is against metastatic disease. Examples include strontium-89, sodium iodide I 131, and chromic phosphate P 32.

*Biological response modifiers:* Biological response modifiers have complex antineoplastic, antiviral, and immunomodulating activities. It is believed that the antitumor activity of interferons is a result of a direct antiproliferative action against tumor cells and modulation of the host immune response. Examples of biological agents include the following:

> aldesleukin (human interleukin-2)
> interferon alfa-2a (recombinant DNA)
> interferon alfa-2b (recombinant DNA)
> interferon alfa-n3 (human leukocyte)
> interferon gamma-1B (recombinant DNA)

*Miscellaneous:* Metabolism of altretamine is required for cytotoxicity, although the mechanisms are not clear. Asparaginase is an enzyme that inhibits protein synthesis of malignant cells by inhibiting asparagine, which is required for protein synthesis. Intravesical BCG is a suspension of *Mycobacterium bovis* that promotes a local inflammatory reaction in the urinary bladder and reduces cancerous lesions. Cladribine inhibits DNA synthesis and repair through a complex mechanism. Levamisole is an immunomodulator with complex effects. Procarbazine produces toxic metabolites that induce chromosomal breakage. Tretinoin is a retinoid related to retinol (vitamin A) that induces cytodifferentiation. Porfimer is a photosensitivity agent. Topotecan and irinotecan are topoisomerase I inhibitors.

*Extravasation:* Extravasation occurs when IV fluid and medication leak into interstitial tissue. Damage resulting from extravasation of certain antineoplastic agents can range from painful erythematous swelling to full-thickness injury with deep necrotic lesions requiring surgical debridement and skin grafting.

*Prevention* – Prevention of extravasation injury is based on careful, accurate IV drug administration. Avoid areas of previous irradiation and extremities with poor venous circulation for IV cannula placement. Dilute drugs properly and give at an appropriate rate.

*Treatment* – Treatment of extravasation includes immediate discontinuation of infusion and appropriate antidote administration. Goals of treatment are palliation and prevention of severe tissue damage. For further information regarding the instillation of a specific antidote, refer to individual product monographs. Consider surgical evaluation if an open wound occurs. Some practitioners recommend leaving the IV cannula in place to aspirate some of the chemotherapeutic agent and administering an antidote to the injured site. Others recommend immediate removal of the cannula and administration of the antidote by intradermal or subcutaneous injections. Immediate removal of the cannula followed by application of ice also has been recommended for all agents except etoposide, vinblastine, and vincristine (warm compresses are recommended for these agents). Apply the ice for 15 to 20 minutes every 4 to 6 hours for the first 72 hours. Elevate the affected area.

Hydrocortisone sodium succinate or dexamethasone sodium phosphate have been used on the extravasated site for their antiinflammatory activity. However, these agents, as well as other drugs (sodium bicarbonate, DMSO), are unproven for antidote use. Specific antidotes that are recommended include sodium thiosulfate for mechlorethamine and hyaluronidase for vincristine and vinblastine.

*Drugs associated with severe local necrosis (vesicants) include the following –*

| | |
|---|---|
| dacarbazine | mechlorethamine |
| dactinomycin | mitomycin |
| daunorubicin | streptozocin |
| doxorubicin | vinblastine |
| epirubicin | vincristine |
| idarubicin | vinorelbine |

*Nausea and vomiting:* Nausea and vomiting may be the most prominent adverse reactions of cancer chemotherapy from the patient's perspective. In clinical trials, 17% to 98% of patients reported emesis. At least 30% of patients experience acute emesis despite antiemetic therapy. Uncontrolled emesis may cause serious complications, including dehydration, malnutrition, metabolic disorders, esophageal injury, and aspiration. In addition, the patient's quality of life may be reduced significantly. Prevention and management of nausea and vomiting is an important aspect of cancer treatment.

Antineoplastics can be categorized according to their emetogenic potential based on the frequency of emesis. Level 1 is the least emetogenic, while Level 5 is the most emetogenic. Combining antineoplastic agents may increase the overall risk for emesis. For example, a combination of drugs with the risks factors of $2 + 2 + 2$ may give a combined emetogenic risk of Level 3 (or $2 + 2 + 3 = 4$ and $3 + 3 + 3 = 5$).

| Emetogenic Potential of Antineoplastics | | |
|---|---|---|
| Level | Frequency of emesis | Chemotherapeutic agent |
| 1 | < 10% | Bleomycin<br>Busulfan (oral, < 4 mg/kg/day)<br>Chlorambucil (oral)<br>Cladribine<br>Doxorubicin, liposomal<br>Estramustine<br>Floxuridine<br>Fludarabine<br>Hydroxyurea | Interferon alfa<br>Melphalan (oral)<br>Mercaptopurine<br>Methotrexate $\leq$ 50 mg/m$^2$<br>Pentostatin<br>Thioguanine (oral)<br>Tretinoin<br>Vinblastine<br>Vincristine<br>Vinorelbine |
| 2 | 10% to 30% | Asparaginase<br>Cytarabine (< 1000 mg/m$^2$)<br>Daunorubicin, liposomal<br>Denileukin diftitox<br>Docetaxel<br>Doxorubicin HCl (< 20 mg/m$^2$)<br>Etoposide<br>Fluorouracil (< 1000 mg/m$^2$) | Gemcitabine<br>Methotrexate (50 to 250 mg/m$^2$)<br>Mitomycin<br>Paclitaxel<br>Pegaspargase<br>Teniposide<br>Thiotepa<br>Topotecan |
| 3 | 30% to 60% | Aldesleukin<br>Altretamine (oral)<br>Capecitabine (oral)<br>Cyclophosphamide ($\leq$ 750 mg/m$^2$)<br>Cyclophosphamide (oral)<br>Dactinomycin ($\leq$ 1.5 mg/m$^2$)<br>Daunorubicin ($\leq$ 50 mg/m$^2$) | Doxorubicin HCl (20 to 60 mg/m$^2$)<br>Epirubicin<br>Idarubicin<br>Ifosfamide ($\leq$ 1500 mg/m$^2$)<br>Methotrexate (250 to 1000 mg/m$^2$)<br>Mitoxantrone (< 15 mg/m$^2$)<br>Temozolomide |
| 4 | 60% to 90% | Carboplatin<br>Carmustine ($\leq$ 250 mg/m$^2$)<br>Cisplatin (< 50 mg/m$^2$)<br>Cyclophosphamide (750 to 1500 mg/m$^2$)<br>Cytarabine ($\geq$ 1000 mg/m$^2$)<br>Dactinomycin (> 1.5 mg/m$^2$)<br>Daunorubicin (> 50 mg/m$^2$) | Doxorubicin HCl (> 60 mg/m$^2$)<br>Irinotecan<br>Lomustine ($\leq$ 60 mg/m$^2$)<br>Melphalan (IV)<br>Methotrexate ($\geq$ 1000 mg/m$^2$)<br>Mitoxantrone ($\geq$ 15 mg/m$^2$)<br>Procarbazine |
| 5 | > 90% | Carmustine (> 250 mg/m$^2$)<br>Cisplatin ($\geq$ 50 mg/m$^2$)<br>Cyclophosphamide (> 1500 mg/m$^2$)<br>Dacarbazine | Ifosfamide (> 1500 mg/m$^2$)<br>Lomustine (> 60 mg/m$^2$)<br>Mechlorethamine<br>Streptozocin |

The incidence of emesis with these and other agents varies greatly among individuals. Dose, schedule, concomitant therapy, other medical complications, and psychologic parameters may affect the incidence as well.

*Prevention and treatment* – Prevention and treatment of nausea and vomiting should include measures such as dietary adjustment, restriction of activity, and positive support. However, if pharmacologic management is necessary, several agents or groups of agents may prove useful. Some drugs that have been used with varying degrees of success, either alone or in combination, include 5-HT$_3$ receptor antagonists (eg, ondansetron, dolasetron, granisetron), phenothiazines, butyrophenones, cannabinoids, corticosteroids, antihistamines, benzodiazepines, metoclopramide, and scopolamine.

# TAMOXIFEN CITRATE

**Tablets:** 10 and 20 mg *(Rx)*                    Various, *Nolvadex* (AstraZeneca)

**Warning:**
*Women with ductal carcinoma in situ (DCIS) and women at high risk for breast cancer:* Serious and life-threatening events associated with tamoxifen in the risk reduction setting (women at high risk for cancer and women with DCIS) include uterine malignancies, stroke, and pulmonary embolism. Incidence rates for these events were estimated from the NSABP P-1 trial. Uterine malignancies consist of endometrial adenocarcinoma (incidence rate per 1000 women-years of 2.2 for tamoxifen vs 0.71 for placebo) and uterine sarcoma (incidence rate per 1000 women-years of 0.17 for tamoxifen vs 0 for placebo) (updated long-term followup data [median length of followup is 6.9 years] from NSABP P-1 study). For stroke, the incidence rate per 1000 women-years was 1.43 for tamoxifen vs 1 for placebo. For pulmonary embolism, the incidence rate per 1000 women-years was 0.75 for tamoxifen vs 0.25 for placebo.

Some of the strokes, pulmonary emboli, and uterine malignancies were fatal.

Health care providers should discuss the potential benefits vs risks of these serious events with women at high risk of breast cancer and women with DCIS considering tamoxifen to reduce their risk of developing breast cancer.

The benefits of tamoxifen outweigh its risks in women already diagnosed with breast cancer.

## Indications
*Breast cancer:*
*Adjuvant therapy* – For treatment of axillary node-negative breast cancer in women following total mastectomy or segmental mastectomy, axillary dissection, and breast irradiation.

For treatment of node-positive breast cancer in postmenopausal women following total mastectomy or segmental mastectomy, axillary dissection, and breast irradiation.

*Advanced disease therapy* – Effective in the treatment of metastatic breast cancer in women and men. In premenopausal women with metastatic breast cancer, tamoxifen is an alternative to oophorectomy or ovarian irradiation. Estrogen receptor positive tumors are most likely to benefit.

*Reduction in breast cancer incidence in high-risk women:* To reduce the incidence of breast cancer in women at high risk for breast cancer. "High risk" is defined as women at least 35 years of age with a 5-year predicted risk of breast cancer at least 1.67% as calculated by the Gail model. (Refer to the Package Insert for examples of risk factor combinations.)

*DCIS:* In women with DCIS, following breast surgery and radiation, tamoxifen is indicated to reduce the risk of invasive breast cancer.

*Unlabeled uses:* Tamoxifen has been used in the treatment of mastalgia (10 mg/day for 4 months).

## Administration and Dosage
*Breast cancer patients:* 20 to 40 mg daily. Give doses greater than 20 mg/day in divided doses (morning and evening).

Some studies have used dosages of 10 mg 2 or 3 times/day for 2 years and 10 mg twice daily for 5 years. The reduction in recurrence and mortality was greater in those studies that used the drug for 5 years or more than in those that used it for a shorter period. There was no indication that doses greater than 20 mg/day were more effective. Current data from clinical trials support 5 years of adjuvant tamoxifen therapy for patients with breast cancer.

*Reduction in breast cancer incidence in high-risk women:* 20 mg daily for 5 years. There are no data to support the use of tamoxifen other than for 5 years.

For sexually active women of childbearing potential, initiate tamoxifen therapy during menstruation. In women with menstrual irregularity, a negative B-HCG immediately prior to the initiation of therapy is sufficient.

*DCIS:* 20 mg/day for 5 years.

### Actions

*Pharmacology:* Tamoxifen is a nonsteroidal agent with potent antiestrogenic properties.

*Pharmacokinetics:* Tamoxifen is extensively metabolized after oral administration. Approximately 65% of an administered dose was excreted from the body over a period of 2 weeks with fecal excretion as the primary route of elimination.

After initiation of therapy, steady-state concentrations for tamoxifen are achieved in about 4 weeks and steady-state concentrations for N-desmethyl tamoxifen are achieved in about 8 weeks, suggesting a half-life of approximately 14 days for this metabolite.

### Contraindications

Hypersensitivity to the drug; women who require concomitant coumarin-type anticoagulant therapy; women with a history of deep vein thrombosis or pulmonary embolus (reduction in breast cancer incidence and DCIS indications).

### Warnings

*Thromboembolic effects:* Consider the risks and benefits of tamoxifen carefully in women with a history of thromboembolic events. Among women receiving tamoxifen, the events appeared between 2 and 60 months from the start of treatment.

*Uterus-endometrial cancer and uterine sarcoma:* An increased incidence of uterine malignancies has been reported in association with tamoxifen treatment.

*Ocular disturbances:* Ocular disturbances, including corneal changes, cataracts, the need for cataract surgery, decrement in color vision perception, retinal vein thrombosis, and retinopathy, have occurred with tamoxifen use.

*Disease of bone:* Increased bone pain, tumor pain, and local disease flare sometimes are associated with a good tumor response shortly after starting tamoxifen and generally subside rapidly. Lesion size may increase suddenly in soft tissue disease, sometimes with new lesions, or with erythema in or around the lesion.

*Hypercalcemia:* Hypercalcemia has occurred in some breast cancer patients with bone metastases within a few weeks of starting therapy with tamoxifen.

*Hepatic effects:* Tamoxifen has been associated with changes in liver enzyme levels and, on rare occasions, fatty liver, cholestasis, hepatitis, and hepatic necrosis.

*Pregnancy: Category D.*

*Lactation:* It is not known whether this drug is excreted in breast milk.

*Children:* The safety and efficacy of tamoxifen for girls 2 to 10 years of age with McCune-Albright syndrome and precocious puberty have not been studied beyond 1 year of treatment. The long-term effects of tamoxifen therapy for girls have not been established.

### Precautions

*Monitoring:* Perform periodic CBCs, including platelet counts, and liver function tests. Perform a breast examination, a mammogram, and a gynecologic examination prior to the initiation of therapy. Repeat these studies at regular intervals while on therapy.

*Leukopenia/Thrombocytopenia:* Use cautiously in patients with existing leukopenia or thrombocytopenia.

*Hyperlipidemias:* Hyperlipidemias have occurred infrequently.

### Drug Interactions

Drugs that may interact with tamoxifen include anticoagulants, bromocriptine, cytotoxic agents, letrozole, medroxyprogesterone, phenobarbital, and rifamycins.

*Drug/Lab test interactions:* $T_4$ elevations occurred in a few postmenopausal patients but were not accompanied by clinical hyperthyroidism. Variations in the karyopyknotic index on vaginal smears and various degrees of estrogen effect on Pap smears have been infrequently seen in postmenopausal patients.

**Adverse Reactions**

Adverse reactions occurring in at least 3% of patients after 5-year therapy include the following: Fluid retention, hot flashes, increased AST, irregular menses, nausea, skin changes, vaginal discharge, and weight loss.

Adverse reactions occurring in at least 3% of patients taking tamoxifen vs ovarian ablation include the following: Altered menses, amenorrhea, bone pain, coughing, edema, fatigue, flushing, menstrual disorder, musculoskeletal pain, nausea, oligomenorrhea, ovarian cyst(s), pain.

# INTERFERON ALFA-2a (rIFN-A; IFLrA)

**Injection Solution**: 3 million units/mL, 6 million units/mL, 9 *Roferon-A* (Roche)
million units per 0.9 mL (*Rx*)
**Powder for Injection**: 6 million units/mL when reconstituted
(*Rx*)

## Indications
*Hairy-cell leukemia:* In select patients 18 years of age and older.

*AIDS-related Kaposi sarcoma:* In select patients 18 years of age and older.

*Chronic myelogenous leukemia (CML):* In chronic phase, Philadelphia chromosome (Ph)
positive CML patients who are minimally pretreated (within 1 year of diagnosis).

## Administration and Dosage
Give subcutaneously or IM. Subcutaneous administration is suggested for, but not limited to, patients who are thrombocytopenic (platelet count less than 50,000/mm$^3$)
or who are at risk for bleeding.

*Hairy-cell leukemia:*
Induction dose – 3 million units daily for 16 to 24 weeks, subcutaneously or IM.
Maintenance dose – 3 million units 3 times/week. Dosage reduction by one-half or
withholding of individual doses may be needed when severe adverse reactions occur.
The use of doses higher than 3 million units is not recommended.

Treat patients for about 6 months before determining whether to continue
therapy. Patients with hairy-cell leukemia have been treated for up to 20 consecutive months. The optimal duration of treatment for this disease has not been
determined.

*AIDS-related Kaposi sarcoma:*
Induction dose – 36 million units daily for 10 to 12 weeks, administered IM or subcutaneously.
Maintenance dose – 36 million units 3 times/week. Dose reductions by one-half or
withholding of individual doses may be required when severe adverse reactions
occur. An escalating schedule of 3, 9, and 18 million units daily for 3 days followed
by 36 million units daily for the remainder of the 10- to 12-week induction period
also has produced equivalent therapeutic benefit with some amelioration of the
acute toxicity in some patients.

When disease stabilization or a response to treatment occurs, treatment should
continue until there is no further evidence of tumor or until discontinuation is
required because of a severe opportunistic infection or adverse effects. The optimal duration of treatment for this disease has not been determined.

If severe reactions occur, modify dosage (50% reduction) or temporarily discontinue therapy until the adverse reactions abate. The need for dosage reduction
should take into account effects of prior x-ray therapy or chemotherapy that may
have compromised bone marrow reserve. Minimum effective doses have not been
established.

*CML:*
Chronic phase Ph-positive CML – Prior to initiation of therapy, make a diagnosis of Ph-
positive CML in chronic phase by the appropriate peripheral blood, bone marrow
and other diagnostic testing. Regularly monitor hematologic parameters (eg, monthly).
Because significant cytogenic changes are not readily apparent until after hematologic response has occurred, and usually not until several months of therapy have
elapsed, cytogenic monitoring may be performed at less frequent intervals. Achievement of complete cytogenic response has been observed up to 2 years following
the start of interferon alfa-2a treatment.
Induction dose – 9 million units daily administered subcutaneously or IM. Based on
clinical experience, short-term tolerance may be improved by gradually increasing
the dose of interferon alfa-2a over the first week of administration from 3 million units daily for 3 days to 6 million units daily for 3 days to the target dose of
9 million units daily for the duration of the treatment period.

*Maintenance* – Optimal dose and duration of therapy have not been determined. Even though the median time to achieve the complete hematologic response was 5 months in clinical studies, hematologic responses have been observed up to 18 months after starting treatment. Continue therapy until disease progression. If severe side effects occur, a treatment interruption or reduction in either the dose or the frequency of injections may be necessary to achieve the individual maximally tolerated dose.

*Children* – Limited data are available on the use of interferon alfa-2a in children with CML. In one report of 15 children with Ph-positive, adult-type CML, doses between 2.5 and 5 million units/m²/day given IM were tolerated. In another study, severe adverse effects including death were noted in children with previously untreated, Ph-negative juvenile CML who received interferon doses of 30 million units/m²/day.

## Actions

*Pharmacology:* Interferon alfa-2a is a sterile protein product manufactured by recombinant DNA technology that employs a genetically engineered *Escherichia coli* bacterium. The mechanism by which interferons exert antitumor activity is not clearly understood. However, direct antiproliferative action against tumor cells and modulation of the host immune response may play important roles.

*Pharmacokinetics:*

*Absorption/Distribution* – In healthy people, interferon alfa-2a exhibited an elimination half-life of 3.7 to 8.5 hours (mean, 5.1 hours), volume of distribution at steady state of 0.223 to 0.748 L/kg (mean, 0.4 L/kg), and a total body clearance of 2.14 to 3.62 mL/min/kg (mean, 2.79 mL/min/kg) after a 36 million units (2.2 x 10$^8$ pg) IV infusion. After IM and subcutaneous administrations of 36 million units, peak serum concentrations ranged from 1500 to 2580 pg/mL (mean, 2020 pg/mL) at a mean time to peak of 3.8 hours and from 1250 to 2320 pg/mL (mean, 1730 pg/mL) at a mean time to peak of 7.3 hours, respectively. Multiple IM doses resulted in accumulation of 2 to 4 times the single dose serum concentrations. The apparent fraction of the dose absorbed after IM injection was greater than 80%.

*Metabolism/Excretion* – Alfa interferons are filtered through the glomeruli and undergo rapid proteolytic degradation during tubular reabsorption, rendering a negligible reappearance of intact alpha interferon in the systemic circulation, suggesting near complete reabsorption of interferon alfa-2a catabolites. Liver metabolism and subsequent biliary excretion are minor pathways of elimination.

## Contraindications

Hypersensitivity to alpha interferon or any component of the product.

## Warnings

*GI hemorrhage:* Infrequently, severe or fatal GI hemorrhage has been reported in association with alfa interferon therapy.

*Laboratory tests:* Prior to initiation of therapy, perform tests to quantitate peripheral blood hemoglobin, platelets, granulocytes, and hairy cells and bone marrow hairy cells. Monitor periodically (eg, monthly) during treatment to determine response to treatment. If a patient does not respond within 6 months, discontinue treatment. If a response occurs, continue treatment until no further improvement is observed and these laboratory parameters have been stable for about 3 months. It is not known whether continued treatment after that time is beneficial.

*Exercise caution in the following:* In patients with severe renal or hepatic disease, seizure disorders, or compromised CNS function or myelosuppression.

Administer with caution to patients with cardiac disease or with any history of cardiac illness. Acute, self-limited toxicities (eg, fever, chills) frequently associated with interferon alfa administration may exacerbate preexisting cardiac conditions.

Exercise caution when administering to patients with myelosuppression.

*CNS reactions:* CNS reactions have occurred in a number of patients and included decreased mental status, exaggerated CNS function, and dizziness. Careful periodic neuropsychiatric monitoring of all patients is recommended.

*Leukopenia and elevation of hepatic enzymes:* Leukopenia and elevation of hepatic enzymes occurred frequently but were rarely dose-limiting. Thrombocytopenia occurred less frequently. Proteinuria and increased cells in urinary sediment also were seen infrequently.

*Neutralizing antibodies:* Neutralizing antibodies were detected in approximately 27% of all patients (3.4% for patients with hairy cell leukemia). No clinical sequelae have been documented.

*Anemia:* In CML patients, a severe or life-threatening anemia was seen in 15% of patients. A severe life-threatening leukopenia and thrombocytopenia were seen in 27% or less. Changes usually were reversible when therapy was discontinued.

*Renal/Hepatic function impairment:* Transient increases in liver transaminases or alkaline phosphatase of any intensity were seen in up to 50% of patients during treatment with interferon alfa-2a. Only 5% of patients had a severe or life-threatening increase in AST.

Dose-limiting hepatic or renal toxicities are unusual.

*Pregnancy: Category C.*

*Lactation:* It is not known whether this drug is excreted in breast milk. Because of the potential for serious adverse reactions in nursing infants, decide whether to discontinue nursing or to discontinue the drug, taking into account the importance of the drug to the mother.

*Children:* Safety and efficacy in children younger than 18 years of age have not been established.

## Precautions

*Monitoring:* Prior to initiation of therapy, perform tests to quantitate peripheral blood hemoglobin, platelets, granulocytes, hairy cells, and bone marrow hairy cells. Monitor periodically (eg, monthly) during treatment to determine response to treatment. If a patient does not respond within 6 months, discontinue treatment. If a response occurs, continue treatment until no further improvement is observed and these laboratory parameters have been stable for about 3 months. It is not known whether continued treatment after that time is beneficial.

Because responses of hairy-cell leukemia generally are not observed for 1 to 3 months after initiation of treatment, very careful monitoring for severe depression of blood cell counts is warranted during the initial phase of treatment.

Patients who have preexisting cardiac abnormalities or who are in advanced stages of cancer should have ECGs taken prior to and during the course of treatment.

## Drug Interactions

Drugs that may be affected by interferon alfa-2a include aminophylline; theophylline; neurotoxic, hematotoxic, or cardiotoxic drugs; interleukin-2; and CNS drugs.

## Adverse Reactions

Most adverse reactions are reversible if detected early. If severe reactions occur, reduce dosage or discontinue the drug; take appropriate corrective measures according to physician's clinical judgment. Reinstitute therapy with caution; consider further need for the drug, and be alert to possible recurrence of toxicity.

Adverse reactions occurring in at least 3% of patients include fever; fatigue; myalgias; headache; chills; arthralgia; coughing; dyspnea; hypotension; edema; chest pain; anorexia; nausea; diarrhea; emesis; abdominal pain; dizziness; decreased mental status; depression; confusion; diaphoresis; paresthesias; numbness; lethargy; visual or sleep disturbances; partial alopecia; rash; dryness or inflammation of the oropharynx; dry skin or pruritus; weight loss; change in taste; reactivation of herpes labialis; transient impotence; night sweats; rhinorrhea; lab test abnormalities including leukopenia; neutropenia; thrombocytopenia; decreased hemoglobin; abnormal AST-alkaline phosphatase, LDH, and BUN; hypocalcemia; elevated fasting serum glucose and elevated serum phosphorus and serum uric acid neutralizing antibodies.

# INTERFERON ALFA-2b (IFN-alpha 2; rIFN-α2; α-2-interferon)

**Powder for injection, lyophilized**: 5, 10, 18, 25, and 50 million units/vial (*Rx*)

**Solution for injection**: 3, 5, 10, 18, and 25 million units/vial (*Rx*)

**Injection**: 3, 5, and 10 million units/dose in multidose pens (*Rx*)

*Intron* A[1] (Schering)

[1] Not all dosage forms and strengths are appropriate for some indications.

---

**Warning:**
> Alpha interferons, including interferon alfa-2b, recombinant, cause or aggravate fatal or life-threatening neuropsychiatric, autoimmune, ischemic, and infectious disorders. Closely monitor patients with periodic clinical and laboratory evaluations. Withdraw patients with persistently severe or worsening signs or symptoms of these conditions from therapy. In many, but not all, cases, these disorders resolve after stopping interferon alfa-2b, recombinant therapy. See Warnings and Adverse Reactions.

---

## Indications

*Hairy-cell leukemia:* In patients 18 years of age and older with hairy-cell leukemia.

*Malignant melanoma:* Adjuvant to surgical treatment in patients 18 years of age and older with malignant melanoma who are free of disease but at high risk for systemic recurrence within 56 days of surgery.

*Follicular lymphoma:* Initial treatment of clinically aggressive follicular non-Hodgkin lymphoma in conjunction with anthracycline-containing combination chemotherapy in patients 18 years of age and older.

*Condylomata acuminata:* Intralesional treatment of external genital or perianal warts in select patients 18 years of age and older.

*AIDS-related Kaposi sarcoma:* In select patients 18 years of age and older with AIDS-related Kaposi sarcoma.

*Chronic hepatitis C:* In patients 18 years of age or older with compensated liver disease who have a history of blood or blood product exposure and/or patients who are hepatitis C virus (HCV)-antibody-positive. (Interferon alfa-2b also is indicated for hepatitis C in combination with ribavirin capsules. Please refer to the interferon alfa-2b/ribavirin capsules combination monograph for more information.)

*Chronic hepatitis B:* In patients 1 year of age and older with compensated liver disease and HBV replication. Patients must be serum HBsAg-positive for at least 6 months and have HBV replication (serum HBeAg-positive) with elevated serum ALT.

*Unlabeled uses:*

| Interferon Alfa Unlabeled Uses | | |
|---|---|---|
| *Neoplastic diseases* | | |
| Significant activity | Limited activity | No activity |
| Bladder tumors (local use for superficial tumors) Chronic myelogenous leukemia Cutaneous T-cell lymphoma Non-Hodgkin lymphoma Essential thrombocytosis Chronic granulocytic leukemia | Melanoma Multiple myeloma Acute leukemias Carcinoid tumor Hodgkin disease | |

| Interferon Alfa Unlabeled Uses | | |
|---|---|---|
| *Neoplastic diseases* | | |
| Significant activity | Limited activity | No activity |
| *Viral infections* | | *Miscellaneous* |
| Cytomegaloviruses<br>Herpes simplex | Papillomaviruses<br>Rhinoviruses<br>Varicella zoster<br>HIV[1] | Behçet syndrome<br>Hypereosinophilic<br>syndrome<br>Polycythemia vera<br>treatment |

[1] Interferons have anti-HIV activity and may be enhanced by foscarnet/zidovudine.

## Administration and Dosage

Do not use interferon alfa-2b solution for injection IV; only powder for injection may be used IV.

The patient may self-administer the dose at bedtime.

*Hairy-cell leukemia:* 2 million units/m² IM or subcutaneously 3 times/week for up to 6 months. Do not use the 50 million unit strength of the powder for injection for the treatment of hairy-cell leukemia.

*Malignant melanoma:* 20 million units/m² IV infusion on 5 consecutive days/week for 4 weeks. Maintenance dosage is 10 million units/m² subcutaneously 3 times/week for 48 weeks.

Perform regular lab testing to monitor abnormalities for the purpose of dose modification. If adverse reactions develop during interferon alfa-2b treatment, particularly if granulocytes decrease to less than 500/mm³ or ALT/AST rises to less than 5 times the upper limit of normal (ULN), temporarily discontinue treatment until adverse reactions abate. Restart interferon alfa-2b at 50% of the previous dose. If intolerance persists, or if granulocytes decrease to less than 250/mm³, or ALT/AST rises to more than 10 times the ULN, discontinue interferon alfa-2b therapy.

*Follicular lymphoma:* 5 million units subcutaneously 3 times/week for up to 18 months in conjunction with an anthracycline-containing chemotherapy regimen.

Discontinue interferon alfa-2b therapy if AST exceeds more than 5 times the upper limit of normal or serum creatinine more than 2 mg/dL.

*Condylomata acuminata:* Inject 1 million units/lesion 3 times/week for 3 weeks on alternate days intralesionally. Use only 10 million unit vials because dilution of other strengths results in a hypertonic solution. Use a tuberculin or similar syringe and a 25- to 30-gauge needle.

The 10 million units vial of interferon alfa-2b powder for injection must be reconstituted with 1 mL of diluent (Bacteriostatic Water for Injection).

Maximum response usually occurs 4 to 8 weeks after therapy initiation. If results are not satisfactory after 12 to 16 weeks, a second course may be instituted. Patients with 6 to 10 condylomata may receive a second (sequential) course. Patients with more than 10 condylomata may receive additional sequences.

*Drug delivery* – Do not go beneath the lesion too deeply or inject too superficially. As many as 5 lesions can be treated at one time. To reduce side effects, give in evening with acetaminophen.

Direct the needle at the center of the base of the wart and at an angle almost parallel to the plane of the skin. This will deliver the interferon to the dermal core of the lesion, infiltrating the lesion and causing a small wheal.

*AIDS-related Kaposi sarcoma:* 30 million units/m² 3 times/week administered subcutaneously or IM. Do not use the 18 and 25 million units multidose strengths of the interferon alfa-2b solution for injection for the treatment of AIDS-related Kaposi sarcoma. Maintain the selected dosage regimen unless the disease progresses rapidly or severe intolerance occurs. If severe adverse reactions develop, modify dosage (50% reduction) or temporarily discontinue therapy until adverse reactions abate. When patients initiate therapy at 30 million units/m² 3 times/week, average dose tolerated at the end of 12 weeks of therapy is 110 million units/week and 75 million units/week at end of 24 weeks of therapy.

When disease stabilization or response to treatment occurs, continue treatment until there is no further evidence of tumor or until discontinuation is required by evidence of a severe opportunistic infection or adverse effect.

*Chronic hepatitis C:* 3 million units 3 times/week subcutaneously or IM. In patients tolerating therapy with normalization of ALT at 16 weeks of treatment, extend therapy to 18 to 24 months at 3 million units 3 times/week to improve the sustained response. Consider discontinuing therapy in nonresponders after 16 weeks. If severe adverse reactions develop, modify the dose (50% reduction) or temporarily discontinue therapy until reactions abate. If intolerance persists after dose adjustment, discontinue therapy. See interferon alfa-2b recombinant and ribavirin combination therapy monograph when used in combination with ribavirin capsules.

*Chronic hepatitis B:*

*Adults* – 30 to 35 million units/week subcutaneously or IM, either as 5 million units daily or 10 million units 3 times/week for 16 weeks.

*Pediatrics* – 3 million units/m$^2$ 3 times/week for the first week of therapy followed by dose escalation to 6 million units/m$^2$ 3 times/week (maximum of 10 million units 3 times/week) administered subcutaneously for a total therapy duration of 16 to 24 weeks.

If serious adverse reactions or lab abnormalities develop during therapy, decrease the dose by 50% or discontinue if appropriate until adverse reactions abate. If intolerance persists after dose adjustment, discontinue the drug.

*Decreased white blood cell, granulocyte, or platelet counts* – Use the following guidelines:

| Interferon Alfa-2b Dose with Decreased White Blood Cell, Granulocyte, or Platelet Counts | | | |
|---|---|---|---|
| Granulocyte count | White blood cell count | Platelet count | Interferon alfa-2b dose |
| < 750/mm$^3$ | < 1500/mm$^3$ | < 50,000/mm$^3$ | Reduce by 50% |
| < 500/mm$^3$ | < 1000/mm$^3$ | < 30,000/mm$^3$ | Permanently discontinue |

When platelet or granulocyte counts return to normal or baseline values, reinstitute therapy at up to 100% of initial dose.

### Actions

*Pharmacology:* Interferon alfa-2b is a protein produced by recombinant DNA techniques. Interferons exert their cellular activities by binding to specific membrane receptors on the cell surface. Once bound to the cell membrane, interferon initiates a complex sequence of intracellular events that includes the induction of certain enzymes. These events include inhibition of virus replication in virus-infected cells, suppression of cell proliferation, and immunomodulating activities.

*Pharmacokinetics:*

*Absorption/Distribution* – Maximum serum concentrations obtained via subcutaneously and IM occurred 3 to 12 hours after administration. Serum concentrations were below the detection limit by 16 hours after the injections.

After IV use, serum concentrations peaked by the end of infusion, then declined at a slightly more rapid rate than after IM or subcutaneous administration, becoming undetectable 4 hours after infusion.

*Metabolism/Excretion* – Elimination half-lives were about 2 to 3 hours. Interferon could not be detected in urine; the kidney may be the main site of interferon catabolism.

### Contraindications

Hypersensitivity to interferon alfa-2b or any components of the product. Interferon alfa-2b and ribavirin must not be used by women who are pregnant or by men whose female partners are pregnant. Extreme care must be taken to avoid pregnancy in female patients and in female partners of patients taking combination interferon alfa-2b/ribavirin therapy. Patients with autoimmune hepatitis must not be treated with combination interferon alfa-2b/ribavirin therapy.

## Warnings

*Hemolytic anemia:* Therapy containing interferon alfa-2b and ribavirin capsules was associated with hemolytic anemia. Hemoglobin less than 10 g/dL was observed in about 10% of patients in clinical trials. Anemia occurred within 1 to 2 weeks of initiation of ribavirin therapy.

*Thrombocytopenia:* Do not give IM to patients with platelet counts less than 50,000/mm$^3$. Instead, give subcutaneously.

*50 million unit vial size:* This vial size is to be used *only* for treatment of patients with AIDS-related Kaposi sarcoma or with malignant melanoma.

*Condylomata acuminata:*
   *Do not use* – Do not use 3, 5, 18, 25, or 50 million units vials of powder for injection or the 3 or 18 million units multidose vials intralesionally to treat condylomata acuminata; concentrations are inappropriate.

*AIDS-related Kaposi sarcoma:* Do not use interferon alfa-2b solution for injection, multidose pens, or the 18 or 25 million units multidose strengths; concentrations are inappropriate. Do not use in patients with rapidly progressive visceral disease. There may be synergistic adverse effects between interferon alfa-2b and zidovudine. Patients have had a higher incidence of neutropenia than that expected with zidovudine alone. Careful monitoring of the WBC count is indicated.

*Malignant melanoma:* Interferon solution for injection is not recommended for the IV treatment of malignant melanoma.

*Preexisting psychiatric condition/history of severe psychiatric disorder:* Depression and suicidal behavior including suicidal ideation, suicidal attempts, and completed suicides have been reported. Patients with a pre-existing psychiatric condition, especially depression, or a history of severe psychiatric disorder should not be treated with interferon alfa-2b.

*Bone marrow toxicity:* Interferon alfa-2b therapy suppresses bone marrow function and may result in severe cytopenias, including very rare events of aplastic anemia. Obtain CBCs pretreatment and monitor routinely during therapy. Discontinue interferon alfa-2b therapy in patients who develop severe decreases in neutrophil (less than $0.5 \times 10^9$/L) or platelet counts (less than $25 \times 10^9$/L).

*Thyroid abnormalities:* Infrequently, patients receiving interferon alfa-2b therapy developed thyroid abnormalities, either hypothyroid or hyperthyroid. Patients developing symptoms consistent with possible thyroid dysfunction of therapy should have their thyroid function evaluated and appropriate treatment instituted. Discontinue therapy if thyroid function cannot be normalized by medication. Discontinuation of therapy has not always reversed thyroid dysfunction occurring during treatment.

*Fever/"Flu-like" symptoms:* Because of fever and other "flu-like" symptoms associated with this drug, use cautiously in patients with debilitating medical conditions, such as a history of pulmonary disease or diabetes mellitus prone to ketoacidosis. Observe caution in coagulation disorders or severe myelosuppression.

*Pulmonary infiltrates:* Pulmonary infiltrates, pneumonitis, and pneumonia, including fatality, have been observed.

*Cardiovascular:* Use therapy cautiously in patients with a history of cardiovascular disease. Cardiovascular adverse experiences include hypotension, arrhythmia, or tachycardia of at least 150 beats/min and, rarely, cardiomyopathy and MI. Hypotension may occur during administration, or up to 2 days posttherapy, and may require supportive therapy, including fluid replacement to maintain intravascular volume.

*Ophthalmologic disorders:* Decrease or loss of vision, retinopathy (including macular edema), retinal artery or vein thrombosis, retinal hemorrhages and cotton wool spots, optic neuritis, and papilledema may be induced or aggravated by treatment with interferon alfa-2b or other alpha interferons. All patients should receive an eye examination at baseline.

*Hepatotoxicity:* Hepatotoxicity, including fatality, has been observed.

*Autoimmune disease:* Rare cases of autoimmune diseases including thrombocytopenia, vasculitis, Raynaud's phenomenon, rheumatoid arthritis, lupus erythematosus, and rhabdomyolysis have been observed.

*Hyperglycemia:* Diabetes mellitus and hyperglycemia have been observed rarely in patients treated with interferon alfa-2b.

*Benzyl alcohol:* The powder for injection for interferon alfa-2b, when reconstituted with the provided diluent (bacteriostatic water for injection) contains benzyl alcohol and is not indicated for use in infants. There have been reports of death in infants associated with excessive exposure to benzyl alcohol.

*Hypersensitivity reactions:* Acute serious hypersensitivity reactions (eg, urticaria, angioedema, bronchoconstriction, anaphylaxis) have been observed rarely in treated patients.

*Hepatic function impairment:* Do not treat patients with decompensated liver disease, autoimmune hepatitis, history of autoimmune disease, or immunocompromised transplant recipients.

*Fertility impairment:* Interferon may impair fertility. Fertile women should not receive interferon alfa-2b unless they are using effective contraception. Use with caution in fertile men.

*Pregnancy:* Category C. (Category X if used with ribavirin).

*Lactation:* It is not known if this drug is excreted in breast milk.

*Children:* Safety and efficacy in children younger than 18 years of age have not been established.

### Precautions

*Monitoring:* Prior to beginning treatment and periodically thereafter perform the following: Standard hematologic tests with complete blood counts and differential, platelet counts, blood chemistries, electrolytes, TSH, liver function tests. Patients with pre-existing cardiac abnormalities or those in advanced stages of cancer should have ECGs taken before and during treatment.

Baseline chest X-rays are suggested; repeat if clinically indicated.

For malignant melanoma patients, monitor differential, WBC count, and liver function tests weekly during the induction phase of therapy and monthly during the maintenance phase of therapy.

*Triglycerides:* Elevated triglyceride levels have been observed in patients treated with interferon therapy. Hypertriglyceridemia may result in pancreatitis.

*Chronic hepatitis B:* Perform a liver biopsy to establish presence of chronic hepatitis and extent of liver damage.

*ALT increase* – A transient increase in ALT at least 2 times baseline (flare) can occur, generally 8 to 12 weeks after therapy initiation, and is more frequent in responders.

*Chronic hepatitis C:* Perform a liver biopsy to establish diagnosis. Test for presence of antibody to HCV. Exclude patients with other causes of chronic hepatitis, including autoimmune hepatitis.

*Psoriasis and sarcoidosis:* There have been reports of interferon exacerbating pre-existing psoriasis and sarcoidosis as well as development of new sarcoidosis.

*Photosensitivity:* Photosensitivity may occur.

### Drug Interactions

Drugs that may be affected by interferon alfa-2b include theophylline and zidovudine.

### Adverse Reactions

The most frequently reported reactions are "flu-like" symptoms, particularly fever, headache, chills, myalgia, and fatigue. Other adverse reactions occurring in more than 5% of patients include the following: abdominal pain; alopecia; amnesia; anorexia; anxiety; arthralgia; asthenia; back pain; chest pain; confusion; constipation; coughing; decreased libido; depression; dermatitis; diarrhea; dizziness; dry mouth; dry skin; dyspepsia; dyspnea; facial edema; gingivitis; herpes simplex; hypesthesia; impaired concentration; increased sweating; injection site inflammation; insomnia; irritability; lab test abnormalities including hemoglobin, WBC count, platelet count, serum creatinine, alkaline phosphatase, lactate dehydrogenase, AST, ALT, serum urea nitrogen, and granulocyte count; loose stools; malaise; moniliasis; muscle pain; nasal congestion; nausea; nervousness; nonproductive cough; pain (unspecified); paresthesia; pharyngitis; pruritus; rash; rigors; sinusitis; somnolence; taste alteration; vomiting; weight loss.

# INTERFERON ALFA-2b, RECOMBINANT AND RIBAVIRIN COMBINATION

**Injection/Capsules**: 3 million units interferon alfa-2b, recombinant per 0.5 mL and 200 mg ribavirin (*Rx*)          *Rebetron* (Schering)

**Warning:**
Combination ribavirin/interferon alfa-2b therapy is contraindicated in women who are pregnant and in the male partners of women who are pregnant. Extreme care must be taken to avoid pregnancy during therapy and for 6 months after completion of treatment in female patients and in female partners of male patients who are taking combination ribavirin/interferon alfa-2b therapy. Women of childbearing potential and men must use 2 reliable forms of effective contraception during treatment and during the 6-month posttreatment followup period. Alpha interferons, including interferon alfa-2b, cause or aggravate fatal or life-threatening neuropsychiatric, autoimmune, ischemic, and infectious disorders.

## Indications
*Hepatitis C:* Treatment of chronic hepatitis C in patients with compensated liver disease previously untreated with alpha interferon or who have relapsed following alpha interferon therapy.
Ribavirin monotherapy is not effective for the treatment of chronic hepatitis C and should not be used for this indication.

## Administration and Dosage
Administer interferon alfa-2b subcutaneously and ribavirin orally without regard to food. Hydrate patients well, especially during initial treatment stages.

The recommended ribavirin dose depends on the patient's body weight. Administer doses of ribavirin and interferon alfa-2b according to the following table for 6 months (24 weeks). The safety and efficacy of the combination therapy has not been established for more than 6 months of treatment.

| Recommended Interferon Alfa-2b/Ribavirin Combination Dosing | | |
|---|---|---|
| Body weight | Ribavirin | Interferon alfa-2b injection |
| ≤ 75 kg | 400 mg am | 3 million units 3 times/week subcutaneously |
|  | 600 mg pm |  |
| > 75 kg | 600 mg am |  |
|  | 600 mg pm |  |

*Dose modifications:* It is recommended that patients who experience moderate depression (persistent low mood, loss of interest, poor self image, or hopelessness) have their interferon alfa-2b dose temporarily reduced or be considered for medical therapy. Discontinue treatment in patients experiencing severe depression or suicidal ideation/attempt from combination therapy and follow closely with appropriate medical management.

| Interferon Alfa-2b/Ribavirin Combination Dose Modification Guidelines | | |
|---|---|---|
| Parameter | Dose reduction[1]<br>Ribavirin - 600 mg daily<br>Interferon alfa-2b - 1.5 million units<br>3 times/week | Permanent discontinuation<br>of combination treatment |
| Hemoglobin | < 10 g/dL (reduce ribavirin) | < 8.5 g/dL |
| | *Cardiac history patients only:*<br>≥ 2 g/dL decrease during any 4-week period during treatment (reduce ribavirin/interferon alfa-2b) | *Cardiac history patients only:*<br>< 12 g/dL after 4 weeks of<br>dose reduction |
| White blood count | < 1.5 × 10⁹/L (reduce interferon alfa-2b) | < 1 × 10⁹/L |
| Neutrophil count | < 0.75 × 10⁹/L (reduce interferon alfa-2b) | < 0.5 × 10⁹/L |
| Platelet count | < 50 × 10⁹/L (reduce interferon alfa-2b) | < 25 × 10⁹/L |

[1] Medication to have a dose reduction is shown in parentheses.

*Administration of interferon alfa-2b injection:* At the discretion of the physician, the patient may self-administer interferon alfa-2b.

Withdraw the appropriate dose from the vial or set on the multidose pen and inject subcutaneously. After administration, follow the procedure for proper disposal of syringes and needles.

| Administration of Interferon Alfa-2b Injection | | |
|---|---|---|
| Vial/Pen label strength | Fill volume | Concentration |
| 3 million units vial | 0.5 mL | 3 million units per 0.5 mL |
| 18 million units multidose vial[1] | 3.8 mL | 3 million units per /0.5 mL |
| 18 million units multidose pen[2] | 1.5 mL | 3 million units per 0.2 mL |

[1] This is a multidose vial that contains 22.8 million units of interferon alfa-2b/3.8 mL in order to provide the delivery of six 0.5 mL doses, each containing 3 million units of interferon alfa-2b (for a label strength of 18 million units).

[2] This is a multidose pen that contains a 22.5 million units of interferon alfa-2b/1.5 mL in order to provide the delivery of six 0.2 mL doses, each containing 3 million units of interferon alfa-2b (for a label strength of 18 million units).

*Treatment duration:* The recommended duration of treatment for patients previously untreated with interferon is 24 to 48 weeks. Consider treatment discontinuation in any patient who has not achieved an HCV RNA below the limit of detection of the assay by 24 weeks.

### Precautions

*Monitoring:* The following laboratory tests are recommended for all patients on combination therapy, prior to beginning treatment and then periodically thereafter: Standard hematologic tests including hemoglobin (pretreatment, week 2 and week 4 of therapy, and as clinically appropriate), complete and differential white blood cell counts, and platelet count; liver function tests and TSH; pregnancy including monthly monitoring for women of childbearing potential.

*Cardiac disease:* Administer therapy with caution to patients with pre-existing cardiac disease. Assess patients before commencement of therapy and appropriately monitor them during therapy. If there is any deterioration of cardiovascular status, stop therapy.

*Renal function impairment:* Administer with caution in patients with Ccr less than 50 mL/min.

# ERLOTINIB

| | |
|---|---|
| **Tablets:** 25, 100, and 150 mg *(Rx)* | *Tarceva* (Genentech/OSI) |

## Indications
*Non-small cell lung cancer (NSCLC):* For the treatment of patients with locally advanced or metastatic NSCLC after failure of at least 1 prior chemotherapy regimen.

## Administration and Dosage
The recommended daily dose of erlotinib is 150 mg once daily taken at least 1 hour before or 2 hours after the ingestion of food. Continue treatment until disease progression or unacceptable toxicity occurs. There is no evidence that treatment beyond progression is beneficial.

*Dose modifications:* When dose reduction is necessary, reduce the erlotinib dose in 50 mg decrements.

*Pulmonary symptoms* – In patients who develop an acute onset of new or progressive pulmonary symptoms, such as dyspnea, cough, or fever, interrupt treatment with erlotinib pending diagnostic evaluation. If interstitial lung disease (ILD) is diagnosed, discontinue erlotinib and institute appropriate treatment as necessary.

*Diarrhea/Skin reactions* – Diarrhea can usually be managed with loperamide. Patients with severe skin reactions and those with severe diarrhea who are unresponsive to loperamide or who become dehydrated may require dose reduction or temporary interruption of therapy.

*Hepatic function impairment* – Use caution when administering erlotinib to patients with hepatic impairment. Consider dose reduction or interruption of erlotinib if severe adverse reactions occur or changes in liver function are severe.

## Actions
*Pharmacology:* Erlotinib inhibits the intracellular phosphorylation of tyrosine kinase associated with the epidermal growth factor receptor (EGFR).

*Pharmacokinetics:*

*Absorption/Distribution* – Bioavailability is approximately 60% and peak plasma levels occur 4 hours after dosing. Approximately 93% is protein bound to albumin and alpha-$_1$ acid glycoprotein (AAG). The apparent volume of distribution of 232 L.

*Metabolism/Excretion* – Half-life is approximately 36 hours. Erlotinib is metabolized primarily by CYP3A4 and, to a lesser extent, CYP1A2 and the extrahepatic isoform CYP1A1. Following a 100 mg oral dose, 91% of the dose was recovered: 83% in feces (1% of the dose as intact parent) and 8% in urine (0.3% of the dose as intact parent). Median half-life of 36.2 hours. Time to reach steady-state plasma concentration is 7 to 8 days. Smokers had a 24% higher rate of erlotinib clearance.

## Contraindications
None known.

## Warnings
*Pulmonary toxicity:* There have been infrequent reports of serious ILD, including fatalities. In the event of acute onset of new or progressive, unexplained pulmonary symptoms, such as dyspnea, cough, and fever, interrupt erlotinib therapy pending diagnostic evaluation. If ILD is diagnosed, discontinue erlotinib and institute appropriate treatment as necessary.

*Hepatic function impairment:* Erlotinib exposure may be increased in patients with hepatic dysfunction.

*Pregnancy: Category D.*

*Lactation:* It is not known whether erlotinib is excreted in human milk.

## Precautions
*Monitoring:*

*Elevated international normalized ratio (INR) and potential bleeding* – Regularly monitor patients taking warfarin or other coumarin-derivative anticoagulants for changes in prothrombin time or INR.

*Hepatotoxicity:* Asymptomatic increases in liver transaminases have been observed. Consider periodic liver function testing.

### Drug Interactions

*CYP450 system:* Use caution when administering or taking erlotinib with ketoconazole and other strong CYP3A4 inhibitors such as atazanavir, clarithromycin, indinavir, itraconazole, nefazodone, nelfinavir, ritonavir, saquinavir, telithromycin, troleandomycin, and voriconazole.

Consider alternate treatments lacking CYP3A4 inducing activity. If an alternative treatment is unavailable, consider an erlotinib dose greater than 150 mg. If the erlotinib dose is adjusted upward, the dose will need to be reduced upon discontinuation of rifampin or other inducers. Other CYP3A4 inducers include rifabutin, rifapentine, phenytoin, carbamazepine, phenobarbital, and St. John's wort.

*Warfarin:* INR elevations and infrequent reports of bleeding events, including GI bleeding, have been reported in clinical studies, some associated with warfarin coadministration.

### Adverse Reactions

Adverse reactions occurring in at least 10% of patients treated with erlotinib and at least 3% more often than in the placebo group in the randomized trial include the following: abdominal pain, anorexia, conjunctivitis, cough, diarrhea, dry skin, dyspnea, fatigue, infection, keratoconjunctivitis sicca, nausea, pruritus, rash, stomatitis, vomiting.

## GEFITINIB

| | |
|---|---|
| **Tablets**: 250 mg (*Rx*) | *Iressa* (AstraZeneca) |

### Indications

*Nonsmall cell lung cancer (NSCLC):* Gefitinib is indicated as monotherapy for the treatment of patients with locally advanced or metastatic non-small cell lung cancer after failure of platinum-based and docetaxel chemotherapies.

### Administration and Dosage

*Dose:* The recommended daily dose of gefitinib is one 250 mg tablet with or without food. Higher doses do not give a better response and cause increased toxicity.

*Dosage adjustment:*

*Diarrhea/Skin reactions* – Patients with poorly tolerated diarrhea or skin adverse drug reactions may be successfully managed by providing a brief (up to 14 days) therapy interruption followed by reinstatement of the 250 mg/day dose.

*Pulmonary* – In the event of acute onset or worsening of pulmonary symptoms, interrupt gefitinib therapy. If interstitial lung disease (ILD) is confirmed, discontinue gefitinib and treat the patient appropriately.

*Ocular* – For patients who develop onset of new eye symptoms such as pain, interrupt gefitinib therapy. After symptoms and eye changes have been resolved, decide on reinstatement of the 250 mg/day dose.

*CYP3A4 inducers:* In patients receiving a potent CYP3A4 inducer such as rifampin or phenytoin, consider a dose increase to 500 mg/day in the absence of severe adverse drug reaction.

### Actions

*Pharmacology:* Gefitinib inhibits the intracellular phosphorylation of numerous tyrosine kinases associated with transmembrane cell surface receptors, including the tyrosine kinases associated with epidermal growth factor receptor (EGFR-TK).

*Pharmacokinetics:*

*Absorption/Distribution* – Gefitinib is slowly absorbed, with peak plasma levels occurring 3 to 7 hours after dosing and mean oral bioavailability of 60%. Mean steady-state volume of distribution is 1400 L following IV administration. It is 90% protein bound.

*Metabolism/Excretion* – Gefitinib undergoes extensive hepatic metabolism in humans, predominantly by CYP3A4.

Total plasma clearance and elimination half-life values of 595 mL/min and 48 hours, respectively, after IV administration. Excretion is predominantly via the feces (86%), with renal elimination of drug and metabolites accounting for less than 4% of the administered dose.

## Contraindications

Severe hypersensitivity to gefitinib or any other component of the product.

## Warnings

*Pulmonary toxicity:* Cases of ILD have been observed in patients receiving gefitinib at an overall incidence of about 1%. Approximately one third of the cases have been fatal. Reports have described the adverse event as interstitial pneumonia, pneumonitis, and alveolitis. Patients often present with the acute onset of dyspnea, sometimes associated with cough or low-grade fever, often becoming severe within a short time and requiring hospitalization.

If ILD is confirmed, discontinue gefitinib and treat the patient appropriately (see Administration and Dosage).

*Renal function impairment:* Treat patients with severe renal impairment with caution when giving gefitinib.

*Hepatic function impairment:* Gefitinib exposure may be increased in patients with hepatic dysfunction.

*Pregnancy: Category D.*

*Lactation:* It is not known whether gefitinib is excreted in human milk. Advise women against breastfeeding while receiving gefitinib.

*Children:* Safety and efficacy of gefitinib in pediatric patients have not been studied.

## Precautions

*Hepatotoxicity:* Asymptomatic increases in liver transaminases have been observed; consider periodic liver function testing.

## Drug Interactions

Drugs that may affect gefitinib include CYP3A4 inducers (eg, rifampin), CYP3A4 inhibitors (eg, ketoconazole), $H_2$ antagonists (eg, cimetidine), sodium bicarbonate, metoprolol, and warfarin.

## Adverse Reactions

Adverse reactions occurring in at least 3% of patients include the following: acne, anorexia, asthenia, diarrhea, dry skin, nausea, pruritus, rash, vomiting, weight loss.

# APPENDIX

# FDA PREGNANCY CATEGORIES

The rational use of any medication requires a risk versus benefit assessment. Among the myriad of risk factors that complicate this assessment, pregnancy is one of the most perplexing.

The FDA has established five categories to indicate the potential of a systemically absorbed drug for causing birth defects. The key differentiation among the categories rests upon the degree (reliability) of documentation and the risk versus benefit ratio. Pregnancy *Category* X is particularly notable in that if any data exists that may implicate a drug as a teratogen and the risk versus benefit ratio does not support use of the drug, the drug is contraindicated during pregnancy. These categories are summarized below:

| FDA Pregnancy Categories | |
|---|---|
| **Pregnancy Category** | **Definition** |
| A | Controlled studies show no risk. Adequate, well-controlled studies in pregnant women have failed to demonstrate risk to the fetus. |
| B | No evidence of risk in humans. Either animal findings show risk, but human findings do not; or if no adequate human studies have been done, animal findings are negative. |
| C | Risk cannot be ruled out. Human studies are lacking, and animal studies are either positive for fetal risk or lacking. However, potential benefits may justify the potential risks. |
| D | Positive evidence of risk. Investigational or post-marketing data show risk to the fetus. Nevertheless, potential benefits may outweigh the potential risks. If needed in a life-threatening situation or a serious disease, the drug may be acceptable if safer drugs cannot be used or are ineffective. |
| X | Contraindicated in pregnancy. Studies in animals or human, or investigational or post-marketing reports have shown fetal risk which clearly outweighs any possible benefit to the patient. |

*Regardless of the designated Pregnancy Category or presumed safety, no drug should be administered during pregnancy unless it is clearly needed and potential benefits outweigh potential hazards to the fetus.*

# CONTROLLED SUBSTANCES

The Controlled Substances Act of 1970 regulates the manufacturing, distribution and dispensing of drugs that have abuse potential. The Drug Enforcement Administration (DEA) within the US Department of Justice is the chief federal agency responsible for enforcing the act.

**DEA Schedules:** Drugs under jurisdiction of the Controlled Substances Act are divided into five schedules based on their potential for abuse and physical and psychological dependence. All controlled substances listed in *Drug Facts and Comparisons®* are identified by schedule as follows:

Schedule I *(c-i)* – High abuse potential and no accepted medical use (eg, heroin, marijuana, LSD).

Schedule II *(c-ii)* – High abuse potential with severe dependence liability (eg, narcotics, amphetamines, dronabinol, some barbiturates).

Schedule III *(c-iii)* – Less abuse potential than schedule II drugs and moderate dependence liability (eg, nonbarbiturate sedatives, nonamphetamine stimulants, limited amounts of certain narcotics).

Schedule IV *(c-iv)* – Less abuse potential than schedule III drugs and limited dependence liability (eg, some sedatives, antianxiety agents, nonnarcotic analgesics).

Schedule V *(c-v)* – Limited abuse potential. Primarily small amounts of narcotics (codeine) used as antitussives or antidiarrheals. Under federal law, limited quantities of certain *c-v* drugs may be purchased without a prescription directly from a pharmacist if allowed under state statutes. The purchaser must be at least 18 years of age and must furnish suitable identification. All such transactions must be recorded by the dispensing pharmacist.

**Registration:** Prescribing physicians and dispensing pharmacies must be registered with the DEA, PO Box 28083, Central Station, Washington, DC 20005.

**Inventory:** Separate records must be kept of purchases and dispensing of controlled substances. An inventory of controlled substances must be made every 2 years.

**Prescriptions:** Prescriptions for controlled substances must be written in ink and include the following: Date; name and address of the patient; name, address, and DEA number of the physician. Oral prescriptions must be promptly committed to writing. Controlled substance prescriptions may not be dispensed or refilled more than 6 months after the date issued or be refilled more than 5 times. A written prescription signed by the physician is required for schedule II drugs. In case of emergency, oral prescriptions for schedule II substances may be filled; however, the physician must provide a signed prescription within 72 hours. Schedule II prescriptions cannot be refilled. A triplicate order form is necessary for the transfer of controlled substances in schedule II. Forms are available for the individual prescriber at no charge from the DEA.

**State Laws:** In many cases, state laws are more restrictive than federal laws and therefore impose additional requirements (eg, triplicate prescription forms).

# MANAGEMENT OF ACUTE HYPERSENSITIVITY REACTIONS

*Type* I hypersensitivity reactions (immediate hypersensitivity or anaphylaxis) are immunologic responses to a foreign antigen to which a patient has been previously sensitized. Anaphylactoid reactions are not immunoogically mediated; however, symptoms and treatment are similar.

## Signs and Symptoms

Acute hypersensitivity reactions typically begin within 1 to 30 minutes of exposure to the offending antigen. Tingling sensations and a generalized flush may proceed to a fullness in the throat, chest tightness, or a "feeling of impending doom." Generalized urticaria and sweating are common. *Severe* reactions include life-threatening involvement of the airway and cardiovascular system.

## Treatment

Appropriate and immediate treatment is imperative. The following general measures are commonly employed:

**Epinephrine:** 1:1000, 0.2 to 0.5 mg (0.2 to 0.5 mL) SC is the primary treatment. In children, administer 0.01 mg/kg or 0.1 mg. Doses may be repeated every 5 to 15 minutes if needed. A succession of small doses is more effective and less dangerous than a single large dose. Additionally, 0.1 mg may be introduced into an injection site where the offending drug was administered. If appropriate, the use of a tourniquet above the site of injection of the causative agent may slow its absorption and distribution. However, remove or loosen the tourniquet every 10 to 15 minutes to maintain circulation.

Epinephrine IV (generally indicated in the presence of hypotension) is often recommended in a 1:10,000 dilution, 0.3 to 0.5 mg over 5 minutes; repeat every 15 minutes, if necessary. In children, inject 0.1 to 0.2 mg or 0.01 mg/kg/dose over 5 minutes; repeat every 30 minutes.

A conservative IV epinephrine protocol includes 0.1 mg of a 1:100,000 dilution (0.1 mg of a 1:1000 dilution mixed in 10 mL normal saline) given over 5 to 10 minutes. If an IV infusion is necessary, administer at a rate of 1 to 4 mcg/min. In children, infuse 0.1 to 1.5 (maximum) mcg/kg/min.

Dilute epinephrine 1:10,000 may be administered through an endotracheal tube, if no other parenteral access is available, directly into the bronchial tree. It is rapidly absorbed there from the capillary bed of the lung.

**Airway:** Ensure a patent airway via endotracheal intubation or cricothyrotomy (ie, inferior laryngotomy, used prior to tracheotomy) and administer oxygen. Severe respiratory difficulty may respond to IV aminophylline or to other bronchodilators.

**Hypotension:** The patient should be recumbent with feet elevated. Depending upon the severity, consider the following measures:
- Establish a patent IV catheter in a suitable vein.
- Administer IV fluids (eg, Normal Saline, Lactated Ringer's).
- Administer plasma expanders.

♦ Administer cardioactive agents (see group and individual monographs). Commonly recommended agents include dopamine, dobutamine, norepinephrine, and phenylephrine.

**Adjunctive therapy:** Adjunctive therapy does not alter acute reactions, but may modify an ongoing or slow-onset process and shorten the course of the reaction.

♦ *Antihistamines: Diphenhydramine* – 50 to 100 mg IM or IV, continued orally at 5 mg/kg/day or 50 mg every 6 hours for 1 to 2 days. For children, give 5 mg/kg/day, maximum 300 mg/day.

*Chlorpheniramine* – (adults, 10 to 20 mg; children, 5 to 10 mg) IM or slowly IV.

*Hydroxyzine* – 10 to 25 mg orally or 25 to 50 mg IM 3 to 4 times daily.

♦ *Corticosteroids*, eg, hydrocortisone IV 100 to 1000 mg or equivalent, followed by 7 mg/kg/day IV or oral for 1 to 2 days. The role of corticosteroids is controversial.

♦ *H₂ antagonists: Cimetidine* – *Children*, 25 to 30 mg/kg/day IV in 6 divided doses; *adults*, 300 mg every 6 hours.

*Ranitidine* – 50 mg IV over 3 to 5 minutes. May be of value in addition to H₁ antihistamines, although this opinion is not universally shared.

# CALCULATIONS

*To calculate milliequivalent weight:* $mEq = \dfrac{\text{gram molecular weight/valence}}{1000}$

$mEq = \dfrac{mg}{eq\ wt}$     *equivalent weight or eq wt* $= \dfrac{\text{gram molecular weight}}{\text{valence}}$

| Commonly used mEq weights | | | |
|---|---|---|---|
| Chloride | 35.5 mg = 1 mEq | Magnesium | 12 mg = 1 mEq |
| Sodium | 23 mg = 1 mEq | Potassium | 39 mg = 1 mEq |
| Calcium | 20 mg = 1 mEq | | |

*To convert temperature* °C ↔ °F: $\dfrac{°C}{°F - 32} = \dfrac{5}{9}$  *or*  $°C = \dfrac{5}{9}\ (°F - 32)$

$$°F = 32 + \dfrac{9}{5}\ °C$$

*To calculate creatinine clearance (Ccr) from serum creatinine:*

Male: $Ccr = \dfrac{\text{weight (kg)} \times (140 - age)}{72 \times \text{serum creatinine (mg/dL)}}$     Female: Ccr = 0.85 × calculation for males

*To calculate ideal body weight (kg):*

Male = 50 kg + 2.3 kg (each inch > 5 ft)     Female = 45.5 kg + 2.3 kg (each inch > 5 ft)

*To calculate body surface area (BSA) in adults and children:*

1) *Dubois method:*

SA $(cm^2)$ = wt $(kg)^{0.425}$ × ht $(cm)^{0.725}$ × 71.84

SA $(m^2)$ = K × $\sqrt[3]{wt^2\ (kg)}$ (common K value
0.1 for toddlers, 0.103 for neonates)

2) *Simplified method:*

$$BSA\ (m^2) = \sqrt{\dfrac{ht\ (cm) \times wt\ (kg)}{3600}}$$

*To approximate surface area $(m^2)$ of children from weight (kg):*

| Weight range (kg) | ≈ Surface area $(m^2)$ |
|---|---|
| 1 to 5 | (0.05 x kg) + 0.05 |
| 6 to 10 | (0.04 x kg) + 0.10 |
| 11 to 20 | (0.03 x kg) + 0.20 |
| 21 to 40 | (0.02 x kg) + 0.40 |

| Suggested Weights for Adults | |
|---|---|
| Height* | Weight in pounds† |
| 4'10" | 91-119 |
| 4'11" | 94-124 |
| 5'0" | 97-128 |
| 5'1" | 101-132 |
| 5'2" | 104-137 |
| 5'3" | 107-141 |
| 5'4" | 111-146 |
| 5'5" | 114-150 |
| 5'6" | 118-155 |
| 5'7" | 121-160 |
| 5'8" | 125-164 |
| 5'9" | 129-169 |
| 5'10" | 132-174 |
| 5'11" | 136-179 |
| 6'0" | 140-184 |
| 6'1" | 144-189 |
| 6'2" | 148-195 |
| 6'3" | 152-200 |
| 6'4" | 156-205 |
| 6'5" | 160-211 |
| 6'6" | 164-216 |

* Without shoes.     † Without clothes.

The higher weights in the ranges generally apply to people with more muscle and bone. Source: Nutrition and Your Health: Dietary Guidelines for Americans, 4th ed, 1995. US Department of Agriculture, US Department of Health and Human Services. At press time, these new guidelines had not been officially released. It is possible some changes to this chart will occur.

# NORMAL LABORATORY VALUES

In the following tables, normal reference values for commonly requested laboratory tests are listed in traditional units and in SI units. The tables are a guideline only. Values are method dependent and "normal values" may vary between laboratories.

| Blood, Plasma, or Serum | | |
|---|---|---|
| | Reference Value | |
| Determination | Conventional Units | SI Units |
| Ammonia (NH₃) – diffusion | 20-120 mcg/dL | 12-70 mcmol/L |
| Ammonia Nitrogen | 15–45 µg/dL | 11–32 µmol/L |
| Amylase | 35-118 IU/L | 0.58-1.97 mckat/L |
| Anion Gap (Na⁺−[Cl⁻+HCO₃⁻]) (P) | 7–16 mEq/L | 7–16 mmol/L |
| Antinuclear antibodies | negative at 1:10 dilution of serum | negative at 1:10 dilution of serum |
| Antithrombin III (AT III) | 80-120 U/dL | 800-1200 U/L |
| Bicarbonate: Arterial | 21–28 mEq/L | 21–28 mmol/L |
| Venous | 22–29 mEq/L | 22–29 mmol/L |
| Bilirubin: Conjugated (direct) | ≤ 0.2 mg/dL | ≤ 4 mcmol/L |
| Total | 0.1-1 mg/dL | 2-18 mcmol/L |
| Calcitonin | < 100 pg/mL | < 100 ng/L |
| Calcium: Total | 8.6-10.3 mg/dL | 2.2-2.74 mmol/L |
| Ionized | 4.4-5.1 mg/dL | 1-1.3 mmol/L |
| Carbon dioxide content (plasma) | 21-32 mmol/L | 21-32 mmol/L |
| Carcinoembryonic antigen | < 3 ng/mL | < 3 mcg/L |
| Chloride | 95-110 mEq/L | 95-110 mmol/L |
| *Coagulation screen:* | | |
| Bleeding time | 3-9.5 min | 180-570 sec |
| Prothrombin time | 10-13 sec | 10-13 sec |
| Partial thromboplastin time (activated) | 22-37 sec | 22-37 sec |
| Protein C | 0.7-1.4 µ/mL | 700-1400 U/mL |
| Protein S | 0.7-1.4 µ/mL | 700-1400 U/mL |
| Copper, total | 70-160 mcg/dL | 11-25 mcmol/L |
| Corticotropin (ACTH adrenocorticotropic hormone) – 0800 hr | < 60 pg/mL | < 13.2 pmol/L |
| Cortisol: 0800 hr | 5-30 mcg/dL | 138-810 nmol/L |
| 1800 hr | 2-15 mcg/dL | 50-410 nmol/L |
| 2000 hr | ≤ 50% of 0800 hr | ≤ 50% of 0800 hr |
| Creatine kinase: Female | 20-170 IU/L | 0.33-2.83 mckat/L |
| Male | 30-220 IU/L | 0.5-3.67 mckat/L |
| Creatine kinase isoenzymes, MB fraction | 0-12 IU/L | 0-0.2 mckat/L |
| Creatinine | 0.5-1.7 mg/dL | 44-150 mcmol/L |
| Fibrinogen (coagulation factor I) | 150-360 mg/dL | 1.5-3.6 g/L |
| Follicle-stimulating hormone (FSH): | | |
| Female | 2-13 mIU/mL | 2-13 IU/L |
| Midcycle | 5-22 mIU/mL | 5-22 IU/L |
| Male | 1-8 mIU/mL | 1-8 IU/L |
| Glucose, fasting | 65-115 mg/dL | 3.6-6.3 mmol/L |

| Glucose Tolerance Test (Oral) | mg/dL | | mmol/L | |
|---|---|---|---|---|
| | Normal | Diabetic | Normal | Diabetic |
| Fasting | 70-105 | > 140 | 3.9-5.8 | > 7.8 |
| 60 min | 120-170 | ≥ 200 | 6.7-9.4 | ≥11.1 |
| 90 min | 100-140 | ≥ 200 | 5.6-7.8 | ≥ 11.1 |
| 120 min | 70-120 | ≥ 140 | 3.9-6.7 | ≥ 7.8 |

| | Conventional Units | SI Units |
|---|---|---|
| (γ) - Glutamyltransferase (GGT): Male | 9-50 units/L | 9-50 units/L |
| Female | 8-40 units/L | 8-40 units/L |
| Haptoglobin | 44-303 mg/dL | 0.44-3.03 g/L |

| Blood, Plasma, or Serum | | |
|---|---|---|
| | Reference Value | |
| Determination | Conventional Units | SI Units |
| *Hematologic tests:* | | |
| Fibrinogen | 200-400 mg/dL | 2-4 g/L |
| Hematocrit (Hct), female | 36%-44.6% | 0.36-0.446 fraction of 1 |
| male | 40.7%-50.3% | 0.4-0.503 fraction of 1 |
| Hemoglobin $A_{1C}$ | 5.3%-7.5% of total Hgb | 0.053-0.075 |
| Hemoglobin (Hb), female | 12.1-15.3 g/dL | 121-153 g/L |
| male | 13.8-17.5 g/dL | 138-175 g/L |
| Leukocyte count (WBC) | 3800-9800/mcL | $3.8-9.8 \times 10^9$/L |
| Erythrocyte count (RBC), female | $3.5-5 \times 10^6$/mcL | $3.5-5 \times 10^{12}$/L |
| male | $4.3-5.9 \times 10^6$/mcL | $4.3-5.9 \times 10^{12}$/L |
| Mean corpuscular volume (MCV) | 80-97.6 mcm³ | 80-97.6 fl |
| Mean corpuscular hemoglobin (MCH) | 27-33 pg/cell | 1.66-2.09 fmol/cell |
| Mean corpuscular hemoglobin concentrate (MCHC) | 33-36 g/dL | 20.3-22 mmol/L |
| Erythrocyte sedimentation rate (sedrate, ESR) | ≤ 30 mm/hr | ≤ 30 mm/hr |
| Erythrocyte enzymes: Glucose-6-phosphate dehydroge nase (G-6-PD) | 250-5000 units/$10^6$ cells | 250-5000 mcunits/cell |
| Ferritin | 10-383 ng/mL | 23-862 pmol/L |
| Folic acid: normal | > 3.1-12.4 ng/mL | 7-28.1 nmol/L |
| Platelet count | $150-450 \times 10^3$/mcL | $150-450 \times 10^9$/L |
| Reticulocytes | 0.5%-1.5% of erythrocytes | 0.005-0.015 |
| Vitamin $B_{12}$ | 223-1132 pg/mL | 165-835 pmol/L |
| Iron: Female | 30-160 mcg/dL | 5.4-31.3 mcmol/L |
| Male | 45-160 mcg/dL | 8.1-31.3 mcmol/L |
| Iron binding capacity | 220-420 mcg/dL | 39.4-75.2 mcmol/L |
| Isocitrate Dehydrogenase | 1.2-7 units/L | 1.2-7 units/L |
| Isoenzymes | | |
| Fraction 1 | 14%-26% of total | 0.14-0.26 fraction of total |
| Fraction 2 | 29%-39% of total | 0.29-0.39 fraction of total |
| Fraction 3 | 20%-26% of total | 0.20-0.26 fraction of total |
| Fraction 4 | 8%-16% of total | 0.08-0.16 fraction of total |
| Fraction 5 | 6%-16% of total | 0.06-0.16 fraction of total |
| Lactate dehydrogenase | 100-250 IU/L | 1.67-4.17 mckat/L |
| Lactic acid (lactate) | 6-19 mg/dL | 0.7-2.1 mmol/L |
| Lead | ≤ 50 mcg/dL | ≤ 2.41 mcmol/L |
| Lipase | 10-150 units/L | 10-150 units/L |
| *Lipids:* | | |
| Total Cholesterol | | |
| Desirable | < 200 mg/dL | < 5.2 mmol/L |
| Borderline-high | 200-239 mg/dL | < 5.2-6.2 mmol/L |
| High | > 239 mg/dL | > 6.2 mmol/L |
| LDL | | |
| Desirable | < 130 mg/dL | < 3.36 mmol/L |
| Borderline-high | 130-159 mg/dL | 3.36-4.11 mmol/L |
| High | > 159 mg/dL | > 4.11 mmol/L |

| Blood, Plasma, or Serum | | |
|---|---|---|
| | Reference Value | |
| Determination | Conventional Units | SI Units |
| HDL (low) | < 35 mg/dL | < 0.91 mmol/L |
| Triglycerides | | |
| Desirable | < 200 mg/dL | < 2.26 mmol/L |
| Borderline-high | 200-400 mg/dL | 2.26-4.52 mmol/L |
| High | 400-1000 mg/dL | 4.52-11.3 mmol/L |
| Very high | > 1000 mg/dL | > 11.3 mmol/L |
| Magnesium | 1.3-2.2 mEq/L | 0.65-1.1 mmol/L |
| Osmolality | 280-300 mOsm/kg | 280-300 mmol/kg |
| Oxygen saturation (arterial) | 94%-100% | 0.94-1 fraction of 1 |
| $PCO_2$, arterial | 35-45 mm Hg | 4.7-6 kPa |
| pH, arterial | 7.35-7.45 | 7.35-7.45 |
| $PO_2$, arterial: Breathing room air[1] | 80-105 mm Hg | 10.6-14 kPa |
| On 100% $O_2$ | > 500 mm Hg | |
| Phosphatase (acid), total at 37°C | 0.13-0.63 IU/L | 2.2-10.5 IU/L or 2.2-10.5 mckat/L |
| Phosphatase alkaline[2] | 20-130 IU/L | 20-130 IU/L or 0.33-2.17 mckat/L |
| Phosphorus, inorganic,[3] (phosphate) | 2.5-5 mg/dL | 0.8-1.6 mmol/L |
| Potassium | 3.5-5 mEq/L | 3.5-5 mmol/L |
| Progesterone | | |
| Female | 0.1-1.5 ng/mL | 0.32-4.8 nmol/L |
| Follicular phase | 0.1-1.5 ng/mL | 0.32-4.8 nmol/L |
| Luteal phase | 2.5-28 ng/mL | 8-89 nmol/L |
| Male | < 0.5 ng/mL | < 1.6 nmol/L |
| Prolactin | 1.4-24.2 ng/mL | 1.4-24.2 mcg/L |
| Prostate specific antigen | 0-4 ng/mL | 0-4 ng/mL |
| Protein: Total | 6-8 g/dL | 60-80 g/L |
| Albumin | 3.6-5 g/dL | 36-50 g/L |
| Globulin | 2.3-3.5 g/dL | 23-35 g/L |
| Rheumatoid factor | < 60 IU/mL | < 60 kIU/L |
| Sodium | 135-147 mEq/L | 135-147 mmol/L |
| Testosterone: Female | 6-86 ng/dL | 0.21-3 nmol/L |
| Male | 270-1070 ng/dL | 9.3-37 nmol/L |
| *Thyroid Hormone Function Tests:* | | |
| Thyroid-stimulating hormone (TSH) | 0.35-6.2 mcU/mL | 0.35-6.2 mU/L |
| Thyroxine-binding globulin capacity | 10-26 mcg/dL | 100-260 mcg/L |
| Total triiodothyronine ($T_3$) | 75-220 ng/dL | 1.2-3.4 nmol/L |
| Total thyroxine by RIA ($T_4$) | 4-11 mcg/dL | 51-142 nmol/L |
| $T_3$ resin uptake | 25%-38% | 0.25-0.38 fraction of 1 |
| Transaminase, AST (aspartate aminotransferase, SGOT) | 11-47 IU/L | 0.18-0.78 mckat/L |
| Transaminase, ALT (alanine aminotransferase, SGPT) | 7-53 IU/L | 0.12-0.88 mckat/L |
| Transferrin | 220-400 mg/dL | 2.20-4.00 g/L |
| Urea nitrogen (BUN) | 8-25 mg/dL | 2.9-8.9 mmol/L |
| Uric acid | 3-8 mg/dL | 179-476 mcmol/L |
| Vitamin A (retinol) | 15-60 mcg/dL | 0.52-2.09 mcmol/L |
| Zinc | 50-150 mcg/dL | 7.7-23 mcmol/L |

[1] Age dependent    [2] Infants and adolescents up to 104 U/L    [3] Infants in the first year up to 6 mg/dL

| Urine | | |
|---|---|---|
| | Reference Value | |
| Determination | Conventional Units | SI Units |
| Calcium[1] | 50-250 mcg/day | 1.25-6.25 mmol/day |
| *Catecholamines:* Epinephrine | < 20 mcg/day | < 109 nmol/day |
| Norepinephrine | < 100 mcg/day | < 590 nmol/day |
| Catecholamines, 24-hr | < 110 μg | < 650 nmol |
| Copper[1] | 15-60 mcg/day | 0.24-0.95 mcmol/day |
| Creatinine: Child | 8-22 mg/kg | 71-195 μmol/kg |
| Adolescent | 8-30 mg/kg | 71-265 μmol/kg |
| Female | 0.6-1.5 g/day | 5.3-13.3 mmol/day |
| Male | 0.8-1.8 g/day | 7.1-15.9 mmol/day |
| pH | 4.5-8 | 4.5-8 |
| Phosphate[1] | 0.9-1.3 g/day | 29-42 mmol/day |
| Potassium[1] | 25-100 mEq/day | 25-100 mmol/day |
| Protein | | |
| Total | 1-14 mg/dL | 10-140 mg/L |
| At rest | 50-80 mg/day | 50-80 mg/day |
| Protein, quantitative | < 150 mg/day | < 0.15 g/day |
| Sodium[1] | 100-250 mEq/day | 100-250 mmol/day |
| Specific Gravity, random | 1.002-1.030 | 1.002-1.030 |
| Uric Acid, 24-hr | 250-750 mg | 1.48-4.43 mmol |

[1] Diet dependent

| Drug Levels† | | |
|---|---|---|
| | Reference Value | |
| Drug Determination | Conventional Units | SI Units |
| *Aminoglycosides* Amikacin | | |
| (trough) | 1-8 mcg/mL | 1.7-13.7 mcmol/L |
| (peak) | 20-30 mcg/mL | 34-51 mcmol/L |
| Gentamicin | | |
| (trough) | 0.5-2 mcg/mL | 1-4.2 mcmol/L |
| (peak) | 6-10 mcg/mL | 12.5-20.9 mcmol/L |
| Kanamycin | | |
| (trough) | 5-10 mcg/mL | nd |
| (peak) | 20-25 mcg/mL | nd |
| Netilmicin | | |
| (trough) | 0.5-2 mcg/mL | nd |
| (peak) | 6-10 mcg/mL | nd |
| Streptomycin | | |
| (trough) | < 5 mcg/mL | nd |
| (peak) | 5-20 mcg/mL | nd |
| Tobramycin | | |
| (trough) | 0.5-2 mcg/mL | 1.1-4.3 mcmol/L |
| (peak) | 5-20 mcg/mL | 12.8-21.8 mcmol/L |

| Drug Levels† | | |
|---|---|---|
| | Reference Value | |
| Drug Determination | Conventional Units | SI Units |
| **Antiarrhythmics** | | |
| Amiodarone | 0.5-2.5 mcg/mL | 1.5-4 mcmol/L |
| Bretylium | 0.5-1.5 mcg/mL | nd |
| Digitoxin | 9-25 mcg/L | 11.8-32.8 nmol/L |
| Digoxin | 0.8-2 ng/mL | 0.9-2.5 nmol/L |
| Disopyramide | 2-8 mcg/mL | 6-18 mcmol/L |
| Flecainide | 0.2-1 mcg/mL | nd |
| Lidocaine | 1.5-6 mcg/mL | 4.5-21.5 mcmol/L |
| Mexiletine | 0.5-2 mcg/mL | nd |
| Procainamide | 4-8 mcg/mL | 17-34 mcmol/mL |
| Propranolol | 50-200 ng/mL | 190-770 nmol/L |
| Quinidine | 2-6 mcg/mL | 4.6-9.2 mcmol/L |
| Tocainide | 4-10 mcg/mL | nd |
| Verapamil | 0.08-0.3 mcg/mL | nd |
| **Anticonvulsants** | | |
| Carbamazepine | 4-12 mcg/mL | 17-51 mcmol/L |
| Phenobarbital | 10-40 mcg/mL | 43-172 mcmol/L |
| Phenytoin | 10-20 mcg/mL | 40-80 mcmol/L |
| Primidone | 4-12 mcg/mL | 18-55 mcmol/L |
| Valproic acid | 40-100 mcg/mL | 280-700 mcmol/L |
| **Antidepressants** | | |
| Amitriptyline | 110-250 ng/mL[3] | 500-900 nmol/L |
| Amoxapine | 200-500 ng/mL | nd |
| Bupropion | 25-100 ng/mL | nd |
| Clomipramine | 80-100 ng/mL | nd |
| Desipramine | 115-300 ng/mL | nd |
| Doxepin | 110-250 ng/mL[3] | nd |
| Imipramine | 225-350 ng/mL[3] | nd |
| Maprotiline | 200-300 ng/mL | nd |
| Nortriptyline | 50-150 ng/mL | nd |
| Protriptyline | 70-250 ng/mL | nd |
| Trazodone | 800-1600 ng/mL | nd |
| **Antipsychotics** | | |
| Chlorpromazine | 50-300 ng/mL | 150-950 nmol/L |
| Fluphenazine | 0.13-2.8 ng/mL | nd |
| Haloperidol | 5-20 ng/mL | nd |
| Perphenazine | 0.8-1.2 ng/mL | nd |
| Thiothixene | 2-57 ng/mL | nd |
| **Miscellaneous** | | |
| Amantadine | 300 ng/mL | nd |
| Amrinone | 3.7 mcg/mL | nd |
| Chloramphenicol | 10-20 mcg/mL | 31-62 mcmol/L |
| Cyclosporine[1] | 250-800 ng/mL (whole blood, RIA) | nd |
| | 50-300 ng/mL (plasma, RIA) | nd |
| Ethanol[2] | 0 mg/dL | 0 mmol/L |
| Hydralazine | 100 ng/mL | nd |
| Lithium | 0.6-1.2 mEq/L | 0.6-1.2 mmol/L |
| Salicylate | 100-300 mg/L | 724-2172 mcmol/L |
| Sulfonamide | 5-15 mg/dL | nd |
| Terbutaline | 0.5-4.1 ng/mL | nd |
| Theophylline | 10-20 mcg/mL | 55-110 mcmol/L |
| Vancomycin | | |
| (trough) | 5-15 ng/mL | nd |
| (peak) | 20-40 mcg/mL | nd |

† The values given are generally accepted as desirable for treatment without toxicity for most patients. However, exceptions are not uncommon.
[1] 24 hour trough values   [2] Toxic: 50-100 mg/dL (10.9-21.7 mmol/L)   [3] Parent drug plus N-desmethyl metabolite
nd – No data available

| Classification of Blood Pressure* | | | |
|---|---|---|---|
| | Reference Value | | |
| Category | Systolic (mm Hg) | | Diastolic (mm Hg) |
| Optimal† | < 120 | and | < 80 |
| Normal | < 130 | and | < 85 |
| High-normal | 130-139 | or | 85-89 |
| Hypertension‡ | | | |
| Stage 1 | 140-159 | or | 90-99 |
| Stage 2 | 160-179 | or | 100-109 |
| Stage 3 | ≥ 180 | or | ≥ 110 |

**Adapted from the Sixth Report of the Joint National Committee on Prevention, Detection, Evaluation, and Treatment of High Blood Pressure, National Institutes of Health**

* For adults age 18 and older who are not taking antihypertensive drugs and not acutely ill. When systolic and diastolic blood pressures fall into different categories, the higher category should be selected to classify the individual's blood pressure status. In addition to classifying stages of hypertension on the basis of average blood pressure levels, clinicians should specify presence or absence of target organ disease and additional risk factors.

† Optimal blood pressure with respect to cardiovascular risk is below 120/88 mm Hg. However, unusually low readings should be evaluated for clinical significance.

‡ Based on the average of two or more readings taken at each of two or more visits after an initial screening.

# GENERAL MANAGEMENT OF ACUTE OVERDOSAGE

Rapid intervention is essential to minimize morbidity and mortality in an acute toxic ingestion. Institute measures to prevent absorption and hasten elimination as soon as possible; however, symptomatic and supportive care takes precedence over other therapy. It is assumed that basic life support measures, (eg, cardiopulmonary resuscitation [CPR]) have been instituted. Specific antidotes are discussed in the overdosage section of individual or group monographs. The discussion below outlines procedures used in the management of acute overdosage of orally ingested systemic drugs.

## Advanced Life Support Measures

**Adequate Airway:** Adequate airway must be established and maintained, generally via oropharyngeal or endotracheal airways, cricothyrotomy, or tracheostomy.

**Ventilation:** Ventilation may then be performed via mouth-to-mouth insufflation, hand-operated bag (ambu bag) or by mechanical ventilator.

**Circulation:** Circulation must be maintained.

♦ *Hypotension:* If hypotension/hypoperfusion occurs, place the patient in shock position (head lowered, feet elevated); specific therapy may include:
Establish IV access and initiate IV fluids (eg, 0.9% or 0.45% Saline, Lactated Ringer's, Dextrose). A maintenance flow rate is generally 100 to 200 mL/hour; individualize as necessary.
Plasma, plasma protein fractions, whole blood or plasma expanders may be required.
Severe hypotension may require judicious use of cardiovascular active agents. The most commonly recommended agents are dopamine, dobutamine and norepinephrine.

♦ *Arrhythmia* treatment is dictated by the offending drug.

♦ *Hypertension,* sometimes severe, may occur. (See Nitroprusside and Diazoxide, Parenteral in the Agents for Hypertensive Emergencies section.)

**Seizures:** Simple isolated seizures may require only observation and supportive care. Repetitive seizures or status epilepticus require therapy. Give IV diazepam or lorazepam followed by fosphenytoin and/or phenobarbital. Pancuronium may also be considered.

## Reduction of Absorption

**Gastric emptying** is generally recommended as soon as possible; however, this is generally not very effective unless employed within the first 1 to 2 hours after ingestion. Syrup of ipecac and gastric lavage are the two most commonly employed methods for gastric emptying.

♦ *Syrup of ipecac* is the method of choice outside the hospital. Do not induce vomiting if the medication is caustic or a petroleum or if the patient is in a coma or having seizures. Syrup of ipecac takes 20 to 30 minutes to work. Consider gastric lavage if response is needed immediately.

*6 months to 1 year* – 10 mL
*1 year to 12 years* – 15 mL
*> 12 years* – 30 mL

May be followed by a glass of water. A second dose may be given if results do not occur within 20 to 30 minutes.

♦ *Gastric lavage* is indicated in the comatose patient or for those in whom syrup of ipecac fails to produce emesis. Gastric lavage is immediate and does not have a delay reaction, and is preferred over forced emesis. Airway protection via endotracheal intubation is appropriate for the patient without a gag reflex or comatose patients. Position the patient on left side, face down and use a large bore tube. Instill warm water or saline 300 to 360 mL for adults. Avoid water for infants and children; use warm saline or 5% to 6% polyethylene glycol solution. Give until lavage solution becomes clear. Add charcoal before removing the tube.

**Adsorption:** Adsorption, using activated charcoal alone or after completion of emesis or lavage, is indicated for virtually all significant toxic ingestions. It adsorbs a wide variety of toxins and there are no contraindications. However, it adsorbs many orally administered antidotes as well, so space dosage properly. Give an adult 50 to 100 g of activated charcoal mixed in 240 mL of water; the pediatric dose is 1 g/kg, or 25 to 50 g in 120 mL of water.

**Cathartics:** Cathartics increase the elimination of charcoal-poison complex. Generally using a saline or osmotic cathartic (eg, magnesium sulfate or citrate or sorbitol) with 3 mL/kg of a 35% to 75% solution of sorbitol has the most rapid effect.

**Whole bowel irrigation (WBI):** Whole bowel irrigation utilizes rapid administration of large volumes of lavage solutions, such as PEG. The dose is 4 to 6 L over 1 to 2 hours for adults and 0.5 L/hr for children. It may be most useful to remove iron tablets, sustained-release capsules or cocaine-containing condoms or balloons.

## Elimination of Absorbed Drug

**Interruption of enterohepatic circulation:** Interruption of enterohepatic circulation by "gastric dialysis" uses scheduled doses of activated charcoal for 1 to 2 days. Gastric dialysis not only interrupts the enterohepatic cycle of some drugs, but also creates an osmotic gradient, drawing drug from the plasma back into the gastrointestinal lumen where it is bound by the charcoal and excreted in the feces.

**Diuresis:** Diuresis may be effective as identified in the individual drug monographs.

♦ *Forced diuresis* is occasionally useful. It may cause volume overload or electrolyte disturbances. Forced diuresis is useful for phenobarbital, bromides, lithium, salicylate, or amphetamines overdoses. Do not use for tricyclic antidepressants, sedative-hypnotics, or highly protein-bound medications. The most common agents employed are furosemide and osmotic diuretics with mannitol.

♦ *Alkaline diuresis* promotes elimination of weak acids (eg, barbiturates, salicylates) and is accomplished by the administration of IV sodium bicarbonate.

♦ *Acid diuresis* may be indicated in overdoses with weak bases (eg, amphetamines, fenfluramine, quinine), but use with caution in patients with renal or liver disease. It is usually accomplished with oral or IV ascorbic acid or ammonium chloride.

**Dialysis:** Dialysis is indicated in a minority of severe overdose cases. Drug factors that alter dialysis effectiveness include volume of distribution, drug compartmentalization, protein binding and lipid/water solubility.

♦ *Hemodialysis* may be used after an overdose and when the patient is having complications (eg, severe metabolic acidosis, electrolyte imbalances, renal failure).

♦ *Peritoneal dialysis* is even less effective than hemodialysis.

♦ *Charcoal hemoperfusion* is useful when a drug can be adsorbed by charcoal (eg, theophylline, barbiturates).

# Poison Control Center

**Poison Center Hotline:** The American Association of Poison Control Centers (AAPCC) has established a national toll-free poison center hotline. Now everyone in the United States can call

**1-800-222-1222**

to reach the local poison center. Poison Center services are available 24 hours a day, 7 days a week.

The phone number can be used for a poison emergency or questions about poisons and poison prevention.

Regardless of where the call is placed, the hotline automatically connects callers to the closest poison control center. Existing local poison center numbers will still connect callers to their poison centers.

Callers who use a TTY/TDD and non-English speaking callers also can use this hotline.

# INDEX